Introduction to
Critical
Care
Nursing

Introduction to
Critical Care Nursing

Fourth Edition

Mary Lou Sole
PhD, RN, CCNS, FAAN
Professor
School of Nursing
College of Health and Public Affairs
University of Central Florida
Orlando, Florida

Deborah G. Klein
MSN, RN, CCRN, CS
Clinical Nurse Specialist
Cardiac ICU and Heart Failure Special Care Unit
Cleveland Clinic Foundation;
Clinical Instructor
Frances Payne Bolton School of Nursing
Case Western Reserve University
Cleveland, Ohio;
Adjunct Clinical Associate
School of Nursing
Kent State University
Kent, Ohio

Marthe J. Moseley
PhD, RN, CCRN, CCNS
Clinical Nurse Specialist, Critical Care
South Texas Veterans Health Care System
Audie Murphy Division;
Adjunct Assistant Professor
University of Texas Health Science Center
San Antonio, Texas

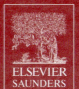

ELSEVIER
SAUNDERS

ELSEVIER
SAUNDERS

11830 Westline Industrial Drive
St. Louis, MO 63146

NOTICE

Nursing is an ever-changing field. Standard safety precautions must be followed, but as new research and clinical experience broaden our knowledge, changes in treatment and drug therapy may become necessary or appropriate. Readers are advised to check the most current product information provided by the manufacturer of each drug to be administered to verify the recommended dose, the method and duration of administration, and contraindications. It is the responsibility of the licensed prescriber, relying on experience and knowledge of the patient, to determine dosages and the best treatment for each individual patient. Neither the publisher nor the authors assume any liability for any injury and/or damage to persons or property arising from this publication.

The Publisher

Previous editions copyrighted 2001, 1997, 1993

International Standard Book Number: 0-7216-0520-6

Executive Publisher: *Barbara Nelson Cullen*
Developmental Editor: *Julie Vitale*
Publishing Services Manager: *John Rogers*
Project Manager: *Doug Turner*
Senior Designer: *Kathi Gosche*

Printed in the United States of America

Last digit is the print number: 9   8   7   6   5   4   3   2   1

*To my critical care colleagues and patients who continue to teach me about
critical care nursing on a daily basis. To my husband, Bob, and daughter,
Erin, for their support and encouragement in all of my endeavors.*

MLS

*To the critical care nurses and patients who are always teaching me.
To my husband, Ron, and my sons, David and Seth, for their support in all that I do.
To my parents Rena Goldenberg, RN, BSN, and Ira Goldenberg, MD,
for their guidance and inspiration. In memory of Diane Fritsch, RN, MSN, CCRN, CS,
for her passion and leadership in the care of the critically ill.*

DGK

*To my friends (especially Michael, Margie, and Denise) and family who teach me
about critical care in and out of the hospital. To my husband, Randy, and my son,
Nicholas, for wanting Momma to take good care of the sick people.
And to Marjory Olson, MSN, RN, who has always provided me support in all that I do.*

MJM

Mary Lou Sole

Mary Lou Sole, PhD, RN, CCNS, FAAN, has extensive experience in critical care practice, education, consultation, and research. She is currently a Professor at the University of Central Florida School of Nursing in Orlando, Florida. She also has a per diem appointment as a Clinical Nurse Specialist at Orlando Regional Medical Center. As part of her teaching assignment, Dr. Sole often teaches the undergraduate critical care elective course. She began her career as a diploma graduate from the Ohio Valley General Hospital School of Nursing in Wheeling, West Virginia. She received a BSN from Ohio University, a master's degree in nursing from The Ohio State University, and a PhD in nursing from the University of Texas at Austin. She has been active locally and nationally in many professional organizations, including the American Association of Critical-Care Nurses. She is past editor of *AACN Clinical Issues: Advanced Practice in Acute and Critical Care*, and serves on the editorial boards of several critical care journals. She has published over 40 articles in peer-reviewed journals; the majority of articles are related to critical care and nursing education. Dr. Sole has received numerous local, state, and national awards for clinical practice, teaching, and research. In 1997, she was inducted as a Fellow of the American Academy of Nursing.

Deborah G. Klein

Deborah G. Klein, MSN, RN, CCRN, CS, has over 27 years of experience in critical care practice, education, consultation, and research. She is currently Clinical Nurse Specialist for the Cardiac ICU and Heart Failure Special Care Unit at the Cleveland Clinic Foundation in Cleveland, Ohio. She is a Clinical Instructor at Frances Payne Bolton School of Nursing, Case Western Reserve University, and Adjunct Clinical Associate at Kent State University School of Nursing. She received her BSN and MSN from Frances Payne Bolton School of Nursing, Case Western Reserve University in Cleveland, Ohio. She is active both locally and nationally in professional organizations, including the American Association of Critical-Care Nurses. She has served on editorial boards of several critical care nursing journals and has published over 30 articles on critical care topics in peer-reviewed journals. Mrs. Klein has received local and national awards for clinical practice and teaching.

Marthe J. Moseley

Marthe J. Moseley, PhD, RN, CCRN, CCNS has over 20 years of experience in critical care practice, education, consultation, and research. She is currently a Clinical Nurse Specialist for Critical Care at the South Texas Veterans Health Care System at Audie Murphy Hospital in San Antonio, Texas. She also has an Adjunct Assistant Professor position at the University of Texas Health Science Center at San Antonio, Texas. As a role component of the Clinical Nurse Specialist, Dr. Moseley regularly teaches the orientation to critical care course. She received a bachelor of arts degree in nursing from Jamestown College in Jamestown, North Dakota, following completion of a BA degree in health, physical education, and biology from Concordia College in Moorhead, Minnesota. She completed her MSN and PhD at the University of Texas Health Science Center in San Antonio, Texas. She has been active locally and nationally in professional organizations, specifically the American Association of Critical-Care Nurses as well as within the VA system. She is on the editorial board for several critical care journals and has published in peer-reviewed journals on critical care topics. Dr. Moseley has received local and national awards for clinical practice and teaching.

Marcia E. Abbott, MSN, RN, CCNS-AC
Clinical Nurse Specialist
Private Practice, Cardiology
San Antonio, Texas
Hemodynamic Monitoring

Karla S. Ahrns, BSN, RN, CCRP
Clinical Research Coordinator
Trauma Burn Critical Care
University of Michigan Health System
Ann Arbor, Michigan
Burns

Pamela J. Bolton, MS, RN, CCRN, CNS
Critical Care Clinical Nurse Specialist
The Christ Hospital
Cincinnati, Ohio
Surgical and Trauma Management

Zara R. Brenner, BSN, MS, APRN, BC
State University of New York at Brockport
Brockport, New York;
Clinical Nurse Specialist, Care Manager
Rochester General Hospital
Rochester, New York
Endocrine Alterations

Jacqueline Fowler Byers, PhD, RN, CNAA
Associate Professor
University of Central Florida
Orlando, Florida
Ethical and Legal Issues in Critical Care Nursing

Lori A. Czekaj, MSN, RN
Director of Education
St. Luke's Baptist Hospital
San Antonio, Texas
Hemodynamic Monitoring

Janet Goshorn, MSN, ARNP, BC
Nurse Practitioner
Nephrology Associates of Central Florida
Orlando, Florida
Acute Renal Failure

Carolyn D. Hix, ASN, BSN, MSN, CNAA
Director
Acute Care Services
Centennial Medical Center
Nashville, Tennessee
Acute Respiratory Failure

Deborah G. Klein, MSN, RN, CCRN, CS
Clinical Nurse Specialist
Cardiac ICU and Heart Failure Special Care Unit
Cleveland Clinic Foundation;
Clinical Instructor
Frances Payne Bolton School of Nursing
Case Western Reserve University
Cleveland, Ohio;
Adjunct Clinical Associate
School of Nursing
Kent State University
Kent, Ohio
Comfort and Sedation; Code Management;
Surgical and Trauma Management

Anne D. Leonard, BSN, RN, MPH, FAHA
Coordinator
UTHSCSA Stroke Program
Department of Medicine/Neurology
The University of Texas Health Science Center
San Antonio
San Antonio, Texas
Nervous Systems Alterations

Susan Loyola, MSN, RN, CCRN
Staff Development Educator
Baptist Health System
San Antonio, Texas
Dysrhythmia Interpretation

Jeffery E. Ludy, EdD, RRT
Assistant Professor and Program Director
Cardiopulmonary Sciences Program
Department of Health Professions
College of Health & Public Affairs
University of Central Florida
Orlando, Florida
Ventilatory Assistance

Maryanne Ludy, MSN, ARNP
Adjunct Clinical Instructor
School of Nursing
University of Central Florida
Orlando, Florida
Ventilatory Assistance

Mary G. McKinley, MSN, RN, CCRN
Partner
Critical Connections
Wheeling, West Virginia
Shock and Sepsis

Debra Michaud, MSN, RN, ARNP, FNP-C
Nurse Practitioner
Facility Administration
DaVitaCare (Kidney Care Services)
Las Vegas, Nevada
Research Analysis (Ethical and Legal Issues in Critical Care Nursing)

Marthe J. Moseley, PhD, RN, CCRN, CCNS
Clinical Nurse Specialist, Critical Care
South Texas Veterans Health Care System
Audie Murphy Division;
Adjunct Assistant Professor
University of Texas Health Science Center
San Antonio, Texas
*Hemodynamic Monitoring;
Nutritional Support*

Sheila A. Myer, MSN, RN
Associate Professor and Chairperson
State University of New York College
   at Brockport
Brockport, New York
Endocrine Alterations

Virginia Oenning, MSN, RN, CSN
Vascular Surgery
South Texas Veterans Health Care System
Audie Murphy Division
San Antonio, Texas
Cardiovascular Alterations

Gaye B. Padayao, BSN, RN, CCRN, OCN
South Texas Veterans Health Care System
Audie Murphy Division
San Antonio, Texas
Hematological and Immune Disorders

Joan Ramirez, BS, RD, CNSD
Dietitian
South Texas Veterans Health Care System
Audie Murphy Division
San Antonio, Texas
Nutritional Support

Janis N. Rice, MSN, RN, CS
Assistant Professor
School of Nursing
The University of Texas Health Science Center
San Antonio
San Antonio, Texas
Nervous Systems Alterations

Catherine McBride Robichaux, PhD, RN, CCRN, BSN, MSN
Assistant Professor, Clinical
The University of Texas Health Science Center
San Antonio, Texas
Nervous System Alterations

Lisa Robinson, MSN, RN, CCRN
Clinical Instructor
University of the Incarnate Word;
Clinical Nurse Educator
Life Care Hospitals of San Antonio;
Staff/Preceptor ICU
Methodist Specialty and Transplant Hospital
San Antonio, Texas
Gastrointestinal Alterations

Mary Lou Sole, PhD, RN, CCNS, FAAN
Professor
School of Nursing
College of Health and Public Affairs
University of Central Florida
Orlando, Florida
*Overview of Critical Care Nursing
Ventilatory Assistance*

Daphne Stannard, PhD, RN, CCRN, CCNS
Assistant Professor
School of Nursing
San Francisco State University
San Francisco, California
Individual and Family Response to the Critical Care Experience

Ross W. Swanson, MSN, RN, CCRN
Clinical Consultant
Corazon Consulting, LP
Pittsburgh, Pennsylvania
Comfort and Sedation

**Linda M. Tamburri, MS, RN, CNS,
C, CCRN**
Clinical Nurse Specialist
Critical Care Medicine
Robert Wood Johnson University Hospital
New Brunswick, New Jersey
Acute Respiratory Failure

**Carol J. Thompson, MSN, RN,
AOCN, CS**
Oncology Supervisor
Nurse Manager, Bone Marrow Transplant Program
South Texas Veterans Health Care System
Audie Murphy Division
San Antonio, Texas
Hematological and Immune Disorders

Beverly Tuomala, BSN, RN, CCRN
CHF Case Manager
University Hospital
San Antonio, Texas
Cardiovascular Alterations

**Jeffrey Williams, MSN, RN, CCRN,
CCNS**
Clinical Nurse Specialist
Critical Care and Cardiology
Presbyterian Hospital of Dallas
Dallas, Texas
Cardiovascular Alterations

Patricia B. Wolff, MSN, APRN, BC
Clinical Nurse Specialist
Medical Oncology
South Texas Veterans Health Care System
Audie Murphy Division
San Antonio, Texas
Hematological and Immune Disorders

Laura C. Bevis, MSN, FNP-C, ACNP-C
Assistant Professor
Department of Nursing
Wichita State University
Wichita, Kansas

Reitha Cabaniss, MSN, RN
Bevill State Community College
Jasper, Alabama

Barbara Chamberlain, MSN, RN, CCRN, CNS
College of Nursing and Health Professions
Drexel University
Philadelphia, Pennsylvania

Judy Crewell, MSN, RN
Critical Care Clinical Specialist
Faculty
Regis University;
Staff Nurse Per Diem
Exempla Lutheran Medical Center
Denver, Colorado

Janet Czermak, MS, RN, APRN-BC
Essex County College
Newark, New Jersey

Luann M. Daggett, DSN, RN
College of Nursing
The University of Southern Mississippi
Meridian, Mississippi

Pam Dulin, MSN, RN, CCRN, Pulmonary CNS
Florida Hospital
Orlando, Florida

Mary E. Farrell, PhD, RN, CCRN
Salem State College
Salem, Massachusetts

Janice Garrison Lanham, MSN, RN, FNP
Greenville Memorial Medical Center
Greenville, South Carolina

Julie Gottemoller-Mueller, MS, RN, ACNP, CNS
University of Chicago
Chicago, Illinois

Diane S. Jedlicka, PhD, RN, CNS
Otterbein College
Westerville, Ohio

Jennifer Kane, BSN, RN
Massachusetts General Hospital
Boston, Massachusetts

Francine R. Margolius, MSN, EdD, RN, BSN, FAAN
College of Nursing
Medical University of South Carolina
Charleston, South Carolina

Carmen T. Ramirez, EdD, RN, CPC, ACNP
University of Arkansas for Medical Services
Little Rock, Arkansas

Marycarol Rossingnol, DNSc, RN
Seton Hall University
South Orange, New Jersey

Donna Routh, RN, MN, CCRN
Linfield College
Portland, Oregon

Bonnie R. Sakallaris, MSN, RN
Washington Hospital Center
Washington, District of Columbia

Lori B. Schumacher, MS, RN, CCRN
School of Nursing
Medical College of Georgia
Augusta, Georgia

Gail A. Vitale, MS, APRN, BC
Assistant Professor
College of Nursing and Health Professions
Lewis University
Romeoville, Illinois

Critical care nursing deals with human responses to life-threatening health problems. Critically ill patients continue to have high levels of acuity and complex care needs. These patients are cared for in critical care units, step-down units, outpatient settings, and at home. The critical care nurse is challenged to provide comprehensive care for these patients and their family members. The demand for critical care nurses who can work across the continuum of care continues to increase.

A solid knowledge foundation in concepts of critical care nursing is essential for practice. Nurses must also learn the assessment and technical skills associated with management of the critically ill patient.

The goal of this 4th edition of *Introduction to Critical Care Nursing* is to facilitate attainment of this foundation for critical care nursing practice. The book continues to provide essential information in an easy-to-learn format for nurses who are new to critical care; it is not intended to be a complete reference on critical care nursing. Information common to all critical care nursing, regardless of setting, is presented. The textbook is targeted to both undergraduate nursing students and experienced nurses who are new to critical care. Both groups have found past editions of the book to be beneficial.

Organization

Introduction to Critical Care Nursing is organized into three sections. Part I, Fundamental Concepts, introduces the reader to critical care nursing; psychosocial concepts related to patients, families, and nurses; and legal/ethical issues related to critical care nursing practice. Part II, Tools for the Critical Care Nurse, remains a unique feature of this text. Chapters in this section provide vital information concerning recognition of dysrhythmias, hemodynamic monitoring, airway management and mechanical ventilation, and management of life-threatening emergencies. Chapters on nutrition and sedation have been added to this section in this edition.

The final ten chapters of the book complete Part III, Nursing Care During Critical Illness. The nursing process is used as an organizing framework for each chapter. Nursing care plans continue to be included so that nurses new to critical care are familiar with nursing diagnoses and interventions common to many critically ill patients. A summary of anatomy and physiology as well as pathophysiology diagrams for common problems seen in critical care are provided. Features of each chapter include drug tables, clinical and laboratory alerts, geriatric considerations, application of current research, critical thinking questions, and case studies. Content on management of the surgical patient has been added to the trauma chapter. Additions and revisions were made based on reader feedback and current trends.

Special Features

This edition features a new two-color design with additional two-color figures to enhance reader understanding. Many new and updated learning aids appear in the fourth edition to highlight chapter content.

- **Clinical Alerts** highlight particular concerns, significance, and procedures in a variety of clinical settings to help students understand the potential problems encountered in that setting.
- **Laboratory Alerts** detail both common and cutting-edge tests and procedures to alert students to the importance of laboratory results.
- **Geriatric Assessments,** formerly *Geriatric Considerations*, alert the user to the special needs of the older patient in the critical care environment.
- Client-specific **Case Studies** with accompanying questions help students apply the chapter's content to real-life situations while also testing their critical-thinking abilities. Discussions for these questions, along with the **Critical Thinking Questions** found at the end of each chapter, are included on the Instructor's Electronic Resource, free to instructors upon adoption.
- **Research Analyses** present summaries of current research articles with accompanying analysis to present new frontiers in critical care nursing.
- **Nursing Care Plans** have been redesigned and updated to describe patient diagnoses, outcomes, nursing interventions, and rationales, a column new to this edition.
- An increased number of **Pathophysiology Flow Charts** expands analysis of the course and outcomes of particular injuries and disorders.
- **Drug Tables** reflect the most current and most commonly used critical care drugs.

TWO NEW CHAPTERS

In addition to the new and updated special features, two new chapters are found in this edition. These new chapters reflect the latest real-world challenges of the critical care nurse.

- *Comfort and Sedation* (Chapter 4) discusses the physical and psychological effects of pain and anxiety and describes the challenges in the assessment of patient comfort in the critically ill patient.
- *Nutritional Support* (Chapter 5) provides a basic understanding of anatomy and physiology of utilization of nutrients in the body and discusses nutritional assessment and types of nutritional therapies.

Ancillary Package

We are pleased to have two new ancillaries, in addition to the Instructor's Resource CD-ROM, in this edition: a new student CD-ROM, which can be found at the back of this book and the Evolve Learning Resources companion Web site for students and instructors.

FOR STUDENTS...

This edition comes with a **new CD-ROM and companion EVOLVE Learning Resources** for students.

The new **Student CD-ROM** packaged with the text contains the following:

- **Open book quizzes** consisting of fill-in-the-blank questions, matching questions, and multiple-choice questions for each chapter.
- **Animations, Images, Video Clips,** and **Audio Clips,** which feature innovative content from supplemental materials.
- More than 250 **Audio Pronunciations** from Dorland's Dictionary.

The Evolve Web site is available at http://evolve.elsevier.com/Sole/ and features a wealth of assets:

- **Open book quizzes** consisting of fill-in-the-blank questions, matching questions, and multiple-choice questions.
- **Online Study Guide** with crossword puzzles and other interactive exercises.
- **Online Concept Map Creator,** a one-of-a-kind program that allows students to create customized concept maps. Students are prompted to enter the following client data: medical diagnosis, pathophysiology, risk factors, clinical manifestations, nursing diagnoses, collaborative problems, expected outcomes, and nursing interventions. The program then generates a concept in two formats: (1) a graphic "map" that clearly illustrates the relationships among various client data and components of the nursing process, and (2) a tabular word processing file that students may print and use to record client response/evaluation data, thereby completing the nursing process.
- Internet resources with **WebLinks** for each chapter.
- **Animations, Images, Video Clips,** and **Audio Clips,** which feature innovative content from supplemental materials.
- More than 250 **Audio Pronunciations** from Dorland's Dictionary.

FOR INSTRUCTORS. . .

The **Instructor's Resource** is available both online and on CD-ROM. Instructors will have access to the student resources.

The **Instructor's Resource CD-ROM** includes the following:

- **Instructor's Manual** includes discussions for the critical thinking questions and case study questions presented in the textbook.
- The **PowerPoint Presentation** collection contains more than 1000 text slides to accompany each chapter.
- The computerized **Test Bank** has more than 500 questions.
- An **Image Collection** contains more than 300 images from the text and additional sources.

Evolve Learning Resources to Accompany *Introduction to Critical Care Nursing,* **fourth edition, Instructor Resources** include all of the components of the Instructor's Resource CD-ROM and all of the Student Resources. You can also use **Evolve** for the following:

- Publish your class syllabus, outline, and lecture notes.
- Set up "virtual office hours" and e-mail communication.
- Share important dates and information through the online class *Calendar.*
- Encourage student participation through *Chat Rooms* and *Discussion Boards.*
- Also available for WebCT and Blackboard systems.

Critical care nursing is an exciting and challenging field. Health care organizations need critical care nurses who are knowledgeable about basic concepts as well as research-based practice, technologically competent, and caring towards patients and families. Our hope is that this edition of *Introduction to Critical Care Nursing* will provide the foundation for critical care nursing practice.

MLS
DGK
MJM

ACKNOWLEDGMENTS

This edition of *Introduction to Critical Care Nursing* would not have been possible without the support of many individuals. We would first like to thank the staff at Elsevier. We were fortunate to work again with Barbara Nelson Cullen as Editor for the textbook. Barbara provided ongoing support, guidance, and motivation for this edition. Her talent for organizing, delegating, and making the editors feel special is noteworthy. Julie Vitale assumed the role of Developmental Editor for this edition. She worked diligently to assist us in meeting deadlines, revising artwork, and systematically organizing and reviewing the manuscripts. She always had a positive "can do" attitude that facilitated the workload. Doug Turner was the Project Manager for the book. He ensured that copyediting was consistent across chapters.

Two new editors joined in the development of this edition. Deborah G. Klein and Marthe J. Moseley provided outstanding clinical input into developing this edition of the textbook. Together the three of us were a great team in planning, organizing, and completing the job.

Our families have been very supportive during this revision. They recognized that many times we had extra work to do to meet deadlines. We appreciate their patience and support.

We would like to acknowledge the support of our superiors and peers in our work settings who endured our discussions about updating the book. We are grateful for the support staff at our institutions who assisted us in completing the project in a timely manner.

Our contributors updated the chapters and added the new features. Since everyone appears to be working harder these days, we are thankful that everyone worked diligently to complete the revisions so that the book would publish on time.

Lastly, we would also like to thank Drs. Jeanette Hartshorn and Marilyn Lamborn for their contributions as past editors of this textbook. Dr. Hartshorn had the vision for this book in the early 1990s. Her past leadership and inspiration have ensured the ongoing success of this textbook. Dr. Lamborn was also involved from the beginning, offering vision, creativity, and a sense of humor. We thank them for providing an excellent foundation on which to build this fourth edition of *Introduction to Critical Care Nursing*.

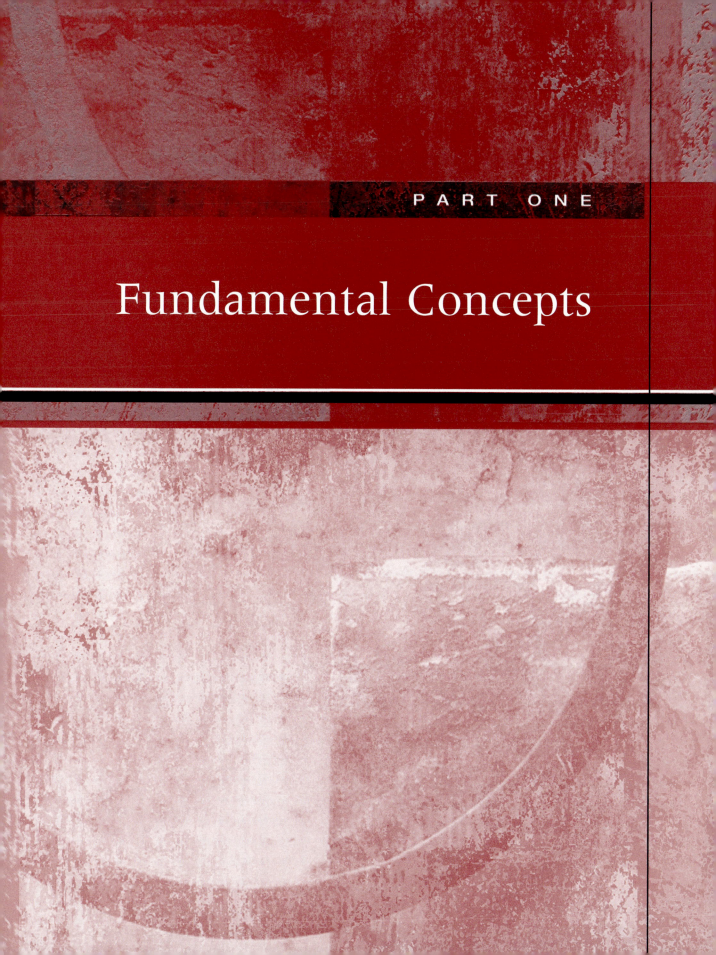

PART ONE

Fundamental Concepts

CHAPTER 1

Overview of Critical Care Nursing

Mary Lou Sole, PhD, RN, CCNS, FAAN

OBJECTIVES

- Define critical care nursing.
- Discuss the purposes and functions of the professional organizations that support critical care practice.
- Describe standards of care and performance for critical care nursing.
- Identify current trends in critical care nursing.

Definition of Critical Care Nursing

Critical care nursing is concerned with human responses to life-threatening problems, such as trauma or major surgery. The human response can be a physiological or psychological phenomenon. The focus of the critical care nurse includes both the patient's and family's responses to illness and involves prevention as well as cure.

The American Association of Critical-Care Nurses (AACN) supports the role of the critical care nurse as patient advocate (AACN, 2003c). These roles are listed in Box 1-1. Desired nursing competencies for critical care practice are listed in Box 1-2.

Evolution of Critical Care

The specialty of critical care has its roots in the 1950s, when polio victims were cared for in specialized units. In the 1960s, recovery rooms were established for the care of patients who had undergone surgery, and coronary care units were instituted for the care of patients with cardiac problems. Improved outcomes were noted for patients cared for in intensive care units. Critical care nursing evolved as a specialty in the 1970s with the development of general intensive care units. Since that time, critical care nursing has become increasingly specialized. Examples of specialized critical care units are cardiovascular, surgical, neurological, trauma, transplantation, burn, pediatric, and neonatal units.

Critical care nursing has expanded beyond the walls of traditional critical care units. For example, critically ill patients are cared for in emergency departments, postanesthesia units, step-down/progressive care units, and interventional radiology and cardiology units. Acutely ill patients with high-technology requirements and/or complex problems, such as patients who are ventilator dependent, may be cared for in medical-surgical units, in long-term acute care hospitals, or at home.

evolve Be sure to check out the bonus material, including free self-assessment exercises, on the Evolve Web site at http://evolve.elsevier.com/Sole/ and on the CD-ROM.

3

BOX 1-1

Role of the Critical Care Nurse as Patient Advocate

- Support the right of the patient or surrogate to autonomous informed decision making.
- Intervene when the best interest of the patient is in question.
- Help the patient to obtain necessary care.
- Respect the patient's values, beliefs, and rights.
- Provide education and support to help the patient or surrogate make decisions.
- Represent the patient in accordance with the patient's choices.
- Support the decisions of the patient or surrogate.
- Intercede for patients who cannot speak for themselves.
- Monitor and safeguard the quality of care.
- Act as liaison with the patient, family, and health care professionals.

American Association of Critical-Care Nurses. (2003). Role of the critical-care nurse (position statement). Aliso Viejo, CA: Author.

BOX 1-2

Desired Competencies of Nurses Caring for the Critically Ill

- Clinical judgment and clinical reasoning skills
- Advocacy and moral agency in identifying and resolving ethical issues
- Caring practices that are tailored to the uniqueness of the patient and family
- Collaboration with health care team members, including family members
- Systems thinking that promotes holistic nursing care
- Response to diversity
- Clinical inquiry and innovation to promote the best patient outcomes
- Role as patient/family educator

Data from the American Association of Critical-Care Nurses. (2003). *AACN Certification Corporation: The AACN synergy model of patient care.* Aliso Viejo, CA: Author.

Critical care nurses practice in varied settings to manage and coordinate care for patients who require in-depth assessment, high-intensity therapies and interventions, and continuous nursing vigilance. Critical care nurses also function in various roles and levels, such as staff nurse, educator, and advanced practice nurse. Nearly one third of nurses employed in hospital settings care for critically ill patients (AACN, 2002a).

Professional Organizations

Two professional organizations specifically support critical care practice. These are the American Association of Critical-Care Nurses (AACN) and the Society of Critical Care Medicine (SCCM).

AMERICAN ASSOCIATION OF CRITICAL-CARE NURSES

Overview

The AACN is a professional organization that was established in 1969; it is the largest nursing specialty organization in the world, with more than 65,000 members. In addition to the national organization, more than 250 chapters are in existence to support critical care nurses at the local level (AACN, 2003a). The mission of the organization is to provide leadership to establish work and patient care environments that are respectful, healing, and humane. The organization provides resources to maximize the contributions of critical care nurses to improve the health care of critically ill patients and their family members. Education of the critical care nurse is the organization's number one priority (AACN, 2002b). The purpose of the organization is to promote the health and welfare of critically ill patients by advancing the art and science of critical care nursing and to support environments that promote professional nursing practice (AACN, 2003a). Values of the organization include accountability, advocacy, integrity, collaboration, leadership, stewardship, life-long learning, quality, innovation, and commitment (AACN, 2002b). These values are supported through education, research, and collaborative practice.

Membership benefits include continuing education offerings, educational advancement scholarships, research grants, and official publications: *Critical Care Nurse*, *American Journal of Critical Care*, and *AACN Clinical Issues: Advanced Practice in Acute and Critical Care*. Membership information and other general information are available by contacting the AACN at 1-800-899-AACN or online at http://www.aacn.org.

Vision

The AACN has adopted a vision to guide critical care nursing practice. The organization supports creating a health care system driven by needs of patients and families in which critical care nurses make their optimal contributions (AACN, 2002b).

Certification

Critical care nurses are eligible for certification. Certification validates knowledge of critical care nursing, promotes professional excellence, and helps nurses to maintain a current knowledge base (AACN, 2002a). The AACN Certification Corporation oversees the critical care certification process.

The certification for nurses in bedside practice is known as CCRN. CCRN certification is available for care of adult, pediatric, or neonatal populations. Nurses who have provided direct care for critically ill patients for at least 1750 hours within 2 years preceding the date of application are eligible to take the CCRN examination. Once they pass the written examination, nurses may use the CCRN credential. Continuing education and ongoing care for critically ill patients are required for recertification (AACN, 2003b).

Advanced practice certification for critical care nurses is also available. Critical care clinical nurse specialists can seek the CCNS credential through the AACN Certification Corporation. Acute care nurse practitioners can become certified as ACNPs. A master's degree in the specialty and clinical practice in the field are required for advanced certification (AACN, 2003b).

Both the CCRN and CCNS credentials are based on a synergy model of practice (Curley, 1998). The synergy model of certified practice states that the needs of patients and families influence and drive competencies of nurses. Each patient and family is unique, with a varying capacity for health and vulnerability to illness. Patients who are more severely compromised have more complex needs (AACN, 2003d). Nursing practice is based on meeting these needs.

SOCIETY OF CRITICAL CARE MEDICINE

Overview

The SCCM is a multidisciplinary scientific and educational organization. The SCCM was founded in 1970 by a group of physicians, and it has grown to nearly 10,000 members. The mission of the organization is to secure the highest-quality care for critically ill patients through a multidisciplinary, multispecialty international group. The SCCM is dedicated to ensuring excellence and consistency in critical care practice through education, research, and advocacy (SCCM, 2003). Membership is open to physicians and other members of the health care team who support critical care. The SCCM publishes *Critical Care Medicine, New Horizons: The Science and Practice of Acute Medicine,* and *Pediatric Critical Care Medicine.* Membership and other information are available online at http://www.sccm.org.

Vision

SCCM's vision is to have a health care system in which all critical care patients obtain care from a multiprofessional health care team under the direction of a physician specializing in intensive care. The system promotes desired outcomes, is consistent with established knowledge, and is humane and respectful (SCCM, 2003).

Standards

Standards serve as guides for clinical practice. They establish goals for patient care and provide mechanisms for nurses to assess the achievement of patient goals, regardless of the setting for practice.

STANDARDS FOR CRITICAL CARE PRACTICE

The AACN *Standards for Acute and Critical Care Nursing Practice* describes practice for nurses who care for critically ill patients (Medina, 2000). The standards describe a level of care or performance so quality can be judged, and they describe expected roles and responsibilities of nurses. They are written as standards of care (competent practice) and standards of professional performance. Boxes 1-3 and 1-4 list the broad standards.

Trends and Issues

As changes in health care delivery evolve, critical care nursing continues to expand and develop to meet patients' needs. Several trends affect current practice. Critical care nurses must be aware of these and

---

BOX 1-3

Standards of Care

The nurse caring for acute and critically ill patients:
- Collects relevant patient health data
- Analyzes the assessment data in determining diagnoses
- Identifies individualized, expected outcomes for the patient
- Develops a plan of care that includes interventions to attain expected outcomes
- Implements interventions identified in the plan of care
- Evaluates the patient's progress toward attaining expected outcomes

Data from Medina, J. (2000). *Standards for acute and critical care nursing practice.* 3rd ed. Aliso Viejo, CA: American Association of Critical-Care Nurses.

BOX 1-4

Standards of Critical Care Professional Practice

The nurse caring for acute and critically ill patients:

- Systematically evaluates the quality and effectiveness of nursing practice
- Reflects knowledge of current professional practice standards, laws, and regulations
- Acquires and maintains current knowledge and competency in the care of acute and critically ill patients
- Interacts with and contributes to the professional development of peers and other health care providers as colleagues
- Acts on behalf of patients in an ethical manner
- Collaborates with the team, which consists of patient, family, and health care providers, to provide care in a healing, humane, and caring environment
- Uses clinical inquiry in practice
- Considers factors related to safety, effectiveness, and cost in planning and delivering patient care

Data from Medina, J. (2000). *Standards for acute and critical care nursing practice.* 3rd ed. Aliso Viejo, CA: American Association of Critical-Care Nurses.

---

other emerging trends when they care for critically ill patients.

Critical illnesses have increased complexity, and critically ill patients are more ill than ever before. The critical care nurse is challenged to provide care for patients who have multisystem organ dysfunction and complex needs. Contributing to this trend is the increasingly aging population. The elderly have more chronic illnesses that contribute to the complexity of their care than do younger patients. They also tend to develop multisystem organ failure, which requires longer hospital stays, increased cost, and increased intensive nursing care.

Costs for critical care services account for a large portion of an institution's budget and a high percentage of total health care costs. Critical care nurses are challenged to provide comprehensive services while reducing costs and lengths of stay. Changing nurse-to-patient ratios and employing unlicensed assistive personnel are strategies being implemented to reduce costs. However, outcomes associated with changes in staffing need to be monitored and evaluated to ensure that outcomes and patient safety are not compromised.

Critical care personnel are expected to evaluate outcomes associated with practice. Many institutions employ clinical nurse specialists or outcomes managers to monitor the quality and the cost of patient care. Critical pathways and care maps are used in many institutions to standardize care and to evaluate outcomes.

Patient safety has emerged as an important issue. Strategies that facilitate patient care, while reducing health care errors, are essential.

Clinical practice guidelines are being implemented to ensure that care is appropriate and based on research. Nurses are encouraged to implement care that is evidence based and to challenge practices that have "always been done" but are not supported by clinical evidence. Advance practice nurses can assist the staff in developing practice guidelines based on research findings.

Today's environment emphasizes collaborative practice teams for the care of patients. The goal of these teams is to provide comprehensive patient care in a cost-effective manner while recognizing and using each others' talents and expertise.

Technology that assists in patient care is growing at a rapid pace. Invasive and noninvasive monitoring systems are employed to facilitate patient assessment and to evaluate responses to treatment. Point-of-care laboratory testing is done at the bedside to provide immediate values and to expedite treatment. Institutions are implementing computerized records to facilitate documentation. Data from monitoring equipment are incorporated into the computerized database. Nurses must become increasingly comfortable with application of technology, troubleshooting, and evaluating accuracy of values. Technology must be balanced with caring and compassion.

As more technological advances become available to sustain and support life, ethical issues have skyrocketed. Termination of life support, organ and cell transplantation, and quality of life are just a few issues that nurses must address in everyday practice. Nurses must be comfortable addressing ethical issues as they arise in the critical care setting.

Palliative care for all patients is an important intervention. Greater emphasis on palliative care in critical care units is an emerging trend.

The use of telemedicine is another emerging trend. Technology allows experts to provide consultation and evaluation of patients who may be a great distance from a tertiary critical care center. Data from monitors can be transferred for evaluation, and the expert can conduct an assessment from a distant location. Although information on such technology has been addressed to physicians and nurse practitioners, critical care nurses may be providing telenursing care to patients at satellite hospitals in the very near future. These telehealth strategies will not replace the high-touch, hands-on care delivered by nurses in the critical care unit, but they will assist health care workers at remote sites in decision making.

The critical care environment itself is changing. Units are being redesigned with the interests of both patients and nurses in mind. Equipment is becoming more portable, thus making transfer of patients for diagnostic testing or to other units easier and safer. Some institutions have adopted a universal care model of patient care. In this setting, patients remain in one unit throughout their hospitalization. The level of nursing care is adjusted to meet the needs of the patient. The universal care model eliminates the need to transfer patients to other units and promotes continuity of care (Joyce & Pandolph, 2001; Mitchell, 2002).

Patients are being transferred from critical care units much earlier than before and are discharged from the hospital often while they are still acutely ill. Nurses must ensure that patients and their family members are able to provide care in the home setting, which may be challenging given the reduced length of hospital stays.

Last, and most important, the United States is facing a shortage of critical care nurses. Many factors are contributing to the shortage: decreased supply and higher demand for critical care nursing services, issues related to retention in the workplace, and greater availability of other career choices for women. Priorities for recruiting, educating, and retaining more nurses to work in critical care settings are essential.

These and other trends will continue to shape the future of critical care practice. Each nurse must continue to monitor trends. Participation in organized nursing is one of the best ways to influence practice in an ever-changing environment.

SUMMARY

Because the boundaries of critical care have expanded, all nurses will be providing care for critically ill patients. Knowledge of professional organizations and of the scope and standards of practice is important for the nurse entering critical care practice. The purpose of this textbook is to provide fundamental information essential to the care of critically ill patients. The reader is challenged to apply the concepts discussed throughout this book to daily practice.

CRITICAL THINKING QUESTIONS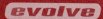

1. Discuss critical care nursing practice and what it means to you.

2. Compare perceptions of critical care from the viewpoints of student, nurse, patient, and family.

3. Give examples of various environments of critical care nursing practice.

4. Discuss the contributions of professional organizations to critical care nursing practice.

5. Debate the pros and cons of hiring new graduates to work in a critical care unit.

6. Envision the critical care unit of the future. Describe the environment and how care could be delivered.

REFERENCES

American Association of Critical-Care Nurses. (2002a). About critical care nursing (press release). Aliso Viejo, CA: Author. Retrieved from http://www.aacn.org. Accessed 1/12/2004.

American Association of Critical-Care Nurses. (2002b). Mission, vision, and values (member services). Aliso Viejo, CA: Author. Retrieved from http://www.aacn.org. Accessed 1/12/2004.

American Association of Critical-Care Nurses. (2003a). Fact sheet. Aliso Viejo, CA: Author. Retrieved from http://www.aacn.org. Accessed 1/12/2004.

American Association of Critical-Care Nurses. (2003b). General information regarding certification. Aliso Viejo, CA: AACN Certification Corporation. Retrieved from http://www.aacn.org/certcorp. Accessed 1/12/2004.

American Association of Critical-Care Nurses. (2003c). Role of the critical-care nurse (position statement). Aliso Viejo, CA: Author.

American Association of Critical-Care Nurses. (2003d). The AACN synergy model of patient care. Aliso Viejo, CA: AACN Certification Corporation. Retrieved from http://www.aacn.org/certcorp. Accessed 1/12/2004.

Curley, M. A. Q. (1998). Patient-nurse synergy: Optimizing patient outcomes. *American Journal of Critical Care, 7,* 64-72.

Joyce, L., & Pandolph, P. (2001). One stop post op cardiac surgery recovery: A proven success. *Journal of Cardiovascular Management, 12*(5), 16-18.

Medina, J. (2000). *Standards for acute and critical care nursing practice.* 3rd ed. Aliso Viejo, CA: American Association of Critical-Care Nurses.

Mitchell, K. (2002). Perspectives in leadership: Universal care puts a premium on growth. *Nursing Spectrum (Florida Edition)*, *12*(5), 6.

Society of Critical Care Medicine. (2003). Guiding the future of critical care: About the Society of Critical Care Medicine. Chicago, IL: Author. Retrieved from http://www.sccm.org. Accessed 1/12/2004.

RECOMMENDED READINGS

American Association of Critical-Care Nurses. (2002). Safeguarding the patient and the profession: The value of critical care certification. Aliso Viejo, CA: AACN Certification Corporation. Retrieved from http://www.aacn.org/certcorp. Accessed 1/12/2004.

American Association of Critical-Care Nurses. (2003). Promoting the value of nursing. Aliso Viejo, CA: Author. Retrieved from http://www.aacn.org. Accessed 1/12/2004.

Bench, S., Crowe, D., Day, T., Jones, M., & Wilebore, S. (2003). Developing a competency framework for critical care to match patient need. *Intensive Critical Care Nursing*, *19*, 136-142.

Molter, N.C. (2003). Creating a healing environment for critical care. *Critical Care Nursing Clinics of North America*, *15*(3), 295-304.

Hodge, M., Kochie, L.D., Larsen, L., & Santiago, M. (2003). Clinician-implemented research utilization in critical care. *American Journal of Critical Care*, *12*(4), 361-366.

evolve **Did you remember to check out the bonus material, including free self-assessment exercises, on the Evolve Web site at http://evolve.elsevier.com/Sole/ and on the CD-ROM?**

CHAPTER **2**

Individual and Family Response to the Critical Care Experience

Daphne Stannard, PhD, RN, CCRN, CCNS

OBJECTIVES

- Describe contextual factors that influence the critical care experience for patients, family members, and critical care nurses.
- Relate the causes of delirium in the critically ill population to selected nursing interventions.
- Discuss the critical care experience from the patient's and family's perspectives.
- Describe common family needs and family-centered nursing interventions.
- Describe the American Association of Critical-Care Nurses synergy model, relating patient and nurse characteristics.

Introduction

The modern hospital came of age in the early part of the twentieth century. The premature station at the Sarah Morris Hospital in Chicago opened in 1922 and is often heralded as the first permanent neonatal critical care unit in the United States (O'Donnell, 1990). One year later, a three-bed adult critical care unit was opened to care for postoperative neurosurgical patients at Johns Hopkins (Hilberman, 1975). Nearly 40 years later, virtually all hospitals in the United States had a critical care unit (Groeger et al., 1992).

Yet not all critically ill patients are cared for in a critical care unit. The American Association of Critical Care Nurses (AACN) defines critically ill patients as those patients who are "at high risk for actual or potential life-threatening health problems" (AACN, 2002). Critical care nurses work wherever critically ill patients and their families are found: critical care units, cardiac catheterization laboratories, emergency departments, hemodialysis units, operating rooms, postanesthesia care units, and progressive care units, to name a few.

Although critical care nurses have been caring for patients and their families since the inception of critical care, researchers have only recently begun to document the experience of critical illness for patients, families, and critical care providers. The purpose of this chapter is to highlight selected literature and to describe the critical illness experience for patients, their families, and the critical care nurses involved in their care.

The Critical Care Environment

Critical care areas are inherently filled with stress. Some obvious stressors related to the typical critical care environment include loss of privacy, artificial lighting 24 hours a day, constant noise from monitoring and life support machines, lack of meaningful stimuli such as the personal touch of family members, and physical pain or discomfort resulting from medical and nursing procedures and the serious illness itself.

The critical care environment provides the backdrop against which all physiological and nonphysiological care of patients and their families occurs. Contextual factors, such as the patient-family care environment and the patient's clinical status, make some interventions and activities possible while prohibiting others (Benner, Hooper-Kyriakidis, & Stannard, 1999). The environment in a busy emergency department on a Friday night, for instance, will not allow for the comparable level of attentiveness and quality of nonphysiological patient and family care that can be provided in that same emergency department on a quiet afternoon.

Other contextual factors that have been identified as influencing nurses' ability to provide quality patient and family care include nurse staffing levels, nurse-physician collaboration, the type of critical care area, and unit culture (Aiken, Clarke, & Sloane, 2002; Baggs et al., 1999; Benner, Hooper-Kyriakidis, & Stannard, 1999; Benner, Tanner, & Chesla, 1996; Chesla & Stannard, 1997; Cho, Ketefian, Barkauskas, & Smith, 2003; Dang, Johantgen, Pronovost, Jenckes, & Bass, 2002; Mitchell, Armstrong, Simpson, & Lentz, 1989; Needleman, Buerhaus, Mattke, Stewart, & Zelevinsky, 2002; Shannon, Mitchell, & Cain, 2002). The tempo, mood, climate, design, and culture of any nursing unit make certain kinds of caring practices possible while discouraging others. These factors, as well as the patient population and unit staff, influence how nurses interact with patients and their families.

A "family-friendly" unit culture, for example, is a unit culture with a socially embedded ethic of family care. This kind of unit culture has been shown to greatly influence nurses' openness to family care practices (Benner, Hooper-Kyriakidis, & Stannard, 1999). However, the opposite is also true. Less than optimal family care or breakdown between nurses and families occurs frequently in critical care units with a "family-restraint" culture (Chesla & Stannard, 1997).

The built environment, or the design and physical layout of the nursing unit, also influences the critical care experience for patients, families, and critical care staff. In particular, critically ill patients who are cared for in windowless environments have less accurate memories of the length of their stay, are less oriented to time during their stay, and experience delusions and hallucinations at more than twice the rate of similar patients who are cared for in units with

windows (Keep, 1977; Keep, James, & Inman, 1980). Additionally, critical care areas that have shared wards are associated with increased infection rates and a greater incidence of patient anxiety and hostility (Bayat, Shaaban, Dodgson, & Dunn, 2003; Leigh, Hofer, Cooper, & Reiser, 1972).

Family members of critically ill patients have consistently reported two recurring needs as they pertain to the environment. The first need is that of proximity, or the need to be close to their critically ill loved one (Leske, 1992). Translating this need into reality requires that there be adequate space around the critically ill patient's bed to accommodate the myriad of health care providers, therapeutic devices and other life-saving technologies, *and* the ill patient's family. The second need that families have consistently reported is the need for comfort (Heyland et al., 2002; Leske, 1992). This need can be conceptualized in many ways, ranging from emotional comfort to the personal comforts often found in family waiting areas, such as comfortable seating, beverages and snacks, access to a telephone, television, and the provision of clean blankets and pillows.

Finally, researchers have determined that critical care nurses typically work under a fairly significant amount of stress (Cartledge, 2001; Fischer, Calame, Dettling, Zeier, & Fanconi, 2000). The typical cramped and crowded critical care areas, coupled with the often inadequate break room, have been cited as sources of stress among critical care nurses (Cassem & Hackett, 1972). Additionally, one study found that the excessive noise in a critical care unit caused tachycardia and annoyance in critical care nurses (Morrison, Haas, Shaffner, Garrett, & Fackler, 2003).

Sustained noise levels louder than 70 decibels (dB) are associated with hearing loss. The Environmental Protection Agency (EPA) recommends that hospital noise levels not exceed 45 dB (EPA, 2004). Yet noise in critical care areas often exceeds recommended levels (Table 2-1). Researchers have demonstrated, however that interventions, such as installing acoustical ceiling tiles, implementing noise reduction protocols and guidelines, and instituting music therapy can decrease noise and nighttime light levels, can decrease procedural pain, anxiety, and annoyance, and can promote sleep (Bally, Campbell, Chesnick, & Tranmer, 2003; Berens & Weigle, 1996; Byers & Smyth, 1997; Olson, Borel, Laskowitz, Moore, & McConnell, 2001; Walder, Francioli, Meyer, Lancon, & Romand, 2000; Wong, Lopez-Nahas, & Molassiotis, 2001). Although noise continues to be a significant problem in many critical care areas, all aspects of the built environment need additional innovation and testing. See the Recommended Readings list for critical care design guidelines and standards.

TABLE 2-1

Noise Levels Associated With Patient Care Devices and Activities

Activity	Sound Level (dB)
Toilet flushing	44-76*
Cardiac monitor alarm	44-78*
Scraping of chairs/stools across floor	46-86*
Call-bell	48-63*
Oxygen/chest tube bubbling, ventilator	49-70*
Adding medication to/adjusting intravenous line	58-60*
Conversations (staff, patients, and family)	59-90*
Voice over intercom	60-70*
Telephone ringing	60-75*
Television (normal volume at 12 feet)	65†
Raising/lowering head of bed	68-78*
Pneumatic tube arrival	88*
Raising/lowering side rails on bed	90*
Shouts among staff	90†
Addressograph machine	100†
Dropping a stainless steel bowl	108*

*Data from Sommargren, C. (1995). Environmental hazards in the technological age. *Critical Care Nursing Clinics of North America*, 7(2), 287-295.
†Data from Grumet, G. (1994). Noise hampers healing and curbs productivity. *Health Facilities Management*, 7(1), 22-25.

BOX 2-1

Patients' Recollection of the Critical Care Experience

- Difficulty communicating
- Pain
- Thirst
- Difficulty swallowing
- Anxiety
- Lack of control
- Depression
- Fear
- Lack of family or friends
- Physical restraint
- Feelings of dread
- Inability to get comfortable
- Difficulty sleeping
- Loneliness
- Thoughts of death and dying

The Critically Ill Patient

Given the environmental backdrop of critical care coupled with the symptoms of critical illness, it is no wonder that critically ill patients have reported impaired cognitive functioning and discomforts such as problems with sleeping, pain, and anxiety (Stein-Parbury & McKinley, 2000).

Several researchers measured and described patients' perceptions of stressors in the critical care unit (Box 2-1). The experience of mechanical ventilation, along with difficulty communicating, pain, dyspnea, fatigue, and the need for arterial blood gas sampling and tracheal suctioning, creates one of the most common stressful scenarios for the critically ill patient (Minnick, Leipzig, & Johnson, 2001; Turner, Briggs, Springhorn, & Potgieter, 1990; Twibell, Siela, & Mahmoodi, 2003). Additional major stressors that have been identified by patients when recalling their critical care experience are listed in Box 2-1 (Jones, Hoggart, Withey, Donaghue, & Ellis, 1979; Koivula, Paunonen-Ilmonen, Tarkka, & Laippala, 2001; Nelson et al., 2001; Rotundi et al., 2002; Simpson, Armstrong, & Mitchell, 1989; Simpson, Lee, & Cameron, 1996; Soehren, 1995; Turner, Briggs, Springhorn, & Potgieter, 1990). The combination of these experiences in critically ill patients often produces anxiety and agitation and, in some cases, severe stress leading to the development of posttraumatic stress disorder and delirium (Schnyder et al., 2000; Szokol & Vender, 2001).

ANXIETY, AGITATION, AND DELIRIUM

Anxiety is a condition characterized by apprehension and autonomic arousal (Szokol & Vender, 2001). *Agitation,* conversely, is associated with increased motor activity on the part of the patient. Anxiety, agitation, and pain are often interrelated (Stannard, Puntillo, Miaskowski, Gleeson, Kehrle, & Nye, 1996). *Delirium* is defined as an acute, reversible condition characterized by disorientation, impaired short-term memory, altered sensory perceptions (hallucinations), abnormal thought processes, and inappropriate behavior (Szokol & Vender, 2001). Delirium can be differentiated from dementia, which is usually chronic and not reversible. When delirium is suspected, underlying and contributing metabolic or physiological processes must be identified and corrected (Box 2-2). Once these processes are ruled out, the next step is to ensure that the patient is receiving adequate analgesia, because pain is a primary cause of agitation in the critically ill patient.

BOX 2-2

Causes of Delirium in Critically Ill Patients

METABOLIC CONDITIONS
- Acid-base disturbance
- Electrolyte imbalance
- Hypoglycemia

INTRACRANIAL CAUSES
- Epidural or subdural hematoma
- Intracranial hemorrhage
- Meningitis
- Encephalitis
- Cerebral abscess, tumor

ENDOCRINE CONDITIONS
- Hyperthyroidism or hypothyroidism
- Addison's disease
- Hyperparathyroidism
- Cushing's syndrome

ORGAN FAILURE
- Liver encephalopathy
- Uremic encephalopathy
- Septic shock

DRUG-RELATED CAUSES
- Alcohol withdrawal
- Drug-induced conditions
- Heavy metal poisoning

PULMONARY CAUSES
- Hypoxemia
- Hypercarbia

Data from Szokol, J., & Vender, J. (2001). Anxiety, delirium, and pain in the intensive care unit. *Critical Care Clinics, 17*(4), 821-842.

Delirium or ICU syndrome was first documented by Blachly and Starr (1964) and by Egerton and Kay (1964), who described the psychosis experienced by patients who had undergone cardiotomy. Since then, many studies have examined delirium. Some of the terms used to describe delirium include *ICU syndrome, ICU psychosis, postcardiotomy delirium, postoperative psychosis, intensive care delirium, acute confusion,* and *impaired psychological response.*

A main nursing goal for patients with delirium is to ensure their safety and to reduce sleep deprivation and noxious sensory overload. Additionally, it is important to increase pleasant sensory input, such as

encouraging familiar voices of the family and family touch, and also to reestablish day-night cycles by positioning the patient by a sunny window during the day and reducing light levels in the patient's room at night. Reorienting the patient every 2 to 4 hours and addressing the patient directly will help to minimize confusion. Instead of repeatedly questioning the patient (e.g., "Do you know what day it is? Do you know where you are?"), a less demeaning and less frustrating way to reorient the patient is to incorporate this content into normal conversation (e.g., "It's 8 o'clock in the morning on the fifth of September. You are still in the critical care unit. Your family will be here to see you in about 10 minutes"). Conversations about other patients and personal issues are conducted outside the patient's hearing range because such information can increase confusion on the part of the patient and can contribute to sensory overload. It is also very helpful to have orienting objects, such as a clock, calendar, and windows within the patient's visual field. Personal and meaningful items brought from home by the family may also help to reorient the patient. Finally, nursing activities and medical procedures should be clustered to maximize a critically ill patient's resting periods. These interventions help to decrease noxious sensory overload and increase pleasant sensory input. Patients with delirium usually have a resolution of the symptoms within 1 to 2 days after treatment and after being transferred out of the critical care area.

PERCEPTIONS OF CARING PRACTICES

Several researchers have examined patients' perceptions concerning the quality of nursing care they received while in a critical care area. The overarching theme that has been described in multiple studies is the need for a critical care patient to feel safe (Hupcey, 2000). Because a critically ill patient is often physiologically and psychologically vulnerable, nursing caring practices that may make a patient feel safe can range from technical competence to attentive and vigilant response-based practice (Baldursdottir & Jonsdottir, 2002; Benner, et al., 1999; Holland, Cason, & Prater, 1997; Holland, et al., 1997). Some patients feel safe when their family is at the bedside (Simpson, 1991). Conversely, patients do not feel cared for when they feel depersonalized, when they are not listened to, when they experience unprofessional behavior, and when they feel forgotten by health care providers (Doering, McGuire, & Rourke, 2002; Fitzsimmons, Parahoo, Richardson, & Stringer, 2003).

Patients have also described to researchers the importance of their informational needs. During the critical illness, patients have reported needing general information and orientation, whereas information about what had happened and piecing together events are important to patients after their critical illness (Hupcey & Zimmerman, 2000). Many patients can hear, understand, and respond emotionally to what is being said even when they are in an unconscious state (Lawrence, 1995). For that reason, nurses and family members should strive to talk to patients, regardless of the patients' ability to interact (Benner, et al., 1999). Nurses must frequently orient critically ill patients to time and place, inform them of their progress, and remind them that they are safe and have family and people nearby who care about their well-being.

QUALITY OF LIFE AFTER CRITICAL CARE

With technological and other therapeutic advances, health care providers can now, in many cases, cure what was once considered incurable. One-year survival rates after critical care vary widely, from 27% to 75% (Eddleston, White, & Guthrie, 2000). Survival, however, is just one aspect of the overall patient and family experience. To appreciate a typical critical illness trajectory fully, it is important briefly to review some of the research that focuses on patients' quality of life after discharge from critical care.

Discharge from a critical care area is often difficult for patients and families. Although it represents progress toward recovery from illness, it also means having to learn new nurses, new routines, a new unit, and in some cases, new roommates when the patient rooms are shared. Patients' mixed feelings regarding the actual transfer from a critical care area to the ward has been referred to as *relocation stress* (McKinney & Deeny, 2002). This stress continues and, in many cases, is exacerbated once the patient is discharged home to be cared for by family and friends. To minimize the stress, careful discharge planning, teaching, and preparation on the part of the patient and family are imperative.

Common patient complaints after critical care include fatigue, muscle weakness, sleep disturbance, pain, poor concentration, short-term memory impairment, and poor appetite (Eddleston, et al., 2000; Fletcher et al., 2003; Frick, Uehlinger, & Zenklusen, 2002; Gardner & Sibthorpe, 2002; Hunt, Hendrata, & Myles, 2000; Shenkman & Stechmiller, 1987). Despite these complaints, research has shown that former critically ill patients and their family members would still be willing to undergo critical care and mechanical ventilation again in most cases to achieve any prolongation of survival (Danis, Jarr, Southerland, Nocella, &

Patrick, 1987; Danis, Patrick, Southerland, & Green, 1988; Mendelsohn, Belle, Fischhoff, Wisniewski, Degenholtz, & Chelluri, 2002).

INDIVIDUALIZED PATIENT RESPONSES

Each individual patient's response to critical illness is influenced by various factors, including age and developmental stage, prior experiences with illness and hospitalization, family relationships and social support, prior stressful experiences and coping mechanisms, and personal philosophies about life, death, and spirituality. Some elderly patients have a diminished ability to adapt and cope with the major physical and psychosocial stressors of critical illness. This is often the result of multiple losses over the years, including loss of physical function, loss of family members, and loss of resources, such as homes and income. Yet some elderly patients with chronic illnesses who have endured multiple critical illnesses demonstrate amazing resilience. Patients who have survived a prior critical illness generally have less anxiety during subsequent admissions. For other patients, their only prior experience with critical illness may have ended with the death of a family member. This scenario can add considerably to the patient's

Geriatric Assessment

- Anxiety disorders are less prevalent in the elderly than in younger adults. New-onset anxiety in elderly persons is often secondary to physical illness, depression, medication side effects, or withdrawal from drugs.
- Dementia greatly increases the risk of delirium, as do advanced age and comorbid physical problems.
- Recognizing and diagnosing late-life depression can be challenging. Elderly persons may complain of lack of energy or other somatic symptoms, may attribute symptoms to old age or other physical ailments, or may fail to mention symptoms to a health care provider.
- Medications that may cause or aggravate sleep problems include alcohol, antidepressants, beta-blockers, bronchodilators, caffeine, clonidine, cortisone, diuretics, levodopa, methyldopa, nicotine, phenytoin, progesterone, quinidine, reserpine, sedatives, and sympathomimetics.

Data from Reuben, D., Herr, K., Pacala, J., Potter, J., Pollock, B., & Semla, T. (2002). *Geriatrics at your fingertips*. New York: American Geriatrics Society.

fears and anxiety. Although the fears and concerns of the geriatric patient are similar to the concerns of younger critically ill patients, in many ways the elderly patient is at greater risk of negative outcomes. For example, most patients are concerned about how long it will take them to regain their previous functional status; yet, for many elders, critical illness will result in some permanent decline or loss of functional abilities. The Geriatric Assessment Box provides an overview.

CULTURAL CONSIDERATIONS

Another factor that influences the responses of both individual patients and their families is cultural orientation. Culture influences values, beliefs about health and illness, preferences for interaction with family members and health care providers, methods of communicating, personal space boundaries and feelings about being touched, time orientation, and roles and obligations (Bushy, 1999). Cultural considerations that are particularly important in the critical care environment are beliefs about health and healing, personal space and touch preferences, and social organization or the role of family. Table 2-2 lists cultural considerations for some of the cultural groups that may be seen in critical care areas.

Family Members of the Critically Ill Patient

Although the experience of being critically ill most directly affects the individual patient, the resulting impact on family members and significant others can be substantial. The illness or injury of one family member influences all members of the family. The burden of an illness can affect families in many ways, ranging from emotional distress and despair to financial bankruptcy (Kleiber et al., 1994; Swoboda & Lipsett, 2002). Likewise, in caring for the critically ill patient, the nurse must recognize the influence of the family on the individual patient's recovery (Benner, et al., 1999).

A reciprocal relationship exists between a patient and her or his family. Nurses who respect this life-long reciprocal relationship understand that caring for a patient's family is simply another way of caring for the patient. By working with patients and their families,

---

TABLE 2-2

Cultural Considerations

Culture of Origin	Health and Healing Beliefs	Space and Touch Preferences	Families and Social Organization
Asian	Traditional health and illness beliefs. May rely on traditional practitioners, such as herbalists.	Prefer minimal physical contact.	Strong family ties. Particularly loyal to elders. Devoted to family traditions.
Anglo-Americans	Reliance on modern health care systems, particularly for illnesses perceived as critical or life threatening.	Prefer minimal physical contact.	Nuclear families are most common.
Black/African American	Belief in traditional folk medicines and healers.	Close personal space.	Large, extended families, often female head of household. Strong church affiliation.
Native American	Belief in traditional folk medicine and healers (e.g., medicine man).	Minimal spatial boundaries. Strive to be at one with the universe and surrounding beings.	Strong, extended family ties. Highly respectful of elders and family traditions.
Latino/Mexican American	Belief in traditional folk medicine and healers (e.g., curandero).	Comfortable with tactile relationships, touching, and embracing.	Nuclear and extended families. Godparents play important role.

Modified from Arnault, D. (1998). Framework for culturally relevant psychiatric nursing. In E. Varcarolis (Ed.), *Foundations of psychiatric mental health nursing* (3rd ed.) Philadelphia: W. B. Saunders; and Bushy, A. (1999). The need for cultural linguistic competent care for families with special health problems. In J. Sebastian & A. Bushy (Eds.). *Special populations in the community: Advances in reducing health disparities.* Gaithersburg, MD: Aspen.

critical care nurses can support and strengthen meaningful relationships during great stress.

FAMILY ASSESSMENT

Once the patient has been admitted to the critical care unit, an assessment of the family will provide valuable information for preparation of the nursing care plan. One of the most widely recognized assessment models is the Calgary Family Assessment Model (Figure 2-1). This model consists of three major categories: structural, developmental, and functional (Wright & Leahey, 2000). Each category contains several subcategories. Not all subcategories, however, need to be assessed with each family during the initial meeting. In fact, some subcategories may never need to be assessed with a particular family. Each nurse should determine which subcategories are appropriate to explore with each family at a given point in the critical illness trajectory (Wright & Leahey, 2000). Just as critically ill patients are continually evaluated and assessed by critical care clinicians, so too should the critically ill patients' family members be evaluated.

According to the Calgary Family Assessment Model, a structural assessment includes the internal structure (who is in the family), the external structure (examining extended family and larger systems), and family context (including ethnicity, race, social class, religion and spirituality, and the environment) (Wright & Leahey, 2000). Assessment of the family structure is the first step and is essential before specific interventions can be designed.

In addition to understanding family structure, the critical care nurse may require an understanding of the developmental life cycle for a particular family. This category is further subdivided into stages, tasks, and attachments (Wright & Leahey, 2000).

Finally, the functional family assessment is concerned with how family members actually function or behave in relation to one another. There are two basic aspects of family functioning: instrumental and expressive (Wright & Leahey, 2000). The instrumental aspect of family functioning refers to activities of daily living, such as eating, sleeping, and cooking. For family members experiencing the critical illness

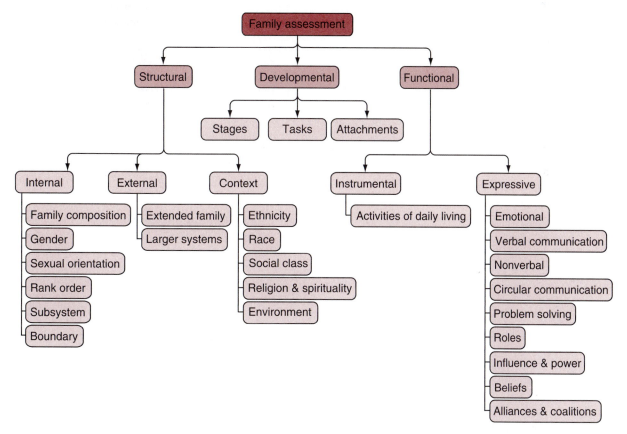

FIGURE 2-1 Calgary Family Assessment Model. (From Wright, L., & Leahy, M. [2000]. *Nurses and families: A guide to family assessment and intervention* [p. 68]. 3rd ed. Philadelphia: F. A. Davis.)

trajectory, this can be a particularly important area, because many of the family's routines and habits are disrupted. The expressive aspect of family functioning refers to communication patterns, problem-solving abilities, beliefs, roles, and alliances within the family. These aspects are extremely important for the critical care nurse to assess, because communication patterns within the family are often altered by the stress of critical illness thus communication has been shown to be a vital component of quality family care (Azoulay et al., 2000).

Although assessment data can be challenging to gather for complex family units, it can be even more daunting to record the collected data in a concise manner on already cramped Kardexes, flowsheets, and care plans. Yet it is imperative to share assessment data with the entire health care team to ensure that care is tailored to the individual patient and family. One concise way to record family assessment data is the family genogram. As information about the structural, developmental, and functional aspects of the family is gathered, the bedside genogram can be modified and developed further (Figures 2-2 and 2-3).

FAMILY NEEDS

Many studies have identified needs of families of the critically ill and have examined family needs across the life span and in a variety of settings (Bass, 1991; Bijttebier, Lee, Chien, & Mackenzie, 2000; Delva, Vanoost, Bobbaers, Lauwers, & Vertommen, 2000; Farrell & Frost, 1992; Fisher, 1994; Leske, 1986;

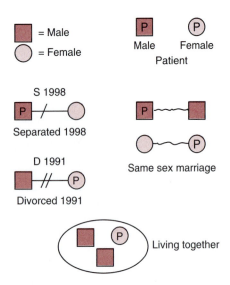

FIGURE 2-2 Genogram symbols. (From Stannard, D. [2001]. Family care. In H. Schell & K. Puntillo (Eds.). *Critical care nursing secrets* [p. 383]. Philadelphia: Hanley & Belfus.)

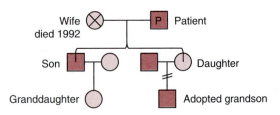

FIGURE 2-3 Sample bedside genogram. (From Stannard, D. [2001]. Family care. In H. Schell & K. Puntillo (Eds.). *Critical care nursing* secrets [p. 383]. Philadelphia: Hanley & Belfus.)

Mi-Kuen, French, Kai-Kwong, 1999; Miracle & Hovekamp, 1994; Molter, 1979). Other variations on the needs studies include studying the relationship between needs and unmet needs (Kosco & Warren, 2000; Mendonca & Warren, 1998) and examining needs over time (Freichels, 1991).

The results of these studies suggest that these family members have predictable sets of needs. The needs experienced by most families can be grouped into five major categories: receiving assurance, remaining near the patient, receiving information, being comfortable, and having support available (Leske, 1992). Meeting these needs has been shown to increase family satisfaction (Azoulay et al., 2001; Johnson, Wilson, Cavanaugh, Bryden, Gudmundson, & Moodley, 1998; Wasser, Pasquale, Matchett, Bryan, & Pasquale, 2001).

FAMILY INTERVENTIONS

A crucial nursing intervention is ensuring that a family can be with their critically ill loved one. Because family access promotes family cohesion, connection, and closure, it fosters patient well-being and provides the family with information (Benner, et al., 1999). Yet, historically, critical care settings have severely restricted family access, thereby limiting nurse-family interactions and, in some cases, nurses' development of family care practices (Chesla & Stannard, 1997). Commonly cited rationales to limit family access include concerns regarding patient stability, infection, rest, and privacy; the effect of visitation on the family; space limitations; and health care providers' performance abilities. Although some of these concerns have merit, numerous studies investigated family visitation and found no adverse effects on patient stability and infection, or negative consequences on the patient or family (Diniaco & Ingoldsby, 1983; Kowba & Schwirian, 1985; LaRosa, Murphy, Wade, & Clasby, 1995; Lewis et al., 1991; Nicholson et al., 1993; Paludetto, Faggiano-Perfetto, Asprea, De Curtis, & Margara-Paludetto, 1981; Ramsey, Cathelyn,

Gugliotta, & Glenn, 1999; Schulte et al., 1993; Solheim & Spellacy, 1988; Tuller et al., 1997; Yu, Jamieson, & Astbury, 1981).

Another critical nursing intervention is nurses' provision of information and support to critically ill patients' families. Information has been identified as a crucial component in family coping and satisfaction in critical care settings, and support, in the form of nurses' caring behaviors and interactions, is enormously influential in shaping the critical care experience for both patients and families (Benner, et al., 1999). Taken together, these two nursing interventions are highly valued by families and are even more meaningful when family access is ensured.

RESEARCH ANALYSIS

ARTICLE REFERENCE
Leur, J., Zwarveling, J., Loef, B., & Schans, C. (2003). Patient recollection of airway suctioning in the ICU: Routine versus a minimally invasive procedure. *Intensive Care Medicine, 29,* 433-436.

REVIEW OF STUDY METHODS AND FINDINGS
The purpose of this prospective, randomized clinical trial was to determine whether critically ill patients perceived minimally invasive airway suctioning (group 1) as less stressful or uncomfortable as compared with patients who received routine endotracheal suctioning (group 2). Routine endotracheal suctioning was accomplished by removing group 2 patients from the ventilator, manually hyperinflating with 100% fraction of inspired oxygen, and suctioning using a standard 49-cm suction catheter. With routine endotracheal suctioning, negative pressure (200 to 400 mm Hg) was applied for a maximum duration of 3 seconds, and the procedure was repeated three to four times. Normal saline was instilled between suctioning cycles for group 2 patients. Additional suctioning was allowed if clinically warranted. Group 1 patients received the same treatment as group 2 patients, except they were suctioned using custom-made 29-cm suction catheters. All group 1 patients had an endotracheal tube of the same length as the suction catheter, so it was impossible to touch the trachea or bronchi with the suction catheter. Group 1 patients did not receive normal saline boluses down their endotracheal tubes. Additionally, patients in group 1 were suctioned on demand, based on their clinical needs. All adult patients admitted to two participating critical care units in the Netherlands were included and were randomized to group 1 or group 2 if they were intubated for longer than 24 hours. Participating patients completed a questionnaire within 3 days of critical care unit discharge (N = 208). No significant difference in level of discomfort was found between group 1 and group 2, although patients in group 1 had a statistically significant decreased prevalence of suctioning recollection as compared with group 2 patients (*P* = .001). Minimally invasive airway suctioning resulted in decreased recollection of airway suctioning when compared with routine endotracheal suctioning, but it did not appear to minimize the discomfort associated with endotracheal suctioning.

BRIEF CRITIQUE OF STUDY STRENGTHS AND WEAKNESSES
This study contributes to the growing body of literature that tests which routine procedures in the critical care unit can accomplish the same desired result while optimizing beneficial outcomes. In this case, patients who were suctioned using the minimally invasive suctioning equipment did not recall the procedures as clearly or vividly as patients in the group receiving routine endotracheal suctioning. The researchers attribute this difference to the treatment regimens, namely, patients in group 1 were suctioned fewer times per day. Additionally, the lack of saline instillation in group 1 patients could have shortened the duration of each suctioning cycle. A shorter suctioning cycle without the added trauma of a saline bolus in one's airway could alone explain the statistical difference found.

IMPLICATIONS OF THE STUDY FOR NURSING PRACTICE
The implications of this study for nursing include the realization that some required procedures may be less noxious to critically ill patients than others. Although this study tested specialized equipment, future research should test whether patients report decreased discomfort when they are suctioned using an in-line suction catheter, as opposed to disconnecting the patient from the ventilator and manually hyperinflating as with routine endotracheal suctioning.

Encouraging family involvement in caregiving activities is another essential family nursing intervention, and it can range from minor involvement (e.g., asking a family member to pass an alcohol wipe) to major involvement (e.g., inviting a family member to assist with the patient's bath). Although numerous obstacles for family participation exist (e.g., hesitancy on the part of nurses, unit policies that prohibit family involvement, inadequate staffing, and lack of time), studies have shown that families both desire and value involvement in their loved ones' care (Chesla, 1996; Coulter, 1989; Glaser & Straus, 1968; Hammond, 1995; Pondelicek, Konigova, & Broz, 1983). Simple acts of helping can facilitate patient-family bonding and togetherness, can promote patient healing and comfort, can decrease a family member's sense of helplessness and anxiety, and can assist family members in understanding their loved one's condition (Benner, et al., 1999).

The Critical Care Nurse

The historical conceptualization of nursing—namely, one that defines clinical practice by the nurse's role, the clinical setting, and the patient's diagnosis—is of limited utility in today's current health care climate because it overlooks patients' and families' unique needs and characteristics as the driving force behind nursing practice (AACN Certification Corporation, 1995). In response to the evolving health care system, AACN and the AACN Certification Corporation designed a model that describes nursing practice based on the needs and characteristics of patients and their families (Curley, 1998). The core concept behind this model, which is called the *synergy model*, is that the unique needs or characteristics of patients and their families influence and drive the competencies of the nurses who care for them (AACN & AACN Certification Corporation, 2003). According to the model, optimal patient outcomes result when patients' and nurses' characteristics are matched (Curley, 1998). The process of matching the needs and characteristics of a particular patient and family with those of the nurse creates synergy or the cooperative activity of two or more agents or people, which, when working together, produce a combined result greater than they would have if they were working alone.

THE SYNERGY MODEL

Seven patient characteristics that span the continuum of health and illness (Table 2-3) and eight nursing competencies (Table 2-4) comprise the synergy model. Patients move among different points along the seven continua. Thus, to create synergy, nurses must

---

TABLE 2-3

American Association of Critical-Care Nurses Synergy Model Patient Characteristics

Resiliency: the capacity to return to a restorative level of functioning using compensatory/coping mechanisms; the ability to bounce back quickly after an insult

Vulnerability: susceptibility to actual or potential stressors that may adversely affect patient outcomes

Stability: the ability to maintain a steady-state equilibrium

Complexity: the intricate entanglement of two or more systems (e.g., body, family, therapies)

Resource Availability: extent of resources (e.g., technical, fiscal, personal, psychological, and social) that the patient/family/community bring to the situation

Participation in Care: extent to which patient/family engages in aspects of care

Participation in Decision Making: extent to which patient/family engages in decision making

Predictability: a characteristic that allows one to expect a certain course of events or course of illness

From *The AACN synergy model for patient care.* (2004). Aliso Viejo, CA: AACN Certification Corporation.

---

be able to bring into play any of the given competencies in order to best meet patient needs. Although all eight nursing competencies are essential for nursing practice, each assumes more or less importance based on the patient's unique characteristics (Curley, 1998). Several assumptions regarding patients, families, and nurses guide the synergy model (Biel, 1997). First, all patient and nurse characteristics must be viewed in context. Second, patients are biological, psychological, social, and spiritual entities who present at a particular developmental stage. The whole patient (body, mind, and spirit) must be considered. Third, the patient, family, and community all contribute to providing a context for the nurse-patient relationship. Finally, patients and nurses can be described by certain characteristics. All characteristics and competencies contribute to each other, and, as such, cannot be understood in isolation. The interrelated dimensions paint the profile of the patient and nurse.

APPLYING THE SYNERGY MODEL TO PRACTICE

A critical care nurse shared a clinical incident involving a patient named Sandy and her family for whom the nurse had cared (Stannard, 1999):

Sandy was [in the hospital] for 5 months. She had four kids and a husband. She was 34 when she

TABLE 2-4

American Association of Critical-Care Nurses Synergy Model Nurse Competencies

Clinical Judgment: clinical reasoning, which includes clinical decision making, critical thinking, and a global grasp of the situation, coupled with nursing skills acquired through a process of integrating education, experiential knowledge, and evidence-based guidelines.

Clinical Inquiry (Innovator/Evaluator): the ongoing process of questioning and evaluating practice and providing informed practice. Creating changes through evidence-based practice, research utilization, and experiential knowledge.

Collaboration: working with others (e.g., patients, families, health care providers) in a way that promotes/ encourages each person's contributions toward achieving optimal/realistic patient/family goals. Involves intra- and inter-disciplinary work with all colleagues and community.

Systems Thinking: the body of knowledge and tools that allow the nurse to manage whatever environmental and system resources exist for the patient/family and staff, within or across healthcare and non-healthcare systems.

Advocacy and Moral Agency: working on another's behalf and representing the concerns of patient/family and nursing staff; serving as a moral agent in identifying and helping to resolve ethical and clinical concerns within outside the clinical setting.

Caring Practices: the constellation of nursing activities that create a compassionate, supportive, and therapeutic environment for patients and staff, with the aim of promoting comfort and healing and preventing unnecessary suffering. Includes, but is not limited to, vigilance, engagement, and responsiveness of caregivers, including family and healthcare personnel.

Response to Diversity: the sensitivity to recognize, appreciate and incorporate differences into the provision of care. Differences may include, but are not limited to, cultural differences, spiritual beliefs, gender, race, ethnicity, lifestyle, socioeconomic status, age, and values.

Facilitation of Learning: the ability to facilitate learning for patients/families, nursing staff, other members of the health care team, and community. Includes both formal and informal facilitation of learning.

From *The AACN synergy model for patient care.* (2004). Aliso Viejo, CA: AACN Certification Corporation.

[developed] a viral syndrome that really affected her heart. . . . Here was this young, beautiful woman who, 3 days ago, was leading an aerobics class, and suddenly was dying. . . . She was on the VAD [ventricular assist device], she was on a balloon pump, she was bleeding, I mean everything! We [the health care team] were very hopeful, but things didn't look good. [And the husband] was so scared of all the technology. [But] he knew that Sandy liked to have her makeup on. So he held her hand through the whole ordeal and stopped getting scared of the machines. A month into [the critical care unit stay], he was putting lipstick on her [endotracheal] tube! He was right in there.

The patient in this clinical incident had a miraculous recovery, was transferred to a cardiac rehabilitation facility, and eventually was discharged to home. Although this is a dramatic story, it also illustrates the synergistic power of the nurse-patient-family relationship that helped to produce optimal patient and family outcomes.

Because this patient required such extensive cardiac and ventilatory support by way of external circulatory assist devices and mechanical ventilation, the patient's condition could be described as extremely vulnerable, highly unstable, and very complex. Sandy was also very resilient, because many other patients could not have survived such massive circulatory collapse. The social support the husband provided the patient during her extended critical care unit stay factored highly into the patient's resource availability, as did the husband's participation in care and decision making. For example, although cosmetics may seem like mere accessorizing to some, Sandy's makeup was an important part of who she was. By taking an active role, the husband helped to preserve Sandy's identity and what was important to her when she was unable to do that for herself. Finally, the patient could be described as very unpredictable because even though the health care team was very hopeful, her condition did not look good. In spite of her often tenuous physiological status, Sandy survived the hospitalization and was eventually discharged home to be with her family.

Because patient characteristics and needs drive nurse competencies according to the synergy model, it is important briefly to examine the competencies of the nurse who cared for Sandy and her husband. The patient's highly vulnerable, unstable, and complex state certainly required keen clinical judgment on the part of the nurse. Finely honed clinical reasoning and expert nursing skills were needed to stabilize and maintain the patient's labile hemodynamic status, as well as to support the patient's husband so he could be there to advocate for and assist his critically ill wife. This particular patient also required the nurse to be a strong moral agent. Listening to the husband's concerns about the pervasive technology surrounding Sandy's bedside and helping him to acclimate to the critical care unit and to Sandy's changing clinical condition illustrates strong advocacy and moral agency skills. Working closely with the patient's husband also required the nurse to be a strong facilitator of learning, with good collaboration skills and well-developed caring practices. Through vigilance, engagement, and responsiveness to Sandy and her husband, the nurse established a trusting relationship, which involved the sharing of information and support. Finally, the way in which this clinical incident was framed by the nurse does not lead one to believe that high levels of systems thinking, response to diversity, or clinical inquiry were required for the nurse to optimally care for this particular patient and her family. It is not difficult, however, to think of other patients whose cases require these particular nurse competencies to be highly developed.

In summary, the nurse, patient, and family developed synergy together through their evolving relationship, which produced greater results than if any one of these parties had worked without the others. Yet the relationship itself is what created the synergy. With the heavy emphasis on outcomes in our current health care environment, it is important to realize that the process, namely, matching patients' and families' needs with nurses' competencies, is essential to achieving optimal outcomes.

SUMMARY

The experience of critical illness has a profound effect on the patient, the critically ill patient's family, and the critical care nurses involved in the care. This chapter provides an overview of the critical care environment, as well as the experience of critical illness from the perspective of the patient, family, and nurse. By understanding the critical care experience from a variety of perspectives, critical care nurses are better able to tailor their responses and interventions to meet what is both desired and required by critically ill patients and families. The resulting synergy is essential to achieving optimal patient, family, and nurse outcomes.

CRITICAL THINKING QUESTIONS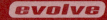

1. If you could design the ideal critical care space, what would it look like and why?
2. Nurse staffing levels, nurse-physician collaboration, and type of critical care area and unit culture have all been identified as critical contextual factors that influence nurses' ability to provide quality patient and family care. List other contextual factors you believe would affect a nurse's ability to achieve optimal patient and family outcomes.
3. You are the nurse caring for an elderly patient who is anxious and agitated. How would you differentiate delirium from dementia, and what interventions would you employ to ensure the patient's safety, comfort, and well-being?
4. You are the critical care nurse caring for two patients, one of Asian descent and another of black/African-American descent. How would you expect the belief systems and preferences of these patients to differ, based on knowledge of these two cultural backgrounds?
5. Research has demonstrated that family needs can be grouped into five categories: receiving assurance, remaining near the patient, receiving information, being comfortable, and having support available. Meeting these needs has also been shown to increase family satisfaction. What specific nursing interventions would you employ to meet these five family need categories?
6. You are the charge nurse in a busy critical care unit. How would you use the synergy model to help make nurse-patient assignments?

REFERENCES

Aiken, L., Clarke, S., & Sloane, D. (2002). Hospital staffing, organization, and quality of care: Cross-national findings. *International Journal for Quality in Health Care, 14*(1), 5-13.

American Association of Critical-Care Nurses (AACN). (2002). AACN fact sheet. Retrieved from http://www.aacn.org. Accessed 7/6/2004.

American Association of Critical-Care Nurses and AACN Certification Corporation (2003). Safeguarding the patient and the profession: The value of critical care nurse certification (white paper). *American Journal of Critical Care, 12*, 154-164.

Azoulay, E., Chevret, S., Leleu, G., Pochard, F., Barboteu, M., Adrie, C., Canoui, P., Le Gall, J. & Schlemmer, B. (2000).

Half the families of intensive care unit patients experience inadequate communication with physicians. *Critical Care Medicine, 28,* 3044-3049.

Azoulay, E., Pochard, F., Chevret, S., Lemaire, F., Mokhtari, M., Le Gall, J., Dhainaut, J., & Schlemmer, B. (2001). Meeting the needs of intensive care unit patient families: A multicenter study. *American Journal of Respiratory and Critical Care Medicine, 163,* 135-139.

Baggs, J., Schmitt, M., Mushlin, A., Mitchell, P., Eldredge, D., Oakes, D., & Hutson, A. (1999). Association between nurse-physician collaboration and patient outcomes in three intensive care units. *Critical Care Medicine, 27*(9), 1991-1998.

Baldursdottir, G., & Jonsdottir, H. (2002). The importance of nurse caring behaviors as perceived by patients receiving care at an emergency department. *Heart and Lung, 31,* 67-75.

Bally, K., Campbell, D., Chesnick, K., & Tranmer, J. (2003). Effects of patient-controlled music therapy during coronary angiography on procedural pain and anxiety distress syndrome. *Critical Care Nurse, 23*(2), 50-58.

Bass, L. (1991). What do parents need when their infant is a patient in the NICU? *Neonatal Network, 10*(4), 25-33.

Bayat, A., Shaaban, H., Dodgson, A., & Dunn, K. (2003). Implications for burns unit design following outbreak of multi-resistant *Acinetobacter* infection in ICU and burns unit. *Burns, 29,* 303-306.

Benner, P., Hooper-Kyriakidis, P., & Stannard, D. (1999). *Clinical wisdom and interventions in critical care: A thinking-in-action approach.* Philadelphia: W. B. Saunders.

Benner, P., Tanner, C., & Chesla, C. (1996). *Expertise in nursing practice: Caring, clinical judgment, and ethics.* New York: Springer.

Berens, R., & Weigle, C. (1996). Cost analysis of ceiling tile replacement for noise abatement. *Journal of Perinatology, 16*(3), 199-201.

Biel, M. (1997). Reconceptualizing certified practice: Envisioning critical care practice of the future (white paper). Aliso Viejo, CA: AACN Certification Corporation.

Bijttebier, P., Delva, D., Vannost, S., Bobbaers, H., Lauwers, P., & Vertommen, H. (2000). Reliability and validity of the critical care family needs inventory in a Dutch-speaking Belgian sample. *Heart and Lung, 29,* 278-286.

Blachly, P., & Starr, A. (1964). Postcardiotomy delirium. *American Journal of Psychiatry, 121,* 371-375.

Bushy, A. (1999). The need for cultural-linguistic competent care for families with special health problems. In J. Sebastian & A. Bushy (Eds.). *Special populations in the community: Advances in reducing health disparities.* Gaithersburg, MD: Aspen.

Byers, J., & Smyth, K. (1997). Effect of a music intervention on noise annoyance, heart rate, and blood pressure in cardiac surgery patients. *American Journal of Critical Care, 6,* 183-191.

Cartledge, S. (2001). Factors influencing the turnover of intensive care nurses. *Intensive and Critical Care Nursing, 17,* 348-355.

Cassem, N., & Hackett, T. (1972). Sources of tension for the CCU nurse. *American Journal of Nursing, 72*(8), 1426-1430.

Chesla, C. A. (1996). Reconciling technologic and family care in critical-care nursing. *Journal of Nursing Scholarship, 28*(3), 199-203.

Chesla, C., & Stannard, D. (1997). Breakdown in the nursing care of families in the ICU. *American Journal of Critical Care, 6*(1), 64-71.

Cho, S., Ketefian, S., Barkauskas, V., & Smith, D. (2003). The effects of nurse staffing on adverse events, morbidity, mortality, and medical costs. *Nursing Research, 52*(2), 71-80.

Coulter, M. (1989). The needs of family members of patients in intensive care units. *Intensive Care Nursing, 5,* 4-10.

Curley, M. (1998). Patient-nurse synergy: Optimizing patients' outcomes. *American Journal of Critical Care, 7,* 64-72.

Dang, D., Johantgen, M., Pronovost, P., Jenckes, M., & Bass, E. (2002). Postoperative complications: Does intensive care unit staff nursing make a difference? *Heart and Lung, 31*(3), 219-228.

Danis, M., Jarr, S., Southerland, L., Nocella, R., & Patrick, D. (1987). A comparison of patient, family, and nurse evaluations of the usefulness of intensive care. *Critical Care Medicine, 15*(2), 138-143.

Danis, M., Patrick, D., Southerland, L, & Green, M. (1988). Patients' and families' preferences for medical intensive care. *JAMA, 260,* 797-802.

Diniaco, M., & Ingoldsby, B. (1983). Parental presence in the recovery room. *AORN Journal, 38*(4), 685-693.

Doering, L., McGuire, A., & Rourke, D. (2002). Recovering from cardiac surgery: What patients want you to know. *American Journal of Critical Care, 11,* 333-343.

Eddleston, J., White, P., & Guthrie, E. (2000). Survival, morbidity, and quality of life after discharge from intensive care. *Critical Care Medicine, 28,* 2293-2299.

Egerton, N., & Kay, J. (1964). Psychological disturbances associated with open-heart surgery. *British Journal of Psychiatry, 110,* 1365-1370.

Environmental Protection Agency (EPA). (2004). EPA Identifies Noise Levels Affecting Health and Welfare. Retrieved from http://www.epa.gov/history1/topics/noise/01.htm. Accessed 7/6/2004.

Farrell, M., & Frost, C. (1992). The most important needs of parents of critically ill children: Parents' perceptions. *Intensive and Critical Care Nursing, 8,* 130-139.

Fischer, J., Calame, A., Dettling, A., Zeier, H., & Fanconi, S. (2000). Experience and endocrine stress responses in neonatal and pediatric critical care nurses and physicians. *Critical Care Medicine, 28,* 3281-3288.

Fisher, M. (1994). Identified needs of parents in a pediatric intensive care unit. *Critical Care Nurse, 14*(3), 82-90.

Fitzsimmons, D., Parahoo, K., Richardson, S., & Stringer, M. (2003). Patient anxiety while on a waiting list for coronary artery bypass surgery: A qualitative and quantitative analysis. *Heart and Lung, 32,* 23-31.

Fletcher, S., Kennedy, D., Ghosh, I., Misra, V., Kiff, K., Coakley, J., & Hinds, C. (2003). Persistent neuromuscular and neurophysiologic abnormalities in long-term survivors of prolonged critical illness. *Critical Care Medicine, 31,* 1012-1016.

Freichels, T. A. (1991). Needs of family members of patients in the intensive care unit over time. *Critical Care Nursing Quarterly, 14*(3), 16-29.

Frick, S., Uehlinger, D., & Zenklusen, R. (2002). Assessment of former ICU patients' quality of life: Comparison of different quality-of-life measures. *Intensive Care Medicine, 28*, 1405-1410.

Gardner, A., & Sibthorpe, B. (2002). Will he get back to normal? Survival and functional status after intensive care therapy. *Intensive and Critical Care Nursing, 18*, 138-145.

Glaser, B., & Strauss, A. (1968). *Time for dying.* Chicago: Aldine.

Groeger, J., Strosberg, M., Halpern, N., Raphaely, R., Kaye, W., Guntupalli, D., Bertram, D., Greenbaum, D., Clemmer, T., Gallagher, T., Nelson, L., Thompson, A., Cerra, F., & Davis, W. (1992). Descriptive analysis of critical care units in the United States. *Critical Care Medicine, 20*(6), 846-863.

Hammond, F. (1995). Involving families in care within the intensive care environment: A descriptive survey. *Intensive and Critical Care Nursing, 1*, 256-264.

Heyland, D., Rocker, G., Dodek, P., Kutsogiannis, D., Konopad, E., Cook, D., Peters, S., Tranmer, J., O'Callaghan, C. (2002). Family satisfaction with care in the intensive care unit: Results of a multiple center study. *Critical Care Medicine, 30*, 1413-1418.

Hilberman, M. (1975). The evolution of intensive care units. *Critical Care Medicine, 3*(4), 159-165.

Holland, C., Cason, C. L., & Prater, L. R. (1997). Patients' recollections of critical care. *Dimensions of Critical Care Nursing, 16*(3), 132-141.

Hunt, J., Hendrata, M., & Myles, P. (2000). Quality of life 12 months after coronary artery bypass graft surgery. *Heart and Lung, 29*, 401-411.

Hupcey, J. (2000). Feeling safe: The psychosocial needs of ICU patients. *Journal of Nursing Scholarship, 32*(4), 361-367.

Hupcey, J., & Zimmerman, H. (2000). The need to know: Experiences of critically ill patients. *American Journal of Critical Care, 9*, 192-198.

Johnson, D., Wilson, M., Cavanaugh, B., Bryden, C., Gudmundson, D., & Moodley, O. (1998). Measuring the ability to meet family needs in an intensive care unit. *Critical Care Medicine, 26*, 266-271.

Jones, J., Hoggart, B., Withey, J., Donaghue, K., & Ellis, B. W. (1979). What the patients say: A study of reactions to an intensive care unit. *Intensive Care Medicine, 5*, 89-92.

Keep, P. (1977). Stimulus deprivation in windowless rooms. *Anaesthesia, 32*, 598-600.

Keep, P., James, J., & Inman, M. (1980). Windows in the intensive therapy unit. *Anaesthesia, 35*, 257-262.

Kleiber, C., Halm, M., Titler, M, Montgomery, L., Johnson, S., Nicholson, A., Craft, M., Buckwalter, K., & Megivern, K. (1994). Emotional responses of family members during a critical care hospitalization. *American Journal of Critical Care, 3*, 70-76.

Koivula, M., Paunonen-Ilmonen, M., Tarkka, M., Tarkka, M, & Laippala, P. (2001). Fear and anxiety in patients awaiting coronary artery bypass grafting. *Heart and Lung, 30*, 302-311.

Kosco, M., & Warren, N. (2000). Critical care nurses' perceptions of family needs as met. *Critical Care Nursing Quarterly, 23*(2), 60-72.

Kowba, M. D., & Schwirian, P. M. (1985). Direct sibling contact and bacterial colonization in newborns. *Journal of Obstetric, Gynecologic, and Neonatal Nursing, 14*(5), 412-417.

LaRosa, P., Murphy, J., Wade, L., & Clasby, L. (1995). Implementing a parent-present induction program. *AORN Journal, 61*(3), 526-531.

Lawrence, M. (1995). The unconscious experience. *American Journal of Critical Care, 4*, 227-232.

Lee, I., Chien, W., & Mackenzie, A. (2000). Needs of families with a relative in a critical care unit in Hong Kong. *Journal of Clinical Nursing, 9*, 46-54.

Leigh, H., Hofer, M., Cooper, J., & Reiser, M. (1972). A psychological comparison of patients in "open" and "closed" coronary care units. *Journal of Psychosomatic Research, 16*, 449-457.

Leske, J. S. (1986). Needs of relatives of critically ill patients: A follow-up. *Heart and Lung, 15*(2), 189-193.

Leske, J. (1992). Needs of family members after critical illness: Prescriptions for interventions. *Critical Care Nursing Clinics of North America, 4*, 587-596.

Lewis, M., Bendersky, M., Koons, A., Hegyi, T., Hiatt, I., Ostfeld, B., & Rosenfeld, D. (1991). Visitation to a neonatal intensive care unit. *Pediatrics, 88*(4), 795-800.

McKinney, A., & Deeny, P. (2002). Leaving the intensive care unit: A phenomenological study of the patients' experience. *Intensive and Critical Care Nursing, 18*, 320-331.

Mendelsohn, A., Belle, S., Fischhoff, B., Wisniewski, S., Degenholtz, H., & Chelluri, L. (2002). How patients feel about prolonged mechanical ventilation 1 year later. *Critical Care Medicine, 30*, 1439-1445.

Mendonca, D., & Warren, N. (1998). Perceived and unmet needs of critical care family members. *Critical Care Nursing Quarterly, 21*(1), 58-67.

Mi-Kuen, T., French, P., & Lueng, K. (1999). The needs of the family of critically ill neurosurgical patients: A comparison of nurses' and family members' perceptions. *Journal of Neuroscience Nursing, 31*(6), 348-356.

Minnick, A., Leipzig, R., & Johnson, M. (2001). Elderly patients' reports of physical restraint experiences in intensive care units. *American Journal of Critical Care, 10*, 168-171.

Mitchell, P., Armstrong, S., Simpson, T., & Lentz, M. (1989). American Association of Critical-Care Nurses Demonstration Project: Profile of excellence in critical care nursing. *Heart and Lung, 18*, 19-37.

Molter, N. (1979). Needs of relatives of critically ill patients: A descriptive study. *Heart and Lung, 8*(2), 332-339.

Morrison, W., Haas, E., Shaffner, D., Garrett, E., & Fackler, J. (2003). Noise, stress, and annoyance in a pediatric intensive care unit. *Critical Care Medicine, 31*, 113-119.

Needleman, J., Buerhaus, P., Mattke, S., Stewart, M., & Zelevinsky, K. (2002). Nurse-staffing levels and the quality of care in hospitals. *New England Journal of Medicine, 346*, 1715-1722.

Nelson, J., Meier, D., Oei, E., Nierman, D., Senzel, R., Manfredi, P., Davis, S., & Morrison, R. (2001). Self-reported symptom experience of critically ill cancer patients receiving intensive care. *Critical Care Medicine, 29*, 277-282.

Nicholson, A., Titler, M., Montgomery, L., Kleiber, C., Craft, M., Halm, M., Buckwalter, K., & Johnson, S. (1993). Effects of child visitation in adult critical care units: A pilot study. *Heart and Lung, 22*, 36-45.

O'Donnell, J. (1990). The development of a climate for caring: A historical review of premature care in the United States from 1900 to 1979. *Neonatal Network, 8*(6), 7-17.

Olson, D., Borel, C., Laskowitz, D., Moore, D., & McConnell, E. (2001). Quiet time: A nursing intervention to promote sleep in neurocritical care units. *American Journal of Critical Care, 10*, 74-78.

Paludetto, R., Faggiano-Perfetto, M., Asprea, A., De Curtis, M., & Margara-Paludetto, P. (1981). Reactions of sixty parents allowed unrestricted contact with infants in a neonatal intensive care unit. *Early Human Development, 5*, 401-409.

Pondelicek, I., Konigova, R., & Broz, L. (1983). Role of "accompanying" relatives in burn care. *Acta Chirurgiae Plasticae, 25*(4), 213-216.

Ramsey, P., Cathelyn, J., Gugliotta, B., & Glenn, L. (1999). Visitor and nurse satisfaction with a visitation policy change in critical care units. *Dimensions of Critical Care Nursing, 18*(5), 42-48.

Rotundi, A., Chelluri, L., Sirio, C., Mendelsohn, A., Schulz, R., Belle, S., Im, K., Donahoe, M., & Pinsky, M. (2002). Patients' recollections of stressful experiences while receiving prolonged mechanical ventilation in an intensive care unit. *Critical Care Medicine, 30*, 746-752.

Schnyder, U., Morgeli, H., Nigg, C., Klaghofer, R., Renner, N., Trentz, O., & Buddeber, C. (2000). Early psychological reactions to life-threatening injuries. *Critical Care Medicine, 28*, 86-92.

Schulte, D., Burrell, L., Gueldner, S., Bramlett, M., Fuszard, B., Stone, S., & Dudley, W. (1993). Pilot study of the relationship between heart rate and ectopy and unrestricted vs. restricted visiting hours in the coronary care unit. *American Journal of Critical Care, 2*, 134-136.

Shannon, S., Mitchell, P., & Cain, K. (2002). Patients, nurses, and physicians have differing views of quality of critical care. *Journal of Nursing Scholarship, 34*(2), 173-179.

Shenkman, B., & Stechmiller, J. (1987). Patient and family perception of projected functioning after discharge from a burn unit. *Heart and Lung, 16*, 490-496.

Simpson, T. (1991). Critical care patients' perceptions of visits. *Heart and Lung, 20*(6), 681-688.

Simpson, T., Armstrong, S., & Mitchell, P. (1989). American Association of Critical-Care Nurses Demonstration Project: Patients' recollections of critical care. *Heart and Lung, 18*, 325-332.

Simpson, T., Lee, E., & Cameron, C. (1996). Patients' perceptions of environmental factors that disturb sleep after cardiac surgery. *American Journal of Critical Care, 5*, 173-181.

Soehren, P. (1995). Stressors perceived by cardiac surgical patients in the intensive care unit. *American Journal of Critical Care, 4*, 71-76.

Solheim, K., & Spellacy, C. (1988). Sibling visitation: Effects on newborn infection rates. *Journal of Obstetric, Gynecologic, and Neonatal Nursing, 17*(1), 43-48.

Stannard, D. (1999). Being a good dance partner: The synergy model in practice. *Critical Care Nurse, 19*(6), 86-87.

Stannard, D., Puntillo, K., Miaskowski, C., Gleeson, S. Kehrle, K., & Nye, P. (1996). Clinical judgment and management of postoperative pain in critical care patients. *American Journal of Critical Care, 5*, 433-441.

Stein-Parbury, J., & McKinley, S. (2000). Patients' experiences of being in an intensive care unit: A select literature review. *American Journal of Critical Care, 9*, 20-27.

Swoboda, S., & Lipsett, P. (2002). Impact of a prolonged surgical critical illness on patients' families. *American Journal of Critical Care, 11*, 459-466.

Szokol, J., & Vender, J. (2001). Anxiety, delirium, and pain in the intensive care unit. *Critical Care Clinics, 17*(4), 821-842.

Tuller, S., McCabe, L., Cronenwett, L., Hastings, D., Shaheen, A., Daley-Faulkner, C., & Wheeler, K. (1997). Patient, visitor, and nurse evaluations of visitation for adult postanesthesia care unit patients. *Journal of Perianesthesia Nursing, 12*(6), 402-412.

Turner, J. S., Briggs, S. J., Springhorn, H. E., & Potgieter, P. D. (1990). Patients' recollections of intensive care unit experience. *Critical Care Medicine, 18*(9), 966-968.

Twibell, R., Siela, D., & Mahmoodi, M. (2003). Subjective perceptions and physiological variables during weaning from mechanical ventilation. *American Journal of Critical Care, 12*, 101-112.

Walder, B., Francioli, D., Meyer, J., Lancon, M., & Romand, J. (2000). Effects of guidelines implementation in a surgical intensive care unit to control nighttime light and noise levels. *Critical Care Medicine, 28*, 2242-2247.

Wasser, T., Pasquale, M., Matchett, S., Bryan, Y., & Pasquale, M. (2001). Establishing reliability and validity of the critical care family satisfaction survey. *Critical Care Medicine, 29*, 192-196.

Wong, H., Lopez-Nahas, V., & Molassiotis, A. (2001). Effects of music therapy on anxiety in ventilator-dependent patients. *Heart and Lung, 30*, 376-387.

Wright, L. & Leahey, M. (2000). *Nurses and families: A guide to family assessment and intervention.* 3rd ed. Philadelphia: F. A. Davis.

Yu, V., Jamieson, J., & Astbury, J. (1981). Parents' reactions to unrestricted parental contact with infants in the intensive care nursery. *Medical Journal of Australia, 1*, 294-296.

RECOMMENDED READINGS

Centers for Disease Control and Prevention and the Health care Infection Control Practices Advisory Committee. (2003). Guidelines for environmental infection control in health-care facilities [Special issue]. *Morbidity & Mortality Weekly Report, 52.*

Consensus Committee, American Academy of Pediatrics. (2003). Recommended standards for newborn ICU design [Special issue]. *Journal of Perinatology, 23,* s3-s21.

Grumet, G. (1994). Noise hampers healing and curbs productivity. *Health Facilities Management, 7*(1), 22-25.

Leur, J., Zwaveling, J., Loef, B., & Schans, C. (2003). Patient recollection of airway suctioning in the ICU: Routine versus a minimally invasive procedure. *Intensive Care Medicine, 29,* 433-436.

Reuben, D., Herr, K., Pacala, J., Potter, J., Pollock, B., & Semla, T. (2002). *Geriatrics at your fingertips.* New York: American Geriatrics Society.

Stannard, D. (2001). Family care. In H. Schell & K. Puntillo (Eds.). *Critical care nursing secrets.* Philadelphia: Hanley & Belfus.

evolve *Did you remember to check out the bonus material, including free self-assessment exercises, on the Evolve Web site at http://evolve.elsevier.com/Sole/ and on the CD-ROM?*

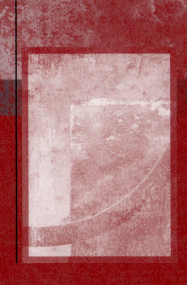

CHAPTER 3

Ethical and Legal Issues in Critical Care Nursing

Jacqueline Fowler Byers, PhD, RN, CNAA

OBJECTIVES

- Discuss nurses' ethical obligations to patients in the critical care setting.
- Compare the components of a systematic, ethical decision-making model.
- Describe the ethical and legal value of established ethical codes and standards of care.
- Define professional negligence and its relationship with legal professional negligence claims.
- Identity three conditions that must be present for patients to give informed consent.
- Explain how advance directives ensure patients' rights to self-determination.
- Discuss the legal and ethical issues that surround organ and tissue transplantation.

Introduction

Critical care nurses are often confronted with ethical and legal dilemmas related to informed consent, withholding or withdrawal of life-sustaining treatment, organ and tissue transplantation, confidentiality, and, increasingly, justice in the distribution of health care resources. Many dilemmas are byproducts of advanced medical technologies and therapies developed over the past several decades. Although technology provides substantial benefits to critically ill patients, extensive public and professional debate occurs over the appropriate use of these technologies, especially those that are life sustaining. One of the primary concerns in critical care is whether patients' values and beliefs about treatment can be overridden by the technological imperative, or the strong tendency to use technology because it is available.

Although many ethical dilemmas are not unique to critical care, they occur with greater frequency in critical care settings. Therefore, it is crucial that nurses examine the nature and scope of their ethical and legal obligations to patients.

The ethical and legal issues that frequently arise in the nursing care of critical care patients are examined in this chapter. The discussion includes problems that surround patients' rights and nurses' obligations, professional negligence, informed consent, withholding and withdrawal of treatment, and organ and tissue transplantation. The elements of ethical decision making and the involvement of the nurse are discussed.

Ethical Obligations and Nurse Advocacy

Critical care nurses' ethical and legal responsibilities for patient care have increased dramatically since the early 1990s. Evolving case law and current concepts

evolve *Be sure to check out the bonus material, including free self-assessment exercises, on the Evolve Web site at http://evolve.elsevier.com/Sole/ and on the CD-ROM.*

of nurse advocacy and accountability indicate that nurses have substantial ethical and legal obligations to promote and protect the welfare of their patients.

The duty to practice ethically and to serve as an ethical agent on behalf of patients is an integral part of nurses' professional practice. The nurse's duty is stated in the *Code for Nurses With Interpretive Statements,* which was adopted by the American Nurses Association (ANA) in 1976 and was revised in 2002 (ANA, 2002) (Box 3-1). The code for nurses delineates the moral principles that guide professional nursing practice. Nurses in all practice arenas, including critical care, must be knowledgeable about the provisions of the code and must incorporate its basic tenets into their clinical practice. The code is a powerful tool that shapes and evaluates individual practice, as well as the nursing profession. Additional ANA position statements related to human rights and ethics are available from the ANA's Web site (http://www.nursingworld.org).

Nurses' ethical obligation to serve as advocates for their patients is derived from the unique nature of the nurse-patient relationship. Critical care nurses assume a significant caregiving role that is characterized by intimate, extended contact with persons who are often the most physiologically and psychologically vulnerable and with their families. Critical care nurses have a

moral and professional responsibility to act as advocates on their patients' behalf because of their unique relationship with their patients and their specialized nursing knowledge. The American Association of Critical Care Nurses (AACN) published *An Ethic of Care* (AACN, 2002) that illustrates the ethical foundations for critical care practice. Ethics involves the interrelatedness and interdependence of individuals, systems and society. When ethical care is practiced, individual uniqueness, personal relationships, and the dynamic nature of life are respected. Compassion, collaboration, accountability and trust are essential characteristics of ethical nursing practice (AACN, 2002).

Ethical Decision Making

As reflected in the ANA code of ethics (ANA, 2002), one of the primary ethical obligations of professional nurses is protection of their patients' basic rights. This obligation requires nurses to recognize ethical dilemmas that actually or potentially threaten patients' rights and to participate in the resolution of those dilemmas.

An ethical dilemma is a difficult problem or situation in which conflicts exist about the making of morally justifiable decisions. Whether to give the one available critical care bed to a patient with cancer

---

BOX 3-1

The American Nurses Association Code of Ethics for Nurses

1. The nurse, in all professional relationships, practices with compassion and respect for the inherent dignity, worth, and uniqueness of every individual, unrestricted by considerations of social or economic status, personal attributes, or the nature of health problems.
2. The nurse's primary commitment is to the patient, whether it is an individual, family, group or community.
3. The nurse promotes, advocates for, and strives to protect the health, safety, and rights of the patient.
4. The nurse is responsible and accountable for individual practice and determines the appropriate delegation of tasks consistent with the nurse's obligation to provide optimum patient care.
5. The nurse owes the same to self as to others, including the responsibility to preserve integrity and safety, to maintain competence, and to continue personal and professional growth.
6. The nurse participates in establishing, maintaining, and improving health care environments and conditions of employment conducive to the provision of quality health care and consistent with the values of the profession through individual and collective action.
7. The nurse participates in the advancement of the profession through contributions to practice, education, administration, and knowledge development.
8. The nurse collaborates with other health professionals and the public in promoting community, national and international efforts to meet health needs.
9. The profession of nursing, as represented by organizations and their members, is responsible for articulating nursing values, for maintaining the integrity of the profession and its practice, and for shaping social policy.

Reprinted with permission from American Nurses Association. (2001). *Code of ethics for nurses with interpretive statements.* Washington, DC: American Nurses Publishing, American Nurses Foundation/American Nurses Association.

who is experiencing hypotension after chemotherapy or to a patient in the emergency department who has an acute myocardial infarction is an example of an ethical dilemma. The conflicting issue in this example is which patient should be given the bed, based on the moral allocation of limited resources.

Rushton and Scanlon (1998) list warning signs that can assist the critical care nurse in recognizing that an ethical dilemma may exist.

- Is the situation emotionally charged?
- Has the patient's condition changed significantly?
- Is there confusion or conflict about the facts?
- Is there increased hesitancy about the right course of action?

- Is the proposed action a deviation from customary practice?
- Is there a perceived need for secrecy around the proposed action?

If these warning signs occur, the critical care nurse must reassess the situation and determine whether an ethical dilemma exists and what additional action is needed.

Arriving at a morally justifiable decision when an ethical dilemma exists can be difficult for patients, families, and health professionals. One helpful way to approach ethical decision making is to use a systematic, structured process, such as the one depicted in Figure 3-1. This model provides a framework for

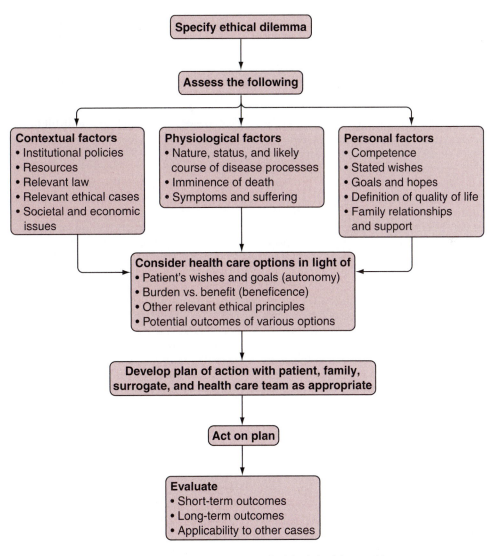

FIGURE 3-1 The process of ethical decision making.

evaluation of the related ethical principles and the potential outcomes, as well as relevant facts concerning the contextual factors and the patient's physiological and personal factors. Using this approach, the patient, family, and health care team members evaluate choices and identify the option that promotes the patient's best interests.

Ethical decision making includes implementing the decision and evaluating the short-term and long-term outcomes. Evaluation provides meaningful feedback about decisions and actions in specific instances, as well as the effectiveness of the decision-making process. The final stage in the decision-making process is assessing whether the decision in a specific case can be applied to other dilemmas in similar circumstances. In other words, is this decision useful in similar cases? A systematic approach to decision making does not guarantee that morally justifiable decisions are reached or that the outcome is beneficial to the patient. However, it ensures that all applicable information is considered in the decision.

Ethical Principles

As reflected in the decision-making model, relevant ethical principles should be considered when a moral dilemma exists. Principles facilitate moral decisions by guiding the decision-making process, but they may conflict with each other and may force a choice among the competing principles based on their relative weight in the situation. Several ethical principles are pertinent in the critical care setting. These principles are intended to provide respect and dignity for all persons.

The principle of *autonomy* states that any person should be free to govern his or her life to the greatest degree possible. The autonomy principle implies a strong sense of self-determination and an acceptance of responsibility for one's own choices and actions. Autonomy is the opposite of *paternalism*, which is interference with one's liberty. The threat of paternalism from health care providers has been reduced somewhat in recent years as the trend moves from unilateral to shared decision making.

The principle of *beneficence* is the duty to provide benefits to others when in a position to do so and to help balance harms and benefits. In other words, the benefits of an action should outweigh the burdens. A related concept is *futility*. Care should not be given if it is futile in terms of improving comfort or the medical outcome. The principle of *nonmaleficence* is the explicit duty not to inflict harm on others intentionally.

The principle of *justice* requires that health care resources be distributed fairly and equitably among groups of people. The principle of justice is particularly relevant to critical care, because most health care resources are expended in this practice setting. This includes all health care technology and pharmaceuticals currently available.

The principle of *veracity* states that persons are obligated to tell the truth in their communication with others. The principle of *fidelity* requires that one has a moral duty to be faithful to the commitments that one makes to others. These two principles, along with *confidentiality*, are the key to the nurse-patient relationship.

Increasing Nurses' Involvement in Ethical Decision Making

Although nurses play a significant role in the care of patients, they often report limited involvement in the formal processes of ethical decision making. Nurses' perception of limited involvement in the resolution of ethical dilemmas may be related to many factors, such as lack of formal educational preparation in ethics, lack of institutional mechanisms for review of dilemmas, perceived lack of administrative or peer support for involvement in decision making, concern about reprisals, and lack of perceived decision-making authority.

If nurses are to fulfill their advocacy obligations to patients, they must become active in the process of ethical decision making at all levels. Ways for nurses to increase their participation in ethical decision making starts with open communication with the health care team, the patient, and the family regarding the patient's wishes and ethical concerns. Some hospitals have established ethics consultation services with nursing and medical ethicists to assist staff, patients, and families in responding to difficult ethical issues. This service should be used when the issues cannot be resolved among the health care team, patient, and family. Nurses can also become more involved with ethical decision making through participation in institutional ethics committees, multidisciplinary ethics forums and ethics roundtables, peer review and quality assurance committees, and institutional research review boards.

The Joint Commission for Accreditation of Health Care Organizations requires that a formal mechanism be in place to address patients' ethical concerns. Bioethics committees are one way to address this need. A multidisciplinary committee of health professionals serves as an education and policy-making body and, in some cases, provides ethics consultation on a case-by-case basis. Typical membership includes physicians, nurses, chaplains, social workers, and, if available, bioethicists.

Nurses can improve and update their knowledge through formal and continuing education courses on bioethics, as well as through telephone and computerized electronic consultation and reference services. Educational programs and ethics consultation services are available through several ethics and law centers in the United States. A few key programs and services are listed in Box 3-2. Additional Internet educational resources are available.

Legal Accountability in Nursing

In addition to ethical obligations, nurses in the critical care setting have legal responsibilities to patients. Legal responsibilities have expanded dramatically since the early 1980s as nursing standards of care have been developed and used as a benchmark for defining professional responsibilities.

Preventing situations that compromise patients is far preferred to defending one's actions in court, but prevention is possible only if nurses have a clear, current knowledge of their legal obligations to patients. This section of the chapter briefly explores theories of professional negligence, as well as other legal doctrines relevant to critical care practice.

PROFESSIONAL NEGLIGENCE

Negligence is a category of tort law. A tort is a legal wrong committed by a person or persons against the person or property of another. To recover monetary damages or other forms of compensation, the law provides that the injured person may bring a civil suit against the person who caused harm.

Negligence is the failure of a person to act in a reasonable and prudent manner. Two types of negligence exist: acts of commission (e.g., giving a wrong medication to a patient) and acts of omission (e.g., failing to raise the side rails on the bed of a sedated patient or missing a critical laboratory test). The professional nurse's conduct is measured against a standard of care, or what other reasonably prudent nurses would do or not do in the same or similar circumstances. When a professional nurse commits negligent acts during the course of duty, the nurse may be liable for professional negligence, commonly referred to as malpractice.

ELEMENTS OF A PROFESSIONAL NEGLIGENCE CLAIM

In medical professional negligence cases, the plaintiff (the person bringing the suit) has the burden of proving that the defendant (the person being sued) is liable, or responsible for, an injury. For a professional negligence claim against a nurse to be successful, the plaintiff must establish proof of the following elements:
- The nurse had a specific professional duty to the patient.
- The nurse did not carry out his or her duty (i.e., breached a duty).
- The nurse caused injury to the patient.
- The patient suffered an injury as a result of the nurse's negligent action.

For example, a patient develops a corneal ulcer while he or she is unconscious. The nurse caring for the patient has a duty to assess and protect an unconscious patient's eyes from injury. If the nurse failed to assess and protect the patient's eyes, he or she breached the standard of care. If the patient and his or her legal team proves the nurse's failure to meet the standard of care resulted in the patient's corneal ulcer (the injury), professional negligence exists.

Professional Standards of Care

One of the most crucial aspects of negligence involving nurses is the determination of standards of care by which the conduct of professional nurses can be evaluated. From a legal perspective, a standard is defined as the general recognition of, and conformity to, established practice. A plaintiff who is able to establish that the nurse's failure to perform to an accepted standard of care caused an injury may win a judgment against the nurse.

Acceptable standards of professional nursing practice are derived from external sources, including expert nurse testimony, state nurse practice acts, the ANA standards of practice, accreditation standards and regulations, authoritative publications, and internal institutional policies and protocols. In addition, courts may review nursing job descriptions and nursing documentation. An acceptable standard of care is the minimum a professional nurse should do in a specific situation. An important standard for critical care nurses is the *Standards for Acute and Critical Care Nursing Practice* (Medina, 2000) (see Chapter 1). Standards generally reflect a growing trend to evaluate nursing practice from national rather than local standards. The underlying assumption in today's technological society is that most nurses have access to similar educational materials and scientific information and can be held to a universal standard. Because baseline standards of care are continuously evolving, the critical care nurse has a responsibility to maintain current knowledge in the field.

DUTY TO TREAT AND ABANDONMENT

Strong ethical and legal justifications support a nurse's duty to treat regardless of personal feelings about the patient or the patient's illness. From a legal perspective, a nurse's duty to provide care is derived from a contract or relationship with the employing agency and the historical tradition that the practice of professional nursing may involve certain acknowledged risks. An ethical obligation exists as well.

However, when a nurse is unwilling to care for a patient because it violates personal ethical or religious beliefs, the situation is different. No nurse is obligated to violate his or her moral beliefs. Examples may include a woman undergoing an abortion or a patient who refuses blood transfusions even though it is putting the patient's life in jeopardy.

In the instance of moral conflict, the required action of a professional nurse who objects to an assignment is to request a reassignment of the patient to another qualified nurse, and to ensure the transfer of care. However, this request may put the nurse's employment at risk if the employer has a policy requiring the nurse to provide care to all patients. A nurse should discuss potential moral conflicts with a potential supervisor before employment, to determine whether the employer has policies regarding situations in which moral conflict may arise. This approach allows both the nurse and the employer to be aware of potential issues and to make informed choices.

Nurses working in critical care settings are responsible for their patients' safe and continuous care. *Abandonment* by the nurse or by other health providers is defined as the unilateral severance of a professional relationship while a patient is still in need of health care. Although professional negligence cases involving abandonment primarily involve physicians, nurses have also been charged with abandonment.

Selected Ethical and Legal Issues

INFORMED CONSENT

Many complex dilemmas in critical care nursing concern informed consent. Consent problems arise because patients are experiencing acute, life-threatening illnesses that interfere with their ability to make decisions about treatment or participation in a clinical research study. The doctrine of informed consent is based on the principle of autonomy; competent adults have the right to self-determination or to make decisions regarding their acceptance or rejection of treatment.

Elements of Informed Consent

Three primary elements must be present for a person's consent or decline of medical treatment or research participation to be considered valid: competence, voluntariness, and disclosure of information. *Competence* (or capacity) refers to a person's ability to understand information regarding a proposed medical or nursing treatment. Competence is a legal term and is determined in court. Health care providers evaluate mental capacity. A patient's ability to understand relevant information is an essential prerequisite to his or her participation in the decision-making process and should be carefully evaluated by physicians and nurses seeking consent. Critically ill patients frequently do not have the mental capacity to provide informed consent because of the severe nature of their illness or their treatment (e.g., sedation). Patients providing informed consent should be free from severe pain and depression. If the patient is not mentally capable to provide consent, informed consent should be obtained from the designated health care surrogate or legal next of kin. State law governs consent issues, and legal counsel should be consulted for specific questions.

Consent must be given voluntarily for the consent to be legally binding. *Voluntariness* requires that a person's consent be given without coercion or fraud. This includes freedom from pressure from family members, health care providers, and payers.

Persons who consent should base their decision on sufficient knowledge. *Disclosure* of basic information considered necessary for decision making includes the following:

- A diagnosis of the patient's specific health problem and condition
- The nature, duration, and purpose of the proposed treatment or procedures
- The probable outcome of any medical or nursing intervention
- The benefits of medical or nursing interventions
- The potential risks that are generally considered common or hazardous
- Alternative treatments and their feasibility
- Short-term and long-term prognoses if the proposed treatment or treatments are not provided

Informed Consent of Adolescents

State law regarding informed consent of adolescents varies considerably. Although an adolescent is still legally a minor, most states have exceptions that allow an adolescent to provide informed consent based on age or condition. Consult your state law for specifics. Good resources to determine state law include risk managers, legal counsel, and the FindLaw Web site.

DECISIONS REGARDING LIFE-SUSTAINING TREATMENT

Care of persons who are terminally ill or in a persistent vegetative state raises profound questions about the constitutional rights of persons or surrogates (one who speaks for the patient) to make decisions related to death or life-sustaining care, as well as the rights of the state to intervene in treatment decisions. Box 3-3 lists definitions for some terms pertinent to these issues.

The issue of treatment for persons whose quality of life is severely compromised, as in irreversible coma or brain death, is often a result of advanced biomedical technology. Technology frequently sustains life in persons who would have previously succumbed to their illnesses. The widespread use of advanced life-support systems and cardiopulmonary resuscitation has changed the nature and context of dying. A "natural death" in the traditional sense is rare; most patients who die in health care facilities undergo resuscitation efforts.

The benefits derived from aggressive technological management often outweigh the negative effects, but the use of life-sustaining technologies for persons with severely impaired quality of life or for those who are terminally ill has stimulated intensive debate and litigation. Two key issues in this debate are the appropriate use of technology and the ability

---

BOX 3-3

Definitions in Critical Care Ethics

Advance Directive: A statement in which competent persons give direction for their care in the event that they lose the capacity to do so. Advance directives may be formal (e.g., living will) or informal (e.g., oral statement).

Brain Death: Complete and irreversible cessation of brain function.

Clinical Death: Irreversible cessation of spontaneous ventilation and circulation.

Do Not Resuscitate (DNR) Order: A medical order that prohibits the use of cardiopulmonary resuscitation and emergency cardiac care to reverse signs of clinical death. The DNR order may or may not be specified in patients' advance directives.

Durable Power of Attorney: A family member or surrogate designated as the legal agent for another should that person become incompetent or incapacitated.

Futility: A medical situation in which important goals of care are not achievable.

Health Care Surrogate: Someone designated by the person (when judged competent) or appointed to make medical decisions for the person in the event that the person loses the capacity to do so.

Living Will: A specific request made by a competent person that directs medical care in the event that the person loses the capacity to do so. The living will is a formalized advance directive that is held to be legally binding in most states.

Persistent Vegetative State: A condition in which a person does not meet any of the criteria for brain death but displays profound neurological impairment with little to no chance of recovering quality of life.

Resuscitation: Intervention with the intent of preserving life, restoring health, or reversing clinical death.

---

of the seriously ill person to retain decision-making rights. These issues are based on the ethical principles of beneficence and autonomy.

At the heart of the technology controversy are conflicting beliefs about the morality and legality of allowing persons who are terminally ill or severely debilitated to request withdrawal or withholding of medical treatment. There are two levels of treatment to consider: ordinary care and extraordinary care. These levels of care are at two ends of a continuum of potential treatment options. Although, based on one's beliefs, some therapies could be put in either category, this distinction is still helpful from a legal and ethical perspective. However, ethicists believe that any treatment can become extraordinary whenever the patient decides that the burdens outweigh the benefits.

Traditionally, extraordinary care includes complex, invasive, and experimental treatments such as resuscitation efforts by cardiopulmonary resuscitation or emergency cardiac care, maintenance of life support through invasive means, or renal dialysis. Experimental treatments such as gene therapy also are extraordinary therapies.

Ordinary care usually involves common, noninvasive, and tested treatments such as providing nutrition, hydration, or antibiotic therapy. In the critical care setting the noninvasive criterion does not apply; ordinary care is defined as usual and customary for the patient's condition.

Cardiopulmonary Resuscitation Decisions

Resuscitation efforts are used to reverse the clinical signs of death: loss of spontaneous respiration and/or loss of cardiac function. No reliable clinical method exists for determining the extent of brain damage that has already occurred at the time that resuscitation efforts are initiated. Ethical questions arise about the use of cardiopulmonary resuscitation and emergency cardiac care. In what situations should resuscitation efforts be used? How long should efforts continue? A generally accepted position is that resuscitation should cease if the physician determines the efforts to be futile or hopeless. Futility constitutes sufficient reason for either withholding or ceasing extraordinary treatments. According to the American Heart Association (AHA, 2000), health care providers may stop resuscitation when 30 minutes (adults and children) or 15 minutes (newborns) of advanced cardiac life support have been attempted without restoration of breathing and heartbeat, unless hypothermia or drug overdose is present.

Withholding or stopping extraordinary resuscitation efforts is ethically and legally appropriate if the patient or surrogate has previously made his or her preferences known through advance directives (see later discussion of advance directives). It is also acceptable if the physician determines the resuscitation to be futile or has discussed the situation with the patient, family, and/or surrogate as appropriate and if there is mutual agreement not to resuscitate in the event of cardiopulmonary arrest. For the nurse not to initiate the resuscitation, a Do Not Resuscitate (DNR) order must be written. Most physicians also write supporting documentation regarding the order in the progress notes, such as conversations with the patient and family members.

Withholding or Withdrawal of Life Support

Withholding and/or withdrawal of life support can range from not initiating hemodialysis (withholding) to terminal weaning from mechanical ventilation (withdrawal). Decisions are made based on consideration of all factors in the ethical decision-making model. In all instances of withholding and withdrawing of life support, comfort measures are maintained, including management of pain, management of pulmonary secretions, and other symptom management as needed.

The health care team or the family can initiate communication regarding withdrawing and withholding life support. Key points to keep in mind as a critical care nurse involved in this conversation include the following:

- Communicate frequently throughout the critical care stay, not just when death is imminent.
- Provide consistent, honest information. Ensure that all health care providers are giving the same message.
- Keep the discussion on withdrawing and withholding of life support based on the patient's wishes and the burdens versus benefits of the various options.
- Recognize that the patient and family are anticipatorily grieving, and provide support.

The Karen Ann Quinlan case (*In re* Quinlan, 1976) dramatically drew attention in the courts and the public arena to the issue of withdrawing life-sustaining treatment. The case raised substantial questions about the criteria used for withdrawal of treatment, as well as the actual process of decision making. The New Jersey Supreme Court recognized the right of incompetent patients to be withdrawn from life-sustaining treatment, if such an act can be determined to be in their best interests. The court interpreted the constitutional right of privacy contained within the Ninth Amendment to be the basis for its decision and held that a person did not lose the right to decide whether or not life-sustaining treatment should be terminated merely because of incompetence.

Since the Quinlan decision, several dozen court cases have grappled with the ethical issue of withdrawing treatment from persons who were either permanently brain damaged or dying. Judicial opinions in these cases tended to support the decisions of competent adult patients and families or surrogates to forego life-sustaining treatment if little chance existed for recovery (Meisel, 1995). The AHA further delineates justification for withholding and withdrawal of life support in the instance of brain death, when the burden of treatment exceeds any benefit (AHA, 2000). Withdrawal of life support is also indicated if the patient has a Glasgow Coma Score of less than five, 2 to 3 days after cardiac arrest, if there is an absence of pupillary and motor response 3 days after the arrest, and if the patient has bilateral absence of cortical response to median somatosensory evoked potentials 1 week after the arrest (AHA, 2000).

The courts endorsed the concept that persons have a limited right to refuse treatment, even if that decision may lead to death. The right to refuse life-sustaining treatment is not an absolute. In consideration of such a request, the decision has typically been weighed against four countervailing state interests: preservation of life, prevention of suicide, protection of innocent third parties, and maintenance of the integrity of the medical profession (Meisel, 1995).

Consensus does exist, however, on the rights of competent adult patients to make treatment decisions for themselves. In some instances, adolescents can also make treatment decisions. Nonetheless, concern exists when surrogates or family members make decisions when the patient is incompetent. The courts and legislatures have established stringent procedural safeguards that must be present before treatment can be terminated. The primary concern has been to protect the interests of patients who are unable to articulate their views about life-sustaining treatment.

Although many cases deal with the removal or withholding of life-support technology, a new group of cases focus attention on the cessation of artificial feeding and hydration. These cases raise two questions: whether prolonged artificial feeding is an ordinary or an extraordinary form of medical treatment and whether nondying patients or their surrogates can decline such nourishment.

The Nancy Cruzan case (Frader et al., 1990) is the most influential case to date regarding the removal of nutrition and hydration. Nancy Cruzan was injured in a motor vehicle accident in 1983, and within several weeks she was determined to be in a chronic vegetative state. She was confined to a hospital for several years with no hope of recovery. In 1988, her parents petitioned the state courts for permission to terminate her enteral nutrition and hydration after hospital employees refused to do so without court approval. The family petitioned on the basis of the standards of substitute judgment and best interest. These standards are based on the ethical principle of beneficence. A substitute judgment is one made by the health care surrogate that reflects what the incompetent patient would have wanted. Best interest is more general, reflecting what a reasonable person would want done in the situation or what is in the person's best interest.

Permission to remove enteral nutrition and hydration was initially granted by the Missouri trial court, based on Nancy's preaccident statement to a friend

that she wished to die if no reasonable quality of life existed. However, on appeal, the Missouri Supreme Court reversed the lower court decision, rejected Nancy's statement as unreliable, and rejected her parents' request for termination of treatment. The court concluded that no one else can make that choice for an incompetent person in the absence of either a formal document such as a living will or "clear and convincing evidence" of the patient's wishes.

The case was appealed to the United States Supreme Court, which upheld the decision of the Missouri Supreme Court. The United States Supreme Court (*Cruzan* v. *Director,* 1990) concluded that the states have the right to adopt their own standards of proof to determine a patient's wishes regarding treatment. It also ruled that states are not required to recognize the right of a family to make decisions for the incompetent patient.

On November 1, 1990, the original trial court in Missouri again heard the case. Three witnesses provided testimony and stated that they recalled specific conversations with Nancy in which she stated that she would not wish to live "like a vegetable." The trial court judge reaffirmed his decision to allow the feeding tube to be removed, based on this new evidence concerning Ms. Cruzan's wishes. The family directed hospital authorities to remove the tube on December 14, and Nancy died 2 weeks later (Guarino & Antoine, 1991).

Several subsequent court decisions have upheld the privacy right of both competent and incompetent patients to have nutrition and hydration withheld based on a stringent test of the best interest standard. The contradictory court decisions regarding withdrawal of nutrition and hydration reflect society's and health care providers' ambivalence and discomfort with this practice.

Maintenance of hydration and nutrition through a tube feeding is an example of a treatment that falls somewhere between ordinary and extraordinary care. The traditional medical ethic has regarded the provision of sustenance as a fundamental act of caring; some may view this shift as a violation of medical and nursing codes.

Most decisions regarding withdrawing and withholding of life support are not made in the courts. They are made based on open communication with the patient, family, and surrogate, as appropriate. An ethical decision-making approach is used to decide on the best actions to take or not take in the situation. If ethical or legal questions arise, ethics consultation services, ethics committees, and risk managers can provide assistance. Based on the legal cases discussed earlier, the value of clearly stating in writing one's end-of-life issues before becoming critically ill *(advance directive)* is key to avoiding having treatment given or not given against one's wishes.

END-OF-LIFE ISSUES
Patient Self-Determination Act

In response to public concern about end-of-life decisions and the overall lack of consistent hospital policies, the United States Congress enacted the Patient Self-Determination Act (Public Law, 1990). This act requires that all health care facilities that receive Medicare and Medicaid funding inform their patients about the patients' right to initiate an advance directive and the right to consent to or refuse medical treatment.

Discussions regarding advance directives and end-of-life wishes should be made as early as possible, preferably before death is imminent. The ideal time to discuss advance directives is when a person is relatively healthy, not in the critical care or hospital setting. This allows more time for discussion, processing, and decision making. Nurses in every practice setting should assess patients regarding their perceptions of quality of life and end-of-life wishes in a caring and culturally sensitive way and should document the patient's wishes. Patients should be strongly encouraged to complete advance directives, including living wills and durable power of attorney, to ensure that their wishes will be followed if they are ever terminally ill or in a persistent vegetative state.

Advance Directives

An *advance directive* is a communication that specifies a person's preference about medical treatment should he or she become incapacitated. Several types of advance directives exist, but the most common are living wills and durable powers of attorney for health care. Forms specific for each state are available at the United States Living Wills Registry. Competent persons can change their mind and update their advance directives at any time.

The *living will* provides a mechanism by which a person diagnosed with a terminal illness can authorize which specific treatments can be withheld in the event that he or she becomes incapacitated. Although living wills provide direction to caregivers, in some states, living wills are not legally binding and are seen as advisory. When completing a living will, a person can add special instructions about end-of-life wishes.

The *durable power of attorney for health* care is more protective of patients' interests regarding medical treatment than is the living will. With a durable power of attorney for health care, patients legally designate an agent whom they trust, such as a family member or friend, to make decisions on their behalf should they become incapacitated. This person is called the *health care surrogate* or proxy. A durable power of

attorney for health care allows the health care surrogate to make decisions whenever the patient is incapacitated, not just at the time of terminal illness. Some legal commentators recommend the joint use of a living will and a durable power of attorney to give added protection to a person's preferences about medical treatment.

Ultimately, if self-determination and informed consent are to have real value, patients or their surrogates must be given an opportunity to consider options and to shape decisions that affect their life or death. Communication and shared decision making among the patient, family, and health care team regarding end-of-life issues are key (Heyland, Tranmer, & Feldman-Stewart, 2000). Unfortunately, this frequently does not happen before admission to a critical care unit. The critical care nurse must be part of the team that educates the patient and family, so they can determine and communicate end-of-life wishes.

Promoting a Good Death

As part of patient advocacy and the ethic of care (AACN, 2002), it is the critical care nurse's responsibility to facilitate a positive experience for patients and their families at the end of life. Steinhauser and colleagues conducted focus groups with patients, families, physicians, nurses, social workers, chaplains, and hospice volunteers to determine what constituted a "good death." All groups were in agreement, except physicians placed more emphasis on the biomedical aspects of death. The identified themes included biomedical, psychological, social, and spiritual aspects. The six identified themes were pain and symptom management, clear decision making, preparation for death, completion, contributing to others, and affirmation of the whole person (Steinhauser et al., 2000). Consideration of these aspects in planning and delivering nursing care at the end of life is key to promoting a good death. End-of-life information and tools are included in the CD resource accompanying this text.

ORGAN AND TISSUE TRANSPLANTATION

Improved surgical methods and increasingly effective immunosuppressive drug therapy have improved the number and the type of successfully transplanted organs and tissues. Table 3-1 lists tissues and organs that are transplanted and the medical indication.

Despite the successes in transplantation, there is a severe shortage of organs to meet the growing demand. The United States Congress enacted the Nation Organ Procurement and Transplantation Network to facilitate fair allocation of organs and tissues for transplantation. This system is administered

TABLE 3-1

Organ and Tissue Transplantation

Material Transplanted	Necessitating Condition
Bone	Conditions requiring facial/ bone reconstruction
Bone marrow	Leukemias
Brain tissue	Parkinson's disease
Cartilage	Conditions requiring facial/ bone reconstruction
Corneas	Corneal damage, agenesis
Fascia	Conditions requiring repair of tendons, ligaments
Heart	End-stage cardiomyopathy
Heart valves	Diseased valves
Kidneys	End-stage renal disease
Liver	End-stage liver disease
Lungs	End-stage lung disease
Pancreas	Diabetes mellitus
Skin	Burns (temporary cover)
Veins	Diseased veins/arteries

BOX 3-4

Tests Used to Determine Brain Death*

- Cessation of spontaneous respiration
- Cessation of spontaneous heartbeat
- Cessation of brain function, including absence of all function of the brainstem and cerebral hemispheres, and verified by:
  - No response on neurological examination
  - Isoelectric electroencephalogram
  - Bilateral absence of cortical response to median somatosensory-evoked potentials
  - Absence of cerebral blood flow in the absence of hypothermia or drug-induced states

*These tests are formalized into criteria for brain death by different institutions or groups, such as the Harvard Medical School Ad Hoc Committee or the National Institute of Health Collaborative Study of Cerebral Survival. No absolute standardization exists for "brain death criteria."

by the United Network of Organ Sharing (UNOS), a group that maintains a list of patients who are awaiting organ and tissue transplantation and helps to coordinate the procurement of organs. In 2003, 82,500 people were on the organ transplantation waiting list for the United States. Approximately 24,000 organ transplantations occurred in 2002 from approximately 12,000 donors (UNOS, 2003).

Potential donors may agree to donate organs or tissues at any time by signing a donor card, but final consent for donation by the patient, family, or surrogate is needed before the transplantation team will harvest the organs. In some situations, removal of the organ to be transplanted is not life threatening and can be accomplished without causing significant harm to a living donor (e.g., kidneys and bone marrow). Other types of organ and tissue removal (e.g., heart) are performed only in donors who meet the legal definition for brain death.

The concept of brain death is distinct from the concept of persistent vegetative state or irreversible coma. In brain death, complete and irreversible cessation of brain function occurs, whereas in irreversible coma or persistent vegetative state, some brain function remains intact. Tests to determine brain death are outlined in Box 3-4. If the patient is brain dead and is a designated donor, perfusion and oxygenation of organs are maintained until the organs can be removed. Even with optimal artificial perfusion and

oxygenation, organs intended for transplantation must be removed and transplanted quickly.

Everyone in the United States has the legal right to donate organs. To uphold that right, family members or significant others must be given the opportunity to donate organs or tissues on behalf of their loved ones. Local organ procurement organizations have designated requestors whose role is to seek consent for organ donation. The role of the critical care nurse is to refer potential organ donors to the organ procurement organization. Because the consent rate for organ donation is only about 50%, it is important to approach potential donors sensitively and with awareness of cultural and religious implications.

Ethical Concerns Surrounding Transplantation

Organ and tissue transplantation involves numerous and complex ethical issues. First consideration is given to the rights and privileges of all moral agents involved: the donor, the recipient, the family or surrogate, and all other recipients and donors. Important ethical principles that are useful in ethical decision making regarding transplantation include respect for persons and their autonomous choices, beneficence and nonmaleficence, justice, and fidelity.

Three of the most controversial issues in transplantation are the moral value that should be placed on the human body part, the just distribution of a human body part, and the complex problems inherent in applying the concept of brain death to clinical situations.

RESEARCH ANALYSIS

Debra Michaud, MSN, ARNP, and Jacqueline F. Byers, PhD, RN, CNAA

ARTICLE REFERENCE

Puntillo, K.A., Benner, P., Drought, T., Drew, B., Stotts, N., Stannard, D., Rushton, C., Scanlon, C., White, C. (2001). End-of-life issues in intensive care units: A national random survey of nurses' knowledge and beliefs. *American Journal of Critical Care, 10*(4), 216-229.

PURPOSE AND METHODS

The purpose of this study was to investigate the knowledge, beliefs, and ethical concerns of nurses caring for patients dying in intensive care units. A survey was mailed to a 4% stratified random sample of members of the American Association of Critical-Care Nurses (3000 surveys). There was a 30% return rate (N = 906). The survey had three sections; the first consisted of four clinical scenarios (pain management, withholding or withdrawing life support, assisted suicide, and euthanasia) involving four different critically ill patients. The nurse was asked to choose which action he or she thought was the scenario represented in each of the examples. The scenarios were designed to elicit the nurses' ability to make ethical distinctions among the various actions. The second section of the questionnaire assessed the knowledge and opinions about pain management and end-of-life practices in their respective critical care units using a four-point Likert scale. The third section collected demographic information about the survey sample.

STUDY FINDINGS

Findings demonstrated that 99% to 100% of respondents correctly identified the pain management and withholding or withdrawing life support scenarios, 17% recognized assisted suicide, 5% recognized voluntary euthanasia, and 2% to 11% recognized nonvoluntary euthanasia; 83% disagreed with assisted suicide. There was an inverse relationship between how religious the respondents considered themselves and their agreement with assisted suicide: 14% of those who considered themselves religious agreed with assisted suicide, whereas 86% of the religious respondents disagreed (*P* < .001). Distinctions were made between agreeing with assisted suicide and agreeing with nonvoluntary euthanasia. Fewer than one third of the 17% of nurses who agreed with assisted suicide agreed with nonvoluntary euthanasia, whereas more than two thirds (69%) of this same group disagreed with nonvoluntary euthanasia (*P* < .001). Ninety-eight percent of respondents agreed or strongly agreed that administering analgesics to decrease pain and suffering at the end of life was appropriate. However, 78% of nurses reported that dying patients frequently or sometimes received inadequate pain medication in this instance; 97% of subjects rated themselves as somewhat or very skillful in nonpharmacologic comfort measures at the end of life. Respondents reported that they acted against their conscience to a great extent (6%) or some (34%) of the time, whereas 59% reported never acting against their conscience. There was a low reported availability of end-of-life consultants including pain management, hospice, and ethics specialists.

STUDY STRENGTHS

The design of the study facilitated understanding of critical care nurses' knowledge, beliefs, and ethical concerns related to practices in caring for dying patients in the critical care unit by providing a detailed, validated survey instrument. The sample size was adequate to answer the research questions.

STUDY WEAKNESSES

The study was limited by the low survey response rate. The sensitive nature of the questions or the extensive length of the survey may have contributed to the low response rate. Generalizability to nurses who are not professional organization members should be made with caution.

IMPLICATIONS FOR PRACTICE

Understanding of the ethical dilemmas posed to nurses on a daily basis can provide insight into current nursing practice and assist with identification of multidisciplinary performance improvement opportunities. This study identifies pain management and access to end-of-life specialists as definite areas of opportunity. Most of the nurses in this study were against assisted suicide and euthanasia. Greater discussion is needed among health care providers and patients to optimize end-of-life care.

SUMMARY

The ethical and legal responsibilities of nurses who work in acute care settings have increased dramatically since the early 1990s. Based on evolving case law and state nurse practice acts, nurses are held to a high standard of care and are also held directly accountable for their individual nursing actions. Nurses must maintain and continually update their knowledge base and clinical competencies. Failure to do so could not only cause harm to patients but could also put nurses and their employers at risk for allegations of professional negligence.

Nurses who care for critically ill patients are challenged by legal and ethical dilemmas on a daily basis. In their role of patient advocate, ethical decision making and open communication must be facilitated. Numerous resources are available to assist with developing the knowledge and skill to do this well. There are no easy answers to ethical dilemmas. A formal decision-making model assists the nurse, but some situations may still remain very ambiguous. Appropriate ethical nursing responses are based on wanting to do the right thing for the patients and families that you care for and initiating the steps to advocate for the patient.

CRITICAL THINKING QUESTIONS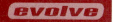

1. You are taking care of Mrs. H., a 90-year-old patient with gastrointestinal bleeding. She has developed numerous complications and requires mechanical ventilation. She is unresponsive to nurses and family members. She has been in the hospital for 2 weeks and requires a transfusion nearly every day to sustain adequate hemoglobin and hematocrit levels. Her prognosis is poor. Before this hospitalization, she lived independently at her own home. Her family tells you they are tired of seeing their mother suffer. How do you respond to the family, and what follow-up do you perform?

2. You are taking care of Mr. J., a 23-year-old man with a closed-head injury. During your shift, you note a change in the level of consciousness at 3:00 AM. You call the physician, who tells you to watch Mr. J. until the physician attends rounds the next morning. He tells you not to call him back. Mr. J.'s neurological status continues to deteriorate. What actions do you take? What are the rationales for your actions?

3. It is 2 days later, and Mr. J., as described earlier, now has a herniated brainstem and is declared brain dead but remains on life support. His wife is at the bedside and is fully aware of the situation. You do not know whether or not Mr. J. signed an organ donor card. What are your ethical and legal obligations regarding organ donation at this point? How would you approach the situation?

4. You are caring for Mrs. M., a 68-year-old woman with an acute myocardial infarction. She is in the coronary care unit after a successful angioplasty. Her husband brought in her living will, which states that Mrs. M. does not desire resuscitation. Mrs. M. is pain free and alert. As you start your beginning-of-shift assessment, Mrs. M. says, "You know, now that I've made it through the angioplasty, I realize that tubes and machines may not be so bad after all. I haven't made it this far to give up now. If I go into cardiac arrest, I want you to do all that you can for me." What ethical principle is Mrs. M. using? As her nurse, what actions should you take and why?

5. You are the charge nurse of a nine-bed critical care unit. You have one open bed. The house supervisor calls and tells you that there are two patients who need a critical care bed. The first is a 23-year-old female patient currently in the operating room after multiple trauma. The second patient is a 78-year-old man who is in the emergency department with severe septic shock. According to the supervisor, both patients are going to need mechanical ventilation and inotropic therapy. What are your decisions and actions at this point? What ethical principles are your actions based on?

Case Study

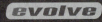

Mr. W. is a 67-year-old patient in the coronary care unit who has severe congestive heart failure and chronic obstructive pulmonary disease. Mr. W. has been in and out of the hospital for 3 years and requires oxygen therapy at night when he is at home. He has severe, chronic chest pain and dyspnea. He suffered respiratory arrest and was put on the ventilator last night. He awakens after the resuscitation and asks that the breathing tube be removed and that he be allowed to die. He is tired of the pain and dyspnea. He asks for medication to make him comfortable after the tube is removed. His family agrees with the plan of care.

Mr. W.'s wishes are followed. He is extubated and is given morphine for sedation and comfort. Mr. W.'s family members all remain at the bedside, taking turns holding his hand and talking to him.

QUESTIONS

1. Apply the ethical decision-making model discussed in this chapter to this case. What are the relevant ethical principles? Are there other areas that must be assessed before proceeding?
2. As the critical care nurse caring for Mr. W., what are your priorities at this point? On what ethical principles are these priorities based?
3. Suppose that you have strong religious beliefs about withdrawal of life support. If you were assigned to Mr. W., what actions should you take?

REFERENCES

American Association of Critical-Care Nurses. (2002). *An ethic of care.* Retrieved from http://www.aacn.org/AACN/memship.nsf/. Accessed 08/25/2003.

American Heart Association. (2000). *Guidelines 2000 for cardiopulmonary resuscitation and emergency cardiovascular care.* Dallas, TX: Author.

American Nurses Association. (2002). *Code of ethics for nurses with interpretive statements.* Retrieved from http://www.nursingworld.org/ethics/code/ethicscode150.htm. Accessed 08/25/2003.

Cruzan v. *Director.* Missouri Department of Health. 58 USLW 49116 (US 1990).

Frader, J., Francis, L., Grodin, M., Hackler, C., & Jennings, B. (1990). Bioethicists' statement on the U.S. Supreme Court's Cruzan decision. *New England Journal of Medicine, 323*(10), 688.

Guarino, K. S., & Antoine, M. P. (1991). The case of Nancy Cruzan: The Supreme Court's decision. *Critical Care Nurse, 11*(1), 32, 34-36, 38-40.

Heyland, D.K., Tranmer, J., & Feldman-Steward, D. (2000). End-of-life decision making in the seriously ill hospitalized patient: An organizing framework and results of a preliminary study. *Journal of Palliative Care, 16,* S31-39.

In re Quinlan, No. 70 NJ 10, 355 A 2d 647 (1976).

Medina, J. (2000). *Standards for acute and critical care.* 3rd ed. Aliso Viejo, CA: American Association of Critical Care Nurses.

Meisel, A. (1995). *The right to die.* 2nd ed. New York: John Wiley & Sons.

Public Law No. 101-508, 4206, 104 Stat. 291. (1990). The Self-Determination Act amends the Social Security Act's provisions on Medicare and Medicaid. Social Security Act 1927, 42 U.S.C. 1396.

Rushton, C. H., & Scanlon, C. (1998). A road map for negotiating end-of-life care. *MedSurg Nursing, 7,* 57-59.

Steinhauser, K. E., , Clipp, E. C., McNeilly, M., Christakis, N. A., McIntyre, L. M., & Tulsky, J. A. (2000). In search of a good death: Observations of patients, families and providers. *Annals of Internal Medicine, 132,* 825-832.

United Network for Organ Sharing. (2003). *Data.* Retrieved from http://www.unos.org/. Accessed 08/25/2003.

RECOMMENDED READINGS

Baggs, J. G. (2002). End-of-life care for older adults in ICUs. *Annual Review of Nursing Research, 20,* 181-229.

Finger, W. (2001). Choices must be informed, voluntary. *Network, 21*(2), 16-19.

Hohenleitner, R. (2002). Critical care nurses' role in code status discussion. *Dimensions of Critical Care Nursing, 21*(4), 140-143.

Robinson, E., M. (2002). An ethical analysis of cardiopulmonary resuscitation for elders in acute care. *AACN Clinical Issues, 13*(1), 132-144.

Vittone, S. B. (2002). Ethics in the ICU. *Critical Care Nursing Clinics of North America, 14*(2), 157-163.

evolve *Did you remember to check out the bonus material, including free self-assessment exercises, on the Evolve Web site at http://evolve.elsevier.com/Sole/ and on the CD-ROM?*

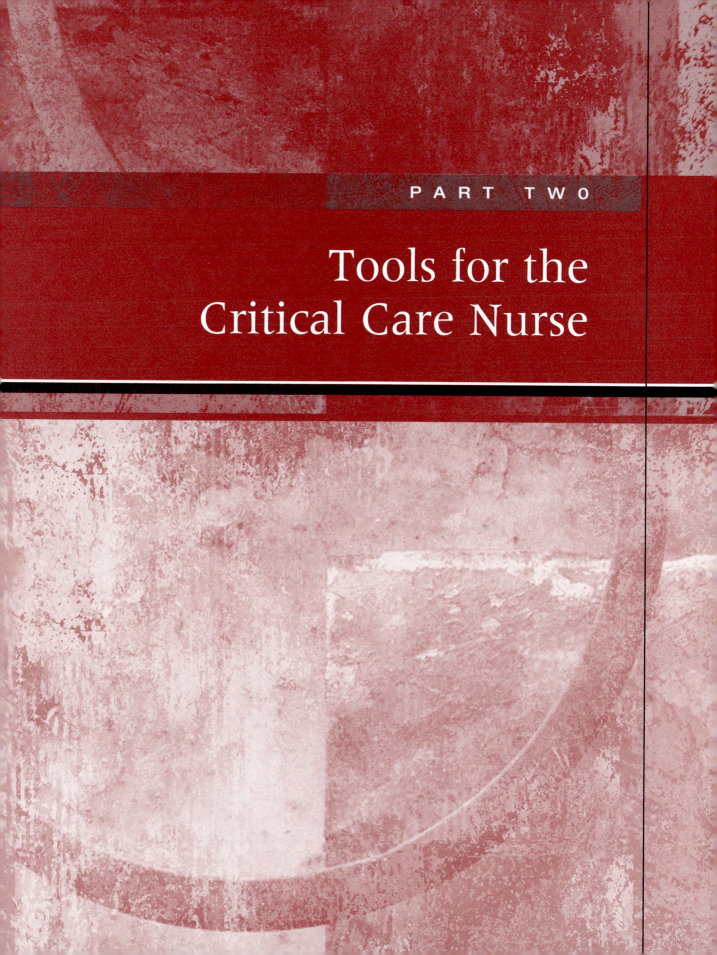

PART TWO

Tools for the
Critical Care Nurse

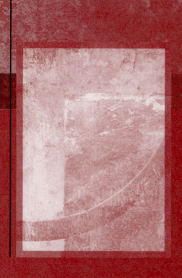

CHAPTER 4

Comfort and Sedation

Ross W. Swanson, MSN, RN, CCRN
Deborah G. Klein, MSN, RN, CCRN, CS

OBJECTIVES

- Describe the relationship between pain and anxiety.
- Identify factors that place the critically ill patient at risk for developing pain and anxiety.
- Discuss the physical and psychological effects of pain and anxiety.
- Describe methods and tools for assessing pain and anxiety in the critically ill patient.
- Describe challenges in the assessment of patient comfort in the critically ill patient.
- Identify nonpharmacological and pharmacological strategies to promote comfort and reduce anxiety.

Introduction

Maintaining an optimal level of comfort for the critically ill patient is a universal goal for physicians and nurses (Jacobi et al., 2002). Patients in the critical care unit experience pain from preexisting diseases, invasive procedures, or trauma. Pain can also be caused by monitoring devices (catheters, drains), noninvasive ventilating devices, and endotracheal tubes, routine nursing care (airway suctioning, dressing changes, and patient mobilization), and prolonged immobility. It is estimated that 22% to 70% of patients after they are discharged recall having experienced pain during their critical care unit stay (Kwekkeboom & Herr, 2001). Unrelieved pain may contribute to inadequate sleep, which may lead to exhaustion, anxiety, and disorientation. Agitation may result from inadequate pain relief.

Hospitals and health care accrediting agencies have recognized that pain and anxiety are major contributors to patient morbidity and length of stay. Pain has become known as the fifth vital sign because the patient's level of pain should be assessed routinely and as needed. Nursing interventions for a critically ill patient in pain include actions that promote comfort. Interventions for patients experiencing anxiety involve measures that promote rest. The treatment of pain and anxiety may include the use of pharmacological agents.

There are many theories about the pathophysiological phenomena thought to induce pain and anxiety. These theories and the pathophysiology of pain and anxiety are discussed in broader detail in most medical-surgical nursing textbooks. This chapter focuses on the assessment and management

evolve Be sure to check out the bonus material, including free self-assessment exercises, on the Evolve Web site at http://evolve.elsevier.com/Sole/ and on the CD-ROM.

strategies for the critically ill patient experiencing acute pain and/or anxiety.

Definitions of Pain and Anxiety

The International Association on Pain (1979) defines *pain* as an unpleasant sensory and emotional experience associated with actual or potential tissue damage. This explanation of pain alludes to the global nature of pain; however, pain may be difficult to assess in the patient who is not exhibiting any expected assessment findings associated with tissue damage. McCaffery (1979) defined pain as "whatever the experiencing person says it is, existing whenever he says it does." Using this definition, the patient becomes the true authority on the pain that is being experienced, and the patient's pain should be managed based on this description. Many critically ill patients have underlying chronic pain, thus making assessment and management more challenging.

There are many theoretical bases for the development of pain. The four most commonly discussed theories are the specificity, intensity, pattern, and gate control theories (Box 4-1).

Anxiety has been defined as a state marked by apprehension, agitation, autonomic arousal, and/or fearful withdrawal (McCartney and Boland, 1994). It is a prolonged state of apprehension in response to a real or perceived fear. Anxiety must be assessed in the same way used to assess pain: the patient's level of anxiety is whatever the patient reports.

Pain and anxiety are often intertwined and may be difficult to differentiate because they have similar subjective and objective findings. The relation between pain and anxiety is cyclical (Figure 4-1), with each exacerbating the other (Cullen, Greiner, & Titler, 2001). If pain and anxiety are unresolved and escalate, the patient may experience feelings of powerlessness, suffering, and psychological changes such as agitation and delirium.

It is understood that inadequately treated pain leads to greater anxiety, and anxiety is associated with higher pain intensity. Anxiety may contribute to pain perception by activating pain pathways, altering the cognitive evaluation of pain, increasing aversion to pain, and increasing the report of pain (Cullen, Greiner, & Titler, 2001). Because interventions to manage pain may differ from those used to manage anxiety, the nurse must be astute to the patient's precipitating problem. If pain is being treated in a patient who is experiencing anxiety only, the anxiety may worsen as potentially ineffective management strategies are employed. For example, the pharmacological agents used to treat pain have very different properties compared with those agents used to treat anxiety. Pain management involves anti-inflammatory and analgesic medications, whereas sedative medications are used to treat anxiety.

Predisposing Factors to Pain and Anxiety

Many factors inherent to the critical care environment place patients at risk of developing pain and anxiety. As stated earlier, pain perception occurs as

---

BOX 4-1

Theoretical Bases for Pain

Theory	Synopsis
Specificity theory	There are four major categories of cutaneous sensation: (1) touch, (2) warmth, (3) cold, and (4) pain. Each sensation is the result of stimulation of specific receptor sites on the skin. A direct relationship exists between the stimulus and the perception of pain.
Intensity theory	Pain results from excessive stimulation of sensory receptors. Pain occurs if the stimulus is applied with enough intensity. A pathological condition that promotes summation of impulses produced by normally nonnoxious stimuli can cause pain.
Pattern theory	The perception of pain is a result of stimulus intensity and the summation of impulses. Nonspecific receptors transmit patterns of nerve impulses from the skin to the spinal cord. Certain patterns of impulses then are perceived as pain.
Gate control theory	Innocuous (nonpainful) stimuli transmitted by large afferent nerve fibers may prevent the transmission of painful stimuli. Stimulation of larger nerve fibers cause synapses in the dorsal horn of the spinal cord to cease firing, thus creating a "closed gate." A closed gate decreases the stimulation of trigger cells, decreases transmission of impulses, and diminishes pain perception. Persistent stimulation of the large fibers may allow for adaptation, allowing pain signals to reach the spinal cord and brain.

Modified from Heuther, S. & Leo, J. (2002). Pain, temperature regulation, sleep, and sensory function In K. L. McCance, and S. E. Heuther, *Pathophysiology: The pathologic basis for disease in adults & children.* 4th ed. [pp. 401-437]. St. Louis: Mosby.

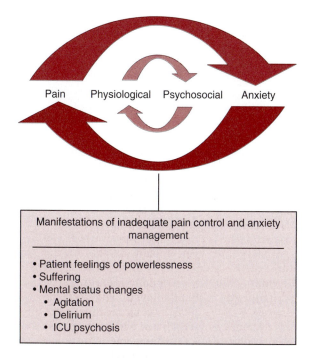

Pain   Physiological   Psychosocial   Anxiety

Manifestations of inadequate pain control and anxiety management

- Patient feelings of powerlessness
- Suffering
- Mental status changes
  - Agitation
  - Delirium
  - ICU psychosis

FIGURE 4-1 The anxiety-pain cycle. (From Cullen, L., Greiner, J., & Titler, M. G. [2001] Pain management in the culture of critical care. *Critical Care Nursing Clinics of North America, 13*[2], 151-166.)

a result of preexisting diseases, invasive procedures, monitoring devices, nursing care, or trauma. The perception of pain can be influenced by the expectation of pain, prior pain experiences, a patient's emotional state, and the cognitive processes of the patient (Carroll et al., 1999).

Anxiety is likely to result from the inability to communicate while one is surrounded by the continuous noise of alarms, equipment, and personnel; continuous ambient lighting; and excessive stimulation from inadequate analgesia, frequent assessments, repositioning, lack of mobility, and uncomfortable room temperature. Sleep deprivation and the circumstances that resulted in an admission may also increase patient anxiety. Efforts to reduce anxiety include frequent reorientation, providing patient comfort, providing adequate analgesia and sedation, and optimizing the environment. For example, a nurse's explanation to the patient and family of the different types of alarms heard in the critical care unit could lessen anxiety levels. Providing information allows the patient and family to anticipate and understand the critical care experience.

Physiology of Pain and Anxiety

PAIN

All pain results from a signal cascade within the body's neurological network. Pain is initiated by signals that travel through the nervous system to the brain for processing. In all forms of acute pain, the sympathetic nervous system (SNS) is usually activated quickly. Several physiological responses typically occur (Table 4-1). In contrast, some forms of chronic pain, may result in less activation of the SNS with a different clinical presentation. The person in chronic pain may exhibit a decreased sense of awareness or a lack of interest in social interaction.

The sensation of pain is carried to the central nervous system on two separate pathways (Figure 4-2). The fast (sharp) pain signals are transmitted to the spinal cord by small type A-delta (δ) fibers at velocities of 6 to 30 m/sec. Type A δ fibers carry well-localized, sharp pain sensations and are important in initiating rapid reactions to stimuli. Conversely, slow (chronic) pain is transmitted by type C fibers at velocities between 0.5 and 2 m/sec (Guyton & Hall, 2000). Because of the size of the large C fiber and the lack of a myelin sheath, pain signal transmission is relatively slow. This type of pain is more susceptible to local anesthesia (Huether & Leo, 2001).

Many nerve receptors are capable of receiving painful stimuli. The most abundant receptors in the nervous system for pain recognition are nociceptors (Guyton & Hall, 2000). Mechanical, chemical, and thermal stimuli activate nociceptors to produce a painful sensation. Examples of mechanical stimuli include crushing of a body structure and a surgical wound. A chemical stimulus is any substance that produces skin irritation, and a thermal stimulus for pain would be a partial-thickness burn injury. Identifying the correct pain-inducing stimulus is important in the effective management of pain. Removal of the

TABLE 4-1
Physiological Responses to Pain and/or Anxiety

Tachycardia	Diaphoresis
Tachypnea	Increased glucose
Hypertension	production
Increased cardiac output	(gluconeogenesis)
Pallor and/or flushing	Nausea
Cool extremities	Urinary retention
Mydriasis (pupillary	Constipation
dilation)	Sleep disturbance

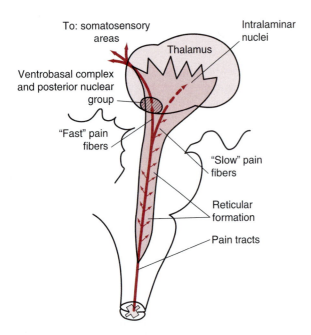

To: somatosensory areas

Intralaminar nuclei

Thalamus

Ventrobasal complex and posterior nuclear group

"Fast" pain fibers

"Slow" pain fibers

Reticular formation

Pain tracts

FIGURE 4-2 Transmission of pain signals into the brainstem, thalamus, and cerebral cortex by way of the "fast" pain pathway and "slow" pain pathway. (From Guyton, A., & Hall, J. (2000). *Somatic sensations: II. Pain, headache, and thermal sensations.* Philadelphia: W. B. Saunders.)

stimulus should always precede other treatment measures in managing pain.

Nociceptors differ from other nerve receptors in the body in that they adapt very little to the pain response. If the stimulus for pain has not been removed, the body will continue to experience pain until the stimulus is discontinued or other interventions (e.g., analgesic agents) are initiated. This is a protective mechanism so the body tissues being damaged will be removed from harm.

Nociceptors usually lie near capillary beds and mast cells. When tissue injury occurs, the nociceptor initiates an inflammatory response near the injured capillary (McHugh & McHugh, 2000). The mast cells in the damaged tissues degranulate, releasing histamine and chemotactic agents that promote infiltration of injured tissues with neutrophils and eosinophils. As neutrophils move into the site of injury, more neurotransmitter-like substances (acetylcholine, bradykinins, substance P, and enkephalins) are released from the neutrophils into the surrounding tissue. These substances act as mediators and may induce or suppress

pain. Endogenous cytokines that suppress pain induction are commonly referred to as the *endorphins*.

ANXIETY

The physiology of anxiety is less clearly understood in comparison with pain. Anxiety differs from pain in that it is confined to neurological processes within the brain. Pain can begin in the body's periphery where the signal is carried to the cerebrum through the spinal cord. Some pain can also originate in the cerebrum, as in migraine headaches. Anxiety is a more complex process in relation to pain because there is no actual tissue injury thought to occur with anxiety alone. Anxiety is a purely psychogenic disorder. Anxiety has multiple complex causes that are debated in the current literature (Crippen, 1995).

Anxiety has been linked to the reward and punishment centers within the limbic system of the brain. Stimulation in the punishment centers can frequently inhibit the reward centers completely (Guyton & Hall, 2000). The punishment center is also responsible for helping a person escape from potentially harmful situations. The punishment center has dominance over the reward center for the person to escape harm.

If anxiety is left untreated, agitation may develop. There is a large body of research that demonstrates that proper anxiety management greatly benefits the patient. For example, by managing anxiety, the patient experiences a decrease in potential injury from dislodging tubes or other invasive equipment (Summer & Puntillo, 2001). Decreasing agitation promotes hemodynamic stability by reducing oxygen consumption and lowering the patient's hyperactive state.

Positive Effects of Pain and Anxiety

In the healthy person, pain and anxiety are adaptive mechanisms used to increase mental and physical performance levels. This allows a person to remove himself or herself from potential harm. Activation of the SNS occurs with pain or anxiety. With this sympathetic activation the person usually becomes more vigilant of the environment, especially to potential dangers. Once dangers are recognized, the person makes a choice whether to flee the situation or combat the possible threat. For this reason, SNS activation has become known as the fight-or-flight response. However, pain and anxiety can induce significant stress. For someone already under stress, such as the critically ill patient, both can produce negative effects.

Negative Effects of Pain and Anxiety

PHYSICAL EFFECTS

Pain increases the activation of the SNS and raises catecholamine levels, which may place a significant burden on the cardiovascular system, especially in a critically ill patient. The physiological response to stress interferes with the healing process and impairs perfusion and oxygen delivery to tissue (Birka, 1999). When a patient presents initially with an unknown cause of illness or is improperly treated for pain or anxiety, tachycardia, hypertension, and tachypnea may result (Roberts, 2001). These physiological phenomena place the critically ill patient at greater risk of hemodynamic instability, immunosuppression, and tissue catabolism, which may lead to poor outcomes (Szokol & Vender, 2001).

Tachycardia and hypertension both lead to increased myocardial oxygen demand. Any large organ that experiences an increase in oxygen consumption places the critically ill patient at risk of increased rates of complications related to end-organ ischemia (Lighthall & Pearl, 2003). Pharmacological support is initiated to decrease the heart rate and blood pressure to acceptable levels. Tachycardia is most commonly treated with medications such as beta-blockers and calcium channel blockers. Both these classes of medications may be difficult to initiate and titrate in the critically ill patient because of the negative inotropic and hypotensive properties of these drugs. If a patient is tachycardic and/or hypertensive from pain or anxiety, the most effective management targets that pain or anxiety while sparing the patient's cardiovascular system.

Hyperventilation (tachypnea) can be stressful to the patient because rapid breathing requires a significant amount of effort with the use of accessory muscles. Hyperventilation may cause respiratory alkalosis. If the patient is mechanically ventilated, increased respiratory rates lead to feelings of breathlessness. As the patient "fights" the mechanical ventilator, further alveolar damage ensues, and the endotracheal or tracheostomy tube creates a "choking" sensation and increased anxiety.

An increase in blood pH (alkalosis) may result in impaired tissue perfusion, and many vasoactive medications become less effective. Even mild increases in respiratory rate can result in alkalosis or failure to wean the patient from mechanical ventilation. Medications used to treat tachypnea include sedatives and opioids. Opioids may cause respiratory depression and sedation, which can be considered an adverse reaction or a desired effect to facilitate mechanical ventilation.

PSYCHOLOGICAL EFFECTS

The critical care environment overloads the patient with sensory stimulation, placing the patient at risk for developing pain and anxiety. Many patients in the critical care unit report feelings of panic and fear related to the loss of body functions. These feelings are likely related to experiences such as being unable to communicate effectively with nurses or visitors and loss of normal sleep-wake cycles (Rotondi et al., 2002). Pain and anxiety further exacerbate reports of lack of sleep, nightmares, and feelings of bewilderment, isolation, and loneliness.

Extreme anxiety, pain, and adverse effects of medications can also lead to agitation. Agitation is associated with inappropriate verbal behavior, physical aggression, and increased movement that may lead to harm to the patient or caregiver. Agitation is common in the critical care unit (Fraser et al., 2000).

The nurse must attempt to manage pain and anxiety so the negative psychological effects of the critical care unit are minimal (see Chapter 2). Nurses can provide information with thorough and frequent explanations of the critical care unit environment (Rotondi et al., 2002). Nurses can alter the physical environment or arrange more liberal visiting hours so the typical stressors are decreased. For example, rotating the bed so the patient can see out the window may have a relaxing effect. Patients in a critical care unit who report anxiety and distress also have an increase in the perception of pain (Summer & Puntillo, 2001). Nurses must appropriately assess and use both nonpharmacological and pharmacological strategies to manage pain and anxiety effectively in this vulnerable patient population.

Assessment

The assessment of pain and anxiety is a continuous process. The nurse must be aware of what procedures may cause pain (Puntillo et al., 2004). In addition, when interventions are used to alleviate pain or anxiety, the effectiveness of the intervention must be evaluated. When patients exhibit signs of anxiety or agitation, the first priority is to identify and treat the underlying cause such as hypoxemia, hypoglycemia, hypotension, pain, and withdrawal from alcohol and drugs. When possible, patients should be questioned about the use of herbal remedies because these products may contribute to medication interactions and adverse effects (Kaye et al., 2000).

Assessment involves the collection of subjective and objective data. Subjective data include asking the patient to describe their pain or anxiety or to provide a numerical score to indicate the level of pain or anxiety. Subjective data also include knowledge of the patient's past medical history and any mechanism of injury or reason for admission. These data are valuable in determining the best management strategies. For example, a trauma patient admitted with a humerus or femur fracture will experience significant pain and will likely require potent analgesic medications such as an opioid and antispasmodics.

In contrast, objective findings of pain are phenomena that are observed. For example, increased blood pressure or a facial grimace or frown may indicate pain or anxiety. Typical physiological responses related to pain are detailed in Table 4-1. In the healthy person, these responses are adaptive mechanisms and result from activation of the SNS in an attempt to ready the individual for the fight-or-flight response. In the critically ill patient, these changes may induce further stress on an already compromised person.

SUBJECTIVE TOOLS

In the assessment of pain, the nurse asks the patient to identify several characteristics associated with the pain. These characteristics include the precipitating cause, severity, location (including radiation to other sites), duration, intensity, and any alleviating or aggravating factors. Any pain assessment should address these pain characteristics or the assessment is not complete. The patient is the best source to describe pain and to share any past strategies, including medications, that have been used to successfully manage pain (Meinhart & McCaffery, 1983). Patients with chronic pain conditions, such as arthritis, may be able to provide a detailed list of effective pain remedies that may be useful during the present hospitalization.

Several tools are available to ensure that the appropriate pain assessment questions are asked. One tool used in assessing the patient with chest pain is the PQRST method. The PQRST method allows the nurse to remember a mnemonic so all the chest pain

characteristics (e.g., duration, intensity) are documented. The letter P represents "provocation or position." What precipitated the chest pain symptoms and where in the chest area is the pain located? The letter Q stands for "quality." Is the pain sharp, dull, crushing? The letter R represents "radiation." Does the pain travel to other parts of the body? The letter S stands for "severity or symptoms associated with the pain." The patient is asked to rate the pain on a numerical scale and to describe what other symptoms are present. The final letter T represents "timing or triggers" for the pain. Is the pain constant or intermittent, and does it occur with certain activities?

One of the most common methods used to determine pain intensity or severity is to ask for a *pain score*. Patients are asked to rate their pain on a numbered scale such as 0 to 10. A score of 0 would indicate no pain, and a score of 10 would be indicative of the worst pain the patient could possibly imagine. Some institutions require nurses to intervene for pain scores greater than a predesignated number. The pain score is reassessed after medications or other pain-relieving measures have been provided. Some institutions have guidelines for how and when the patient's pain intensity is assessed. The pain score method should be used only with patients who are cognitively aware of their surroundings and are able to follow simple commands. This would not be an appropriate method to use to assess pain in nonverbal or disoriented patients.

A second tool is known as the FACES scale. Patients are asked to describe how they feel by pointing to a series of "smiling" faces. Each face represents a different level of pain (Figure 4-3). The FACES method involves a higher level of emotional intellect because the patient must be able to process different yet similar visual stimuli accurately (Kwekkeboom & Herr, 2001). The most common versions of the FACES scale use between five and seven different faces.

Another widely used subjective pain measurement tool is the Visual Analog Scale (VAS). When using the VAS, the nurse holds up the scale, and the patient points to the level of pain on a linear scale that looks similar to a timeline. The scale may be

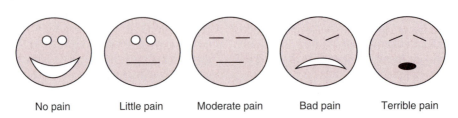

No pain   Little pain   Moderate pain   Bad pain   Terrible pain

FIGURE 4-3 A version of the FACES scale.

drawn horizontally or vertically, and it may or may not be numbered. The number 0 indicates no pain, whereas the number 10 indicates the most pain (Figure 4-4). This measurement tool is effective for awake nonverbal patients such as those patients who are being supported by mechanical ventilation. Another benefit of the VAS is that it can also be used to evaluate a patient's level of anxiety. Like the pain score, the VAS must be used for patients who are fully alert and able to follow directions. Patients can provide a score on the VAS by simply pointing to a number on the scale, or they can place on "X" on an actual copy using a pencil. Some patients may not be able to provide a score on the VAS because of an inability to lift their extremities or limited visual acuity.

One final subjective pain assessment tool that has been extensively studied is the McGill-Melzack Pain Questionnaire (MPQ) (Melzack, 1975). The MPQ has four separate parts (Figure 4-5). The distinct parts of the MPQ ask the patient to identify where the pain is located, what it feels like, how it changes with time, and how intense or strong the pain feels. This tool may not be appropriate for the critically ill patient because it involves a high level of visual acuity and it takes more time to complete the questionnaire than the other pain scoring methods. In addition, the overwhelming stimulation from the critical care environment may make completion of the MPQ technically difficult, if not impossible. The MPQ may be more useful for patients who are ambulatory (Kwekkeboom & Herr, 2001).

OBJECTIVE TOOLS

Objective assessment tools are used for patients who are unable to communicate their current state of pain and anxiety. These tools are especially important for the critical care nurse because patients in this setting are likely to be receiving therapies (mechanical ventilation and medications) that may affect their level of arousal.

There is no objective tool that will completely reflect a patient's pain level. Pain may or may not be measured effectively using objective tools because the patient may not exhibit expected findings such as restlessness, grimacing, wincing, or moaning or these assessment findings may be delayed. A delayed assessment picture is common in patients with chronic pain syndromes (migraines, arthritis).

PAIN MEASUREMENT

Few pain measurement tools are available for use in the nonverbal adult population. One scale that has been developed to assess pain in the critically ill adult is the Behavioral Pain Scale (BPS) (Payen et al., 2001). The BPS was developed to assist with pain assessment in critically ill patients who are nonverbal or unable to communicate (Table 4-2). This tool consists of three categories: facial expression, upper limb movement, and compliance with ventilation. The patient is scored in each of the three categories. The points are added from each of the three categories for a minimum score of 3 and a maximum score of 12. Any total score greater than 6 necessitates a need for pain intervention. The BPS has been found to provide critical care nurses with an objective and reliable pain measurement tool for adult nonverbal patients (Payen et al., 2001). The BPS has been researched only in the mechanically ventilated patient and therefore may not be appropriate in those patients who do not require ventilator support.

In the pediatric population, the FLACC tool has been developed to assess pain in children who lack the verbal and cognitive skills to provide pain intensity reports. The acronym FLACC (face, legs, activity, cry, and consolability) was developed to remind users of the five different categories of the scale (Merkel et al., 1997). Similar to the BPS, the FLACC scale (Table 4-3) is scored in each of the five categories, with scores ranging from 0 to 2. Cumulative scores can range between 0 and 10. Pediatric critical care nurses currently assess and treat children using the FLACC score as though the patient were able to provide a subjective number similar to the VAS scale (Merkel et al., 1997). Scores greater than 4 to 5 necessitate intervention. The FLACC tool may have promising usefulness in the critically ill adult, but the tool has yet to be researched in this patient population.

SEDATION MEASUREMENT

No objective tool is considered the gold standard for determining a patient's level of anxiety.

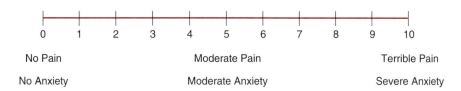

FIGURE 4-4 The Visual Analog Scale.

McGill-Melzack
PAIN QUESTIONNAIRE

Patient's name _____ Age _____

File No. _____ Date _____

Clinical category (e.g., cardiac, neurologic)

Diagnosis: _____

_____

_____

Analgesic (if already administered):

1. Type _____

2. Dosage _____

3. Time given in relation to this test ___

Patient's intelligence: circle number that represents best estimate.

1(low)   2   3   4   5 (high)

****

This questionnaire has been designed to tell us more about your pain. Four major questions we ask are

1. Where is your pain?
2. What does it feel like?
3. How does it change with time?
4. How strong is it?

It is important that you tell us how your pain feels now. Please follow the instructions at the beginning of each part.

_____

© R. Melzack, Oct. 1970

Part 2. What Does Your Pain Feel Like?

Some of the words below describe your *present* pain. Circle *ONLY* those words that best describe it. Leave out any category that is not suitable. Use only a single word in each appropriate category—the one that applies best.

1	6	11	16
Flickering	Tugging	Tiring	Annoying
Quivering	Pulling	Exhausting	Troublesome
Pulsing	Wrenching	**12**	Miserable
Throbbing	**7**	Sickening	Intense
Beating	Hot	Suffocating	Unbearable
Pounding	Burning	**13**	**17**
2	Scalding	Fearful	Spreading
Jumping	Searing	Frightful	Radiating
Flashing	**8**	Terrifying	Penetrating
Shooting	Tingling	**14**	Piercing
3	Itchy	Punishing	**18**
Pricking	Smarting	Grueling	Tight
Boring	Stinging	Cruel	Numb
Drilling	**9**	Vicious	Drawing
Stabbing	Dull	Killing	Squeezing
Lancinating	Sore	**15**	Tearing
4	Hurting	Wretched	**19**
Sharp	Aching	Blinding	Cool
Cutting	Heavy		Cold
Lacerating	**10**		Freezing
5	Tender		**20**
Pinching	Taut		Nagging
Pressing	Rasping		Nauseating
Gnawing	Splitting		Agonizing
Cramping			Dreadful
Crushing			Torturing

Part 1. Where Is Your Pain?

Please mark, on the drawings below, the areas where you feel pain. Put E if external, or I if internal, near the areas you mark. Put EI if both external and internal.

Part 3. How Does Your Pain Change With Time?

1. Which word or words would you use to describe the *pattern* of your pain?

1	2	3
Continuous	Rhythmic	Brief
Steady	Periodic	Momentary
Constant	Intermittent	Transient

2. What kind of things *relieve* your pain?

3. What kind of things *increase* your pain?

Part 4. How Strong Is Your Pain?

People agree that the following 5 words represent pain of increasing intensity. They are:

1	2	3	4	5
Mild	Discomforting	Distressing	Horrible	Excruciating

To answer each question below, write the number of the most appropriate word in the space beside the question

1. Which word describes your pain right now?_____
2. Which word descibes it at its worst?_____
3. Which word describes it when it is least?_____
4. Which word describes the worst toothache you ever had?_____
5. Which word describes the worst headache you ever had?_____
6. Which word describes the worst stomach ache you ever had?_____

FIGURE 4-5 The McGill-Melzack Questionnaire. (From Melzack, R. (1975). The McGill Pain Questionnaire: Major properties and scoring methods. *Pain, 1,* 277-299.)

TABLE 4-2

The Behavioral Pain Scale

Item	Description	Score
Facial expression	Relaxed	1
	Partially tightened (e.g., brow lowering)	2
	Fully tightened (e.g., eyelid closing)	3
	Grimacing	4
Upper limbs	No movement	1
	Partially bent	2
	Fully bent with finger flexion	3
	Permanently retracted	4
Compliance with ventilation	Tolerating movement	1
	Coughing but tolerating ventilation most of the time	2
	Fighting ventilator	3
	Unable to control ventilation	4

Each of the three categories—facial expression, upper limbs, and compliance with ventilation—is scored from 1 to 4. The values are added together for a total score between 3 and 12. From Payen, J-F., Bru, O., Bosson, J-L., Lagrasta, A., Novel, E., Deschaux, I., Lavagne, P., & Jacquot, C. (2001). Assessing pain in critically ill sedated patients by using a behavioral pain scale. *Critical Care Medicine, 29*(12), 2258-2263.

Anxiety typically produces hyperactive psychomotor functions including tachycardia, hypertension, and movement. Patients are typically sedated to limit this hyperactivity. The level of sedation can be measured by using objective tools or scales. An ideal sedation scale provides data that are simple to compute and record, accurately describes the degree of sedation or agitation within well-defined categories, guides the titration of therapy, and has validity and reliability in critically ill patients (Jacobi et al., 2002). These scales may have a moderate level of interrater variability depending on how nurses have been trained in its use.

One of the most frequently used objective tools to measure levels of sedation in a critically ill patient is the Ramsay Sedation Scale (RSS) (Ramsay et al., 1974). The RSS has the nurse make a visual and cognitive assessment of the patient (Table 4-4). One nurse could rate a patient as having a score of 3, whereas another nurse would rate the same patient as receiving a score of 2. This variability in scores is particularly important because sedative medications may be titrated based on the RSS score. When using medications to sedate a patient, the goal is to achieve a certain level of sedation using the lowest dose. By using lower doses of medications, the patient is less likely to experience drug accumulation or adverse effects. These adverse effects include increased hospital stay, delayed ventilator weaning, immobility, and increased rates of ventilator associated pneumonia. Conversely, not enough sedation may lead to

TABLE 4-3

The FLACC Scale

Categories	Scoring		
	0	1	2
Face	No particular expression or smile	Occasional grimace or frown, withdrawn, disinterested	Frequent to constant quivering chin, clenched jaw
Legs	Normal position or relaxed	Uneasy, restless, tense	Kicking, or legs drawn up
Activity	Lying quietly, normal position, moves easily	Squirming, shifting back and forth, tense	Arched, rigid or jerking
Cry	No cry (awake or asleep)	Moans or whimpers; occasional complaint	Crying steadily, screams or sobs, frequent complaints
Consolability	Content, relaxed	Reassured by occasional touching, hugging or being talked to, distractable	Difficult to console or comfort

Each of the five categories (F) Face; (L) Legs; (A) Activity; (C) Cry; (C) Consolability is scored from 0 to 2. The values added together for a total score between 0 and 10.
Reprinted from *Pediatric Nursing*, 1997, Volume 23, Number 3, pp. 293-297. Reprinted with permission of the publisher, Jannetti Publications, Inc., East Holly Avenue, Box 56, Pitman, NJ 08071-0056; Phone (856) 256-2300; Fax: (856) 589-7463. For a sample copy of the journal, please contact the publisher.

TABLE 4-4

The Ramsay Sedation Scale

Level	Scale
1	Patient awake, anxious and agitated or restless, or both
2	Patient awake, cooperative, oriented, and tranquil
3	Patient awake; response to commands only
4	Patient asleep; brisk response to light glabellar tap or loud auditory stimulus
5	Patient asleep; sluggish response to light glabellar tap or loud auditory stimulus
6	Patient asleep; no response to light glabellar tap or loud auditory stimulus

From Ramsay, M. A., Savege, T. M., Simpson, B. R., et al. (1974). Controlled sedation with alphalalone-alphadolone. *British Medical Journal, 2*(90), 656-659.

(Table 4-5) is becoming more widely used because it describes very specific patient behaviors seen in the continuum of sedation to agitation (Riker et al., 2001). The MAAS (Table 4-6) is similar to the SAS and uses clear and concise descriptors to assess the sedation level of the patient. Nurses have found that the MAAS appears to reflect the patient's true level of sedation adequately and is very easy to use (Devlin et al., 1999). The key is to use one tool consistently within the critical care unit and to ensure that the nursing staff understand how to use it. The critical care nurse should always use tools that have been shown to be valid and reliable, with acceptable inter-rater reliability (McGaffigan, 2002; Quirke et al., 1997).

The appropriate target level of sedation depends on the patient's disease process and therapeutic or support interventions required. A common target level of sedation is a calm patient who can be easily aroused; however, deeper levels of sedation may be needed to facilitate mechanical ventilation. The desired level of sedation should be determined at the start of therapy and reevaluated regularly, based on the patient's clinical condition.

agitation, inappropriate use of paralytics, increased metabolic demand, and an increased risk of myocardial ischemia (McGaffigan, 2002).

Other tools available to score patient levels of sedation are the Sedation-Agitation Scale (SAS) and the Motor Activity Assessment Scale (MAAS). The SAS

TECHNOLOGICAL DEVICES

No technological device can provide the bedside nurse with an absolute measurement of the patient's pain or anxiety. However, some devices can assist the nurse in determining a patient's level of consciousness. Pain and anxiety are likely to result in a heightened level of consciousness as a result of activation of the SNS.

TABLE 4-5

Sedation-Agitation Scale

Score	Characteristic	Examples of Patient's Behavior
7	Dangerously agitated	Pulls at endotracheal tube, tries to remove catheters, climbs over bed rail, strikes at staff, thrashes from side to side
6	Very agitated	Does not calm despite frequent verbal reminding of limits, requires physical restraints, bites endotracheal tube
5	Agitated	Is anxious or mildly agitated, attempts to sit up, calms down in response to verbal instructions
4	Calm and cooperative	Is calm, awakens easily, follows commands
3	Sedated	Is difficult to arouse, awakens to verbal stimuli or gentle shaking but drifts off again, follows simple commands
2	Very sedated	Arouses to physical stimuli but does not communicate or follow commands, may move spontaneously
1	Unarousable	Has minimal or no response to noxious stimuli, does not communicate or follow commands

From Riker, R. R., Fraser, G. L., Simmons, L. E., & Wilkins, M. L. (2001). Validating the sedation-agitation scale with the bispectral index and visual analog scale in adult ICU patients after cardiac surgery. *Intensive Care Medicine, 27*(5), 853-858.

TABLE 4-6		
The Motor Activity Assessment Scale		
Score	**Description**	**Definition**
0	Unresponsive	Does not move with noxious stimulus
1	Responsive only to noxious stimuli	Opens eyes OR raises eyebrows OR turns head toward stimuli OR moves limbs with noxious stimulus
2	Responsive to touch or name	Opens eyes OR raises eyebrows OR turns head toward stimuli OR moves limbs when touched or name is loudly spoken
3	Calm and cooperative	No external stimulus is required to elicit movement AND patient is adjusting sheets or clothes purposefully and follows commands
4	Restless and cooperative	No external stimulus is required to elicit movement AND patient is picking at sheets or tubes OR uncovering self and follows commands
5	Agitated	No external stimulus is required to elicit movement AND attempting to sit up OR moves limbs out of bed AND does not consistently follow commands (e.g., will lie down when asked but soon reverts back to attempts to sit up or move limbs out of bed)
6	Dangerously agitated, uncooperative	No external stimulus is required to elicit movement AND patient is pulling at tubes or catheters OR thrashing side to side OR striking at staff OR trying to climb out of bed AND does not calm down when asked

From Devlin, J., Boleski, G., Mlynarek, M., Nerenz, D., Peterson, E., Jankowski, M., Horst, H. M., & Zarowitz, B. J. (1999). Motor Activity Assessment Scale: A valid and reliable sedation scale for use with mechanically ventilated patients in an adult surgical intensive care unit. *Critical Care Medicine, 27*(7), 1271-1275.

Technological devices have been used in the operating room to measure a patient's level of consciousness in order to verify that proper anesthesia dosing has been achieved. These devices are now being introduced into the critical care unit. Two of these devices are the electroencephalogram (EEG) and bispectral index (BIS) monitoring.

The EEG records spontaneous brain activity that originates from the cortical pyramidal cells on the surface of the brain. Any major brain activity produces a resultant peak in activity on the EEG monitor. EEG sedation measures have been developed based on the observation that the EEG generally changes from a low-amplitude, high-frequency signal while the patient is awake to a large-amplitude, low-frequency signal when the patient is deeply anesthetized (Aspect Medical Systems, 1999).

The EEG monitor receives data from 21 electrodes that are placed in key positions on the patient's head. The number of electrodes may be decreased depending on the patient's head size and the purpose for the EEG procedure (Malarkey, McMorrow, & Eoyang, 2000). The EEG is used infrequently to detect levels of sedation because it takes significant time (up to 60 minutes) to acquire proper electrode

placement and a high level of skill to interpret the EEG recording. Advances in digital EEG acquisition have made continuous EEG monitoring in the critical care unit more technically feasible and useful (Scheuer, 2002). An EEG is more commonly used to assess a patient for physiological brain dysfunction.

More devices are becoming available that provide "conscious" monitoring by analyzing continuous EEG signals without the use of the traditional 21-electrode system. An example of one such technological device is the BIS monitor. The BIS monitor has simple steps for application, with results displayed as a numerical score. This score provides an objective analysis of the level of wakefulness (Kruskamp, 2003). The BIS monitor and electrode are shown in Figure 4-6. The electrode is placed across the patient's forehead and is attached to a monitor. The monitor displays the raw EEG and the BIS value.

The BIS value is an empirical, statistically derived number ranging from 0 to 100 that is correlated with the hypnotic level of the patient (McGaffigan, 2002). The BIS value correlates directly with the amplitude and frequency of the EEG signal. If the monitoring system detects an isoelectric EEG signal, then a value of 0 will be displayed (Riker et al., 2001). A BIS value

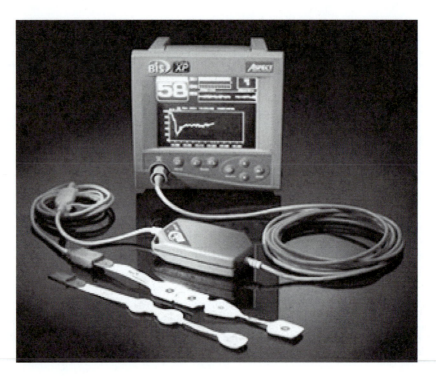

FIGURE 4-6 The Bispectral Index (BIS) monitor and electrode. (Courtesy of Aspect Medical Systems, Newton, MA.)

with a score greater than 90 typically indicates full consciousness, and a score of less than 60 indicates profound sedation. BIS scores in the 40 to 60 range have frequently been observed in the operating room when patients are under general anesthesia (Simmons et al., 1999). A BIS score near 70 indicates a light hypnotic state with a low probability of recall (Kruskamp, 2003).

The BIS values must be correlated with the patient's clinical assessment and correct electrode placement. The BIS score is usually documented with each set of vital signs. The monitoring device attempts to filter any ambient artifact, such as patient movement, that may artificially elevate BIS scores. The BIS monitor is ideal for critically ill patients who are treated with medications that produce deep sedation or neuromuscular blockade (Simmons et al., 1999).

Pain and Anxiety Assessment Challenges

There are situations that may lead to an incomplete assessment and/or management of pain or anxiety. These include delirium, nonverbal patients, and the use of neuromuscular blocking (NMB) agents.

DELIRIUM

A relationship exists among acute delirium, pain, and anxiety. Acute delirium is common in a critical care unit; more than 8 of 10 patients will develop some form of delirium during their stay (Truman & Ely, 2003). Delirium is characterized by an acutely changing or fluctuating mental status, inattention, disorganized thinking, and altered levels of consciousness.

Delirium is categorized according to the level of alertness and level of psychomotor activity. It is divided into three clinical subtypes: hyperactive, hypoactive, and mixed (Table 4-7). Patients with hyperactive delirium are agitated, combative, and disoriented. They may try to remove catheters or tubes, hit, bite, cry, yell, and even fall out of bed (Truman & Ely, 2003). These patients can place themselves or others at risk for injury because of their altered thought processes and resultant behaviors (Arbour, 2000). These behaviors may be frightening because they are typically associated with psychotic features such as hallucinations, delusions, and paranoia. Patients may believe that members of the nursing or medical staff are attempting to harm them.

Hypoactive delirium is often referred to as *quiet delirium.* The mixed subtype describes the fluctuating

TABLE 4-7

Clinical Subtypes of Delirium

Subtype	Characteristics
Hyperactive	Agitation
	Restlessness
	Attempts to remove catheters or tubes
	Hitting
	Biting
	Emotional lability
Hypoactive	Withdrawal
	Flat affect
	Apathy
	Lethargy
	Decreased responsiveness
Mixed	Concurrent or sequential appearance of some features of both hyperactive and hypoactive delirium

From Truman, B., & Ely, E. W. (2003). Monitoring delirium in critically ill patients: Using the confusion assessment method for the intensive care unit. *Critical Care Nurse, 23*(2), 25-36.

TABLE 4-8

Risk Factors for Delirium

Age more than 70 years
Transfer from a nursing home
History of depression, dementia, stroke
Alcohol or substance abuse
Electrolyte imbalance
Hypothermia or fever
Renal failure
Liver disease
Cardiogenic or septic shock
Human immunodeficiency virus infection
Rectal or bladder catheters
Tube feedings
Central venous catheters
Malnutrition
Presence of physical restraints
Visual or hearing impairment

Modified from Truman, B., & Ely, E. W. (2003). Monitoring delirium in critically ill patients: Using the confusion assessment method for the intensive care unit. *Critical Care Nurse, 23*(2), 25-36.

nature of delirium. Some agitated patients with hyperactive delirium may receive sedatives in the critical care unit to calm them and then may emerge from sedation in a hypoactive state.

The exact pathophysiological mechanisms involved with the development and progression of delirium are unknown. However, they may be related to imbalances in the neurotransmitters that modulate the control of cognitive function, behavior, and mood (Truman & Ely, 2003). Risk factors for the development of delirium include hypoxia, metabolic disturbances, electrolyte imbalances, head trauma, the presence of catheters and drains, and certain medications. Neurotransmitter levels are affected by medications with anticholinergic properties.

Benzodiazipines, opioids, and other psychotropic medications have all been associated with an increased risk of development of delirium (Table 4-8).

All critically ill patients should be monitored for level of sedation and delirium (Jacobi et al., 2002). The level of sedation can be assessed using one of the sedation scales described earlier. There are several tools available for assessing the mental status of a critically ill patient, including the Glasgow Coma Scale, the Cognitive Test for Delirium, and the Confusion Assessment Method (Box 4-2).

Management of delirium focuses on keeping the patient safe. The least restrictive measures are used because unnecessary use of restraints or medication may precipitate or exacerbate delirium. If the patient

BOX 4-2

Common Tools for Patient Mental Assessment

Tool	Description
Glasgow Coma Scale	A rough measurement of the status of consciousness altered by external circumstances
Cognitive Test for Delirium	Assessment of orientation, attention span, memory, comprehension, and vigilance obtained by using nonverbal responses
Confusion Assessment Method	Assessment of change in mental status from baseline or a status that fluctuates, inattention, disorganized thinking, and altered level of consciousness

Modified from Roberts, B. L. (2001). Managing delirium in adult intensive care patients. *Critical Care Nurse, 21*(1), 48-55.

is pulling at catheters, drains, or dressings, splints or binders may be used to restrict movement. Any type of tubing should be removed as soon as possible, particularly nasogastric tubes, which are irritating to agitated patients (Justic, 2000). If these measures are not successful, medication may be necessary, not to sedate the patient but to clear cognition. Haloperidol, a neuroleptic agent, is the recommended medication for delirium because it has few anticholinergic and hypotensive effects. In the critically ill patient, the intermittent intravenous route of delivery is preferred because it is more reliably absorbed and has fewer side effects than the oral or intramuscular formulations. Haloperidol produces mild sedation without analgesia or amnesia. Prolongation of the QT interval on the ECG may be seen and can result in torsades de pointes. Patients with cardiac disease are at higher risk for this dysrhythmia. Other side effects include neuroleptic syndrome, as evidenced by extreme anxiety, tachycardia, tachypnea, diaphoresis, fever, muscle rigidity, increased creatine phosphokinase levels, and hyperglycemia.

NONVERBAL PATIENTS

Critically ill patients may not be able to verbalize because of the presence of an artificial airway, sedative medications, NMB agents, or brain injury. The most frequent reason that critically ill patients are unable to speak is due to the presence of an endotracheal or tracheostomy tube. One of the greatest anxiety-provoking situations for these patients is being unable to communicate effectively with hospital staff or family members (Rotondi et al., 2002). The nurse must find alternative ways for the patient to communicate.

The simplest method is to ask the patient yes/no questions that require only a simple nod of the head. Many facilities also have communication boards, which contain several different illustrations that indicate common patient concerns, such as toileting, pain, and being hot or cold. One of the most useful tools that the nurse can provide the patient is a paper and pencil. However, some patients may find writing difficult due to the effects of medications; the presence of hand edema, intravenous catheters, and dressings; and prolonged bed rest, and/or sleep deprivation. For other patients, the most effective way to assess for pain and anxiety is to use the FACES scale or VAS, as discussed earlier.

NEUROMUSCULAR BLOCKADE

NMB agents, historically used in the operating room, are being used more in the critical care unit to facilitate endotracheal intubation and mechanical ventilation, to control increases in intracranial pressure (ICP), and to facilitate procedures at the bedside (bronchoscopies, tracheostomies). The goal of neuromuscular blockade is complete chemical paralysis.

During a difficult endotracheal intubation, the use of a rapid-acting NMB agent allows the airway to be secured quickly and without trauma. In addition, some patients are unable to tolerate mechanical ventilation despite adequate sedation. Long-acting NMB agents may improve chest wall compliance, reduce peak airway pressures, and prevent the patient from "fighting" the ventilator. Neuromuscular blockade promotes tolerance of newer modes of mechanical ventilation, including inverse ratio, pressure control, and permissive hypercapnea (Luer, 2002). The result is improved gas exchange with increased oxygen delivery and decreased oxygen consumption.

In patients with elevated ICP, suctioning, coughing, and agitation can provoke dangerous elevations in ICP. NMB agents diminish ICP elevations during these activities. In some patients, complete immobility may be required for a short period for minor surgical and diagnostic procedures (bronchoscopy, tracheostomy) performed at the bedside.

NMB agents do not possess any sedative or analgesic properties. Any patient who is receiving effective neuromuscular blockade will not be able to communicate or to produce any voluntary muscle movement, including breathing. Therefore, any patient receiving these agents must also be sedated. Many institutions start continuous infusions of analgesic and/or sedative medications before they initiate an NMB agent.

Patients receiving NMB therapy are closely monitored for respiratory problems, skin breakdown, corneal abrasions, and the development of venous thrombi. If a patient is experiencing pain or anxiety while receiving an NMB agent, an increase in heart rate or blood pressure may indicate pain or anxiety. Nursing care for patients receiving NMB therapy is presented in Box 4-3.

One important nursing intervention is assessing the level or degree of paralysis using a train-of-four (TOF) monitoring device. The TOF device delivers four low-energy impulses over a nerve that results in a muscular twitch. The ulnar nerve and the facial nerve are the most frequently used sites for peripheral nerve stimulation. The TOF evaluates the level of neuromuscular blockade to ensure that the greatest amount of neuromuscular blockade is achieved with the lowest dose of NMB medication. When the ulnar nerve is used, twitches of the thumb are observed. Four twitches of the thumb indicate incomplete neuromuscular blockade. The absence of thumb twitches indicates complete neuromuscular blockade. The TOF goal is two out of four twitches. An example of a TOF device is shown in Figure 4-7.

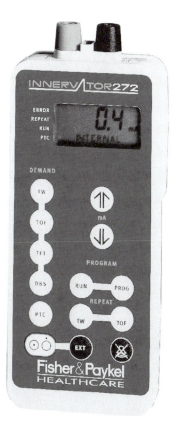

FIGURE 4-7 A train-of-four peripheral nerve stimulator. (Courtesy of Fisher & Paykel Healthcare, Auckland, New Zealand.)

No tools or devices can adequately assess pain and/or sedation in patients receiving NMB agents. The patient is monitored for physiological changes (see Table 4-1), and if changes do occur, the nurse must determine whether pain or anxiety is the potential cause. These patients may be the best candidates for assessment by nontraditional means such as the BIS monitoring system.

Although several NMB agents are available, the most frequently used are outlined on Table 4-9. Succinylcholine (paralytic), when administered with etomidate (sedative), is frequently used for rapid intubation because of its short half-life. However, succinylcholine should not be used in the presence of hyperkalemia because ventricular arrhythmias and cardiac arrest may occur. Pancuronium is a long-acting NMB agent. When it is given in bolus doses, tachycardia and hypertension may result. The effects of pancuronium are prolonged in patients with liver disease and renal failure. Atracurium is the most frequently used NMB in the critically ill because it can be used safely in patients with liver or renal failure. However, prolonged weakness has been described after long-term use in critically ill patients. Dosing of NMB agents should be titrated to provide the minimal level of neuromuscular blockade to achieve beneficial effects (Murphy & Vender, 2001).

Management of Pain and Anxiety

NONPHARMACOLOGICAL MANAGEMENT

Nonpharmacological approaches to manage pain and/or anxiety are early strategies because many medications used for sedation or analgesia have potentially negative hemodynamic effects. Many of these nonpharmacological approaches are clustered under the heading *complementary or alternative medicine*. These therapies are rapidly being integrated into the critical care environment. The three most commonly used complementary or alternative medicine therapies in the critical care are environmental manipulation, guided imagery, and music or art therapy.

Environmental Manipulation

The nurse may decrease patient anxiety and pain by changing the *environment* so it appears less hostile. Explanations of the monitoring equipment, alarms, and nursing care will help to decrease anxiety.

TABLE 4-9

DRUGS FREQUENTLY USED IN THE TREATMENT OF ANXIETY, PAIN, OR FOR NEUROMUSCULAR BLOCKADE*

Indication	Class	Drug	Common Route(s)/Dosage(s)	Common Side Effects	Nursing Implications
Anxiety/ Sedation	Benzodiazepines	Midazolam (Versed)	IM: 0.07-0.08 mg/kg IV: 1-8 mg over 1 minute, may require redosing q10min to a maximum of 20 mg	Central nervous system depression Hypotension Respiratory depression Paradoxical agitation	Increase doses slowly in increments with titration. Monitor blood pressure and respiratory status. Administer fluids as indicated. Slowly wean drug after prolonged therapy.
		Diazepam (Valium)	PO: 2-10 mg tid-qid IV: 2.5-10 mg; may require 2.5-5 mg q10min	Hypotension Respiratory depression Paradoxical agitation	
		Lorazepam (Ativan)	PO: 2-6 mg/day in bid-tid IV: 0.25-2 mg 0.5-1 mg (mild anxiety) 2-4 mg (moderate-severe anxiety) may repeat 1-2 mg in 10 min	Hypotension (less than midazolam) Respiratory depression Paradoxical agitation Hyperosmolar metabolic acidosis (IV prolonged infusion)	
	Nonbenzodiazepine sedative/anesthetic	Propofol (Diprivan)	IV: 5-50 mcg/kg/min (continuous infusion) Premixed solution	Hypotension Hyperlipidemia Respiratory depression	Patient should be intubated and receiving mechanical ventilation. Monitor blood pressure and hemodynamic status. Change infusion set every 12 hours using aseptic technique. Monitor plasma lipid levels.
	Selective alpha$_2$-adrenoreceptor agonist/anesthetic	Dexmedetomidine (Precedex)	IV: loading dose: 1 mcg/kg over 10 min Infusion: 0.2-0.7 mcg/kg/hr (continuous) Must dilute before administration	Hypotension Nausea Bradycardia	Give only by continuous infusion, not to exceed 24 hours. Evaluate hepatic and renal function.
Pain	Opioids	Fentanyl (Sublimaze [IV]/ Duragesic [patch])	TD: initially 25 mcg/hr, titrate as needed, change patch q72hr 25 mcg/hr or size: 10 cm^2 50 mcg/hr or size: 20 cm^2 75 mcg/hr or size: 30 cm^2 100 mcg/hr or size: 40 cm^2 IV: 50-100 mcg q1-2hr PRN Infusion: 1-3 mcg/kg/hr (continuous)	Hypotension Decreased gastric motility Respiratory depression Bradycardia Itching	Increase doses slowly in increments with titration. Monitor blood pressure, heart rate, and respiratory status. Administer fluids as indicated. Give as an infusion if extended therapy is required.

Category	Drug	Dose	Adverse Effects	Nursing Considerations
	Hydromorphone (Dilaudid)	PO/IM/IV/Subcutaneous: 1-4 mg q4-6hr PRN	Hypotension Decreased gastric motility Respiratory depression	Increase doses slowly in increments with titration. Monitor blood pressure, heart rate, and respiratory status. Administer fluids as indicated.
	Morphine (Duramorph/MS Contin/Roxanol)	Subcutaneous/IM: 4-15 mg q4hr PRN PO: 5-30 mg q4hr PRN Extended release: 15-60 mg q8-12hr IV: 2-10 mg q2-4hr PRN	Hypotension Decreased gastric motility Respiratory depression Nausea and vomiting Histamine release with itching or rash Urinary retention	Increase doses slowly in increments with titration. Monitor blood pressure, heart rate, and respiratory status. Administer fluids as indicated.
	Meperidine (Demerol)	PO/IM/IV/Subcutaneous: 50-150 mg q3-4hr PRN	Hypotension Decreased gastric motility Respiratory depression Tachycardia Seizures Urinary retention	Increase doses slowly in increments with titration. Monitor blood pressure, heart rate, and respiratory status. Administer fluids as indicated. Avoid using high doses in the critically ill
Nonsteroidal antiinflammatory drugs (NSAIDs)	Aspirin (Ecotrin/Bayer)	PO/PR: 325-650 mg q4-6hr PRN, not to exceed 4 g/day (analgesic)	Bleeding Gastrointestinal ulcers Thrombocytopenia Tinnitus	Administer with food if taking PO. Do not exceed recommended doses. Monitor complete blood count and renal function.
	Ketorolac (Toradol)	IV/IM: 30 mg q6hr (maximum, 120 mg); duration should not exceed 5 days PO: 20 mg followed by 10 mg q4-6hr	Headache Dyspepsia, pain Nausea Acute renal failure	Monitor complete blood count. Monitor renal and liver function.
Nonnarcotic analgesic	Acetaminophen (Tylenol)	PO/PR: 325-1000 mg q4-6hr PRN, not to exceed 4 g/day	Renal failure with chronic overdosage Blood dyscrasias Hepatic toxicity	Assess other drugs for acetaminophen content (Percocet 325 mg tablet). Monitor renal and liver function.
Delirium Neuroleptic	Haloperidol (Haldol)	PO: 0.5-5 mg bid or tid maximum; 30 mg/day IM: 2-5 mg q1-8hr PRN IV: 2-5 mg q1-8hr 0.5-2 mg (mild agitation) 5 mg (moderate agitation) 10 mg (severe agitation) may require dosing q30min (maximum single dose, 40 mg)	Drowsiness Prolonged QT interval Extrapyramidal symptoms Euphoria/agitation Paradoxical agitation Neuroleptic malignant syndrome Tachycardia	Measure QT interval at start of therapy and periodically. Use with caution when patient is receiving other proarrhythmic agents. Administer anticholinergic if extrapyramidal symptoms occur. Monitor blood pressure with initial treatment or change in the dose.

Continued

TABLE 4-9

DRUGS FREQUENTLY USED IN THE TREATMENT OF ANXIETY, PAIN, OR FOR NEUROMUSCULAR BLOCKADE*—cont'd

Indication	Class	Drug	Common Route(s)/Dosage(s)	Common Side Effects	Nursing Implications
	Antipsychotic	Olanzapine (investigational) (Zyprexa/Zyprexa Zydis [orally disintegrating tablet])	PO: 5-10 mg/day; maximum 20 mg/day	Agitation Headache Insomnia Somnolence Postural hypotension Dry mouth (xerostomia) Rhinitis	Maintain adequate hydration. Avoid exposure of extreme heat. Periodically assess liver enzymes in patients with significant hepatic disease.
Paralysis	Neuromuscular blockade	Atracurium (Tracurium)	IV: loading dose: 0.4-0.5 mg/kg Maintenance infusion: 5-10 mcg/kg/min to a maximum of 17.5 mcg/kg/min	Hypotension	Ensure adequate airway. This is safer than other neuromuscular blocking agents in patients with hepatic or renal failure.
		Pancuronium (Pavulon)	IV: intermittent dosing: 0.05-0.1 mg/kg q2hr PRN	Renal dysfunction Tachycardia Hypertension	Use intermittent boluses. Avoid continuous infusion because of long half-life and duration.
		Succinylcholine	IV: loading dose: 1-1.5 mg/kg Maximum: 2 mg/kg	Hyperkalemia	Avoid in patients with elevated serum potassium.

*This table does not account for typical dose adjustments used with the geriatric population.
bid, Two times per day; *g,* gram; *IM,* intramuscular; *IV,* intravenous; *PO,* by mouth; *PR,* per rectum; *PRN,* as needed; *qid,* four times per day; *tid,* three times per day; *TD,* transdermal.
Data from Arbour, R. (2000). Sedation and pain management in critically ill adults. *Critical Care Nurse, 20,* 39-56; Ellsworth, A. J., Witt, D., Dugdale, D. C., & Oliver, L.M. (2002). *Mosby's medical drug reference.* St. Louis: Mosby; Lacy C., Armstrong. L, Goldman. M., & Lance, L. (2000-2001). *Drug information handbook.* 8th ed. Lexi-Comp, Inc.: Hudson, OH; Gora-Harps, M. L. (1998). *The injectable drug reference.* Princeton, NJ: Bioscientific Resources; and Lober, C. (2003). *Oral communication.* Cleveland, OH: Cleveland Clinic Foundation Department of Pharmacy.

The presence of calendars and clocks is helpful. For a patient experiencing delirium, continual reorientation and repetition of explanations and information is helpful. Family members often benefit from role modeling as nursing staff members offer support and reassurance to patients while avoiding arguments with patients who have irrational ideas or misperceptions.

Another effective strategy is altering the patient's room. Patients and families should be encouraged to bring in personal items from home. Pictures of family members and other small keepsakes provide diversions from the stressful critical care environment. In some critical care units, it may be possible to move the patient's bed so it faces a window, or the patient could be moved to a completely different bed space. Physically moving the patient to a different location prevents the patient from becoming tired of the surroundings, and it may provide some sense of clinical improvement for the patient and family. There are also critical care units in which the monitoring equipment can be concealed behind cabinetry to provide a homelike atmosphere.

Family involvement is one of the most important strategies that can decrease the patient's anxiety or pain. A breadth of research has revealed the importance of family presence during critical illness (Lange, 2001). Patients need to be surrounded by familiar sights and sounds. In addition, the patient's family is often able to interpret patient behaviors, especially those associated with pain or anxiety, to the nursing staff. Data also show that as families feel more involved with their loved one's care, their levels of anxiety and frustration decrease (Lange, 2001). Families should be asked to participate in the care whenever the patient's condition allows it. Examples of family participation include coaching during breathing exercises and assisting with passive range of motion.

Guided Imagery

Guided imagery is a mind-body intervention intended to relieve stress and to promote a sense of peace and tranquility at a stressful time (Tusek & Cwynar, 2000). It involves a form of directed daydreaming. It is a way of purposefully diverting and focusing thoughts. Guided imagery has been used in Lamaze training during childbirth. The laboring mother focuses on a picture or object when labor pains are the most intense. This focus technique is coupled with rhythmic breathing exercises to create a state of relaxation. Guided imagery is a very powerful technique in controlling pain and anxiety.

Patients in the critical care unit may be instructed in the use of guided imagery during painful procedures. For example, when performing a needlestick puncture, the nurse may tell the patient to think about his or her children or imagine walking on a beach.

Patients undergoing gastrointestinal endoscopies were studied with guided imagery as an intervention. Those patients educated in guided imagery had significantly lower diastolic blood pressures throughout the procedure (Salmore & Nelson, 2000). Studies have also shown that guided imagery decreases hospital length of stay, decreases medication costs, and increases patient satisfaction (Beyea, 2002).

One study demonstrated the benefits of guided imagery for the patient undergoing open heart surgery. Patients were instructed on the use of guided imagery during preoperative education. Patients were then given a free videocassette or compact disc that contained relaxing sounds. Patients would wear small headphones and listen to the videocassette during the surgical procedure and in the critical care unit. The researchers found that the guided imagery program (1) reduced stress and anxiety, (2) decreased pain and narcotic consumption, (3) decreased surgical side effects, (4) decreased length of stay, (5) reduced hospital costs, (6) enhanced patient's sleep, and (7) increased patient satisfaction (Tusek & Cwynar, 2000). Guided imagery is a very simple and inexpensive strategy that all nurses can easily incorporate into their daily practice.

Music Therapy

Similar to guided imagery, a music therapy program offers patients a diversionary technique for pain and anxiety relief. Some medical institutions may have staff members dedicated solely to music therapy. When appropriate, a music therapist comes to the patient's bedside in the critical care unit and offers one-on-one therapy.

Music therapy may be effective in reducing pain and anxiety if patients are able to participate. Patients who are heavily sedated, chemically paralyzed, or physically restrained may not benefit from this type of therapy. Music therapy is an ideal intervention for patients with low energy states who fatigue easily, such as those who require ventilatory support, because it does not require the focused concentration necessary for guided imagery.

Music therapy research has shown that musical selections without lyrics that contain slow, flowing rhythms that duplicate pulses of 60 to 80 beats per minute decrease anxiety in the listener (Chlan, 2000). Music can also provide an alternative focus on a pleasant, comforting stimulus, rather than on stressful environmental stimuli or thoughts. Careful scrutiny of musical selections and of personal preferences of what is considered relaxing is important for success.

PHARMACOLOGICAL MANAGEMENT

Even with the most aggressive nonpharmacological therapies, many critically ill patients require medications to relieve anxiety and/or pain. The appropriate management of pain may result in improved pulmonary function, earlier ambulation and mobilization, decreased stress response with lower catecholamine concentrations, and lower oxygen consumption (Szokol & Vender, 2001). Table 4-9 summarizes pharmacological therapies used in managing pain and anxiety.

Common medications for managing pain include opioids and nonsteroidal antiinflammatory drugs (NSAIDs). The most commonly used opioids in the critically ill are fentanyl, morphine, and hydromorphone. The selection of an opioid is based on its pharmacology and potential for adverse effects. The benefits of opioids include rapid onset, ease of titration, lack of accumulation, and low cost. Fentanyl has the fastest onset and the shortest duration, but repeated dosing may cause accumulation and prolonged effects. Morphine has a longer duration of action, and intermittent dosing may be given. However, hypotension may result from vasodilation, and its active metabolite may cause prolonged sedation in patients with renal insufficiency. Hydromorphone is similar to morphine in its duration of action. Meperidine has an active metabolite that causes excitability, including apprehension, tremors, delirium, and seizures, and it may interact with antidepressants. Therefore, it is not recommended for repetitive use.

Renal or hepatic insufficiency may alter opioid and metabolite elimination. Titration to the desired response and assessment of prolonged effects are necessary. Elderly patients may have reduced opioid requirements.

Adverse effects of opioids are common in critically ill patients. Respiratory depression is a concern in nonintubated, spontaneously breathing patients. Hypotension may occur in hemodynamically unstable patients or in hypovolemic patients. Depressed level of consciousness and hallucinations leading to increased agitation may be seen in some patients. Gastric retention and ileus may occur as well.

The use of a reversal agent, such as naloxone, is not recommended after prolonged analgesia. It can induce withdrawal and may cause nausea, cardiac stress, and arrhythmias (Jacobi et al., 2002).

Fentanyl may also be administered by a transdermal patch in hemodynamically stable patients with chronic pain. The patch provides consistent drug delivery, but the extent of absorption varies depending on permeability, temperature, perfusion, and thickness of the skin. Fentanyl patches are not recommended for acute analgesia because it takes 12 to 24 hours to achieve peak effect and, once the patch is removed, another 12 to 24 hours until the medication is no longer present in the body.

NSAIDs provide analgesia by inhibiting cyclooxygenase, a critical enzyme in the inflammatory cascade. NSAIDs have the potential to cause significant adverse effects including gastrointestinal bleeding, bleeding secondary to platelet inhibition, and renal insufficiency. The risk of developing NSAID-induced renal insufficiency is higher in patients with hypovolemia or renal hypoperfusion, in the elderly, and in patients with preexisting renal impairment. NSAIDs should not be administered to patients with asthma and aspirin sensitivity.

Administration of NSAIDs may reduce opioid requirements, although the analgesic benefits of NSAIDs have not been studied in critically ill patients. Oral agents are available, and ibuprofen and naproxen are available in liquid form. Ketorolac is the only NSAID available in intravenous form.

Acetaminophen is used to treat mild to moderate pain, such as pain associated with prolonged bed rest, or as an antipyretic. In combination with an opioid, acetaminophen has a greater analgesic effect than higher doses of an opioid alone. Acetaminophen is administered cautiously in patients with renal or hepatic dysfunction.

Preventing pain is more effective than treating established pain. When patients are administered opioids on an "as needed" basis, they may receive less than the prescribed dose and there may be delays in treatment. Analgesics should be administered on a continuous or scheduled intermittent basis, with supplemental bolus doses as required (Acute Pain Management Guidelines Panel, 1992). Intravenous administration usually requires lower and more frequent doses than intramuscular administration to achieve patient comfort. Intramuscular administration is not recommended in hemodynamically unstable patients because of altered perfusion and variable absorption (Jacobi, 2002). A pain management plan should be established for each patient and reevaluated as the patient's clinical condition changes.

Anxiety in the critical care setting is typically treated with benzodiazepines, propofol, or dexmedetomidine (Covington, 1998). Both pain and anxiety may exist with evidence of psychotic features (as manifested in delirium). In this situation, neuroleptic agents, antidepressants, and anesthetic agents are frequently used as additional medications (Arbour, 2000).

Benzodiazepines are sedatives and hypnotics that block new information and potentially unpleasant experiences at that moment. Although they are not considered an analgesic, they do moderate the anticipatory pain response. Benzodiazepines vary in their potency, onset and duration of action, distribution, and metabolism. The patient's age, prior alcohol abuse, concurrent drug therapy, and current medical condition affect the intensity and duration of activity and therefore require individual titration. Elderly patients and patients with renal or hepatic insufficiency exhibit slower clearance of benzodiazepines, a feature contributing to a significant delay in elimination.

Benzodiazepines should be titrated to a predefined end point, for example, a specific level of sedation using the RSS, the SAS, or the MAAS. Hemodynamically unstable patients may become hypotensive with the initiation of sedation. Sedation may be maintained with a series of intermittent doses of lorazepam, diazepam, or midazolam; however, patients requiring frequent doses to maintain the desired effect may benefit from a continuous infusion by using the lowest effective infusion dose. Patients receiving continuous infusions must be monitored for the effects of oversedation.

Propofol is an intravenous general anesthetic; however, sedative and hypnotic effects can be achieved at lower doses. Propofol has no analgesic properties. It has a rapid onset and short duration of sedation once it is discontinued. Adverse effects include hypotension, bradycardia, and pain when the drug is infused through a peripheral intravenous site. Propofol is available as an emulsion in a phospholipid substance, which provides 1.1 kcal/mL from fat, and it should be counted as a caloric source (Jacobi et al., 2002). Long-term or high-dose infusions may result in hypertriglyceridema, metabolic acidosis, or arrhythmias. Propofol requires a dedicated catheter for continuous infusion because of the risk of incompatibility and infection. Bottles should not hang for more than 12 hours.

Dexmedetomidine is an anesthetic agent with selective alpha-2 agonist properties that has been approved by the United States Food and Drug Administration for use as a sedative for short-term use (less than 24 hours) in patients receiving mechanical ventilation. It reduces concurrent analgesic and sedative requirements and produces anxiolytic effects comparable to those of the benzodiazepines. Transient

THE CLEVELAND CLINIC FOUNDATION CICU SEDATION GUIDELINES

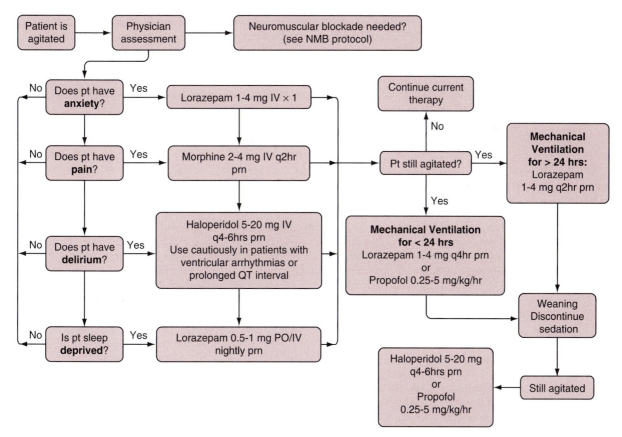

FIGURE 4-8 Sample algorithm of sedation guidelines. (Courtesy of The Cleveland Clinic Foundation, Cleveland, OH.)

elevations in blood pressure may be seen with rapid administration. Bradycardia and hypotension may develop, especially in the presence of hypovolemia, in patients with severe ventricular dysfunction, and in the elderly. The role of this medication in the sedation of critically ill patients is being determined.

Patients exposed to more than 1 week of high-dose opioid or sedative therapy may develop physiological dependence. Stopping these medications abruptly could lead to withdrawal symptoms. Opioid withdrawal symptoms include pupillary dilation, sweating, rhinorrhea, tachycardia, hypertension, tachypnea, vomiting, diarrhea, increased sensitivity to pain, restlessness, and anxiety. Signs of benzodiazepine withdrawal include tremor, headache, nausea, sweating, fatigue, anxiety, agitation, increased sensitivity to light and sound, muscle cramps, sleep disturbances, and seizures. Doses should be tapered slowly and systematically. Multidisciplinary development and implementation of sedation guidelines have been shown to reduce sedation medication cost, number of hours on the ventilator, and length of time in the critical care unit (Jacobi et al., 2002). The use of an algorithm assists in this process (Figure 4-8).

RESEARCH ANALYSIS

ARTICLE REFERENCE
Reimer-Kent, J. (2003). From theory to practice: Preventing pain after cardiac surgery. *American Journal of Critical Care, 12*(2), 136-143.

REVIEW OF STUDY METHODS AND FINDINGS
The purpose of this study was to determine the effectiveness of a new pain management guideline to prevent pain after cardiac surgery. The guideline was based on a wellness model and used a proactive treatment approach in which analgesic nonsteroidal antiinflammatory drugs (NSAIDs) were administered postoperatively around the clock. In addition, opioid medications were used as adjunct medications to treat procedural or breakthrough pain. In contrast, many existing pain guidelines treat the patient's pain reactively once the patient reports pain. Consequently, treatment takes place after pain occurs, thus causing some patients to experience severe pain. The new pain management guideline was evaluated through retrospective chart review of 133 patient records. The type and dose of analgesics administered for the first 6 days after surgery, the effectiveness of the pain management plan, the occurrence of adverse effects, time to extubation, and postoperative lengths of stay were determined. Pain management was considered effective if the patient did not numerically rate pain higher than a verbal score of 3 for a period of 12 hours or more. Ninety-five percent of patients were found to have effective pain relief. Almost all patients received acetaminophen around the clock. A total of 89% received indomethacin. All patients received opioids intermittently. This proactive, low-risk, well-tolerated pain management approach is cost-effective, simple, and feasible to use.

CRITIQUE OF STUDY STRENGTHS AND WEAKNESSES
This study appeared well designed in looking at the multiple variables (e.g., nausea, gut motility, time to extubation) that could be affected through proper pain management. The authors did reevaluate their earlier pain treatment guidelines (drafted in 1996) when they implemened the new and improved treatment regimen. The pain management treatment guideline follows a simple algorithmic approach that is depicted well in the study. The limiting factors in this study included the use of a retrospective approach. Data would have been obtained using more scientific rigor if this study had been conducted by a randomized-blinded approach in which patient (control versus treatment) groups have been compared. The other limitation in this study involved the collection of many of the variables. The number of patients who experienced nausea, time to first postoperative bowel movement, time to extubation, and length of stay were obtained from the clinical pathway. Because this documentation system was new, some data were missing.

IMPLICATIONS OF THE STUDY FOR NURSING PRACTICE
The strongest implication of this study for nursing practice is the effectiveness of proactive pain treatment. This study reveals the need for pain medications to be given on a scheduled basis so patients do not have to experience pain to be medicated. This study also reveals that different medication classes (opioids and NSAIDs) may provide synergistic effects such that pain is more effectively treated than with one medication alone.

Patient-Controlled Analgesia

Patient-controlled analgesia (PCA) is a medication delivery system in which the patient is able to control when medication is given. PCA involves a special type of infusion pump (Figure 4-9), which has a "locked" supply of opioid medication. When the patient feels pain or just before any pain-inducing therapy, the patient can depress a button on the pump that will deliver a prescribed bolus amount of medication.

The PCA pump will only allow a single dose of a narcotic to be delivered each time the button is depressed; however there is a time limit before the next dose can be delivered. These special safety features within the pump decrease the risk of receiving too much medication. Opioids delivered by PCA pump result in stable drug concentrations, good quality of analgesia, less sedation, less opioid consumption, and potentially fewer side effects, and PCA has been proven to be a safe and effective method of pain management (Pasero & McCaffery, 2001).

PCA management is rarely appropriate for critically ill patients, because most patients are unable to depress the button, or they are too ill to manage their pain effectively (Pasero & McCaffery, 2001). However, some patients in the surgical critical care unit after an elective operation may benefit from PCA therapy to manage postoperative incisional pain. Typical patient criteria for PCA therapy are listed in Box 4-4.

Epidural Analgesia

Opioids or local anesthetics can be delivered through an epidural or intrathecal (subarachnoid space) catheter. The discovery of opioid receptors in the spinal cord is considered a major breakthrough in

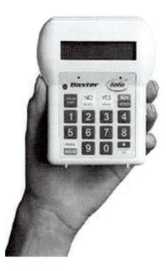

FIGURE 4-9 A patient-controlled analgesia infusion pump. (Courtesy of Baxter Healthcare, Deerfield, IL.)

BOX 4-4

Typical Patient Criteria for Patient-Controlled Analgesia Therapy

- An elective surgical procedure
- Large surgical wounds likely to result in pain (e.g., thoracotomy incisions)
- Large traumatic wounds
- Normal cognitive function
- Normal motor skills (able to depress the medication delivery button)

---

the management of pain associated with traumatic injury of the chest and abdomen. Blunt or penetrating trauma to the chest can cause rib fractures, pulmonary contusions, pneumothorax, hemothorax, and tracheobronchial tree injury. These injuries result in tremendous pain that causes suboptimal chest expansion. Patients do not want to cough, breathe deeply, ambulate, or participate in pulmonary exercises that clear secretions because it is too painful. Eventually, atelectasis, hypoxia, respiratory failure, and pneumonia result. Similar complications may be seen in patients with upper abdominal injuries requiring surgical intervention.

The use of epidural agents in this population of patients has demonstrated improvements in pulmonary function, fewer days spent on the ventilator, earlier ambulation, and decreased critical care and hospital stays (Alpen & Morse, 2001). Box 4-5 describes further potential benefits of epidural analgesia.

The patient is carefully assessed to determine the appropriateness of spinal analgesia. Contraindications include coagulopathies, cardiovascular instability, sepsis, spine injury, infection or injury to the skin at the proposed insertion site, patient refusal, inability to lie still during catheter insertion, and alcohol or drug intoxication (Alpen & Morse, 2001). Potential side effects of spinal analgesia using opioids include respiratory depression, sedation, nausea and vomiting, and urinary retention. Potential side effects of spinal analgesia using local anesthetics include sympathetic blockade (hypotension, venous pooling), motor weakness, sensory block, and urinary retention.

Management Challenges

INVASIVE PROCEDURES

Many invasive procedures, including nasogastric tube insertion, tracheal suctioning, central venous catheter insertion, chest tube insertion, wound care, femoral sheath removal, and cardioversion, take place in the critical care unit. All these invasive procedures have the likelihood of inducing pain or anxiety

BOX 4-5

Potential Benefits of Epidural Analgesia

System	Response
Pulmonary	↑ Vital capacity
	↑ Functional residual capacity
	Improved airway resistance
Cardiac	Coronary artery vasodilation
	↓ Blood pressure, heart rate
Gastrointestinal	Less nausea and vomiting
	Faster return of gastrointestinal function
Neurological	↓ Total opioid requirement
	↓ Sedation
Activity	Earlier extubation
	Earlier mobilization
	Decreased length of stay

↑, Increased; ↓, decreased,
Modified from Alpen, M. A., & Morse, C. (2001). Managing the pain of traumatic injury. *Critical Care Nursing Clinics of North America, 13*(2), 243-257.

(Puntillo et al., 2004). If symptoms of pain or anxiety occur during any critical procedure, the length and difficulty of the procedure may be increased, inaccurate data may be obtained from the procedure, and physical harm could result (Moline, 2000).

To avoid negative outcomes, the patient's comfort must be appropriately assessed and managed. Many times, the patient is kept in a conscious state during the procedure because full anesthetization is not necessary and it would increase the risk of complications such as respiratory depression and hypotension. Therefore, sedative and/or analgesic agents are given in a way that the patient appears sedate yet is able to verbalize. This type of sedation has been referred to as *procedural sedation* or *conscious sedation.*

Typical nursing care during these procedures usually involves monitoring vital signs including pulse oximetry, ensuring a patent airway, and observing for the adverse effects of medications. Many institutions use specialized flowsheets or forms in which assessment findings are documented during invasive procedures (Figure 4-10). Pain or sedation scales are often included as part of an ongoing assessment so the patient's level of pain and/or anxiety can be quantified at different intervals.

SUBSTANCE ABUSE

Patients who have a history of substance abuse pose special challenges in the critical care unit. Several studies have shown that alcoholism increases hospital length of stay because of an increased number of complications. These complications include higher infection rates, increased use of restraints, increased incidence of acute respiratory distress syndrome, and acute delirium (Moss et al., 1996).

The pharmacological management of patients in the critical care unit typically involves the administration of sedative and hypnotic medications. Patients with a history of substance abuse may have a higher than normal dosage threshold to achieve therapeutic actions with many of these pharmacological agents. If alcoholism or drug abuse is suspected, it may be beneficial to start with higher than normal doses of sedative and analgesic medications. There are times when it may be necessary to exceed the recommended maximum dosage of a medication, based on the patient's response.

Alcoholism continues to be an underrecognized problem in many medical centers. Chronic alcoholism that is not recognized, and therefore not treated on hospital admission, predisposes the patient to alcohol withdrawal syndrome (AWS). Symptoms of AWS usually present within 72 to 96 hours after the patient's last alcohol intake. The symptoms may begin as delirium tremens (shaking of the extremities or digits) and can progress to paranoid-like behavior, seizures, convulsions, and even death. Folic acid and thiamine are frequently given to patients with a history of alcoholism to prevent Wernicke's encephalopathy.

RESTRAINING DEVICES

Restraining or immobilizing devices are commonly used in the critical care setting to ensure that the patient is unable to disrupt invasive lines or pull at lifesaving devices. The purpose of restraints is to assist with maintaining patient safety; however, there is evidence that restraints can actually be dangerous if the patient is not oriented (Evans, Wood, & Lambert, 2003). The goal of applying restraints is to use the least restrictive device so the patient still has some movement. Commonly used restraining devices are listed in Table 4-10.

The most common adverse events associated with restraints involve complications associated with immobility. Patients with restraining devices must be repositioned, and the areas where the restraints are applied are assessed for perfusion and sensation at least every hour. This assessment is often documented on a special part of the critical care flowsheet. Patients who are restrained are monitored continuously for complications and potential disruption of therapy.

Nursing Assessment:

Prep: _____

NPO since: _____

I.D. Band check (if applicable): _____

Dentures ❑ yes ❑ no ❑ N/A

Glasses ❑ yes ❑ no ❑ N/A

Other: _____

Patient Education re: procedure ❑ yes ❑ no ❑ N/A

Nursing Plan of care initiated: ❑ yes ❑ no ❑ N/A

Transportation home verified? ❑ yes ❑ no ❑ N/A

IV site: _____

_____ Initials _____

INTAKE

TIME	SOLUTION - ml's/hr	ABSORBED	CREDIT

Patient Assessment Score	pre	post
Moves 4 extremities voluntarily on command	2	2
Moves 2 extremities voluntarily on command	1	1
Moves 0 extremities voluntarily on command	0	0
Able to breathe deeply & cough freely	2	2
Dyspnea or limited breathing	1	1
Apneic	0	0
Fully awake	2	2
Arousable on calling	1	1
Not responding	0	0
Able to maintain O_2 saturation > 90% on RA	2	2
Needs O_2 to maintain O_2 sat > 90%	1	1
O_2 sat < 90% with O_2	0	0
Able to stand up and walk upright	2	2
Vertigo when erect	1	1
Dizziness when supine	0	0
Non-ambulatory	0	0
TOTAL		

OUTPUT

TIME	URINE	EBL		

Procedure Start Time: _____

Procedure Finish Time: _____

Total fluoroscopy time: _____

Dressing: _____

Bovie pad site: _____

Condition of skin upon removal of Bovie: _____

PRE-PROCEDURAL VASCULAR ASSESSMENT ❑ No deferred/ not indicated

PALPABLE: 4+= BOUNDING 3+= normal 2+= decreased 1+= weak 0= absent

Pulses: Pre	F	P	DP	PT	OTHER
RL					
LL					

Pre-Procedure Vital Signs: Time: _____ BP: _____ P: _____ R: _____ T: _____ O_2 Sat: _____

TIME	BP	P	R	O_2 SAT	LOC*	MEDS / O_2	NOTES/PAIN ASSESSMENT	INITIALS

*Modified Ramsay Score LOC 1=Anxious 2=Awake, tranquil, 3=Drowsy, responds easily to verbal commands 4=Asleep, brisk response to tactile or loud auditory stimulus 5=Asleep, minimal response to tactile or loud auditory stimulus 6=Asleep, no response
Patients should not remain below level 4 for longer than 15 minutes in conscious sedation. Patients with a Ramsey score of 5 or 6 are in deep sedation.

FIGURE 4-10 The Cleveland Clinic Foundation Procedural Sedation Record: Nursing Assessment Page. (Courtesy of The Cleveland Clinic Foundation, Cleveland, OH.)

TABLE 4-10

Common Restraining Devices

Restraint type	Description
Soft wrist restraints	Constructed from padded foam with Velcro or tie straps. Typically applied around the wrist and tied to the bed frame. Prevents the patient from pulling at items on the upper torso or near the face.
Soft mitts	Constructed from a padded foam material with mesh. Slipped over the hand so the palm rests on a pillow foam. Allows the patient full range of motion with the upper extremities but does not allow a grasping motion with the fingers. Ideal for patients who are "picking" at items such as dressings, intravenous infusion sites, or feeding tubes.
Elbow immobilizer	Large plastic sheath that is soft but does not have any flexion. Slipped over the forearm and placed over the elbow joint. Allows full range of motion at the shoulder and wrist but does not allow the elbow to bend. The patient cannot bring their forearm towards their head. Works well for patients who are attempting to remove an endotracheal tube.
Posey vest	Made from a Teflon-mesh material with straps that can be tied. Typically worn around the upper torso and can be tied to a bed frame or a chair. Keeps the patient bound to the bed or chair. Full range of motion in the lower extremities is possible. Ideal for patients who are sitting in chairs. Prevents the patient from standing unassisted.

ELDERLY PATIENTS

As the population ages, the number of elderly patients admitted to a critical care unit continues to increase. Patients who are older than 65 years pose special concerns because of comorbidities, multiple medications, physical frailty, and cognitive/sensory deficits. The elderly patient is also more vulnerable to alcohol and/or substance abuse.

Older patients generally receive less analgesia or sedation compared with younger adults, perhaps because of elderly patients' beliefs about their pain and/or anxiety. Some elderly patients believe that pain is a normal process of aging and is something that they must learn to accept as normal. Elderly patients often believe that complaining of pain to nursing staff will label them as "problem" patients. Finally, elderly patients may comment to their family and friends that the nurse is too busy to listen to their complaints, and they do not want to be a "bother." Refer to Geriatric Assessment for strategies for managing pain or anxiety in the elderly patient.

Geriatric Assessment: Strategies for Managing Pain and Anxiety

- Speak slowly and clearly.
- Verify any underlying cognitive deficits (e.g., dementia, Alzheimer's disease, cerebrovascular accident).
- Ensure that scales or other assessment tools have a large font/text.
- Stoic behavior may be the patient's normal baseline; therefore, assess for nonverbal cues to pain (facial grimace or withdrawal).
- Observe for changes in behavior, such as confusion or agitation. Elderly patients are at risk of developing delirium.
- Elderly patients may be resistant to taking additional medications; therefore, offer nonpharmacological strategies to manage anxiety or pain.
- Elderly patients may not ask for as-needed medications in a timely fashion. Pain medications should be routinely scheduled.
- Medication dosages may be reduced because of decreased renal and liver clearance.
- Certain medications may have paradoxical effects in the elderly (e.g., benzodiazepines causing agitation).

WITHDRAWAL OF MEDICAL THERAPY

At times, patients and/or their families may choose to end aggressive medical treatment to hasten a comfortable death. Patients may state their end-of-life wishes before their hospital admission if advance directives (e.g., a living will) have been completed. The patient is the ultimate authority regarding his or her medical care. Allowing the critically ill patient to die naturally has become known as *withdrawing medical therapy support.* This practice has become more common and acceptable in the critical care unit because of the aging population, patients with greater comorbidities, the high prevalence of multiple organ dysfunction, and the complexity of disease (Francis, 2002).

As discussed in the previous chapter, many ethical and cultural factors should be considered when medical efforts appear futile. Because of the holistic nature of nursing care, the critical care nurse is well suited to facilitate the patient's peaceful and dignified death. Nursing care during this process should be comprehensive, inclusive of all the patient domains (physical, psychosocial, and spiritual), and inclusive of all the specialties and disciplines that can be helpful at this complex time (Kirchhoff, 2002). The provision of patient comfort is the focus of care.

The bedside nurse should respect the patient's decision even if that decision is in conflict with the nurse's own values or beliefs. The patient's family should be given the option to be at the bedside during the patient's dying process.

Limited data are available regarding palliative or end-of-life care in the critical care unit (Nelson & Danis, 2001). Many published reports indicate that nurses and physicians are not comfortable in dealing with conversations that involve death, and they do not feel adequately trained in this realm (Levy, 2001). Therefore, the transition to provide only supportive and comfort measures may be difficult. For the critical care nurse, the respect of patient autonomy and the provision of comfort should be the driving factors in delivering care at the end of the patient's life. Francis (2002) outlines interventions that are helpful in preparing the patient in the critical care unit for a natural death (Box 4-6). Because of the complexity of patients and their illness, there is no one single method used to discontinue medical support. In addition, the time from the discontinuation of medical therapies to death can range from a few minutes to several hours, and in rare cases death may not occur for 1 to 2 days (Francis, 2002).

BOX 4-6

Steps in the Withdrawal of Medical Therapy

1. A final decision regarding persistence of treatment is made after careful discussion with the patient (if appropriate), the family, and the hospital staff.
2. A do-not-resuscitate (DNR) order is written. If the patient is not intubated, a do-not-intubate order is written.
3. Family support is provided (consider contacting a social worker if available).
4. A narcotic analgesic (morphine, fentanyl) drip is started. This can help to alleviate any symptoms of dyspnea or "air-hunger."
5. Conscious patients are treated for potential anxiety, preferably with benzodiazepine medications. Consider the use of haloperidol and/or propofol for more severe anxiety.
6. All chemical neuromuscular blockade is stopped, and neuromuscular function is restored.
7. If the patient is ventilated, then gradually decrease the ventilator rate, positive end-expiratory pressure, inspired oxygen content, and tidal volume until the patient is spontaneously breathing room air.
8. Some patients or families will ask that the endotracheal tube be removed. This can be done after appropriate suctioning.
9. Vasoactive medications are stopped.
10. Intraaortic balloon pumps and other forms of mechanical circulatory support are disconnected.
11. Antibiotic therapy is stopped.
12. Artificial nutrition is stopped.
13. Blood draws and other laboratory collection methods are discontinued.
14. Restraints are removed, monitors are discontinued, and alarms are silenced.
15. Excessive secretions are suctioned.

Modified from Francis, G. S. (2002). End-of-life care. In E. J. Topol (Ed.). *Textbook of cardiovascular medicine.* 2nd ed. Philadelphia, PA: Lippincott Williams & Wilkins.)

Case Study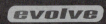

MB is a 52-year-old man in the surgical intensive care unit (SICU) after liver transplantation the previous day. He has a 15-year history of hepatic cirrhosis secondary to a history of remote alcohol abuse. He is intubated and is receiving multiple vasopressor medications for low blood pressure. At 6:30 AM, he is following simple commands and is denying pain or anxiety with simple head nods. At 7:00 AM, MB is kicking his legs and placing his arms outside the side rails. Attempts by the nurse to reorient him result in his pulling at his endotracheal tube. His wrists are restrained with soft restraints. At this time, he is not following any simple commands. He continually shakes his head back and forth. Facial grimacing is noted, and he is biting down on the endotracheal tube, which is causing the ventilator to sound the high-pressure alarm. His blood pressure is now 185/110 mm Hg, with a mean arterial pressure of 135 mm Hg. The monitor displays sinus tachycardia at a rate of 140 beats per minute. Medication infusions include epinephrine (3 mcg/min), norepinephrine (15 mcg/min), dopamine (2 mcg/kg/min), and fentanyl (100 mcg/hr). His only other medications are his immunosuppressive drug regimen.

DISCUSSION QUESTIONS

1. Score MB's pain and/or anxiety using the objective tools listed below:

Tool	Score
Behavioral Pain Scale (BPS)	
Ramsay Sedation Scale (RSS)	
Sedation-Agitation Scale (SAS)	
Motor Activity Assessment Scale (MAAS)	

2. Would complementary or alternative medicine therapies be appropriate at this time? If not, what therapies would be appropriate?
3. What type of medication is MB receiving for pain?
4. Is this an appropriate dose of medication for MB? If not, what is the correct dose?

SUMMARY

Patients admitted to the critical care unit are at an increased risk of developing pain and/or anxiety. The critical care environment and medical interventions may be the greatest contributing factors in the development of pain or anxiety. The assessment of both may be a challenge for the critical care nurse because patients may not be able to communicate. The use of assessment tools designed to recognize pain and anxiety are helpful. Nonpharmacological and pharmacological strategies to relieve pain and anxiety should be used so critical care patients have the best possible outcomes.

CRITICAL THINKING QUESTIONS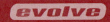

1. Describe factors that place patient a risk for pain and anxiety in the critical care unit.
2. Differentiate between subjective and objective tools when assessing pain and provide examples of each.
3. What is delirium? What are some of the behaviors seen in the hyperacute subtype?

REFERENCES

Acute Pain Management Guidelines Panel. (1992). *Acute pain management: Operative or medical procedures and trauma. Clinical practice guideline.* Rockville, MD: Agency for Health Care Policy and Research. AHCPR publication no. 92-0032.

Alpen, M. A., & Morse, C. (2001). Managing the pain of traumatic injury. *Critical Care Nursing Clinics of North America, 13*(2), 243-257.

Arbour, R. (2000). Sedation and pain management in critically ill adults. *Critical Care Nurse, 20*(5), 39-56.

Aspect Medical Systems. (1999). Overview: The effects of electromyography (EMG) and other high-frequency signals on the Bispectral Index (BIS) [pamphlet]. Newton, MA: Aspect Medical Systems, Inc.

Beyea, S. (2002). Guided imagery; intervention for smoking; pagers and bacteria; scissors; abdominal wound separation [compendium]. *AORN Journal, 76*(3), 520-522.

Birka, A. (1999). New perspectives on the use of propofol [commentary]. *Critical Care Nurse, 19*(4), 18-19.

Carroll, K. C., Atkins, P. J., Herold, G. R., et al. (1999). Pain assessment and management in critically ill postoperative and trauma patients: A multisite study. *American Journal of Critical Care,* 8, 105-107.

Chlan, L. L. (2000). Music therapy as a nursing intervention for patients supported by mechanical ventilation. *AACN Clinical Issues,* 11(1), 128-138.

Covington, H. (1998). Use of propofol for sedation in the ICU. *Critical Care Nurse,* 18(4), 34-39.

Crippen, D. (1995). Treating anxiety effectively in the intensive care unit. *Journal of Critical Illness,* 10(10), 708-710, 713-714, 717.

Cullen, L., Greiner, J., Titler, M. G. (2001) Pain management in the culture of critical care. *Critical Care Nursing Clinics of North America,* 13(2), 151-166.

Devlin, J., Boleski, G., Mlynarek, M., Nerenz, D., Peterson, E., Jankowski, M., Horst, H. M., & Zarowitz, B. J. (1999). Motor Activity Assessment Scale: a valid and reliable sedation scale for use with mechanically ventilated patients in an adult surgical intensive care unit. *Critical Care Medicine,* 27(7), 1271-1275.

Ely, E. W., Inouye, S. K., Bernard, G. R., Gordon, S., Francis, J., May, L., Truman, B., Speroff, T., Gautam, S., Margolin, R., Hart, R. P., & Dittus, R. (2001). Delirium in mechanically ventilated patients: Validity of the confusion assessment method for the intensive care unit (CAM-ICU). *JAMA,* 286, 2703-2710.

Evans, D., Wood, J., & Lambert, L. (2003). Patient injury and physical restraint devices: A systematic review. *Journal of Advanced Nursing,* 41(3), 274-282.

Francis, G. S. (2002). End-of-life care. In Topol, E. J. (Ed.). *Textbook of cardiovascular medicine.* Philadelphia, PA: Lippincott Williams & Wilkins.

Fraser, G. I., Prato, S., Berthiaume, D., et al. (2000). Evaluation of agitation in ICU patients: Incidence, severity, and treatment in the young versus the elderly. *Pharmacotherapy, 20,* 75-82.

Guyton, A. C., & Hall, J. E. (2000). Somatic sensations: II. Pain, headache, and thermal sensations. In A. C. Guyton & J. E. Hall. *Textbook of medical physiology.* 10th ed. Philadelphia, PA: W. B. Saunders.

Huether, S. E., & Leo, J. (2001). Pain, temperature regulation, sleep, and sensory function. In K. L. McCance & E. E. Heuther (Eds.). *Pathophysiology: The biologic basis for disease in adults and children.* St. Louis, MO: C. V. Mosby.

International Association on Pain, Mersky, H. (Chairman), Subcommittee on taxonomy. (1979). Pain terms: A list with definitions and notes on usage. *Pain,* 6, 249.

Jacobi, J., Fraser, G. L., Coursin, D. B., et al. (2002). Clinical practice guidelines for the sustained use of sedatives and analgesics in the critically ill adult. *Critical Care Medicine,* 30(1), 119-141.

Justic, M. (2000). Does "ICU psychosis" really exist? *Critical Care Nurse,* 20(3), 28-39.

Kaye, A. D., Clarke, R. C., Sabar, R., et al. (2000). Herbal medicines: Current trends in anesthesiology practice — A hospital survey. *Journal of Clinical Anaesthesia, 12,* 468-471.

Kirchhoff, K. T. (2002). Promoting a peaceful death in the ICU. *Critical Care Nursing Clinics of North America,* 14(2), 201-206.

Kruskamp, T. (2003). The changing face of sedation: Goal-directed care. *AACN News,* 20(11), 12-16.

Kwekkeboom, K. L., & Herr, K. (2001). Assessment of pain in the critically ill. *Critical Care Nursing Clinics of North America,* 13(2), 181-194.

Lange, P. (2001). Family stress in the intensive care unit. *Critical Care Medicine,* 29(10), 2025-2026.

Levy, M. (2001). End-of-life care in the intensive care unit: Can we do better? *Critical Care Medicine,* 29(2)[suppl], N56-N61.

Lighthall, G. K, & Pearl, R. G. (2003). Volume resuscitation in the critically ill: Choosing the best solution — how do crystalloid solutions compare with colloids? *Journal of Critical Illness,* 18(6), 252-260.

Luer, J. M. (2002). Sedation and neuromuscular blockade in patients with acute respiratory failure: Protocols for practice. *Critical Care Nurse,* 22(5), 70-75.

Malarkey, L. M., McMorrow, M. E., & Eoyang, T. (2000). *Nurse's manual of laboratory tests and diagnostic procedures.* Philadelphia, PA: W. B. Saunders.

McCaffery, M. (1979). *Nursing management of the patient with pain.* 2nd ed. Philadelphia, PA: J. B. Lippincott.

McCartney, J., & Boland, R. (1994). Anxiety and delirium in the intensive care unit. *Critical Care Clinics,* 10, 673-680.

McGaffigan, P. (2002). Advancing sedation assessment to promote patient comfort. *Critical Care Nurse [suppl],* 29-36.

McHugh, J. M., & McHugh, W. B. (2000). Pain: Neuroanatomy, chemical mediators, and clinical implications. *AACN Clinical Issues,* 11(2), 168-178.

Meinhart, N. T., & McCaffery, M. (1983). *Pain: A nursing approach to assessment and analysis.* Norwalk, CT: Appleton-Century-Crofts.

Melzack, R. (1975). The McGill Pain Questionnaire: Major properties and scoring methods. *Pain, 1,* 277-299.

Merkel, S. I., Shayevitz, J. R., Voepel-Lewis, T., & Malviya, S. (1997). The FLACC: A behavioral scale for scoring postoperative pain in young children. *Pediatric Nursing,* 23(3), 293-297.

Moline, L. R. (2000). Patient psychologic preparation for invasive procedures: An integrative review. *Journal of Vascular Nursing,* 18(4), 117-122.

Moss, M., Bucher, B., Moore, F. A., Moore, E. E., & Parsons, P. E. (1996). The role of chronic alcohol abuse in the development of acute respiratory distress syndrome in adults. *JAMA,* 275(1), 50-54.

Murphy, G. S., & Vender, J. S. (2001). Neuromuscular-blocking drugs: Use and misuse in the intensive care unit. *Critical Care Clinics,* 17(4), 925-942.

Nelson, J. E., & Danis, M. (2001). End-of-life care in the intensive care unit: Where are we now? *Critical Care Medicine,* 29(2)[suppl], 2-9.

Pasero, C., & McCaffery, M. (2001). Multimodal balanced analgesia in the critically ill. *Critical Care Nursing Clinics of North America,* 13(2), 195-206.

Payen, J-F., Bru, O., Bosson, J-L., Lagrasta, A., Novel, E., Deschaux, I., Lavagne, P., & Jacquot., C. (2001). Assessing pain in critically ill sedated patients by using a behavioral pain scale. *Critical Care Medicine,* 29(12), 2258-2263.

Puntillo, K. A., Morris, A. B., Thompson, C. L., Stanik-Hutt, J., White, C. A., & Wild, L. R. (2004). Pain behaviors observed during six common procedures: Results from Thunder Project II. *Critical Care Medicine 32*(2):421-427.

Quirke, S., Bowyer, J., Buxton, E., Clarke, R., Hart, P., & Thruston, I. (1997). Development of a sedation scoring protocol. *Intensive and Critical Care Nursing, 13*(3), 130-134.

Ramsay, M. A., Savege, T. M., Simpson, B. R., & Goodwin, R. (1974). Controlled sedation with alphaxalone-alphadolone. *British Medical Journal, 2*(920), 656-659.

Riker, R. R., Fraser, G. L., Simmons, L. E., & Wilkins, M. L. (2001). Validating the Sedation-Agitation Scale with the Bispectral Index and Visual Analog Scale in adult ICU patients after cardiac surgery. *Intensive Care Medicine, 27*(5), 853-858.

Roberts, B. L. (2001). Managing delirium in adult intensive care patients. *Critical Care Nurse, 21*(1), 48-55.

Rotondi, A. J., Chelluri, L., Sirio, C., Mendelsohn, A., Schulz, R., Belle, S., Im, K., Donahoe, M., & Pinsky, M. (2002). Patient's recollections of stressful experiences while receiving prolonged mechanical ventilation in an intensive care unit. *Critical Care Medicine, 30*(4), 746-752.

Salmore, R. G., & Nelson, J. P. (2000). The effect of preprocedure teaching, relaxation instruction, and music on anxiety as measured by blood pressures in an outpatient gastrointestinal endoscopy laboratory. *Gastroenterology Nursing, 23*(3), 102-110.

Scheuer, M. L. (2002). Continuous EEG monitoring in the intensive care unit. *Epilepsia, 43*[suppl 3], 114-127.

Simmons, L. E., Riker, R. R., Prato, B. S., & Fraser, G. L. (1999). Assessing sedation during intensive care unit mechanical ventilation with the Bispectral index and the Sedation-Agitation Scale. *Critical Care Medicine, 27*(8), 1499-1504.

Summer, G. J., & Puntillo, K. A. (2001). Management of surgical and procedural pain in a critical care setting. *Critical Care Nursing Clinics of North America, 13*(2), 233-242.

Szokol, J. W., & Vender, J. S. (2001). Anxiety, delirium, and pain in the intensive care unit. *Critical Care Clinics, 17*(4), 821-842.

Truman, B., & Ely, E. W. (2003). Monitoring delirium in critically ill patients: Using the Confusion Assessment Method for the intensive care unit. *Critical Care Nurse, 23*(2), 25-36.

Tusek, D. L., & Cwynar, R. E. (2000). Strategies for implementing a guided imagery program to enhance patient experience. *AACN Clinical Issues, 11*(1), 68-76.

RECOMMENDED READINGS

Abbott, American Association of Critical Care Nurses, & Saint Thomas Health Care System Sedation Expert Panel Members (2004). Consensus conference on sedation assessment. *Critical Care Nurse, 24*(2), 33-41.

Olson, D. M., Chioffi, S. M., Macy, G. E., Meek, L. G., & Cook, H. A. (2003). Potential benefits of Bispectral Index monitoring in critical care. *Critical Care Nurse, 23*(4), 45-51.

Puntillo, K. A., Stannard, D., Miaskowski, C., et al. (2002). Use of a pain assessment and intervention notation (P.A.I.N.) tool in critical care nursing practice: Nurses' evaluations. *Heart and Lung, 31*(4), 303-314.

Truman, B., & Ely, E. W. (2003). Monitoring delirium in critically ill patients: Using the Confusion Assessment Method for the intensive care unit. *Critical Care Nurse, 23*(2), 25-36.

evolve *Did you remember to check out the bonus material, including free self-assessment exercises, on the Evolve Web site at http://evolve.elsevier.com/Sole/ and on the CD-ROM?*

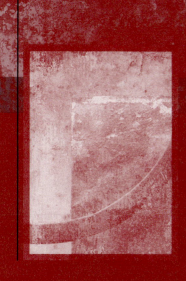

CHAPTER 5

Nutritional Support

Joan Ramirez, BS, RD, CNSD
Marthe J. Moseley, PhD, RN, CCRN, CCNS

OBJECTIVES

- Review the anatomy and physiology of utilization of nutrients in the body.
- Discuss nutritional assessment and types of therapies used to provide nutritional therapy.
- Implement adult hospitalized patient nutrition support standards.
- Formulate a nutrition care plan.
- Monitor and evaluate the nutrition plan of care.
- Make the transition from total parenteral/enteral feeding to an oral diet or long-term enteral feeding.

Introduction

All patients admitted to the critical care unit are assumed to be at nutritional risk. Any time the body is placed in a "stress" situation (e.g., sepsis, surgery, trauma, organ failure), nutritional support is required as an important component of the overall care plan. Without nutritional support, the risk of malnutrition is increased. Malnutrition can lead to immunocompromise and decreased respiratory ability, and it can also lead to wasting of muscle and adipose tissue.

This chapter provides a physiological review of the sites of absorption in the gastrointestinal (GI) system, drug-nutrient interactions, the basic assessment of a patient's nutritional status, the typical nutritional problems found in the critical care unit, and the types of nutrition therapy most often encountered in the critical care setting.

Utilization of Nutrients

The body uses nutrition in a variety of ways; each cell requires carbohydrates, proteins, fats, water, electrolytes, vitamins, and trace elements to provide fuel for energy necessary to maintain body function. When nutrients are ingested orally, they are first broken down by the mouth through mastication and then mixed with enzymes (salivary amylase, which digests starch) secreted by the salivary glands. Saliva is rich in mucus and helps to coat foods. The food bolus stimulates peristalsis, involving the contraction and relaxation of esophageal muscles, a process that continues until the bolus reaches the esophageal sphincter, at which point peristalsis causes the sphincter to relax so the bolus can pass into the stomach. The stomach is divided into four areas: the cardia, the fundus, the body, and the antrum. One of the functions of the stomach is to store food. While in

evolve *Be sure to check out the bonus material, including free self-assessment exercises, on the Evolve Web site at http://evolve.elsevier.com/Sole/ and on the CD-ROM.*

71

the stomach, food is mixed with gastric secretions until it forms a mixture called chyme. Once this occurs, the chyme is slowly emptied into the small intestine at a rate that allows for proper digestion and absorption. Gastric secretions are produced by the mucus-secreting cells that line the inner surface of the stomach; these cells secrete pepsinogen and hydrochloric acid. Mucous cells also secrete alkaline mucus that coats the stomach and provides for protection and lubrication.

One protein that is secreted only by the stomach is intrinsic factor, which is necessary for the absorption of vitamin B_{12} in the ileum. Vitamin B_{12} is critical for the formation of red blood cells. The stomach secretes fluid that is high in sodium and potassium and other electrolytes. If excessive fluid is lost from the stomach, either from vomiting or from gastric suction, the patient will be at risk for fluid and electrolyte imbalance.

The first part of the small intestine is the duodenum, the area where the pancreatic juices and the bile from the liver empty. The duodenum contains mucus-secreting glands called Brunner's glands that help to protect the duodenal wall from the gastric juices. Minerals such as chloride, sulfate, iron, calcium, and magnesium are absorbed here. The next segment is called the jejunum; monosaccharides (sugars), glucose, galactose, and fructose are absorbed in the first part of the jejunum. The water-soluble vitamins thiamine, riboflavin, pyridoxine, folic acid, and vitamin C are also absorbed in the jejunum.

At the end of the jejunum is the ileum. Protein is broken down into amino acids and is absorbed in the first part of the ileum. The fat-soluble vitamins (A, D, E, and K), fat, cholesterol, bile salts, and vitamin B_{12} are absorbed at the end of the ileum. The ileoceal valve located at the end of the ileum helps to prevent reflux of colonic contents of the large intestine back into the ileum. The colon is further divided into the ascending, transverse, and descending colon and the rectum. Sodium and potassium are absorbed in the first part of the colon. Vitamin K is formed by bacterial action and is absorbed toward the distal portion of the colon. Water is reabsorbed at the end of the colon. The colon is also a major site for generation and absorption of short-chain fatty acids. These fatty acids are the products of bacterial metabolism of undigested complex carbohydrates such as fruits and vegetables.

The pancreas aids in digestion. It secretes bicarbonate and enzymes into the first part of the duodenum and is also responsible for both exocrine and endocrine functions. Exocrine digestive enzymes (trypsinogen and chymotrypsinogen) are secreted in an inactive form to prevent autodigestion of the pancreas. Bicarbonate is also secreted by the pancreas and aids in neutralizing the pH of gastric chyme. The endocrine function produces insulin and glucagon.

The largest solid organ in the body is the liver. It aids in digestion by filtering out bacteria and foreign material and by secreting bile. Bile is composed of water, electrolytes, bile salts, phospholipids, cholesterol, and bilirubin. It plays an important role in carbohydrate metabolism by maintaining normal blood glucose concentrations in the blood. The liver has a role in the utilization of glucose, fructose, and galactose, and it stores glucose in the form of glycogen, which can be readily used if needed. Gluconeogenesis is carried out only in the liver and the renal cortex. This organ is essential for the protein metabolism of all nonessential amino acids.

The liver synthesizes the majority of circulating proteins and albumin. It detoxifies ammonia (a by-product of the breakdown of amino acids) by combining it with carbon dioxide (CO_2), producing urea and releasing it into the bloodstream. It is important in lipid metabolism. Fatty acids are synthesized in the liver from carbohydrate precursors and are generally stored in the form of triglycerides. The liver also plays a role in vitamin A metabolism.

The gallbladder contributes bile salts, which are secreted into the duodenum. The contraction of the gallbladder and the relaxation of the sphincter of Oddi control the bile flow. Bile salts help to emulsify fats and play a role in the absorption of fatty acids.

Assessment of Patient's Nutritional Status

Nutritional assessment is a comprehensive approach to defining nutritional status that uses medical, nutrition, and medication histories, physical examination, anthropometric measurements, and laboratory data (August et al., 2002a). It includes the organization of data and the evaluation of information to declare a professional judgment. The purpose of a nutritional assessment in the critically ill patient is to document baseline subjective and objective nutritional parameters, determine nutritional risk factors, identify nutritional deficits, establish nutritional needs for patients, and identify medical, psychosocial, and socioeconomic factors that may influence the administration of specialized nutritional support (Russell, Andrews, Brewer, Rogers, & Seidner, 2002). Malnutrition is a common occurrence in hospitalized patients, with an incidence of 30% to 55% (Shopbell, Hopkins, & Shronts, 2001).

Assessment of the patient in the critical care unit begins first with the subjective assessment of data. The subjective global assessment is a valid measure to evaluate nutritional status and severity of illness (August et al., 2002a). Once the determination has been made that the patient can communicate, determine orientation by asking whether the patient knows who he or she is and where he or she is. If the critically ill patient is intubated or sedated or has an altered mental status, then determine whether the patient has an adequate gag reflex and whether the patient can swallow without complaints of dysphagia. If the patient is able to tolerate an oral diet, the ability to tolerate a variety of textures is determined in part by adequate dentition. Assess for the presence of adequate saliva production by checking the oral mucosa for dryness; it should be pink and moist. Extra fluids may be required to facilitate easier swallowing if dryness is apparent. Evaluate the patient for muscle and/or adipose tissue loss, most notably in assessing for the appearance of wasting associated with chronic disease (e.g., cancer, multiple sclerosis). In addition, assess whether the patient is retaining fluid, as is associated with an edematous state.

Objective data include the evaluation of the patient's medical history. Assess for the presence of a malabsorptive syndrome that could impair the patient's ability to use nutrients such as short bowel syndrome, a history of radiation to the bowel, the presence of persistent ileus, intestinal pseudoobstruction, persistent vomiting, Crohn's disease, diverticulosis, or gastroparesis.

A patient who is not able to meet his or her needs orally may require enteral or parenteral nutrition. Enteral nutrition refers to the delivery of nutrients into the GI tract and is the preferred route of administration unless contraindicated. Various oral supplements or formulas are administered using different feeding tubes (e.g., nasogastric, nasojejunal, jejunostomy, or gastrojejunostomy). Nasally placed tubes predispose a patient to nasopharyngeal ulcers, nasal septum necrosis, sinusitis, otitis, hoarseness, and vocal cord paralysis if they are used on a long-term basis (August et al., 2002d).

Parenteral nutrition refers to the infusion of nutrient solutions into the bloodstream by a peripherally inserted central catheter, a centrally inserted external catheter, or a centrally inserted tunneled catheter or subcutaneous port. Parenteral nutrition is a successful way to provide nutrients to patients who are unable to tolerate enteral therapy or must have "nothing by mouth" as part of their treatment.

Large-bore nasogastric tubes can be used for medication administration, decompression of the gut, gastric suction, or drainage. A smaller, more flexible small-bore tube (usually 5 to 12 French) can be used in place of large-bore tubes. The small-bore tube is better tolerated because of its size and flexibility; it can reduce the risk of necrosis of the nasal tissue. Patients requiring long-term access can receive a percutaneous endoscopic gastrostomy (August et al., 2002d). This tube placement does not require general anesthesia and allows for feedings to begin soon after placement. A jejunostomy can be placed during laparotomy and gastrojejunotomy. These tubes have jejunal extensions added to access the small bowel. However, these tubes have a high rate of mechanical dysfunction and dislodgment, and are not advocated for long-term use (Shapiro, Minard, & Kudsk, 1997).

Parenteral solutions require access of the central venous system because of the high concentration of nutrients. It is possible to provide parenteral solutions through a peripheral vein if the concentration of carbohydrate does not exceed vein tolerance. The carbohydrate concentration is the limiting factor because of its high osmolarity. Factors for deciding which therapy to use are based on the length of time the patient will receive parenteral nutrition, as well as the patient's vascular access history, venous anatomy, and coagulation state. The hospitalized patient commonly receives a temporary percutaneously placed central venous catheter. Specialized nutritional support is initiated in patients whose oral intake has been inadequate for 7 to 14 days or in those patients in whom inadequate oral intake is expected over a 7- to 14-day period (August et al., 2002b).

Review current laboratory values such as the chemistry 20 panel. If possible, assess trends from several days of laboratory values and take note of the patient's inputs and outputs and the types of fluids that are being administered (e.g., 5% dextrose in water, half-normal saline, normal saline). In addition, assess whether any types of medications that the patient is receiving are available in a fluid solution. The sum of this information is used to determine the presence of adequate hydration or overhydration. Considering specifically the outputs, assess for the adequacy of urine output and for the presence of constipation or diarrhea. Validate other sources of output such as nasogastric suction, vomiting, ostomy, or wound drainage output. These other outputs are summed to look for possible trends such as those associated with refeeding syndrome, electrolyte alterations (phosphorus, magnesium, potassium), and overhydration or underhydration. In the review of medications, check for drug-nutrient interactions such as those commonly found in patients receiving warfarin (Coumadin), phenytoin (Dilantin), laxatives, antacids, antibiotics, neoplastics, alcohol, or potassium-wasting drugs such as furosemide (Lasix).

Nutritional Therapy Goal

The goal of nutritional therapy is to provide nutritional support consistent with specific metabolic needs and disease processes, to avoid complications of feedings, and ultimately to improve patient outcomes.

TABLE 5-1

Estimation of Nutrient Needs

Caloric Requirements	Protein Requirements	Fluid Requirements
Normal nonstressed 25 kcal/kg/day	0.8 g/kg/day	30-40 mL/kg/day
Mildly stressed 25-30 kcal/kg/day	0.8-1 g/kg/day	Patient specific
Moderately stressed 30-35 kcal/kg/day	1-1.5 g/kg/day	Patient specific
Severely stressed 35 kcal/kg/day	1-2 g/kg/day	Patient specific

The nutrition care plan then provides a template for nutritional therapy and is created by the analysis of information from many aspects of care, including consultations, therapies, and assessments. The nutrition care plan includes nutrient requirements and intake targets, the route of specialized nutritional support administration, and measurable short- and long-term goals of care and intervention (Russell, Andrews, Brewer, Rogers, & Seidner, 2002).

The first step in formulating the nutrition care plan is to estimate the patient's calorie, protein, and fluid requirements (Table 5-1). Normal caloric intake includes a 25 kcal/kg/day intake given no presence of metabolic stress, adequate weight, good hydration, and normal laboratory values. This type of patient can meet his needs by oral intake.

A moderately stressed patient who is malnourished requires 30 to 35 kcal/kg/day. This type of patient typically appears malnourished and may or may not be able to meet his or her needs adequately with intake only by mouth. In addition, the patient may have trouble with absorption, may have signs of sepsis, or may have had recent major surgery.

Severely stressed patients require 35 kcal/kg/day for adequate intake. These patients are likely to be underweight and unable to meet their needs by oral intake alone, and they may have had a major procedure with a septic event. Most patients in the intensive care unit are under metabolic stress, meaning that they are usually catabolic (patients are breaking down tissue for energy, not building or repairing it).

Nitrogen requirements for maintenance include an intake of 0.8 to 1 g protein/kg/day. This value is used for the patient who has adequate albumin and prealbumin levels. A moderately stressed patient requires a protein intake of 1 to 1.5 g/kg/day. These patients have moderate protein depletion, usually are third spacing, and have an increased protein need mostly for wound healing. The severely stressed patient's protein requirements are 1 to 2 g/kg/day. This patient has severe protein depletion because of a prolonged illness, inadequate protein intake, nonresolving sepsis, and/or the presence of extensive wounds. If the patient has hepatic failure with encephalopathy or renal insufficiency and if there is evidence of protein intolerance, then 25 g of protein per day is recommended (4 g nitrogen) (protein requirements: 6.25 = nitrogen requirements per gram).

Parenteral nutrition support is determined by initial recommendations that can be individualized (Table 5-2). The recommendations regarding fatty acids are that 1% to 2% of daily energy requirements are provided in the form of lipids to prevent essential fatty acid deficiency (August et al., 2002c). Sources of amino acids for parenteral nutrition are synthetic crystalline essential and nonessential amino acids. Electrolyte supplementation for parenteral solutions follows the recommended dietary allowances

TABLE 5-2

Parenteral Nutrition Initial Recommendations

Item	Requirement	Units
Volume	30-35 mL/kg/day	mL/day
Carbohydrate	4-7 mg/kg/min/day*	g/day
Protein	0.8-2 g/kg/day*†	kg/day
Fat	1-2.5 g/kg/day‡	g/day

*Assuming the patient is nonstressed. If the patient is stressed, requirements need to be individualized.
†If patient has hepatic encephalopathy and/or renal dysfunction, nitrogen initially should not exceed 4 g/day. To convert protein to grams of nitrogen, divide protein by 6.25.
‡Some data support a maximum of lipid of 1 g/kg/day intravenously to minimize adverse reactions.

Nursing Care Plan

NURSING DIAGNOSIS *Imbalanced Nutrition: less than body requirements: body weight ≥20% under ideal weight; weakness of muscles required for swallowing or mastication, inability to ingest food; related to inability to ingest or digest food or absorb nutrients because of biological or psychological factors.*

Nursing Outcomes	Nursing Interventions	Rationales
Demonstrates improved nutritional status as evidenced by progressively gaining weight toward desired goal.	Assess the patient's ability to obtain and use essential nutrients. Maintain a high index of suspicion of malnutrition as a contributing factor in infections. Be alert for food-nutrient-drug interactions.	Cases of vitamin deficiency and decreased caloric intake are prevalent in adult populations, specifically the elderly. Impaired immunity is a critical adjunct factor in malnutrition-associated infections in all age groups in all populations of the world. Patients at greatest risk are those who are malnourished, consume alcohol, receive many drugs on a long-term basis for chronic diseases, or take medications with meals or through a feeding tube. Case reports still appear describing scurvy in persons with alcoholism.
	Assess for recent changes in physiological status that may interfere with nutrition.	The consequences of malnutrition can lead to a further decline in the patient's condition that then becomes self-perpetuating if not recognized and treated. Extreme cases of malnutrition can lead to septicemia, organ failure, and death. Diarrhea in patients receiving warfarin has been suggested as possibly, causing lower intake and/or malabsorption of vitamin K.
	Weigh patient daily under the same circumstances. Assess for protein-energy malnutrition in the elderly. Interpret laboratory findings cautiously.	Protein-energy malnutrition in older persons is rarely recognized and is even more rarely treated appropriately. Compromised kidney function makes reliance on urine samples for nutrient analysis less reliable in the elderly than in younger persons.

From Ackley, B. J., & Ladwig, G. B. (2002). *Nursing diagnosis handbook: A guide to planning care.* 5th ed. St. Louis: Mosby.

and dietary reference intakes (RDA/AI). The standard dosing ranges for parenteral electrolytes assume normal organ function without abnormal losses. Electrolyte content of parenteral nutrient stock solutions is taken into consideration.

Enteral nutrition is preferred to parenteral nutrition to the greatest extent possible to preserve gut mucosa (August et al., 2002b). It is commonly selected for patients with neuromuscular impairment, patients who cannot meet their nutritional needs by oral intake alone, patients who are hypercatabolic, or patients who are unable to eat as a result of their underlying illness, such as those on ventilators or with hypoperfusion states. Enteral feeding is associated with significantly lower risk for infection; it is relatively inexpensive and easy to place (August et al., 2002d). If enteral access is to be used, a formula is selected that most closely meets the patient's current requirements for type of tube and location of tube placement. Consideration of how the gut is functioning is weighed along with other underlying medical problems such as diabetic gastroparesis. The use of enteral feedings, even if the gut cannot handle a full enteral feeding schedule, is advantageous because it prevents bacterial overgrowth and potential bacterial migration across the intestinal wall and into the bloodstream (August et al., 2002g). These benefits are crucial in critically ill patients. Enteral feedings have been used successfully in almost all situations including the presence of ileus and pancreatitis. Total parenteral nutrition is used in combination with enteral nutrition to meet the nutritional needs of the patient whose GI tract cannot accommodate the full caloric load.

Various formulas are on the market (Table 5-3). Standard formulas are typically 1 calorie per milliliter and are not designed for any specific purpose. Protein sources include soy protein isolate, calcium caseinate, sodium caseinate, and milk protein concentrate. The proteins typically are in a polymeric form and are the original complete form. The protein may be prepared as a form of hydrolyzed protein, which is broken down into smaller components to aid in digestion. In addition, the protein can be in the form of an elemental protein, which is completely broken down and ready for absorption. Fat sources include canola oil, a medium-chain triglyceride oil, sunflower oil, safflower oil, soy, and lecithin. Lipids provide 30% to 50% of the total kilocalories. There are two primary

forms, the long-chain triglycerides (a major source of essential fatty acids and fat-soluble vitamins) and the medium-chain triglycerides, which foster the absorption of fat better than the long-chain triglycerides but have side effects of nausea, vomiting, abdominal distention, and diarrhea (Heitz & Horne, 2001). Carbohydrates are the most easily digested and absorbed component of enteral formulas (Heitz & Horne, 2001). Sources include corn syrup, hydrolyzed cornstarch, and maltodextrin. The carbohydrates are not usually from lactose because lactose intolerance is a common problem.

Vitamins and trace elements are essential nutrients that act as coenzymes and cofactors involved in metabolism. For enteral nutrition, recommendations are based on the RDA/AI levels. Dosing beyond the RDA/AI values near the tolerable upper intake level is not generally supported by experimental data for most patients requiring specialized nutritional support. The dosing guidelines for parenteral vitamins and trace elements are considered as approximations of need.

TABLE 5-3

Enteral Formulas

Generic Description	Sample Product	Indications for Use
Elemental/predigested 1 kcal/mL 45 g Pro/L Free amino acids	Vivonex Plus	GI dysfunction, minimal residual
Standard isotonic 1 kcal/mL 37 37 g Pro/L	Osmolite	Normal GI function
High protein 1 kcal/mL 62.5 g Pro/L	Promote	Normal GI fuction Need for increased protein
Fiber enriched 1 kcal/mL 44 g Pro/L	Jevity	Normal GI function
Calorie dense 2 kcal/mL 70 g Pro/L	NutriRenal	Need for increased fiber Normal GI function
Oral supplement 1.06 kcal/mL 38 g Pro/L	Ensure	Renal dysfunction, decreased fluid volume Oral supplement
Oral supplement; high calorie 1.5 kcal/mL 54.9 g Pro/L	Ensure Plus	Normal GI function Oral supplement Normal GI function Need for increased calories and protein

GI, Gastrointestinal; *Pro*, protein.

Formulas have a variety of additives. Fiber is added for the benefit of blood glucose control and to reduce hyperlipidemia and diarrhea. Wound-healing formulas have added additional L-arginine and L-glutamine because they tend to be higher in protein content per liter than are standard formulas.

The next group of formulas comprises the elemental and semielemental formulas; their protein sources are enzymatically hydrolyzed casein and free amino acids. The carbohydrate and fat sources are the same as those of the standard formulas. These are used primarily for patients with impaired gut function, such as diabetic gastroparesis or short bowel syndrome.

Pulmonary formulas are designed for patients with impaired pulmonary function. The protein, fat, and carbohydrate sources are similar to those of the standard formula, with the exception of the fat content, which is higher. Renal formulas are also similar in content to the standard formula, except they tend to be more concentrated: 2 kcal/mL, with higher protein, carbohydrate, and fat content per liter than the standard formula. Diabetic formulas have protein, fat, and carbohydrate sources similar to those of the standard formula, with the differences of a decreased amount of carbohydrate per mL and an increase in fat per mL as compared with the standard formulas. Immune-enhancing formulas have carbohydrate and protein sources similar to those of the standard formula.

Practice Guidelines for Enteral Access

Decisions regarding access for enteral nutrition should take into account the effectiveness of gastric emptying, GI anatomy, and aspiration risk. In addition, enteral nutrition depends on an intact bowel that is able to absorb nutrients. The mouth is the ideal route of intake for enteral nutrition, but for patients who are unable to consume food orally, various routes are available for the administration of enteral nutrition.

Short-term enteral feeding routes include nasogastric, nasoduodenal, and nasojejunal. A gastrostomy or jejunostomy is done for long-term enteral nutrition. Feedings into the small bowel are often initiated within 24 hours of the onset of injury or illness. Nutrients are usually well absorbed in the small bowel.

Nasoenteric tube placement initially is attempted using a bedside placement technique; if this is unsuccessful, fluoroscopic or endoscopic guidance is used. Radiographic confirmation of the feeding tube tip position is obtained after placement of a nasogastric or nasojejunal access tube.

Feeding schedules are either intermittent or continuous. The stomach is normally a reservoir for intermittent feedings. Therefore, most authorities recommend an intermittent schedule. Feedings delivered in this manner are delivered by gravity and are regulated with a roller clamp to infuse over the course of 60 minutes. Delivery of tube feeding by use of a syringe is not recommended because of the risk of pulmonary aspiration.

Feedings delivered into the small intestine are delivered by constant infusion because the intestinal mucosa normally receives nutrients from the stomach in peristaltic waves. Enteral feeding pumps are used for delivery.

In terms of care for the patient with an enteral access, the gastric residuals are checked frequently when feedings are initiated. Clinical judgment is used when assessing for residual of feeding. First, determine whether a patient needs to have residuals assessed. A residual is a large volume of fluid obtained from the GI tract (30 to 300 mL or greater, depending on the hourly rate of the enteric feeding). If no signs of GI intolerance exist, then there is no clinical reason to assess residuals frequently. Tolerance of feedings includes the auscultated presence of bowel sounds in four quadrants, the presence of bowel motility, palpation of a soft abdomen, and percussion of the abdomen revealing tympanic findings. Signs of intolerance include the presence of nausea, vomiting, abdominal distention, or cramping; presence of these signs requires frequent reassessment for GI residual. Feedings are held if residual volumes exceed the hourly rate of administration, and each hour the patient is reassessed to determine whether the feeding is moving through the GI tract. As long as the residual remains equal to or greater than the infusion rate per hour, the feeding is held, and the physician is notified. Complications of enteral feedings are summarized in Table 5-4.

Feeding tubes are routinely flushed with 20 to 30 mL of warm water every 4 hours during the continuous feedings and before and after intermittent feedings and medication administration. Standardized protocols for enteral nutrition ordering, administration, and monitoring are used (August et al., 2002d).

Practice Guidelines for Parenteral Access

Parenteral nutrition is delivered through a catheter located with its distal tip in the superior vena cava or right atrium (August et al., 2002d). A chest radiograph is obtained after catheter insertion unless internal jugular or upper extremity intravenous access is obtained by an interventional radiology technique.

TABLE 5-4

Tube Feeding Complications and Nursing Interventions

Complication	Nursing Interventions
MECHANICAL	
Tube obstruction	Flush feeding tube with at least 30 mL of water every 4 hr during continuous feeding, after medications, after intermittent feedings, and before and after gastric residuals are checked. Use polyurethane tube. Use medications in elixir form whenever possible. If the tube becomes obstructed, irrigate it with either water or cola; some protocols use enzymes to relieve the obstruction.
PULMONARY	
Improper tube placement	Verify the position of all small-bore feeding tubes by x-ray study. Note: Air insertion into tube with auscultation can be misleading. Identify patients at risk for malposition such as those with impaired gag/cough reflex, those who are obtunded, those who are heavily sedated, or those receiving neuromuscular blocking agents. Attempting to aspirate gastric contents may be difficult because small-bore tubes collapse easily.
Aspiration	Monitor residuals every 4 hr and temporarily discontinue feedings if volume is greater than 100-150 mL/hr for 2 consecutive hours, or exceeds the hourly rate. Monitor for abdominal distention with abdominal girth measurements. Assess bowel sounds. Monitor for tube position every 4 hr by aspirating fluid. Note the appearance of the aspirate and check pH (should be acidic unless patient is taking histamine blockers or antacids). Mark feeding tube at exit site. To prevent reflux, keep head of bed elevated 30-40 degrees during feedings. Discontinue feedings for 10-15 min before patient's head is turned for therapies.
GASTROINTESTINAL	
Diarrhea	Review medications the patient is receiving. Administer fiber-enriched formulas or bulking agents to normalize stool consistency (e.g., Metamucil). Prevent bacterial contamination: • When possible, use full-strength, ready-to-use formula. • Use meticulous hand-washing techniques in the handling of all formulas and supplies. • Avoid touching the inside of delivery sets. • Wash delivery sets with soapy water and rinse after intermittent feedings. Change delivery set every 24 hr. • Limit hanging time of formulas at room temperature to 8 hr. Exception: prefilled sets; read manufacturer recommendtions.
Dumping syndrome	Limit bolus feedings to <300 mL. Slow the rate and frequency of bolus if abdominal distention or cramping persists.
METABOLIC	
Hyperglycemia	Monitor blood glucose level by fingerstick every 6 hr until stable. Observe for signs and symptoms of hyperglycemia. Administer insulin as ordered, usually per sliding scale. Use delivery methods that ensure administration of feeding at a constant rate.
Hypercapnia	Use formulas with lower carbohydrate and higher fat content for respiratory-compromised and ventilator-dependent patients. Monitor arterial carbon dioxide tension.
Electrolyte imbalance	Monitor fluid status closely. Monitor serum sodium, potassium, and phosphate levels.

RESEARCH ANALYSIS

ARTICLE REFERENCE

Marshall, A. P., & West, S. H. (2003). Gastric tonometry and enteral nutrition: A possible conflict in critical care nursing practice. *American Journal of Critical Care, 12*(4), 349-356.

STUDY PURPOSE, METHODS, AND FINDINGS

The purpose of this study was to examine the effect of enteral feeding on the tonometric measurement of gastric mucosal carbon dioxide (CO_2). Gastric tonometers were placed in 20 critically ill patients, and the tonometric pressure of CO_2 ($PtCO_2$) of the gastric mucosa was measured in both the full and the empty stomach during a 48-hour period. The $PtCO_2$ measured by the tonometer increased after enteral feeding, and a significant difference in the $PtCO_2$ of the full versus the empty stomach was evident at 24 and 48 hours. $PtCO_2$ at 4, 24, and 48 hours differed significantly in the full stomach and in the empty stomach. However, the data did not reveal a significant difference in either the full stomach or the empty stomach between $PtCO_2$ at 24 hours and $PtCO_2$ at 48 hours. After 24 hours of feeding, the initial increase in $PtCO_2$ observed at 4 hours was not evident, a finding suggesting stabilization of the intragastric environment. However, a higher $PtCO_2$ was evident in the empty stomach, a finding indicating that the presence of the feeding solution may reduce the diffusion of CO_2 into the tonometer balloon. Consequently, measurements of intragastric $PtCO_2$ obtained after 24 hours of feeding may be reliable if the stomach is emptied by aspiration through the tonometer immediately before measurement.

STRENGTHS AND LIMITATIONS

One of the strengths of the study was that an instrument was used that is subject to less operator error, can measure the desired parameter more often, and is less time-consuming to use. In addition, readings in triplicate were obtained at each time period. Another strength of this study was that it offered a change in practice for optimizing nutritional support in that the withholding of enteral nutrition for a minimum of 1 hour was recommended because of a suspected influence of enteral feeding on tonometric measurements, and this approach delayed nutritional support or provided inadequate nutritional support. With the recommendation not to hold feedings, patients are afforded optimal nutrient intake.

A limitation of the study was sample size: only 10 men and 10 women participated in this study; thus, one cannot generalize these findings to the population. In addition, the sample demographics were not normally distributed.

IMPLICATIONS FOR PRACTICE

Because of the findings that the $PtCO_2$ in the full and the empty stomach stabilized after 24 to 48 hours of enteral feeding, the recommended practice of withholding enteral feeding for 1 hour prior to $PtCo_2$ measurement may be unnecessary. Once enteral feeding is established for 24 hours, the $PtCO_2$ can be obtained without stopping enteral feeding if the measurements are consistently obtained in the same intragastric environment, that is, with enteral feeding solution in the stomach or after aspiration of the gastric tonometer to empty the stomach.

Although $PtCO_2$ appeared to stabilize after 24 hours of enteral feeding, at 24 and 48 hours, measurements obtained in the full stomach differed significantly from those obtained in the empty stomach. The findings suggest that the presence of enteral feeding solution does interfere with the measurement of $PtCO_2$. The differences between $PtCO_2$ in the full stomach and $PtCO_2$ in the empty stomach may be related to the ability of CO_2 to diffuse into the tonometer balloon when enteral feeding solution is in the stomach. Enteral feeding solution in the stomach causes the tonometer balloon to move away from the gastric mucosa and may cause a decrease in measured $PtCO_2$. In addition, when enteral feeding solution is present in the stomach, the CO_2 must travel through the solution to the tonometer balloon. The ability of CO_2 to diffuse through this type of liquid is unknown.

Several strategies have been investigated to determine the decreased risk of catheter-associated sepsis (August et al., 2002d). Full barrier precautions are used during the insertion of central lines, including skin preparation before catheter insertion using chlorhexidine. The use of antimicrobial-impregnated catheters is recommended in high-risk patients and high-risk care settings. Often, low-dose anticoagulant therapy is used in the inpatient setting for those patients requiring long-term catheterization. Some institutions use specialized nursing teams to provide care for venous access devices in patients receiving parenteral nutrition.

Nurses are responsible for the administration of parenteral nutrition. Practice guidelines in monitoring for complications of specialized nutritional support are discussed in a later section of this chapter (August et al., 2002d). Major complications include fluid and electrolyte imbalances and sepsis. Maintaining the sterility of the setup is essential. All tubing is changed every 24 hours. No intravenous push or infusion medications are given in the same line. Intravenous site care is meticulous. Because parenteral nutrition is hyperosmolar, it usually has a high potential for infection. Monitoring for fluid and electrolyte imbalance and early signs of infection are important aspects of nursing care. Serum chemistries and glucose levels are monitored. Patients receiving parenteral nutrition undergo blood glucose monitoring by fingerstick every 6 hours until glucose tolerance is assessed. Insulin therapy occasionally is administered with parenteral nutrition, especially in patients in whom insulin secretion and regulation is impaired. Patients receiving this form of nutritional therapy are weaned from it slowly to prevent hypoglycemic reactions.

Practice Guidelines Regarding Drug-Nutrient Interactions

Medication profiles of patients receiving specialized nutritional support are reviewed for potential effects on nutritional and metabolic status (August et al., 2002e). Medications that are coadministered with enteral nutrition are reviewed periodically for potential incompatibilities. Whenever medications are administered by an enteral feeding tube, the tube should be flushed before and after each medication is administered. Liquid medication formulations are used, when available, for administration by enteral feeding tube. Patients receiving enteral nutrition who develop diarrhea are evaluated for antibiotic-associated causes,

including *Clostridium difficile*. The coadministration of an admixture of medications known to be incompatible with parenteral nutrition is prevented. In the absence of reliable information concerning compatibility of a specific drug with an specialized nutritional support formula, the medication is administered separately from the specialized nutritional support. Each parenteral nutrition formulation that is compounded is inspected for signs of gross particulate contamination, discoloration, particulate formation, and phase separation at the time of compounding, and this same check is repeated before medication administration (August et al., 2002e).

Monitoring and Evaluating the Nutrition Care Plan

Monitoring of the effects of nutritional therapy is decided at the initiation of nutritional support. Factors that influence optimal outcomes are the degree of malnutrition present, the type of therapy, tolerance, and the patient's level of metabolic stress. Stable patients can be monitored weekly or more often as indicated. Patients who are critically ill or who have refeeding syndrome or sepsis require more frequent monitoring. When one is monitoring patients who are receiving nutritional support, the patient's physical status is reviewed to determine whether the patient is moving toward achievement of the outcome objectives. Trending of objective data, noting inputs, outputs, and vital signs including blood pressure, pulse,

 Geriatric Assessment

- Elderly patients (older than 65 years old) are at nutritional risk and need to undergo nutritional screening to identify those who require formal nutritional assessment with the development of a nutrition care plan by the health care team.
- Age and lifestyle considerations are considered in the elderly.
- Potential drug-nutrient interactions are assessed in all elderly patients.
- Dietary and specialized nutritional support prescriptions are considered in this age group because altered nutrient requirements are observed.

Data from August, D., Teitelbaum, D, Albinas, J., et al. (2002g). Section XI: Specific guidelines for disease: Adults. Guidelines for the use of parenteral and enteral nutrition in adult and pediatric patients. *Journal of Parenteral and Enteral Nutrition, 26*(1), 61SA-96SA.

respiratory status, and temperature, is determined along with routine tracking of the patient's weight. Documentation of tolerance to eating, evaluation of enteral or parenteral intake, assessment of laboratory values, including complete blood count, glucose, blood urea nitrogen, creatinine, and electrolytes (sodium, chloride, potassium, magnesium, and phosphorus), and monitoring of liver function, specifically triglycerides, albumin, and prealbumin levels, are imperative. Any changes in medications are reviewed, and decisions are made regarding whether the patient is meeting intermediate outcomes toward the goals of nutritional support set for that patient. If goals are not being met, for example, if the patient has consistent weight loss or an elevated glucose concentration, or appears dehydrated or overhydrated, then reassessment of the plan is necessary to help the patient to achieve the nutritional goals. The transition from parenteral nutrition to enteral nutrition or to oral feeding is monitored and documented according to the adequacy of intake. Adequacy of energy and nutrient intake, approximately 60% of estimated requirements, is assessed before discontinuing the previous form of nutritional support (Russell, et al., 2002).

Practice Guidelines for the Monitoring of Complications

Malnourished patients are at risk for refeeding syndrome and thus are monitored closely for adequate serum phosphorus, magnesium, potassium, and glucose levels at initiation of SNS. In patients with diabetes or in those who have risk factors for

---

 ## Case Study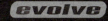

Mr. Howard is at postoperative day 7 after coronary artery bypass graft surgery. He has not eaten any significant calories since the operation because he does not like hospital food and has some trouble chewing his foods because of poor dentition. He appears depressed. He has lost 15 pounds since admission. Objective data include the following: height, 6 feet; weight, 135 pounds; and a history of a 20-pound weight loss in the last month. Laboratory data include a prealbumin level of less than 7.4 (normal values, 16.4 to 38 g/dL) and an albumin level of 1.6 (normal values, 3.5 to 5 g/dL); urine output has been adequate, and he has hypoactive bowel sounds.

Estimation of the patient's calorie, protein, and fluid needs are noted in Table 5-1. Based on the subjective and objective data presented, Mr. Howard is a combination of moderately stressed to severely stressed. His kilocalorie intake requirements are 35 kcal/kg/day. In addition, because Mr. Howard is a combination of moderate to severely stressed, his nitrogen requirements will be approximately 1.5 to 2 g/kg/day.

Another patient, Mr. Johnson, is a 67-year-old man admitted for pneumonia who has a history of chronic obstructive pulmonary disease. He is alert and oriented. He has not eaten for the past 10 days and says that when he tries to swallow, food gets caught in his throat. His physical appearance is of a man who appears older than his stated age. He has extensive muscle wasting and poor skin turgor, his oral mucosa appears dry, and he is missing teeth. Currently, he has faint bowel sounds. His current diet order is nothing by mouth, and he is being assessed for potential for aspiration. He is 6 feet tall and weighs 120 pounds. Current medications include furosemide (Lasix), potassium chloride, and phenytoin (Dilantin). He is admitted to the intensive care unit. Within the first 24 hours, he is unable to breathe adequately despite 100% oxygen on a nonrebreather, and he subsequently requires intubation.

His initial serum chemistries appear normal. Of note, his albumin level is at 4.0 g/dL, and his sodium concentration is 148 mg/dL. Intake and output reveal a trend of greater intake than output despite having intravenous hydration of 5% dextrose and half-normal saline with 20 mEq of potassium chloride running at 75 mL/hour. He now has edema in his extremities. The health care team decides to start nutritional support, and they have a small-bore feeding tube placed with x-ray verification. Just as with the previous patient, Mr. Johnson is evaluated as a combination of moderately to severely stressed and will require the kilocalorie and nitrogen requirements of those patient populations to optimize his nutritional intake needs.

QUESTIONS

1. What combination of assessment findings determines the patient's nutritional status for either case study?
2. How do you justify the preferred route of intake in the critically ill patient?
3. What laboratory data best determine the patient's state within a nutritional context?
4. What is the overall goal of nutritional therapy?

glucose intolerance, SNS is initiated with a low dextrose infusion rate, and blood and urine glucose concentrations are monitored closely. Serum electrolytes (sodium, potassium, chloride, and bicarbonate) are monitored frequently on initiation of SNS until measurements are stable. Patients receiving intravenous fat emulsion require serum triglyceride levels to be determined and monitored until stable and when changes are made in the amount of fat administration. Liver function tests are performed, and values are trended periodically in patients receiving parenteral nutrition. Bone densitometry is sometimes performed on initiation of long-term SNS and again as a reevaluation measure. In specific reference to enteral feeding, postpyloric placement of feeding tubes is recommended for patients who are considered at high risk for aspiration (August et al., 2002d).

SUMMARY

Patients with critical illness are at nutritional risk. specialized nutritional support is initiated when it is anticipated that critically ill patients will be unable to meet nutrient needs orally for 5 to 10 days. Enteral nutrition is the preferred route for specialized nutritional support, and parenteral nutrition is reserved for patients in whom enteral nutrition is not possible (August et al., 2002f). Nutritional support is critical for optimal outcomes and successful management of critically ill patients. Adequate nutrition aids in wound healing and tissue repair, improving immune function, and minimizing muscle wasting. Assessment of patients' nutritional status by the critical care nurse and timely intervention by the interdisciplinary health care team optimize patients' outcomes and transition through their critical care phase.

CRITICAL THINKING QUESTIONS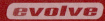

1. What factors are considered when selecting a type of enteral tube for feedings?
2. What assessment findings are indicative of a patient's tolerance to feedings, both enteral and parenteral?
3. What factors would you consider in selecting an enteral formula?
4. Do any drug interactions form potential complications with either enteral or parenteral formulas?

REFERENCES

Ackley, B. J., & Ladwig, G. B. (2002). *Nursing diagnosis handbook: A guide to planning care.* 5th ed. St. Louis: Mosby.

August, D., Teitelbaum, D., Albinas, J., et al. (2002a). Section III: Nutrition assessment: Adults. Guidelines for the use of parenteral and enteral nutrition in adult and pediatric patients. *Journal of Parenteral and Enteral Nutrition, 26*(1), 9SA-11SA.

August, D., Teitelbaum, D., Albinas, J., et al. (2002b). Section V: Administration of specialized nutrition support. Guidelines for the use of parenteral and enteral nutrition in adult and pediatric patients. *Journal of Parenteral and Enteral Nutrition, 26*(1), 18SA-21SA.

August, D., Teitelbaum, D., Albinas, J., et al. (2002c). Section VI: Normal requirements: Adults. Guidelines for the use of parenteral and enteral nutrition in adult and pediatric patients. *Journal of Parenteral and Enteral Nutrition, 26*(1), 22SA-24SA.

August, D., Teitelbaum, D., Albinas, J., et al. (2002d). Section VIII: Access for administration of nutrition support. Guidelines for the use of parenteral and enteral nutrition in adult and pediatric patients. *Journal of Parenteral and Enteral Nutrition, 26*(1), 33SA-41SA.

August, D., Teitelbaum, D., Albinas, J., et al. (2002e). Section IX: Drug-nutrient interactions. Guidelines for the use of parenteral and enteral nutrition in adult and pediatric patients. *Journal of Parenteral and Enteral Nutrition, 26*(1), 42SA-44SA.

August, D., Teitelbaum, D Albinas, J., et al. (2002f). Section X: Life cycle and metabolic conditions. Guidelines for the use of parenteral and enteral nutrition in adult and pediatric patients. *Journal of Parenteral and Enteral Nutrition, 26*(1), 52SA.

August, D., Teitelbaum, D Albinas, J., et al. (2002g). Section XI: Specific guidelines for disease: Adults. Guidelines for the use of parenteral and enteral nutrition in adult and pediatric patients. *Journal of Parenteral and Enteral Nutrition, 26*(1), 61SA-96SA.

Heitz, U. E., & Hone, M. M. (2001). *Mosby's fluid, electrolyte, and acid-base balance.* 4th ed. St. Louis: Mosby.

Russell, M. K., Andrews, M.R., Brewer, C.K., Rogers, J. Z., & Seidner, D. L. (2002). Standard for specialized nutrition support: Adult hospitalized patients. *Nutrition in Clinical Practice, 16*, 385-386.

Shapiro, T., Minard, G., & Kudsk, K. A. (1997). Transgastric jejunal feeding tubes in critically ill patients. *Nutrition in Clinical Practice 12*, 164-167.

Shopbell, J. M., Hopkins, B., & Shronts, E. P. (2001). Nutrition screening and assessment. In M.M. Gottschlich (ed.). *The science and practice of nutrition support.* Dubuque, IA: Kendall/Hunt.

RECOMMENDED READINGS

Enteral Product Reference Guide. (2001). Novartis.

Marik, P. E., & Zaloga, G. P. (2003). Gastric versus post-pyloric feeding: A systematic review. *Critical Care Medicine*, 7(3), R46-51.

McClave, S. A., & Dryden, G. W. (2003). Critical care nutrition: Reducing the risk of aspiration. *Seminars in Gastrointestinal Disease*, 14(1), 2-10.

Williams, D. T., & Harding, K. (2003). Healing responses of skin and muscle in critical illness. *Critical Care Medicine*, 31(8), S547-57.

evolve *Did you remember to check out the bonus material, including free self-assessment exercises, on the Evolve Web site at http://evolve.elsevier.com/Sole/ and on the CD-ROM?*

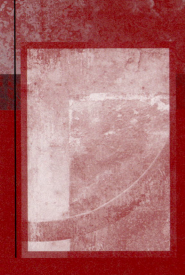

CHAPTER 6

Dysrhythmia Interpretation

Susan Loyola, MSN, RN, CCRN

Introduction

The ability to analyze and interpret dysrhythmias is a fundamental skill that is required of the critical care nurse. The goal of this chapter is to provide a basic understanding of electrocardiography for the purpose of analyzing and interpreting cardiac dysrhythmias. Electrocardiography is the process of creating a visual tracing of the electrical activity of the cells in the heart. This tracing is called the *electrocardiogram* (ECG).

The critical care nurse must have a clear understanding of cardiac monitoring, lead selection, and rhythm interpretation. Distinguishing and assessing the patient for potential or actual hemodynamic-compromising ECG changes become crucial for early nursing and medical intervention and thereby affect patient outcomes.

Basic Electrophysiology

AUTOMATICITY

The ECG tracing provides evidence that the cardiac muscle is generating electrical activity. The basis for this electrical activity is automaticity. *Automaticity* means that the cardiac muscle can generate its own electrical activity, even during brief times when blood supply or nervous stimulation is absent. Special groups of cells generate automatic impulses for the purpose of exciting the remainder of the heart's muscle cells. Although this process is facilitated by blood flow from the coronary arteries and stimulation from the sympathetic and parasympathetic nervous systems, the heart can continue to generate electrical activity for a brief time after blood and nervous supply have ceased.

evolve *Be sure to check out the bonus material, including free self-assessment exercises, on the Evolve Web site at http://evolve.elsevier.com/Sole/ and on the CD-ROM.*

The Cardiac Cycle

The cardiac cycle is composed of both the electrical activity caused by automaticity and the mechanical, or muscular, response known as *contraction*. The electrical activity can be divided into two phases that are called *depolarization* and *repolarization*. The mechanical response is divided into systole and diastole. Depolarization is the active phase of electrical activity and is associated with systole. Repolarization is the resting phase and is associated with diastole. Electrical activity precedes mechanical activity.

Cardiac Action Potential

Cardiac muscle cells are capable of generating an electrical current. This mechanism is known as the cardiac action potential. This is especially noted in a small group of special cardiac cells located in the posterior wall of the right atrium—the sinoatrial node (SA node). Depolarization and repolarization occur as a result of an exchange of electrolytes across the cell membrane. Before depolarization, sodium is outside the cell, and potassium is found inside the cell. This initial state causes the myocardial cell to be negatively charged, thus setting up the cardiac action potential. The initial phase is known as the cardiac cells' resting potential. It begins at −90 mV for the cardiac conduction system. However, the resting membrane potential for the SA and atrioventricular (AV) nodes is −65 mV. This allows these special cells to initiate the electrical impulse earlier than the other cells. These specialized cells are referred to as pacemaker cells. When a cell is stimulated, the permeability of the myocardial cell membrane changes. Large amounts of sodium enter the cell and cause it to have a more positive value, thus initiating the electrical process known as depolarization. Additionally, calcium ions slowly enter the cell through special calcium channels. This prolongs depolarization and allows for cardiac muscle contraction. Toward the end of depolarization, sodium ceases its movement into the cardiac cell. Potassium continues to leak to the outside of the cardiac cell. To return to the resting membrane potential fully, sodium moves back out of the cell and potassium back into the cell by means of a pump. The pump requires energy in the form of adenosine triphosphate. The energy generated by this pump aids in removing calcium from the cell. The net result is restoration of the normal resting membrane potential of −90 mV for nonpacemaker cells and −65 mV for pacemaker cells, and the resting phase, or repolarization, begins. This state of repolarization stimulates the next depolarization. This process continues over a lifetime, thereby providing automatic excitation of the SA node (Figure 6-1).

Normally, a cardiac action potential originates in the SA node, spreads through the heart, and thereby

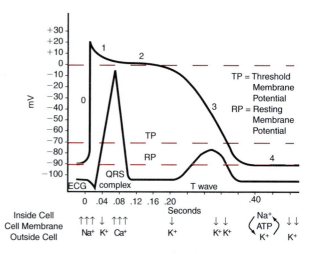

FIGURE 6-1 Cardiac action potential with the electrocardiogram and movement of electrolytes. *ATP,* Adenosine triphosphate; *Ca$^+$,* calcium; *K$^+$,* potassium; *Na$^+$,* sodium. (From American Heart Association. [1997]. *Advance cardiac life support textbook.* Dallas: Author.)

initiates the electrical activity of the heart. However, if the SA node fails to generate an electrical impulse, another area of the cardiac muscle will generate an impulse and take control of the heart beat, as discussed more fully in this chapter. Many antidysrhythmic drugs affect the cardiac action potential by altering the sodium, potassium, and calcium gradients across the cardiac cell membrane (Table 6-1).

RELATIONSHIP BETWEEN ELECTRICAL ACTIVITY AND MUSCULAR CONTRACTION

Under normal circumstances, depolarization is followed by contraction of a cardiac muscle fiber. The term *systole* refers to this contraction. Repolarization of the cardiac cell leads to a resting state for the muscle. During repolarization the ventricles fill with blood from the atria. A sufficient time of rest is necessary for the ventricles to be adequately filled before the next depolarization and subsequent systole occur.

The ECG tracing, or ECG, is evidence of electrical activity only. The presence of an ECG pattern does not necessarily ensure that the patient's heart is also contracting. For confirmation that cardiac contraction is occurring, a clinically detectable pulse and the presence of adequate blood pressure are sought.

If the situation arises suddenly in which no pulse is detected, the nurse begins cardio-pulmonary resuscitation, unless the patient has "do not resuscitate" status. When the patient lacks cardiac contractility but displays electrical activity on the cardiac monitor,

TABLE 6-1

ANTIDYSRHYTHMIC DRUG CLASSIFICATIONS

Class	Description	Examples
IA	Inhibits the fast sodium channel Prolongs repolarization time Used to treat atrial and ventricular dysrhythmias	Quinidine, disopyramide, procainamide
IB	Inhibits the fast sodium channel Shortens the action potential duration Used to treat ventricular dysrhythmias only	Lidocaine, phenytoin, mexiletine, tocainide
IC	Inhibits the fast sodium channel Shortens the action potential duration of only Purkinje fibers Controls ventricular tachyarryhthmias resistant to other drug therapies Has proarrhythmic effects	Flecainide, propafenone
II	Causes beta-adrenergic blockade	Esmolol, propranolol, sotalol
III	Lengthens the action potential Acts on the repolarization phase	Amiodarone, sotalol, bretylium
IV	Blocks the slow inward movement of calcium to slow impulse conduction, especially in the atrioventricular node Used for treatment of supraventricular tachycardias	Diltiazem, verapamil
IVb-like	Opens the potassium channel	Adenosine, ATP

Modified from Opie, L. H. & Gersh, B. J. (2001). *Drugs for the heart.* 5th ed. Philadelphia: W. B. Saunders.

the condition is known as pulseless electrical activity. For the best chance of survival, the cause must be quickly identified and treated. The most common conditions impairing contractile function include hypovolemia, hypoxia, electrolyte imbalances, hypothermia, tension pneumothorax, cardiac tamponade, massive myocardial infarction, drug overdose, acidosis, and pulmonary emboli (AHA, 2002).

Even though the heart is no longer contracting and pumping blood to the coronary arteries and the nervous tissues, the patient's heart may continue to generate electrical impulses, thereby creating an ECG tracing after a patient is pronounced dead. This is often observed after exhausting all efforts of resuscitation or in patients dying of terminal illnesses. Once the patient has expired, the cardiac monitor can be turned off. The length of time that the heart can continue to create an electrical activity varies, but it usually ceases within minutes.

NORMAL CARDIAC CONDUCTION PATHWAY

Theoretically, any cardiac cell can generate an electrical impulse. However, under normal conditions, special groups of cardiac cells are responsible for impulse generation and conduction. These special cells make up the cardiac conduction pathway (Figure 6-2). The cardiac cells are networked so depolarization can spread easily from cell to cell. Depolarization normally begins in the SA, or sinoatrial, node, a special group of cardiac cells located high in the right atrium. The SA node is often referred to as the "master," or "dominant," pacemaker of the heart. This dominance results from the SA node's anatomical position and its intrinsic ability to generate 60 to 100 beats per minute under normal circumstances. Once the impulse is formulated in the SA node, it is conducted through the atria by the internodal pathways. These pathways connect the SA and AV nodes and are responsible for conducting the impulse throughout the right and left atria.

The atria serve as reservoirs that collect blood returning from the head, body, and lungs. The right atrium receives deoxygenated blood from the head through the superior vena cava and from the body through the inferior vena cava. The left atrium receives oxygenated blood that is returning from the lungs through the pulmonary veins.

Atrial depolarization precedes atrial contraction. The time during which atrial depolarization occurs correlates with the time when the atria drain their blood into the ventricles. Most of this process occurs as a result of gravity flow. However, as depolarization ends, the atria contract, sending any remaining blood down into the ventricles. Contraction of the atria results in roughly a 30% increase in the volume of blood sent to the ventricles, thereby dramatically affecting stroke volume and cardiac output for the next ventricular systole. The final phase of atrial systole is known as the *atrial kick.*

From the atria, depolarization proceeds to the AV node, which is located between the atria and the ventricles. The AV node has two important functions. First, the AV node delays entry of the electrical impulse into the ventricles. If the impulse immediately proceeds into the ventricle, contraction occurs before the ventricles have had adequate time to fill with blood from the atria. The result is a decreased stroke volume for the next systole and therefore a decrease in cardiac output. This delay in impulse conduction is very short, only 0.02 seconds; however, it allows for adequate ventricular filling.

A second important function of the AV node is to act as a back-up pacemaker for the heart should the SA node fail. When acting as the back-up pacemaker, the AV node generates 40 to 60 beats per minute under normal conditions. The AV node can emerge as the dominant pacemaker when the SA node's rate falls to less than 40 beats per minute or when automaticity is increased in the AV node. Stress, caffeine, and nicotine are common causes of increased automaticity.

Once ventricular filling has been accomplished, the impulse leaves the AV node and moves down into the ventricles through the common bundle of His. The bundle of His is a thick cord of nerve fibers that runs down the first third of the ventricular septum. The common bundle then divides into the right and left bundle branches. The right bundle branch runs down the right side of the ventricular septum, and the left bundle branch runs down the left side. The bundle branches have divisions known as *fascicles.* The right bundle branch has one fascicle. The left bundle branch divides into two fascicles, the anterior-superior and the posterior-inferior fascicles. The large muscle mass of the left ventricle requires two fascicles for adequate depolarization, whereas the smaller, right ventricle requires only one (see Figure 6-2).

The impulse first enters the left ventricle through the left bundle branch and then moves across the septum for conduction down the right bundle branch. The impulse enters the left ventricle first, to allow

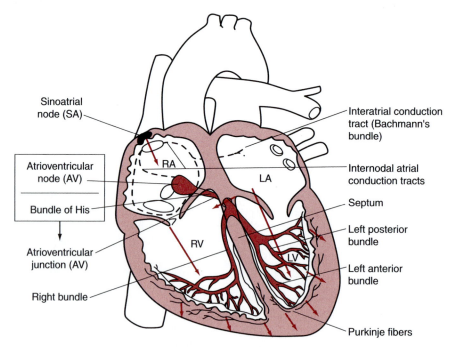

FIGURE 6-2 The electrical conduction system of the heart. Arrows indicate direction of electrical currents. The ECG represents the net sum of these currents. *LA,* Left atrium; *LV,* left ventricle; *RA,* right atrium; *RV,* right ventricle. (Modified from Paul, S., & Hebra, J. [1998]. *The nurse's guide to cardiac rhythm interpretation: Implications for patient care.* Philadelphia: W. B. Saunders.)

more time for its depolarization. However, despite this slight lead time, the overall effect is virtually simultaneous depolarization of both ventricles. From the bundle branches, the electrical impulse is carried deep within the ventricular muscle by fine conductive fibers known as *Purkinje fibers*. The Purkinje fibers also act as a final back-up pacemaker for the heart. Should both the SA and the AV nodes fail, the Purkinje fibers can generate an intrinsic rhythm of 15 to 40 beats per minute.

The speed or velocity of conduction is known as *dromotropy*. Many medications have dromotropic effects and increase or decrease the speed of conduction. Drugs affecting the heart rate are referred to as chronotropic, whereas drugs affecting contractility are described as inotropic.

Any change in the normal generation or conduction of impulses leads to the development of dysrhythmias. Therefore, a thorough understanding of the normal conduction pathway and of its intrinsic capabilities is prerequisite knowledge.

The 12-Lead Electrocardiograph System

The 12-lead ECG system includes 3 standard limb leads, 3 augmented limb leads, and 6 precordial leads. It is useful to think of the 12-lead ECG as depicting the cardiac rhythm from 12 different views. Waveforms, particularly the QRS complex, vary according to the lead monitored. In some leads, the QRS complex is normally upright, whereas in others it is negative. The summation of the electrical current of the heart depolarizes leftward and inferiorly, with the exception of the septum, which depolarizes left to right (see Figure 6-2). Therefore, the QRS complex is upright in leads at which depolarization is in the direction of the positive electrode, such as leads II and V_5 and is negative in leads at which depolarization is going away from the positive electrode, such as aVR and V_1.

STANDARD LIMB LEADS

The three limb leads are designated leads I, II, and III. Limb leads are placed anywhere on the arms and legs, with leg leads placed below the level of the umbilicus. These leads are bipolar, meaning that a positive lead is placed on one limb and a negative lead on another.

Electricity flows from negative to positive. Lead I records the flow of electricity from a negative lead on the right arm to a positive lead on the left arm. Lead II records activity between a negative lead on the right arm and a positive lead on the left leg. Lead III records activity between a negative lead on the left arm and a positive lead on the left leg (Figure 6-3). The normal ECG waveforms are upright in the limb leads, with lead II producing the most upright waveforms.

AUGMENTED LIMB LEADS

The augmented limb leads are designated aVR, aVL, and aVF. These leads are unipolar, meaning that they record electrical flow in only one direction. A reference point is established in the center of the heart, and electrical flow is recorded from that reference point toward the right arm (aVR), the left arm (aVL), and the left foot (aVF) (Figure 6-4). The *a* in the names of these leads means augmented, and

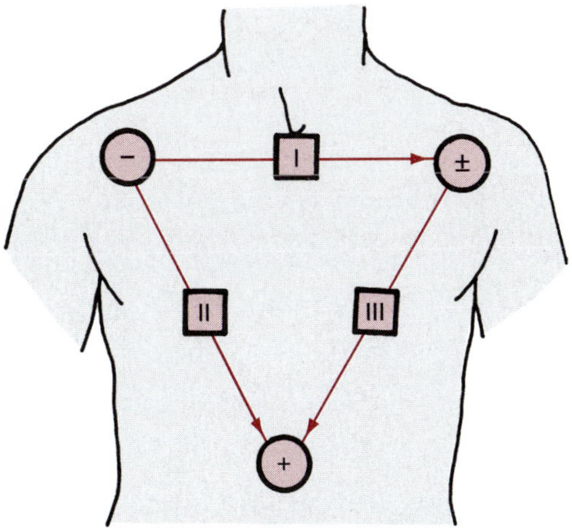

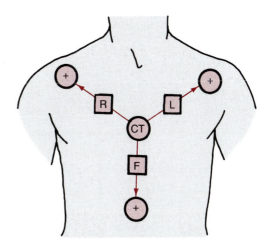

FIGURE 6-3 The bipolar limb leads. (From Abedin, Z., & Conner, R. [1989]. *Twelve-lead ECG interpretation.* Philadelphia: W. B. Saunders.)

FIGURE 6-4 The unipolar limb leads. (From Abedin, Z., & Conner, R. [1989]. *Twelve-lead ECG interpretation.* Philadelphia: W. B. Saunders.)

because these leads produce small ECG complexes, they must be augmented or enlarged for analysis. The ECG machine increases the size of these complexes 1.5-fold. Normally, the ECG complexes are upright, or positive, in lead aVF and downward, or negative, in aVR. Lead aVL usually produces an equiphasic biphasic QRS complex, meaning that half of the complex rises above the baseline and half falls below the baseline (Figure 6-5). The augmented leads are monitored by use of the limb leads already in place.

PRECORDIAL LEADS

The six precordial leads (also called chest leads) are positioned on the chest wall directly over the heart. The landmarks for placement of these leads are the intercostal spaces, the sternum, and the clavicular and axillary lines. Positions for these six leads are as follows (Figure 6-6):

V_1: Fourth intercostal space, right sternal border
V_2: Fourth intercostal space, left sternal border
V_3: Halfway between V_2 and V_4
V_4: Fifth intercostal space, left midclavicular line
V_5: Fifth intercostal space, left anterior axillary line
V_6: Fifth intercostal space, left midaxillary line

The precordial leads are unipolar, with a postive electrode and the heart as a center reference. The precordial leads are useful in the localization of septal, anterior, and lateral myocardial ischemia, injury, and infarction of the left ventricle. Because these leads lie directly over the surface of the heart, changes in the normal ECG can indicate which areas of the heart have sustained insult. V_1 lies over the anterior or frontal surface of the right ventricle and septum. V_2 lies over the septum and the anterior part of the left ventricle. V_3 and V_4 lie over the anterior, or frontal, surface of the left ventricle, and V_5 and V_6 lie

over the lateral, or side, surface of the left ventricle. None of the 12 leads records activity directly over the posterior, or back side, of the heart.

CONTINUOUS CARDIAC MONITORING

In most settings a 6-second strip of the patient's rhythm is obtained and documented in the patient's chart every 4 hours. In addition to scheduled times, a rhythm strip should be obtained when a different nurse assumes care of a patient and when a patient

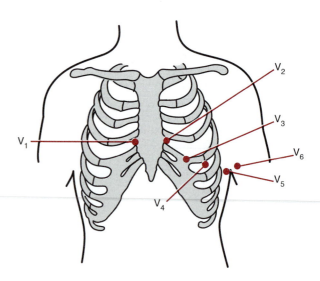

FIGURE 6-6 The precordial leads.

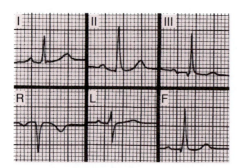

FIGURE 6-5 Note the positive QRS complex in aVF and the negative QRS complex in aVR. The QRS in aVL is equiphasic. (From Abedin, Z., & Conner, R. [1989]. *Twelve-lead ECG interpretation.* Philadelphia: W. B. Saunders.)

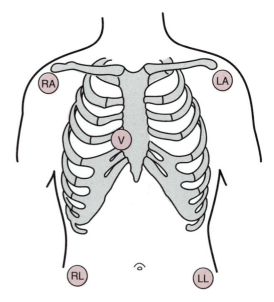

FIGURE 6-7 Lead placement when using a five-lead cable. The chest lead is shown in the V_1 position.

experiences any change in cardiac rhythm or has chest pain.

Whatever type of monitoring system is used, proper lead placement is necessary for the production of high-quality ECG tracings. Limb leads are placed on the body close to where the limbs join the torso. The right and left arm leads are placed at the shoulder where the arms join the body. The right and left leg leads are placed on the lower abdomen closer to where the legs join the torso below the umbilicus.

Most critical care units use five-lead systems capable of monitoring multiple leads. Electrodes to monitor limb leads are placed on each shoulder and on the left and right sides of the abdomen below the umbilicus. The chest lead (V lead) can be placed to monitor any of the V leads (Figure 6-7). Other units,

such as telemetry units or emergency departments, may use a three-lead system for cardiac monitoring. Figure 6-8 shows correct lead placement for leads I, II, III, or V_1 using five leads.

In the clinical setting, monitors are capable of viewing two leads simultaneously. Many monitors have ST-segment monitoring capabilities to identify ischemia, assess effectiveness of therapy such as thrombolytics or percutaneous coronary intervention, and facilitate rapid intervention should acute changes occur. It is recommended that nurses use both lead V_3 and III to detect acute ischemic changes (Drew, 2002).

Some newer monitors have the capability of performing 12-lead ECGs. Research recommends continuous ST-segment monitoring of all 12 leads to

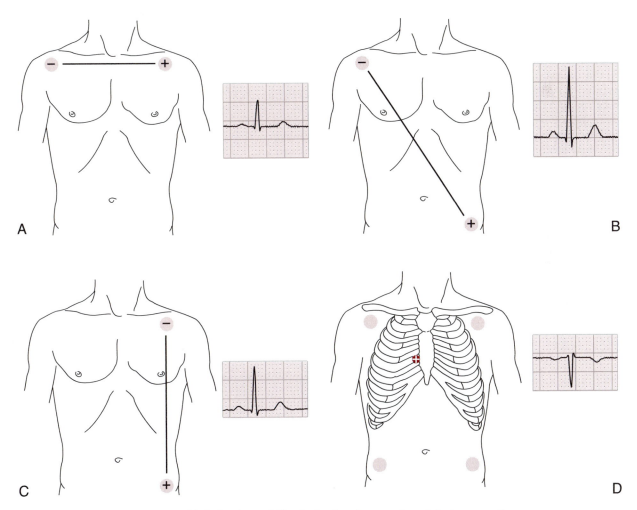

FIGURE 6-8 Limb leads and V_1 electrode placement and their respective waveforms: **A,** Lead I ; **B,** lead II ; **C,** lead III ; and **D,** lead V_1. (From Paul, S, & Hebra, J. [1998]. *The nurse's guide to cardiac rhythm interpretation: Implications for patient care.* Philadelphia: W. B. Saunders.)

detect ischemia accurately (Drew, 2002). A complete 12-lead ECG is usually obtained daily in patients with cardiac disease and when the patient experiences a change in cardiac status, particularly chest pain.

Analyzing the Basic Electrocardiographic Tracing

MEASUREMENTS

ECG paper has standard measures, whether a single-lead or a 12-lead rhythm strip is obtained (Figure 6-9). The horizontal boxes measure time, and the vertical boxes measure voltage or amplitude.

When ECG paper is used to measure time, the least unit of measure is the small box, which is equal to 0.04 seconds, or 40 milliseconds. The next greater unit of measure is the large box, which contains five small boxes. One large box represents 0.20 seconds, or 200 milliseconds. Five large boxes represents 1 second, or 1000 milliseconds.

The largest unit of measure is in seconds and is marked off at the top of the ECG paper by vertical hatch marks (see Figure 6-9). There may be 1, 2, or 3 seconds between two hatch marks. Five large boxes between hatch marks equal 1 second. Ten large boxes between hatch marks equal 2 seconds. Fifteen large boxes between hatch marks equal 3 seconds. In the clinical setting, it is standard for 6-second rhythm strips to be obtained for analysis and mounting in the patient's chart. To obtain a 6-second strip, the clinician counts off the appropriate number of hatch marks. The value of measuring time on the ECG tracing is that speed of depolarization and repolarization in the atria and ventricles can be determined.

Amplitude is measured on the vertical axis of the ECG paper (see Figure 6-9). Each small box is equal to 0.1 mV in amplitude. Waveform amplitude indicates the amount of electrical voltage being generated in the various areas of the heart. When waveforms are small, voltage is low. When waveforms are large, voltage is high. Low voltage and small waveforms are expected from the small muscle mass of the atria. High voltage and large waveforms are expected from the larger muscle mass of the ventricles.

WAVEFORMS AND INTERVALS

The normal ECG tracing is composed of P, Q, R, S, and T waves (Figure 6-10). These waveforms emerge from a flat baseline called the *isoelectric line. Isoelectric* means neither positive nor negative, that is, a flat line. Any waveform that projects above the isoelectric line is considered positive, and any that projects below the line is considered negative.

P Wave

The P wave is an indication of atrial depolarization. It is usually upright in leads I and II and has a rounded configuration. The amplitude of the P wave is measured at the center of the waveform and should not exceed three boxes, or 3 mm, in height.

Normally, a P wave indicates that the SA node initiated the impulse that depolarized the atrium. However, a change in the form of the P wave can indicate that the impulse did not come from the SA node, but rather from an abnormal pacemaking site, such as the atria or AV node.

PR Interval

The P wave is connected to the next set of waveforms, the QRS complex, by the PR interval. The interval is measured from the beginning of the P wave, in which the positive deflection of the P wave leaves the isoelectric line, to where the QRS complex begins.

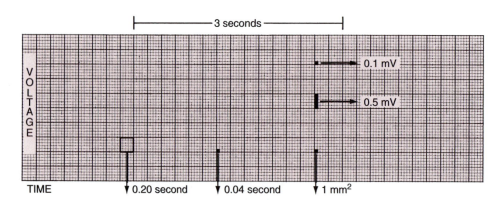

FIGURE 6-9 Standard electrocardiographic paper. (From Patel, J., McGowan, S., & Moody, L. [1989]. *Arrhythmias: Detection, treatment, and cardiac drugs.* Philadelphia: W. B. Saunders.)

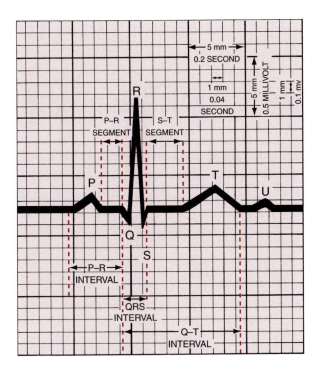

FIGURE 6-10 Electrocardiographic grid with waveforms and intervals. (From Foster, D. [1996]. *Twelve-lead electrocardiography for ACLS providers.* Philadelphia: W. B. Saunders.)

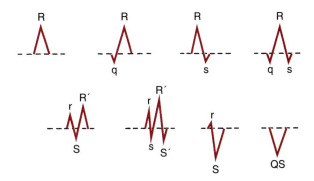

FIGURE 6-11 Different types of QRS complexes. An R wave is a positive waveform. A negative deflection before the R wave is a Q wave. The S wave is a negative deflection after the R wave. (From Kinney, M. R., Packa, D. R., [1996.]. *Andreoli's Comprehensive Cardiac Care* [8th ed]. St. Louis: Mosby.

The PR interval measures the time it takes for the impulse to depolarize the atria, travel to the AV node, and then dwell there briefly before entering the bundle of His. The normal PR interval is 0.12 to 0.20 second, which is three to five small boxes wide (see Figure 6-10). When the PR interval is longer than normal, the speed of conduction is abnormally slow. When the PR interval is shorter than normal, the speed of conduction is abnormally fast.

QRS Complex

The QRS complex is a set of three distinct waveforms that are indicative of ventricular depolarization (see Figure 6-10). The "textbook" normal QRS complex begins with a negative, or downward, deflection immediately after the P wave. This negative deflection is the Q wave.

The first positive, or upright, waveform that follows the P wave is the R wave. A Q wave may or may not be present before the R wave. The R wave is normally tall and positive in lead II. The amplitude of the R wave varies across leads. Leads V_4 to V_6 usually have the tallest R waves because they measure electricity in the large muscle mass of the left ventricle. Some patients may have a second positive waveform in

their QRS complex. If so, then that second positive waveform is called *R prime (R')*.

The S wave is a negative waveform that follows the R wave. In an S wave, the waveform must go below the isoelectric line. The amplitude of the S wave is measured from the point at which it leaves the isoelectric line to its deepest point.

The term *QRS complex* is imprecise. QRS complex is a generic term for the waveforms that indicate ventricular depolarization. However, many people do not have all three distinct waveforms, Q, R, and S, in their QRS complex. Figure 6-11 depicts variations of the QRS complex.

If present, the Q wave is assessed for abnormalities. When a Q wave is 0.04 seconds in width and measures more than one fourth of the R wave amplitude, it is abnormal. This is referred to as *pathological Q wave* or *significant Q wave*. Pathological Q waves are found on ECGs of patients who have had myocardial infarctions. The deep Q wave in these patients indicates that an area of myocardial tissue has died. The ECG machine reads no electrical activity in the area and creates a deep, negative waveform (Figure 6-12).

QRS Interval

The QRS interval is measured from the beginning to the end of the QRS complex (see Figure 6-10). Whichever waveform begins the QRS complex (whether it is a Q or an R) marks the beginning of the interval. Therefore, the *first* deflection, either positive or negative, that follows the P wave indicates the beginning of the interval. The QRS interval is (abnormal Q wave) 0.04 seconds wide and at least one fourth the height of the R wave measured from the point of first deflection to where the *final* deflection returns to baseline. The final deflection may be an R or an S wave.

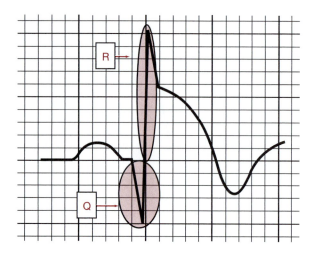

FIGURE 6-12 Pathological Q wave (abnormal Q wave) 0.04 seconds wide and at least one fourth the height of the R wave.

	Lead V$_1$	Leads I and V$_6$
Typical RBBB		
Typical LBBB		

FIGURE 6-13 Right and left bundle branch blocks as shown in leads V$_1$ or I and V$_6$. (From Foster, D. [1996]. *Twelve-lead electrocardiography for ACLS providers*. Philadelphia: W.B. Saunders.)

Sometimes it is difficult to determine the QRS interval. One tip is that the line of the QRS tracing is thinner than the rest of the tracing because the stylet on the printer has to move fast to trace the ventricular depolarization.

The normal width of the QRS complex is 0.06 to 0.10 seconds. This figure equates to 1.5 to 2.5 small boxes in length.

When the QRS width is greater than 0.10 second, the patient is said to have a bundle branch block (BBB), or an intraventricular conduction delay. The delay in conduction is most commonly caused by coronary artery disease. Either or both of the bundle branches can be blocked. A BBB causes a change in the normal conduction of impulses through the ventricles, hence the prolonged interval. BBBs also result in a change in the QRS complex morphology.

A right BBB produces a QRS that has two distinct R waves in V$_1$, rSR' (Figure 6-13). The second R wave results from delayed conduction through the right ventricle. Normally, the QRS complex is evidence of biventricular depolarization. However, in right BBB, the first R wave is evidence of left ventricular depolarization, and the second R wave is evidence of the delayed right ventricular depolarization.

A left BBB usually produces a wide, negative QRS complex in V$_1$. The widening of the QRS complex occurs as a result of delay of the impulse's entry into the left ventricle (see Figure 6-13).

T Wave

The T wave represents ventricular repolarization (see Figure 6-10). Note that a waveform indicating atrial repolarization is not described in this chapter. Such a waveform probably exists, but it would be obscured by the large QRS complex.

Some beginning students of electrocardiography state that they have problems differentiating the P wave from the T wave. This differentiation should not be a problem, because the P wave normally precedes the QRS complex, and the T wave normally follows the QRS complex. Additionally, the T wave is usually of greater size and amplitude than the P wave. This is because the atria are smaller muscle masses and therefore produce smaller waveforms than do the larger ventricles. T-wave amplitude is measured at the center of the waveform and should be no greater than five small boxes, or 5 mm, high. Changes in T-wave amplitude can indicate electrical disturbances resulting from electrolyte imbalance or myocardial infarction. For example, hyperkalemia can cause tall, peaked T waves.

ST Segment

The ST segment connects the QRS complex to the T wave. The ST segment is usually isoelectric, or flat. However, in some conditions the segment may be depressed (falling below baseline) or elevated (rising above baseline). The point at which the QRS complex ends and the ST segment begins is called the *J (junction) point*. ST-segment change is measured 0.04 second following the J point. It is imperative that ST displacement above or below the isoelectric line be reported and documented. To identify ST-segment elevation, use the PR segment as a reference for baseline. Next, check to see whether the ST segment is level with the PR segment (see Figure 6-10). If the ST segment is above or below the baseline, count the number of small boxes 0.04 seconds after the J point. A displacement in the ST segment can indicate myocardial ischemia or injury as seen in the acute coronary syndromes (AHA, 2002). ECG monitors should be set to alarm to detect ST-segment changes. Current bedside monitors have the software capability to monitor continuously for ST-segment changes. The leads identified to best monitor for ST-segment changes are both V_3 and III when the ideal continuous 12-lead technology is not available (Table 6-2) (Drew, 2002).

QT Interval

The QT interval is measured from the beginning of the QRS complex to the end of the T wave (see Figure 6-10). This interval measures the time taken for ventricular depolarization and repolarization. No standard QT interval exists. Normal QT intervals are based on heart rate. The slower the heart rate is, the longer the normal QT, and the faster the rate is, the shorter the normal QT. QT intervals are normally longer in female patients. A QT chart is used to determine the outer limits for normal intervals.

A final waveform that may be noted on the ECG is the U wave. The U wave is a small waveform of unknown origin. If present, it immediately follows the T wave and is of the same deflection (see Figure 6-10). In other words, if the T wave is positive, the U wave is also positive. U waves may be seen in patients with electrolyte imbalance, particularly hypokalemia, and in those who have had a myocardial infarction. However, the U wave is sometimes a normal finding;

therefore, diagnosis of disease should be dependent on more specific indicators.

Systematic Interpretation of Dysrhythmias

This section proposes a systematic approach for the analysis and interpretation of dysrhythmias (Box 6-1). Systematic analysis focuses attention on the following areas:
- Assessment of rhythmicity, both atrial and ventricular
- Assessment of rate, both atrial and ventricular
- Assessment of waveform configuration and location
- Assessment of intervals

RHYTHMICITY

Rhythmicity refers to the regularity or pattern of the heart beats. P waves are used to establish atrial rhythmicity, and R waves establish ventricular rhythmicity. When an atrial rhythm is perfectly regular, each P wave is an equal distance from the next P wave. When a ventricular rhythm is perfectly regular, each R wave is an equal distance from the next R wave. Systematic interpretation of rhythm strips requires looking at both atrial and ventricular rhythmicities.

Rhythmicity can be established through the use of calipers or paper and pencil and must be analyzed in both the atria and the ventricle. Establishing atrial rhythmicity requires placing one caliper point on one P wave and the other caliper point on the next consecutive P wave. The second point is left stationary, and the calipers are flipped over. If the first caliper

---

TABLE 6-2

Recommended Electrocardiographic Monitoring Leads for Specific Clinical Incidents

Clinical Incident	ECG Monitoring Leads
Atrial flutter	II, III, aVF
New-onset bundle branch blocks	V_1, V_6
Acute myocardial ischemia	III, V_3 (ideally, continuous 12-lead ST-segment monitoring is recommended)
Dysrhythmias	V_1
Broad QRS tachycardia, cardiac dysrhythmias	V_1, V_2, V_6

From Drew, B. (2002). Celebrating the 100th birthday of the electrocardiogram: Lessons learned from research in cardiac monitoring. *American Journal of Critical Care, 11,* 378-386.

BOX 6-1

Systematic Approach for Rhythm Interpretation

1. Is the underlying rhythm regular or irregular? Look at the atrial and ventricular rhythms.
2. What is the atrial rate? What is the ventricular rate?
3. Are there P waves? Do the P waves precede the QRS complex? What is the PR interval? Are the P waves consistent in appearance?
4. What is the QRS complex duration and configuration? Is the QRS complex consistent in appearance?
5. Examine the ST segment and T waves for signs of myocardial injury or ischemia.
6. Using rules for interpretation, what is the rhythm?

point lands exactly on the next P wave, the atrial rhythm is perfectly regular. If the point lands one small box or less away from the next P or R wave, the rhythm is essentially regular. If the point lands more than one small box away, the rhythm is considered irregular.

The same process is followed for assessing ventricular rhythmicity, *except* that the caliper points are placed on R waves. For establishment of ventricular rhythmicity, one caliper point is placed on one R wave and the other caliper point on the next consecutive R wave. The second point is left stationary, and the calipers are flipped over. If the first caliper point lands exactly on the next R wave, the ventricular rhythm is perfectly regular (Figure 6-14).

Rhythmicity can also be established by use of paper and pencil. A piece of blank paper is slid over the rhythm strip, and the straight edge is placed along the peak of the P wave to assess atrial rhythmicity or along the peak of the R wave to assess ventricular rhythmicity. With the pencil, the peak of either the P or the R wave is marked on the paper. Without moving the paper, another mark is made on the next P or R wave. The paper is then slid over to the next P or R waveform. If the pencil mark lands exactly on the next P or R wave, the rhythm is perfectly regular. If the pencil mark is one small box or less away from the next P or R wave, the rhythm is essentially regular. If the pencil mark lands more than one small box away from the next P or R wave, the rhythm is irregular (Figure 6-15).

Irregular rhythms can be regularly irregular or irregularly irregular. Regularly irregular rhythms have a pattern. In other words, the irregularity occurs in a predictable fashion, for example, every second beat (Figure 6-16). Irregularly irregular rhythms have no pattern and no predictability.

RATE

The rate equals how fast the heart is depolarizing. Under normal conditions, the atria and the ventricles depolarize at the same rate. However, each can depolarize at a different rate. An important part of systematic analysis is calculation of both the atrial and the ventricular rates. P waves are used for calculation of the atrial rate, and R waves are used for

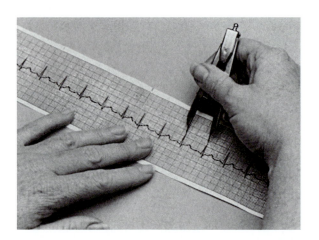

FIGURE 6-14 Establishing ventricular rhythmicity with calipers.

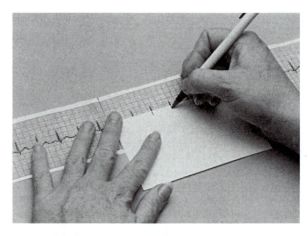

FIGURE 6-15 Establishing ventricular rhythmicity with paper and pencil.

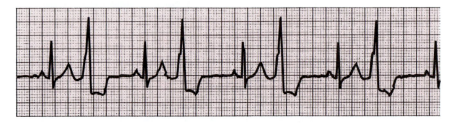

FIGURE 6-16 The irregularity in rhythm is predictable. The abnormal complexes occur every other beat. (From Patel, J., McGowan, S., & Moody, L. [1989]. *Arrhythmias: Detection, treatment, and cardiac drugs.* Philadelphia: W. B. Saunders.)

calculation of the ventricular rate. Rate can be assessed in various ways. Although many methods for assessing heart rate exist, this text addresses the following two popular methods:

1. The rule of 1500 is used to calculate the *exact* rate of a *regular* rhythm. In this method, 2 consecutive P or R waves are located. P waves are used to calculate the atrial rate, and R waves are used to calculate the ventricular rate. The tallest point of either the P wave or the R wave is located. The number of small boxes between the highest points of 2 consecutive P or R waves is counted, and that number of small boxes is divided into 1500 to determine the exact heart rate in beats per minute (Figure 6-17). This method is accurate only if the rhythm is regular. Charts are available for the calculation of heart rate based on the rule of 1500.

2. The rule of 10 is a popular method for calculating the *approximate* rate. This method can be used for either regular or irregular rhythms. The rule of 10 is accomplished by counting the number of P or R waves in a 6-second strip and then multiplying that number by 10. This equation yields an approximate heart rate for 60 seconds, or 1 minute. For example, if 6 R waves are found on a 6-second strip, those 6 complexes are multiplied by 10 for an approximate rate of 60 ventricular beats per minute. This method is used when a quick assessment of rate is needed or when a patient is having an irregular rhythm.

Cardiac monitors display heart rates, usually in digital form. However, these monitor-calculated rates may be inaccurate and should *always* be verified by one of the aforementioned rate-calculation methods.

WAVEFORM CONFIGURATION AND LOCATION

In the systematic analysis of ECG rhythms, configuration and location of the normal P, Q, R, S, and T waveforms are very important.

Configuration

Each cardiac cell, once depolarized, creates a distinct waveform configuration that manifests on the ECG rhythm strip. Changes in the shape and appearance of a waveform are often the first clue in the assessment of dysrhythmias. Once a clinician is knowledgeable regarding normal waveform configuration, he or she can easily discern abnormal waveforms. No systematic analysis and interpretation are complete without careful study and comparison of each waveform on the 6-second strip, in which both normal and abnormal configurations are assessed.

Location

Location of waveforms is very important for a systematic analysis of dysrhythmias. The normal waveforms P, Q, R, S, and T should occur in their natural order. A P wave should precede each QRS; QRS complexes should be followed by T waves; and T waves should be followed by the next subsequent P wave.

In the analysis of rhythm strips, it is very important to note whether waveforms occur in this order. In the later discussion of the basic dysrhythmias, several rhythms are characterized by abnormal location or sequencing of waveforms (Figure 6-18).

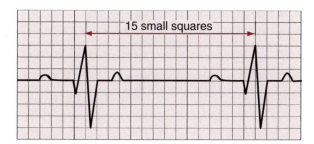

FIGURE 6-17 Calculating ventricular rate with the rule of 1500. Count the number of small boxes between QRS complexes. In this strip there are 15 small squares between QRS complexes; 1500 divided by 15 equals a heart rate of 100. (From Paul, S., & Hebra, J. D. [1998]. *The nurse's guide to cardiac rhythm interpretation: Implications for patient care.* Philadelphia: W. B. Saunders.)

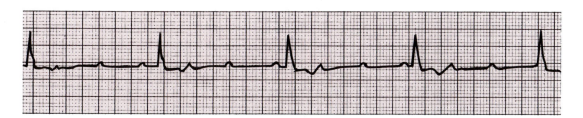

FIGURE 6-18 Note how P, Q, R, S, and T waves are out of normal sequence and location. (From Patel, J., McGowan, S., & Moody, L. [1989]. *Arrhythmias: Detection, treatment, and cardiac drugs.* Philadelphia: W. B. Saunders.)

INTERVALS

A final important aspect of the systematic analysis of rhythm strips is the assessment of the intervals discussed previously in the section on analysis of the normal ECG tracing. No rhythm strip analysis is complete and no interpretation is possible without the assessment of the PR, QRS, and QT intervals.

Basic Dysrhythmias

The word *dysrhythmia* refers to an abnormal cardiac rhythm. People also speak of cardiac arrhythmias. The word *arrhythmia* means no rhythm. Therefore, *dysrhythmia* is a more useful and descriptive term.

The basic dysrhythmias can be grouped under the following anatomical areas:

- Dysrhythmias of the SA node
- Dysrhythmias of the atria
- Dysrhythmias of the AV node
- Dysrhythmias of the ventricles
- AV blocks

A section has been developed for each anatomical area and includes rhythm strip examples of common dysrhythmias associated with that anatomical area or structure. However, of more importance is the description of characteristics that make each dysrhythmia unique and recognizable to the practitioner. These characteristics are listed as the criteria for the diagnosis of that particular dysrhythmia. The most critical criteria for diagnosis are listed first.

These critical criteria eliminate the confusion surrounding dysrhythmia analysis and interpretation. The practitioner must learn the criteria for each rhythm and then make a diagnosis based on the criteria.

Those beginning the study of basic electrocardiography should memorize these critical criteria or keep them in a notebook for easy reference. Initially, the task seems overwhelming, and a great deal of information must be learned. Focusing on the critical criteria helps one to organize the information for easier analysis and interpretation.

The criteria become easier to use and remember as the clinician encounters patients with the dysrhythmia.

Dysrhythmia analysis and interpretation are skills that develop through practice.

Each dysrhythmia has an impact on the body's ability to maintain a normal hemodynamic status and adequate cardiac output. The hemodynamic effects of each dysrhythmia are discussed. The treatments for the dysrhythmias are discussed at the end of the chapter.

NORMAL SINUS RHYTHM

The most important rhythm of this chapter, normal sinus rhythm, is the rhythm against which all others are compared (Figure 6-19). Without a thorough understanding of what is normal, abnormal cannot be understood. Initial analysis of a rhythm strip should determine whether the rhythm is normal sinus rhythm or a dysrhythmia that requires further analysis.

The SA node is the master pacemaker of the heart. This special group of cardiac cells generates an electrical impulse that is conducted down the normal conduction pathway, thereby depolarizing all cardiac cells.

Critical Criteria for Diagnosis of Normal Sinus Rhythm

- Upright, small, rounded P waves are present in lead II.
- P waves precede each QRS complex.
- Both the atrial rate and the ventricular rate are the same, and that rate is between 60 and 100 beats per minute.
- Rhythm is regular or essentially regular.
- The PR interval is 0.12 to 0.20 second in duration.
- The QRS interval is 0.06 to 0.10 second in duration.

Hemodynamic effects. The normal sinus rhythm is the optimal cardiac rhythm for the maintenance of adequate cardiac output and blood pressure.

DYSRHYTHMIAS OF THE SINOATRIAL NODE

Sinus Tachycardia

Tachycardia is defined as a rapid heart rate. Sinus tachycardia results when the SA node generates

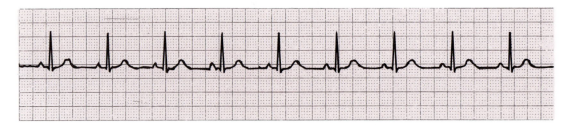

FIGURE 6-19 Normal sinus rhythm. Rhythm strip generated by the AA-700 Rhythm Simulator. (Courtesy of Armstrong Medical Industries, Lincolnshire, IL.)

more than 100, but fewer than 150, beats per minute (Figure 6-20). Sinus tachycardia is a normal response to stimulation of the sympathetic nervous system. Sinus tachycardia is also a normal finding in children under the age of 6 years. Several other processes can lead to sinus tachycardia, including exercise, use of stimulants, increased body temperature, and alterations in fluid status.

Exercise. Exercise is a natural stimulant to the heart. Heart rate increases as the body's oxygen demand and consumption increase.

Stimulants. Many types of stimulants can increase the heart rate. Commonly used and abused drugs such as caffeine and nicotine stimulate the heart rate. Additionally, drugs such as decongestants and appetite suppressants can markedly increase the heart rate. Stress and pain stimulate the sympathetic nervous system, resulting in a faster heart rate.

Increased body temperature. Elevation in body temperature causes an increase in heart rate.

Alterations in fluid status. Both hypovolemia and hypervolemia can result in an increased heart rate. When the circulating blood volume is low, such as in dehydration or after hemorrhage, the heart must beat faster to maintain adequate cardiac output and blood pressure. When the circulating blood volume is increased, such as in fluid overload, the heart must beat faster to compensate for the increased blood coming into the heart.

Critical Criteria for Diagnosis of Sinus Tachycardia

- Same criteria as for normal sinus rhythm *except* the heart rate is greater than 100 beats per minute.

Hemodynamic effects. Sinus tachycardia leads to a decrease in ventricular filling time, less blood volume in the ventricle for the next systole, and consequently lower cardiac output and arterial blood pressure. Another consequence of sinus tachycardia is increased myocardial oxygen consumption. This condition is especially detrimental in the patient with inadequate coronary artery perfusion.

Sinus Bradycardia

Bradycardia is defined as a slowed heart rate. Sinus bradycardia results when the SA node generates fewer than 60 beats per minute (Figure 6-21). The following sections discuss several processes that can lead to sinus bradycardia.

Bradycardia as a normal finding. Athletes and others who are physically fit may have a slower than

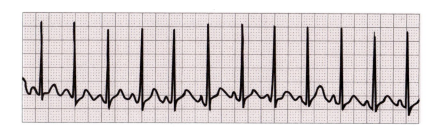

FIGURE 6-20 Sinus tachycardia. (From Paul, S., & Hebra, J. D. [1998]. *The nurse's guide to cardiac rhythm interpretation: Implications for patient care.* Philadelphia: W. B. Saunders.)

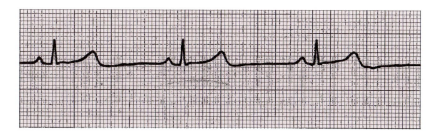

FIGURE 6-21 Sinus bradycardia. (From Conover, M. B. [1996]. *Understanding electrocardiography.* 7th ed. St. Louis: Mosby.)

normal heart rate. Physical conditioning leads to increased strength of the cardiac muscle and therefore increased effectiveness of the heart as a pump. An effective pump can deliver adequate amounts of blood to the body at a slower heart rate.

Increased vagal stimulation. The parasympathetic nervous system influences the heart rate through the vagus nerve. When the vagus nerve is stimulated, an impulse is sent to the heart, and the heart rate is decreased. The Valsalva maneuver, as well as coughing, gagging, suctioning, and vomiting, can stimulate the vagus nerve and can cause sinus bradycardia.

Drug effects. Many of the drugs administered to patients with cardiac disease decrease the heart rate. This slowing in heart rate is often a desired result of treatment. When a patient's heart beats at a slower rate, oxygen demands are lessened. When bradycardia occurs as a side effect of a drug, the drug is said to have a negative chronotropic effect.

Sinoatrial node ischemia. When the patient has myocardial ischemia, injury, or infarction in the area surrounding the SA node, the node may become less able to generate impulses. Bradycardia can result.

Effects of hypoxia. Sinus bradycardia can occur during episodes of hypoxia. Hypoxia may result from both acute and chronic conditions.

Increased intracranial pressure. Cushing's reflex is a hemodynamic response to increased intracranial pressure. Blood pressure increases, and heart rate decreases and often becomes irregular.

Critical Criteria for Diagnosis of Sinus Bradycardia

- Same criteria as for normal sinus rhythm *except* that the heart rate is less than 60 beats per minute.

Hemodynamic effects. Patients demonstrate various hemodynamic responses to sinus bradycardia.

BOX 6-2

Symptoms of Decreased Cardiac Output

- Decreased level of consciousness
- Hypotension
- Chest pain
- Shortness of breath
- Pulmonary congestion; crackles
- Syncope
- Possible consequense of shock or acute myocardial infarction

---

Many patients continue to maintain adequate cardiac output and blood pressure, despite a lowered heart rate. This ability to compensate is better in patients with a healthy heart. Other patients experience a decrease in cardiac output and related symptoms and require treatment (Box 6-2).

Sinus Dysrhythmia

Sinus dysrhythmia is a cardiac rhythm disturbance that is associated with normal respiration. During inspiration, air is brought into the lungs by a negative intrathoracic pressure. Because the heart lies within the thoracic cavity, this negative intrathoracic pressure causes more blood to be brought into the right atrium from the superior and inferior vena cava. As compensation for this increased amount of blood coming to the heart, the heart rate is increased.

With exhalation, the pressure in the thoracic cavity is changed to positive, and air is forced from the lungs. During exhalation, the flow of blood into the heart returns to normal, as does the heart rate.

The ECG tracing demonstrates an alternating pattern of faster heart rate, which is associated with inspiration, then slower heart rate, which is associated with exhalation (Figure 6-22). This rhythm is considered a normal phenomenon; however, certain conditions, such as increased intracranial pressure, increased vagal tone, and myocardial ischemia, can cause the rhythm changes.

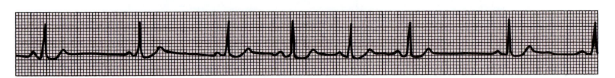

FIGURE 6-22 Sinus dysrhythmia. (From Kinney, M. R., & Packa, D. R. [1996]. *Andreoli's comprehensive cardiac care.* 8th ed. St. Louis: Mosby.)

Critical Criteria for Diagnosis of Sinus Dysrhythmia

- Same criteria as for normal sinus rhythm *except* for a cyclical increasing and decreasing of the heart rate.
- Changes in heart rate are associated with respiration.
- The rhythm is usually regularly irregular.

Hemodynamic effects. Significant changes in cardiac output and blood pressure rarely occur with this rhythm. It is normally tolerated well unless it is associated with bradycardia or tachycardia.

Sinus Arrest and Sinus Exit Block

Occasionally, the sinus node temporarily fails as the dominant pacemaker. This failure may be caused by an inability of the sinus node to generate an electrical impulse (sinus arrest), or the impulse may be generated but blocked from exiting the SA node (sinus exit block). The end result is that no atrial or ventricular depolarization occurs for one heart beat or more (Figure 6-23).

This loss of the normal waveforms creates a pause of varying length on the ECG tracing. A pause is a long flat line between two beats that exceeds the normal amount of space found between other beats. If this pause is long enough to drop the heart rate to less than 60 beats per minute, then the AV node or the Purkinje fibers may serve as a back-up pacemaker and may generate an escape beat or escape rhythm. The escape beat is so named because it allows the patient to escape the slowed heart rate, thus preventing further compromise. Sinus arrest or sinus exit block may be caused by enhanced vagal tone, coronary artery disease, or use of certain drugs.

Enhanced vagal tone. The Valsalva maneuver, coughing, gagging, or vomiting may temporarily suppress impulse generation in, or conduction from, the SA node.

Coronary artery disease. Coronary artery disease can lead to decreased perfusion of the SA node, resulting in impaired performance.

Effects of drugs. Administration of various cardiac drugs that slow heart rate can lead to episodes of sinus arrest and exit block.

Critical Criteria for Diagnosis of Sinus Arrest and Sinus Exit Block

- The heart rate can be normal (60 to 100 beats per minute) or slower than normal.
- Pauses caused by missed beats are noted on the ECG.
- The rhythm is irregular as the result of missed beats.
- Pauses may be interrupted by an escape beat from the AV node or the Purkinje fibers.

Hemodynamic effects. The hemodynamic effects of sinus arrest and/or exit block depend on the number of sinus beats that are arrested or blocked and the length of the resulting pause. Changes in cardiac output and blood pressure depend on how low the heart rate falls. When multiple beats are arrested or blocked, asystole results. The patient ceases to have any cardiac output.

DYSRHYTHMIAS OF THE ATRIA

Increased automaticity in the right, the left, or both atria can result in abnormal cardiac rhythms. These dysrhythmias are most often caused by increased automaticity from a wide variety of processes.

Stress. The stress response causes the liberation of epinephrine and norepinephrine. This phenomenon can cause increased automaticity in the atria. Drugs that stimulate the sympathetic nervous system, such as amphetamines, cocaine, and decongestants, can also cause atrial dysrhythmias (AHA, 2002).

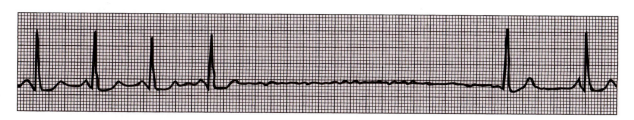

FIGURE 6-23 Sinus arrest/sinus exit block. Note the junctional escape beat at the end of the pause. (From Kinney, M. R., & Packa, D. R. [1996]. *Andreoli's comprehensive cardiac care.* 8th ed. St. Louis: Mosby.)

Electrolyte imbalances. Electrolyte imbalances, particularly hypokalemia, can result in increased automaticity in the atria.

Hypoxia. The atria become irritable when they are deprived of oxygen. Patients with chronic obstructive pulmonary disease are at high risk for atrial dysrhythmias.

Injury to the atria. When the atria are injured, such as with trauma related to cardiac surgery, they are more prone to generate ectopic beats.

Digitalis toxicity. Administration of digitalis in toxic doses can be stimulating to the myocardium, particularly to the atria. Digitalis may convert atrial dysrhythmias to sinus rhythm, or it may only slow the ventricular response to atrial tachycardias.

Hypothermia. Lowered body temperature predisposes a patient to atrial dysrhythmias.

Hyperthyroidism. The state of hyperthyroidism places a patient in a metabolic state that is very similar to the stress response. The hormones produced by the thyroid gland have a stimulating effect on the heart.

Alcohol intoxication. Alcohol is a cardiac stimulant that has an irritating effect on the heart.

Pericarditis. When the pericardial lining surrounding the heart is inflamed or infected, the atria become more irritable. Atrial dysrhythmias may be one of the first signs of pericarditis.

Premature Atrial Contractions

Premature atrial contractions (PACs) are common dysrhythmias and are usually seen in the setting of normal sinus rhythm (Figure 6-24). PACs are generated very near the SA node. This situation frequently leads to depolarization of the tissue surrounding the SA node and causes a pause on the ECG. This pause is usually

---

> **BOX 6-3**
>
> ## Compensatory Versus Noncompensatory Pause
>
> - A rhythm strip with a premature beat is analyzed using calipers or paper and pencil.
> - Two consecutive normal beats are located just before the premature beat, and the caliper points or pencil marks are placed on the R wave of each normal beat.
> - The calipers are flipped over, or the paper is slid over, to where the next normal beat should have occurred. The premature beat occurs early.
> - Now, with care taken not to lose placement, the calipers are flipped, or the paper is slid over, one more time. If the point of the calipers or the mark on the paper lands exactly on the next normal beat's R wave, the sinus node compensated for the one premature beat and kept its normal rhythm (see Figure 6-25).
> - If the caliper point or pencil mark does not land on the next normal beat's R wave, then the sinus node did not compensate and had to establish a new rhythm, resulting in a noncompensatory pause.

noncompensatory. Box 6-3 discusses determining compensatory versus noncompensatory pauses.

Critical Criteria for Diagnosis of Premature Atrial Contractions

- The ectopic beats are premature.
- The PR interval is usually normal but often differs from the PR interval seen during normal sinus rhythm.
- PACs are *usually* followed by a noncompensatory pause.
- The P wave of the premature beat may be found in the T wave just before the premature beat. When this occurs, the T wave of the preceding

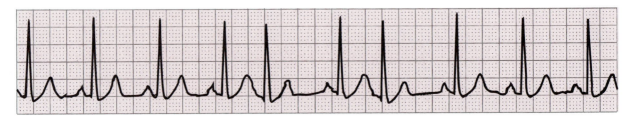

FIGURE 6-24 Premature atrial contractions shown in the fifth and seventh beats. The P wave occurs on the T wave for these premature atrial contractions. (From Paul, S., & Hebra, J. D. [1998]. *The nurse's guide to cardiac rhythm interpretation: Implications for patient care.* Philadelphia: W. B. Saunders.)

beat is distorted. The T wave of the beat preceding the premature beat can be compared with other, normal, T waves on the ECG strip.

Occasionally, a PAC is generated and conducted down to the AV node just after a normal impulse has been conducted. The PAC arrives at the AV node when the bundle of His and its branches are refractory to, or unable to conduct, the premature impulse. The impulse is blocked and is not allowed to enter the ventricle. This blocked PAC can be detected as a pause on the ECG. Before the pause, a different-looking T wave can usually be noted (Figure 6-25). The unusual T wave is caused by the PAC's premature P wave imposed on the normal T wave (Figure 6-26).

Critical Criteria for Diagnosis of Blocked Premature Atrial Contraction

- A pause is noted on the ECG tracing.
- A premature P wave, which differs from the normal P wave, is found in the T wave or just after the T wave of the last normal beat before the pause.

Hemodynamic effects. PACs do not usually alter cardiac output or blood pressure in a significant way. However, many patients do report having palpitations.

Increasing numbers of PACs may herald the development of atrial fibrillation or flutter.

Wandering Atrial Pacemaker

Wandering atrial pacemaker is a dysrhythmia characterized by varied pacemaking activity throughout the atria. For the criteria for this rhythm to be met, at least three sites of atrial pacemaking must be documented.

When impulses are generated from different pacemaking sites, different P-wave morphologies are present on the ECG. Varying waveform morphology is another way of saying that the P waves look different in shape, slope, or orientation. P waves in wandering atrial pacemaker can be upright, inverted, flat, pointed, notched, and/or slanted in different directions. The PR interval varies because the impulses originate from different locations within the atria, taking various times to reach the AV node (Figure 6-27).

Critical Criteria for Diagnosis of Wandering Atrial Pacemaker

- At least three different-looking P waves must be seen.
- The heart rate must not be greater than 100 beats per minute.
- The PR intervals vary.
- The rhythm is usually irregular.

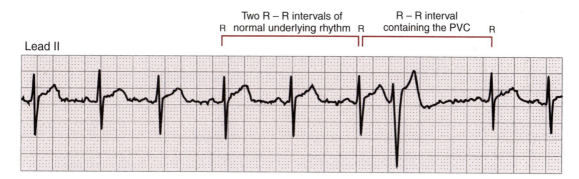

FIGURE 6-25 Compensatory pause. *PVC*, Premature ventricular contraction. (From Paul, S., & Hebra, J. D. [1998]. *The nurse's guide to cardiac rhythm interpretation: Implications for patient care.* Philadelphia: W. B. Saunders.)

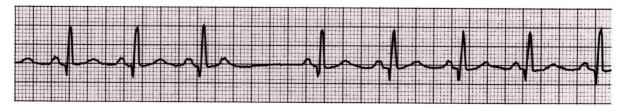

FIGURE 6-26 Blocked premature atrial contraction (PAC). Note the unusual looking T wave following the third beat. (Modified from Patel, J., McGowan, S., & Moody, L. [1989]. *Arrhythmias: Detection, treatment, and cardiac drugs.* Philadelphia: W. B. Saunders.)

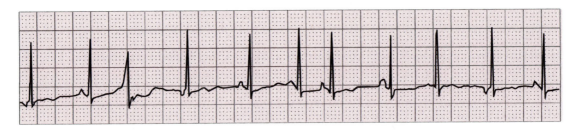

FIGURE 6-27 Wandering atrial pacemaker. Note the varying P-wave morphologies. (From Paul, S., & Hebra, J. D. [1998]. *The nurse's guide to cardiac rhythm interpretation: Implications for patient care.* Philadelphia: W. B. Saunders.)

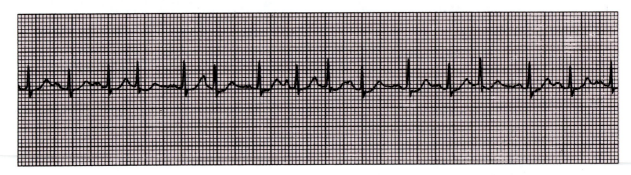

FIGURE 6-28 Multifocal atrial tachycardia. (From Patel, J., McGowan, S., & Moody, L. [1989]. *Arrhythmias: Detection, treatment, and cardiac drugs.* Philadelphia: W. B. Saunders.)

Hemodynamic effects. Wandering atrial pacemaker may result in less effective atrial depolarization. Ventricular filling may be affected, thus decreasing cardiac output and blood pressure.

Multifocal Atrial Tachycardia

Multifocal atrial tachycardia is essentially the same as wandering atrial pacemaker, except the heart rate exceeds 100 beats per minute. It is almost exclusively found in the patient with chronic obstructive pulmonary disease. The cause of the dysrhythmia is thought to be right atrial dilation secondary to increased pulmonary pressures (Porth, 2002) (Figure 6-28).

Critical Criteria for Diagnosis of Multifocal Atrial Tachycardia

- These criteria are the same as for wandering atrial pacemaker *except* the heart rate is greater than 100 beats per minute.

Hemodynamic effects. The hemodynamic effects of multifocal atrial tachycardia are the same as those for wandering atrial pacemaker. The faster the rate is, the less time there is for ventricular filling, resulting in lowered blood pressure.

Paroxysmal Atrial Tachycardia

Paroxysmal atrial tachycardia is a rapid rhythm that arises from the atria without warning. Because of the fast rate, paroxysmal atrial tachycardia can be a life-threatening dysrhythmia. It is usually seen in patients with cardiac disease; however, it may also occur in healthy patients. In some instances, increased numbers of PACs precede the onset of paroxysmal atrial tachycardia.

When the atria generate impulses more rapidly than the AV node can conduct, AV block may result. AV block on the ECG is evidenced by P waves that are not followed by QRS complexes. P waves may merge with T waves. Sometimes, the AV node blocks impulses in a set pattern, such as every third or fourth beat. When diagnosing the rhythm, the nurse notes the number of P waves in proportion to the number of QRS complexes. For example, when the AV node conducts every second atrial impulse, a 2:1 block exists. In other words, for every two atrial impulses, or every two P waves, only one is conducted (Figure 6-29).

The degree of block may be fixed or varied. *Varied* means that the number of P waves being conducted through to the ventricles is unpredictable versus patterned.

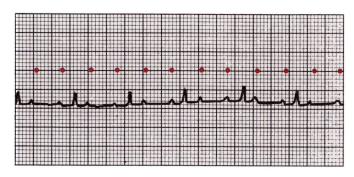

FIGURE 6-29 Paroxysmal atrial tachycardia with a fixed degree of block. Note the dots over the P waves. Every second P wave is conducted. (American Heart Association. [1987]. *Textbook of advanced cardiac life support.* Dallas, TX: Author.)

BOX 6-4

Supraventricular Tachycardia

Definition: Supraventricular tachycardia describes any tachycardia that originates from a site above the ventricles, usually the atria, at a rate of greater than 150 beats per minute.
Paroxysmal: Refers to supraventricular tachycardia that starts and ends suddenly.

Some clinicians refer to an atrial tachydysrhythmia as a supraventricular tachycardia. When the rate is greater than 150 beats per minute, it becomes difficult to make an accurate diagnosis; therefore, clinicians often use the term *supraventricular tachycardia* (Box 6-4).

Critical Criteria for Diagnosis of Paroxysmal Atrial Tachycardia

- It occurs suddenly, usually without warning.
- The heart rate is usually 150 to 250 beats per minute.
- The rhythm is absolutely regular.

- P waves, if present, usually merge with the preceding T waves, thereby altering the appearance of the T wave.
- AV block that may be of a fixed or varying degree is present.
- The width of the QRS complex is usually normal.

Hemodynamic effects. The hemodynamic effects of paroxysmal atrial tachycardia can vary from none to shock. The faster the rate is, the less time there is for ventricular filling. At faster rates, cardiac output and blood pressure can be severely compromised.

Atrial Flutter

Atrial flutter is a dysrhythmia that arises from a single irritable focus in the atria. Atrial flutter is most commonly seen in patients with heart disease. Patients who have valvular disease seem particularly susceptible to its development (AHA, 2002).

The waveforms associated with atrial flutter are flutter, or F, waves. Flutter waves are best seen in leads II, III, and aVF. They are biphasic: the first part of the waveform is negative, and it is followed by an upright, or positive, waveform (Figure 6-30). This waveform has an appearance much like the teeth of a saw's

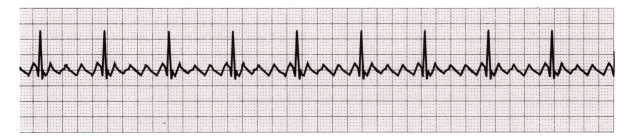

FIGURE 6-30 Atrial flutter with a fixed degree of block. Note the sawtooth configuration and the negative orientation of the flutter waves. Rhythm generated by the AA-700 Rhythm Simulator. (Courtesy of Armstrong Medical Industries, Lincolnshire, IL.)

blade. To calculate the atrial flutter rate, find the sharpest point of two consecutive flutter waves. Mark the points with a pencil mark or with the point of a caliper. Count the number of small boxes between the two points, and divide the number of small boxes into 1500.

Flutter waves occur incessantly and with perfect regularity. The irritable focus in the atria never stops firing. This means that the flutter waves continue throughout the ECG strip and often alter the appearance of the QRS complex and the T wave (see Figure 6-30).

Flutter waves are usually generated at a rate of 250 to 350 beats per minute. However, the AV node is physiologically unable to conduct all these impulses. Therefore, as in paroxysmal atrial tachycardia, the AV node selectively conducts a given number of flutter waves down to the ventricle. If, for example, the atrial focus generates 300 beats per minute, the AV node may be able to conduct every third beat. This would be a 3:1 ratio of conduction, and the resultant ventricular rate would be 100 beats per minute (300 ÷ 3 = 100). As in paroxysmal atrial tachycardia, the degree of block may be fixed and predictable (2:1, 3:1, 4:1) (see Figure 6-30) or unpredictable and varied (Figure 6-31).

Critical Criteria for Diagnosis of Atrial Flutter

- Flutter waves are present in leads II, III, and aVF.
- The atrial rate is usually 250 to 350 beats per minute. The ventricular rate varies with the degree of AV block.
- The onset is usually rapid.

Hemodynamic effects. The hemodynamic effects of atrial flutter are dependent on the ventricular rate, sometimes called the *ventricular response*. Patients who sustain atrial flutter with a fast ventricular response often have symptoms of low cardiac output. Patients whose AV nodes are blocking greater numbers of the atrial impulses and who maintain a heart rate between 60 and 100 beats per minute tend to maintain a more normal cardiac output and blood pressure.

Atrial Fibrillation

Atrial fibrillation is a dysrhythmia that is characterized by erratic impulse formation throughout the atria. Widespread irritability and increased automaticity lead to a chaotic state of impulse formation (Figure 6-32). Atrial fibrillation produces a wavy baseline with no discernible P waves. As the AV node is bombarded with rapidly fired atrial impulses, it conducts impulses to the ventricles in an unpredictable fashion, and the result is an irregularly irregular ventricular rhythm.

As the AV node attempts to regulate the movement of impulses into the ventricle, it may conduct an atrial impulse before the bundle of His and the branches are able to conduct. The right bundle branch requires a longer time to repolarize than the left bundle does. If the right bundle branch is still repolarizing, the impulse must cross the ventricular septum and move down the left bundle branch first and then cross back over the septum and depolarize the right ventricle. Depolarization of the ventricles takes longer, resulting in a widened QRS complex. When this event occurs, the impulse is said to be aberrantly conducted (Figure 6-33).

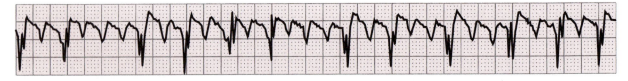

FIGURE 6-31 Atrial flutter with varying degrees of block. (From Paul, S., & Hebra, J. D. [1998]. *The nurse's guide to cardiac rhythm interpretation: Implications for patient care.* Philadelphia: W. B. Saunders.)

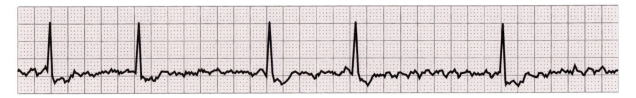

FIGURE 6-32 Atrial fibrillation. (From Paul, S., & Hebra, J. D. [1998]. *The nurse's guide to cardiac rhythm interpretation: Implications for patient care.* Philadelphia: W. B. Saunders.)

In atrial fibrillation, aberrantly conducted beats are referred to as *Ashman's beats.* Ashman's beats are more likely to occur when an atrial impulse arrives at the AV node just after a previously conducted impulse (Figure 6-34). Ashman's beats are often seen when the rate changes from slower to faster, which is referred to as a long-short cycle. Ashman's beats are not clinically significant.

One complication of atrial fibrillation is thromboembolism. The blood that collects in the atria is agitated by fibrillation, and normal clotting is accelerated. Small thrombi, called *mural* thrombi, begin to form along the walls of the atria. These clots may dislodge, resulting in pulmonary embolism or stroke.

For this reason, if a patient has been in atrial fibrillation for an unknown amount of time, and if the blood pressure is stable, the patient should receive anticoagulation therapy before any attempt is made to convert atrial fibrillation to normal sinus rhythm.

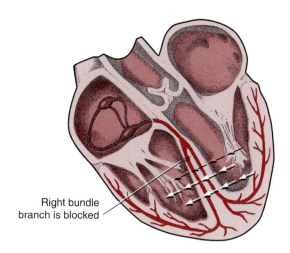

FIGURE 6-33 Aberrancy is most likely to result when the right bundle branch blocks. The impulse must depolarize the left side of the heart first. The impulse then crosses the septum and abnormally depolarizes the right side of the heart. This results in a widened QRS complex.

Right bundle branch is blocked

Intravenous heparin is the drug of choice for anticoagulation. If the atrial fibrillation persists or is recurrent, long-term warfarin (Coumadin) therapy is usually prescribed to diminish the risk of thromboembolism.

Critical Criteria for Diagnosis of Atrial Fibrillation

- A wavy baseline exists with no discernible P waves.
- An irregularly irregular ventricular rhythm exists.
- The width of the QRS complex may vary between normal and slightly widened.
- Ashman's beats may be present.

Hemodynamic effects. In atrial fibrillation, the atria are never fully depolarized and therefore do not contract. Therefore, patients lose the atrial kick. The hemodynamic effects of atrial fibrillation also relate to the ventricular response. Patients with markedly slower or faster rates are more likely to experience a decrease in cardiac output and blood pressure (see Research Analysis).

DYSRHYTHMIAS OF THE ATRIOVENTRICULAR NODE

Junctional Rhythm

Dysrhythmias of the AV node are called *junctional rhythms.* The term *nodal rhythms* is also used. The AV node is located in the middle of the heart between the atria and the ventricles. The tissue immediately surrounding the AV node is referred to as *junctional tissue.* Both the AV node itself and the junctional tissue are capable of generating cardiac rhythms.

The following are the two primary causes of junctional rhythms:

1. Dysrhythmias can originate in the AV node or the junctional tissue surrounding it. When a singular beat or ongoing rhythm originates in an area other than the sinus node, that beat or rhythm is considered ectopic. *Ectopic* means out of the normal place. Ectopic rhythms are usually caused by increased automaticity. Increased automaticity is commonly caused by stress or the use of nicotine or caffeine. It can also result from myocardial ischemia, injury,

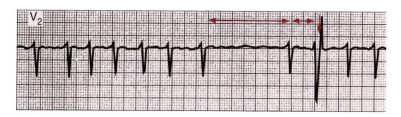

FIGURE 6-34 Atrial fibrillation. Note Ashman's beat, following a long-short cycle. (From Laver, J. [1992]. Electrical activity of the heart and dysrhythmias. In C. Guzzetta & B. Dossey [Eds.], *Cardiovascular nursing: Bodymind tapestry.* St. Louis: Mosby.)

RESEARCH ANALYSIS

ARTICLE REFERENCE

Wyse, D. G., Waldo, A. L., et al., & Affirm Investigators (2002). A comparison of rate control and rhythm control in patients with atrial fibrillation. *New England Journal of Medicine*, 347(23), 1825-1832.

STUDY PURPOSE, METHODS, AND FINDINGS

The relative benefits and risks of rate control versus rhythm control are currently the most controversial issues in treating atrial fibrillation. The purpose of this study was to compare these two common approaches in treating atrial fibrillation: cardioversion and treatment with antiarrhythmic drugs versus rate-controlling drugs, allowing the atrial fibrillation to persist. The investigators conducted a randomized prospective, multicenter comparison of these two treatment strategies using a total of 4060 patients. The Atrial Fibrillation Follow-up Investigation of Rhythm Management (AFFIRM) investigators found that patients receiving the rhythm-control drugs were significantly more likely to be hospitalized than those receiving rate-control drugs. The benefits of rate control over rhythm control were established in this study. The investigators concluded that medical management of atrial fibrillation with the rhythm-control strategy (cardioversion and the use of antiarrhythmic drugs) offered no survival advantage over the rate-control strategy. Additionally, antiarrhythmic drug therapy has some adverse effects such as proarrhythmic tendencies.

STRENGTHS AND LIMITATIONS

This study was well designed. Graphs and tables provided visual illustrations of the characteristics of the patients such as cumulative mortality, adverse effects, and hazard ratio for death in prespecified subgroups (age, sex, rhythm at randomization, coronary artery disease, hypertension, heart failure, left ventricular ejection fraction). The researchers noted that the results could not be generalized to younger patients, but were representative of the majority of patients with atrial fibrillation.

IMPLICATIONS FOR PRACTICE

Implications for this study are primarily prevention. Atrial fibrillation is the most common sustained dysrhythmia and can lead to stroke, heart failure, and cardiomyopathy and their associated risk of death. Therefore, therapy aimed at prevention remains key. Rate control and anticoagulation therapy should be considered a primary approach to therapy. This study confirmed no added benefit of rhythm control (cardioversion with an antiarrhythmic agent). A greater number of adverse effects, such as bradycardia and torsades de pointes, occurred in the rhythm-control group owing to the adverse effects of antiarrhythmic drug used to maintain sinus rhythm. If cardioversion and treatment with antiarrhythmic drugs to maintain sinus rhythm comprise the strategy selected to treat atrial fibrillation, the nurse must emphasize to the patient the importance of continuous anticoagulation because it was noted that antiarrhythmic drug therapies frequently fail to maintain the sinus rhythm. Patients with atrial fibrillation will need preventive treatment for a lifetime.

---

or infarction. Digitalis toxicity can produce all forms of junctional rhythms. At toxic levels, digitalis can suppress the heart rate or can act as a myocardial stimulant.

2. Escape rhythms can be generated from the AV node should the sinus node fail. The AV node is capable of generating 40 to 60 beats per minute as a back-up pacemaker.

Several ECG changes are common to all the junctional dysrhythmias. These changes include P-wave abnormalities and PR-interval changes.

P-wave changes. Because of the location of the AV node—in the center of the heart—impulses generated may be conducted forward, backward, or both. Like ripples from a rock thrown into a pool of water, the impulse can radiate both forward and backward. With the potential of forward, backward, or bidirectional impulse conduction, three different P wave-forms may be associated with junctional rhythms, as follows:

1. When the AV node impulse moves forward, *P waves are absent* because the impulse enters the ventricle

first. The atria do not receive the wave of depolarization; therefore, no P wave exists. Without depolarization, the atria do not contract (Figure 6-35).

2. When the AV node impulse is conducted backward, the impulse enters the atria first. Conduction back toward the atria allows for at least partial depolarization of the atria. When depolarization occurs in a backward fashion, an inverted P wave is created. Once the atria have been depolarized, the impulse then moves down the bundle of His and depolarizes both ventricles normally (Figure 6-36). A short PR interval (<0.12 second) is noted.

3. When the impulse is conducted in both a forward and a backward fashion, *P waves may be present after the QRS.* In this type of conduction, the impulse first moves into the ventricles, depolarizing them and creating a QRS complex. Because the impulse is also conducted backward, some

atrial depolarization occurs, and a late P wave is noted after the QRS complex (Figure 6-37).

Critical Criteria for Diagnosis of Junctional Rhythm

- P waves may be absent or inverted or may follow the QRS complex.
- The heart rate is 40 to 60 beats per minute.
- The PR interval is at the low end of normal or shorter than normal.
- The rhythm is usually regular.
- The QRS complex is of normal width.

Hemodynamic effects. In junctional rhythms, atrial depolarization (atrial kick) is usually less effective or absent, resulting in decreased ventricular filling. Diminished cardiac output and blood pressure may occur.

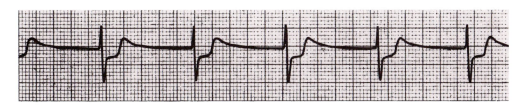

FIGURE 6-35 Junctional (nodal) rhythm. Note absence of P waves. (From Lewis, S., Collier, I. C., & Heitkemper, M. M. [1996]. *Medical-surgical nursing: Assessment and management of clinical problems.* 4th ed. St. Louis: Mosby.)

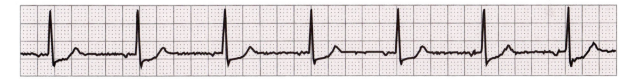

FIGURE 6-36 Junctional (nodal) rhythm. Note the shortened PR interval. (From Paul, S., & Hebra, J. D. [1998]. *The nurse's guide to cardiac rhythm interpretation: Implications for patient care.* Philadelphia: W. B. Saunders.)

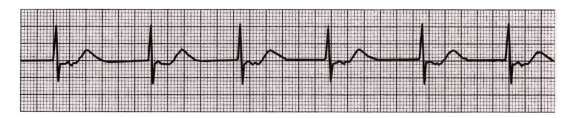

FIGURE 6-37 Junctional (nodal) rhythm. Note the P waves after the QRS complex. (From Patel, J., McGowan, S., & Moody, L. [1989]. *Arrhythmias: Detection, treatment, and cardiac drugs.* Philadelphia: W. B. Saunders.)

Accelerated Junctional Rhythm and Junctional Tachycardia

The normal intrinsic rate for the AV node and junctional tissue is 40 to 60 beats per minute, but rates can accelerate. Accelerated junctional rhythms have a rate between 60 and 100 beats per minute, whereas junctional tachycardia (rates faster than 100 beats per minute) can reach the upper rate capability for the AV node of 150 (Figure 6-38).

Critical Criteria for Diagnosis of Accelerated Junctional and Junctional Tachycardia

These criteria are the same as for junctional rhythm except for the following:
- The heart rate is between 60 and 100 beats per minute for an accelerated junctional rhythm.
- The heart rate is between 100 and 150 for a junctional tachycardia.

Hemodynamic effects. The hemodynamic effects of junctional tachycardia are the same as for a junctional rhythm. However, ventricular filling may be further compromised by the faster heart rate. Conversely, the acceleration in heart rate may actually improve cardiac output. If stroke volume is decreased, then an increase in heart rate may increase cardiac output.

Premature Junctional Contractions

Irritable areas in the AV node and junctional tissue can generate beats that are earlier than the next expected beat (Figure 6-39). These premature beats most often occur in normal sinus rhythm and temporarily upset rhythmicity.

Either a compensatory or noncompensatory pause may occur after a premature junctional contraction. The closer the site of premature impulse generation is to the sinus node, the less likely it is that the SA node will compensate. When a premature impulse fires close to the SA node, a wave of depolarization moves backward toward the sinus node and excites the tissue of the SA node. After depolarization has occurred, the sinus node requires time for repolarization before generating the next beat. This delay usually creates a noncompensatory pause on the ECG.

Critical Criteria for Diagnosis of Premature Junctional Contractions

- The ectopic beats are premature.
- If a P wave is present before the QRS complex, the PR interval is usually shorter than normal.
- P waves may be absent or inverted or may occur after the QRS complex.
- Premature junctional contractions are *usually* followed by a noncompensatory pause.

Hemodynamic effects. Premature junctional contractions do not usually alter the cardiac output or blood pressure in a significant way. However, many patients do report having palpitations. Increasing numbers of premature junctional contractions may herald the development of junctional tachycardia.

DYSRHYTHMIAS OF THE VENTRICLE

Because impulses for ventricular dysrhythmias originate in the lower portion of the heart, depolarization occurs in an abnormal way. The impulse must travel in a backward or sideways fashion to depolarize the ventricles. This abnormal flow of electricity lengthens the time interval in which depolarization of the ventricles occurs. The result is a widened QRS complex. The QRS interval extends beyond the normal interval of 0.06 to 0.10 second.

Depolarization from abnormal ventricular beats rarely moves as far backward as the atria. Therefore, most ventricular dysrhythmias have no evident P

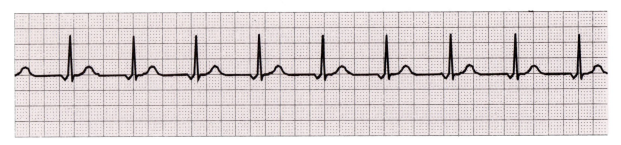

FIGURE 6-38 Junctional tachycardia. Note the short PR interval and heart rate of 70 beats per minute. Rhythm generated by the AA-700 Rhythm Simulator. (Courtesy of Armstrong Medical Industries, Lincolnshire, IL.)

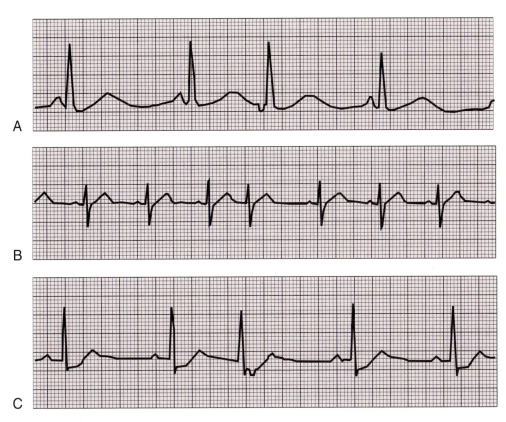

FIGURE 6-39 Premature junctional contractions. **A,** Third beat with a shortened PR interval and an inverted P wave; **B,** Fourth beat, no P waves visible; **C,** third beat with a retrograde P wave. (From Conover, M. B. [1996]. *Understanding electrocardiography.* 7th ed. St. Louis: Mosby.)

waves. However, if a P wave is present, it is usually seen in the T wave of the previous beat. Two types of ventricular dysrhythmias, ectopic and escape, exist:

1. *Ectopic* means occurring outside of the normal place. The ectopic rhythms are abnormal and disturb or override the normal sinus rhythm. These ectopic rhythms are capable of firing at fast rates and may be life-threatening.
2. The Purkinje fibers can act as a site for back-up pacemaking should the SA and AV nodes fail. The Purkinje fibers can generate an escape rhythm of 15 to 40 beats per minute. Although this is a very slow intrinsic rate, some patients are able to maintain an adequate cardiac output and blood pressure with rates that are close to 40 beats per minute.

   Generation of ventricular dysrhythmias can be secondary to myocardial ischemia, injury, or infarction or to hypokalemia, hypomagnesemia, hypoxia, or acid-base imbalances (AHA, 2002).

Myocardial ischemia, injury, and infarction. When blood supply is decreased to an area of the ventricle, the blood-deprived area becomes irritable and is more likely to have increased automaticity. Prolonged ischemia can lead to permanent injury to the area, creating an even greater potential for ectopic impulse formation.

Hypokalemia. Low serum potassium levels can facilitate the development of ventricular dysrhythmias. As discussed earlier, potassium plays an important role in the normal depolarization/repolarization process.

Hypomagnesemia. Low serum magnesium levels have been correlated with the development of ventricular dysrhythmias, in particular torsades de pointes (AHA, 2002). Torsades de pointes is a type of ventricular tachycardia in which the QRS complex changes polarity from negative to positive.

Hypoxia. Inadequate amounts of oxygen are irritating to the ventricles and often stimulate ectopic and escape beats.

Acid-base imbalances. Both alkalosis and acidosis can stimulate ventricular ectopy.

Premature Ventricular Contractions

Premature ventricular contractions (PVCs) are a common ventricular dysrhythmia. The beats can be generated anywhere in the ventricles. When only one focus of ventricular irritability exists, all the ectopic beats appear the same. Ventricular beats coming from one area are called *unifocal PVCs* (Figure 6-40). Because PVCs are generated in the ventricles, a considerable distance from the SA node, the SA node is usually able to compensate for the premature beat. This compensation is noted on the ECG tracing as a compensatory pause that follows the PVC.

There can also be multiple areas, or foci, of ventricular irritability. When ventricular ectopic beats come from multiple areas, each QRS looks different (Figure 6-41). These PVCs are called *multifocal.*

PVCs may also occur in a predictable pattern. For example, PVCs may occur every other beat, every third beat, or every fourth beat. When PVCs occur every other beat, the pattern is referred to as *bigeminy* (Figure 6-42). When the PVCs occur every third beat, the pattern is called *trigeminy,* and every fourth beat, *quadrigeminy.* PVCs can also occur sequentially. Two PVCs in a row are termed a *couplet* (Figure 6-43). Three PVCs in a row are termed a *triplet* or *salvo* (Figure 6-44).

The downslope of the T wave is called the *vulnerable period.* If a PVC is generated during this time, ventricular fibrillation may occur. This is referred to as *R-on-T phenomenon;* the R wave of a PVC falls on the T wave of a normal beat (Figure 6-45). R-on-T phenomenon occurs frequently in the clinical setting, often without significant consequence (Conover, 2003).

Isolated (fewer than six PCVs per minute) PVCs are rarely treated. Rather, PVCs are considered signs of underlying disease that requires attention, for example, hypoxia, ischemia, or electrolyte imbalance. PVCs in the patient with myocardial infarction are treated

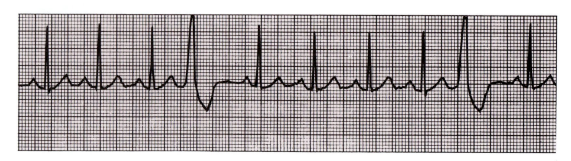

FIGURE 6-40 Unifocal premature ventricular contractions. (From Patel, J., McGowan, S., & Moody, L. [1989]. *Arrhythmias: Detection, treatment, and cardiac drugs.* Philadelphia: W. B. Saunders.)

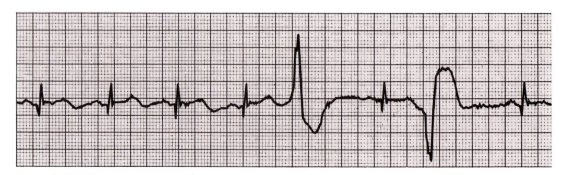

FIGURE 6-41 Multifocal premature ventricular contractions. Note the compensatory pause. (From Patel, J., McGowan, S., & Moody, L. [1989]. *Arrhythmias: Detection, treatment, and cardiac drugs.* Philadelphia: W. B. Saunders.)

when associated with such symptoms as angina or hypotension (AHA, 2002).

PVCs, couplets, R-on-T phenomenon, and multifocal ventricular ectopy should be considered warning dysrhythmias. The nurse should assist in identification of causative factors and be alert for development of worsening dysrhythmias.

Critical Criteria for Diagnosis of Premature Ventricular Contractions

- Ectopic beat occurs prematurely, before the next anticipated sinus beat.
- The QRS complex of the premature beat is wider than 0.10 second.
- The rhythm is irregular as a result of the premature beats. However, the premature beats may occur in a regular pattern.
- The premature beat is usually followed by a compensatory pause.
- The ST segment of the PVC is in the opposite direction of the QRS of the PVC. In other words, if the QRS complex of the PVC is upright, or positive, then the ST segment is downward, or negative (see Figure 6-41).

- P waves are usually absent before the ectopic beat.
- PVCs may be unifocal or multifocal and may occur in tandem as couplets or triplets.

Hemodynamic effects. The hemodynamic effects associated with PVCs are varied. Some patients may be asymptomatic, whereas others may report having palpitations and lightheadedness. Symptoms usually worsen with an increase in the number of PVCs.

Ventricular Tachycardia

Ventricular tachycardia is a rapid, life-threatening dysrhythmia that originates in the ventricles. It is characterized by at least three premature ventricular complexes in a row. Ventricular tachycardia occurs at a rate greater than 100 beats per minute. The site of irritability in the ventricle is unifocal; therefore, all waveforms appear the same. Depolarization of the ventricles occurs in an abnormal way, producing a widened QRS complex (Figure 6-46).

The wave of depolarization associated with ventricular tachycardia rarely reaches the atria. Therefore, P waves are usually absent. If P waves are present, they have no association with the QRS complex.

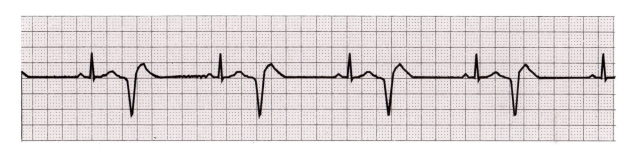

FIGURE 6-42 Premature ventricular contractions in a bigeminal pattern. Rhythm strip generated by the AA-700 Rhythm Simulator. (Courtesy of Armstrong Medical Industries, Lincolnshire, IL.)

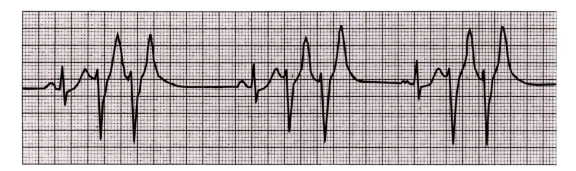

FIGURE 6-43 Two premature ventricular contractions in a row (couplet). (From Patel, J., McGowan, S., & Moody, L. [1989]. *Arrhythmias: Detection, treatment, and cardiac drugs.* Philadelphia: W. B. Saunders.)

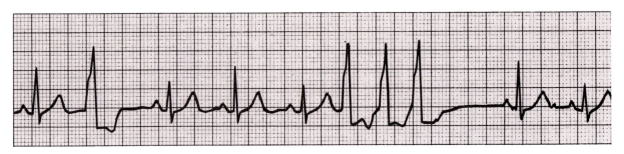

FIGURE 6-44 Three premature ventricular contractions in a row (triplet). (From Patel, J., McGowan, S., & Moody, L. [1989]. *Arrhythmias: Detection, treatment, and cardiac drugs.* Philadelphia: W. B. Saunders.)

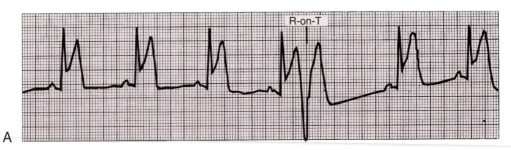

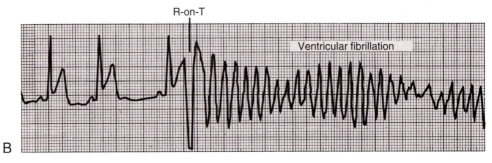

FIGURE 6-45 A, R-on-T phenomenon in a patient with an acute myocardial infarction; **B,** in the same patient, the R-on-T phenomenon causes ventricular fibrillation. (From Conover, M. B. [1996]. *Understanding electrocardiography.* 7th ed. St. Louis: Mosby.)

The sinus node may continue to depolarize at its normal rate, unaware that the ventricle is being depolarized abnormally by an ectopic pacer. P waves may appear to be randomly scattered throughout the rhythm, but the P waves are actually being fired at a consistent rate from the sinus node.

Critical Criteria for Diagnosis of Ventricular Tachycardia

- The occurrence of more than three PVCs in a row is considered ventricular tachycardia.
- The heart rate is faster than 100 beats per minute.
- The QRS complex width is greater than 0.10 second.

- P waves may or may not be visible. If visible, P waves appear to be scattered throughout the rhythm and have no relationship with the QRS complex.

Hemodynamic effects. Hemodynamic effects associated with ventricular tachycardia may vary. Most patients have a significant loss of cardiac output, with a resultant low blood pressure. Many patients become pulseless, with no obtainable blood pressure. However, in rare instances, some patients maintain a pulse and a blood pressure while experiencing ventricular tachycardia. Treatment of the

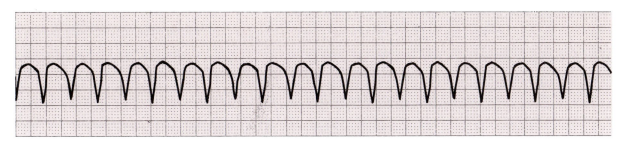

FIGURE 6-46 Ventricular tachycardia. Rhythm strip generated by the AA-700 Rhythm Simulator. (Courtesy of Armstrong Medical Industries, Lincolnshire, IL.)

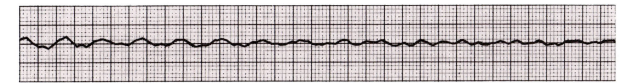

FIGURE 6-47 Fine ventricular fibrillation. (From Patel, J., McGowan, S., & Moody, L. [1989]. *Arrhythmias: Detection, treatment, and cardiac drugs.* Philadelphia: W. B. Saunders.)

dysrhythmia is dependent on the presence or absence of a pulse and blood pressure (AHA, 2002).

Ventricular Fibrillation

Ventricular fibrillation is a chaotic rhythm characterized by a quivering of the ventricles that results in total loss of cardiac output. Patients experiencing ventricular fibrillation are in a state of clinical death. Clinical death means that the patient's heart has stopped contracting; therefore, there is no blood flow to the vital organs.

Ventricular fibrillation can occur without a known cause. Ventricular fibrillation that occurs without the presence of cardiac disease or other explainable cause is referred to as *primary ventricular fibrillation.* More commonly, however, fibrillation occurs secondary to the processes listed under the discussion of PVCs.

The electrical energy created by ventricular fibrillation varies in amplitude. When voltage is low in the fibrillating ventricle, the result is a small-amplitude waveform. This form of ventricular fibrillation is referred to as *fine* (Figure 6-47).

When voltage is greater in the fibrillating ventricle, the result is a larger-amplitude waveform. This form of ventricular fibrillation is referred to as *coarse* (Figure 6-48). Coarse ventricular fibrillation responds better to defibrillation than does fine ventricular fibrillation (AHA, 2002).

Because a loose lead or electrical interference can produce a waveform similar to ventricular fibrillation, it is always important to confirm ventricular fibrillation in at least two leads and to assess the patient's condition.

Critical Criteria for Diagnosis of Ventricular Fibrillation

- A fluctuating, jagged baseline exists. No discernible P, Q, R, S, and T waves are present.
- Ventricular fibrillation may be coarse or fine.

Hemodynamic effects. All atrial and ventricular contractions cease, leading to total loss of cardiac output. No palpable pulse is present, and no blood pressure can be obtained. Brain death occurs within 4 to 6 minutes if life support is not instituted.

Idioventricular Rhythm

Idioventricular rhythm is an escape rhythm that is generated by the Purkinje fibers. This rhythm emerges only when the SA and AV nodes have failed. The Purkinje fibers are capable of an intrinsic rate of 15 to 40 beats per minute. Because this rhythm originates in the deepest portion of the ventricles, normal depolarization is impossible, and aberrant conduction results. Therefore, the QRS of the idioventricular rhythm is wider than normal. Because of the distance of the impulse formation from the atria, atrial depolarization is not likely to occur. Usually, no evidence of P waves is present on the ECG strip (Figure 6-49).

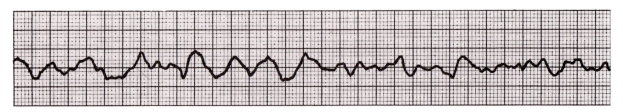

FIGURE 6-48 Coarse ventricular fibrillation. (From Patel, J., McGowan, S., & Moody, L. [1989]. *Arrhythmias: Detection, treatment, and cardiac drugs.* Philadelphia: W. B. Saunders.)

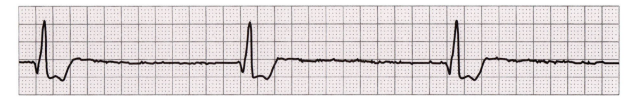

FIGURE 6-49 Idioventricular rhythm. (From Paul, S., & Hebra, J. D. [1998]. *The nurse's guide to cardiac rhythm interpretation: Implications for patient care.* Philadelphia: W. B. Saunders.)

Some patients with cardiac disease may experience idioventricular rhythm while they are sleeping. During deep sleep the metabolic demands of the body are diminished, and the heart rate decreases. If the patient is in sinus bradycardia to begin with, this further slowing can encourage competition between the SA node and the Purkinje fibers, resulting in an idioventricular rhythm. The rhythm disappears on awakening as the release of epinephrine and norepinephrine causes an increase in heart rate.

Critical Criteria for Diagnosis of Idioventricular Rhythm

- The heart rate is 15 to 40 beats per minute and regular.
- A widened QRS interval is present, usually 0.12 second or greater.
- P waves are not usually visible.

Hemodynamic effects. Hemodynamic effects vary with the idioventricular rhythm. Some patients are able to maintain adequate cardiac output and blood pressure, whereas others become hypotensive.

Accelerated Idioventricular Rhythm

Accelerated idioventricular rhythm is the same as that discussed for idioventricular rhythm, except the rate exceeds 40 beats per minute. The faster rate is the result of increased automaticity in the Purkinje fibers. This effect is most often caused by myocardial ischemia, injury, or infarction, but it can also be caused by hypokalemia, digitalis toxicity, or various forms of heart disease (Figure 6-50).

Critical Criteria for Diagnosis of Accelerated Idioventricular Rhythm

- These criteria are the same as for idioventricular rhythm, except the heart rate is greater than 40 beats per minute but less than 100 beats per minute (Fenstermacher, 1998).

Hemodynamic effects. The hemodynamic effects of accelerated idioventricular rhythm correspond to the heart rate.

Ventricular Standstill (Asystole)

Ventricular standstill is characterized by complete cessation of all electrical activity. A flat baseline is seen, without any evidence of P, Q, R, S, or T waveforms. Ventricular standstill is also called *asystole* because all contraction of the heart muscle stops (Figure 6-51).

Asystole may occur as the end result of a severe bradycardia or sinus arrest. In the evaluation of asystole, the nurse should *always* check to see that the patient's electrodes and ECG connections are intact. For patient safety, asystole should be confirmed in two leads.

Critical Criteria for Diagnosis of Ventricular Standstill (Asystole)

- A flat baseline is observed, with no evidence of P, Q, R, S, or T waveforms in two leads.

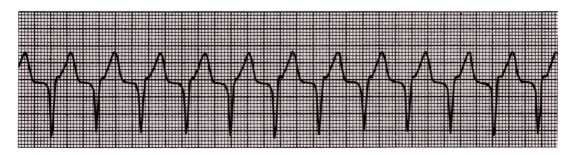

FIGURE 6-50 Accelerated idioventricular rhythm. (From Patel, J., McGowan, S., & Moody, L. [1989]. *Arrhythmias: Detection, treatment, and cardiac drugs.* Philadelphia: W. B. Saunders.)

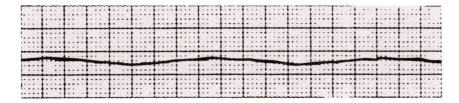

FIGURE 6-51 Ventricular standstill or asystole. (From Fenstermacher, K. [1989]. *Dysrhythmia recognition and management.* Philadelphia: W. B. Saunders.)

Hemodynamic effects. The hemodynamic effects are the same as for ventricular fibrillation. The patient loses all cardiac output, and death occurs without intervention.

ATRIOVENTRICULAR BLOCKS

AV block refers to an impairment in the conduction of impulses from the atria to the ventricles. This impairment may cause slowed conduction of impulses, intermittent blockage of impulses, or complete blockage of impulse conduction from the atria to the ventricles. The following discussion describes the most common causes of impaired impulse conduction.

Coronary artery disease. Coronary artery disease robs the AV node conduction pathway of its normal blood supply, thereby impairing impulse generation and conduction.

Infectious and inflammatory processes. Infectious and inflammatory processes can damage the AV node conduction pathway and can lead to impairment or blockage of impulses. These processes include systemic lupus erythematosus and myocarditis.

Enhanced vagal tone. When the vagus nerve is stimulated, the heart rate decreases, and a transient impairment in AV node impulse conduction may occur.

Effects of drugs. Many cardiac drugs have a negative dromotropic effect; that is, they slow down conduction of impulses from the atria to the ventricles. This is often a desired effect, in that a slower heart rate decreases the myocardial oxygen demand. However, bradycardia may cause a decrease in cardiac output.

Types. Four types of AV block exist, each categorized in terms of degree. The four types of block are first-degree, second-degree type I, second-degree type II, and third-degree. The higher the degree of block is, the more severe are the consequences. First-degree block has minimal consequences, whereas third-degree block may be life-threatening.

First-Degree Block

First-degree AV block is delayed conduction through the AV junction. It is shown on the ECG as a prolonged PR interval.

First-degree block is a common dysrhythmia in the elderly and in patients with cardiac disease. As the normal conduction pathway ages or becomes diseased, impulse conduction becomes slower than normal (Figure 6-52).

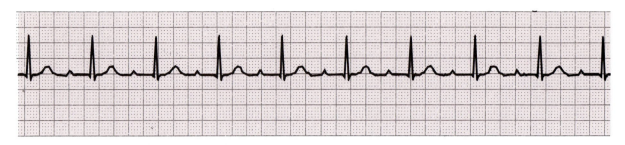

FIGURE 6-52 First-degree block. Rhythm strip generated by the AA-700 Rhythm Simulator. (Courtesy of Armstrong Medical Industries, Lincolnshire, IL.)

 Geriatric Assessment

- The sinoatrial node becomes fibrotic with aging.
- The number of pacemakers located in the sinoatrial node decreases with age.
- By age 75 years, only 10% of the normal number of pacemaker cells may remain.
- The PR interval, QRS complex, and QT interval are increased.
- The amplitude of the QRS complex is increased because of left ventricular wall thickening.
- Atrial fibrillation occurs frequently in the elderly as a result of fibrosis and cellular alteration.
- Elderly persons are susceptible to dysrhythmias.
- Peak heart rate declines with age, and elderly persons must rely on increased stroke volume to increase cardiac output.
- Elderly persons are less dependent on rapid filling of the heart, but they are more dependent on active filling (atrial kick) to maintain stroke volume and cardiac output.

Critical Criteria for the Diagnosis of First-Degree Block

- The underlying rhythm is usually normal sinus rhythm.
- The PR interval is longer than 0.20 second.
- The PR interval of each beat is the same.
- First-degree block is often accompanied by sinus bradycardia.

Hemodynamic effects. Usually, no hemodynamic changes are associated with first-degree block.

Second-Degree Block

Second-degree block refers to AV conduction that is intermittently blocked. Two types of second-degree block exist. Both types are characterized by distinctive criteria for diagnosis.

Second-Degree Block Type I: Mobitz I or Wenckebach's Phenomenon

Second-degree AV block type I usually occurs at the level of the AV node and is characterized by a steadily lengthening PR interval. The AV node becomes progressively more fatigued as it conducts each beat. Therefore, each beat takes longer to conduct through the AV node, resulting in a longer PR interval. Ultimately, the AV node is unable to conduct one or more beats. When conduction fails, a P wave is seen on the ECG that is not followed by a QRS complex. By not conducting this one beat, the AV node is able to recover and then conduct the next atrial impulse (Figure 6-53).

Critical Criteria for Diagnosis of Second-Degree Block Type I

- The PR interval progressively lengthens on a beat-by-beat basis until a P wave is not conducted. The lengthening of the PR may occur over three to four beats, or it may occur over fewer beats.
- Pauses are noted on the ECG after the nonconducted P waves.
- A pattern or group of beats appears before each missed beat.
- P to P intervals are usually regular.
- R to R intervals are usually irregular.
- QRS width is usually normal.

Hemodynamic effects. Second-degree block type I is considered a self-limiting rhythm and rarely progresses to a higher or more severe degree of block (AHA, 2002). Hemodynamic effects rarely occur unless the underlying rhythm is slow. Bradycardia with this block may result in decreased cardiac output.

Second-Degree Block Type II: Mobitz II

Second-degree block type II is a more severe form of AV block. The conduction delay occurs below the AV node, often at the level of the bundle branches. The SA node generates impulses, so P waves occur at regular intervals. In Mobitz II block, impulses are occasionally blocked, resulting in a P wave with no QRS after it (Figure 6-54). Mobitz II block is often associated with a BBB abnormal conduction through the ventricles. Second-degree block type II may progress to the more clinically significant third-degree block.

Critical Criteria for Diagnosis of Second-Degree Block Type II

- Occasional P waves are not followed by a QRS complex. These unconducted P waves may occur in a regular pattern, such as every other beat, or they may occur randomly, without a pattern.
- The PR interval of conducted beats is consistently the same, or fixed.
- The P to P interval is regular.
- The condition may be associated with a BBB.

Hemodynamic effects. The hemodynamic effects of second-degree block type II correspond to the decrease in rate caused by the nonconducted beats. The greater the number is of nonconducted beats, the greater is the impact on the cardiac output and blood pressure. Patients with second-degree block type II may require transvenous or permanent pacemaking. Patients must be observed for progression to third-degree block.

Third-Degree Block (Complete Heart Block)

Third-degree block is often called complete heart block because *no* atrial impulses are conducted down to the ventricles. The block in conduction can occur at the level of the AV node, the bundle of His, or the bundle branches.

With complete heart block, the atria and ventricles beat independently of each other. The atria beat at one rate, and the ventricles beat at a different rate. No communication exists between the two. For this reason, third-degree block is sometimes called *AV dissociation.*

In third-degree block, the atria are paced by the SA node, usually at a rate of 60 to 100 beats per minute. However, the atrial impulses are blocked from entering the ventricles. When the ventricles do not receive an impulse from the atria, either the AV node or the Purkinje fibers can generate an escape rhythm.

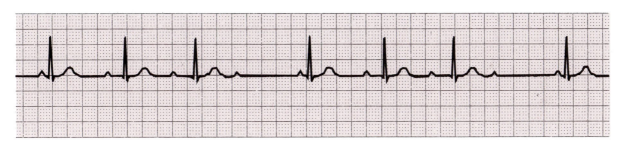

FIGURE 6-53 Second-degree block, Mobitz type I, or Wenckebach's phenomenon. Note the steadily lengthening PR interval. Rhythm strip generated by the AA-700 Rhythm Simulator. (Courtesy of Armstrong Medical Industries, Lincolnshire, IL.)

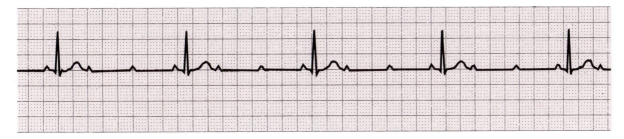

FIGURE 6-54 Second-degree block, Mobitz type II. Note the fixed PR interval. Rhythm strip generated by the AA-700 Rhythm Simulator. (Courtesy of Armstrong Medical Industries, Lincolnshire, IL.)

If the AV node becomes the secondary pacemaker, a junctional escape rhythm will be noted (Figure 6-55). A third-degree block may also be associated with a ventricular escape rhythm (Figure 6-56).

One hallmark of third-degree heart block is an abnormal sequencing of the P wave, QRS complex, and T wave. P waves are not related to the QRS complex because of the blocked conduction. Whenever a strip appears to have no consistent, predictable relationship between P waves and QRS complexes, third-degree block should be considered.

Critical Criteria for Diagnosis of Third-Degree Block (Complete Heart Block)

- A difference exists between the atrial and ventricular heart rates. The atrial rate is usually greater than the ventricular rate.
- The P to P intervals are regular.
- The R to R intervals are regular.
- No true PR interval exists.
- P waves are not related to the QRS complex.
- Either a junctional or a ventricular escape rhythm is present.

Hemodynamic effects. The hemodynamic effects of third-degree block depend on the ventricular rate.

Transcutaneous pacing is often warranted for symptomatic third-degree block.

Interventions for Dysrhythmias

Rhythms must be treated if the patient has symptoms of decreased cardiac output. Serious signs and symptoms include chest pain, shortness of breath, decreased level of consciousness, hypotension, shock, pulmonary congestion, and heart failure. Treatments for dysrhythmias are addressed in depth in Chapter 11.

TACHYDYSRHYTHMIAS

Treatment of symptomatic tachycardia may include the following:

1. The effects of the sympathetic nervous system are mediated through stress reduction techniques, avoiding caffeine and nicotine, and relief of pain.
2. Vagal maneuvers are used to stimulate the parasympathetic nervous system (and slow the heart rate). Carotid massage and the Valsalva maneuver are two strategies for stimulating the vagus nerve. To perform carotid massage, the physician exerts gentle, downward pressure on one carotid artery. The procedure can lead to cerebral insufficiency in patients with carotid occlusive

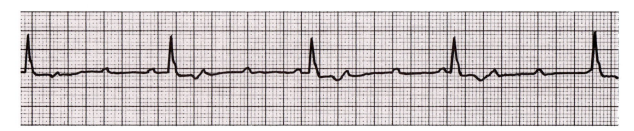

FIGURE 6-55 Third-degree block with junctional escape. (From Patel, J., McGowan, S., & Moody, L. [1989]. *Arrhythmias: Detection, treatment, and cardiac drugs.* Philadelphia: W. B. Saunders.)

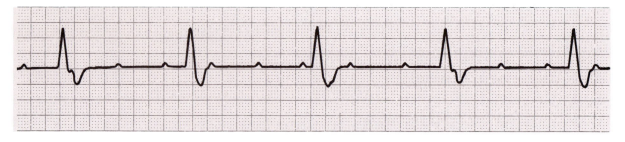

FIGURE 6-56 Third-degree block with ventricular escape. Rhythm strip generated by the AA-700 Rhythm Simulator. (Courtesy Armstrong Medical Industries, Lincolnshire, IL.)

disease, so the patient's neurological status must be closely monitored. The Valsalva maneuver is performed by asking the patient to "bear down." Vagal maneuvers are done under the order of a physician. As vagal maneuvers are performed, the cardiac rhythm is closely monitored for the rhythm to return to a more normal rate. If the rhythm does not respond to vagal stimulation, medications and or electrical cardioversion may be needed.

3. Intervention with appropriate cardiac drugs (See Table 6-1; also see Chapter 11).
4. Electrical energy (cardioversion or defibrillation) is used to convert the rhythm to a slower, more normal rhythm. Recurrent life-threatening tachycardia may need to be treated with an implantable cardioverter-defibrillator (ICD), a permanent device.
5. Overdrive cardiac pacing is used to interrupt a rapid rhythm.
6. Radiofrequency ablation is used to destroy abnormal pathways in the conduction system.

BRADYDYSRHYTHMIAS

Treatment of symptomatic bradycardia may include the following:

1. The parasympathetic nervous system is suppressed (and the heart rate is increased). Strategies include avoiding activities that increase vagal tone, such as vomiting, gagging, Valsalva maneuver, or endotracheal suctioning.
2. Intervening with appropriate cardiac drugs, such as atropine and epinephrine.
3. Cardiac pacing is used.

ELECTRICAL PACEMAKERS

An electrical pacemaker delivers electrical current to stimulate depolarization. A pacemaker may be required to treat symptomatic bradycardia; second-degree block type II and third-degree block often require the use of pacemakers. Pacemakers can also be set at a fast rate to overdrive or interrupt a symptomatic tachycardia. The need for the pacemaker may be temporary (e.g., after an acute myocardial infarction or cardiac surgery) or permanent. Battery-operated, external pulse generators are used to provide electrical energy for temporary pacemakers. Internal pulse generators with long-life batteries provide electrical stimulation for permanent pacing.

Methods for temporary pacing include the following:

- Transthoracic: Electrical stimulation is delivered through external electrode pads connected to an external pacemaker or pacemaker-defibrillator (see Chapter 9).

- Transvenous: A pacemaker catheter is inserted into the right ventricle, where it contacts the endocardium near the ventricular septum; it is connected to a small external pulse generator.
- Epicardial: Pacing wires are inserted into the epicardial wall of the heart during cardiac surgery; wires are brought through the chest wall and can be connected to a pulse generator if needed.

Methods for permanent pacing include transvenous and epicardial. Transvenous pacing is more commonly used. Some implantable cardioverter-defibrillators also have pacemaker capabilities and are known as pacemaker cardioverter-defibrillators.

Pacemakers may be used to stimulate the atrium, ventricle, or both chambers (dual-chamber pacemakers). Atrial pacing is used to mimic normal conduction and to produce the atrial kick. Ventricular pacing stimulates ventricular contraction; it is commonly used in emergency situations. Dual-chamber pacing allows for stimulation of both atria and ventricle as needed to produce a near-normal cardiac contraction.

Permanent pacemakers have the ability to be programmed in a variety of ways. The International Commission on Heart Disease Code is a method for programming pacemakers; it is described in Chapter 11. It is important to know the programming information for the pacemaker to assess proper functioning on the rhythm strip. Other terms used in describing pacemaker function are *rate, mode, electrical output, sensitivity, sense-pace indicator*, and *AV interval*.

1. The rate control determines the number of impulses delivered per minute to the atrium and/or the ventricle. The rate is set to produce effective cardiac output and to reduce symptoms.
2. Pacemakers can be operated in a demand mode or asynchronous mode. The demand mode paces the heart based on need. For example, the rate control is set at 60 beats per minute. The pacemaker will generate a beat only if the patient's rate drops to less than 60. The asynchronous mode paces the heart at a set rate, independent of any activity the patient's heart generates. The asynchronous mode may compete with the patient's own rhythm and deliver an impulse on the T wave (R on T), with the potential for producing ventricular tachycardia or fibrillation. The demand mode is safer and is the mode of choice.
3. The electrical output is the amount of electrical energy needed to stimulate depolarization. The output is measured in milliamperes (mA). The numbers of milliamperes varies. Transthoracic pacing requires many more milliamperes than transvenous or epicardial pacing, because the electrical energy must be delivered through the chest wall.

4. The sensitivity is the ability of the pacemaker to recognize the body's intrinsic electrical activity (heartbeat). It is measured in millivolts (mV). Some temporary generators have a sense-pace indicator. When the generator delivers a paced beat, the "pace" light comes on. If the generator detects the patient's own beat, the "sense" indicator should light. Temporary generators have dials for adjusting sensitivity.

5. The AV indicator is used to determine the interval between atrial and ventricular stimulation. It is used only in dual-chamber pacemakers.

Pacemaker rhythms. Pacemaker rhythms are usually easy to note on the cardiac monitor or rhythm strip. The electrical stimulation is noted by an electrical artifact called the pacer spike. If the atrium is paced, the spike appears before the P wave (Figure 6-57). If the ventricle is paced, the spike appears before the QRS complex (Figure 6-58). If both the atrium and ventricle are paced, spikes will be noted before both the P wave and the QRS complex (Figure 6-59). The heart rate is carefully assessed on the rhythm strip. The rate should not be lower than the rate set on the pacemaker.

The pacemaker spike is followed by a larger than normal P wave in atrial pacing or a widened QRS complex in ventricular pacing. Because the heart is paced in an artificial or abnormal fashion, the path of depolarization is altered, resulting in waveforms and intervals that are also altered.

Pacemaker malfunction. Three primary problems can occur with a temporary pacemaker. These problems include failure to pace, failure to capture, and failure to sense.

Failure to pace. Failure to pace occurs when the pacemaker fails to initiate an electrical stimulus when the pacemaker is due to fire. It is noted by absence of pacer spikes on the rhythm strip. Causes of failure to pace include battery or pulse generator failure, fracture or displacement of pacemaker wire, loose connections, or electromagnetic interference.

Failure to capture. When the pacemaker generates an electrical impulse (pacer spike) and no depolarization is noted, it is known as failure to capture. On the ECG, a pacer spike is noted, but it is not followed

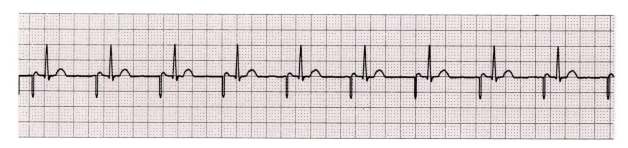

FIGURE 6-57 Paced rhythm: atrial. Note the spike in front of the P wave. Rhythm strip generated by the AA-700 Rhythm Simulator. (Courtesy of Armstrong Medical Industries, Lincolnshire, IL.)

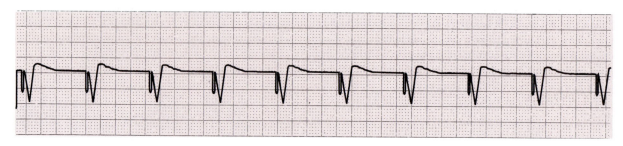

FIGURE 6-58 Paced rhythm: ventricular. Note the spike in front of the QRS complex. Rhythm strip generated by the AA-700 Rhythm Simulator. (Courtesy of Armstrong Medical Industries, Lincolnshire, IL.)

by a P wave (atrial pacemaker) or a QRS complex (ventricular pacemaker) (Figure 6-60). Common causes of failure to capture include output (mA) set too low or displacement of pacing lead wire from the myocardium (transvenous or epicardial leads). Other causes of failure to capture include battery failure, fracture of the pacemaker wire, or increased pacing threshold as a result of drugs or electrolyte imbalance. Adjusting the milliamperes and placing the patient on his or her left side are nursing interventions to treat failure to capture. Turning the patient onto the left side facilitates contact of a transvenous pacing wire with the endocardium and septum.

Failure to sense. When the pacemaker does not sense the patient's own cardiac rhythm and initiates an electrical impulse, it is called failure to sense. Failure to sense manifests as pacer spikes that fall too closely to the patient's own rhythm, earlier than the programmed rate (Figure 6-61). The most common

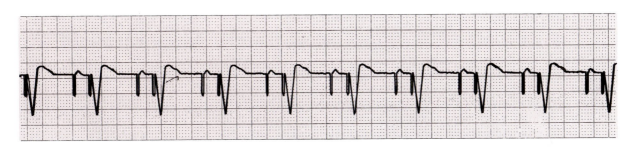

FIGURE 6-59 Paced rhythm: dual chamber. Note the spikes before the P wave and the QRS complex. Rhythm strip generated by the AA-700 Rhythm Simulator. (Courtesy of Armstrong Medical Industries, Lincolnshire, IL.)

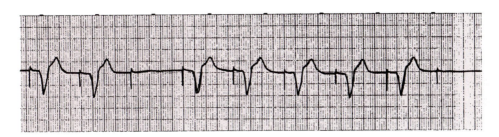

FIGURE 6-60 Paced rhythm with failure to capture. (From Smith, L. F., & Fish, F. H. [1995]. *Pure practice for ECGs.* Philadelphia: W. B. Saunders.)

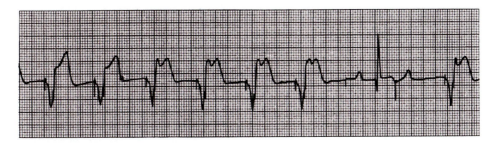

FIGURE 6-61 Paced rhythm with failure to capture (seventh spike) and failure to sense (eighth spike). (From Smith, L. F., & Fish, F. H. [1995]. *Pure practice for ECGs.* Philadelphia: W. B. Saunders.)

cause is displacement of the electrode. Repositioning the patient (left side) and adjusting the sensitivity are nursing interventions when failure to sense occurs.

Biventricular Pacemaker

Biventricular pacemaker implantation, also known as *cardiac resynchronization therapy,* can produce dramatic results in patients who suffer from advanced congestive heart failure. Those with advanced heart failure can exhibit interventricular conduction delay also known as *ventricular dyssnychrony.* This results in an abnormal contraction of the heart along with abnormal septal wall motion, reduced cardiac contractility, decreased diastolic filling time, and mitral regurgitation. Increased morbidity and mortality have been reported with these abnormalities. In addition, these patients have a high propensity for conduction disturbances that can result in sudden cardiac death from ventricular tachycardia or ventricular fibrillation.

Right and left pacemaker wires are placed in the heart. One pacing wire is placed in the right ventricle. The other is skillfully placed in the outside of the left posterior ventricular wall by way of the tortuous coronary sinus (Figure 6-62). Results are often immediate, with patients experiencing improvement within a day of the procedure (Figure 6-63). This

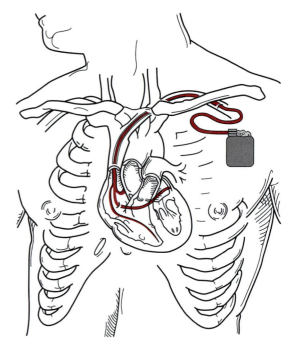

FIGURE 6-62 Biventricular pacing with wires of the right atrium/ventricle and left ventricle. (Courtesy of Guidant Corporation, St. Paul, MN.)

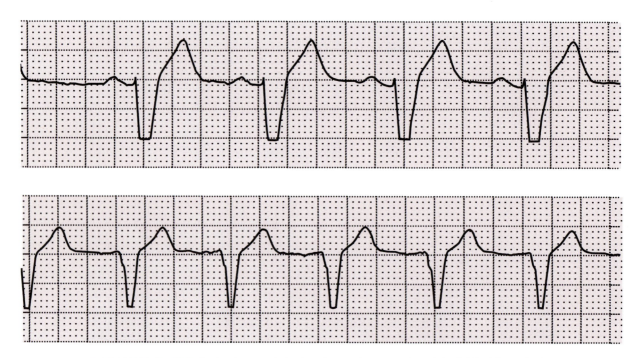

FIGURE 6-63 Patient's actual rhythm (top strip, note the wide QRS). Biventricular pacing of left and right ventricle (bottom strip, note the QRS is not as wide as the top strip). (Courtesy of Guidant Corporation, St. Paul, MN.)

device not only helps the heart to pump more effectively, but it also treats life-threatening heart rhythms.

SUMMARY

ECG interpretation is a basic skill that develops only through practice. For the beginning student, the critical criteria for diagnosis provide the structure by which rhythms are analyzed. Initial effort should be the memorization of these criteria. It is hoped that this chapter will be a valuable reference in the delivery of high-quality care to patients with cardiac dysrhythmias and to their families.

Nursing Care Plan

NURSING DIAGNOSIS: *Alteration in Tissue Perfusion Related to Dysrhythmia*

Patient Outcomes	Interventions	Rationales

Adequate tissue perfusion as evidenced by usual mental status, normal vital signs, urine output greater than 30 mL/hr, warm and dry skin, and absence of dysrhythmias.	Monitor for signs and symptoms of dysrhythmias:
	  Abnormal rate, rhythm
	  Palpitations, syncope
	  Hemodynamic compromise, hypotension
		Myocardial ischemia reduces oxygen to myocardial tissue. Ischemic tissue is electrically unstable tissue causing dysrhythmias that could potentially lead to lethal dysrhythmias and death. Additionally, dysrhythmias can occur secondary to reperfusion of ischemic tissue after medical intervention.

	Monitor:
	  Fluids and electrolytes: potassium, magnesium, phosphorus, and calcium as ordered
	  Acute ST-segment changes
		Electrolytes are crucial in electrophysiology; abnormalities can result in dysrhythmias.
		Patients with acute coronary syndrome do not always exhibit classic symptoms of myocardial tissue compromise; therefore, early acute ST-segment changes can be picked up on the electrocardiographic monitor for early intervention (time is muscle).

	Cardiac enzymes	These enzymes are diagnostic markers that injury to myocardial tissues has occurred.
	Continued electrocardiographic monitoring in the appropriate leads	Early detection and intervention of dysrhythmias and ST-segment changes are the goals.
	Maintain oxygen therapy as ordered	Increase the supply of oxygen to myocardial tissue.

CRITICAL THINKING QUESTIONS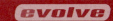

1. You are working in the intensive care unit, and your patient's heart rate suddenly decreases from 88 to 50 beats per minute. What may be some of the reasons for decreased heart rate? What assessments will you make?

2. Discuss why patients with pulmonary disease are prone to atrial dysrhythmias.

3. A 65-year-old woman with type 2 diabetes presents to the emergency department; she is short of breath and complaining of neck and shoulder pain. Her blood pressure is 185/95, and her heart rate is 155.
   a. How will you initially manage this patient?
   b. What medical intervention would you anticipate?
   c. List serious signs and symptoms of hemodynamic instability in a patient with a tachycardia dysrhythmia.

4. Why does tachycardia sometimes lead to heart failure?

REFERENCES

American Heart Association. (2002). *Textbook of advanced cardiac life support.* Dallas, TX: Author.

Conover, M. B. (2003). *Understanding electrocardiography: Arrhythmias and the 12-lead ECG.* 8th ed. St. Louis: Mosby.

Drew, B. (2002). Celebrating the 100th birthday of the electrocardiogram: Lessons learned from research in cardiac monitoring. *American Journal of Critical Care, 11,* 378-386.

Fenstermacher, K. (1998). *Dysrhythmia recognition and management.* Philadelphia, PA: W. B. Saunders.

McKinley, M. G., Pelter, M. M., & Adams, M. G.(2001). *AACN procedure manual for critical care.* 4th ed. Philadelphia: W. B. Saunders.

Porth, C. M. (2002). *Pathophysiology: Concepts of altered health states.* 6th ed. Philadelphia: Lippincott Williams & Wilkins.

Wyse, D. G., Waldo, A. L, et al., & AFFIRM Investigators (2002). A comparison of rate control and rhythm control in patients with atrial fibrillation. *New England Journal of Medicine, 347*(23), 1825-1832.

RECOMMENDED READINGS

Aehlert, B. (2001). *ECGs made easy.* St. Louis, MO: Mosby.

Albert, N. M. (2003). Biventricular pacing in patients with heart failure and ventricular dyssynchrony. *Critical Care Nurse, 23*(3), 2-15.

Copstead, L. C., & Banasik, J. L. (2003). *Pathophysiology: Biological and behavioral perspectives.* Philadelphia: W. B. Saunders.

Drew, B. J., & Krucoff, M. W. (1999). Multilead ST-segment monitoring in patients with acute coronary syndromes: A consensus statement for healthcare professionals. ST-Segment Monitoring Practice Guideline International Working Group. *American Journal of Critical Care, 8,* 372-386.

Leeper, B. (2003). Continuous ST-segment monitoring. *AACN Clinical Issues, 14*(2), 145-154.

Shlafer, M. (2002). *The nurse, pharmacology, and drug therapy: A prototype approach.* 2nd ed. New York: Addison-Wesley Nursing.

evolve *Did you remember to check out the bonus material, including free self-assessment exercises, on the Evolve Web site at http://evolve.elsevier.com/Sole/ and on the CD-ROM?*

CHAPTER 7

Hemodynamic Monitoring

Marthe J. Moseley, PhD, RN, CCRN, CCNS
Lori A. Czekaj, MSN, RN
Marcia E. Abbott, MSN, RN, CCNS-AC

OBJECTIVES

- Identify the physiological basis for hemodynamic monitoring in critically ill patients.
- Describe the indications, measurement, complications, and nursing implications associated with invasive monitoring of right atrial, left atrial, pulmonary artery, and intraarterial pressures and those associated with noninvasive monitoring of hemodynamic indices.
- Identify the normal values of the aforementioned pressures.
- Analyze the conditions that alter hemodynamic values.
- Articulate appropriate nursing actions for patients with alterations in hemodynamic values.
- Discuss the rationale and methods for continuous monitoring of mixed venous oxygen saturation.
- Explain the clinical relevance and methods of measuring cardiac output.

Introduction

An initial exposure to the critical care environment may be rather mystifying. The complicated equipment, including digital readouts, waveforms, and ever-changing sequences of alarms and the tangle of wires, tubings, and cables may at first seem impossible to comprehend. However, even when the technical equipment and data obtained are well understood, technology serves only to augment patient care and does not detract from a holistic perspective. Viewing the patient as a person first and using the equipment as merely an adjunct should be the focus in critical care.

Much of the equipment used in the critical care setting is for the purpose of hemodynamic monitoring. The term *hemodynamics* refers to the interrelationship of the various dynamic forces that affect the blood's circulation through the body. Development of a working knowledge of the concepts of *pressure, flow,* and *resistance* provides the foundation for this understanding. Insight into the factors affecting the heart's ability to pump effectively is also essential. This chapter discusses the basic principles of hemodynamics, the role of the heart as a pump, and hemodynamic monitoring. Essential nursing considerations for patients who are being hemodynamically monitored are also introduced.

Review of Anatomy and Physiology

CARDIOVASCULAR SYSTEM

The cardiovascular system is a closed, fluid-filled system consisting of the heart, blood vessels, and blood. This system allows for the transport of oxygen,

evolve **Be sure to check out the bonus material, including free self-assessment exercises, on the Evolve Web site at http://evolve.elsevier.com/Sole/ and on the CD-ROM.**

nutrients, and hormones to the tissues, and for the removal of metabolic waste, in direct response to the metabolic needs of the body (Darovic, 2002).

- The heart pumps the blood forward through the vasculature.
- The arteries provide a conduit to carry oxygenated blood from the heart to the rest of the body. Based on the metabolic need of the tissue, arteries and their smaller arteriole branches constrict and dilate to regulate the amount of blood flow delivered.
- Capillaries are microscopic vessels that allow for exchange of gases, nutrients, and metabolic waste products between the plasma and the body cells.
- Veins are vessels that return deoxygenated blood back to the heart. Approximately 70% of the circulating blood volume is in the venous system at any one time. Venous constriction or dilation affects the amount of blood returned to the heart.
- Blood has both a fluid and a cellular component. About 60% of the blood is plasma. Plasma provides the liquid medium in which respiratory gases, nutrients, metabolic waste, and hormones are dissolved. The remainder of blood consists of cellular components, such as erythrocytes (red blood cells), leukocytes (white blood cells), and platelets. Erythrocytes make up approximately 99% of the cellular components and transport oxygen, in the form of oxyhemoglobin, to the tissues. An increase in blood cells in relation to the amount of plasma causes the blood to be "thicker," or more viscous. Increased viscosity makes blood flow through small vessels more difficult.

PRESSURE, FLOW, AND RESISTANCE

To understand hemodynamics and hemodynamic monitoring, it is important to understand a basic law of physics:

$$Pressure = Flow \times Resistance$$

Pressure in a liquid system is the force exerted on the liquid per unit of area. It is measured in dynes per square centimeter (dynes/cm^2), millimeters of mercury (mm Hg), or torr. In the body, blood flow depends partly on the difference in pressure between arterial and venous vessels. One example is the way that blood moves from areas of higher pressure on the arterial side to areas of lower pressure on the venous side. Another example is how blood flows from the atria to the ventricles during the cardiac cycle.

Blood flow is the amount of fluid moved per unit of time. It is usually measured in liters or milliliters per minute (L/min or mL/min) or in cubic centimeters per second (cm^3/sec).

Resistance is the opposition to force or flow. Resistance is influenced by the size (radius) of the vessel, the length of the vessel, and the viscosity (thickness) of the fluid traveling through the vessel. The way blood vessels are aligned, end to end—as occurs with the arteries, or parallel—or in a series, as in the capillary beds, will also influence resistance and flow.

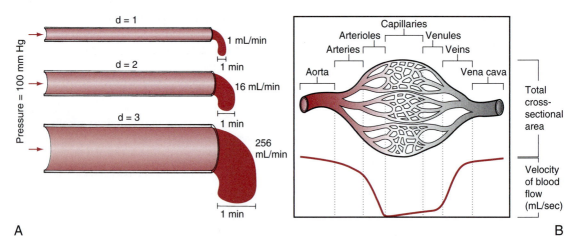

FIGURE 7-1 Lumen diameter, blood flow, and resistance. **A,** Effect of lumen diameter on flow through vessel. d, Diameter. **B,** Blood flows with great speed in the large arteries. However, branching of arterial vessels increases the total cross-sectional areas of the arterioles and capillaries, thus reducing the flow rate. (**A,** From McCance, K., & Huether, S. [2002]. *Pathophysiology: The biologic basis for disease in adults and children* [p. 959]. 4th ed. St. Louis: Mosby. **B,** From Thibodeau, G., & Patton, K. [2004]. *Anatomy and physiology.* 5th ed. St. Louis: Mosby.)

The lumen size of the blood vessels, constricting or dilating in response to sympathetic nervous system innervation, chemical mediators, and hormones, will also affect size. Small changes in the size of the lumen can lead to large changes in vascular resistance and blood flow (Figure 7-1). Additionally, a change in blood viscosity will affect flow. For example, conditions that increase hematocrit increase resistance and decrease flow.

The human circulatory system is actually one continuous circuit (Figure 7-2). Under normal conditions, the system contains a volume of blood that remains relatively constant. When the body's metabolic demands increase, blood needs to be circulated more quickly through the circuit to meet those demands. Likewise, when the body is at rest and its demands are reduced, some of the blood volume is stored (in veins) within the circulatory system itself.

REGULATION OF BLOOD FLOW

To meet metabolic demands, the body uses several mechanisms to regulate the flow of blood (Figure 7-3). The first mechanism involves the ability of blood vessels to change their diameter or lumen size. The walls of the vessels, particularly the veins, have the ability to constrict or dilate according to need. For example, in response to increased demands, the veins constrict. As a result, more blood is forced back to the heart. It then passes through the lungs, where it is reoxygenated, and it is returned to the heart to be pumped out to the tissues. Likewise, when the body is at rest and demands are reduced, the veins become dilated. As their diameter increases, the veins are able to accommodate a larger volume of blood. In this way, veins serve as a reservoir, and a smaller volume of blood is returned to the heart, reducing the cardiac workload. Circulation is accomplished efficiently because only the amount of blood required to meet the demand is being pumped by the heart.

Two other mechanisms that control blood flow involve the heart's ability to control heart rate (HR) and strength of contraction (contractility). These mechanisms are regulated by a complex interaction between the autonomic and central nervous systems in conjunction with input from the circulatory and endocrine systems. The kidneys also play a role in regulating circulation by mechanisms that adjust blood pressure and blood volume through the renin-angiotensin system.

CARDIAC CYCLE

Knowledge of the cardiac cycle assists in understanding how the heart, as a pump, moves blood forward through the body. The heart is a four-chambered

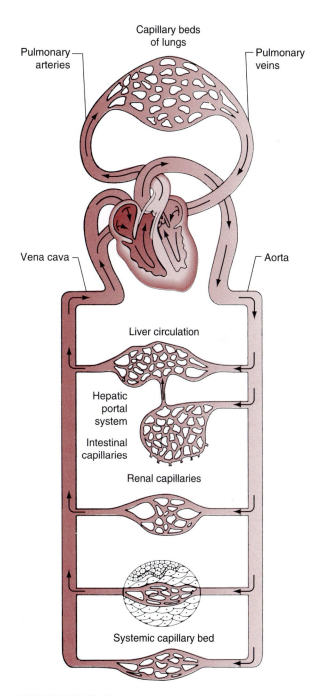

FIGURE 7-2 Illustration depicting the closed circuit, composed of the pulmonary circulation and systemic circulation, which includes portal, intestinal, and renal circulations. (From Hansen, M. [1998]. *Pathophysiology* [p. 340]. Philadelphia W. B. Saunders.)

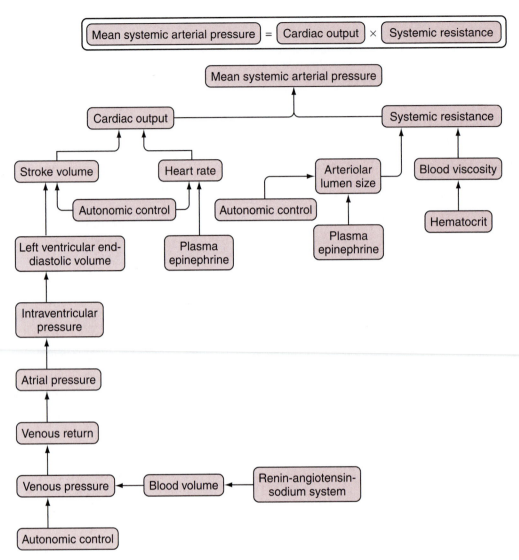

FIGURE 7-3 Mechanisms that regulate systemic arterial pressure. (Data from Widmaier, E. P., Raff, H., Strang, K. T. [2003]. *Vander, Sherman, & Luciano's Human physiology.* 9th ed. New York: McGraw-Hill.)

pump, consisting of two atria and two ventricles. Functionally, the right side of the heart and the left side of the heart serve as two pumps in a series, each with a separate and distinct circulation (Darovic, 2002). Although both the atria and the ventricles have phases of filling (diastole) and contraction (systole), it is most meaningful to look at the cardiac cycle in relation to the ventricles. During ventricular *diastole,* the left and right ventricles receive blood from the atria. During ventricular *systole,* the ventricles contract, squeezing blood out of the heart through the aorta and pulmonary artery (PA). Diastole occurs

simultaneously in the left and right sides of the heart, as does systole. The flow of blood through the heart, and normal intrachamber pressures during systole and diastole, are illustrated in Figure 7-4.

After supplying oxygen to the tissues, deoxygenated blood is collected by the systemic veins. Venous blood from the peripheral circulation enters the right atrium of the heart through the superior and inferior vena cava. During diastole, as the right atrium begins to fill with blood, the tricuspid valve is closed. As the right atrium fills more completely, right atrial pressure (RAP) becomes higher than right

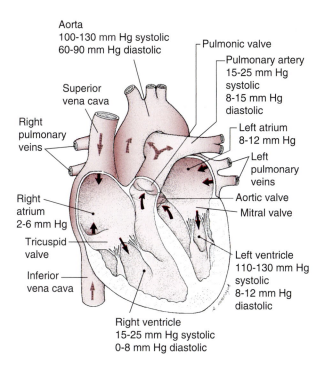

Aorta
100-130 mm Hg systolic
60-90 mm Hg diastolic

Pulmonic valve

Pulmonary artery
15-25 mm Hg
systolic
8-15 mm Hg
diastolic

Superior
vena cava

Right
pulmonary
veins

Left atrium
8-12 mm Hg

Left
pulmonary
veins

Aortic valve

Mitral valve

Right
atrium
2-6 mm Hg

Tricuspid
valve

Inferior
vena cava

Left ventricle
110-130 mm Hg
systolic
8-12 mm Hg
diastolic

Right ventricle
15-25 mm Hg systolic
0-8 mm Hg diastolic

FIGURE 7-4 Normal blood flow through the heart and intrachamber pressures; *arrows* indicate the normal direction of blood flow. This schematic representation of the heart shows all four chambers and valves visible in the anterior view to facilitate conceptualization of blood flow. (From Darovic, G. [2002]. *Hemodynamic monitoring: Invasive and noninvasive clinical application* [p. 64]. 3rd ed. St. Louis: Mosby.)

ventricular pressure (RVP). This pressure difference forces the tricuspid valve to open. Blood then rushes from the right atrium into the right ventricle.

As the right ventricle fills with blood from the right atrium, pressure within the atrium drops, whereas pressure within the ventricle rises. The final phase of right atrial systole occurs and the right atrium contracts, (referred to as *atrial kick*), ejecting blood into the right ventricle to fill it. As this occurs, RVP surpasses RAP and causes the tricuspid valve to snap closed, thus preventing additional blood from entering the right ventricle.

During ventricular systole, the right ventricle begins to contract, increasing intraventricular pressure. When the pressure rises sufficiently to overcome the pressure exerted distally on the pulmonic valve, the valve opens. Blood is ejected out of the right ventricle into the PA. In turn, blood travels through the pulmonary circulation and is oxygenated at the level of the capillaries and alveoli. Oxygenated blood is transported back to the heart through the pulmonary veins.

Oxygenated blood from the pulmonary circulation enters the left atrium during atrial diastole. At this time, the mitral valve is closed. As the left atrium fills, left atrial pressure (LAP) exceeds left ventricular pressure. The pressure difference forces the mitral valve to open, and blood then rushes into the left ventricle. As the left ventricle begins to fill, the final phase of left atrial systole occurs (atrial kick) and the left atrium contracts, ejecting blood to fill the left ventricle.

Left ventricular pressure (LVP) now transcends LAP, and it causes the mitral valve to snap closed and prevents additional blood from entering the left ventricle. The amount of blood in the left ventricle at this phase in the cardiac cycle is known as the *left ventricular end-diastolic volume.* This volume is significant because it determines the amount of blood that is ejected into the systemic circulation. The left ventricular end-diastolic volume is commonly referred to as *preload* and is described in further detail in a later section.

During systole, the left ventricle contracts, elevating the LVP to such a degree that it overcomes the pressure exerted on the aortic valve from the systemic circulation. Oxygenated blood is ejected from the left ventricle through the aorta into the systemic circulation, where it ultimately supplies the tissues with oxygen.

The volume of blood that is ejected with each heart beat is referred to as the *stroke volume* (SV). The volume that remains in the left ventricle at the end of diastole is the left ventricular end-diastolic volume. The left ventricle never ejects its entire end-diastolic volume. It merely ejects a fraction of this volume, known as the *ejection fraction* (EF), which is normally 60% to 70% of the total ventricular volume.

CARDIAC OUTPUT AND SYSTEMIC VASCULAR RESISTANCE

In the body, the relationship among pressure, flow, and resistance can be explored by looking at the relationship of systemic arterial blood pressure with cardiac output (CO; flow) and systemic vascular resistance (SVR).

Arterial blood pressure = CO (flow) × SVR (resistance)

Arterial blood pressure is a measure of the force that is exerted on the arterial walls by the blood contained within the arterial system (Darovic, 2002). Arterial tone and characteristics of the blood determine the resistance to blood flow. The pulsatile nature of the blood flow is created by the systolic and diastolic cycles of the heart. Normal systolic pressures for an adult range from 100 to 130 mm Hg. Normal adult diastolic pressure ranges from 60 to 90 mm Hg. The mean arterial pressure indicates the average perfusion pressure throughout the cardiac cycle.

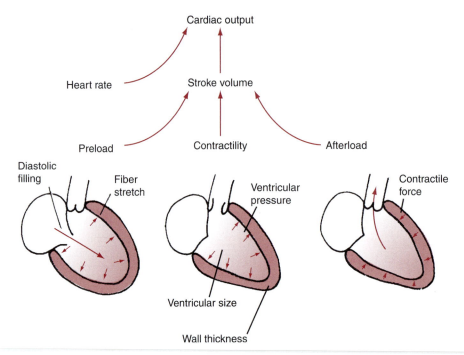

FIGURE 7-5 Factors affecting cardiac output. (From Price, S., & Wilson, L. [2003]. *Pathophysiology: Clinical concepts of disease processes.* 6th ed. St. Louis: Mosby.)

CO is the volume of blood ejected from the heart per minute. Anything that can affect the HR, the SV, or both, affects the CO. A normal range for CO at rest is 4 to 8 L/min. Cardiac index (CI) is the CO divided by body surface area. It is often used because it takes into consideration a person's body size. The normal range is 2.5 to 4.0 L/min/m². Figure 7-5 illustrates factors that affect CO. Physiologically, the CO is equal to the HR times the SV. HR is the number of beats per minute.

SV is defined as the volume of blood ejected by the heart per contraction (each beat). SV is influenced by three variables: (1) preload, (2) afterload, and (3) contractility.

Preload. *Preload* is defined as the amount of muscle fiber stretch before the next contraction. This muscle fiber stretch (also known as the *presystolic fiber length*) is directly affected by the end-diastolic volume in the ventricles. Increased volume, which leads to increased pressure, increases the stretch of the muscle fibers. Thus, preload is defined clinically in terms of either the ventricular end-diastolic volume or pressure. Another important factor that influences SV is that within physiological limits, ventricular contraction is stronger as the muscle fiber stretch (preload) increases. This phenomenon, referred to as the *Frank-Starling principle,* describes the influence of

presystolic fiber length on CO and SV. Clinically, a decrease in a patient's preload (decrease in end-diastolic volume) decreases stretch on the left ventricular wall, often resulting in decreased contractility, decreased SV, and decreased CO.

Afterload. *Afterload* is the pressure or resistance to blood flow out of the ventricle. This pressure or resistance must be overcome for the ventricle to eject its SV. Arterial blood pressure is the principal factor that offers resistance to this blood flow out of the ventricles. If the arterial blood pressure is high, the left ventricle must exert more force to pump blood out of its chamber effectively. Additional energy is required to generate enough pressure or force to eject this blood. This additional energy requirement also increases the oxygen requirements of the myocardial tissue. Clinically, an increase in afterload may cause a decrease in SV, especially if the left ventricle is unable to generate enough force to overcome this resistance.

Contractility. *Contractility,* the third variable affecting SV, is a measure of how forcefully the ventricle contracts to eject its SV. Contractility is the intrinsic ability of the muscle fibers to shorten. How much (extent) and how fast (velocity) these fibers shorten also affect SV. For example, if the ventricular fibers can shorten effectively and rapidly, the rate of pressure rise in the ventricle during systole is able to exceed the arterial blood pressure, resulting in a rapid forceful ejection of SV. Conversely, if the ventricular fibers lose their strength of contraction, the SV decreases.

Systemic vascular resistance (often referred to as *SVR*) is the opposition to blood flow exerted by the blood vessels. SVR is affected by blood viscosity, vascular tone, and friction imposed by the inner lining of the blood vessels. In the clinical setting, a patient's blood pressure may decrease from 136/70 to 80/50 mm Hg. The decrease in blood pressure has occurred because either the flow (CO) has been reduced or the resistance (SVR) has decreased. Conversely, if this patient's blood pressure increases to 190/90 mm Hg, either the CO or the SVR has increased.

A major factor that influences SVR is the lumen size (diameter) of the vessel. For example, if the lumen size narrows, the SVR increases, and vice versa. In the critical care setting, vasoactive drugs are often used to alter the lumen size of the systemic vessels (predominantly the arterioles), with the aim of either decreasing or increasing blood pressure. SVR also changes as a compensatory response to changes in blood pressure. For example, a perceived drop in blood pressure will initiate a sympathetic response, which causes systemic vasoconstriction and increases the SVR. Systemic vasodilation (decreased SVR) occurs in a resting state in response to decreased metabolic and cardiac demands.

Patient Assessment Using Hemodynamic Monitoring

EQUIPMENT

All hemodynamic monitoring equipment contains the following basic components: (1) transducer, (2) monitor, and (3) fluid-filled catheter, tubing, and flush system (Figure 7-6).

The *transducer* is an instrument that is used to sense physiological events and to transform them into electrical signals. Transducers come in many shapes and sizes and are disposable. Some of the physiological events commonly measured by a transducer are pressure, flow, temperature, light intensity, and sound. Housed within the pressure monitor are the amplifier and the display instrument. The *amplifier* connects to the transducer by an electrical cable. It functions by picking up the electrical signal from the transducer and amplifying it while also filtering out interference signals. The improved signal is then transmitted to an instrument where it can be displayed.

Monitors or display instruments are used to record or provide a display of the original signal. The signal may be seen as a waveform or a digital readout. The method generally used to monitor hemodynamic pressures is to display a pressure waveform and a digital reading of the pressure values on a multichannel bedside monitor.

The third component for hemodynamic monitoring is the *fluid-filled catheter, tubing, and flush system.* This system is composed of a catheter that may be inserted into an artery, a vein, or a heart chamber, depending on the type of hemodynamic monitoring required. The catheter is attached to rigid, noncompliant tubing that is ideally less than 48 inches long, which is then attached to some type of flush device that controls flow of solution through the tubing. A flush solution of normal saline that may contain heparin is used to keep the tubing and catheter patent and free of blood clots. This solution is delivered through a tubing system surrounded by an inflatable pressure bag (to 300 mm Hg). The pressure bag is necessary to drive the flow of fluid through the tubing and catheter at a continuous flow rate of 3 to 5 mL/hour.

The use of heparin to avoid clot formation and to promote catheter patency was investigated by the American Association of Critical-Care Nurses (AACN) in the Thunder Project I, a national multicenter nursing research study that was designed to evaluate the effect of heparinized and nonheparinized flush solutions on the patency of arterial pressure lines. The results of this study showed that heparin significantly affects the patency of arterial pressure lines. Variables that were found to promote patency in this study included (1) heparinized flush solutions, (2) arterial catheters longer than 2 inches, (3) femoral placement of arterial catheters, (4) anticoagulant or thrombolytic therapy, and (5) male gender (AACN, 1993).

The equipment must be standardized to obtain reliable measurements. For this purpose, the transducers used for monitoring hemodynamic pressures must be zeroed and leveled.

"Zero referencing" is performed to eliminate the influence of surrounding air pressure on the monitoring system. To control for this variable, the stopcock (air-fluid interface on the flush system) is turned so the patient's pressure is no longer being displayed, and the equipment senses only environmental pressures. Once a straight line appears on the display screen, the *zero* button is depressed to balance the system. In this manner, atmospheric pressure is negated, even though it actually measures about 760 mm Hg at sea level. The critical care nurse often says the phrase "off to the patient, open to air" and then depresses the zero button on the monitor as the procedure steps are completed when "zero referencing."

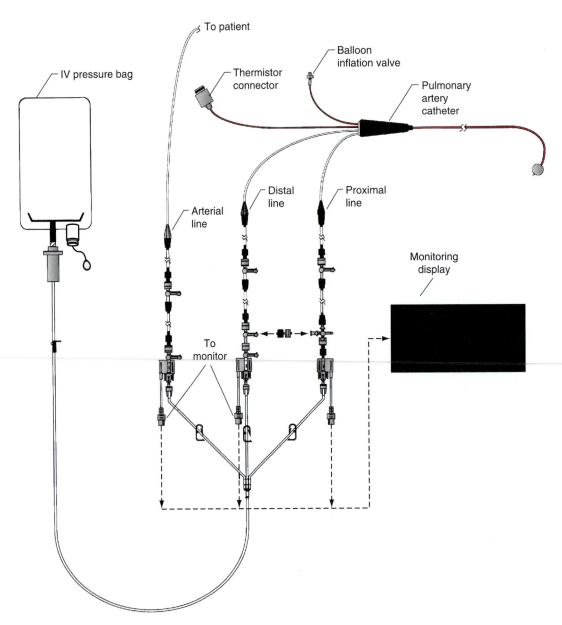

FIGURE 7-6 Pressure system setup. (Courtesy of Edwards Lifesciences, Irvine, CA.)

To level, the nurse positions the stopcock (air-fluid interface) at approximately the level of the patient's right atrium. This area is known as the *phlebostatic axis* and is located at the fourth intercostal space, midway between the anterior and posterior aspects of the chest (often referred to as the *midaxillary position;* Figure 7-7). The transducer may be placed directly on the patient's chest, or it may be attached to an intravenous line pole positioned near the patient. A leveling instrument may be used for ensuring the proper height of the transducer when it is mounted on a pole.

Dynamic Response Testing (Square Wave Test)

Obtaining accurate hemodynamic values is dependent on accurate waveform transmission (PACEP, 2001-2003). Pressures are transmitted through a fluid-filled system. Accuracy depends on the system's natural or resonant frequency, which is the frequency at which

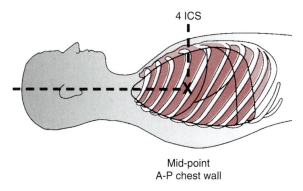

4 ICS

Mid-point
A-P chest wall

FIGURE 7-7 Midpoint anteroposterior chest wall. 4 ICS, fourth intercostal space. (Courtesy of Edwards Lifesciences, Irvine, CA.)

the system oscillates maximally, and the damping coefficient, which is how quickly an oscillating system comes to rest and is determined by the size, shape, and material of components in the fluid-filled system. There are usually one of three responses when obtaining a dynamic response test: damped response, adequate response, or underdamped response (Figure 7-8). If the dynamic response test is a damped response, the greater the damping, the less accurate the waveform becomes. This factor is important if the natural frequency of the system is not optimal or adequate. Fluid-filled systems that are underdamped require some damping.

The desired response for this test is the adequate response. If the dynamic response test reveals a damped response, then the critical care nurse assesses the line for presence of an air bubble, blood clot or fibrin, kink in the tubing, and use of soft, compliant tubing and removes the source of the problem that causes the alteration in the integrity of the line. Damped waveforms falsely decrease systolic pressures and increase diastolic pressures.

If the dynamic response test reveals an underdamped response, the action of the critical care nurse is to add a damping device to the line. The most common reason for an underdamped line is use of a pressurized line that is longer than recommended and use of numerous stopcocks. Underdamped waveforms falsely increase systolic pressures and decrease diastolic pressures.

The assessment of the dynamic response test obligates the critical care nurse to identify and fix the problem with the waveform prior to documenting hemodynamic variables and implementing treatment plans.

The actual procedure for obtaining a dynamic response test is to use the fast flush device and thereby expose the system to a rapid change in pressure, expose the system to a high pressure (300 mm Hg), and evaluate the system's response (see Figure 7-8). As the recording paper is graphing the waveform, rapidly activate and release the fast flush device. The square wave produced by the fast flush activation should have an undershoot followed by one small overshoot then quickly return to baseline (assessment of the damping coefficient). The second bounce should be less than or equal to one-third the height of the first bounce. Next, measure the distance between the bounces. The ideal system is one to two blocks between bounces (assessment of frequency response).

INTRAARTERIAL MONITORING

Intraarterial monitoring is an invasive technique of monitoring arterial blood pressure. This method allows for continuous and accurate measurement of arterial pressure.

Although the sphygmomanometer method of determining arterial pressure is simple and accessible, the manual cuff may be too cumbersome and time-consuming for use with a critically ill patient who may require many other interventions as well. Another method of noninvasive blood pressure

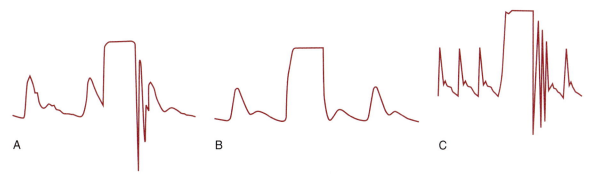

A   B   C

FIGURE 7-8 Dynamic response testing. **A,** Normal response. **B,** Overdamped response. **C,** Underdamped response. (Courtesy of Edwards Lifesciences, Irvine, CA.)

measurement uses an electronic indirect blood pressure device that automatically displays blood pressure at prescribed time intervals using a mechanical sphygmomanometer. However, for very unstable patients, neither of the sphygmomanometer methods is the most accurate. Therefore, the intraarterial method is preferred in unstable patients because it is accurate and continuous and, in addition, allows for painless sampling of blood.

Indications

Most critically ill patients can benefit from intraarterial monitoring. Ideally, an arterial line is placed in any patient receiving intravenous vasoactive infusions to evaluate the response to therapy on an ongoing basis. Other patient populations that benefit from this method of monitoring include the following:

- Patients who require frequent arterial blood gas sampling or laboratory work
- Patients with low-flow states, hypotensive due to unknown causes
- Patients with severe hypertension
- Patients with conditions resulting in severe vasoconstriction or vasodilation

Equipment

The following components are required for the monitoring of intraarterial pressure:

1. A catheter that is percutaneously placed into an artery, often the radial, brachial, or femoral. If the catheter is placed into the radial artery, a modified Allen's test should be performed to assess the patency of the radial and ulnar arteries (Figure 7-9). In patients whose radial ulnar arch is not patent, a radial line should not be placed, because any thrombosis could result in circulatory compromise to the hand, leading to possible limb loss.

2. A pressurized fluid source, which is attached by pressure tubing to the arterial catheter to keep the catheter patent. The fluid is pressurized to 300 mm Hg by use of an inflatable bag to prevent backflow of arterial blood into the tubing-catheter system. Sufficient pressure must be exerted to force the solution to flow against the patient's systolic pressure.

3. The transducer, which is attached to the hub of the catheter by the connecting tubing. Once the transducer is attached to the monitor, it should be zeroed, leveled, and evaluated for appropriate dynamic response.

4. The bedside monitor, which amplifies the signal from the transducer and displays the arterial waveform on an oscilloscope. This arterial waveform is displayed continuously along with numerical values of systole, diastole, and mean pressure readings.

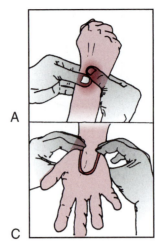
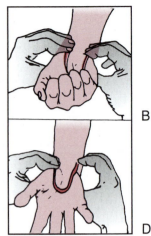

A   B   C   D

FIGURE 7-9 Modified Allen's test. When the patient's hand is held above the head with the fist clenched, both the radial and ulnar arteries are compressed **(A)**. The hand is lowered **(B)** and opened **(C)**. Pressure is then released over the ulnar artery **(D)**. Color should return to the hand within 6 seconds, a finding indicating a patent ulnar artery and an intact superficial palmar arch. (From Kaye, W. [1983]. Invasive monitoring techniques: Arterial cannulation, bedside pulmonary artery catheterization, and arterial puncture. *Heart and Lung*, 12[4], 400.)

Arterial Pressure Waveform and Measurements

The normal arterial waveform consists of a steep ascent during systole followed by a gradual descent during diastole. As the left ventricle contracts, the systolic pressure wave is transmitted to the transducer and then is depicted as a sharp rising wave. The systolic pressure is measured at the peak of the waveform (Figure 7-10). This pressure reflects the function of the left ventricle. Thus, if the left ventricle contracts poorly, the systolic pressure decreases to reflect this decrease in function. The normal value of the systolic pressure is 100 to 130 mm Hg.

The end-diastolic pressure is shown as the lowest point on the arterial waveform. This pressure reflects systemic resistance. The normal diastolic pressure is 60 to 90 mm Hg.

The dicrotic notch is a small notch on the downstroke of the waveform. It occurs as a result of the closure of the aortic valve. This closure is commonly considered the reference point between the systolic and the diastolic phases of the cardiac cycle.

The mean arterial pressure is a calculated pressure that closely estimates the perfusion pressure in the aorta and its major branches. It represents the

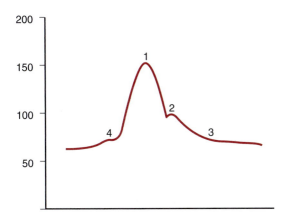

FIGURE 7-10 Normal arterial pressure tracing: *1*, peak systolic pressure; *2*, dicrotic notch; *3*, diastolic pressure; and *4*, anacrotic notch. (Courtesy of Edwards Lifesciences, Irvine, CA.)

average pressure in the systemic arterial system during the entire cardiac cycle. Display monitors continuously record the mean arterial pressure, but it can also be calculated by using the following formula:

[(Systolic blood pressure − Diastolic blood pressure)/3] + Diastolic blood pressure

The bedside monitoring systems use a slightly different formula to calculate the mean pressure. Thus the critical care nurse's calculation may not be the exact same number as the one displayed on the monitor. The normal mean arterial pressure is 70 to 100 mm Hg. The mean arterial pressure must be maintained at greater than 60 mm Hg for the vital organs of the body to be perfused. The pulse pressure is defined as the arithmetic difference between the systolic and diastolic pressure. For example:

If systolic pressure = 130 mm Hg

And diastolic pressure = 70 mm Hg

Then pulse pressure = 60 mm Hg

The pulse pressure widens when the systolic and diastolic pressures become farther apart. As these pressures become closer, the pulse pressure narrows. The pulse pressure is divided by 3 and then is added to the diastolic pressure to determine the mean pressure.

Complications

The major complications of arterial pressure monitoring include thrombosis, embolism, blood loss, and infection. Embolism may occur as a result of small clot formation around the tip of the catheter or from air entering the system. Thrombosis (blood clot) may

occur if a continuous flush solution is not used. Blood loss is usually a result of sudden dislodgment of the catheter from the artery or from disconnection of the tubing. Rapid blood loss may occur (because this is in an artery, not a vein) if either of these occurrences is not promptly recognized.

Infection is usually the result of a catheter's being left in place for a prolonged period, yet routine replacement of the catheter is no longer recommended. Yet the longer a catheter is in place in the critically ill patient, the greater the incidence of infection (CDC, 2002). Radial artery catheters are changed on an as needed basis (CDC, 2002). Replace disposable or reusable transducers at approximately 96-hour intervals. Replace other components of the system (including the tubing, continuous-flush device, and flush solution) at the time the transducer is replaced (CDC, 2002).

Clinical Considerations

The invasive method of obtaining blood pressure is considered to be more accurate than noninvasive methods because it gives beat-by-beat information instead of measuring vibrations (Korotkoff's sounds) of the arterial wall over several beats. In patients who are hypotensive, a serious discrepancy may exist between the blood pressures obtained by invasive and noninvasive means. The cuff pressure may be significantly lower, leading to dangerous mistakes in the treatment of such a patient. Under normal circumstances, a difference of 5 mm Hg or more between invasive and noninvasive blood pressure is expected, with the invasive blood pressure generally greater than the noninvasive value. This difference may vary up to 37 mm Hg from the invasive blood pressure determination, and, for this reason, treatment should never be based on the measurement of a single determination of noninvasive blood pressure alone (Darovic, 2002).

When the noninvasive value is higher than the invasive number, one must become suspicious of equipment malfunction or technical error. Box 7-1 lists the possible causes. Signs of possible problems are waveforms that appear to decrease in amplitude, loss of the dicrotic notch on the downslope, and/or waveforms that depict low systolic pressures (Figure 7-11). This phenomenon is referred to as a *damped waveform* and indicates the presence of interference with the transmission of the pulse through the fluid-filled catheter to the transducer. To make sure that this damped waveform does not indicate that the patient is becoming acutely hypotensive, the nurse obtains a cuff pressure immediately and compares that value with the intraarterial value. If the noninvasive value is higher, the nurse is then alerted to a possible technical problem. Damping caused by catheter obstruction may be corrected by aspiration of any visible clots or by careful repositioning of the catheter if it seems to be lodged against the arterial wall.

BOX 7-1

Causes of Higher Noninvasive Versus Invasive Blood Pressure

- Air bubbles
- Improper cuff size
- Improper cuff placement
- Failure to "zero" the transducer
- Blood in the catheter system
- Blood clot at the catheter tip
- Kinking of the tubing system
- Loose or open connections
- Catheter tip lodging against the arterial wall
- Soft, compliant tubing
- Long tubing (>4 ft)
- Too many stopcocks (>3)

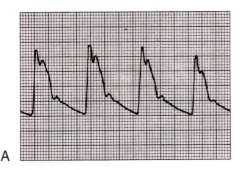

A

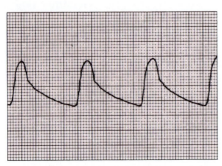

B

FIGURE 7-11 A, Arterial waveform depicting a sharp upstroke and a dicrotic notch. **B,** Damped waveform depicting slow upstroke, lower systolic pressure, and poor dicrotic notch. (From Jackle, M., & Halligan, M. [1980]. *Cardiovascular problems: A critical care nursing focus.* Bowie, MD: Robert J. Brady.)

Nursing Implications

Any nurse caring for a patient with an arterial line must try to prevent or reduce the incidence of complications such as thrombosis, embolism, blood loss, and infection. Nursing interventions include the following:

1. Maintain a continuous flush solution through the catheter to prevent clot formation.
2. Document the insertion date of the catheter and keep the health care team aware of placement time. The longer the catheter is in place, the greater the risk of clot formation.
3. Keep the tubing free of kinks.
4. Maintain a pressure of 300 mm Hg on the flush solution using a pressure bag.
5. Avoid intermittent flushing by hand to minimize the risk of embolism.
6. Document assessment of the extremity every 2 hours for perfusion: color, temperature, sensation, pulse, and capillary refill.
7. Keep the patient's wrist in a neutral position and place it on an armboard.
8. Check for a damped waveform, and, if noted, reposition the catheter or aspirate for air or clots.
9. Tighten all connections (finger tighten) and make sure that these connections remain tight to minimize possible blood loss.
10. Reorient an agitated patient to prevent sudden dislodgment of the catheter or disconnection of the tubing.
11. Set high and low alarms on the monitor.
12. Keep sterile caps over the openings of the stopcocks.
13. Change the dressing by use of aseptic technique (per hospital policy).
14. Change the pressure tubing, flush bag, and transducer every 96 hours or with every change of the catheter (CDC, 2002).
15. When the catheter is removed, ensure that adequate pressure is applied to the site of insertion until hemostasis is obtained (for a minimum of 5 minutes for radial artery catheters). The time required will vary, depending on the type, size, and location of the catheter and the patient's coagulation status.

RIGHT ATRIAL PRESSURE MONITORING

RAP, sometimes referred to as a *central venous pressure* (CVP), is a direct measurement of the pressure of the right atrium, but it may also be measured from the superior or inferior vena cava. Because no valves are present between the right atrium and the vena cava, the pressures within these areas are essentially equal. However, the clinical importance of RAP measurement lies in its ability to also reflect *right ventricular diastolic pressure*. During right ventricular diastole, the heart's tricuspid valve is open, thereby allowing a clear passage for blood to flow from the right atrium to the right ventricle. Because of this, the RAP measurement is a reliable reflection of right ventricular preload or right ventricular end-diastolic volume or pressure.

Pathophysiological Processes Affecting Right Atrial Pressure

The RAP measurement is valuable for helping to reflect right ventricular diastolic pressure and right ventricular end-diastolic pressure. Abnormalities in RAP measurement are generally caused by any condition that alters venous tone, blood volume, or right ventricular contractility. For example, a patient with a low RAP may be experiencing hypovolemia because of dehydration, traumatic blood loss, or *relative* hypovolemia as a result of extreme vasodilation seen in sepsis. In all these conditions, RAP reflects blood return to the heart that is insufficient to meet the body's requirements. Conversely, a high RAP measurement may indicate any condition that reduces the right ventricle's ability to eject blood, thereby increasing RVP and hence RAP. Such conditions include hypervolemia (seen with aggressive intravenous infusions), severe vasoconstriction, or any condition that overloads the ventricle so it is unable to eject properly. Other examples include pulmonary hypertension (heralded by an elevated PA pressure [PAP] because high PAPs prevent blood from flowing freely from the right ventricle to the pulmonary circulation), and right-sided heart failure (seen in right-sided ischemia, which reduces the contractile ability of the right ventricle during systole, thereby causing a backup of blood into the right ventricle and likewise the right atrium).

Methods of Measuring Right Atrial Pressure

Catheters used for RAP measurement are generally stiff and radiopaque. They vary in length and diameter depending on the vein that is used: shorter catheters are generally used for subclavian insertion, and longer catheters are used for upper extremity vein insertion. They generally are triple-lumen catheters.

Several sites may be used for RAP line insertion. The internal jugular site is often preferable because it allows the patient a high degree of mobility, and the risks of infection and thrombophlebitis are relatively low. The subclavian vein is another commonly used site, but it subjects the patient to an additional risk of pneumothorax during insertion. Other veins that may be suitable include the cephalic, femoral, antecubital, and occasionally the basilic and saphenous veins, but to read RAP accurately, these catheters need to be longer in length.

The insertion procedure for central lines is analogous to that for the PA artery catheter and is described in detail later in this chapter. RAP is usually measured by use of a conventional pressure transducer, and it requires all the standard equipment illustrated in Figure 7-6. The normal value for RAP measurement is 2 to 6 mm Hg.

The typical RAP tracing consists of three upwardly deflected waves that correspond to various phases in the cardiac cycle. The "a" wave is produced by atrial contraction, and the "c" wave is produced by closure of the tricuspid valve. The "v" wave depicts volume filling into the right atrium against a closed tricuspid valve. Figure 7-12 illustrates a typical RAP tracing, even though this illustration is from the PA distal port in the right atrial chamber. Identification of the RAP waveform components is done by using the ECG tracing (Box 7-2).

Complications & Interventions of Right Atrial Pressure Monitoring

An important nursing consideration in the care of a patient undergoing RAP monitoring is close observation for complications. Because insertion of a RAP catheter involves a disruption of skin integrity, a risk of infection exists. Although uncommon,

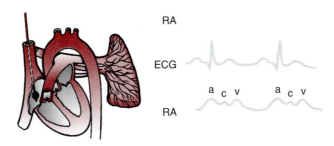

FIGURE 7-12 Right atrial (RA) pressure waveform. A right atrial pressure waveform is the same as the pulmonary artery distal port waveform when it is first inserted into the right atrium. (Courtesy of Edwards Lifesciences, Irvine, CA.)

BOX 7-2

Identifying the RAP Waves: Using the ECG

a wave is found in the PR interval.
c wave, if found, is in the mid to end of the QRS complex.
v wave is located after the T wave.

---

sepsis resulting from central line insertion represents a potentially fatal complication for any patient, particularly one who is critically ill. This risk is greatly reduced if strict attention to hand washing and sterile technique during insertion and site care is observed. Signs of infection include elevated body temperature and pain, warmth, redness, and purulent drainage at the insertion site.

Other complications may occur during the insertion itself. These include carotid puncture, pneumothorax, hemothorax, perforation of the right atrium or ventricle, and disturbances in cardiac rhythm, generally either atrial or ventricular dysrhythmias.

The critical care nurse is responsible for collecting and recording patient data, ensuring the accuracy of the data, and reporting to the physician any data outside the realm of acceptable limits. At that point, analyzing the various hemodynamic parameters is a collaborative responsibility between the medical and nursing staff so that prompt and *appropriate* treatment measures may occur. Measurements of RAP are most valuable when they are compared with other physiological parameters and physical assessment.

Patient positioning. RAP measurements should be taken when the patient is in the supine position, either flat or with the head of the bed elevated up to no more than 60 degrees (Keckeisen, 1998). For accurate RAP measurements to be obtained, the air-fluid interface of the transducer must be properly placed at the phlebostatic axis.

Respiratory variation. A second consideration for obtaining accurate RAP readings is the effect of the respiratory cycle. Any situation that alters intrathoracic pressure, such as spontaneous inspiration or mechanical ventilation, affects the waveform. RAP is obtained at the end of expiration. At end expiration, the pleural pressure remains relatively constant, and the effects of atmospheric pressure are minimal, thus facilitating accurate measurements.

Effect of positive end-expiratory pressure. A third consideration in obtaining accurate RAP

measurements is during mechanical ventilation when using PEEP. The patient may receive PEEP for the correction of hypoxemia. The RAP reading is obtained regardless of the level of PEEP, because removing the PEEP can be detrimental to the patient's oxygen level. While the patient is receiving PEEP, the readings are assessed for any trends from the patient's baseline taken when PEEP was first initiated. Recording of the RAP measurements should indicate that the patient is receiving PEEP. The strip/chart recording can be used to ascertain the RAP.

Another method of recording RAP is analysis of the RAP waveform from a printout on a bedside or central station recorder. All hemodynamic waveforms can be obtained by printout recording. Information derived from this method is more precise than the numerical display. These printout recordings should be examined and evaluated thoroughly whenever serious alterations in hemodynamic values occur. Doing so permits the clinician to take into account the influence of confounding factors such as respiratory variation.

LEFT ATRIAL PRESSURE MONITORING

LAP is the pressure of the blood as it returns to the left side of the heart. LAP is a reflection of left ventricular preload. On the left side of the heart during ventricular diastole, the mitral valve is opened, allowing for communication between the left atrium and the left ventricle. Thus, at the end of diastolic filling under normal circumstances, the LAP is nearly identical to the left ventricular end-diastolic pressure. Normal LAP is 8 to 12 mm Hg (see Figure 7-4). Because the left atrium does not generate significant pressure during atrial contraction, the atrial pressure is recorded as an average (mean) pressure rather than as a systolic or diastolic pressure. Measurement techniques and consideration of patient positioning and use of PEEP are analogous to those described for RAP monitoring.

A patient's clinical condition may affect LAP. A low LAP is found in the following conditions: hypovolemia, massive vasodilation, and excessive PEEP (10 cm H_2O). Increases in LAP may be found in the following conditions: hypervolemia, massive vasoconstriction, pulmonary congestion, mitral stenosis, mitral regurgitation, cardiac tamponade, constrictive pericarditis, and depressed contractile states, such as in myocardial infarction, cardiomyopathy, and hypothermia.

A series of LAP readings depicting trends is more informative than a single abnormal reading. Like other hemodynamic parameters, the LAP is correlated with other assessment data before any changes in therapy are instituted.

Catheter Insertion

The left atrial catheter is composed of a polyvinyl material and is approximately 6 inches long. Although infrequently used, it may offer unique monitoring advantages for some cardiac surgical procedures when close observation of LAP is warranted. It is typically inserted during cardiac surgery, the proximal end is then brought out through an incision in the chest wall. The catheter is connected to a standard pressurized tubing system and is displayed on the monitor. A sterile dressing is placed over the insertion site on the chest wall where the catheter was placed and is changed daily. The LAP catheter is normally used for 24 to 72 hours and then is removed by a physician or other credentialed person.

Complications of Left Atrial Pressure Monitoring

A major danger of LAP catheters is introducing air or debris into the system, thus causing an embolism into the coronary or cerebral circulation. The nurse must ensure that all connections are tightly fitted and all stopcocks have been dead-end capped. Medications or fluids (except for flush solution) are *not* administered through this catheter, to reduce the risk of embolus.

Small clots can pose the same danger as air bubbles. If a clot is suspected, the nurse should manually try to aspirate the clot back into the syringe. However, if this attempt is unsuccessful, the physician is notified, and the catheter should be removed.

Another potential complication with LAP monitoring is infection. The LAP catheter is a direct access into the heart, and any microorganism that invades the cardiac tissue may directly affect the heart's performance. Constant surveillance of the insertion site is essential, and adherence to dressing changes per hospital policy is maintained.

PULMONARY ARTERY MONITORING

The introduction of the PA catheter in 1970 by Drs. Swan and Ganz represented a major breakthrough in hemodynamic monitoring. Before this time, the RAP catheter was the only method by which cardiac function could be monitored. No matter how important the RAP is in the monitoring of right-sided parameters, it is of little help in detecting left-sided problems.

The PA catheter allows the clinician to indirectly monitor valuable information regarding left ventricular function. Any alterations in left ventricular function can severely compromise blood flow to the tissues. Because left ventricular SV is influenced by the blood volume and contractility of the left ventricle

during systole, the PA catheter is helpful in identifying conditions that contribute to abnormalities.

Types of Catheters

The PA catheter is a long, hollow, pliable catheter that is radiopaque and is constructed with a variable number of lumina that extend to several points (measured in centimeters) along the length of the catheter. Distal (PA) and proximal (RAP) lumina are for pressure monitoring, and these are filled with fluid. Medications or fluids are not administered through the distal lumen of the PA catheter. A *thermistor lumen* is used during CO monitoring, and it houses temperature-sensitive wires. The balloon inflation lumen is equipped with a valve that enables a tiny balloon on the tip of the catheter to be inflated with a syringe. This balloon is inflated during insertion of the catheter to allow the catheter tip to flow through the various cardiac structures without causing damage to the cardiac tissue. The balloon is also inflated to measure *pulmonary artery occlusion pressure (PAOP)*.

Several types of PA catheters are available, with varying numbers of lumina and features. *Four-lumen* catheters contain one proximal hub, one distal hub, one balloon-inflation valve, and a thermistor wire connector that is used for obtaining CO measurements. The proximal hub is used for monitoring RAP, as well as for intravenous administration of solutions, and the distal hub is for measuring PAP.

Five-lumen catheters (Figure 7-13) contain an additional fifth port called the *proximal infusion lumen hub*, which is situated high in the right atrium. It is used solely for infusion purposes and is sometimes referred to as the *venous infusion port*. Five-lumen catheters have several advantages over four-lumen catheters. First, they provide a mechanism for continuous monitoring of RAP pressure without interruption of the intravenous infusion. Second, because blood flows through the right atrium at a high velocity, two medications can be infused simultaneously, one through the right atrial lumen and another through the venous infusion port lumen, without fear of drug incompatibility.

Some PA catheters are also designed for the purpose of transvenous pacing. This technique involves the insertion of pacemaker wires through additional lumina in the PA catheter, which exit the catheter into the right ventricle to provide ventricular pacing. Other PA catheters have *continuous CO* (CCO) capabilities. This type of catheter was developed to provide ongoing monitoring of CO. Some catheters also have capability of measuring *mixed venous oxygen saturation* (SvO_2). Continuous monitoring of SvO_2 is through a fiberoptic network housed inside a conventional PA catheter. The concepts of CCO and SvO_2 are discussed later in this chapter.

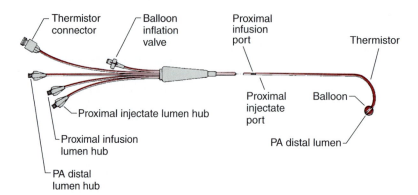

FIGURE 7-13 A five-lumen pulmonary artery (PA) catheter containing the four-lumen components in addition to a second proximal lumen for infusion of fluid or medications. (Courtesy of Edwards Lifesciences, Irvine, CA.)

Nursing Responsibilities Before Insertion

Despite the differences in the types of PA catheters available, the nursing responsibilities before the catheter is inserted are similar. The differences depend on the patient's condition, as well as the personal preference of the physician and the brand of equipment used.

Of primary importance is the need for patient teaching before the catheter is inserted. Patients are often anxious and uncertain about this procedure and can benefit from simple, straightforward explanations. Informed consent is required for the procedure. The physician explains the procedure briefly, along with the risks and benefits of the procedure, but the critical care nurse is able to reinforce necessary information while providing emotional support. The following is a sample of the information that is presented to the patient when the decision has been made to insert a PA catheter:

"Hello, Mrs. Smith. The doctor has discussed the pulmonary artery catheter with you. I can help to clarify some points. The pulmonary artery catheter will give us valuable information about how your heart is working and will help us to decide the best possible treatment. The procedure will probably take about 30 minutes. It won't be too painful, but it will involve the insertion of a small catheter through your skin and into your heart. The skin will be numbed with a local anesthetic. It will be important for you to remain still while the catheter is being placed, but I'll be with you during the entire procedure to make sure you'll be as comfortable as possible."

As the physician continues the procedure, the nurse provides additional reinforcement to help decrease the patient's anxiety. Special attention by the nurse regarding the patient's comfort level and need for emotional support contributes to the well-being of the patient.

Equipment

The equipment required for PA monitoring is similar to the pressure transducer system discussed in the section on RAP monitoring: a transducer, tubing and flush system, an amplifier, and a monitor. Variations from this method are needed when catheters contain both a right atrial port (proximal port) and a PA port (distal port). Two sections of tubing are needed for continuous flushing of both ports of the catheter, and two transducers are necessary for simultaneous monitoring of RAP and PAP.

Because of certain risks involved in this procedure, emergency medications and equipment must be readily available. Complications include hemothorax, pneumothorax, perforation of the vein or cardiac chamber, and cardiac rhythm disturbances. The PA catheter is passed from the right atrium through the right ventricle before it enters the PA. As the catheter passes through the ventricle, it can irritate the ventricle, causing rhythm disturbances, such as premature ventricular contraction and/or ventricular tachycardia. For this reason, intravenous lidocaine may be kept available to be infused on an emergency basis should these rhythm disturbances become hemodynamically significant.

Insertion Method

Subclavian, internal jugular, or external jugular sites are the most common. The patient's bed is placed in Trendelenburg's position to promote venous filling in the upper body for easier insertion of the catheter. This position can also prevent air embolism during insertion. If Trendelenburg's position is contraindicated, such as in a patient with pulmonary edema, a blanket roll can be placed between the patient's shoulder blades to facilitate insertion. The skin is cleaned and draped and is then injected with a local anesthetic. A needled syringe is used to puncture the vessel and to confirm placement by backward flow of blood into the syringe. The syringe is removed, and a guidewire is threaded through the needle into the vessel. The needle is then removed so a hollow tube, called an introducer, may be passed over the guidewire. The wire is then removed, and the PA catheter is passed freely into the vessel through the introducer. Several variations of this method of insertion exist, and physicians may have their own preferences. Technique may also vary according to the brand of equipment used and the patient's anatomy. A chest radiograph is obtained after the procedure to verify catheter placement if fluoroscopy was not used during the insertion. Catheter malposition can be reliably excluded (negative predictive value, 99%) by close observation of specific clinical criteria, so routine daily chest radiographs are not justified (Houghton, Cohn, Schell, Cohn, & Varon, 2002).

Nursing responsibilities during insertion. As the catheter is passed through the cardiac chambers, the nurse monitors and records HR, heart rhythm, and blood pressure. Any dysrhythmias that occur during the procedure are documented, and the usual emergency equipment and medications are made available.

As the tip of the catheter passes through each chamber, the waveform changes and the pressures displayed are recorded. These waveforms appear as follows: right atrial, right ventricular, PA systolic and diastolic, and PA wedge pressure (PAWP) (Figure 7-14). The last waveform signals the end of insertion, at which time the balloon is deflated. Once the balloon is deflated, the tip of the catheter falls back in position in the PA.

The nurse reinflates the balloon to monitor PAWPs as ordered or according to unit protocol. The balloon should not be inflated for more than 8 to 10 seconds, so ischemia is not caused by obstruction of blood flow. Additionally, no more than 1.5 mL of air should ever be used to inflate the PAOP balloon. After the PA catheter is inserted, the measurement of catheter length in centimeters is documented to provide the clinician with an assessment clue should the catheter be accidentally pulled out or advanced.

Patients with prolonged PA catheterization must be carefully examined for signs or symptoms of infection. The time until PA catheter replacement can be extended to 7 days if there is no evidence of catheter-related infection (Chen et al., 2003).

Clinical Significance of Pulmonary Artery Catheter Values

The PAP consists of systolic, diastolic, and mean pressures. The systolic pressure is the peak pressure attained as the right ventricle ejects its SV.

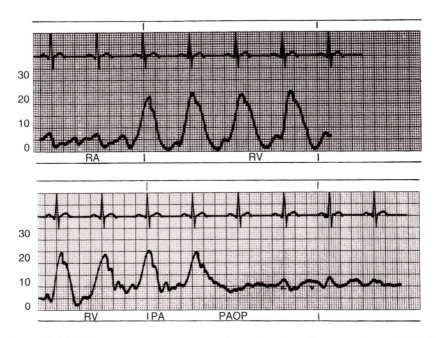

FIGURE 7-14 Waveform depicting the insertion of a pulmonary artery catheter from the right atrium (RA) into the right ventricle (RV) as it is floated into the pulmonary artery and when it becomes wedged (pulmonary artery occlusion pressure [PAOP]). (Courtesy of Edwards Lifesciences, Irvine, CA.)

The diastolic pressure reflects the movement of blood from the PA out into the lung capillaries. The third parameter, the mean pressure, is the average pressure exerted on the pulmonary vasculature (Figure 7-15). The normal PAP is approximately 25/10 mm Hg, and the mean pressure is 15 mm Hg.

The fourth parameter is the PAOP (Figure 7-16). It is also known as the *pulmonary capillary wedge pressure (PCWP)* or *pulmonary artery wedge pressure (PAWP)*. PCWP is a mean pressure with a normal value of 8 to 12 mm Hg (see Figure 7-4). When the balloon is inflated, the PCWP reflects the pressure ahead of the catheter, which is both the LAP and the left ventricular end-diastolic pressure when the mitral valve is open. Thus, the PCWP is a reliable indirect measurement of left ventricular function. In the absence of valvular disease and pulmonary vascular congestion, the PA diastolic pressure also closely approximates left ventricle function because the mitral valve is open during end diastole, thereby providing an open circuit for the free movement of blood from the PA to the lungs and forward into the left atrium and the left ventricle.

An understanding of the PCWP and its relationship with left ventricular end-diastolic pressure is a valuable guide to therapy. In patients with normal ventricles, an increase in left ventricular end-diastolic pressure (and therefore PCWP) indicates an increase in left ventricular blood volume that will be ejected with

the next systole. Likewise, a decrease in left ventricular end-diastolic pressure (and a subsequently low PCWP) signals a reduction in left ventricular blood volume that will be available for the next contraction. Increased PCWP may occur in patients who have fluid volume excess resulting from overzealous administration of intravenous fluid, as well as in those with renal disease who cannot produce adequate urine output. Conditions causing a low PCWP include those that cause fluid volume deficit, such as dehydration, excessive diuretic therapy, and hemorrhage.

An increase in PCWP can also provide the clinician with early information about impending left ventricular failure, as may be seen with myocardial infarction. Through monitoring of changes and trends, the PCWP can be invaluable in determining appropriate therapy, as well as the effectiveness of that therapy.

The PCWP can also be used as a physiological indicator of left ventricular failure and blood volume alterations. However, because the balloon of the catheter is inflated for only a few seconds at a time, the PCWP is not used for continuous monitoring. The nurse never forces the balloon to inflation if resistance is met and makes sure that the balloon is deflated if resistance is met on inflation. Periodic comparisons of the PA diastolic pressure and PCWP are helpful in assessing the accuracy of the PCWP measurement, especially in patients experiencing

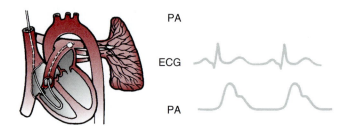

FIGURE 7-15 A pulmonary artery (PA) waveform as it correlates to placement of the catheter in the PA. (Courtesy of Edwards Lifesciences, Irvine, CA.)

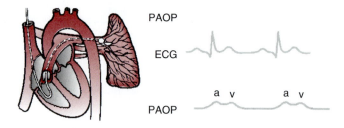

FIGURE 7-16 A pulmonary artery occlusion pressure (PAOP) waveform depicting the wedge position of the pulmonary artery catheter when the balloon port is inflated. (Courtesy of Edwards Lifesciences, Irvine, CA.)

acute hemodynamic changes. Identification of the PCWP waveform components is done by using the ECG tracing (Box 7-3).

Complications of Pulmonary Artery Monitoring

Complications that may occur with PA monitoring are uncommon. Table 7-1 lists the most common complications and implications for the nurse in these situations.

Nursing Implications for Pulmonary Artery Pressure Measurement

Patient positioning. Several studies determined the effects of varying backrest positions up to 60 degrees on PAP, PCWP, and LAP. These studies found little effect on these hemodynamic measurements, provided the phlebostatic axis and proper leveling to the air-fluid interface (stopcock) are used as the zero reference level (Wilson, Bermingham-Mitchell, Wells, & Zachary, 1996).

The effect of the 30-degree lateral recumbent position was studied on PA pressure and PAOP in critically ill adult patients who had undergone cardiac surgical procedures (Bridges, Woods, Brengelmann, Mitchell, & Laurent-Bopp, 2000). Despite demonstrated benefits of lateral positioning, critically ill patients may require prolonged supine positioning to obtain reproducible hemodynamic measurements. The 30-degree right and left lateral positions were studied to determine the effect on PA pressure and PAOP after cardiac surgery in critically ill adult patients. In 35 patients with stable hemodynamics during the first 12 to 24 hours after cardiac surgery, measurements of PA pressure and PAOP obtained in the 30-degree lateral and supine positions were clinically interchangeable.

Respiratory variation. PAPs are measured at the end of expiration because of changes in intrathoracic pressure associated with both mechanical ventilation and spontaneous breathing. End expiration most closely approximates atmospheric pressure and is therefore least likely to produce fluctuations on

recording devices. PAP readings are noted by graphic (hard copy) printout, and measurements from the digital display on the monitor are documented in the medical record. Currently, the literature supports the graphic printout to be the most accurate method of determining PAPs (Lundstedt, 1997).

MIXED VENOUS OXYGEN SATURATION
Monitoring System

SvO_2 is another hemodynamic parameter that can be monitored, either using a special fiberoptic PA catheter or by blood sampled from the distal port of the PA catheter. Blood from the PA catheter is known as *mixed venous* blood because blood returns to the PA from various body organs and tissues that have different needs for metabolic functioning. This venous blood is then "mixed" in the PA, where it reflects an overall picture of the oxygen used by these organs and tissues. The sample of blood is analyzed in the laboratory and is expressed as a *percentage* of oxygen used in body metabolism.

The fiberoptic PA catheter (Figure 7-17) is inserted in the same manner previously described in the section on PA catheters. However, three distinct components exist that enable continuous SvO_2 monitoring: (1) a fiberoptic catheter, which transmits and receives light waves; (2) an optical module, which sends and receives light to the end of the catheter through a fiberoptic channel; and (3) a microprocessor, which interprets SvO_2 values by changing the light signal into an electrical signal that is then displayed as a digital numerical display. Continuous SvO_2 monitoring allows for an assessment of the adequacy of cardiac and pulmonary function. It provides for the calculation of other important parameters, namely *oxygen consumption* (VO_2) and *oxygen delivery* (DO_2).

Clinical Significance of Mixed Venous Oxygen Saturation Value

The SvO_2 is a measurement that reflects the degree to which the tissues of the body are consuming oxygen (oxygen consumption or VO_2) and the adequacy of the oxygen delivery at the tissue level (DO_2). In other words, it helps to evaluate whether the oxygen supply can meet the oxygen demands of the tissues of the body. Oxygen delivery is determined by several variables, such as the content of oxygen in the arterial blood (assessed by the hemoglobin), the partial pressure of arterial oxygen (assessed by the PaO_2), the arterial oxygen saturation (assessed by the SaO_2), and the delivery of this oxygen-rich blood to the tissues of the body (assessed by the CO). Oxygen consumption is determined by the patient's condition. Factors that increase the oxygen consumption include shivering, exercise, fever, pain, anxiety,

---

BOX 7-3

Identifying the PAOP Waves: Using the ECG

a wave is found near the end or after the QRS.
c wave is not visible.
v wave is located after the T wave.

TABLE 7-1

Complications of Pulmonary Artery Catheters

Complication	Cause	Clinical Presentation	Nursing Implications
Infection	Violation of aseptic technique	Redness, pain, irritation, warmth, purulent drainage at insertion site; ↑ body temperature	Observe daily for clinical signs of infection
	Catheter not secured to the surrounding skin	As above; the nonsterile section of the catheter can slip forward into the vessel	Adhere to aseptic technique during dressing changes
Dysrhythmias	Irritation to the endocardium caused when the balloon is deflated and also possibly when the catheter tip migrates back into the right ventricle	Premature ventricular contractions, ventricular tachycardia Reduced perfusion with ventricular dysrhythmias may cause hypotension, mental status changes, ↓ CO, and other problems	Have emergency medication available to treat lethal dysrhythmias Never advance the catheter without inflating the balloon Use continuous ECG monitoring
Air embolization	Balloon rupture Poor technique during insertion Disconnected infusion line	Signs of shock (low BP, ↑ HR) Neurological changes (change in level of consciousness, possibly seizures, motor weakness)	If embolization occurs, position the patient with head down (20 degrees and on left side) During catheter insertion, the patient should be positioned head down (Trendelenburg's position) Notify physician immediately; this is an emergency situation
Pulmonary thromboembolism	Thrombus formation on the catheter caused by inadequate flushing, using nonheparinized flush solution	Sudden onset of dyspnea, chest pain, tachycardia, possibly leading to pulmonary infarction (see below)	Notify physician immediately of suspected PE Use preventive measures: use heparinized flush solution, ensure adequate flushing of lines

Complication	Causes	Signs	Nursing Interventions
Pulmonary artery rupture	Overinflation of the balloon Perforation by catheter tip during insertion Frequent inflation of balloon	Signs of hemorrhage: low BP, low CO, ↑ HR, ↓ pulmonary blood flow	Use no more than 1.5 mL of air to inflate balloon Never flush catheter when it is in the wedge position If the waveform appears dampened, never force flush the line; instead, aspirate the clot
Pulmonary infarction	Catheter movement into the wedged position Balloon left inflated Thrombus formation around the catheter, causing occlusion	Cough, hemoptysis (bloody sputum), pleuritic pain, high fever, bronchial breathing, and pleural friction rub Hypoxemia, hypocarbia, and respiratory alkalosis	Inflate the balloon with no more than 1.5 mL of air, and deflate it immediately after wedge tracing appears on monitor Monitor amount of air necessary to inflate balloon If tracing appears to be wedged and balloon is deflated, notify physician A chest radiograph may be necessary to confirm position

↑, Increased; ↓, decreased; *BP*, blood pressure; *CO*, cardiac output; *ECG*, electrocardiogram; *HR*, heart rate; *PE*, pulmonary embolism.

Data compiled from Gardner, P. J., & Bridges, E. J. (1995). Hemodynamic monitoring. In S. L. Woods, E. S. Sivarajan-Froelicher, C. J. Halpenny, & S. L. Underhill, (Eds.). *Cardiac nursing*, 3rd ed. Philadelphia, PA: J. B. Lippincott; and Keckeison, M. (1998). Pulmonary artery pressure monitoring. *Protocols for practice: Hemodynamic monitoring series*. Aliso Viejo, CA: American Association of Critical-Care Nurses.

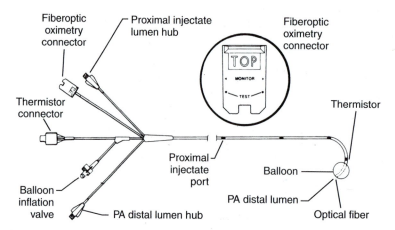

FIGURE 7-17 A mixed venous oxygen saturation fiberoptic pulmonary artery (PA) catheter. (Courtesy of Edwards Lifesciences, Irvine, CA.)

increased work of breathing, turning, activity, bathing or showering, back care, vasoactive drug therapy, and endotracheal suctioning (Table 7-2). Therefore, if the oxygen delivery cannot meet the increase in the oxygen consumption, this condition is reflected in the changing SvO_2 measurement.

The normal SvO_2 measurement is 60% to 75%. Whenever the oxygen delivery fails to meet the oxygen consumption, the SvO_2 decreases to less than 60%, a value that alerts the nurse that either the oxygen delivery is too low or the oxygen consumption is too high. Interventions are then aimed at either increasing the oxygen delivery (increasing CO

or increasing oxygen saturation by blood transfusion or increasing inspired oxygen mixture) or decreasing the oxygen consumption (determining the factor that is increasing the demand and then alleviating or decreasing it).

Several studies have found that changes in body position may affect SvO_2 in critically ill patients. Lewis and colleagues (1997) found that among critically ill men, two consecutive nursing interventions (turning and giving a backrub) produced a greater drop in SvO_2 than each intervention separated by a 5-minute rest period. Gawlinski and Dracup (1998) found that changes in SvO_2 occurred with position

TABLE 7-2

Alterations in Mixed Venous Oxygen Saturation

Alteration	Cause	Possible Cause
Low SvO_2 (<60%)	↓ O_2 delivery	Hypoxia or hemorrhage, anemic states, hypovolemia, cardiogenic shock, dysrhythmias, myocardial infarction, congestive heart failure, cardiac tamponade, massive transfusions of stored blood, restrictive lung disease, ventilation/perfusion abnormalities
	↑ O_2 consumption	Strenuous activity, hyperthermia, pain, anxiety or stress, hormonal imbalances, increased work of breathing, bathing, pheochromocytoma, thiamine/vitamin deficiency, septic shock, seizures, shivering
High SvO_2 (>75%)	↑ O_2 delivery	Increase in FiO_2, hyperoxia
	↓ O_2 consumption	Hypothermia, anesthesia, hypothyroidism, pharmacological paralysis (e.g., pancuronium bromide or vecuronium bromide), early stages of sepsis
High SvO_2 (>80%)	Technical error	PA catheter in wedged position, fibrin clot at end of catheter, noncalibrated monitor

FiO₂, Fractional concentration of oxygen in inspired gas; *O₂,* oxygen; *PA,* pulmonary artery; *SvO₂,* venous oxygen saturation.

changes in critically ill patients with poor cardiac ejection fraction. These investigators attributed these changes to increases in oxygen consumption, rather than decreases in oxygen delivery. Both studies found that the left lateral position was associated with the largest drop in SvO_2. Although these changes may be transient and may not always be clinically significant, the results from these and other studies suggest the importance of close monitoring of individual SvO_2 patterns, especially among critically ill patients with hemodynamic instability.

Increases in SvO_2 may occur when the oxygen delivery exceeds the oxygen consumption or when a decrease in consumption occurs. This may be seen with the following conditions: hypothermia, anesthesia, or the early stages of septic shock. Technical errors may also result in high SvO_2. Nursing interventions for patients receiving SvO_2 monitoring include the following:

1. Before recording SvO_2, allow sufficient time to elapse after treatments such as endotracheal suctioning, vasoactive medication titration, or nursing activities.
2. Avoid excessive manipulation or kinking of the fiberoptic catheter that may impair light transmission to and from the blood.
3. When using a fiberoptic SvO_2 catheter, calibrate the system by comparing the continuous measurement with a blood sample obtained from the PA port every 24 hours, if damage to the system is suspected, or if values appear erroneous (Jesurum, 1998).

CARDIAC OUTPUT MONITORING

CO is an important hemodynamic parameter to monitor in critically ill patients. It is used to assess whether the heart is pumping enough blood to supply oxygen to all the body tissues. Although CO may now be measured continuously, the intermittent thermodilution method is still used. The thermodilution method involves injecting a known amount of solution or *injectate*, at a known temperature (room temperature) through the proximal port (right atrial port) of a PA catheter (the right ventricular port may also be used if the proximal port is not available). The resultant drop in temperature downstream is measured by the thermistor, and the computer calculates the CO by determining the change in temperature over a change in time (Figure 7-18). Although this CO is a reflection of right ventricular blood flow, the CO of the left ventricle closely equals that of the right side. The iced injectate method, using 10 mL of fluid and a series of three injectates, may be more accurate for patients who are hypothermic, have variable CO measurements, or have very high or low CO.

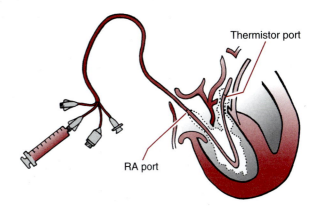

FIGURE 7-18 Illustration depicting injection into right atrium (RA) for cardiac output measurement. (Modified from Gardner, P. J., & Bridges, E. J. [1995]. Hemodynamic monitoring. In S. L. Woods, E. S. Sivarajan-Froelicher, C. J. Halpenny, & S. L. Underhill [eds.]. *Cardiac nursing*, 3rd ed. Philadelphia: J. B. Lippincott.)

Equipment for Intermittent Thermodilution

The equipment needed for intermittent thermodilution CO includes (1) a PA catheter with a thermistor, (2) an injectate (3, 5, or 10 mL of 5% dextrose in water or saline solution) that is room temperature, and (3) a CO module. This *closed injectate delivery* method involves use of a completely closed setup of a sterile injectate solution, tubing coils, and a syringe attached near the proximal injectate port for the instillation of the predetermined amount of solution (Figure 7-19).

Thermodilution Cardiac Output Measurement

Care must be exercised in obtaining accurate CO measurements. Box 7-4 depicts causes of incorrect CO measurements. The following points are important for accurately obtaining this information:

1. The correct position of the PA catheter is verified by the waveform because malposition of the catheter causes erroneous CO values.
2. The appropriate computation or calibration constant (per manufacturer's instruction) must be displayed on the computer to obtain accurate CO measurements. Catheter size and type and the volume and temperature of the injectate are factors that will determine which constant is required.
3. Injection should be smooth and rapid (within 4 seconds) at the end of expiration.
4. The proximal port is assessed for the patency and type of intravenous fluid infusing through this

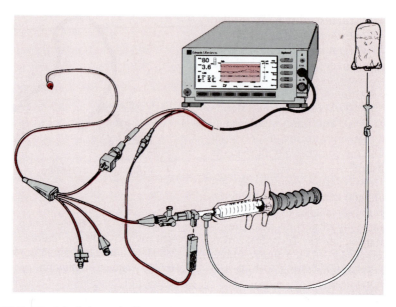

FIGURE 7-19 Schematic illustration of the closed injectate delivery system for use with room temperature injectate. (Courtesy of Edwards Lifesciences, Irvine, CA.)

BOX 7-4

Causes of Errors in Cardiac Output Measurement

- Faulty technique
- Slow injection (>4 sec)
- Incorrect computation constant set on the computer
- Incorrect position of the pulmonary artery catheter
- Faulty thermistor
- Catheter not properly connected to the computer
- Changes in patient position or movement
- Dysrhythmias
- Mechanical ventilation with positive end-expiratory pressure
- Intracardiac shunts (atrial/ventricular septal defect)

---

line during CO injectates. Vasoactive drugs are not administered through this line if it is the port for CO, because harmful effects could result from rapid CO instillations.

5. The patient is positioned in the supine position in a backrest elevation of 0 to 30 degrees.

6. Three CO measurements should be obtained, and an average CO should be calculated. The first CO measurement may be erroneous. Values should be within 10% of each other. Measurements outside this range are not used in averaging the CO.

Continuous Cardiac Output

CCO PA catheters allow clinicians to obtain continuous readings of CO (Figure 7-20). This catheter has a copper filament at the more distal end that delivers pulses of energy at prescribed time intervals and warms the blood in the right ventricle. This temperature change is detected by the thermistor at the tip of the PA catheter, whereas a display monitor interprets the temperature change and averages the CO over several seconds. No boluses are infused, thus eliminating issues related to type and amount of injectate. There are no delays between readings, no need to change the computation constant, and no extra fluid to be given to the patient. Some manufacturers have combined CCO and SvO_2, so both parameters can be obtained simultaneously. A study to compare the effects of varying degrees of backrest elevation on CCO measurements in critically ill patients was conducted at head-of-bed angle of 0 degrees, 30 degrees, and 45 degrees and at time points of 0 minutes, 5 minutes, and 10 minutes after each position change (Giuliano, Scott, Brown, & Olson, 2003). No differences in the continuous CI values across the nine different measurement conditions were found. An examination of the determinants of CO (HR and SV) indicated that the lack of change in continuous CI was not a result of a compensatory change in either HR or SV. These data indicate that, in daily clinical practice with critical medical surgical patients, it may be unnecessary to reposition patients solely for the purpose of obtaining continuous CI

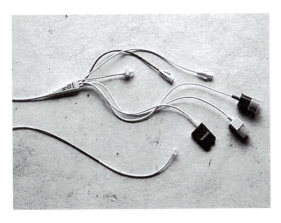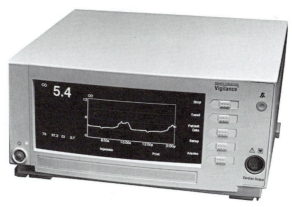

FIGURE 7-20 Continuous cardiac output catheter and monitor. (Courtesy of Edwards Lifesciences, Irvine, CA.)

measurements. The measurements were reproducible at head-of-bed angles up to 45 degrees.

Clinical Relevance

In the critically ill patient, the CO determination has gained widespread acceptance because of its accuracy, ease of use, safety, and reproducibility. The normal CO value is in the range of 4 to 8 L/min. Body size accounts for wide CO variability; for this reason, the CI is frequently used clinically, which takes into account the body size of a patient and is considered to be a more precise measurement of CO. The normal CI is 2.5 to 4.0 L/min/m². The formula is as follows:

$$CI = CO \ (L/min)/Body \ surface \ area$$

CO computers automatically calculate the body surface area based on the height and weight of the patient entered into the computer; thus, CI is a calculated parameter. The ability to obtain the CI enables health care personnel to assess patients' responses to pharmacological agents or fluid administration.

Alterations in the CI result from variations in HR or SV. Causes of a low CI include the following:
1. Abnormally fast or slow HR that causes poor filling of the left ventricle
2. Low SV resulting from a decrease in preload that is caused by the following:
   a. Diuresis
   b. Dehydration
   c. Third-space fluid shifts
   d. Hypovolemia
   e. Vasodilation
3. Low SV caused by an increase in afterload as a result of the following:
   a. Vasoconstriction caused by hypothermia or low-flow states
   b. Compensatory vasoconstriction seen in left ventricular failure

c. Increased blood viscosity
4. Low SV caused by a decrease in contractility (decreased cardiac function) as a result of the following:
   a. Myocardial ischemia or infarction
   b. Heart failure
   c. Cardiomyopathies
   d. Cardiogenic shock
   e. Cardiac tamponade
   f. Valvular disorders

Causes of a high CI can result from the following:
1. Increased physical activity (exercise)
2. Increased anxiety
3. Compensatory cardiac response seen in pulmonary edema
4. Increased metabolic states (e.g., hyperthyroid, fever, tachycardia, adrenal disorders)
5. Anemia resulting in a compensatory elevated HR
6. Sepsis
7. Mild hypertension with a wide pulse pressure

Treatment of a low CI in the critical care patient is often aimed at correcting the underlying problem. Thus, the following therapies may be instituted:
1. Increase the SV by increasing contractility through the use of a positive inotropic agent, for example, dobutamine, dopamine, milrinone, or amrinone. Dobutamine also helps to reduce SVR through vasodilation and therefore may reduce myocardial workload and SV.
2. Increase the SV by increasing the preload through fluid administration (either crystalloid or colloid solutions) and use of blood products based on hemoglobin values or by avoiding diuretic use.
3. Increase the SV by decreasing afterload through the use of afterload-reducing agents, such as sodium nitroprusside (Nipride) or nitroglycerin.
4. Correct the abnormal HR by use of a pacemaker, pharmacological agents (beta-blockers, calcium

RESEARCH ANALYSIS

ARTICLE REFERENCE

Currey, J. Botti, M. & Browne, J. (2003). Hemodynamic team decision making in the cardiac surgical intensive care context. *Heart Lung, 32*(3), 181-189.

STUDY PURPOSE/METHODS/FINDINGS

The purpose of this study was to explore the extent and sources of variability of critical care nurses' hemodynamic decision making as a function of contextual factors in the immediate 2-hour period after cardiac surgery. A qualitative exploratory design with observation and interview was used. Eight critical care nurses were observed on different occasions in clinical practice for a 2-hour period. A brief interview immediately followed each observation to clarify observation data. Analysis of the data revealed that patient management decisions were made both by individual nurses and by a team of nurses and health professionals. During displays of integrated team decision making (TDM), the primary nurse made most hemodynamic decisions and nurses who assisted the primary nurse deferred to the primary nurse's decision. During nonintegrated TDM, nurses assisting the primary nurse assumed responsibilities for most patient-related decisions. Nonintegrated TDM occurred more frequently when inexperienced cardiac surgical intensive care nurses were in the role of primary nurse, whereas integrated TDM was more common among experienced cardiac surgical intensive care nurses. This observed variability can occur in multiple ways and in hemodynamic decision making has implications for patient outcomes as behaviors of nonintegrated TDM led to nurses sensing a loss of control of patient management.

STRENGTHS/LIMITATIONS

The small sample size is a limitation in the study, especially given that the observations and interviews were performed in 3 critical care units of 2 hospitals. Although the nurses were equally split in terms of having experience and being inexperienced, all four of the inexperienced nurses had less than 1 year of full-time cardiac surgical intensive care (CSIC) experience and between 1 and 7 years of critical care experience.

One strength of the study was that the data collection included observation, performed by one data collector, and an interview. The use of the audiotape to record observations allowed the data collector to keep her eyes on the nurse who was caring for the patient, thus not missing data entry due to time recording an observation with pen and paper. In addition, the observation time period also included taking brief field notes. Another strength is that the authors addressed threats to validity with their study findings.

IMPLICATIONS FOR PRACTICE

In this study, once handover was completed, other nurses who assisted did not simply offer technical support to the primary nurse during the first hour of the admission period; rather, they formed a team with the primary nurse to make decisions regarding the patient's recovery from surgery. Team decision making lasted from 20 to 90 minutes and consequently accounted for a high level of decision-making variability. In integrated TDM, communication between the primary nurse and the assistant nurses was open and prompt. During nonintegrated TDM, the primary nurse did not perform all hemodynamic assessment such as establishing hemodynamic monitoring or setting monitor alarm parameters. Nonintegrated TDM activity has the potential for adverse patient outcomes. The decision making that was influenced by colleagues contributed to patient management decisions. For TDM to be effective, it is not sufficient that each individual possesses skills and knowledge; rather, success depends upon such information being communicated between members.

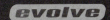

J.S. is a 77-year-old Caucasian male with a known history of coronary artery disease, acute myocardial infarction (AMI), and heart failure and is 1 year status post pacemaker/defibrillator (PC/ICD) implant for ventricular tachycardia. He had a positive thallium stress test that showed slight ischemic changes; a 2D echocardiogram showed normal pulmonary artery pressures; and heart catheterization showed single-vessel disease and cardiomyopathy, with a left ventriculogram exhibiting poor contractility of the inferior wall and a left ventricular ejection fraction of less than 30%. Medical management was recommended.

One month later, Mr. S. came to the clinic complaining of loss of appetite, periodic shortness of breath with no specific pattern, and trace pedal edema. There were no other signs of acute heart failure. He was classified as having New York Heart Association Class II heart failure or Stage B Heart Failure, as classified by the ACC/AHA (2001) as evaluated by activity tolerance. His chemistries and complete blood count were normal and his pulmonary function tests were also normal. He is AV paced at a base rate of 80 bpm and there were no episodes of SVT or VT found upon interrogation of his PC/ICD. Heart rate response to exercise was appropriate. At this point his medication regimen had already been maximized.

Despite reports of proper adherence to medication, diet, and exercise regimens, Mr. S. continued to require frequent visits to the clinic for complaints of periodic shortness of breath and activity intolerance that was not reproducible in the clinic. At each visit, a thoracic electrical bioimpedance (TEB) measurement was taken, along with a 6-minute walk test. Serial measurements were taken for comparison and were used as trending tools (Table 7-3).

Ultimately Mr. S. responded to gentle diuresis (see the decrease in thoracic fluid content, the increase in stroke volume and cardiac output, and the decrease in systemic vascular resistance), but he continued to complain of periodic shortness of breath, although he did report a slight improvement in activity tolerance. At this time, it was believed that more information was necessary to evaluate his shortness of breath. A blood volume analysis was performed, and a brain natriuretic peptide level was determined. He was also sent for a sleep study.

Mr. S. lost 9 lbs in 1 month; his blood volume analysis showed excess in total blood volume of 400 mL, which represents only mild hypervolemia, and the brain natriuretic peptide level was greater than 1300, which the New York Heart Association classifies as class IV heart failure. His sleep study was positive for severe sleep apnea and since treatment with CPAP he has had a more stable heart failure course. Mr. S. has not been admitted to the hospital due to close follow-up of his condition to include optimizing hemodynamic status in the clinic. Trending of values over time assists the practitioner to complete a comprehensive plan of care.

It is important to use various techniques to assess the patient. Noninvasive modalities are becoming routine in many critical care areas and because TEB is often used in the outpatient setting, obtaining data from the outpatient clinic may be helpful in guiding the treatment of each individual patient.

QUESTIONS

1. Which of the parameters in the case study give the indication of optimizing volume therapy?
2. Which comparable parameter would be treated if invasive measures were used to treat this patient?
3. If this patient had presented in the critical care environment having ischemic changes as he originally had in his stress test, what findings could you expect to identify?
4. What is the key in monitoring the patient's hemodynamic status?

TABLE 7-3

Serial Thoracic Bioimpedance Measurements

Parameter	January 16	February 6	February 14
Height	5'8"	5'8"	5'8"
Weight	155 lb	147 lb	146 lb
Heart rate	80 beats/min	80 beats/min	80 beats/min
Systolic blood pressure	94 mm Hg	86 mm Hg	103 mm Hg
Diastolic blood pressure	66 mm Hg	56 mm Hg	59 mm Hg
Cardiac output	4.7 L/min	5.8 L/min	5.6 L/min
Stroke volume	57 mL/beat	72 mL/beat	75 mL/beat
Systemic vascular resistance	846 dynes/sec/cm^{-5}	829 dynes/sec/cm^{-5}	800 dynes/sec/cm^{-5}
Thoracic fluid content	44.8 kW^{-1}	40.6 kW^{-1}	39.2 kW^{-1}
Systolic time ratio	0.54	0.45	0.42

channel blockers, antidysrhythmic drugs), or elective cardioversion.

5. Replace a severely diseased cardiac valve that is causing the problem.

TRENDS IN HEMODYNAMIC MONITORING

The development of tissue hypercapnia is a global phenomenon and occurs in every organ during circulatory failure. The use of gastric tonometry as an indicator of splanchnic perfusion is based on the measurement of luminal carbon dioxide pressure (PCO_2) as a reflection of intramucosal PCO_2 ($PiCO_2$).

Gastric Tonometry

Gastric tonometry is a based on the premise that the gastric (splanchnic) circulation, because of its anatomical features, is the first body system to be affected by inadequate perfusion. With gastric tonometry, ischemic changes within the gastric mucosa produce acidosis during the early stages of circulatory compromise. Mucosal acidosis is determined by intramucosal pH measurements, which may be obtained by use of a fiberoptic nasogastric tube. The nasogastric tube is attached to a bedside display monitor that automatically calculates and displays a gastric pH value. Lower gastric pH values, indicative of a more acidic environment, signal the clinician to possible ischemia within the gastric mucosa as a result of inadequate perfusion.

Sublingual Tonometry

Sublingual PCO_2 ($PslCO_2$) is measured using a disposable CO_2 sensor. It incorporates a CO_2-specific fluorescent dye in a buffer solution encased in a silicone capsule that is permeable to CO_2 gas. The sensor is attached to an instrument that measures the amount of CO_2 present by projecting light onto the sensor with an optical fiber. Changes in the projected light are used to calculate the amount of CO_2 present. For clinical measurements, the sensor is placed under the tongue with the sensor element facing the sublingual mucosa. Before each measurement, the sensor is calibrated against a known standard.

$PslCO_2$ yielded measurements that correlated well with those of gastric tonometry and served as a technically simple and noninvasive clinical measurement of tissue dysoxia in critically ill and injured patients (Marik, 2001). The baseline $PslCO_2$-differential and $PslCO_2$ were better predictors of outcome than were traditional markers of tissue hypoxia and were more responsive to therapeutic interventions (Marik & Bankov, 2003). The $PslCO_2$-differential and $PslCO_2$ may prove to be useful markers for goal-directed therapy and for assessing the response to clinical interventions aimed at improving tissue oxygenation.

Thoracic Electrical Bioimpedence

Thoracic electrical bioimpedance (TEB) is a method of noninvasive hemodynamic monitoring being used in hospital settings to provide practitioners with a "quick look" at hemodynamic measurements at the patient's bedside (Figure 7-21). "This technology has been developed largely in response to economic considerations and the increasing risk of invasive catheters" (Lasater, 2000). A few parameters that are commonly being measured are CO, CI, SVR, and thoracic fluid content (Table 7-4).

In the 1960s, Kubicek introduced TEB to the space program in response to the need to measure SV and CO of astronauts during space travel (Lasater, 2000). This technology has been refined and is being used to guide medical therapies for patients who are treated for hypertensive cardiovascular disease and heart failure. The system works by emitting a low-grade electrical current through skin electrodes that send and receive electrical signals (Figure 7-22). Impedance to current flow through the aorta is calculated; the data are displayed (Figure 7-23) and are then printed (Figure 7-24). Certain conditions that limit the accuracy of measurement are listed in Box 7-5.

TEB is an easy, noninvasive, and painless diagnostic test that gives data that are used to determine interventions that improve patient satisfaction and quality of life (Von Reuden, 2002). The timely trending and treatment of the patient allow for a reduction in the number of hospital admissions, decreasing health care costs.

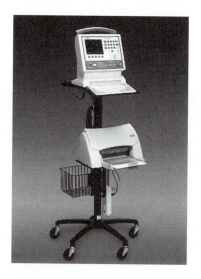

FIGURE 7-21 Thoracic electrical bioimpedance device. (Courtesy of Cardio Dynamics International Corporation, San Diego, CA.)

TABLE 7-4

Parameters Measured with Thoracic Electrical Bioimpedance

	Parameter	Flow
SV/SI	Stroke volume/index	Amount of blood pumped by the left ventricle each heart beat based on BSA
CO/CI	Cardiac output/index	Amount of blood pumped by the left ventricle each minute based on BSA
		Resistance
SVR/ SVRI	Systemic vascular resistance/index	The force the left ventricle must overcome to expel blood into the body (afterload) based on BSA
		Contractility
ACI	Acceleration index	Indicator of aortic blood acceleration
VI	Velocity index	Indicator of aortic blood velocity
PEP	Preejection period	Electrical systole: time interval from the beginning of electrical stimulation of the ventricles to the opening of the aortic valve
LVET	Left ventricular ejection time	Mechanical systole: time interval from the opening to the closing of the aortic valve
STR	Systolic time ratio	The ratio of the electrical and mechanical systole, PEP/LVET
		Fluid Status
TFC	Thoracic fluid content	Indicator of chest fluid status, including interstitial, intraalveolar, and intravascular fluid
		Cardiac Work
LSWI*	Left stroke work index	The amount of work the left ventricle must perform to pump blood each beat
LCW/ LCWI	Left cardiac work/index	The amount of work the left ventricle must perform to pump blood each minute
		Oxygen Transport
DO_2I*	Delivered oxygen index	Amount of oxygen delivered to tissues and organs, the product of cardiac index, arterial saturation, and hemoglobin

*Only available with BioZ ICG Module for GE Medical Systems *Information Technologies* patient monitoring systems; *Solar* 7000, 8000, and 8000M; *Dash* 3000, and 4000. *Dash* and *Solar* are registered trademarks of the General Electric Company. Modified from Cardio Dynamics International Corporation, San Diego, CA.

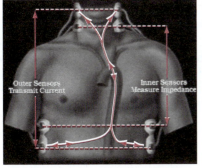

- Diposable sensors transmit a small electrical signal through the thorax.

- Impedence (resistance) to the electrical signal is measured and displayed as the ICG waveform.

- As volume and velocity of blood in the aorta change with each heartbeat, DISQ® (Digital Impedance Signal Quantifier) Technology processes the changes in impedance.

- The changes in impedance are applied to the innovative Z MARC™ (Modulating AoRtic Compliance) Algorithm to provide hemodynamic parameters, including stroke volume, cardiac output, systemic vascular resistance, and trending indices of contractility and fluid status.

FIGURE 7-22 Electrode placement for thoracic electrical bioimpedance by Cardio Dynamics. (Courtesy of Cardio Dynamics International Corporation, San Diego, CA.)

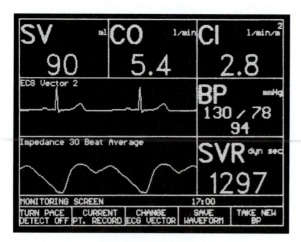

FIGURE 7-23 Monitor display of waveforms and values obtained when assessing noninvasive hemodynamics using Cardio Dynamics. (Courtesy of Cardio Dynamics International Corporation, San Diego, CA.)

MEMORIAL HOSPITAL

1200 MAIN ST., SAN DIEGO, CA 92121

Hemodynamic Status Report

Name:		Age:	63	Height:	5 ft 2 in
ID:		Sex:	Female	Weight:	145 lb
				BSA:	1.67 m²

30 Beat Average   Page 1 of 1

Parameter	Description	Value	Low	Normal	High
HR	Heart Rate	70	58		86
SBP	Systolic Blood Pressure	135	100		140
DBP	Diastolic Blood Pressure	90	60		90
MAP	Mean Arterial Pressure	105	84		100
CI	Cardiac Index	2.2	2.5		4.7
CO	Cardiac Output	3.7	4.2		7.8
SI	Stroke Index	32	35		65
SV	Stroke Volume	52	58		108
SVRI	Systemic Vascular Res. Index	3562	1337		2483
SVR	Systemic Vascular Resistance	2159	742		1378
ACI	Acceleration Index	106	90		170
VI	Velocity Index	48	33		65
TFC	Thoracic Fluid Content	64.6	21.0		37.0
LCWI	Left Cardiac Work Index	3.0	3.0		5.5
LCW	Left Cardiac Work	5.0	5.4		10.0
STR	Systolic Time Ratio	0.45	0.30		0.50
PEP	Pre-Ejection Period	121			
LVET	Left Ventricular Ejection Time	265			

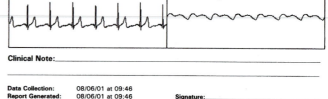

ECG Vector 4   ICG 30 Beat Average

Clinical Note:_____

| Data Collection: | 08/06/01 at 09:46 | |
| Report Generated: | 08/06/01 at 09:46 | Signature:_____ |

FIGURE 7-24 Example of a status report for the noninvasive indices printed with electrocardiograms and waveforms. (Courtesy of Cardio Dynamics International Corporation, San Diego, CA.)

SUMMARY

This chapter is designed as an introduction to the basic principles of hemodynamics and the technological aspects of hemodynamic monitoring. The discussion focuses on the various types of hemodynamic monitoring used in the critical care setting, such as monitoring SvO₂, CO, PAOP, RAP, LAP, PAP, and arterial pressures. In addition, nursing considerations in the care of a patient undergoing each of these types of monitoring are highlighted.

Hemodynamic monitoring is an important physiological assessment tool in the care of critically ill patients. Data obtained from this modality serve as a guide to the health care team in determining and evaluating interventions for such patients.

Geriatric Assessment (In the Absence of Clinical Disease)

Area Affected	Age-Related Changes	Implications
Myocardium and valves	The elderly heart relies more on increased stretch than increased heart rate to increase contractility Collagen increases and elastin decreases in the heart muscle Heart valves become stiffer and thicker Contraction time is slightly prolonged, and relaxation is slower	Little change in cardiac output occurs in disease-free hearts Diastolic time is shortened Filling in early stages of diastole is decreased Atrial kick (filling from atrial contraction) plays an important role in compensating for shortened filling time
Conduction system	Accumulation of fibrosis and fat around the sinoatrial node occurs The number of pacemaker cells is decreased	Sinus node dysfunction occurs Conduction time is increased; heart rate is slightly decreased Atrial fibrillation occurs
Vessels	Calcification of vessels occurs Elastin in vessel walls is decreased Arterial distensibility is lost Vessels become more tortuous Baroreceptor sensitivity decreases	Thickening and rigidity occur, especially in the coronary arteries Systolic blood pressure increases; diastolic blood pressure is the same or slightly increased Pulse pressure widens Blood pressure fluctuates
Response to stress and exercise	Beta-receptor response is diminished Maximal heart rate decreases	Patient cannot rely on increased heart rate to increase cardiac output Patient relies on increased end-diastolic volume and increased stroke volume to increase cardiac output

Data from Eaton, L. (2000). Cardiovascular function. In A. Leukenotte (Ed.). *Gerontologic nursing.* 2nd ed. St. Louis: Mosby; Hamm, R., Sloane, P., & Warshaw, G. (2002). *Primary care geriatrics: A case-based approach.* 4th ed. St. Louis: Mosby; and Silverhorn, D. (2001). *Human physiology: An integrated approach.* 2nd ed. Austin, TX: University of Texas.

CRITICAL THINKING QUESTIONS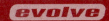

1. How does SV affect CO?
2. Describe how CO affects the delivery of oxygen to tissues. What parameters would be the best to monitor in a patient to assess this influence?
3. If a patient's mean arterial pressure continues to rise significantly, indicating an increase in resistance and a altered ability of the heart to eject blood, what parameters would also be affected as a result?
4. A patient who has undergone surgery has received a bed bath with back care and then undergoes suctioning and is turned. During these care activities, the patient experiences pain. What consequences does this pain have on the patient's SvO_2 status?
5. A patient is bleeding significantly and receives a transfusion of packed red blood cells. You note that the PAOP remains low, and the CI drops again. What is the significance of these alterations? What additional interventions would you expect?
6. You are caring for a patient who requires monitoring of the CI every 2 hours. What technical factors would you consider in obtaining accurate intermittent readings?

REFERENCES

American Association of Critical-Care Nurses. (1993). Evaluation of the effects of heparinized and non-heparinized solutions on the patency of arterial pressure monitoring: The Thunder project. *American Journal of Critical Care, 2*(1), 3-15.

Bridges, E. J., Woods, S. L., Brengelmann, G. L., Mitchell, P., & Laurent-Bopp, D. (2000). Effect of the 30 degree lateral recumbent position on pulmonary artery and pulmonary artery wedge pressures in critically ill adult cardiac surgery patients. *American Journal of Critical Care, 9*(4), 262-275.

Centers for Disease Control and Prevention. (2002). Guidelines for the prevention of intravascular catheter-related infections. *MMWR, 51*(RR10), 1-26. Retrieved from http://www.cdc.gov/mmwr/preview/mmwrhtml/rr5110a1.htm (Accessed 3/22/2004.)

Chen, Y. Y., Yen, D. H., Yang, Y. G., Liu, C. Y., Wang, F. D., & Chou, P. (2003). Comparison between replacement at 4 days and 7 days of the infection rate for pulmonary artery catheters in an intensive care unit. *Critical Care Medicine, 31*(5), 1353-1358.

Darovic, G. (2002). *Hemodynamic monitoring. Invasive and noninvasive clinical application.* 3rd ed. Philadelphia: W. B. Saunders.

Gawlinski, A., & Dracup, K. (1998). Effect of positioning on SvO_2 in the critically ill patient with a low ejection fraction. *Nursing Research, 47,* 293-299.

Giuliano, K. K., Scott, S. S., Brown, V., & Olson, M. (2003). Backrest angle and cardiac output measurement in critically ill patients. *Nursing Research, 52,* 242-248.

Hamm, R., Sloane, P., & Warshaw, G. (2002). *Primary care geriatrics: A case-based approach.* 4th ed. St. Louis: Mosby.

Houghton, D., Cohn, S., Schell, V., Cohn, K., & Varon, A. (2002). Routine daily chest radiography in patients with pulmonary artery catheters. *American Journal of Critical Care, 11*(3), 261-265.

Jesurum, J. T. (1998). SvO_2 monitoring. *Protocols for practice: Hemodynamic monitoring series.* Aliso Viejo, CA: American Association of Critical-Care Nurses.

Keckeisen, M. (1998). Pulmonary artery pressure monitoring. *Protocols for practice: Hemodynamic monitoring series.* Aliso Viejo, CA: American Association of Critical-Care Nurses.

Lasater, M. (2000) Impedance cardiography: A method of non-invasive cardiac output monitoring. *AACN News, 17*(5), 12-14.

Lewis, P., Nichols, E., Mackay, G., et al. (1997). The effect of turning and backrub on mixed venous oxygen saturation in critically ill patients. *American Journal of Critical Care, 6*(2), 132-140.

Lundstedt, J. L. (1997). Comparison of measurements of measuring pulmonary artery pressure. *American Journal of Critical Care, 6*(4), 324-332.

Marik, P. E . (2001). Sublingual capnography: A clinical validation study. *Chest, 120*(3), 923-927.

Marik, P. E., & Bankov, A. (2003). Sublingual capnometry versus traditional markers of tissue oxygenation in critically ill patients. *Critical Care Medicine, 31*(3), 818-822.

PACEP, Pulmonary Artery Catheter Education Project. 2001-2004, PACEP Collaborative. Retrieved from http://www.pacep.org/pages/start/ref.html?xin=sccm. Accessed 3/22/2004.

Von Reuden, K. T. (2002). Outpatient hemodynamic monitoring of patients with heart failure. *Journal of Cardiovascular Nursing, 16*(3), 62-71.

Wilson, A. E., Bermingham-Mitchell, K., Wells, N., & Zachary, K. (1996). Effect of backrest position on hemodynamic and right ventricular measurements in critically ill adults. *American Journal of Critical Care, 5,* 264-270.

RECOMMENDED READINGS

Chittock, D. R., Dhinga, V. K., Ronco, J. J., Russell, J. A., Forrest, D. M., Tweeddale, M., & Fenwick, J. C. (2004). Severity of illness and risk of death associated with pulmonary artery catheter use. *Crit Care Med, 32*(4): 911-915.

Rackow, E. C., O'Neil, P., Astiz, M. E., & Carpati, C. M. (2001). Sublingual capnometry and indexes of tissue perfusion in patients with circulatory failure. *Chest, 120,* 1633-1638.

evolve *Did you remember to check out the bonus material, including free self-assessment exercises, on the Evolve Web site at http://evolve.elsevier.com/Sole/ and on the CD-ROM?*

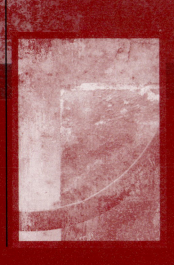

CHAPTER 8

Ventilatory Assistance

Jeffery E. Ludy, EdD, RRT
Mary Lou Sole, PhD, RN, CCNS, FAAN
Maryanne Ludy, MSN, ARNP

OBJECTIVES

- Review the anatomy and physiology of the respiratory system.
- Describe methods for assessing the respiratory system, including physical assessment, interpretation of arterial blood gases, and noninvasive techniques.
- Compare commonly used oxygen delivery devices.
- Discuss methods for maintaining an open airway.
- Identify indications for initiation of mechanical ventilation.
- Describe types and modes of mechanical ventilation.
- Relate complications associated with mechanical ventilation.
- Explain methods for weaning patients from mechanical ventilation.
- Formulate a plan of care for the mechanically ventilated patient.

Introduction

Maintaining an adequate airway and ensuring adequate breathing, or ventilation, are nursing interventions that are essential for all patients. These nursing interventions provide the framework for this chapter. Respiratory anatomy and physiology are reviewed to provide a basis for discussing ventilatory assistance. Assessment of the respiratory system is discussed, including physical examination, arterial blood gas (ABG) interpretation, and noninvasive methods for assessing gas exchange. Airway management and mechanical ventilation are also discussed.

Review of Respiratory Anatomy and Physiology

The primary function of the respiratory system is gas exchange. Oxygen and carbon dioxide are exchanged via the respiratory system to provide adequate oxygen to the cells and to remove excess carbon dioxide from the cells. The respiratory system can be divided into (1) the upper airway, (2) the lower airway, and (3) the lungs. The upper airway provides gas exchange to and from the lower airway, and the lower airway provides gas exchange to the alveoli. The anatomical structure of the respiratory system is shown in Figure 8-1.

evolve *Be sure to check out the bonus material, including free self-assessment exercises, on the Evolve Web site at http://evolve.elsevier.com/Sole/ and on the CD-ROM.*

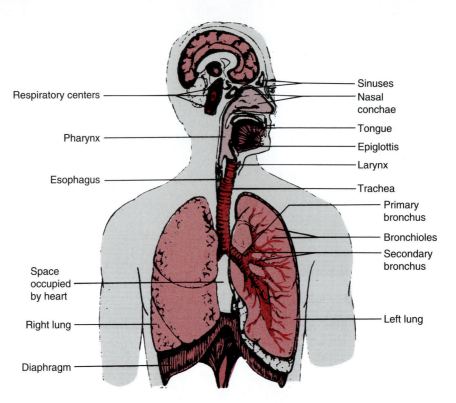

Respiratory centers

Pharynx

Esophagus

Space occupied by heart

Right lung

Diaphragm

Sinuses

Nasal conchae

Tongue

Epiglottis

Larynx

Trachea

Primary bronchus

Bronchioles

Secondary bronchus

Left lung

FIGURE 8-1 Anatomy of the respiratory system. The lungs are located in the thoracic cavity. The diaphragm forms the floor of the thoracic cavity and separates it from the abdominal cavity. The internal view of one lung shows air passages. (From Solomon, E. P. [2003]. *Introduction to human anatomy and physiology.* [p. 220]. 2nd ed. Philadelphia: W. B. Saunders.)

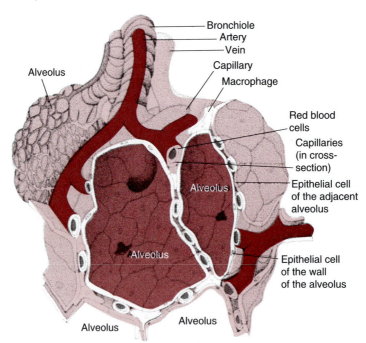

Bronchiole

Artery

Vein

Capillary

Macrophage

Alveolus

Red blood cells

Capillaries (in cross-section)

Epithelial cell of the adjacent alveolus

Alveolus

Alveolus

Epithelial cell of the wall of the alveolus

Alveolus

Alveolus

FIGURE 8-2 Structure and function of the alveolus. (From Solomon, E. P. [2003]. *Introduction to human anatomy and physiology.* [p. 222]. 2nd ed. Philadelphia: W. B. Saunders.)

UPPER AIRWAY

The upper airway consists of the nasal cavity and the pharynx. The bony structure of the nasal cavity is referred to as the nasal conchae. The nasal cavity conducts air, filters large foreign particles, and warms and humidifies air. The nasal cavity also is responsible for voice resonance, smell, and sneeze reflexes. The throat, or pharynx, transports both air and food. Air enters the superior part of the pharynx (the nasopharynx) and then passes behind the mouth through the oropharynx.

LOWER AIRWAY

The lower airway consists of the larynx, trachea, right and left mainstem bronchi, bronchioles, and alveoli. The larynx is the narrowest part of the conducting airways in adults and contains the vocal cords. The larynx is partly covered by the epiglottis, which prevents aspiration of food, liquid, or saliva into the lungs during swallowing. The passage through the vocal cords is the glottis.

The windpipe, or trachea, warms, humidifies, and filters air. Cilia in the trachea propel mucus and foreign material upward through the airway. At about the level of the fifth thoracic vertebra (sternal angle, or angle of Louis), the trachea branches into the bronchi. This bifurcation is referred to as the carina.

The trachea divides into the right and left mainstem bronchi, which conduct air to the respective lungs. The right mainstem bronchus is shorter, wider, and straighter than the left. Mucosal cells in the bronchi trap foreign materials. The bronchi branch into the bronchioles, which, in turn, branch into the alveoli.

The alveoli are the distal airway structures and are responsible for gas exchange at the capillary level. More than 300 million of these tiny air sacs are present in the lungs. The alveoli consist of a single layer of epithelial cells and fibers that permit expansion and contraction. A network of capillaries covers the alveoli. Gas exchange occurs between the alveoli and these capillaries. The inner surface of the alveoli is coated with surfactant, which prevents them from collapsing. The structure of the alveolus is shown in Figure 8-2. The large combined surface area and single cell layer of the alveoli promote diffusion of gases.

LUNGS

The lungs consist of lobes; the left lung has two lobes, and the right lung has three lobes. Each lobe consists of lobules, or segments, that are supplied by one bronchiole. The top, or pointed part, of each lung is the apex, and the lower part of the lung is the base.

The lungs are covered by pleura. The visceral pleura covers the lung surfaces, whereas the parietal pleura covers the internal surface of the thoracic cage.

Between these two tissues a pleural space is formed containing approximately 2 mL of pleural fluid. This fluid layer is quite thin and holds together and lubricates the pleural layers as they slide across each other during the act of breathing (Guyton & Hall, 2000). The intrapleural pressure in the pleural space is always negative (less than atmospheric), so lung expansion can be maintained and inspiration facilitated.

PHYSIOLOGY OF BREATHING

Changes in intrapleural pressure and intraalveolar pressure (the pressure in the lungs) cause the act of breathing (Figure 8-3). At rest, intrapleural pressure is less than atmospheric pressure, whereas the intraalveolar pressure equals atmospheric pressure. During inspiration, the diaphragm lowers and flattens and the intercostal muscles contract, lifting the

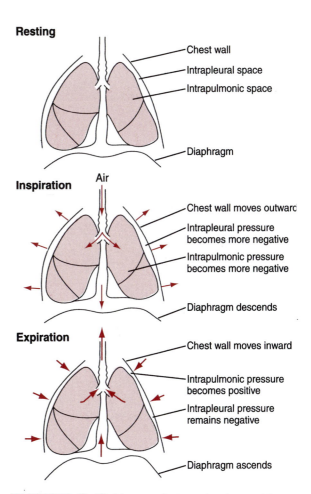

Resting
— Chest wall
— Intrapleural space
— Intrapulmonic space
— Diaphragm

Inspiration — Air
— Chest wall moves outward
— Intrapleural pressure becomes more negative
— Intrapulmonic pressure becomes more negative
— Diaphragm descends

Expiration
— Chest wall moves inward
— Intrapulmonic pressure becomes positive
— Intrapleural pressure remains negative
— Diaphragm ascends

FIGURE 8-3 Changes in intraalveolar and intrapleural pressures and position of diaphragm during the respiratory cycle. (From Hansen, M. [1998] *Pathophysiology* [p. 451]. Philadelphia: W. B. Saunders.)

chest up and outward to increase the size of the chest cavity. Subsequently, intrapleural pressure becomes even more negative, and the intraalveolar pressure becomes negative relative to atmospheric pressure. With this change air begins to flow into the lungs because atmospheric pressure is now greater than both intraalveolar and intrapleural pressure. Expiration is a passive process. After inspiration, the diaphragm and intercostal muscles relax and the lungs recoil. This recoil generates positive alveolar pressure relative to atmospheric pressure, and air flows out of the lungs (expiration).

GAS EXCHANGE

The process of gas exchange (Figure 8-4) consists of four steps: (1) ventilation, (2) diffusion at pulmonary capillaries, (3) perfusion (transportation), and (4) diffusion to the cells (Scanlan & Wilkins, 2003a).

1. *Ventilation* is the movement of gases (oxygen and carbon dioxide) in and out of the alveoli.
2. *Diffusion* of oxygen and carbon dioxide occurs at the pulmonary capillary level. Figure 8-5 illustrates diffusion of oxygen and carbon dioxide at the alveolar-capillary membrane. The alveoli contain higher levels of oxygen than exist in the capillaries, thus causing oxygen to diffuse from the alveoli into the capillaries. Carbon dioxide levels are higher in the capillaries, thus causing carbon dioxide to diffuse into the alveoli for elimination through the lungs.
3. The oxygenated blood in the pulmonary capillary is transported via the pulmonary vein to the left

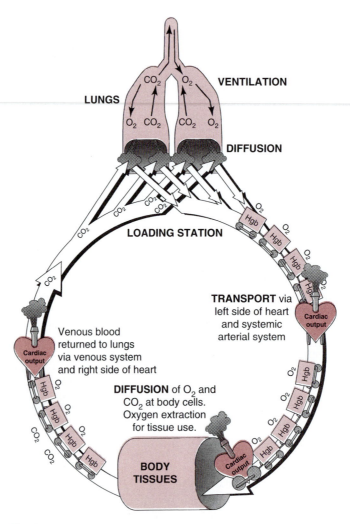

FIGURE 8-4 Schematic view of the process of gas exchange. Hgb, hemoglobin. (Modified from Alspach, J. [1992]. *AACN instructor's resource manual for AACN core curriculum for critical care nursing.* 4th ed. [Transparency 29] Philadelphia: W. B. Saunders.)

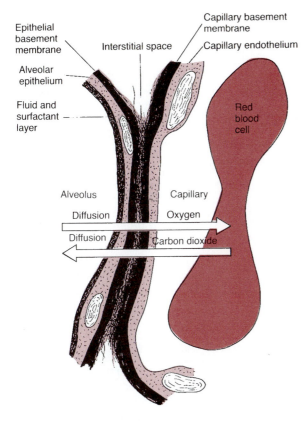

FIGURE 8-5 Diffusion of oxygen and carbon dioxide at the alveolar-capillary membrane. (From Guyton, A. C., & Hall, J. E. [2000]. *Textbook of medical physiology* [p. 459]. 10th ed. Philadelphia: W. B. Saunders.)

side of the heart. The oxygenated blood is *perfused* or transported to the tissues.

4. *Diffusion* of oxygen and carbon dioxide occurs at the cellular level based on concentration gradients. Oxygen enters the cells, and carbon dioxide leaves the cells. Carbon dioxide is transported via the vena cava to the right side of the heart for elimination through the lungs.

Numerous physiological features must be present for optimal gas exchange to occur. These include an intact nervous system, compliant lungs, a sufficient number of functioning alveoli, unencumbered alveolar-capillary membranes, adequate level of normal hemoglobin, good cardiac output, and patent pulmonary vessels (Scanlan & Wilkins, 2003a).

REGULATION OF BREATHING

The rate, depth, and rhythm of ventilation are controlled by respiratory centers in the medulla and pons. When the carbon dioxide level is high or the oxygen level is low, chemoreceptors in the respiratory center, carotid arteries, and aorta send messages to the medulla to regulate respiration. In persons with normal lung function, high levels of carbon dioxide stimulate respiration. However, patients with chronic obstructive pulmonary disease (COPD) maintain higher levels of carbon dioxide as a baseline, and their ventilatory drive in response to increased carbon dioxide levels is blunted. In these patients, the stimulus to breathe is the lower level of oxygen and the hypoxemia it causes.

Work of Breathing

The work of breathing (WOB) is the amount of effort required for the maintenance of a given level of ventilation. The respiratory pattern changes automatically to assist in the WOB, depending on lung compliance and resistance. As the WOB increases, more energy is expended for adequate ventilation to be obtained; this increased energy expenditure requires proportionately more oxygen and glucose. If the WOB becomes too high, mechanical ventilatory support may be needed.

Compliance

Compliance is a measure of the distensibility, or stretchability, of the lung and chest wall. It is defined as the change in volume per unit of pressure change (Levitzky, 2002). Compliance is primarily determined by the amount of elastic recoil that must be overcome before lung inflation can occur. Elastic recoil, or elastance, refers to the ability of the lung to return to a resting position after stretching during inspiration.

Elastic recoil and compliance are inversely related. For example, in pulmonary fibrosis, acute respiratory distress syndrome (ARDS), and pulmonary edema, lung tissue has greater elastic recoil that decreases distensibility. In these situations, compliance is low, and the lungs are stiff and difficult to distend. High pressures are required for inflation of the lungs. Severe obesity also decreases compliance because inflating the lungs in the presence of increased chest wall mass is more difficult.

In emphysema, destruction of lung tissue and enlarged air spaces cause the lungs to lose their elasticity. The decrease in elastic recoil causes compliance to be increased, or high. The lungs are more distensible in this situation and require lower pressures for ventilation.

Static compliance refers to the measurement of thoracic compliance taken during a period of no airflow (e.g., while the patient holds his or her breath). Static compliance is an indicator of elastic recoil. Static compliance in patients with normal lung function usually ranges from 50 to 170 mL/cm H_2O (Pilbeam, 1998).

This means that for every 1 cm H_2O change of pressure in the lungs, the volume of gas increases by 50 to 170 mL. Lung function is altered in most patients requiring mechanical ventilation resulting in decreased compliance. Compliance varies based on the severity of the patient's pulmonary condition, positioning, and level of consciousness. Compliance in the mechanically ventilated patient ranges from 40 to 50 mL/cm H_2O in male patients and 35 to 45 mL/cm H_2O in female patients (Pilbeam, 1998).

Dynamic compliance is measured during breathing and is an indicator of both elastic recoil and airway resistance. Static compliance and dynamic compliance usually range below static compliance values. Dynamic compliance is easier to measure because it does not require breath holding or an inspiratory hold.

The respiratory therapist or nurse measures compliance in the mechanically ventilated patient to identify trends developing in the patient's condition, not for diagnosing lung disease. Poor compliance is an indication of decreased lung elasticity, increased airway resistance, or both, and requires higher ventilatory pressures for adequate ventilation. Higher ventilatory pressures place the patient at increased risk of complications such as volutrauma. Improved compliance reflects improved pulmonary status.

Resistance

Resistance refers to the opposition to gas flow in the airways. Resistance is increased with airway spasms (bronchoconstriction) and the presence of mucus or edema. The small internal diameter of artificial airways increases resistance to airflow (Levitzky, 2002). Normal airway resistance ranges from 0.6 to 2.4 cm H_2O/L/sec in a nonventilated person with normal lung function. Resistance increases to 5 to 7 cm H_2O/L/sec in patients who have an artificial airway. Values are even higher for patients with obstructive pulmonary disease.

LUNG VOLUMES AND CAPACITIES

The lungs have several volumes and capacities that are important for determining adequate pulmonary function. The lung volumes and capacities are shown graphically in Figure 8-6. Descriptions of the lung volumes are provided in Table 8-1. A *spirometer* is used to measure lung volumes. Measurements of lung volumes and capacities allow the practitioner to assess baseline pulmonary function and to monitor the improvement or progression of pulmonary diseases. The volumes and capacities are for healthy men; the values are approximately 20% to 25% less in women (Guyton & Hall, 2000). Lung capacities decline gradually with aging.

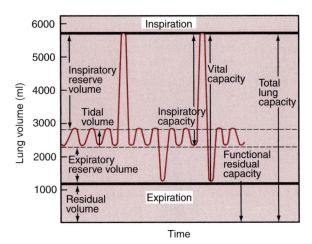

FIGURE 8-6 Lung volumes and capacities. (From Guyton, A. C., & Hall, J. E. [2000]. *Textbook of medical physiology* [p. 437]. 10th ed. Philadelphia: W. B. Saunders.)

Respiratory Assessment

Physical assessment of the respiratory system is an essential tool for the critical care nurse. Assessment skills assist in identifying potential patient problems and in evaluating patient response to interventions. See the Geriatric Assessment box for information related to assessment of elderly patients.

HEALTH HISTORY

Critically ill patients are frequently unable to provide health history information because of their physical and/or cognitive condition. Information is usually obtained from significant others who know the patient's history. Several questions should be asked when a patient's health history is obtained, including the following:

1. Tobacco use: type, amount, and number of years used (or pack-years): pack-years = packs cigarettes/day × years smoked
2. Occupational history, such as coal mining, asbestos work, farming
3. History of sputum production: type, amount, color, consistency, time of day, and whether its appearance is chronic or acute
4. History of shortness of breath, dyspnea, cough, anorexia, weight loss, or chest pain
5. Use of oral and inhalant respiratory medications, such as bronchodilators and steroids
6. Use of over-the-counter drugs
7. Allergies: medication and environmental
8. Date of last chest x-ray study and/or tuberculosis screening

TABLE 8-1

Lung Volumes and Capacities

Name	Definition	Average	Formula
VOLUMES			
Tidal volume (V_T)	Volume of a normal breath	500 mL or 5-10 mL/kg	
Inspiratory reserve Volume (IRV)	Maximum amount of gas that can be inspired at the end of a normal breath (over and above the V_T)	3000 mL	
Expiratory reserve volume (ERV)	Maximum amount of gas that can be forcefully expired at the end of a normal breath	1100 mL	
Residual volume (RV)	Amount of air remaining in the lungs after maximum expiration	1200 mL	
CAPACITIES			
Inspiratory capacity (IC)	Maximum volume of gas that can be inspired at normal resting expiration; the IC distends the lungs to their maximum amount	3500 mL	IC = V_T + IRV
Functional residual capacity (FRC)	Volume of gas remaining in the lungs at normal resting expiration	2300 mL	FRC = ERV + RV
Vital capacity (VC)	Maximum volume of gas that can be forcefully expired after maximum inspiration	4600 mL	VC = V_T + IRV + ERV
Total lung capacity (TLC)	Volume of gas in the lungs at end of maximum inspiration	5800 mL	TLC = V_T + ERV + RV

Geriatric Assessment

Physiological Changes With Aging

- ↓ Alveolar surface area
- ↓ Alveolar elasticity
- ↓ Chest wall distensibility
- ↓ Physiological compensatory mechanisms (respiratory, renal, cardiac, immune)

Assessment Changes

Normal Findings Because of Aging Process
- Kyphosis
- Barrel chest
- ↓ Chest expansion
- Lower PaO_2 levels on ABG

Increased Risk For
- Poor gas exchange
- Respiratory distress
- Respiratory failure

ABG, Arterial blood gas; *PaO₂,* partial pressure of oxygen in arterial blood.

PHYSICAL EXAMINATION

Inspection

Inspection provides an initial clue for potential acute and chronic respiratory problems. The head, neck, fingers, and chest are inspected for abnormalities.

Several assessments are made in the inspection of the head, neck, and fingers. Signs of acute respiratory distress include labored respirations with the use of accessory muscles, sternal retraction, nasal flaring, asymmetrical chest movements, open-mouthed breathing, or gasping breaths. Cyanosis is a late sign of hypoxemia and should not be relied on as an early indicator of distress. Other indications of respiratory abnormalities include pallor or rubor, pursed-lip breathing, jugular venous distention, prolonged expiratory phase of breaths, poor capillary refill, clubbing of fingers, or barrel-shaped chest.

The chest is observed for abnormal breathing patterns, use of chest and abdominal accessory muscles, asymmetrical chest wall movement, and abnormal chest excursion. The normal respiratory rate is 12 to 20 breaths per minute, and expiration is usually twice as long as inspiration (I:E ratio of 1:2). Alterations from normal should be documented and reported.

The normal breathing pattern is regular and even, with an occasional sigh. Normal breathing is referred to as *eupnea*. Alterations from this normal pattern should be noted. *Tachypnea* is defined as a respiratory rate of greater than 20 breaths per minute. Tachypnea may occur with anxiety, fever, pain, anemia, and blood gas abnormalities. *Bradypnea* is a respiratory rate of less than 10 breaths per minute. Bradypnea may occur in central nervous system disorders; it may also result from administration or ingestion of certain central nervous system depressant medications or alcohol, blood gas abnormalities, and fatigue.

Several abnormal breathing patterns (Figure 8-7) are possible and should be reported. *Cheyne-Stokes respirations* have a cyclical respiratory pattern. The patient has deep respirations that become increasingly shallow, followed by a period of apnea that lasts approximately 20 seconds. The cycle repeats after each apneic period. The apneic period may vary and progressively lengthen; therefore, the duration of the apneic period is timed for trending. Cheyne-Stokes respirations may occur in central nervous system disorders and congestive heart failure. *Kussmaul's respirations* are deep, regular, and rapid (usually more than 20 breaths per minute). Kussmaul's respirations commonly occur in diabetic ketoacidosis and other disorders that cause metabolic acidosis. *Biot's respirations,* or cluster breathing, are cycles of breaths that vary in depth and have varying periods of apnea. Biot's respirations are seen with some central nervous system disorders. *Apneustic respirations* are gasping

Cheyne-Stokes Respirations gradually become faster and deeper than normal, then slower; alternates with period of apnea

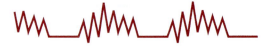

Biot's Respiration faster and deeper than normal with abrupt pauses between efforts; breaths have equal depth

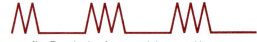

Kussmal's Respiration faster and deeper without pauses

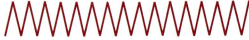

Apneustic Respirations prolonged, gasping, followed by extremely short, inefficient expiration

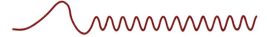

FIGURE 8-7 Breathing patterns. (From Hansen, M. [1998]. *Pathophysiology* [p. 456]. Philadelphia: W. B. Saunders.)

inspirations followed by short, ineffective expirations. They are often associated with brain lesions.

The patient is observed for signs of COPD. Clues that might indicate COPD include wheezing, productive cough, pursed-lip breathing, barrel chest, and muscle wasting. The patient with COPD may also prefer to sit in a chair and lean forward, rather than lie in bed.

Palpation

Palpation is frequently performed simultaneously with inspection. Palpation is used to evaluate chest wall excursion, tracheal deviation, chest wall tenderness, subcutaneous crepitus, and tactile fremitus.

During inspiration, chest wall excursion should be symmetrical. Asymmetrical excursion is usually associated with unilateral ventilation problems. The trachea is normally in a midline position; a tracheal shift may occur in tension pneumothorax. The chest wall should not be tender to palpation; tenderness is usually associated with inflammation or trauma. *Subcutaneous crepitus* or *subcutaneous emphysema* is the presence of air beneath the skin surface. The fingertips are used to palpate for air under the skin. Subcutaneous crepitus may occur around chest tube and tracheostomy sites. It may also result from chest trauma, such as rib fractures, and from barotrauma.

Tactile fremitus is assessed by palpating the patient's chest wall with the palmar or ulnar surface of the hand and noting vibrations transmitted through the chest wall while having the patient recite sounds that vibrate, such as "ninety-nine." The intensity of vibrations is compared bilaterally. Tactile fremitus may be increased over consolidated areas of the lungs; vibrations may be decreased in pleural effusion and pneumothorax.

Percussion

The chest may be percussed to identify respiratory disorders, such as hemothorax, pneumothorax, and consolidation. In percussion, the middle finger of one hand is tapped twice by the middle finger of the opposite hand. The vibrations produced by tapping produce different sounds, depending on the density of the area being percussed.

Five sounds may be audible on percussion: resonance, dullness, flatness, hyperresonance, and tympany. *Resonance* is the sound produced by percussion of normal lung tissue. Resonance is described as sounding like a muffled drum. *Dullness* is heard when tissue that is denser than normal is percussed and consists of a dull thud. Clinical conditions associated with dullness include pleural effusion, hemothorax, consolidation, atelectasis, tumors, and pulmonary fibrosis. *Flatness* is noted when air is absent in lung tissues. The sound heard with flatness is extreme dullness. Clinical conditions that may cause flatness include massive pleural effusion and lung collapse. *Hyperresonance* produces a slight musical sound, like a hollow drum, heard over tissue that has an increased amount of air. Clinical conditions associated with hyperresonance include emphysema, pneumothorax, and acute asthma. *Tympany* is a musical, drum-like sound produced by a large, air-filled area. Clinical conditions that produce tympany include tension pneumothorax and an air-filled cavity caused by an infection or abscess. Gastric distention may also produce tympany over the chest wall.

Auscultation

Lung sounds are routinely assessed, often every 1 to 4 hours, in critically ill patients. Quality of breath sounds, presence of adventitious lung sounds, and character of voice sounds are assessed.

A good stethoscope is essential for proper auscultation. The stethoscope should have both a diaphragm and a bell so both high-pitched (diaphragm) and low-pitched (bell) sounds can be identified. Some stethoscopes are designed for auscultating both high- and low-pitched sounds with a single head by adjusting the amount of pressure placed on the stethoscope head. Sounds are transmitted best through tubing that is thick and short; tubing that is too long decreases the transmission of sound. The earpieces of the stethoscope should fit comfortably.

Several additional techniques facilitate auscultation. A quiet environment is essential. It may be necessary to turn off television, radios, and noise-producing equipment during auscultation. The stethoscope should be placed directly on the patient's chest; sounds are difficult to distinguish if they are auscultated through the patient's gown or clothing. When auscultation is performed over chest hair, the stethoscope head should be held firmly against the skin to minimize a crackling sound that is produced by the hair. If auscultation must be performed over hairy areas, the chest hair should be wet with water before auscultation. Additionally, the stethoscope tubing should not rest against skin or objects such as sheets and bed rails during auscultation.

Auscultation is performed systematically. The anterior, posterior, and lateral aspects of the chest are auscultated (Figure 8-8). Auscultation is best performed with the patient sitting in an upright position. The patient is asked to breathe deeply in and out through the mouth. The stethoscope is moved

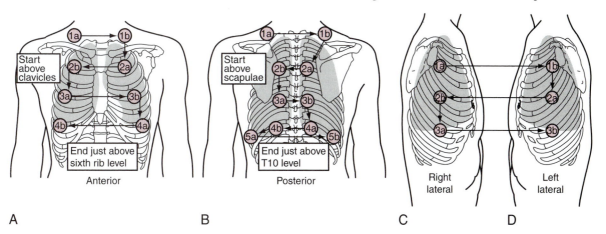

FIGURE 8-8 Systematic method for palpation, percussion, and auscultation of the lungs in anterior (**A**), posterior (**B**), and lateral regions (**C** and **D**). The techniques should be performed systematically to compare right and left lung fields.

back and forth across each side of the chest for comparison of sounds. Lung sounds must be evaluated both anteriorly and posteriorly so all lobes are assessed.

It may not be feasible for a critically ill patient to assume a sitting position for auscultation. In this circumstance, auscultation of the posterior and lateral chest is performed when the patient is turned to the side.

Breath Sounds

Types of normal breath sounds include bronchial, bronchovesicular, and vesicular. Abnormal breath sounds are called adventitious sounds, and include crackles, wheezing, and pleural friction rubs. At times, breath sounds may be decreased. The presence of fluid, air, or increased tissue can cause decreased breath sounds. Shallow respirations can also mimic decreased breath sounds; therefore, the patient must take deep breaths during auscultation. Table 8-2 reviews types of breath sounds.

Bronchial sounds. *Bronchial* sounds are normally heard over the larger airways, that is, over the trachea and mainstem bronchus. Bronchial sounds have a hollow, tubular quality and are not normally heard over the periphery, so their adventitious presence may reflect a disease process such as pneumonia at that location.

Bronchovesicular sounds. *Bronchovesicular* sounds are normally heard over large central airways (e.g., over the sternum) and between the scapulae. They have a hollow, breezy quality.

Vesicular sounds. *Vesicular* sounds are normal breath sounds that are heard over the peripheral lung fields. They are heard throughout the chest, except over the central airways. Vesicular breath sounds have a breezy quality, a moderate intensity, and a low pitch. Although the normal inspiration-to-expiration (I:E) ratio is 1:2, vesicular breath sounds have an audible I:E ratio of 3:1. This occurs because nearly all the air heard during expiration is expelled quickly.

Crackles. *Crackles* are short, explosive, nonmusical, and discontinuous sounds. They are defined as fine to coarse, based on pitch. Crackles are heard primarily in the inspiratory phase but may be noted during either inspiration or expiration. The presence of crackles usually indicates the presence of fluid in the alveoli and airways. Atelectasis is another cause of crackles. Crackles may be audible when previously deflated airways are reinflated on inspiration; therefore, they sometimes disappear after coughing, suctioning, or deep inspiration.

Wheezes. *Wheezes* are continuous sounds resulting from rapid passage of air through narrow airways.

TABLE 8-2

Types of Breath Sounds

	Normal Location	Intensity	Pitch	Quality	I:E Ratio (Audible)	Graphic Representation
Vesicular	Throughout chest except over central airways	Moderate	Low	Breezy, rustling	3:1	
Decreased	Left	Soft	Low	Breezy	3:1	
Bronchovesicular	Over large, central airways (sternal area in first and second intercostal space, between scapulae, right upper lobe posteriorly in some people)	Moderate to loud	Medium to high	Hollow, breezy	1:1	
Bronchial (tracheal)	Over manubrium (trachea and larnyx)	Loud	High	Harsh, hollow, tubular	2:3	

I:E, Inspiration to expiration.

They are high-pitched and musical when they origi-nate in smaller airways *(sibilant wheeze)* and low-pitched with a snoring sound when they originate in larger airways *(sonorous wheeze)*. Wheezes are more commonly heard on expiration, but the sounds may occur during both inspiration and expiration. Airway secretions sometimes produce wheezes; in this situation, wheezes should decrease after coughing or suctioning.

Pleural friction rub. A *pleural friction rub*, or pleu-ral rub, is a grating sound that occurs in the presence of inflammation of the pleura. Pleural rubs are usu-ally heard during inspiration and expiration. If a rub is heard, a pleural rub must be distinguished from a pericardial rub because they sound similar. A pleural rub is audible during respirations, whereas a pericar-dial rub is audible with each heartbeat. A useful way to differentiate is to ask the patient to hold his or her breath; if the rub is no longer heard, it is a pleural friction rub. Adventitious lung sounds are reviewed in Table 8-3.

ARTERIAL BLOOD GAS INTERPRETATION

The ability to interpret ABG results rapidly is an essen-tial critical care skill. ABG results reflect oxygenation, adequacy of gas exchange in the lungs, and acid-base status. Blood for ABG analysis is obtained from either a direct arterial puncture (radial, brachial, or femoral artery) or an arterial line. Traditionally, ABGs are assessed periodically to aid in patient assessment. However, noninvasive measures of gas exchange and continuous ABG monitoring via fiberoptic sensors threaded through an arterial catheter have reduced the frequency of ABG measurements. All blood gas findings must be interpreted in conjunction with the patient's previous ABG values, clinical history, and physical assessment findings.

Oxygenation

The ABG values that reflect oxygenation include the partial pressure of oxygen dissolved in arterial blood (PaO_2) and the arterial oxygen saturation of hemo-globin (SaO_2). Approximately 3% of the available

---

TABLE 8-3

Adventitious Breath Sounds

Type	General Location	Associated Problem(s)	Characteristics	Graphic Illustration
Crackles	Peripheral airways and alveoli	Atelectasis Inflammation Excess fluid (HF) Excess mucus (COPD, pneumonia)	Group of discrete crackles or popping sound Discontinuous sound Usually inspiratory, may be inspiratory and expiratory	Fine Coarse
Sonorous wheeze (rhonchi)	Large airways	Inflammation Excess fluid Excess mucus	Coarse, low-pitched snoring sounds Continuous sound Usually expiratory, may be inspiratory and expiratory	
Sibilant wheeze	Large and/or small airways	Bronchoconstriction (airway narrowing) from broncho-spasm, fluid, mucus, inflammatory by-products, obstructive lesion Airway instability	High-pitched musical sound Continuous sound Usually expiratory, may be inspiratory and expiratory	
Pleural friction rub	Pleural surfaces	Inflamed or roughened pleural surfaces (pleuritis)	Low-pitched grating sound with continuous and discontinuous qualities May appear intermittently Sounds the same or louder with coughing	

COPD, Chronic obstructive pulmonary disease; *HF*, heart failure.

oxygen is dissolved in plasma. The remaining 97% of the oxygen attaches to hemoglobin in red blood cells, forming oxyhemoglobin.

Partial pressure of arterial oxygen. The normal PaO_2 is 80 to 100 mm Hg at sea level. The PaO_2 decreases in the elderly; the value for persons 60 to 80 years of age usually ranges from 60 to 80 mm Hg.

Arterial oxygen saturation of hemoglobin. The SaO_2 refers to the amount of oxygen bound to hemoglobin. The normal saturation of hemoglobin ranges from 93% to 99%. The SaO_2 is very important because most oxygen supplied to the tissues is transported via hemoglobin.

Both the PaO_2 and the SaO_2 are used to assess oxygenation. Decreased oxygenation of arterial blood (PaO_2 lower than 80 mm Hg) is referred to as *hypoxemia.* Hypoxemia is different from *hypoxia,* which is a decrease in oxygen at the tissue level. Symptoms of hypoxemia are described in Box 8-1. A patient with a PaO_2 of less than 60 mm Hg requires immediate controlled and supervised intervention with supplemental oxygen to treat the hypoxemia. A PaO_2 of less than 40 mm Hg is life-threatening because oxygen is not available for cellular metabolism (Huang, 2002; Scanlan & Wilkins, 2003b).

The relationship between the PaO_2 and the SaO_2 is shown in the S-shaped oxyhemoglobin dissociation curve (Figure 8-9). The upper portion of the curve (PaO_2 greater than 60 mm Hg) is flat. In this area of the curve, large changes in the PaO_2 result in only small changes in SaO_2. For example, the normal PaO_2 is 97 mm Hg and is associated with an SaO_2 of 97%. If the PaO_2 decreases to 80 mm Hg, the SaO_2 only decreases to 95%. Likewise, if the PaO_2 decreases from 80 to 60 mm Hg, the SaO_2 decreases from 95% to 90%. Although these examples reflect a drop in PaO_2, the patient is not immediately compromised, because the hemoglobin is still well saturated with oxygen.

The critical zone of the oxyhemoglobin dissociation curve occurs when the PaO_2 decreases to less than 60 mm Hg. At this point, the curve slopes sharply, and small changes in PaO_2 are reflected in large changes in the oxygen saturation. These changes in SaO_2 may cause a significant decrease in oxygen delivered to the tissues.

The oxyhemoglobin dissociation curve may shift in certain conditions (Figure 8-10). When the curve

---

BOX 8-1

Signs and Symptoms of Hypoxemia

INTEGUMENTARY SYSTEM
Pallor
Cool, dry
Cyanosis (late)
Diaphoresis (late)

RESPIRATORY SYSTEM
Dyspnea
Tachypnea
Use of accessory muscles

CARDIOVASCULAR SYSTEM
Tachycardia
Dysrhythmias
Chest pain
Hypertension with increased heart rate
Hypotension with decreased heart rate

CENTRAL NERVOUS SYSTEM
Anxiety
Restlessness
Confusion
Fatigue
Combativeness
Coma

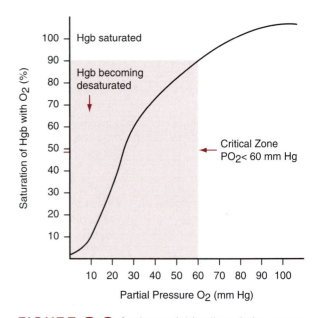

FIGURE 8-9 Oxyhemoglobin dissociation curve. The critical zone of the curve is noted. When the PaO_2 falls below 60 mm Hg, small changes in PaO_2 are reflected in large changes in oxygen saturation. (Redrawn from Kersten L. D. [1989]. *Comprehensive respiratory nursing* [p. 48]. Philadelphia: W. B. Saunders.)

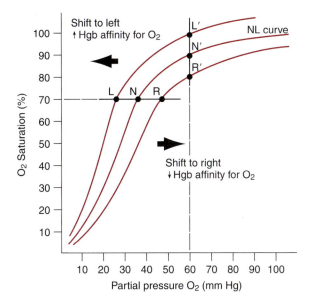

FIGURE 8-10 Shifts in the oxyhemoglobin curve. L, left shift; N, normal shift; R, right shift. (From Alspach, J. [2001]. *AACN instructors resource manual for AACN core curriculum for critical care nursing*, 5th ed. Philadelphia: Saunders.)

shifts to the right, a decreased hemoglobin affinity for oxygen exists. This means that oxygen is more readily released to the tissues. Conditions that cause a right shift include acidemia, increased metabolism (e.g., fever), and increased levels of 2,3-diphosphoglycerate (2,3-DPG), which is a glucose metabolite. Levels of 2,3-DPG are increased in anemia, chronic hypoxemia, and low cardiac output states.

When the curve shifts to the left, hemoglobin affinity for oxygen increases, and hemoglobin clings to oxygen. Conditions that cause a left shift include alkalemia, lowered metabolism, high altitude, carbon monoxide poisoning, and a decreased 2,3-DPG level. Common causes of decreased 2,3-DPG include administration of stored bank blood, septic shock, and hypophosphatemia (Scanlan & Wilkins, 2003b).

Ventilation and Acid-Base Status

Blood gas values that reflect ventilation and acid-base or metabolic status include the pH, partial pressure of carbon dioxide ($PaCO_2$), and bicarbonate (HCO_3^-) (Huang, 2002; Scanlan & Wilkins, 2003b).

pH. The concentration of hydrogen ions (H^+) in the blood is referred to as the *pH*. The pH is the negative logarithm of the H^+ concentration. The normal pH is 7.40; the normal range for pH is 7.35 to 7.45. If the H^+ increases, the pH falls, resulting in acidemia.

Conversely, a decrease in H^+ level results in a high pH and alkalemia. (The suffix *emia* is used to refer to the alteration in pH. The suffix osis is used to refer to the condition or process that causes the alteration in pH.) A pH value less than or equal to 7.2 or greater than 7.6 is considered a panic value that needs to be reported immediately (Chernecky, & Berger, 2001).

PaCO_2. $PaCO_2$ is the partial pressure of carbon dioxide dissolved in arterial plasma. The normal $PaCO_2$ is 35 to 45 mm Hg. The $PaCO_2$ is regulated in the lungs. A $PaCO_2$ of greater than 45 mm Hg indicates respiratory acidosis, whereas a $PaCO_2$ of less than 35 mm Hg indicates respiratory alkalosis. If a patient hypoventilates, carbon dioxide is retained, leading to respiratory acidosis. Conversely, if a patient hyperventilates, excess carbon dioxide is excreted by the lungs, resulting in respiratory alkalosis. A helpful way to remember this concept is to think of carbon dioxide as an "acid" that is regulated by the lungs. Conditions that cause respiratory acidosis and alkalosis are noted in Box 8-2.

Sodium bicarbonate. The HCO_3^- is the concentration of sodium bicarbonate in the blood. The normal HCO_3^- level is 22 to 26 mEq/L. HCO_3^- is regulated by the kidneys. An HCO_3^- level greater than 26 mEq/L indicates metabolic alkalosis, whereas an HCO_3^- level less than 22 mEq/L indicates metabolic acidosis. It may be useful to think of HCO_3^- as a substance that neutralizes acids. Therefore, a high HCO_3^- value indicates the presence of metabolic alkalosis, and a low HCO_3^- value indicates the presence of metabolic acidosis. Conditions that cause metabolic acidosis and alkalosis are noted in Box 8-2.

Buffer System

The body regulates acid-base balance through the buffer system. The buffer system can be described as a mechanism for the neutralization of acids. Three buffer systems exist for maintaining acid-base status: the buffer system in the blood, that in the respiratory system, and that in the renal system (Figure 8-11).

The *blood buffer system* is activated as the H^+ concentration changes. As H^+ level increases, the pH falls, resulting in acidosis. HCO_3^- then combines with H^+ to form carbonic acid (H_2CO_3). Carbonic acid then breaks down into carbon dioxide (which is excreted through the lungs) and water (H_2O). The equation for this mechanism is as follows:

$$H^+ + HCO_3^- \rightarrow H_2CO_3 \rightarrow H_2O + CO_2$$

The *respiratory buffer system* works by excreting excess carbon dioxide from the lungs. The respiratory buffer system begins to work immediately after

BOX 8-2

Causes of Common Acid-Base Abnormalities

RESPIRATORY ACIDOSIS: RETENTION OF CARBON DIOXIDE
Central nervous system depression (anesthesia, narcotics, sedatives, drug overdose)
Neuromuscular disorders
Trauma: spine, brain, chest wall
Restrictive lung diseases
Chronic obstructive pulmonary disease
Acute airway obstruction (late phases)

RESPIRATORY ALKALOSIS: HYPERVENTILATION
Anxiety, fear
Pain
Fever
Stimulants
Central nervous system disorders
Hypoxemia-causing lung conditions
Pneumonia
Atelectasis
Asthma (early stage)
Acute respiratory distress syndrome
Congestive heart failure, pulmonary edema
Pulmonary vascular disease

METABOLIC ACIDOSIS: GAIN OF METABOLIC ACIDS OR LOSS OF BASE
Increased Acids
Renal failure
Diabetic ketoacidosis
Lactic acidosis
Drug overdose (salicylates, methanol, ethylene glycol)

Loss of Base
Diarrhea

METABOLIC ALKALOSIS: GAIN OF BASE OR LOSS OF METABOLIC ACIDS
Gain of Base
Excess ingestion of antacids
Excess administration of sodium bicarbonate

Loss of Metabolic Acids
Vomiting
Nasogastric suctioning
Low potassium and/or chloride
Diuretics (loss of chloride and/or potassium)
Increased levels of aldosterone

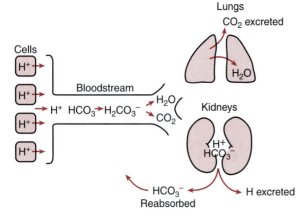

FIGURE 8-11 Buffer systems that regulate the body's acid-base balance. HCO_3^-, Bicarbonate; H_2CO_3, carbonic acid. (Modified from Harvey, M. A. [2000]. *Study guide to the core curriculum for critical care nursing* [p. 11]. 3rd ed. Philadelphia: W. B. Saunders.)

an acid-base alteration is noted. The *renal buffer system* works by excreting excess H^+ and retaining bicarbonate. The renal buffer system activates more slowly and may take up to 2 days to regulate acid-base balance.

Steps in Arterial Blood Gas Interpretation

ABG gas results should be interpreted systematically. The oxygenation status is evaluated first. Second, the acid-base status is determined. Third, the primary cause of the acid-base imbalance is determined. Last, an assessment is made for a compensatory response, if any, that originates from the lungs or kidneys attempting to bring the pH back into balance. Critical ABG values are noted in the Laboratory Alerts box.

Step 1: evaluate oxygenation. Oxygenation is analyzed by evaluating the PaO_2 and the SaO_2. Hypoxemia is considered to be a significant problem

LABORATORY ALERTS: ARTERIAL BLOOD GAS CRITICAL VALUES*

PaO_2 <60 mm Hg

$PaCO_2$ >50 mm Hg

pH <7.25 or >7.6

*These are critical values only if they differ from baseline values (i.e., an acute change). Some patients with pulmonary disease tolerate highly "abnormal" arterial blood gas values.
$PaCO_2$, Partial pressure of carbon dioxide in arterial blood; *PaO_2*, partial pressure of oxygen in arterial blood.

when the PaO_2 falls to less than 60 mm Hg or the SaO_2 falls to less than 90%. A complete assessment must take into account the level of supplemental oxygen a patient is receiving when the ABG is drawn. If the PaO_2 is less than expected for a patient receiving no supplemental oxygen, hypoxemia is classified as follows (Chang, 2001):

Mild	PaO_2 60 to 79 mm Hg
Moderate	PaO_2 40 to 59 mm Hg
Severe	PaO_2 less than 40 mm Hg

When supplemental oxygen is used to treat hypoxemia, the classification of hypoxemia is modified (Shapiro, Peruzzi, & Templin, 1994):

Uncorrected	PaO_2 less than 60 mm Hg
Corrected	PaO_2 60 to 100 mm Hg
Excessively corrected	PaO_2 greater than 100 mm Hg

Age and disease conditions are considered when evaluating oxygenation. Elderly patients normally have a lower PaO_2 because of the progressive changes in pulmonary physiology associated with the natural process of aging. A "normal" baseline can be estimated for a person between the ages of 60 and 90 years by subtracting 1 mm Hg for year of age from the minimal PaO_2 value of 80 mm Hg (Scanlan & Wilkins, 2003a). Patients with COPD have chronic hypoxemia.

Step 2: evaluate acid-base status. For evaluation of acid-base status, the following ABG values are assessed individually:
1. *Evaluate the pH.* A pH of less than 7.35 indicates the presence of acidemia; a pH greater than 7.45 indicates the presence of alkalemia.
2. *Evaluate the $PaCO_2$.* A $PaCO_2$ of less than 35 mm Hg indicates the presence of respiratory alkalosis; a $PaCO_2$ greater than 45 mm Hg indicates the presence of respiratory acidosis.
3. *Evaluate the HCO_3^-.* An HCO_3^- value of less than 22 mm Hg indicates the presence of metabolic acidosis; an HCO_3^- greater than 26 mm Hg indicates the presence of metabolic alkalosis.

Step 3: determine primary acid-base imbalance. The ABG results may reflect only one disorder. However, two acid-base disorders may occur simultaneously. Table 8-4 provides interpretations of acid-base status based on findings. Usually, one is a primary disorder, and the other is a compensatory process aimed at restoring the acid-base balance. The *primary* cause of the acid-base imbalance is determined by evaluation of the pH. If the pH is less than 7.4, the primary disorder is acidosis. If the pH is greater than 7.4, the primary disorder is alkalosis. Occasionally, two primary disorders may occur simultaneously (*mixed acid-base imbalance*). For example, during cardiac arrest, both respiratory acidosis and metabolic acidosis commonly occur because of hypoventilation and lactic acidosis. A mixed acid-base imbalance is suspected. Figure 8-12 illustrates the concepts of acid-base imbalances.

TABLE 8-4

Interpretation of Arterial Blood Gas Results

	$PaCO_2$ <35 mm Hg	$PaCO_2$ 35 to 45 mm Hg	$PaCO_2$ >45 mm Hg
HCO_3^- < 22 mEq/L	Respiratory alkalosis Metabolic acidosis	Metabolic acidosis	Respiratory acidosis Metabolic acidosis
HCO_3^- = 22-26 mEq/L	Respiratory alkalosis	Normal	Respiratory acidosis
HCO_3^- > 26 mEq/L	Respiratory alkalosis Metabolic alkalosis	Metabolic alkalosis	Respiratory acidosis Metabolic alkalosis

HCO_3^-, Bicarbonate; *$PaCO_2$,* partial pressure of carbon dioxide in arterial blood.

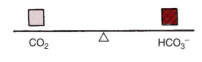

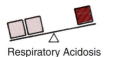
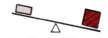

ACIDOSIS   ALKALOSIS

Respiratory System at Fault

Respiratory Acidosis
(too much CO_2)

Respiratory Alkalosis
(too little CO_2)

Metabolic System at Fault

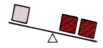

Metabolic Acidosis
(too little HCO_3^-)

Metabolic Alkalosis
(too much HCO_3^-)

FIGURE 8-12 Acid-base imbalances. (From Harvey, M. A. [2000]. *Study guide to the core curriculum for critical care nursing* [p. 11]. 3rd ed. Philadelphia: W. B. Saunders.)

Step 4: determine whether any form of compensatory response has taken place.

The body has three buffer systems that maintain a constant acid-base balance. If an abnormality is present, the buffer system is activated to normalize the pH. The kidneys attempt to compensate for respiratory abnormalities, whereas the lungs attempt to compensate for metabolic problems. For example, if a patient has respiratory acidosis, such as occurs in COPD (low pH, high $PaCO_2$), the kidneys respond by retaining more HCO_3^- and excreting H^+ (metabolic alkalosis). Conversely, if a patient is in metabolic acidosis, such as occurs in diabetic ketoacidosis (low pH, low HCO_3^-), the lungs respond by hyperventilation and excretion of carbon dioxide (respiratory alkalosis). A summary of compensatory mechanisms is shown in Table 8-5.

Compensation may be absent, partial, or complete. Compensation is absent if the usual compensatory mechanisms do not occur as expected to correct acid-bases disturbances. If a compensatory mechanism has occurred but the pH is still abnormal, compensation is referred to as partial. Compensation is complete if compensatory mechanisms are present and the pH is within normal range. Examples of ABG compensation are shown in Box 8-3.

TABLE 8-5	
Compensatory Mechanisms in Acid-Base Disturbances	
Acid-Base Disturbance	**Usual Compensatory Mechanism**
Respiratory acidosis	Metabolic alkalosis
Respiratory alkalosis	Metabolic acidosis
Metabolic acidosis	Respiratory alkalosis
Metabolic alkalosis	Respiratory acidosis

NONINVASIVE ASSESSMENT OF GAS EXCHANGE

Intermittent ABG results have been the "gold standard" for the monitoring of gas exchange and acid-base status. Improvements in technology for non-invasive assessment of gas exchange by pulse oximetry and capnography have reduced the numbers of ABG samples obtained in critically ill patients.

BOX 8-3

Examples of Arterial Blood Gases and Compensation

EXAMPLE 1

PaO_2	80 mm Hg (normal)
pH	7.30 (low; acidosis)
$PaCO_2$	50 mm Hg (high; respiratory acidosis)
HCO_3^-	22 mEq/L (normal)

Interpretation: Respiratory acidosis; no compensation.

EXAMPLE 2

PaO_2	80 mm Hg (normal)
pH	7.32 (low; acidosis)
$PaCO_2$	50 mm Hg (high; respiratory acidosis)
HCO_3^-	28 mEq/L (high; metabolic alkalosis)

Interpretation: Partly compensated respiratory acidosis. The arterial blood gases are only partly compensated because the pH is not yet within normal limits.

EXAMPLE 3

PaO_2	80 mm Hg (normal)
pH	7.36 (normal)
$PaCO_2$	50 mm Hg (high; respiratory acidosis)
HCO_3^-	29 mEq/L (high; metabolic alkalosis)

Interpretation: Completely (fully) compensated respiratory acidosis. The pH is now within normal limits; therefore, complete compensation has occurred.

HCO_3^-, Bicarbonate; $PaCO_2$, partial pressure of carbon dioxide in arterial blood; PaO_2, partial pressure of oxygen in arterial blood.

Assessment of Oxygenation

Pulse oximetry. Pulse oximetry measures a value called SpO$_2$ and reflects the arterial oxygen saturation (SaO$_2$). Pulse oximetry uses a light-emitting diode to measure pulsatile flow and light absorption of the hemoglobin. A sensor that measures SpO$_2$ is placed on the patient's finger, toe, ear, or forehead. Accurate readings are obtained from warm, well-perfused areas. In the critical care unit, most patients have continuous pulse oximetry. SpO$_2$ values are sometimes "spot checked" in patients who are less acutely ill.

The oxyhemoglobin dissociation curve (see Figure 8-9) shows the relationship between SaO$_2$ and PaO$_2$ and provides the basis for pulse oximetry. An SaO$_2$ of 95% is equivalent to a PaO$_2$ of 80 mm Hg, whereas an SaO$_2$ of 90% is equivalent to a PaO$_2$ of 60 mm Hg. In general, SpO$_2$ values of less than 90% require further assessment and clinical intervention if the patient is exhibiting symptoms of hypoxemia. Table 8-6 assists in interpretation of SpO$_2$ values.

Pulse oximetry values are used to monitor a patient's response to treatment (e.g., ventilator changes, suctioning, weaning from mechanical ventilation) by following trends in oxygen saturation. However, SpO$_2$ only measures fluctuation in oxygenation caused by changes in a patient's ventilation, and cannot be used to assess carbon dioxide levels.

Several factors affect SpO$_2$ values. Artifact from patient motion and edema at the sensor site may prevent an accurate measurement. The SpO$_2$ measurements may be lower than the actual SaO$_2$ if the perfusion to the sensor site is reduced, or in the presence of sunlight, fluorescent light, nail polish or artificial nails, and intravenous dyes. The SpO$_2$ measurements may read higher than the actual SaO$_2$ in clinical conditions that alter the hemoglobin such as methemoglobin, sulfmethemoglobin, or carboxyhemoglobin (Chang, 2001).

Assessment of Ventilation

End-tidal carbon dioxide monitoring. End-tidal carbon dioxide monitoring (ETCO$_2$) is done to monitor the patient's ventilatory status. Disposable ETCO$_2$ detectors are routinely used after intubation to differentiate tracheal from esophageal intubation. Continuous capnography uses infrared light to measure exhaled carbon dioxide at the end of inspiration. The equipment samples expired gas from a mainstream or sidestream sensor that is attached to an adaptor on the endotracheal tube (ETT) or tracheostomy (Chang, 2001). A nasal cannula with a sidestream capnometer can be used in patients without an artificial airway.

The ETCO$_2$ values correlate moderately with the PaCO$_2$ in patients with normal lung and cardiac function; ETCO$_2$ values consistently underestimate PaCO$_2$ from 1 to 5 mm Hg and are less exact than values obtained by ABG measurement (Rozycki, Sysyn, Marshall, Malloy, & Wiswell, 1998). The device must be calibrated periodically for accurate results.

ETCO$_2$ monitoring is used to evaluate ventilation when precision is not essential and for trending data. Clinical applications of ETCO$_2$ monitoring include assessment of the patient's response to ventilator changes and respiratory treatments, determining the proper position of the ETT, weaning the patient from mechanical ventilation, detecting disconnection from the ventilator, and detecting disconnection from anesthesia equipment intraoperatively. Decreased values may not be indicative of improvement in gas exchange because some conditions that cause an increase in dead space ventilation result in lower ETCO$_2$ values. Examples include pulmonary embolism, hypotension, and high intrathoracic pressure (Chang, 2001; Scanlan & Wilkins, 2003b).

Oxygen Administration

Oxygen is administered to treat or prevent hypoxemia. Oxygen may be supplied by various sources such as piped into wall devices, oxygen tanks, or oxygen concentrators. Common oxygen delivery devices include the low-flow devices (nasal cannula), reservoir systems (simple face mask, a partial-rebreather mask, and nonrebreather mask), and high-flow systems (air-entrainment or Venturi mask) (Saposnick & Hess, 2002; Heuer & Scanlan, 2003). Table 8-7 lists devices and oxygen flow rates.

Humidified oxygen is recommended when high-liter flows are administered to prevent the mucous

TABLE 8-6

Interpretation of Pulse Oximetry Values (SpO$_2$)

Value on Pulse Oximeter (%)	Probable PaO$_2$ Value (mm Hg)
97	100
95	80
94	70
90	60
85	50
75	40
57	30
32	20
10	10

PaO$_2$, Partial pressure of oxygen in arterial blood; *SpO$_2$,* pulse oximetry.

TABLE 8-7

Oxygen Delivery Devices

Device	Oxygen Flow Rate (L/Min)	Approximate FiO₂
Nasal cannula	1	0.24
	2	0.28
	3	0.32
	4	0.36
	5	0.40
	6	0.44
Face mask	5-6	0.40
	6-7	0.50
	7-8	0.60
Masks with reservoirs	6	0.60
	7	0.70
	8	0.80
	9	0.80-1.00
	10	0.80-1.00
Venturi mask	4	0.24
	5	0.28
	6	0.31
	7	0.35
	8	0.40
	10	0.50

FiO₂, Fractional concentration of oxygen in inspired gas.

membranes from drying. However, oxygen delivery at low flows (typically less than 4 L/min) is often provided without a secondary humidification source. At lower flow rates, the patient's natural humidification system provides adequate humidity (Fink & Hess, 2002).

PICKING THE BEST DEVICE: FIT, FUNCTION, AND TOTAL FLOW

The successful administration of oxygen therapy is important in treating hypoxemia. When administering oxygen, it important to consider these two components of oxygen therapy: fit and function of a device, and the total flow delivered by a device to the patient.

Fit and Function

Assessing proper fit and functioning of an oxygen device may be forgotten during a clinical crisis. To ensure proper fit and function, the nurse or respiratory care practitioner inspects the patient's face and concentrates on the location of the oxygen delivery device and how well it is positioned on the patient's face. While doing this, the caregiver determines whether the patient is breathing through an unobstructed airway. The oxygen-connecting tubing is then traced back to the gas source origin to ensure that it is connected. Finally, it is important to ensure that the gas source is oxygen and that it is turned on.

Total Flow

Flow is determined by two factors: how much oxygen the device can deliver and whether the delivered oxygen remains fixed or varied under changing patient demands (Wissing, 2004). Terms used to describe delivery include fraction of inspired oxygen (FiO₂) or fraction of delivered oxygen (FdO₂). In this text, we use the FiO₂ abbreviation. Devices can deliver low (less than 35%), moderate (35% to 60%), or high (more than 60%) oxygen concentrations.

The delivery of fixed or variable oxygen depends on how much of the patient's inspired gas the device supplies. If a device provides all the patient's inspired gas, the FiO₂ remains fixed or stable, even if demands change. Variable-flow devices provide only some of the inspired gases; the patient draws the remainder of inspired gases from the ambient air. In this case, the air dilutes the oxygen and lowers the FiO₂. Conversely, if a patient breathes more slowly, less air dilutes the oxygen, and the FiO₂ rises. The FiO₂ provided by variable-flow systems changes widely from minute to minute and from breath to breath (Heuer & Scanlan, 2003; Wissing, 2004).

OXYGEN DELIVERY DEVICES

Nasal Cannula (Variable Performance)

A nasal cannula is commonly used to deliver oxygen. The device is relatively comfortable to wear and is easy to secure on the patient. In adult patients, nasal cannulas provide between 24% and 44% oxygen at flow rates up to 6 L/min (Heuer & Scanlan, 2003; Hunt, 1999). An increase in oxygen flow rate by 1 L/min generally increases oxygen delivery by 4% (e.g., 2 L/min nasal cannula delivers 28% of oxygen, whereas 3 L/min provides 32%). Administering oxygen through a nasal cannula at flow rates higher than 6 L/min is not effective in increasing oxygenation because the capacity of the patient's anatomical reservoir in the nasopharynx is surpassed. Gas flowing into the nasopharynx beyond 6 L/min is diverted away from the patient's anatomical reservoir and is lost to the surrounding environment.

Simple Face Mask (Variable Performance)

The simple facemask delivers oxygen directly from an oxygen flowmeter to the patient. A simple mask is chosen to fit the appropriate size of the patient's face for patient comfort and delivery capacity. A simple mask creates an additional "reservoir" beyond what the patient's natural anatomical reservoir can hold. Oxygen is delivered at flow rates of 5 to 10 L/min, which provides an FiO_2 of 0.30 to 0.50. Because this mask is tight fitting (ideally) and rests on the face, it is important that the flow rate for this device be set to at least 5 L/min to avoid rebreathing carbon dioxide (Heuer & Scanlan, 2003; Hunt, 1999).

Face Masks with Reservoirs (Variable Performance)

The partial rebreathing and nonrebreathing reservoir masks provide oxygen concentrations of 60% or more dependent on the flowmeter setting, the fit of the mask, and the patient's respiratory pattern. The reservoir in both masks increases the amount of oxygen available to the patient during inspiration. The reservoir is more effective if it remains at least partially inflated during each respiratory cycle (Heuer & Scanlan, 2003; Hunt, 1999). The main difference between these two devices is that the nonrebreather mask has a one-way valve between the reservoir bag and the fitting attaching the reservoir to the mask. This one-way valve prevents the patient from rebreathing exhaled carbon dioxide and maximizes FiO_2. Either mask may be used in the critically ill patient presenting with severe hypoxemia in an effort to prevent the need for endotracheal intubation and mechanical ventilation.

Venturi or Air-Entrainment Mask (Fixed Performance)

The Venturi or air-entrapment mask delivers an increased total flow of oxygen at a fixed FiO_2. These masks are usually ordered to deliver 24% to 40% of oxygen to the patient. Air entrapment devices direct high-pressure oxygen through a small nozzle or jet surrounded by air-entrapment ports. The FiO_2 is regulated by selecting the appropriate jet adaptor for the desired oxygen delivery. These devices provide an accurate delivery of prescribed oxygen to the patient and are commonly used in the patient with pulmonary disease so the level of oxygen can be closely regulated (Heuer & Scanlan, 2003; Hunt, 1999).

Air Entrainment with Aerosol and Humidity Delivery (Variable or Fixed Performance)

The same air-entrainment functions provided by a mask can provide oxygen to patients who require controlled levels of oxygen and additional humidity. These devices are usually pneumatically powered air-entrainment nebulizers that deliver a fixed FiO_2, added humidity in the form of an aerosol mist, and a temperature-controlled aerosol if needed. These devices provide a fixed or variable oxygen delivery function based on whether enough source gas is used to power the nebulizer. These devices are powered by oxygen flows between 12 and 15 L/min. At higher desired FiO_2 settings, it is possible that too little ambient oxygen is entrained to meet the patient's total inspiratory demand. In this case, an air-entrainment nebulizer should be considered as a variable-performance device (unable to meet expected inspiratory demand), and additional sources of oxygen may need to be provided to meet the patient's FiO_2 needs (Heuer & Scanlan, 2003).

Bag-Valve Devices (Variable Performance)

A bag-valve device is used to ventilate a patient manually while also providing supplemental oxygen (see Chapter 7). The bag-valve device is also referred to as a *manual resuscitation bag*, a self-inflating bag, or *Ambu bag*. The device is attached to a facemask or connected directly to an ETT tube or tracheostomy to ventilate the patient. When used on an emergency basis, the bag-valve device should have a reservoir attached to increase the FiO_2. The oxygen flowmeter attached to the bag is set at 15 L/min to provide adequate flow of oxygen to meet the inspiratory demands of assisted manual ventilation.

Airway Management

POSITIONING

A primary nursing intervention with any patient is to maintain an open airway. The first method for maintaining a patent airway is proper head position. The head-tilt/chin-lift method or jaw thrust is recommended for the maintenance of an open airway.

ORAL AIRWAYS

Methods for maintaining an open airway include oral and nasopharyngeal airways (Figure 8-13). Oral airways are tubes that prevent the tongue from falling into the pharynx (Figure 8-14). Oral airways are used for many reasons: to facilitate secretion removal from the oropharynx, to maintain an open airway when using a bag-valve device and face mask, to prevent a patient from biting on an ETT, and to maintain an open airway in patients during seizure activity.

Sizes of oral airways vary from small adult (80 mm long) to medium adult (90 mm) to large adult (100 mm). Several brands are available. Some oral airways are made of rigid plastic, whereas others are made of softer plastic. The configuration of the tubes also varies.

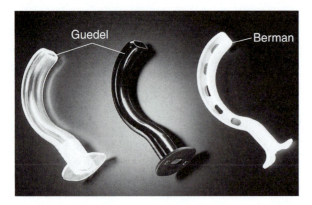

FIGURE 8-13 Oropharyngeal airways: Guedel **(A)** and Berman **(B)**. (From Durbin, C. G. [2004]. Airway management. In J. M. Cairo & S. P. Pilbeam (eds.). *Mosby's respiratory care equipment* [p. 156]. 7th ed. St. Louis: Mosby.)

> **BOX 8-4**
>
> **Insertion of Oral Airway**
>
> 1. Choose the proper size. The length is determined by measuring from the corner of the mouth to the ear lobe.
> 2. Suction mucus from the mouth using a tonsil (Yankauer) tip catheter.
> 3. Turn the airway upside down to facilitate insertion, and open the patient's mouth. (An alternative method is to use a tongue blade to depress the patient's tongue while the airway is inserted.)
> 4. When the posterior wall of the pharynx is reached, turn (rotate) the airway into the proper position.
> 5. After insertion, assess the patency of the airway: air movement through the airway, clear breath sounds, and chest movement. Noises indicating upper airway obstruction should be absent.
> 6. Maintain the patient's proper head alignment after airway insertion.

The technique for inserting an oral airway is described in Box 8-4. Complications of oral airways include airway obstruction if the airway is too long, trauma to the lips and tongue, gagging in a conscious patient, and accumulation of secretions in the oropharynx if oral suctioning is not done.

NASOPHARYNGEAL AIRWAYS

Nasopharyngeal airways, also known as *nasal airways* or *nasal trumpets,* are soft rubber or latex tubes inserted into the nares and nasopharynx (Figure 8-15). Nasopharyngeal airways are better tolerated than oral airways in the conscious patient, are more comfortable, and facilitate nasotracheal suctioning.

The procedure for inserting a nasotracheal airway is described in Box 8-5. Complications of nasopharyngeal airways include insertion into the esophagus if the airway is too long, nosebleeds, and ulceration of the nares. Extended use of nasopharyngeal airways is not recommended because sinusitis or otitis may occur.

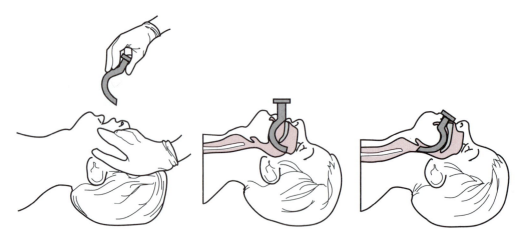

FIGURE 8-14 Maintaining an open airway with an oral airway. (From Durbin, C. G. [2004]. Airway management. In J. M. Cairo & S. P. Pilbeam (eds.). *Mosby's respiratory care equipment* [p. 157]. 7th ed. St. Louis: Mosby.)

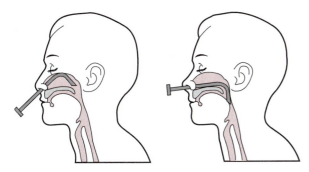

FIGURE **8-15** Maintaining an open airway with a nasopharyngeal airway. (From Durbin, C. G. [2004]. Airway management. In J. M. Cairo & S. P. Pilbeam (eds.). *Mosby's respiratory care equipment* [p. 160]. 7th ed. St. Louis: Mosby.)

ESOPHAGEAL OBTURATORS AND LARYNGEAL MASK AIRWAYS

Endotracheal intubation is the preferred method to sustain the patient's ventilation and to prevent aspiration. If immediate endotracheal intubation is unavailable or unsuccessful, it may become necessary to provide airway protection with either an esophageal obturator airway (EOA) or a laryngeal mask airway (LMA) (Hunt, 1999; Hazinski, Cummins, & Field, 2000). Both these airway devices require special training to insert properly, and they are most often used in prehospital settings.

The EOA device has an opening at the top (proximal) end with several small openings, a distal end without an opening, and a cuff (Figure 8-16). The EOA is inserted into the esophagus, and the cuff is inflated to prevent air from entering the stomach. A mask and bag-valve device are attached to the prox-

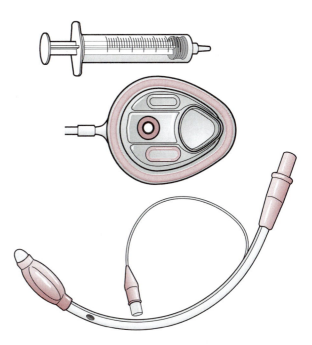

FIGURE **8-16** Esophageal obturater airway. (Redrawn from Durbin, C. G. [2004]. Airway management. In J. M. Cairo & S. P. Pilbeam (eds.). *Mosby's respiratory care equipment.* 7th ed. St. Louis: Mosby.)

imal end of the tube to ventilate the patient. Air is forced through the upper openings into the airway, resulting in ventilation. An ETT should be inserted as soon as possible. To prevent aspiration of gastric contents, the EOA is left in place until the ETT is inserted and placement is verified. Suction should be readily available in case the patient vomits during removal of the EOA.

The LMA is a tube with a small cushioned mask on the distal end (Figure 8-17). The LMA is advanced into the oral cavity until the soft mask at the distal end fits into the posterior pharynx. Once this mask is place, it is inflated until it "caps" or seals the esophagus (Hunt, 1999; Durbin, 2004). The patient is then ventilated with a bag-valve device. The LMA does not protect the patient from regurgitation and aspiration. The LMA can easily become displaced; therefore, the patient's head and alignment of the LMA should be checked frequently to ensure ventilation (Chang, 2001). In addition, if the patient's peak airway pressures are greater than 20 cm H_2O, the mask may not provide an adequate seal.

A Combitube is a variation of the EOA. It is a double-lumen tube that has two cuffs: one to seal the esophagus, and another to seal the pharynx. It also has an opening at the distal end. The tube is

---

BOX 8-5

Insertion of Nasal Airway

1. Choose the proper size. The length is determined by measuring from the nares to the ear lobe and adding 1 inch.
2. Lubricate the tip and sides of the nasal airway with a water-soluble lubricant.
3. If needed, lubricate the nasal passage with a topical anesthetic.
4. Insert the airway medially and downward. It may be necessary to rotate the airway slightly.
5. After insertion, assess the patency of the airway: air movement through the airway and chest movement.

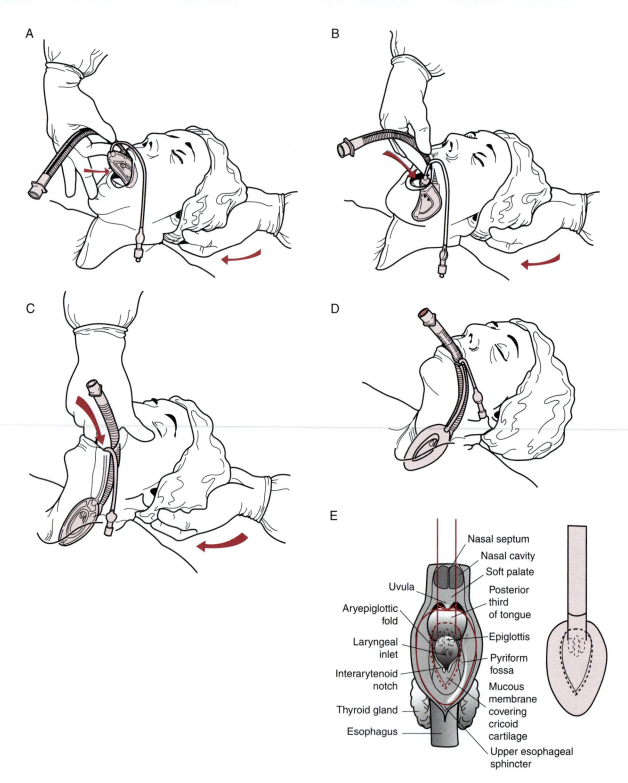

Labels in panel E:
- Nasal septum
- Nasal cavity
- Soft palate
- Uvula
- Posterior third of tongue
- Aryepiglottic fold
- Epiglottis
- Laryngeal inlet
- Pyriform fossa
- Interarytenoid notch
- Mucous membrane covering cricoid cartilage
- Thyroid gland
- Esophagus
- Upper esophageal sphincter

FIGURE 8-17 Laryngeal mask airway. **A,** The laryngeal mask airway (LMA) is held like a pencil and inserted into the open mouth with only the slightest neck extension. **B,** The LMA is directed posterior and down to the oropharnx. **C,** The LMA is advanced with the opposite hand and guided into the posterior pharynx. **D,** The final location of the LMA after correct placement. **E,** Image of the LMA in relation to anatomical structures. (Redrawn from Gensia Automedics. [1992]. San Diego.)

inserted blindly until depth marks are at the lip line or resistance is met. The esophageal cuff is inflated with 15 mL of air, and the pharyngeal cuff is inflated with 100 mL of air. Most of the time, the tube is inserted into the esophagus and functions as an EOA. Occasionally, it is inserted into the trachea. Because the end of the tube is open, it functions as an ETT in this situation (Durbin, 2004).

ENDOTRACHEAL INTUBATION

Intubation refers to the insertion of an ETT into the trachea through either the mouth or the nose. Advantages of oral versus nasal endotracheal intubation are listed in Box 8-6.

The ETT (Figure 8-18) is typically made of a polyvinyl chloride or silicone material with a distal

cuff that is inflated via a one-way valve pilot balloon to facilitate ventilation of the patient by sealing the trachea and allowing only for air passage through the ETT. Standard ETT cuffs are the high-volume, low-pressure type, and most cuffs are inflated with air.

Some ETTs (e.g., Kamen Wilkinson Fome-Cuff) have a distal cuff made of polyurethane foam encased in a silicone case that passively inflates with ambient air pressure once the ETT has been successfully placed in the trachea (Hunt, 1999). If a foam-cuff ETT is used, the manufacturer's instructions must be followed for safe placement of the device as well as maintenance of the cuff while this specialty ETT remains in the patient's airway.

ETTs capable of continuous suctioning of subglottic secretions are used in some facilities. These tubes (e.g., Hi-Lo Evac tube) have an extra suction port just above the cuff for removal of subglottic secretions that accumulate above the cuff. Some evidence

---

BOX 8-6
Oral Versus Nasotracheal Intubation

ORAL INTUBATION
Advantages
Easily and quickly performed
Larger tube facilitates suction and procedures such as bronchoscopy
Less kinking of tube

Disadvantages
Not recommended in patients with suspected cervical injury
Discomfort
Mouth care more difficult to perform
Impairs ability to gag and swallow
May increase salivation
May cause irritation and ulceration of the mouth
Greater risk of self-extubation

NASOTRACHEAL INTUBATION
Advantages
Greater patient comfort and tolerance
Better mouth care possible
Fewer oral complications
Less risk of accidental extubation
Facilitates swallowing of secretions

Disadvantages
May be more difficult to perform
May cause nasal hemorrhage and sinusitis
Secretion removal more difficult because of smaller tube diameter and longer tube length
Increased work of breathing associated with smaller diameter tube

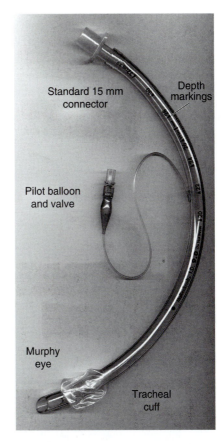

FIGURE 8-18 Endotracheal tube. (From Durbin, C.G. [2004]. Airway management. In J. M. Cairo & S. P. Pilbeam (eds.). *Mosby's respiratory care equipment* [p. 164]. 7th ed. St. Louis: Mosby.)

shows a decrease in ventilator-associated pneumonia when these tubes are used (Collard, Saint, & Matthay, 2003).

In the critical care unit, intubation is performed to maintain an open airway, assist in secretion removal, prevent aspiration, and provide mechanical ventilation. Personnel who are trained and skilled in intubation perform the procedure: anesthesiologists, nurse anesthetists, emergency department physicians, respiratory therapists, and some paramedics (Levitan & Ochroch, 2000). Intubation may be performed on an emergency basis on a patient in cardiopulmonary arrest or electively in a patient with impending respiratory failure.

Nurses must be familiar with equipment used for intubation and be able to gather equipment quickly. Nurses also need to know how to connect the laryngoscope blade to the handle and check to see that it illuminates properly. Necessary equipment is frequently kept together on a crash cart or a special procedures box to facilitate emergency intubation (Box 8-7; Figure 8-19). Oral and endotracheal suctioning equipment must also be readily available.

BOX 8-7

Equipment for Endotracheal Intubation

- Endotracheal tube of proper size
  Average female size, 7.5-8 mm
  Average male size, 8-9 mm
- Stylet
- Laryngoscope and blade
  Straight blade (Miller)
  Curved blade (MacIntosh)
- Suction
  Tonsil tip (Yankauer)
  Suction kit
- Syringe to inflate balloon (usually 10-mL slip-tip)
- Topical anesthetic (optional)
- Water-soluble lubricant
- Tape or device to secure tube
- Stethoscope
- Bag-valve device with reservoir connected to oxygen at 15 L/min
- Optional equipment
  Magill forceps
  Oropharyngeal airway

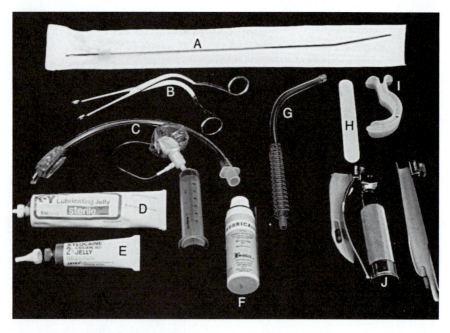

FIGURE 8-19 Equipment used for endotracheal intubation: **A,** stylet (disposable); **B,** Magill forceps; **C,** soft cuffed endotracheal tube with syringe for inflation; **D,** water-soluble lubricant; **E,** anesthetic jelly (optional); **F,** topical anesthetic with spray stick attached to right side of canister; **G,** Yankauer pharyngeal suction tip (disposable); **H,** tongue blade; **I,** oral airway; **J,** laryngoscope handle with a curved blade (attached) and straight blade (right). (From Kersten, L. D. [1989]. *Comprehensive respiratory nursing* [p. 640]. Philadelphia: W. B. Saunders.)

Procedure for Oral Endotracheal Intubation

To facilitate intubation, the patient is placed in a "sniffing" position to align the airway structures. Placing a folded towel or bath blanket under the head may help to achieve this position. If the procedure is performed electively, a topical anesthetic and/or premedication with a sedative or paralytic agent may be administered so the patient better tolerates the procedure.

Before intubation is performed, the patient is hyperoxygenated and hyperventilated with 100% oxygen using a bag-valve device connected to a face mask. The proper size ETT is chosen; it is important that the ETT not be too small, because a smaller diameter ETT substantially increases airway resistance and the patient's WOB. Increased WOB will later negatively affect the patient's efforts to breathe spontaneously and may make mechanical ventilation and weaning difficult.

The average-sized ETT ranges from 7.5 to 8.0 mm for female patients and from 8.0 to 9.0 mm for male patients (Henneman, Ellstrom, & St. John, 1999). After the proper size ETT is selected, the cuff is inflated to check for proper functioning and any leaks. A stylet may be used to stiffen the ETT and to facilitate insertion, but it should be carefully placed inside the ETT to avoid its protrusion beyond the end of the ETT. The ETT is lubricated with a water-soluble lubricant to facilitate passage through the structures of the oropharynx.

The laryngoscope is attached to the appropriate size and type of blade (straight or curved). The choice of blades varies based on the patient's anatomy and the preference of the individual clinician performing the intubation. Blade sizes range from 0 to 4. The average-sized adult is intubated with a size 3 blade (Durbin, 2004). The straight blade (Miller) elevates the epiglottis anteriorly to expose the vocal cords. The tip of the curved blade (Macintosh) fits into the vallecula. When upward traction is placed on the laryngoscope, the epiglottis is displaced anteriorly. Use of the straight versus curved blade is shown in Figure 8-20.

The person doing the intubation, while taking care not to damage the patient's teeth or other structures, inserts the laryngoscope blade into the patient's mouth to visualize the vocal cords. If secretions and vomitus are present, the oral cavity is suctioned to facilitate visualization of the vocal cords. Oral suctioning can be done with a rigid tonsil tip suction (or Yankauer) that is very efficient in removing thick secretions. Once the vocal cords have been exposed and the trachea is visualized, the ETT is inserted 5 to 6 cm beyond the vocal cords, above the carina, and the cuff is inflated.

The intubation procedure should be performed within 30 seconds. If the intubation is difficult, and additional attempts are required to secure the airway, the patient must be manually ventilated between each intubation attempt.

Frequently, a patient requires endotracheal suctioning for removal of excess secretions immediately after intubation. If the patient needs assistance with breathing, ventilation is achieved with either the bag-valve device or a mechanical ventilator. If the patient is breathing spontaneously after intubation, then supplemental oxygen can be delivered to the ETT via a T-piece or Briggs' device (Figure 8-21).

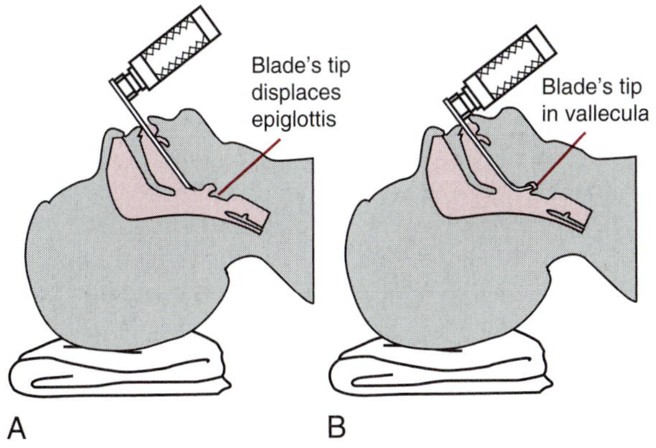

FIGURE 8-20 Positioning and use of a straight **(A)** versus curved **(B)** blade for endotracheal intubation. (Redrawn from Kersten, L. D. [1989]. *Comprehensive respiratory nursing* [p. 643]. Philadelphia: W. B. Saunders.)

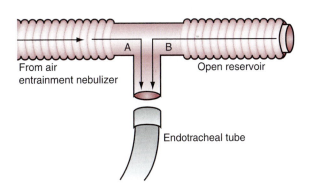

FIGURE 8-21 T-piece. The T-piece is used to provide supplemental oxygen through an endotracheal tube. (In R. L. Wilkins [ed.]. [2004]. *Egan's fundamentals of respiratory care.* 8th ed. St. Louis: Mosby.)

Verification of endotracheal tube placement.
Correct placement of the ETT is verified by primary
and secondary confirmation. Primary confirmation is
done by assessing for bilateral chest rise/fall with each
ventilation, and by five-point auscultation of the chest
and abdomen while the patient is ventilated with a
bag-valve device: left and right anterior chest, left and
right midaxillary line, and the epigastrium (Hazinski,
Cummins, & Field, 2000). These primary measures
assist in verifying tracheal versus esophageal intubation. Failure to hear breath sounds in the chest while
hearing air over the epigastrium represents esophageal
rather than tracheal intubation. Intubation of the right
mainstem bronchus is also common, because the right
mainstem is straighter than the left, and the ETT is
occasionally placed deeper in the trachea during intubation than necessary. Right mainstem bronchus intubation is suspected when unilateral expansion of the
right chest is observed during ventilation.

Secondary confirmation of ETT placement is
assessed by either a bulb aspiration device (esophageal
detector device) or a disposable $ETCO_2$ detector. The
bulb aspiration device is similar to a bulb syringe.
The device is compressed and deflated and then is
attached to the ETT. If the tube is in the trachea, the
bulb inflates rapidly. If the tube is in the esophagus,
filling is delayed. Another option is to attach a disposable $ETCO_2$ detector to the end of the ETT. This
device changes color when carbon dioxide is detected
(Cummins & Hazinski, 2000; Durbin, 2004).

Once a patient is stabilized, ETT placement is
verified by chest radiograph. The tip of the ETT
should be approximately 3 to 4 cm above the carina
(Henneman, Ellstrom, & St. John, 1999). Once proper
tube placement is verified, the ETT is secured with
tape or a commercial device to prevent dislodging.
Figure 8-22 shows one method for securing an ETT
with tape. The length of the tube at the lip line (i.e.,
the cm marker on the ETT) should be documented in
a readily available reference in the medical record.
An indelible marker can be used to mark the ETT at
the lip line. These nursing measures help to ensure
proper tube position.

Rapid sequence intubation. Rapid sequence intubation (RSI) is the rapid administration of both a neuromuscular blocking agent and a potent sedative agent
to facilitate intubation. The goal of RSI is to provide
emergency airway management while decreasing risks
of aspiration, combativeness, and injury to the patient.
RSI is not needed for intubation of the deeply comatose patient or in cardiac arrest situations. It should
be considered for emergency intubation of all other
patients, including children. Assumptions for performing RSI are that patient has a full stomach, the health

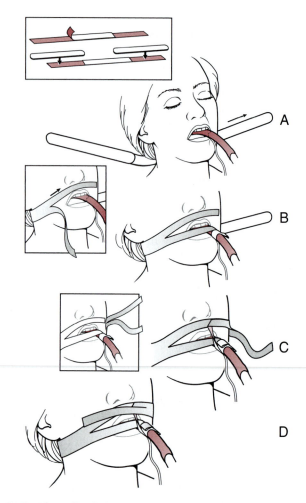

FIGURE 8-22 Steps *A* through *D* indicate technique for taping an endotracheal tube. (From Mims, B.,
Toto, K., Luecke, L., Roberts, M., Brock, J., Tyner, T.
[2004]. *Critical care skills.* 2nd ed. [p. 30] Philadelphia:
W. B. Saunders.)

care provider can secure an airway, and the provider
can resuscitate the patient (Stewart, 2001).

The procedures for inserting the ETT during RSI
are the same as previously discussed. The only difference with RSI is that the patient is premedicated to
reduce the physiological responses to the procedure
and paralyzed to prevent movement. Drugs for premedication may include fentanyl, 2 to 3 mcg/kg at a
rate of 1 to 2 mcg/kg/min intravenous (IV) for analgesia; lidocaine, 1.5 to 2 mg/kg IV over 30 seconds;
and an additional sedative if needed. After 3 minutes,
anesthesia is induced with one of several possible
agents (thiopental, methohexital, fentanyl, ketamine,
etomidate, or propofol). Succinylcholine, 1.5-2 mg/kg
(or other neuromuscular blocking agent), is given by

IV push. The patient is then observed for apnea, jaw relaxation, and decreased resistance to manual ventilation. Cricoid pressure (Sellick's maneuver) is applied to decrease the risk of vomiting by pressing the cricoid cartilage firmly against the esophagus. Intubation is attempted while cricoid pressure is maintained. If intubation can not be accomplished within 20 seconds, manual ventilation for 30 to 60 seconds is recommended between intubation attempts to support the patient's ventilation and oxygenation. Tube placement is verified after the procedure (Hazinski, Cummins, & Field, 2000; Stewart, 2001).

Intubation options. A lighted stylet may facilitate intubation when the patient's vocal cords cannot be visualized, or when the neck cannot be moved. The lighted stylet is lubricated and inserted into a standard ETT that has been shortened to 25 cm. The patient is hyperoxygenated and hyperventilated. The tongue is grasped and pulled forward while the stylet and tube are slid past the epiglottis. When the tube is in correct position, a bright glow is noted in the midline at the level of the Adam's apple (Durbin, 2004). The stylet is removed, and tube placement is verified. The lighted stylet is also useful for nasotracheal intubation.

A fiberoptic laryngoscope is another tool for endotracheal intubation. This laryngoscope allows the operator to intubate a patient either orally or nasally without flexing the neck. Fiberoptic laryngoscopy is most useful in intubating patients with suspected cervical spine trauma, assessing severity of laryngotracheal trauma, and assessing for thermal injury to the trachea and bronchi in a patient with a burn injury (Stewart, 2001). Bleeding into the airway, excess secretions, and vomitus are contraindications to the fiberoptic technique because they obscure vision through the device.

NASOTRACHEAL INTUBATION

Two approaches to nasal intubation are possible: blind and direct visualization (Finucane & Santora, 2003). The equipment for nasotracheal intubation is the same as for oral intubation, with fiberoptic laryngoscopy preferred. The nasal intubation procedure differs from oral intubation in that the naris selected for the ETT passage is prepared with topical agents to provide vasoconstriction and anesthesia to the nasal passage. It may also be more effective to lubricate the ETT with a water-soluble gel containing 2% lidocaine.

After the patient's naris and the ETT have been prepared, the ETT is inserted through the naris and usually is passed "blindly" as the intubator listens to the intensity of the patient's breathing as the ETT is advanced toward the glottis. Blind intubation can be performed only in the patient who is capable of spontaneous respirations. The closer the intubator comes to the glottis, the more intense the sounds of air movement become until the ETT passes the vocal cords and moves into the trachea. The passage of the ETT beyond the vocal cords usually elicits a cough from the patient and a noticeable increase in expired air via the ETT.

Because some patients cease breathing during nasotracheal intubation or present with atypical upper airway anatomy, nasal intubation can also be performed through direct visualization. In this method, the practitioner uses a laryngoscope and Magill forceps, or fiberoptic bronchoscopy, for the procedure. With nasal intubation, the correct placement level of the ETT is usually 23 to 25 cm for male patients and 21 to 23 cm for female patients (Finucane & Santora, 2003; Durbin, 2004).

TRACHEOSTOMY

A tracheostomy tube may be needed if the patient requires long-term mechanical ventilation, frequent suctioning for the management of secretions, or bypassing of an airway obstruction (e.g., a tumor). Under ideal circumstances, the high-volume, low-pressure cuffed ETT can be left in place for up to 3 to 4 weeks. However, if the patient requires long-term ventilatory management (e.g., high-level spinal cord injury) or high ETT cuff pressures to sustain ventilation, then a tracheostomy should be performed sooner. The tracheostomy tube will reduce the patient's WOB associated with the ETT (Vallverdu & Mancebo, 2000).

The tracheostomy has traditionally been a surgical technique performed in the operating room or by a surgical team at the bedside. However, a percutaneous dilatational tracheostomy technique is often performed easily and safely at the bedside by a physician trained in the procedure (Vallverdu & Mancebo, 2000). A percutaneous tracheostomy is performed by making a small incision into the anterior neck down to the anterior wall of the trachea. This incision is made at the level of the cricoid cartilage and the first tracheal ring, or the first and second tracheal rings. Once this location has been reached, the physician inserts a needle and sheath into the trachea. The needle is removed, and a guidewire is passed through the sheath. Progressively larger dilators are introduced over the guidewire until the patient's stoma is large enough to accommodate a tracheostomy tube (Durbin, 2004).

Critically ill patients who need mechanical ventilation require cuffed tubes. However, many other types of tracheostomy tubes are available (Simmons & Scanlan, 2003). Several of these tubes are described in the following sections.

Cuffed Tracheostomy Tube

A cuffed tracheostomy tube has a cuff that is similar to that of the ETT to ensure adequate ventilation and to prevent aspiration. The cuff may be a conventional low-pressure, high-volume type, or it may be constructed of foam. The foam-cuff tube may prevent trauma to the airway because of the low pressure exerted to the airway, and it is sometimes used for patients who have difficulty maintaining a good seal with conventional cuffed tracheostomy tubes. Cuffed tubes may or may not have an inner cannula, depending on the manufacturer. Cuffed tracheostomy tubes with disposable inner cannulas are commonplace in the critical care unit.

Fenestrated Tracheostomy Tube

The fenestrated tracheostomy tube has a hole in the outer cannula that allows air to flow above the larynx. The tube functions as a standard tracheostomy tube when the inner cannula is in place. When the inner cannula is removed, the fenestrated tracheostomy tube assists in weaning a patient from the tracheostomy by gradually allowing the patient to breathe through the natural upper airway. The fenestrated tube also allows the patient to emit vocal sounds, thereby facilitating communications. To use a cuffed fenestrated tracheostomy tube, the inner cannula is carefully removed, the cuff is deflated, and a decannulation plug provided by the manufacturer is inserted into the tube (Simmons & Scanlan, 2003). The inner cannula must be reinserted and the cuff reinflated for suctioning, mechanical ventilation, or use of a bag-valve manual resuscitation device.

Cuffless Tracheostomy Tube

A cuffless tracheostomy tube is used for long-term airway management in a patient who does not require positive-pressure mechanical ventilation and is at low risk of aspiration. For example, a patient with a neurological injury may require a tracheostomy for airway management and secretion removal.

Speaking Tracheostomy Valves

One-way speaking valves are available to allow patients with tracheostomies an opportunity to speak. These valves can be used in both ventilated and non-ventilated patients. However, they can be used only in patients capable of initiating and maintaining spontaneous ventilation (Henneman, Ellstrom, & St. John, 1999; Durbin, 2004). Examples of these adjunctive devices include the Passy-Muir valve and the Olympic Trach-Talk.

For the speaking valve to work correctly, the valve is connected to the tracheostomy tube, the cuff on the tracheostomy tube is deflated, and the patient is allowed to breath and exhale through the natural airway. The valve itself is a one-way device allowing gas to pass through it, into the tracheostomy tube, and then to the patient. However, because this is a one-way valve, exhaled gas exits the trachea via the natural airway, past the deflated cuff of the tracheostomy tube (Durbin, 2004). Careful assessment for immediate problems with exhalation is essential when a speaking valve is used.

If a speaking valve is used in conjunction with volume mechanical ventilation, it must be used with a tracheostomy tube, not an ETT. The delivered tidal volume (V_T) must be increased to ensure an adequate volume to ventilate the patient. This increase in V_T is necessary because a portion of the delivered V_T is lost via the deflated tracheostomy cuff (Passy, 1986; Simmons & Scanlan, 2003).

Endotracheal Suctioning

Patients with an artificial airway need to be suctioned to ensure airway patency because they lose the normal protective ability to cough up secretions. Suctioning is performed according to a standard protocol to prevent complications such as hypoxemia, increased intracranial pressure, airway trauma, and infection. Suctioning also stimulates the cough reflex and increases mucus production.

Because suctioning is associated with complications, it is performed only as indicated by physical assessment and *not* according to a predetermined schedule. Indications for endotracheal suctioning include visible secretions in the tube, frequent coughing, presence of rhonchi, oxygen desaturation, a change in vital signs (e.g., increased or decreased heart rate or respiratory rate), dyspnea, restlessness, increased peak inspiratory pressure (PIP), or high-pressure ventilator alarms (Henneman, Ellstrom, & St. John, 1999). The number of suction passes varies; the patient is usually suctioned until secretions are removed. Suction duration is limited to 10 to 15 seconds.

Key points related to endotracheal suctioning are discussed in Box 8-8. Several techniques are implemented to reduce complications associated with suctioning. Hyperoxygenation with 100% oxygen should be performed for 30 seconds before suctioning, during the procedure, and immediately after suctioning (Henneman, Ellstrom, & St. John, 1999). Newer ventilators have a built-in suction mode that delivers 100% oxygen for a short period (e.g., 2 minutes). Hyperoxygenation can also be administered with a bag-valve device.

If the patient does not tolerate suctioning with hyperoxygenation alone, hyperinflation may be used. Hyperinflation involves the delivery of breaths 1.0 to 1.5 times the V_T and is performed by giving the patient three to five quick breaths before and

BOX 8-8

Key Points for Endotracheal Suctioning

- Suction only as indicated by patient assessment.
- Assemble equipment (suction kit with two gloves, sterile water or saline for rinsing the catheter).
- Use sterile technique.
- Set suction vacuum at 80 to 150 mm Hg.
- Hyperoxygenate the patient via the ventilator circuit before, between, and after suctioning.
- Gently insert suction catheter until resistance is met, then pull back 1 cm.
- Suction the patient no longer than 10 to 15 seconds while applying intermittent or constant suction.
- Repeat endotracheal suctioning until the airway is clear.
- After endotracheal suctioning is performed, rinse the catheter.
- Suction the mouth and oropharynx.
- Auscultate the lungs to assess effectiveness of suctioning.
- Document the amount, color, and consistency of secretions.

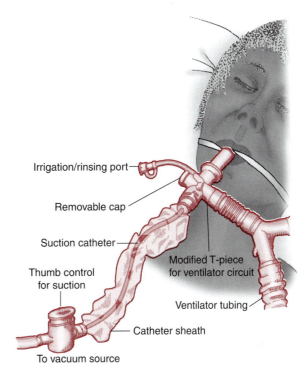

Irrigation/rinsing port

Removable cap

Suction catheter

Thumb control for suction

Modified T-piece for ventilator circuit

Ventilator tubing

Catheter sheath

To vacuum source

FIGURE 8-23 Closed tracheal suction device. (In R. L. Wilkins [ed.]. [2004]. *Egan's fundamentals of respiratory care.* 8th ed. St. Louis: Mosby.)

between suctioning attempts using either the ventilator or bag-valve device.

The closed tracheal, or in-line, suction catheter is an alternative to conventional suctioning. The closed tracheal suction system consists of a suction catheter enclosed in a plastic sheath that is attached to the patient's ventilator circuit (Figure 8-23). The closed system can also be attached to a T-piece adapter. The closed tracheal suction system assists in maintaining oxygenation during suctioning, reduces symptoms associated with hypoxemia, maintains positive end-expiratory pressure (PEEP), permits administration of respiratory medications, protects staff from patient's secretions, and reduces patient anxiety; it is also usually cost-effective (DePew & Noll, 1994; Johnson et al., 1994). Most institutions use closed suctioning for mechanically ventilated patients. At many institutions, all ventilated patients are treated with closed-suction devices. Other institutions use these devices for specific patient indications, such as clinically unstable patients receiving high levels of PEEP and those requiring frequent suctioning (Sole et al., 2003). Key points for use of the closed tracheal suction system are discussed in Box 8-9.

Saline instillation into the trachea during suctioning should not be routinely performed. Although use of saline has been a common practice for many years, more recent studies have found saline instillation to be associated with problems such as oxygen desaturation and patient discomfort (Ridling, Martin, & Bratton, 2003; Kinloch, 1999; O'Neal, Grap, Thompson, & Dudley, 2001; Raymond, 1995). Adequate patient hydration and airway humidification, rather than saline instillation, facilitate secretion removal.

Mechanical Ventilation

Major technological innovations related to mechanical ventilation are being developed and tested. However, the purpose of this chapter is to discuss mechanical ventilation as supportive therapy to facilitate gas exchange, rather than to review a growing list of different machines. Most ventilatory support requires an artificial airway, but some noninvasive methods for ventilatory support exist. The modes of mechanical ventilation are numerous, and the discussion in this chapter focuses on the most common applications. Additional information on mechanical ventilation can be found on the Internet and among the Recommended Readings at the end of this chapter.

INDICATIONS

Mechanical ventilation is warranted for patients who have acute respiratory failure and are unable to maintain normal gas exchange. Such support is indicated

---

BOX 8-9

Key Points for Suctioning with a Closed Tracheal (or In-Line) Suction System

- Choose the proper-size device. The diameter of the suction catheter should be no more than half the diameter of the artificial airway.
- Attach the device to the ventilator circuit. (This step is frequently performed by a respiratory therapist.)
- Set the suction regulator at 80 to 150 mm Hg *while depressing the suction control* on the device.
- Hyperoxygenate the patient via the ventilator circuit before, between, and after suctioning.
- Using the dominant hand, insert the closed-suctioning device into the airway until resistance is met. At the same time, use the nondominant hand to stabilize the artificial airway. Withdraw the suction catheter, using a steady motion while applying intermittent or constant suction for no longer than 10 to 15 seconds.
- Ensure that the catheter has been completely withdrawn from the airway. A marking is visible on the suction catheter when it is properly withdrawn.
- Turn the suction control knob to the "off" position (depends on the brand used).
- Rinse the suction catheter after each use. Connect a small vial or syringe of normal saline for tracheal instillation (without preservatives) to the irrigation port, and simultaneously instill the saline into the port while depressing the suction control.
- Change the system according to manufacturer's recommendations or hospital policy.
- Document the effectiveness of suctioning.
- Keep the suction catheter out of the patient's reach to avoid accidental self-extubation.
- Suction the oropharynx with a tonsil suction device or disposable suction swab.

---

when progressive physiological deterioration is noted, ABG results worsen, infiltrates and other abnormalities appear on chest radiograph, and the patient develops clinical signs of hypoxemia. Physiological parameters indicating the need for mechanical ventilation are presented in Table 8-8. As life-saving therapy, mechanical ventilation is more of a temporary intervention than a means of reversing the acute medical problem (Mutlu & Factor, 2000). Ongoing assessment is essential in determining the need for mechanical ventilation.

NONINVASIVE METHODS OF VENTILATION

Noninvasive ventilation techniques do not require an artificial airway (ETT or tracheostomy). Negative-pressure ventilation and different forms of noninvasive positive-pressure ventilation (NPPV) are among these noninvasive techniques.

Negative-Pressure Ventilation

Negative-pressure ventilation is used for patients with chronic respiratory failure who require assisted ventilation for short periods. Patients with central sleep apnea or other neuromuscular problems who require ventilatory support during sleep are often candidates for negative-pressure ventilation (Corrado & Gorini, 2002). Negative-pressure devices typically enclose the thorax of the patient and allow the head (and airway) access to the ambient atmosphere. The device

TABLE 8-8

Indications for Mechanical Ventilation

Parameter	Normal	Ventilation
ARTERIAL BLOOD GASES		
PaO_2 (mm Hg)	>80	<60
$PaCO_2$ (mm Hg)	35-45	>50
pH	7.35-7.45	<7.25
$PaO_2 = PaCO_2$		
OTHER PARAMETERS		
Respiratory rate/min	12-16	>35
V_T (mL/kg)	6-8	<3.5
VC (mL/kg)	50-60	<10-15
NIF/NIP (cm H_2O)*	>-25	< -25

*Negative inspiratory force (NIF) or negative inspiratory pressure (NIP) is the amount of negative pressure that a patient is able to generate to initiate spontaneous respirations. Normally NIF is – 25 cm of H_2O or greater (e.g., – 30 cm, –40 cm). *PaCO₂,* Partial pressure of carbon dioxide in arterial blood; *PaO₂,* partial pressure of oxygen in arterial blood; *VC,* vital capacity; *V_T,* tidal volume.

creates cyclical increases and decreases in pressure around the chest wall and causes brief changes in intrathoracic pressure. Negative intrathoracic pressure changes prompt inspiration to occur (Figure 8-24), whereas brief positive pressure exerted against the

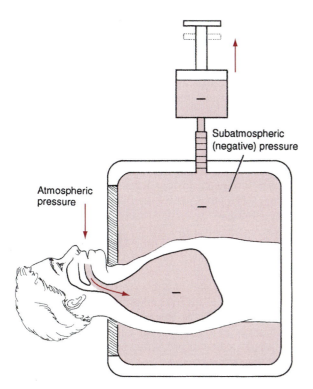

FIGURE 8-24 Concept of negative-pressure ventilation. (From Cairo, J. M., & Pilbeam, S. P. [2004]. *Mosby's respiratory care equipment*, [p. 322]. 7th ed. St. Louis: Mosby.)

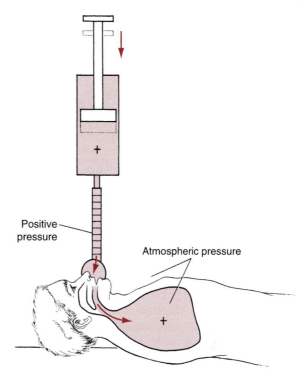

FIGURE 8-25 Concept of positive-pressure ventilation. (From Cairo, J. M., & Pilbeam, S. P. [2004]. *Mosby's respiratory care equipment* [p. 322]. 7th ed. St. Louis: Mosby.)

chest wall facilitates expiration. Examples of negative-pressure ventilators include the iron lung or tank ventilator, chest cuirass, poncho, and body wrap devices (Vines, 2003).

Noninvasive Positive-Pressure Ventilation

NPPV is a therapy to manage chronic respiratory failure or acute respiratory insufficiency that is expected to resolve quickly, such as postextubation hypercapnia or pulmonary edema. NPPV may also be ordered to support ventilation in a patient who refuses intubation (Wedzicha, 2002). NPPV provides ventilation via a face mask that covers the nose and mouth, a nasal mask or pillow, or a mouthpiece with a tight seal. A portable ventilator provides either volume-cycled or flow-cycled breaths through the mask or mouthpiece. NPPV provides low levels of continuous positive airway pressure (CPAP) and pressure support to facilitate gas exchange. Some devices apply positive pressure during both inspiration and expiration and are referred to as bilevel positive airway pressure devices (Vines, 2003).

INVASIVE METHODS OF VENTILATION—POSITIVE-PRESSURE VENTILATION

Invasive ventilation techniques require a stable artificial airway. The most common method for ventilating patients in the acute care setting is positive-pressure ventilation. This method uses positive pressure to force air into the lungs via an artificial airway. Figure 8-25 illustrates the concept of positive-pressure ventilation. Some degree of positive-pressure ventilation or forward flow of inspired gas is necessary to deliver V_T and/or manipulate the patient's airway pressure during the act of ventilation (Hess & Kacmarek, 2002). Positive-pressure ventilation can be categorized as *volume-targeted ventilation* and *pressure-targeted ventilation* (Pierce, 1998). Multifunctional ventilators incorporate microprocessor technology that allows adjustment of time (length of inspiration and expiration), volume, and pressure.

Volume-Targeted Ventilation

In volume-targeted ventilation, a specific volume for delivery of inspiration is set. The ventilator is set to allow airflow into the lungs until a preset volume has been reached. A major advantage of these ventilators is that they deliver the V_T regardless of changes in lung compliance or resistance. This type of ventilation is commonly used to treat adults. Assist/control (A/C) and intermittent mandatory ventilation are types of volume-targeted ventilation.

Pressure-Targeted Ventilation

In pressure-targeted ventilation, a specific PIP is set for delivery of inspiration. The ventilator is set to allow air to flow into the lungs until a preset pressure has been reached. Once the pressure is reached, a valve closes and expiration begins. Pressure-support and pressure-control ventilation are types of pressure-targeted ventilation. A disadvantage of pressure-targeted ventilation is that delivered V_T varies according to compliance and resistance of the patient's pulmonary system, and hypoventilation and respiratory acidosis may occur.

Ventilators with Flexible Capabilities

Microprocessor ventilators offer flexibility in the types of ventilation they provide. Many patients receive a combination of volume-targeted and pressure-targeted modes of mechanical ventilation (Pierce, 1998; Pilbeam, 1998; Pilbeam, 2004). Newer ventilators can often alter modes of delivery based on changes in the patient's respiratory parameters and preset ventilator controls.

VOLUME-TARGETED MODES OF MECHANICAL VENTILATION

Settings on volume-targeted ventilators are adjusted to ensure adequate ventilation and oxygenation of the patient. Modes include *controlled ventilation, A/C ventilation,* and *synchronized intermittent mandatory ventilation* (SIMV). Waveforms depicting these various modes are shown in Figure 8-26.

Controlled Ventilation

The control mode of mechanical ventilation delivers a preset V_T at a preset respiratory rate and provides an expected minute ventilation. This mode ventilates the patient regardless of inspiratory effort. This effectively "locks out" the patient's effort to breathe. The control mode may be ordered for patients who have no inspiratory effort, such as those with high cervical spine injuries. Patients who receive chemical paralysis as part of their medical treatment (e.g., flail chest or head injury) may also be candidates for controlled ventilation. Control is rarely used because A/C control modes achieve similar results and cause the patient less anxiety and hemodynamic instability if recovery of ventilatory function occurs.

Assist/Control Ventilation

The A/C mode of mechanical ventilation delivers a preset V_T whenever the patient exerts a negative inspiratory effort. A preset respiratory rate ensures that the patient receives adequate ventilation, regardless of spontaneous efforts, and helps to decrease WOB. For example, the A/C respiratory rate may be set at 10 breaths per minute at a V_T of 800 mL. If the patient initiates a negative inspiratory effort 16 times per minute, he or she receives 800 mL of air for each of the 16 efforts. If the patient does not initiate any inspiratory effort (e.g., during sleep), he or she receives 800 mL V_T 10 times per minute. The A/C mode is useful in patients with normal respiratory drive who are unable to sustain a normal V_T. It also helps to preserve pulmonary muscle tone and reduces patient-ventilator dyssynchrony, or "fighting the ventilator" (Pilbeam, 1998).

One complication of A/C ventilation is respiratory alkalosis, especially if the patient's spontaneous respiratory rate is high, or the triggering function of the ventilator is set to too sensitive a position. Respiratory alkalosis is treated or prevented by adjusting the ventilator's sensitivity setting or V_T, sedating the patient (if needed), or changing to intermittent mandatory ventilation.

Synchronized Intermittent Mandatory Ventilation

The SIMV mode of mechanical ventilation delivers a preset V_T at a preset mandatory respiratory rate and permits the patient to breathe spontaneously at his or her own respiratory rate and depth between the ventilator breaths. The preset breaths are synchronized with the patient's spontaneous efforts and help to prevent patient-ventilator dyssynchrony. The SIMV mode helps to prevent respiratory muscle weakness and the hyperventilation that can occur in the A/C mode. Like the A/C mode, the SIMV mode guarantees a minimum number of breaths to the patient.

The SIMV mode is often ordered as a method for weaning patients from mechanical ventilation. However, based on individual patient response, SIMV can sometimes increases muscle fatigue associated with spontaneous breathing efforts (Pierce, 1998).

PRESSURE-TARGETED MODES OF MECHANICAL VENTILATION

Pressure-targeted (or pressure-limited) ventilation provides ventilation based on preset inspiratory pressure levels. The delivery of V_T is controlled by the preset inspiratory pressure, the flow rate of gas to the patient, respiratory rate, and the length of inspiratory

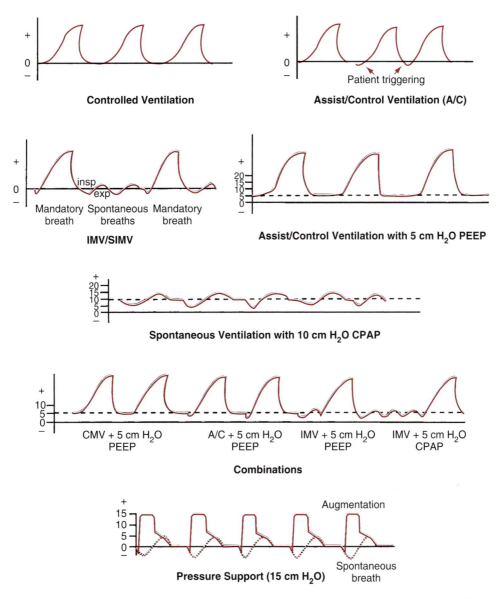

Controlled Ventilation

Assist/Control Ventilation (A/C)

Patient triggering

IMV/SIMV

Mandatory breath   Spontaneous breaths   Mandatory breath

insp
exp

Assist/Control Ventilation with 5 cm H₂O PEEP

Spontaneous Ventilation with 10 cm H₂O CPAP

Combinations

CMV + 5 cm H₂O PEEP   A/C + 5 cm H₂O PEEP   IMV + 5 cm H₂O PEEP   IMV + 5 cm H₂O CPAP

Pressure Support (15 cm H₂O)

Augmentation

Spontaneous breath

FIGURE 8-26 Waveforms of ventilator modes and adjuncts to ventilation. *IMV/SIMV,* Intermittent mandatory ventilation/synchronized IMV; *PEEP,* positive end-expiratory pressure; *CPAP,* continuous positive airway pressure.

time per breath. Once a breath is triggered, a rapid inspiratory flow of gas occurs until the set pressure is reached. At that point, flow decreases, and the breath ends with the patient's receiving a V_T determined by the patient's overall lung compliance. Patients with normal lung compliance will have better delivery of V_T for the amount of pressure-controlled ventilation in use (Pilbeam, 2004). Several examples of pressure-targeted ventilation are described.

Pressure-Support Ventilation

In pressure-support ventilation (PSV), a preset level of positive pressure is applied for the duration of a spontaneous breath and allows a more even distribution of inspired gas. PSV augments a patient's spontaneous V_T and decreases the WOB associated with spontaneous breathing through an artificial airway (Chang, 2001; Pilbeam, 2004). PSV may also increase patient comfort and provide conditioning of the diaphragm, both of which facilitate weaning from the ventilator. PSV is used to enhance other modes of ventilation or as a stand-alone mode to ventilate a spontaneously breathing patient. PSV is typically used in the SIMV mode to promote weaning from mechanical ventilation (Chang, 2001).

Pressure-Controlled Ventilation

In PCV, pressure-controlled breaths are time triggered by a preset respiratory rate. The PCV mode is usually indicated for patients with severe ARDS who require extremely high PIPs during traditional volume ventilation. PCV reduces the risk of barotrauma associated with high PIPs while maintaining adequate oxygenation and ventilation. Patients needing PCV should be sedated to promote comfort and to avoid ventilator dyschrony.

Automode

This hybrid ventilator mode is a combination of volume support during patient spontaneous ventilation and PCV if the patient is not breathing (Hess & Kacmarek, 2002). The ventilator recognizes the patient's actions (spontaneous ventilation) or inactions (apnea) and provides the appropriate level of support based on preestablished parameters of V_T and minute ventilation.

Proportional Assist Ventilation

Proportional assist ventilation is accomplished with a positive feedback control that evaluates a patient's inspiratory efforts. As the patient's inspiratory pressures and volumes change during ventilation, airway support is automatically adjusted. Patient effort ultimately determines ventilating pressures. This mode is thought to provide a more physiological breathing pattern (Hess & Kacmarek, 2002).

Pressure-Controlled Inverse-Ratio Ventilation

With pressure-controlled inverse-ratio ventilation (PC-IRV), the ventilator is set to provide longer inspiratory times to increase the mean airway pressure while maintaining peak inspiratory airway pressures at lower levels than conventional volume ventilation. Lower PIPs are less damaging to the lung, and the longer inspiratory time improves oxygenation. Similar to PCV, PC-IRV may be indicated in patients with severe ARDS. Because PCV reverses the normal I:E ratio, patients must be sedated, and possibly paralyzed, to avoid dyssynchrony with the ventilator (Chang, 2001).

Airway Pressure–Release Ventilation

Airway pressure–release ventilation is a relatively new mode of ventilation that provides two levels of CPAP during the inspiratory and expiratory phases of breathing. During spontaneous inspiration, the patient receives a preset level of CPAP; this level is periodically released to facilitate expiration (Chang, 2001). Airway pressure–release ventilation assists in providing adequate oxygenation while lowering peak inspiratory airway pressures. It is indicated as an alternative to conventional volume ventilation for patients with significantly decreased lung compliance, such as in ARDS. Sedation may be needed with airway pressure–release ventilation to promote patient comfort (Chang, 2001; Hess & Kacmarek, 2002).

ADJUNCT SETTINGS FOR MECHANICAL VENTILATION

Several additional settings can be added to the list of mechanical ventilator control settings to enhance the oxygenation and/or ventilation. These include *PEEP, CPAP*, and *pressure support*. Representative waveforms of these settings are shown in Figure 8-26.

Positive End-Expiratory Pressure

With PEEP, positive airway pressure (higher than ambient) is added to mechanically assisted breaths. Higher than atmospheric pressure keeps the patient's airway open at the end of expiration and increases the functional residual capacity. PEEP increases oxygenation by preventing collapse of small airways and maximizing the number of alveoli available for gas exchange (Figure 8-27). The range for PEEP is 3 to 20 cm H_2O, although levels up to 50 cm H_2O have been ordered to treat severe refractory hypoxemia.

PEEP is often ordered to decrease the FiO_2 needed for optimal oxygenation. For example, a patient may require an FiO_2 of 0.80 to maintain a PaO_2 of 85 mm Hg. If PEEP is added, the FiO_2 may be lowered while still maintaining an adequate PaO_2. In addition, many

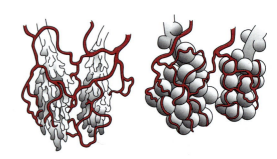

FIGURE 8-27 Effect of application of PEEP on the alveoli. (From Pierce, L. N. B. [1995]. *Guide to mechanical ventilation and intensive respiratory care* [p. 170]. Philadelphia: W. B. Saunders.)

patients routinely receive 3 to 5 cm H_2O of PEEP, a value often referred to as physiological PEEP. This small amount is thought to preserve a more normal functional residual capacity in patients with artificial airways (Pilbeam, 2004).

Sometimes, a phenomenon known as auto-PEEP occurs when residual pressure in the alveoli at the end of exhalation cannot escape the lung. Auto-PEEP is more likely to occur when the ventilator delivers prolonged inspiration, such as in inverse-ratio ventilation (Pilbeam, 2004).

PEEP is associated with several complications: a decrease in cardiac output secondary to decreased venous return, an increased risk of volutrauma, increased intracranial pressure resulting from impedance of venous return from the head, and alterations in renal function caused by reduced renal blood flow (Chang, 2001). Volutrauma may be reduced by reducing the V_T on the ventilator to less than the usual 10 to 15 mL/kg.

The nurse monitors for the presence of PEEP or auto-PEEP by observing the pressure level displayed on the ventilator's analog and graphic displays. When no PEEP is present, the pressure reading should return to zero on the analog display or return to the "zero point" on the graphic display at the end of expiration. The presence of PEEP or auto-PEEP is determined by observing the amount of pressure at end expiration that remains on the ventilator analog or graphic display. When PEEP is ordered, the display will show the amount of PEEP present at the end of expiration. If auto-PEEP occurs, a higher than expected PEEP reading will be noted at the end of expiration.

Continuous Positive Airway Pressure

CPAP is the concept of PEEP applied to the airway used to augment the patient's functional residual capacity and oxygenation during spontaneous breathing (Chang, 2001). CPAP can be administered via a nasal mask, by a face mask, or through an artificial airway. CPAP may be administered with a stand-alone CPAP-type device or a mechanical ventilator capable of providing CPAP, depending on the equipment. Typically, a nasal CPAP system is used to treat symptoms seen in obstructive sleep apnea. CPAP is often administered via a face mask to delay intubation or to support a patient after extubation if needed. Mechanical ventilation can also provide CPAP to patients, usually in the SIMV mode, to assist in weaning from mechanical ventilation. When a spontaneously breathing patient is being ventilated with SIMV, the PEEP delivered during the SIMV (mechanical) breaths is considered PEEP, whereas the pressure delivered during unassisted spontaneous breathing is considered CPAP.

Pressure-Support Ventilation

PSV can be used as a stand-alone mode to ventilate a spontaneously breathing patient. It is commonly ordered in conjunction with SIMV (see previous discussion).

ADVANCED METHODS AND MODES OF MECHANICAL VENTILATION

Microprocessor ventilators offer a wide range of options for mechanical ventilation. However, other forms of ventilatory and oxygenation support are available. These advanced techniques are usually ordered to treat patients with respiratory failure that is refractory to conventional treatment. These techniques include, but are not limited to, high-frequency jet or oscillation ventilation, extracorporeal membrane oxygenation, liquid ventilation, and inhaled nitric oxide. Specialized equipment and training are essential for these advanced treatments.

TYPICAL VENTILATOR SETTINGS AND TERMINOLOGY

In most institutions, the ventilators (Figure 8-28) are set up and managed by respiratory therapy personnel.

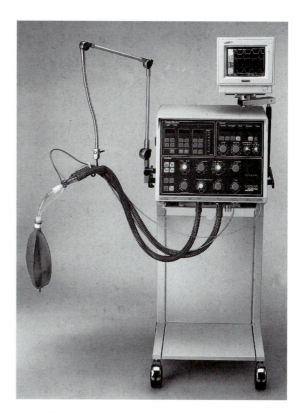

FIGURE 8-28 Example of a mechanical ventilator. (Courtesy of Hamilton Medical, Inc., Reno, NV.)

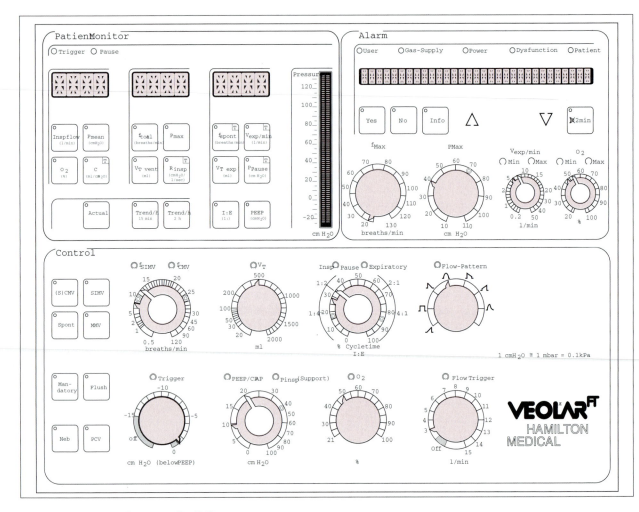

FIGURE 8-29 Mechanical ventilator control panel. (Courtesy of Yvon Dupuis.)

However, the nurse should be familiar with selected dials and values on the control panel so essential ventilator settings and alarm functions can be verified at least once per shift. A representative control panel of a ventilator is shown in Figure 8-29. Although the control panel of a microprocessor-type ventilator can be overwhelming, it is important for the nurse to learn how to identify the common settings that are integral to the assessment of the patient.

Tidal Volume

The amount of air delivered with each preset breath is the V_T. The ventilator has traditionally been set to deliver a V_T between 10 and 15 mL/kg (Chang, 2001). Thus, a patient who weighs 70 kg would have the V_T set between 700 and 1050 mL. However, recent research has found that lower V_T levels (4 to 8 mL/kg) can provide adequate ventilation while reducing

complications associated with mechanical ventilation (ARDS Network, 2000). When lower V_T levels are administered, the patient's carbon dioxide level may rise above normal values, referred to as *permissive hypercapnia*. Adjustments in oxygen levels and PEEP are made to optimize patient oxygenation and ventilation (Hickling, 2002; ARDS Network, 2000). Permissive hypercapnia reduces peak airway pressures and may reduce ventilator-associated lung injury (volutrauma). It is contraindicated in patients with head injuries, because increased intracranial pressure may occur secondary to vasodilation that occurs with higher levels of carbon dioxide.

Respiratory Rate

Respiratory rate is the frequency of breaths (f) set to be delivered by the ventilator to the patient. The respiratory rate multiplied by the V_T determines the patient's minute ventilation. The typical goal is to set the minute ventilation according to the body surface area: 4 times body surface area in men and 3.5 times body surface area in women (Pilbeam, 1998). This minute ventilation calculation assumes a desire to maintain normal physiology. Adjustments are necessary to achieve an ideal minute ventilation.

Fraction of Inspired Oxygen

The FiO_2 is the fraction (or percentage) of inspired oxygen delivered to the patient by the ventilator. FiO_2 may be set from 0.21 (21% or room air) to 1.00 (100% oxygen). The initial FiO_2 setting is based on the patient's immediate physiological need. The equation used to establish a starting FiO_2 value if an ABG is done to guide treatment is

$$\text{Desired } FiO_2 = \frac{PaO_2 \text{ (desired)} \times FiO_2 \text{ (known)}}{PaO_2 \text{ (known)}}$$

In an emergency situation (e.g., mechanical ventilation after emergency intubation), the initial FiO_2 is set between 0.5 and 1.0 to meet the patient's physiological needs. The setting is then adjusted based on ABG and/or noninvasive assessment of gas exchange.

Peak Inspiratory Pressure

The peak inspiratory pressure (PIP) is the maximal pressuring that occurs during ventilation and is usually measured at the end of expiration. The PIP necessary to ventilate the patient increases with changes in airway resistance (e.g., secretions in the airway or biting the ETT) and decreased lung compliance (e.g., ARDS). Baseline values of PIP are needed to determine pressure alarm limits. Respiratory therapists also use the PIP to adjust the ventilator settings. The patient's PIP is monitored, and intervention may be needed. For example, higher PIPs occur with obstruction and may indicate a need for suctioning. PIP rises in clinical conditions such as a pneumothorax.

Sensitivity

Sensitivity determines the amount of patient effort needed to initiate an assisted breath. It is normally set at -1 cm H_2O or less than the patient's recorded baseline pressure on the mechanical ventilator. If the sensitivity is set too low, the patient must generate more work to trigger gas flow. If it is set too high, auto-cycling of the ventilator and patient-ventilator dysynchrony may occur (Pilbeam, 1998).

Inspiratory-to-Expiratory Ratio

In spontaneous ventilation, inspiration is shorter than expiration. When a patient undergoes mechanical ventilation, the I:E ratio is usually set at 1:2. The I:E ratio can be controlled by the ventilator within preset limits or adjusted to maximize gas exchange. For example, inverse-ratio ventilation may be used to treat patients with ARDS.

Sigh

A sigh is a mechanically set breath with greater volume than the preset V_T, usually 1.5 to 2.0 times the V_T. The rationale for using a sigh is to prevent atelectasis, because a ventilated patient is not able to take a deep spontaneous breath, a natural sigh. The sigh mechanism is infrequently used, especially if higher V_T settings are ordered, and other adjuncts to mechanical ventilation reduce the need for artificial sighs.

Humidification

Providing humidification is an important element of ventilator management. It is essential to maintain the inspired gas reaching the patient's airway at as close to 37°C and 100% relative humidity as possible (Hess & Kacmarek, 2002; Wissing, 2004). Two approaches are used to supply supplemental humidification with mechanical ventilation. One method functions by actively passing the dry inspired gas through a water-based humidification system before it reaches the patient's airway. This method is often ordered for patients requiring long-term mechanical ventilation. It is important to monitor the temperature of the water humidification system.

The second method is to attach a heat-moisture-exchanger (HME) to the ventilator circuit. The HME functions as an artificial "nose" to warm and humidify the patient's inspired breath with his or her own expired moisture and body heat. The HME must also be monitored because excess patient secretions can accumulate in the HME device, thus increasing the WOB.

ALARM SYSTEMS

Alarms are an integral part of mechanical ventilation. Because this equipment provides vital life support functions for the patient it is essential that it be fully equipped with alarm systems (Pilbeam, 2004). All modern mechanical ventilators provide an array of alarm systems. The nurse must be familiar with the alarm functions of each ventilator. Examples of alarms include the following:

1. Increased V_T, minute ventilation, or respiratory rate alarms
2. Decreased V_T, minute ventilation, or respiratory rate alarms
3. High and low inspiratory pressure alarms
4. High and low PEEP or CPAP alarms

5. Special mode activation alarms (e.g., I:E ratio activation), apnea alarm
6. Loss of power or loss of gas pressure alarms

RESPIRATORY MONITORING DURING MECHANICAL VENTILATION

Nurses and respiratory therapists routinely monitor numerous physiological and respiratory parameters while a patient receives mechanical ventilation. Monitoring is done to assess the patient's response to treatment and anticipate and to plan for the ventilator weaning process. The respiratory parameters include spontaneous V_T, the vital capacity, negative inspiratory force or pressure, airway resistance, and compliance. These values, along with ABGs, PaO_2/PAO_2, dead space, pulse oximetry, and $ETCO_2$ monitoring, allow assessment of oxygenation and ventilation (Epstein, 2000; Hess & Kacmarek, 2002). The caregiver must monitor all of these parameters as well as assess the patient's overall physical condition.

COMPLICATIONS OF MECHANICAL VENTILATION

Numerous complications are associated with intubation and mechanical ventilation. Many complications can be prevented and/or treated rapidly through vigilant nursing care (Hess & Kacmarek, 2002; Mutlu & Factor, 2000).

Pulmonary System

Volutrauma. Originally known as barotrauma, volutrauma is lung injury or alveolar rupture that occurs from overdistention of the alveoli causing parenchymal damage (Mutlu & Factor, 2000). Injury may cause air to escape into various parts of the thoracic cavity, thus causing pneumothorax or tension pneumothorax, pneumomediastinum, pneumopericardium, pneumoperitoneum, or subcutaneous crepitus. Volutrauma may occur when the alveoli are overdistended, such as with positive-pressure ventilation, PEEP, and high V_T. An increased incidence of barotrauma is likely if the patient is older, has a history of COPD, or has an infection that destroys the alveoli. Volutrauma is typically associated with ARDS in which $PaCO_2$ is difficult to stabilize, and higher V_T is delivered to manage $PaCO_2$ (Gillette & Hess, 2001). Signs and symptoms of barotrauma include high peak inspiratory and mean airway pressures, decreased breath sounds, tracheal shift, subcutaneous crepitus, and symptoms associated with hypoxemia.

A life-threatening complication is *tension pneumothorax* (Figure 8-30). When tension pneumothorax occurs, pressurized air enters the pleural space. Air is unable to exit the pleural space and continues to accumulate. Collapse of the cardiopulmonary system

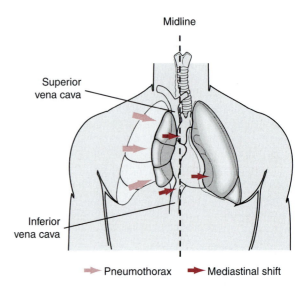

Midline

Superior vena cava

Inferior vena cava

➡ Pneumothorax ➡ Mediastinal shift

FIGURE 8-30 Tension pneumothorax. (From Crimlisk, J. [2004]. Lower respiratory problems. In S. M. Lewis, M. M. Heitkemper, & S. R. Dirksen (Eds.). *Medical-surgical nursing* [p. 621]. 6th ed. St. Louis: Mosby.)

occurs rapidly. Treatment consists of immediate insertion of a chest tube or a needle thoracostomy. Whenever a pneumothorax is suspected in a patient receiving mechanical ventilation, the patient should be removed from the ventilator and ventilated with a bag-valve device until a chest tube is inserted.

Intubation of right mainstem bronchus. The right mainstem bronchus is straighter than the left. If the ETT is manipulated, such as occurs during changing of the tape, it may slip into the right mainstem bronchus. Symptoms include absent or diminished breath sounds in the left lung. Whenever the ETT is manipulated, the nurse must assess for bilateral chest excursion, auscultate the chest for bilateral breath sounds after the procedure, and reassess tube position at the lip.

Endotracheal tube out of position or an unplanned extubation. The ETT can become dislodged if it is not secured properly, during procedures such as changing the tape on the ETT, during transport, or if the patient is anxious or agitated and attempts to pull out the tube. The ETT may end up in the back of the throat, in the esophagus, or completely removed. Auscultation of bilateral breath sounds and use of capnography are helpful in verifying ETT placement. Strategies for preventing an unplanned extubation are described in Box 8-10.

BOX 8-10

Strategies for Preventing Accidental or Unplanned Extubation

- Provide adequate patient sedation and comfort.
- Apply protective devices (e.g., soft wrist restraints) according to hospital protocol.
- Adequately secure the endotracheal tube.
- Cut the end of the endotracheal tube to 2 inches beyond the fixation point.
- Mark the lip line on endotracheal tube with an indelible marker; assess tube position routinely.
- Maintain adequate volume in the cuff of the artificial airway.
- Provide support for the ventilator tubing and closed suction systems; keep these items out of the patient's reach.
- Use two staff members when repositioning an endotracheal tube.
- Educate the patient and family.

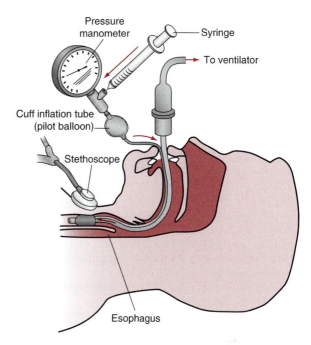

FIGURE 8-31 Monitoring endotracheal tube cuff pressures. (From Lewis, S. M. [2000]. Lower respiratory problems. In S. M. Lewis, M. M. Heitkemper, & S. R. Dirksen, *Medical-surgical nursing* [5th ed.]. St. Louis: Mosby.)

Tracheal damage. Damage to the trachea can occur because of pressure from the cuff. However, this risk is low because all ETT and tracheostomy tubes now have low-pressure cuffs. An intervention for preventing tracheal damage is monitoring cuff pressures on a routine basis; pressures should not exceed 30 cm H_2O (Henneman, Ellstrom, & St. John, 1999). Various commercial devices that measure cuff pressures quickly and easily are available (Figure 8-31).

Damage to the oral or nasal mucosa. Tape or commercial devices that secure the ETT can cause breakdown of the lip and oral mucosa. Nasal intubation may result in skin breakdown on the nares and also a higher risk of sinusitis. Ongoing assessment and skin care can assist in preventing damage to the mouth and nose.

Associated with oxygen administration. Nitrogen is needed to prevent collapse of the airway. If 100% oxygen is administered, a lack of nitrogen in the distal air spaces predisposes the patient to absorption atelectasis. Other complications associated with oxygen administration include tracheobronchitis, acute lung injury (ARDS), and chronic pulmonary dysplasia. As a rule, oxygen concentrations up to 1 can be tolerated for up to 48 hours. After that, the goal is to lower the FiO_2 to less than 0.60 to prevent further lung damage (Heuer & Scanlan, 2003).

Respiratory acidosis or alkalosis. Acid-base disturbances may occur secondary to VT and respiratory rate settings on the ventilator. For example, if a patient is receiving A/C ventilation and is breathing 30 times per minute, respiratory alkalosis usually occurs. If the ventilator is set at a low respiratory rate (e.g., 2 to 6 breaths per minute) and the patient does not have additional spontaneous breathing effort, respiratory acidosis may occur. Acid-base status is also altered when permissive hypercapnia is employed. Ventilator adjustments may be made to alter acid-base status therapeutically (e.g., head injury).

Aspiration. Most patients who require mechanical ventilation also require tube feedings. Gastric distention, impaired gastric emptying with large amounts of gastric residual, and esophageal reflux predispose patients to aspiration. Keeping the head of bed elevated to 30 degrees is warranted to prevent aspiration (Burns, 1998).

Infection. Patients with artificial airways are at an increased risk of pulmonary infection (ventilator-associated pneumonia) because normal defense mechanisms in the nose are bypassed. Procedures such as endotracheal suctioning also predispose the patient to an increased risk of infection. Bacteria that frequently cause nosocomial infections include *Streptococcus* species, *Staphylococcus* species, *Pseudomonas* species, *Escherichia coli*, and *Serratia* species. Because of their debilitated state, patients may also acquire fungal infections, such as from *Candida albicans*. Infections with antibiotic-resistant bacteria are also increasing. Hand washing, sterile technique for suctioning, adequate pressure in the ETT or tracheostomy cuff, and adherence to protocols such as ventilator tubing changes are essential in prevention of infection. Sputum characteristics are monitored, and cultures are obtained when infection is suspected.

Frequent oral hygiene every 2 to 6 hours with fluoride toothpaste, soft-bristled baby toothbrushes, and tap water or normal saline have been shown to keep the oral tissues in good condition and free from plaque buildup with its potentially lethal growth of gram-negative bacteria that could be aspirated or enter the systemic circulation at a compromised gumline (Stiefel, Damron, Sowers, Velez, 2000). Infections are discussed in more detail in Chapter 13.

Ventilator dependence or inability to wean.

Patients who require long-term mechanical ventilation are usually very challenging to wean from the ventilator. Examples of patients in this category include those with underlying COPD and neuromuscular disease.

Cardiovascular System

Decreased cardiac output may occur with mechanical ventilation and PEEP, secondary to increased intrathoracic pressure and a decreased venous return. Patients who are hemodynamically unstable may need a pulmonary artery catheter inserted to monitor the hemodynamic effects of mechanical ventilation.

Gastrointestinal System

Stress ulcers and gastrointestinal bleeding may occur in patients who undergo mechanical ventilation. Another possible complication is a paralytic ileus. Inadequate nutrition may occur if the patient is not started on early nutritional support or receives inadequate supplemental nutrition.

Endocrine System

Fluid retention may occur from increased humidification provided by the ventilator. Another reason for fluid retention is that increased pressure on the baroreceptors in the thoracic aorta from positive-pressure ventilation stimulates the release of antidiuretic hormone. This hormone causes water retention and stimulates the renin-angiotensin-aldosterone mechanism, which causes further fluid retention.

Psychosocial Complications

Several psychosocial hazards may occur as the result of mechanical ventilation. The patient may experience stress and anxiety because he or she requires a machine for breathing. If the ventilator is not set properly or if the patient resists breaths, patient-ventilator dyssynchrony may occur. The noise of the ventilator and the need for frequent procedures, such as suctioning, may result in alteration in sleep and wake patterns. In addition, the patient can become psychologically dependent on the ventilator.

Communication. Communication difficulties are common because of the artificial airway. The lack of vocal expression has been identified by patients as a major stressor that elicits feelings of panic, isolation, anger, helplessness, and decreased self-esteem. Even though the American Association of Critical-Care Nurses singled out communication with the ventilated patient as one of its top 10 research priorities in the 1980s, relatively few studies have been done and/or implemented (Lewandowski & Kositsky, 1983; Menzel, 1994). Barriers to research include high acuity and instability of the patient, nurse frustration associated with lack of training in nonvocal methods of communication such as lip reading, and lack of use of augmentative aids in communication such as speaking valves (Happ, 2001). Patients express a need to know, as well as to make themselves understood (Hupcey, 2000). They need constant reorientation, reassuring words emphasizing a caregiver's presence, and point-of-care information that painful procedures done to them are indeed necessary and helpful. In addition, therapeutic touch, eye contact, and positive facial expressions are beneficial in relieving anxiety (Menzel, 1999). Caregivers who attempt to individualize communication with intubated patients by using a variety of methods will give these patients a greater sense of control, encourage participation in their own care, and minimize cognitive disturbances (Criner, 1995). Enhancing communication ensures a better quality of life during mechanical ventilation and decreases the occurrence of posttraumatic stress after an episode of critical illness (Adler, 1997). For these reasons, it is vital that more research in this area be undertaken.

Nursing Care

Nursing care of the patient who requires mechanical ventilation is a challenge. The nurse must provide care in a holistic approach, along with use of technology. A detailed plan of care is described in the Nursing Care Plan for the Mechanically Ventilated Patient.

Text continued on page 204

Nursing Care Plan for the Mechanically Ventilated Patient

NURSING DIAGNOSIS: *Inability to sustain spontaneous ventilation related to respiratory muscle fatigue, metabolic factors*

Patient Outcomes	Interventions	Rationales
Patient will maintain normal ABG values, maintain airway, mobilize secretions, and remain free of dyspnea or restlessness	Monitor oxygenation and ventilation and respond to changes: ABGs Pulse oximetry End-tidal carbon CO_2	Ensure adequate oxygenation and acid-base balance
	Maintain ETT or tracheostomy; secure tube with tape or other devices	Maintain an adequate airway to facilitate mechanical ventilation
	Suction as needed according to protocol (see Boxes 8-8, 8-9)	Remove secretions and maintain an open airway
	Collaborate with physician to develop a sedation plan if agitation impairs ventilation	Promote effectiveness of mechanical ventilation
	Prevent unplanned extubation (see Box 8-10)	Protect the airway and promote patient safety
	Reposition ETT from side to side every 24 hr; assess and document skin condition Note placement of tube at lip line Use two staff members for procedure Suction secretions above the ETT cuff before repositioning tube Auscultate chest after repositioning tube	Prevent skin breakdown, reduce aspiration of oral secretions and ventilator-associated pneumonia, and ensure that tube remains in proper position after manipulation
	Assess respiratory status every 4 hr; respond to changes: Breath sounds anteriorly and posteriorly Chest excursion Patient's ability to initiate a spontaneous breath Signs and symptoms of hypoxemia	Provide cues of condition improvement or worsening; may indicate need for suctioning
	Monitor respiratory rate and ventilator-assisted and patient-initiated breaths	Assess effectiveness of mechanical ventilation
	Assess tolerance to ventilatory assistance and monitor for asynchronous chest movement, subjective report of breathlessness, or high-pressure alarms; if symptomatic, remove patient from ventilator and manually ventilate and prepare for chest tube insertion	Assess effectiveness of mechanical ventilation and be alert for complications, such as volutrauma; to respond quickly to treat volutrauma
	Have bag-valve device and suctioning equipment readily available	Manually ventilate patient in response to ventilator alarms or other emergencies and maintain a patent airway
	Maintain integrity of mechanical ventilator circuit; monitor ventilator settings; respond to ventilator alarms; keep tubing free of moisture by draining *away* from the patient and using devices such as water traps to facilitate drainage of moisture	Maximize effectiveness of mechanical ventilation and promote patient safety

Continued

Nursing Care Plan for the Mechanically Ventilated Patient—cont'd

Patient Outcomes	Interventions	Rationales

Patient will maintain normal ABG values, maintain airway, mobilize secretions, and remain free of dyspnea or restlessness—*cont'd*	Monitor cuff pressure of ETT or tracheostomy:
	    Inflate cuff with the minimum amount of air needed to prevent leak of air around the cuff and provide ordered tidal volume
	    Use commercial devices to monitor cuff pressure
	    Notify the physician if cuff pressure exceeds 30 cm H_2O or if cuff does not maintain adequate pressure
	Suction oral secretions every 4 hr and as needed
	Monitor serial chest x-ray studies
	Collaborate with the health care team to develop strategies to maximize effectiveness of mechanical ventilation: changes in settings, sedation, analgesia, relaxation techniques, neuromuscular blockade
	Collaborate with the health care team to treat and respond to underlying respiratory failure
	Monitor readiness to wean from mechanical ventilation (see Box 8-11)
	Support patient and family involvement in plan of care and treatment goals
	Implement a plan of care to maintain patient comfort, mobility, nutrition, and skin integrity
		Maximize ventilation and prevent aspiration of oral secretions
		
		Prevent aspiration of oral secretions; improve patient comfort
		Assess for correct positioning of ETT and improvement or worsening of pulmonary conditions
		Therapies may be needed to facilitate mechanical ventilation to optimize ventilation and gas exchange
		
		Treating underlying cause will promote weaning from mechanical ventilation
		Identify indicators that patient is ready to begin the weaning process
		Foster patient and family well-being
		Prevent functional losses associated with mechanical ventilation and bed rest

NURSING DIAGNOSIS: *Airway clearance ineffective, related to artificial airway; decreased ability to cough; thick secretions*

Patient Outcomes	Interventions	Rationales
The patient will maintain an open airway free of secretions; secretions are easily removed	Assess need for ETT suctioning: pressure alarm on ventilator, audible secretions, harsh breath sounds Suction according to hospital protocol (see Boxes 8-8 and 8-9) Assess breath sounds after suctioning If tracheal secretions are thick, assess hydration of patient and humidification of ventilator; avoid instillation of normal saline Reposition the patient frequently	Indications of need for suctioning Prevent complications associated with suctioning Determine effectiveness; breath sounds should improve Assist in thinning secretions for easier removal; saline has not shown to be effective and is associated with hypoxemia Mobilize secretions

Nursing Care Plan for the Mechanically Ventilated Patient—cont'd

NURSING DIAGNOSIS: *Communication impaired, verbal, related to artificial airway and mechanical ventilation*

Patient Outcomes	Interventions	Rationales

Patient will be able to communicate needs to caregiver; patient will be able to communicate with family members	Establish method for communication that is appropriate for the patient's native language
	    Yes/no questions
	    Clipboard with paper and pencil
	    Picture communication boards
	    Devices such as MagnaDoodle
	    Computerized systems
	Attempt lip reading
	Speak slowly and clearly to patient; do not shout
	Explain procedures
	Use significant others to assist with communication
	Consider use of tubes and devices that allow the patient to speak
	Expect frustration
		All strategies promote communication with the patient and help to identify needs, assess responses to treatment, and reduce anxiety. Strategies must be culturally appropriate to facilitate patient understanding

NURSING DIAGNOSIS: *Oral mucous membranes, altered, related to artificial airway*

Patient Outcomes	Interventions	Rationales

Moist oral mucous membranes; absence of ulceration or other lesions	Assess oral mucous membranes for ulcerations or other lesions
	Carefully inspect the mouth around and under the tape or devices used to secure the ETT
	Provide good mouth care at least once per shift:
	    Use oral swabs specifically designed for mouth care
	    Brush teeth; use soft toothbrush, syringe to rinse mouth, and tonsil suction to remove secretions.
	    A toothbrush that attaches to suction is also available
	    Lubricate lips with water-soluble emollients
	    Consider use of disposable versus reusable oral suction devices
		All strategies promote patient comfort; to remove bacteria from the oropharynx and reduce likelihood of ventilator-associated pneumonia

NURSING DIAGNOSIS: *Pulmonary infection, risk of, related to artificial airway*

Patient Outcomes	Interventions	Rationales
Patient will remain free of infection	Maintain head of bed at 30 degrees Monitor temperature every 4 hr; amount, color, consistency, and odor of secretions; notify physician if secretions change	Prevent aspiration of gastric secretions Identify symptoms of infection

Continued

Nursing Care Plan for the Mechanically Ventilated Patient—cont'd

Patient Outcomes	Interventions	Rationales
Patient will remain free of infection—*cont'd*	Use good hand washing techniques; wear gloves for procedures; use aseptic technique for suctioning Suction oral cavity at least every 4 hr; provide oral care; maintain integrity of ETT cuff	Prevent transmission of bacteria to the patient Remove bacteria from the oropharynx, and prevent aspiration of bacteria-laden secretions that can cause ventilator-associated pneumonia

NURSING DIAGNOSIS: *Anxiety and fear, related to need for mechanical ventilation, inability to communicate needs, psychological ventilator dependence*

Patient Outcomes	Interventions	Rationales
Relief of anxiety and fear	Talk to patient frequently Provide simple explanations before and during procedures Establish communication Keep call light within reach Facilitate family visitation Provide diversionary activities, such as radio, television Consider complementary and alternative therapies, such as music therapy, guided imagery, pet therapy, massage Administer anti-anxiety medications as warranted	All are strategies that may assist in preventing and/or relieving fear and anxiety

NURSING DIAGNOSIS: *CO, decreased related to effects of positive-pressure ventilation*

Patient Outcomes	Interventions	Rationales
Adequate cardiac output	Measure CO at least every shift, if pulmonary artery catheter is in place Assess for hypotension, tachycardia, dysrhythmias, decreased level of consciousness Alert the physician to changes in CO	Assess actual cardiac output and identify trends Symptoms of decreased cardiac output Ventilator settings, especially PEEP, may need to be adjusted

NURSING DIAGNOSIS: *Nutrition, altered, related to inability to take oral feedings, increased nutritional needs, impaired gastrointestinal function. Nutrition, altered: less than body requirements*

Patient Outcomes	Interventions	Rationales
Patient will achieve adequate nutritional status	Assess bowel sounds and gastric distention at least once per shift; monitor bowel elimination	Assess for adequate functioning of gastrointestinal system and be alert for complications

Nursing Care Plan for the Mechanically Ventilated Patient—cont'd

Patient Outcomes	Interventions	Rationales
Patient will achieve adequate nutritional status—*cont'd*	Monitor daily weight	Assess for adequate nutritional support
	Obtain nutritional evaluation and provide early and ongoing nutritional support	Dieticians and/or other nutritional experts can ensure that appropriate nutritional support is ordered according to the patient's condition

	Administer parenteral or enteral feedings:
	   Elevate head of bed to 30 degrees
	   Check gastric residual every 4 hr
	   Nasoenteric feedings preferred to decrease risk of aspiration and promote absorption
		Reduce risks associated with enteral nutrition

	Monitor CO_2 levels if high carbohydrate formulas are given; formula may need to be changed	Many formulas are high in carbohydrates; to reduce likelihood of respiratory acidosis secondary to feedings

NURSING DIAGNOSIS: *Fluid volume excess, risk for, related to ventilator humidification, stimulation of renin-angiotensin-aldosterone mechanism*

Patient Outcomes	Interventions	Rationales
Patient will not experience fluid overload	Monitor intake and output every shift, and daily weight	Assess for trends in fluid volume status; weight is the best indicator of fluid gains or losses
	Assess breath sounds every 4 hr	Changes in breath sounds may indicate fluid volume excess
	Assess vital signs every 2 to 4 hr; assess for increased heart rate, respiratory rate, or blood pressure	Assess for symptoms of fluid volume excess

NURSING DIAGNOSIS: *Injury, risk of, gastrointestinal bleeding related to positive-pressure ventilation, stress of critical illness*

Patient Outcomes	Interventions	Rationales
Patient will not experience bleeding	Assess gastric contents and stools for bleeding; guaiac secretions and stools	Assess for bleeding; bleeding may be obvious or hidden
	Monitor serial hemoglobin and hematocrit values	Assess for trends that may indicate bleeding
	Monitor gastric pH; administer antacids, sucralfate, or histamine antagonists as ordered	Reduce gastric acidity; note that long-term administration of histamine antagonists is associated with a higher rate of ventilator-associated pneumonia

Continued

Nursing Care Plan for the Mechanically Ventilated Patient—cont'd

NURSING DIAGNOSIS: *Dysfunctional ventilatory weaning response related to ineffective airway clearance, sleep-pattern disturbances, inadequate nutrition, pain, and psychological factors*

Patient Outcomes	Interventions	Rationales
Patient will wean from mechanical ventilation with adequate ABGs, remain free of dyspnea or restlessness, effectively clear secretions, tolerate extubation after ventilatory support is removed	Assess patient's readiness to wean (see Box 8-11)	Identify readiness to begin the weaning process
	Provide weaning based on protocols and research evidence (see Box 8-12)	Protocol-driven weaning is an effective strategy for systematic weaning
	Collaborate with the health care team to provide mechanical ventilation and coaching that supports respiratory muscle training	Promote respiratory conditioning that will facilitate weaning
	Promote rest and comfort throughout the weaning process; assist in identifying strategies that result in relaxation and comfort; ensure that environment is safe and comfortable	Comfort will facilitate weaning
	Support patients in setting goals for weaning	Goals promote rehabilitation and give patients some control in the process
	Implement strategies that maximize tolerance of weaning:	Strategies assist in ensuring that patient is rested, with an adequate level of consciousness, and decreased anxiety; weaning efforts will be maximized
	Avoid narcotics	
	Give analgesia with minimal sedative effects	
	Schedule when patient is rested	
	Avoid other procedures during weaning	
	Promote normal sleep-wake cycle	
	Limit visitors to supportive persons	
	Coach through periods of anxiety	
	Terminate weaning if patient is unable to tolerate the process (see Box 8-13)	Adequate ventilation and gas exchange must be maintained
	Collaborate with the health care team to determine the most effective strategies for weaning those with severe dysfunctional weaning; the process may need to be slowed down	Various strategies may be needed to wean the patient; ongoing assessment is essential to determine the most effective strategy
	Consider referring patients with prolonged ventilator dependence to an alternative setting	These settings specialize in weaning patients who are "difficult to wean"

ABG, Arterial blood gas; *CO,* cardiac output; *CO₂,* carbon dioxide; *ETT,* endotracheal tube; *PEEP,* positive end-expiratory pressure.

MEDICATIONS

Intubation, mechanical ventilation, advanced methods for ventilation (e.g., inverse-ratio ventilation), and suctioning contribute to patient discomfort. Nonpharmacological methods, such as imagery or music therapy, may be used to manage discomfort and to treat anxiety. However, many patients need medications to facilitate ventilatory support.

Commonly used medications include analgesics, sedatives, and neuromuscular blocking agents. Medications are chosen based on the hemodynamic stability of the patient, the diagnosis, and the desired patient outcomes. Patients often need a combination of drugs. Many institutions use decision trees or algorithms to determine drug therapy. Decision making is guided by assessment of sedation, agitation, and pain. Medications are tapered or discontinued when the patient is ready to be weaned from mechanical ventilation (Luer, 1998).

Chapter 4 discusses sedation and comfort in depth. *Analgesics*, such as morphine and fentanyl, are administered to provide pain relief and sedation. *Sedatives*, such as benzodiazepines, neuroleptics, and propofol, are given to sedate the patient and to promote comfort. Patients who have acute lung injury or increased intracranial pressure or who require nontraditional modes of mechanical ventilation may require therapeutic paralysis. Various *neuromuscular blocking agents* are available for chemical paralysis. Patients receiving neuromuscular blocking agents require the administration of sedative agents and meticulous skin and eye care. Chemical paralysis must be discontinued before one attempts to wean patients from mechanical ventilation.

NUTRITIONAL SUPPORT

Nutritional support is required for all patients who require mechanical ventilation. Support should be provided as soon as possible (Heyland, Dhaliwal, Drover, Gramlich, & Dodek, 2003). See Chapter 5 for an in-depth discussion of nutritional support. Nursing interventions include monitoring gastric residual volumes to assess absorption and keeping the head of bed elevated to reduce the risk of aspiration. Although many nurses routinely put blue food color in feedings to assess for aspiration, this practice has not been substantiated by research (Parrish, Krenitsky, & McCray, 1998). Other nursing interventions include monitoring bowel function, checking serial glucose levels for hyperglycemia, and measuring daily weight.

Various formulas are prescribed depending on the patient's underlying disease process. The carbon dioxide level is monitored in all patients because excess carbon dioxide production may occur with high-carbohydrate feedings. If hypercarbia occurs, a formula with a higher fat content may be ordered.

After extubation or tracheostomy, the patient may be allowed to make the transition to oral feedings. A speech therapy evaluation for swallowing is recommended before oral feedings are initiated because many patients have difficulty with swallowing and are prone to aspiration after prolonged intubation (Parrish, Krenitsky, & McCray, 1998).

RESEARCH ANALYSIS

ARTICLE REFERENCE
Sole, M. L., Byers, J. F., Ludy, J. E., Zhang, Y., Banta, C. M., & Brummel, K. (2003). A multi-site survey of suctioning techniques and airway management practices. *American Journal of Critical Care, 12,* 220-230.

OVERVIEW
Sole and colleagues conducted a study to describe institutional policies and procedures related to closed-system suctioning and airway management of intubated patients, and to compare practices of registered nurses (RNs) and respiratory therapists (RTs). Their assumption was that suctioning and airway management practices may contribute to ventilator-associated pneumonia, a common problem in critically ill patients. Most ventilator-associated pneumonia is associated with microaspiration of oropharyngeal secretions. These investigators conducted a descriptive comparative multisite study of facilities that use closed-system suction (CSS) devices on most adult intubated patients. They recruited sites and staff members via network sampling. Site coordinators provided data about institutional policies. RNs and RTs at each site completed surveys related to their practices. The study followed a pilot study of three sites to develop the data collection instrument. Content validity for both instruments was established by a panel of three persons with nursing, respiratory care, and survey methodology expertise. Test-retest reliability was 0.82.[1]

FINDINGS
Twenty-seven sites provided institutional data, and 1665 RNs and RTs participated in the survey: 1186 RNs (79%) and 479 RTs (21%). The institutions ranged from 84 to 960 beds (median, 500). The majority of RNs and RTs who responded had at least 6 years' experience with ventilated patients (61%) and a baccalaureate degree or higher (54%). The following are summary data reported in the article:
- Institutional data
  - Most sites changed the CSS devices every 24 to 48 hours
  - A single suction tubing and canister set was used for both CSS and oral suctioning at most sites

Continued

RESEARCH ANALYSIS—cont'd

- 93% had policies for endotracheal cuff management
- 88% had policies for hyperoxygenation with CSS
- 74% included saline instillation for thick secretions in policies
- 70% recommended that gloves be worn for CSS
- 37% had toothbrushes available for oral care
- 48% had policies for oral care
- 39% had policies for oral suctioning

- Comparison of practice of RNs versus RTs
  - RTs rinsed the CSS device more often than RNs
  - RTs were twice as likely as RNs to report saline instillation
  - Most respondents reported hyperoxygenating patients before CSS
  - 72% of RNs stated that they performed mouth care every 4 hours with oral swabs
  - 39% of RNs brushed patients' teeth on a routine basis
  - RTs were less likely than nurses to suction oral secretions
  - 72% of staff members stated that they suctioned above the ET cuff most of the time before repositioning an oral ET tube
  - RNs were not aware of how cuff pressures are monitored and maintained

These investigators concluded that policies varied widely from institution to institution. In several cases, policies for routine care, such as oral care and suctioning, were lacking. Most procedures were not based on research evidence. Some airway management procedures need to be followed more consistently by the RNs and RTs who care for ventilator-dependent patients, such as wearing gloves for oral care and suctioning and monitoring and maintaining endotracheal tube cuff pressures. They emphasized the importance of RNs and RTs working together to develop collaborative, evidence-based policies and procedures for airway management.

STRENGTHS

Power analysis was done to determine sample size. The desired sample size was exceeded. Various-sized institutions were represented. The instrument was pilot-tested during a preliminary study. The response rate of RNs and RTs was high. Findings have the potential for generating change in practices and additional research on the topic.

WEAKNESSES

Results are limited to the 27 sites. Although all areas of the United States were geographically represented, generalizability is potentially limited because the sample was obtained via network sampling. Although more than 50% of staff members completed the survey, the practices of those who did not participate is not known. The findings provide many descriptive data; however, relationship to ventilator-associated pneumonia is not directly linked to the practices reported in the study and warrants additional study.

IMPLICATIONS FOR PRACTICE

Collaborative practice teams are needed to address suctioning and airway management practices. Comprehensive airway management protocols are needed that involve both RNs and RTs as accountable for airway management and oral care. Glove use for CSS and airway management needs to be emphasized.

[1]Sole, M.L., Byers, J.F., Ludy, J.E., & Ostrow, C.L. (2002). Suctioning techniques and airway management practices (STAMP): Pilot study and instrument evaluation. *American Journal of Critical Care*, 11, 363-368.

Troubleshooting the Ventilator

Those who care for patients receiving mechanical ventilation must be knowledgeable about the equipment and competent at troubleshooting. For the prevention of errors, *two important rules must be followed:*

1. *Never shut off alarms.* It is acceptable to silence alarms for a preset delay while working with a patient, such as during suctioning. However, alarms should *never* be shut off.
2. Manually ventilate the patient with a bag-valve device if you are unable to troubleshoot alarms quickly or if you suspect equipment failure. A bag-valve device must be readily available at the bedside of every patient who is mechanically ventilated.

Ventilator alarms vary from machine to machine; therefore, nurses must be familiar with the ventilators used in their institution. Several examples of alarms have been discussed. The nurse quickly assesses possible causes of any alarm situation to correct the problem causing the alarm immediately. If the cause is not assessed in seconds, the nurse manually ventilates the patient while a second caregiver further assesses the problem. Most alarms alert the nurse to changes in volume, pressure, or respiratory rate, such as apnea. Three examples are presented.

VOLUME ALARMS

A low-exhaled-volume alarm sounds if the patient does not receive the preset V_T. Causes of volume alarms include disconnection of the ventilator circuit from the artificial airway, a leak in the ETT or tracheostomy cuff, displacement of the ETT or tracheostomy tube, and disconnection of any part of the ventilator circuit.

PRESSURE ALARMS

A high-pressure alarm occurs if the amount of pressure needed for ventilating a patient exceeds the preset pressure limit. Several patient factors can cause high-pressure alarms: excess secretions; biting on the ETT, coughing, gagging, attempting to talk, pulmonary edema, bronchospasm, and pneumothorax or hemothorax. Kinks in the ventilator circuit can also cause a high-pressure alarm.

APNEA ALARMS

An apnea alarm occurs if the ventilator does not detect spontaneous respiration within a preset interval. This alarm is very important when the patient is receiving breaths at a very low rate. For example, a patient is ventilated on SIMV at 2 breaths/min, and his total respiratory rate is 20 breaths/min. The patient is given morphine sulfate, and his respiratory rate drops to 4 breaths/min. The apnea alarm alerts the nurse to this potentially dangerous situation. If this alarm sounds, the nurse must immediately assess the patient. The ventilator settings may need to be adjusted. The nurse manually ventilates the patient with a bag-valve device while the settings are adjusted.

Weaning Patients From Mechanical Ventilation

Once the decision is made to ventilate a patient mechanically, caregivers should begin to plan for weaning or "liberating" the patient from the ventilator (Manthous, 2000). Generally, patients who require short-term ventilatory support, defined as 3 days or less of mechanical ventilation, can be weaned quickly (Hanneman, 1998). Conversely, weaning is usually a slow, tedious process for patients who require ventilatory support for longer periods.

ASSESSMENT FOR READINESS TO WEAN

Several physiological parameters are monitored to determine patient readiness to be weaned from the ventilator and are noted in Box 8-11. Patients are usually able to wean when the underlying disease process is resolving, they are hemodynamically stable, and they have an adequate level of consciousness. Box 8-12 summarizes evidence-based guidelines for weaning patients from mechanical ventilation. Several weaning indices are available to assist in identifying when patients are ready to wean. These tools are useful in assessing a patient's strengths and factors that may interfere with successful weaning. The Burns Wean Assessment Program is one example of a weaning assessment tool that has been scientifically tested in critically ill patients. It is a 28-item tool that provides a systematic assessment of readiness to wean (Burns, 1998; Epstein, 2000). Researchers recommend assessment of several indicators of readiness to be weaned for timely, efficient weaning. Assessments include physiological variables related to gas exchange, hemodynamic status, diaphragmatic expansion, and airway clearance (Twibell, Siela, & Mahmoodi, 2003).

The weaning process is challenging for many patients. Patients are assessed and monitored throughout the weaning process. In addition to monitoring serial measurements of negative inspiratory force and forced vital capacity, caregivers must ensure that the patient does not become overtaxed by the weaning effort and become dyspneic or compromised in some other manner (Shelledy, 2003). Box 8-13 provides a list of physiological changes that may indicate that the patient is not tolerating the weaning process.

BOX 8-11

Assessment Parameters Indicating Readiness to Wean

Underlying Cause for Mechanical Ventilation Resolved
Improved chest x-ray findings
Minimal secretions
Normal breath sounds

Hemodynamic Stability; Adequate Cardiac Output
Adequate respiratory muscle strength
Respiratory rate <25 breaths/min
Negative inspiratory pressure or force > –20 cm H_2O
Spontaneous tidal volume 4-5 mL/kg
Vital capacity 10-15 mL/kg
Minute ventilation 5-10 L/min

Adequate ABG Results Without a High FiO$_2$ and/or a High PEEP
PaO_2 > 60 mm Hg with FiO_2 0.4–0.5
$PaCO_2$ < 45 mm Hg
PaO_2/FiO_2 >150-200
pH ≥ 7.25
PEEP ≤ 5 cm H_2O

Adequate Level of Consciousness; Protective Reflexes Intact (e.g., cough)
Good nutritional status and hydration
Absence of factors that impair weaning
  Infection
  Anemia
  Fever
  Fatigue
  Sleep deprivation
  Pain
  Abdominal distention; bowel abnormalities
    (diarrhea or constipation)

Mental Readiness to Wean: Calm, Minimal Anxiety, Motivated

Minimal Need for Sedatives and Other Medications That May Cause Respiratory Depression

ABG, Arterial blood gas; *FiO$_2$,* fractional concentration of oxygen in inspired gas; *PaCO$_2$,* partial pressure of carbon dioxide in arterial blood; *PaO$_2$,* partial pressure of oxygen in arterial blood, *PEEP,* positive end-expiratory pressure.

BOX 8-12

Evidence-Based Guidelines for Ventilatory Weaning

1. In patients requiring mechanical ventilation for more than 24 hours, search for all the causes that may contribute to ventilator dependence. Reversing all possible ventilatory and nonventilatory issues is an integral part of ventilator weaning. (B*)
2. Conduct a formal assessment of potential for weaning if the following criteria are met (B):
   - Evidence of reversal of underlying cause of respiratory failure
   - Adequate oxygenation (PaO_2/FiO_2 >150-200; positive end-expiratory pressure ≤5-8 cm H_2O; FiO_2 ≤0.4-0.5) and pH (≥7.25)
   - Hemodynamic stability
   - Able to initiate an inspiratory effort
3. Formally assess weaning potential during spontaneous breathing. An initial brief period of spontaneous breathing can assess the patient's capability of a spontaneous breathing trial (SBT). Assess the following during SBTs: respiratory pattern, adequacy of gas exchange, hemodynamic stability, and subjective comfort. Patients who tolerate SBTs lasting 30 to 120 minutes should be considered for permanent ventilator discontinuation. (A)
4. Assess airway patency and the ability of the patient to protect the airway to determine whether to remove the artificial airway from a patient who has been successfully weaned. (C)

Continued

BOX 8-12

Evidence-Based Guidelines for Ventilatory Weaning—cont'd

5. If a patient fails an SBT, determine the cause for the failed trial. Correct reversible causes, and attempt SBTs every 24 hours if the patient meets weaning criteria. (A)
6. Provide a stable, nonfatiguing, comfortable form of ventilatory support for a patient who fails an SBT. (B)

7. In postsurgical patients, provide anesthesia/sedation strategies and ventilator management aimed at early extubation. (A)
8. Develop and implement weaning protocols that nonphysician health care providers can implement. (A)
9. Consider a tracheostomy when it becomes apparent that the patient will require prolonged ventilator assistance. Patients with the following conditions may benefit most from early tracheostomy:
   - High levels of sedation to tolerate endotracheal tube
   - Marginal respiratory mechanics (e.g., tachypnea) associated with work of breathing
   - Psychological benefit from ability to eat and speak, and from enhanced mobility
   - Enhanced mobility as a possible aid to physical therapy efforts. (B)
10. Unless evidence of irreversible disease exists (e.g., high cervical spine injury), do not consider a patient to be ventilator dependent until 3 months of weaning attempts have failed. (B)
11. Learn about local facilities that specialize in managing patients who require prolonged mechanical ventilation. Transfer patients in whom weaning attempts have failed to these facilities when these patients are medically stable. (C)
12. Conduct slow-paced weaning with gradual increase in SBT time in patients requiring prolonged mechanical ventilation. (C)

*Grades of Evidence:
A. Scientific evidence provided by well-designed, controlled trials with statistically significant results that consistently support the recommendation
B. Scientific evidence provided by observational studies or by controlled trials with less consistent results to support the guideline recommendation
C. Expert opinion supported the guideline recommendation, but scientific evidence either provided inconsistent results or was lacking.
Modified from MacIntyre et al. (2001). Evidence-based guidelines for weaning and discontinuation of ventilatory support. *Chest*, *120*(6 Suppl), 375S-484S.

BOX 8-13

Criteria for Discontinuing Weaning

- Respiratory rate >30 breaths/min or <8 breaths/min
- Blood pressure changes more than 20% from baseline
- Heart rate changes more than 20% from baseline
- Pulse oximetry less than 90%
- Dysrhythmias (e.g., premature ventricular contractions or bradycardia)
- ST-segment elevation
- Significant decrease in spontaneous tidal volume
- Use of accessory muscles
- Labored respirations
- Diaphoresis
- Decreased level of consciousness
- Restlessness
- Anxiety

SHORT-TERM MECHANICAL VENTILATION

Short-term mechanical ventilation is initiated to treat various patient conditions: drug overdose, cardiovascular and complex surgical cases, exacerbation of asthma, pulmonary edema, and minor trauma (Hanneman, 1998). Numerous methods assist in weaning patients from short-term mechanical ventilation. One method is a *T-piece trial,* whereby the patient is disconnected from the ventilator and is connected to supplemental oxygen via a T-piece for periods of time. Oxygen through the T-piece is often set at an FiO_2 0.10 higher than what is set on the ventilator (Hanneman, 1998). Breathing through the T-piece encourages muscle strengthening.

SIMV is another common method for weaning these patients. The SIMV rate is decreased by 2 to

6 breaths every hour until the patient is assuming most of the WOB. An advantage of using the SIMV method is that it is performed on a continuous basis. A disadvantage is that it may promote muscle fatigue. *PSV* and *CPAP* are also methods for weaning patients, often in conjunction with SIMV.

Most patients can be extubated if they can sustain 1 hour of spontaneous breathing (Hanneman, 1998). Indications for extubation include resolution of the underlying condition requiring mechanical ventilation, hemodynamic stability, ability to manage secretions, and minimal risk of aspiration (Henneman, Ellstrom, & St. John, 1999). Once extubated, the patient is assessed for stridor, hoarseness, changes in vital signs, or low SpO_2 that may indicate complications.

LONG-TERM MECHANICAL VENTILATION

Patients who require ventilation for longer than 3 days are challenging to wean. A collaborative approach is essential for weaning these patients from the ventilator. Team members include nurses, physicians, respiratory therapists, dietitian, physical therapist, occupational therapist, social worker, pastoral ministers, and family members. Each team member has a unique and important role in providing physical and psychological support during the weaning.

Methods for Weaning from Long-Term Mechanical Ventilation

Protocols are effective in weaning patients who require long-term ventilation. For progress to occur, the level of ventilatory support must be decreased. Respiratory muscle work along with adequate rest must be included in the weaning plan (Burns, 1998; Burns, 1999).

Weaning can be classified into two strategies: (1) high-pressure, low-volume work and (2) low-pressure, high-volume work (Burns, 1998). High-pressure, low-volume work requires that the patient breathe spontaneously without support for periods of time. These strategies include T-piece trials that gradually increase the amount of time off of the ventilator, low SIMV rates, and CPAP trials. The goal is to promote respiratory muscle strengthening. The patient must be closely observed for fatigue during these weaning trials.

Low-pressure, high-volume work promotes patient endurance. PSV may be tried, to augment inspiration, thus promoting an adequate spontaneous V_T.

Some physicians order both SIMV and PSV to wean patients from the ventilator. However, this combination may actually prolong the amount of time needed to wean patients (Burns, 1998).

STEPS FOR WEANING

During any weaning attempt, several steps are followed. The procedure is explained to the patient and family in a manner that reduces anxiety. The patient must be adequately rested and positioned comfortably. Baseline parameters, including vital signs, heart rhythm, and ABGs or pulse oximetry/$ETCO_2$ values, are obtained. The patient is monitored during the weaning process for tolerance or intolerance to the procedure.

WHEN WEANING SHOULD BE DISCONTINUED

The weaning process should be stopped if adverse physiological changes occur (Box 8-13). If a patient exhibits signs of not tolerating the weaning process, ABGs or noninvasive measures of gas exchange are assessed, and the patient is placed back on the ventilator at the previous settings.

CAUSES OF IMPAIRED WEANING

Several factors may impair weaning: increased oxygen demand, decreased lung function, psychological factors, and equipment or technique factors. Increased oxygen demands may be caused by anemia, fever, or pain. Decreased lung function may result from malnutrition, overuse of sedatives or hypnotics, and sleep deprivation. Psychological causes include apprehension and fear, helplessness, and depression. Equipment and technique problems include the time of day or inadequate weaning periods.

WEANING THE TERMINALLY ILL PATIENT

Occasionally, ventilatory support is gradually withdrawn from a terminally ill patient. This is referred to as *terminal weaning*. During this period, it is important for the nurse to provide relief of symptoms and patient comfort. The patient may experience dyspnea, pain, anxiety, agitation, or excessive secretions during this time. Medications, such as morphine sulfate, lorazepam, haloperidol, and scopolamine, can be administered for the reduction of symptoms (Weatherill, 1995). Researchers have found that patients with altered consciousness or coma can be kept comfortable during a rapid terminal weaning procedure with morphine and benzodiazepines in low doses (Campbell, Bizek, & Thill, 1999). The nurse must be aware of legal and ethical issues associated with terminal weaning and should provide psychosocial support to the family.

Case Studies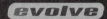

CASE STUDY 1

Miss M., age 19, with type 1 diabetes, came to the hospital in diabetic ketoacidosis after contracting gastrointestinal influenza 2 days ago. Laboratory values included a serum glucose of 652 mg/dL, urine positive for ketones, serum potassium 5.6 mEq/dL, and carbon dioxide 14. Vital signs were: temperature, 100.8°F; blood pressure, 90/50 mm Hg, pulse, 126 beats/min, respirations, 30/min with a rapid and deep (Kussmaul's) pattern. Blood gases were as follows: pH, 7.31; $PaCO_2$, 27 mm Hg; HCO_3^-, 14 mEq/L. Blood urea nitrogen was elevated because of dehydration from vomiting and diarrhea. She had not been eating or taking her insulin since the symptoms of influenza started, and she was comatose, with flushed skin and fruity breath odor on admission. After treatment with insulin, glucose, fluids, and electrolytes, along with antiemetics and antidiarrheals, her values normalized, and she became alert and oriented. Before discharge, teaching was instituted regarding diabetic maintenance regimens during illness and when to call the physician.

CASE STUDY 2

Mr. P. was admitted to the hospital with acute exacerbation of chronic obstructive pulmonary disease after an upper respiratory infection. His family had found him confused and in respiratory distress 2 days after the onset of a cold. He was brought into the emergency department with 5 L of nasal oxygen via cannula, but oxygen saturation was only 91%. A Venturi mask set at FiO_2 of 50% was ordered to replace the cannula, and oxygen saturation increased to 93%. Initial blood gases showed: pH, 7.33; $PaCO_2$, 58 mm Hg; and HCO_3^-, 33 mEq/L. The patient had labored respirations. Vital signs: temperature, 99.2°F; blood pressure, 104/50 mm Hg; pulse, 110 beats/min; respirations, 26/min. Intravenous fluids were infusing at 125 mL/hr, and antibiotics were started. Updraft treatments with bronchodilators were also initiated, as well as intravenous steroids (SoluMedrol). Wheezes and rhonchi were noted on auscultation, along with diminished breath sounds at the bases. Over the next few days,

Mr. P. improved and was discharged on oral steroids, inhalers, and antibiotics. His discharge arterial blood gas values were "normal" for him: pH, 7.36; $PaCO_2$, 50 mm Hg; and HCO_3^-, 29 mEq/L. Why?

CASE STUDY 3

A trauma victim presented to the emergency department with a blunt chest injury after a motor vehicle crash. On admission, he was alert, had right-sided chest pain with shortness of breath, absent breath sounds in the right upper lobe, and increased respiratory effort despite being on 100% oxygen via nonrebreather mask (14 L/min). Oxygen saturation was 91%. His arterial blood gases showed values of: pH, 7.51; $PaCO_2$, 30 mm Hg; and HCO_3^-, 21 mEq/L. After fluid resuscitation and chest tube insertion to treat a pneumothorax, he improved and was admitted to the critical care unit.

CASE STUDY 4

In report you are told that an elderly patient with an intestinal obstruction had 2000 mL of output through the nasogastric tube during the night shift. Your assessment notes that she states she has weakness, shakiness, tingling in her fingers. She is also questioning where she is and why is she "tied down." These are changes in her condition from the previous shift. Her morning laboratory values reveal: serum potassium, 3.1 mEq/L; serum chloride, 88 mEq/L; and serum calcium, 7.7 mg/dL. Her arterial blood gases reveal: pH, 7.54; HCO_3^-, 35 mEq/L; and $PaCO_2$, 52 mm Hg. Her respirations are slow and shallow. Immediate treatment includes correcting fluid and electrolyte losses with potassium, chloride, and calcium solutions and preparation for exploratory surgery to correct the obstruction.

CASE STUDY 5

A critically ill patient admitted with a traumatic injury develops multisystem organ failure, acute respiratory distress syndrome, and septic shock. His blood gases show the following parameters: pH, 7.22; $PaCO_2$, 65 mm Hg; and HCO_3^-, 12 mEq/L.

SUMMARY

Skills in establishing and maintaining an open airway, initiating mechanical ventilation, and on-going patient assessment are essential critical care nursing skills.

Care of the patient requiring mechanical ventilation is an everyday assignment in the critical care unit; therefore, it is essential that the nurse apply knowledge and skills to care for these patients effectively.

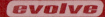

1. Based on your knowledge of clinical disorders, identify different clinical conditions that could cause problems with the following steps in gas exchange:
   a. Ventilation
   b. Diffusion
   c. Perfusion (transportation)

2. Your patient has the following ABG results: pH, 7.28; PaO_2, 52 mm Hg; SaO_2, 84%; $PaCO_2$, 55 mm Hg; HCO_3^-, 24 mEq/L.
   a. What is your interpretation of these ABGs?
   b. What clinical condition or conditions could cause the patient to have these ABG results?

3. Acid-base case studies: Determine which acid-base imbalance is present in the Case Studies (p. 211) and state the possible underlying cause of the disorder.

4. Your patient requires mechanical ventilation for treatment. The pressure alarm keeps going off for a few seconds at a time, even though you have just suctioned the patient. What nursing actions are warranted at this time?

5. You are caring for a patient who has been mechanically ventilated for 2 weeks. Physically, the patient meets all the criteria to begin weaning from mechanical ventilation. How can you provide psychological support during the weaning process?

6. Many hospitals now care for mechanically ventilated patients outside the intensive care unit. What special considerations are necessary for the care of these patients?

REFERENCES

Adler, D. C. (1997). The experience and caring needs of critically ill, mechanically ventilated patients. Doctoral dissertation, University of Pennsylvania, Philadelphia, p. 107.

ARDS Network. (2000). Ventilation with lower tidal volumes compared with traditional tidal volumes for acute lung injury and the acute respiratory distress syndrome. *New England Journal of Medicine, 342,* 1301-1308.

Burns, S. M. (1998). Weaning from long-term mechanical ventilation. In *Care of the mechanically ventilated patient: Protocols for practice.* Aliso Viejo, CA: American Association of Critical-Care Nurses.

Burns, S. M. (1999). Making weaning easier: Pathways and protocols that work. *Critical Care Clinics of North America, 11,* 465-479.

Campbell, M. L., Bizek, K. S., & Thill, M. (1999). Patient responses during rapid terminal weaning from mechanical ventilation: A prospective study. *Critical Care Medicine, 27,* 9-10.

Chang, D. W. (2001). *Clinical application of mechanical ventilation.* 2nd ed. Albany, NY: Delmar.

Chernecky, C. C., & Berger, B. J. (2001). *Laboratory tests and diagnostic procedures.* 3rd ed. Philadelphia: W. B. Saunders.

Collard, H. R., Saint, S., & Matthay, M. A. (2003). Prevention of ventilator-associated pneumonia: An evidence-based systematic review. *Annals of Internal Medicine, 138,* 494-501.

Corrado, A. C., & Gorini, M. (2002). Long-term negative pressure ventilation. *Respiratory Care Clinics of North America, 8,* 545-557.

Criner, G. J. (1995). Psychological issues in the ventilator-dependent patient. *Respiratory Care, 40,* 855-865.

Cummins, R. O., & Hazinski, M. F. (2000). Guidelines based on the principle "first do no harm": New guidelines on tracheal tube confirmation and prevention of dislodgement. *Circulation, 102*[8 suppl], 1380-1384.

DePew, C., & Noll, M. L. (1994). Closed system suctioning: A research analysis. *Dimensions of Critical Care Nursing, 13,* 73-83.

Durbin, C. G. (2004). Airway management. In J. M. Cairo & S. P. Pilbeam. *Mosby's respiratory care equipment* [pp. 153-188]. 7th ed. St. Louis: Mosby.

Epstein, S. K. (2000). Weaning parameters. *Respiratory Care Clinics of North America, 6,* 253-301.

Fink, J. B., & Hess, D. R. (2002). Humidity and aerosol therapy. In D. R. Hess, N. R. MacIntyre, S. C. Mishoe, W. F. Galvin, A. B. Adams, & A. B. Saposnick (Eds.). *Respiratory care principles and practice* [pp. 633-664]. Philadelphia: W. B. Saunders.

Finucane, B. T., & Santora, A. H. (2003). *Principles of airway management.* 3rd ed. St. Louis: Mosby.

Gillette, M. A., & Hess, D. R. (2001). Ventilator-induced injury and evolution of lung-protective strategies in acute respiratory distress syndrome. *Respiratory Care, 46,* 130-148.

Guyton, A. C., & Hall, J. E. (2000). *Textbook of medical physiology.* 10th ed. Philadelphia: W. B. Saunders.

Hanneman, S. K. (1998). Weaning from short-term mechanical ventilation. In *Care of the mechanically ventilated patient: Protocols for practice.* Aliso Viejo, CA: American Association of Critical-Care Nurses.

Happ, M. B. (2001). Communicating with mechanically ventilated patients: State of the science. *AACN Clinical Issues: Advanced Practice in Acute and Critical Care, 12,* 247-258.

Hazinski, M. F., Cummins, R. O., & Field, J. M. (2000). *2000 handbook of emergency cardiovascular care.* Dallas, TX: American Heart Association.

Henneman, E. A., Ellstrom, K., & St. John, R. (1999). Airway management. In *Care of the mechanically ventilated patient: Protocols for practice.* Aliso Viejo, CA: American Association of Critical-Care Nurses.

Hess, D. R., & Kacmarek, R. M. (2002). *Essentials of mechanical ventilation.* 2nd ed. New York: McGraw-Hill.

Heyland, D. K., Dhaliwal, R., Drover, J. W., Gramlich, L., & Dodek, P. (2003). Canadian clinical practice guidelines for nutrition support in mechanically ventilated, critically ill adults. *Journal of Parenteral and Enteral Nutrition, 27,* 355-373.

Heuer, A. J., & Scanlan, C. L. (2003). Medical gas therapy. In R. L. Wilkins, J. K. Stoller, & C. L. Scanlan (Eds.). *Egan's fundamentals of respiratory care* [pp. 827-861]. 8th ed. St. Louis: Mosby.

Hickling, K. G. (2002). Permissive hypercapnia. *Respiratory Care Clinics of North America, 8,* 155-169.

Huang, Y. T. (2002). Arterial blood gases. In D. R. Hess, N. R. MacIntyre, S. C. Mishoe, W.F. Galvin, A. B. Adams, & A. B. Saposnick (Eds.). *Respiratory care principles and practice.* [pp. 362-396]. Philadelphia: W. B. Saunders.

Hunt, G. E. (1999). Gas therapy. In J. B. Fink & G. E. Hunt (Eds.). *Clinical practice in respiratory care* [pp. 249-286]. Philadelphia: Lippincott Williams & Wilkins.

Hupcey, J. E. (2000). The need to know: Experiences of critically ill patients. *American Journal of Critical Care, 9,* 192-198.

Johnson, K. L, et al. (1994). Closed versus open endotracheal suctioning: Costs and physiologic consequences. *Critical Care Medicine, 22,* 658-666.

Kinloch, D. (1999). Instillation of normal saline during endotracheal suctioning: Effects on mixed venous oxygen saturation. *American Journal of Critical Care, 8,* 231-240.

Levitan, R. M., & Ochroch, E. A. (2000). Airway management and direct laryngoscopy: A review and update. *Critical Care Clinics, 16,* 373-388.

Levitzky, M. G. (2002). *Pulmonary physiology.* 6th ed. New York: McGraw-Hill.

Lewandowski, L.A., & Kositsky, A. M. (1983). Research priorities for critical care nursing: A study by the American Association of Critical-Care Nurses, *Heart & Lung, 12,* 35-44.

Luer, J. M. (1998). Sedation and neuromuscular blockade in patients with acute respiratory failure. In *Care of the mechanically ventilated patient: Protocols for practice.* Aliso Viejo, CA: American Association of Critical-Care Nurses.

Manthous, C. A. (Ed.). (2000). Summarizing the logistics of liberation from mechanical ventilation. *Respiratory Care Clinics of North America, 6,* 463-468.

Menzel, L. (1994). Need for communication-related research in mechanically ventilated patients. *American Journal of Critical Care, 3,* 165-167.

Menzel, L. (1999). Ventilated patients' self-esteem during intubation and after extubation. *Clinical Nursing Research, 8,* 51-68.

Mutlu, G. M., & Factor, P. (2000). Complications of mechanical ventilation. *Respiratory Care Clinics of North America, 6,* 213-252.

O'Neal, P. V., Grap, M. J., Thompson, C., & Dudley, W. (2001). Level of dyspnoea experienced in mechanically ventilated adults with and without saline instillation prior to endotracheal suctioning. *Intensive and Critical Care Nursing, 17,* 356-63.

Parrish, C. R., Krenitsky, J., McCray, S. (1998). Nutrition support for the mechanically ventilated patient. In *Care of the mechanically ventilated patient: Protocols for practice.* Aliso Viejo, CA: American Association of Critical-Care Nurses.

Passy, V. (1986). Passy-Muir tracheostomy speaking valve. *Otolaryngology Head and Neck Surgery, 95,* 247-248.

Pierce, L. N. B. (1998). Traditional and nontraditional modes of mechanical ventilation. In *Care of the mechanically ventilated patient: Protocols for practice.* Aliso Viejo, CA: American Association of Critical-Care Nurses.

Pilbeam, S. P. (1998). *Mechanical ventilation: Physiological and clinical applications.* 3rd ed. St. Louis: Mosby.

Pilbeam, S. P. (2004). Introduction to ventilators. In J. M. Cairo & S. P. Pilbeam. *Mosby's respiratory care equipment* [pp. 318-390]. 7th ed. St. Louis: Mosby.

Raymond, S. J. (1995). Normal saline instillation before suctioning: Helpful or harmful? A review of the literature. *American Journal of Critical Care, 4,* 267-271.

Ridling, D. A., Martin, L. D., & Bratton, S. L. (2003). Endotracheal suctioning with or without instillation of isotonic sodium chloride solution in critically ill children. *American Journal of Critical Care, 12,* 212-219.

Rozycki, J. J., Sysyn, G. D., Marshall, M. K., Malloy, R., & Wiswell, T. E. (1998). Mainstream end-tidal carbon dioxide monitoring in the neonatal intensive care unit. *Pediatrics, 101,* 648-653.

Saposnick, A. B., & Hess, D. R. (2002). Oxygen therapy: Administration and management. In D. R. Hess, N. R. MacIntyre, S. C. Mishoe, W.F. Galvin, A.B. Adams, & A. B. Saposnick (Eds.). *Respiratory care principles and practice* [pp. 592-611]. Philadelphia: W. B. Saunders.

Scanlan, C. L., & Wilkins, R. L. (2003a). Gas exchange and transport. In R. L. Wilkins, J. K. Stoller, & C. L. Scanlan (Eds.). *Egan's fundamentals of respiratory care* [pp. 229-254]. 8th ed. St. Louis: Mosby.

Scanlan, C. L., & Wilkins, R. L. (2003b). Analysis and monitoring of gas exchange. In R. L. Wilkins, J. K. Stoller, & C. L. Scanlan (Eds.). *Egan's fundamentals of respiratory care* [pp. 355-389]. 8th ed. St. Louis: Mosby.

Shapiro, B. A., Peruzzi, W. T., & Templin, R. (1994). *Clinical applications of blood gases.* 5th ed. St. Louis: Mosby.

Shelledy, D. C. (2003). Discontinuing ventilatory support. In R. L. Wilkins, J. K. Stoller, & C. L. Scanlan, (Eds.). *Egan's fundamentals of respiratory care* [pp. 1121-1154]. 8th ed. St. Louis: Mosby.

Simmons, K. F., & Scanlan, C. L. (2003). Airway management. In R. L. Wilkins, J. K. Stoller, & C. L. Scanlan (Eds.). *Egan's fundamentals of respiratory care* [pp. 653-704]. 8th ed. St. Louis: Mosby.

Sole, M. L., Byers, J. F., Ludy, J. E., Zhang, Y., Banta, C. M., & Brummel, K. (2003). A multi-site survey of suctioning techniques and airway management practices. *American Journal of Critical Care, 12,* 220-230.

Stewart, C. E. (2001). Verification of endotracheal tube placement. *Emergency Medical Services, 30*(5), 120-125.

Stiefel, K. A., Damron, S., Sowers, N., & Velez, L. (2000). Improving oral hygiene for the seriously ill patient: Implementing research-based practice. *MEDSURG Nursing, 9*(1), 40-44.

Twibell, R., Siela, D., & Mahmoodi, M. (2003). Subjective perceptions and physiological variables during weaning from mechanical ventilation. *American Journal of Critical Care, 12,* 101-112.

Vallverdu, I., & Mancebo, J. (2000). Approach to patients who fail initial weaning trials. *Respiratory Care Clinics of North America, 6,* 365-384.

Vines, D. L. (2003). Noninvasive positive-pressure ventilation. In R. L. Wilkins, J. K. Stoller, & C. L. Scanlan (Eds.). *Egan's fundamentals of respiratory care* [pp. 1059-1080]. 8th ed. St. Louis: Mosby.

Weatherill, G. G. (1995). Pharmacologic symptom control during the withdrawal of life support: Lessons in palliative care. *AACN Clinical Issues: Advanced Practice in Acute and Critical Care, 6,* 344-351.

Wedzicha, J. A. (2002). Outcome of long-term noninvasive positive pressure ventilation. *Respiratory Care Clinics of North America, 8,* 559-573.

Wissing, D. R. (2004). Humidity and aerosol therapy. In J. M. Cairo & S. P. Pilbeam (Eds.). *Mosby's respiratory care equipment* [pp. 87-129]. 7th ed. St. Louis: Mosby.

RECOMMENDED READINGS

Ahrens, T., & Sona, C. (2003). Capnography application in acute and critical care. *AACN Clinical Issues: Advanced Practice in Acute and Critical Care, 14,* 123-132.

Burns, S.M. Working with respiratory waveforms: How to use bedside graphics. *AACN Clinical Issues: Advanced Practice in Acute and Critical Care, 14,* 133-144.

Cairo, J. M., & Pilbeam, S. P. (2004). *Mosby's respiratory care equipment.* 7th ed. St. Louis: Mosby.

Parrish, C. R., & McCray, S. F. (2003). Nutrition support for the mechanically ventilated patient. *Critical Care Nurse, 23*(1), 77-80.

Wilkins, R. L., Stoller, J. K., & Scanlon, C. I. (2003). *Egan's fundamentals of respiratory care.* 7th ed. St. Louis: Mosby.

St. John, R. E. (2004). Airway management. *Critical Care Nurse, 24*(2), 93-96.

Thomas, L. A. (2003). Clinical management of stressors perceived by patients on mechanical ventilation. *AACN Clinical Issues: Advanced Practice in Acute and Critical Care, 14,* 73-81.

evolve *Did you remember to check out the bonus material, including free self-assessment exercises, on the Evolve Web site at http://evolve.elsevier.com/Sole/ and on the CD-ROM?*

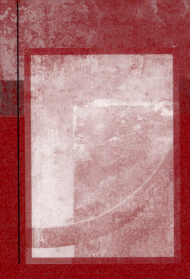

CHAPTER 9

Code Management

Deborah G. Klein, MSN, RN, CCRN, CS

OBJECTIVES

- Compare roles of caregivers in managing cardiopulmonary arrest situations.
- Identify equipment used during a code.
- Differentiate basic and advanced life support measures used during a code.
- Identify medications used in code management, including use, action, side effects, and nursing implications.
- Discuss treatment of special problems that can occur during a code.
- Describe special concerns related to the geriatric population during a code.
- Identify information to be documented during a code.
- Describe care of patients after resuscitation.
- Identify psychosocial, legal, and ethical issues related to code management.

Code, code blue, code 99, and *Dr. Heart* are terms frequently used in hospital settings to refer to emergency situations that require lifesaving resuscitation and interventions. Codes are called when patients suffer a cardiac and/or respiratory arrest or a life-threatening cardiac dysrhythmia that has caused loss of consciousness. (The generic term *arrest* is used in this chapter to refer to these conditions.) Whatever the cause, patient survival and positive outcome depend on prompt recognition of the situation and immediate institution of basic and advanced life support measures. *Code management* refers to the initiation of a code and the lifesaving interventions performed when a patient arrests.

Introduction

This chapter discusses the roles of the personnel involved in a code and identifies the equipment that must be readily available during a code. Basic and advanced life support measures are presented, including medications commonly used during a code. The chapter concludes with a brief discussion of psychosocial, legal, and ethical implications of code management. For the most up-to-date information, the reader should contact the American Heart Association for current recommendations for basic and advanced cardiac life support (www.cpr-ecc.org).

All personnel involved in hospital patient care should have basic cardiac life support (BCLS) training,

evolve *Be sure to check out the bonus material, including free self-assessment exercises, on the Evolve Web site at http://evolve.elsevier.com/Sole/ and on the CD-ROM.*

including how to operate an automated external defibrillator (AED). This training is also recommended for the lay public through the "Heartsaver" course. Advanced cardiac life support (ACLS) provider training is available through the American Heart Association and is strongly recommended for anyone working in critical care.

Roles of Caregivers in Code Management

Prompt recognition of a patient's arrest and rapid initiation of cardiopulmonary resuscitation (CPR) and ACLS measures are essential for improved patient outcomes. The first person to recognize that a patient has suffered an arrest should call for help, instruct someone to "call a code," call for a defibrillator, and begin CPR. One-person CPR is continued until additional help arrives.

CODE TEAM

Key personnel are notified to assist with code management. An overhead paging system or individual pagers may be used for contacting personnel, depending on hospital policies.

Most hospitals have code teams that are designated to respond to codes (Table 9-1). The code team usually consists of a physician, a critical care or emergency department nurse, a nursing supervisor, an anesthetist or anesthesiologist, a respiratory therapist, a pharmacist or pharmacy technician, an electrocardiogram (ECG) technician, and a chaplain. The code team responds to the code and works in conjunction with the patient's nurse and primary physician, if present.

TABLE 9-1

Roles and Responsibilities of Code Team Members

Team Member	Primary Role
Leader of the code (usually a physician)	Directs code Makes diagnoses and treatment decisions
Primary nurse	Provides information to code leader Measures vital signs Assists with procedures Administers medications
Second nurse	Coordinates use of the crash cart Prepares medications Assembles equipment (intubation, suction)
Nursing supervisor	Controls the crowd Contacts the attending physician Assists with medications and procedures Ensures that a bed is available in critical care unit Assists with transfer of patient to critical care unit
Nurse or assistant	Records events on designated form
Anesthesiologist, nurse anesthetist, or emergency physician	Intubates patient Manages airway and oxygenation
Respiratory therapist	Assists with ventilation Obtains blood sample for ABG analysis Sets up respiratory equipment
Code management pharmacist or technician	Assists with medication administration Prepares intravenous infusions
ECG technician	Obtains 12-lead ECG
Chaplain	Supports family

ABG, Arterial blood gas; *ECG*, electrocardiogram.

If a code team does not exist, any available personnel usually respond.

LEADER OF THE CODE

The person who directs, or "runs," the code is responsible for making diagnoses and treatment decisions. The leader is usually a physician who is preferably experienced in code management, such as an emergency department physician. However, the leader may be the patient's primary physician or another physician who is available and qualified for the task. If several physicians are present, one should assume responsibility for being the code team leader and should be the only person giving orders for interventions, to avoid confusion and conflict. In some small hospitals, codes may be directed by a nurse trained in ACLS. In this situation, standing physician orders are needed for guiding and supporting the nurse's decision making.

The leader of the code needs as much information about the patient as possible to make treatment decisions. Necessary information includes the reason for the patient's hospitalization, the patient's current treatments and medications, the patient's code status, and the events that occurred immediately before the code.

If possible, the code leader should not be performing CPR or other tasks. The leader should give full attention to assessment, diagnosis, and treatment decisions to direct resuscitative efforts.

CODE NURSES

Primary Nurse

The patient's primary nurse should be free to relate information to the person directing the code. The primary nurse may also start intravenous (IV) lines, measure vital signs, administer emergency medications, assist with procedures, or defibrillate the patient as directed by the code leader (if the primary nurse is qualified).

Second Nurse

The major task of the second nurse present is to coordinate the use of the crash cart. This nurse must be thoroughly familiar with the layout of the cart and the location of items. This nurse locates, prepares, and labels medications and IV fluids. He or she also assembles equipment for intubation, suctioning, and other procedures, such as central line insertion. An additional nurse or assistant records the code events on a designated form.

Nursing Supervisor

The nursing supervisor responds to the code to assist in whatever manner is needed. Frequently, more people respond to a code than are needed. One job of the supervisor is to limit the number of people in the code to only those necessary and those there for learning purposes. This approach decreases crowding and confusion. Other responsibilities may include contacting the patient's primary physician, relaying information to the staff and family, and ensuring that all the necessary equipment is present and functioning. If the patient must be transferred to the critical care unit, the supervisor may also ensure that a critical care bed is available and coordinate the transfer.

ANESTHESIOLOGIST OR NURSE ANESTHETIST

The anesthesiologist or anesthetist assumes control of the patient's ventilation and oxygenation. This team member intubates the patient to ensure an adequate airway and to facilitate ventilation. The primary or second nurse assists with the setup and checking of intubation equipment.

RESPIRATORY THERAPIST

The respiratory therapist usually assists with manual ventilation of the patient before and after intubation. The therapist may also obtain a blood sample for arterial blood gas analysis, set up oxygen and ventilation equipment, and suction the patient. In some institutions, the respiratory therapist performs intubation.

PHARMACIST OR PHARMACY TECHNICIAN

In some hospitals, a pharmacist or pharmacy technician responds to codes. This person may prepare medications and mix IV infusions for administration during the code. The pharmacist may also calculate appropriate medication doses based on the patient's weight. Frequently, pharmacy staff members are also responsible for bringing additional medications. At the termination of the code, pharmacy staff may replenish the crash cart medications and ensure pharmacy charges to the patient's account.

ELECTROCARDIOGRAM TECHNICIAN

In some hospitals, an ECG technician responds to codes. This person is available to obtain 12-lead ECGs that may be ordered.

CHAPLAIN

Another person who may respond to a code is the hospital chaplain. The chaplain can be very helpful in comforting and waiting with the patient's family. The chaplain or other support person usually takes the family to a quiet, private area for waiting and remains with them during the code. This person may also be able to check on the patient periodically to provide the family a progress report.

OTHER PERSONNEL

Other personnel should be available to run errands, such as taking blood samples to the laboratory or obtaining additional supplies. Meanwhile, other patients need monitoring and care. Only staff members necessary for the code should remain; others should attend to the other patients.

Equipment Used in Codes

While the first person to recognize a code calls for help and begins life support measures, another team member immediately brings the crash cart and defibrillator to the patient's bedside (Figure 9-1). Crash carts vary in organization and layout, but they all contain the same basic emergency equipment and medications. Many hospitals have standardized crash carts, so anyone responding to a code is familiar with the location of the items on the cart. In other hospitals, the makeup and organization of the crash cart are unique to each unit. Whether carts are standardized or unique to an individual unit, nurses responding to codes must be familiar with them.

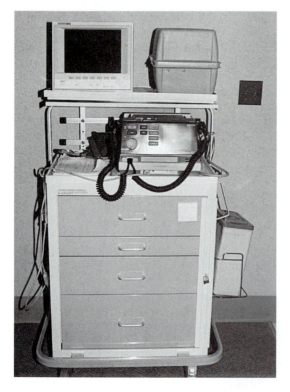

FIGURE 9-1 A typical crash cart.

Most carts have equipment stored on top and in several drawers. Table 9-2 lists equipment on a typical crash cart. Equipment such as back boards and portable suction machines may be attached to the cart. Larger equipment is stored on the top of the cart or in a large drawer; smaller items, such as medications and IV equipment, are in the smaller drawers.

A back, or "cardiac," board is usually located on the back or side of the cart. It is placed under the patient as soon as possible to provide a hard, level surface for the performance of chest compressions. Alternatively, some hospital bed headboards are removable for use as a cardiac board. The patient is either lifted up or log-rolled to one side for placement of the board. Care should be taken to protect the patient's cervical spine if injury is suspected.

A monitor-defibrillator is located on top of the cart or on a separate cart. The patient's cardiac rhythm is monitored via the leads and electrodes on this machine. Placing the defibrillation paddles on the chest by use of the "quick-look" method enables monitoring of cardiac rhythm. In the hospital setting, continuous monitoring via the electrodes is preferable to intermittent use of the defibrillation paddles for "quick looks." The monitor must have a recorder for documenting the patient's ECG rhythm for the cardiac arrest record.

A transcutaneous pacemaker may be stored on the crash cart or may be part of the monitor/defibrillator unit. Some patient care units may use an AED for initial code management.

A bag-valve device (BVD) with an attached face mask and oxygen tubing is usually kept on the crash cart. The tubing is connected either to a wall oxygen inlet or to a portable oxygen tank on the crash cart. Supplemental oxygen is always used with the BVD.

Airway management supplies are located in one of the drawers. Some institutions have a separate box or kit containing airway management supplies.

Another drawer contains IV supplies and IV solutions. Normal saline (NS) and Ringer's lactate solution are the IV fluids most often used. Five percent dextrose in 250- and 500-mL bags is used for preparing vasoactive infusions.

Emergency medications fill another drawer or may be located in a separate box. These include IV push medications and medications that must be added to IV fluids for continuous infusions. Most IV push medications are available in prefilled syringes. Several drugs that are given via a continuous infusion (e.g., lidocaine, dopamine) are also available as premixed bags. Medications are discussed in more depth in the section on pharmacological intervention.

Other important items on the cart include a suction setup and suction catheters, nasogastric tubes,

TABLE 9-2	
Typical Contents of a Crash Cart	
Main Items	**Specific Supplies**
BACK Cardiac board	
SIDE Portable suction machine, bag-valve device, and oxygen tank	Suction canister and tubing, face mask, and oxygen tubing
TOP Monitor-defibrillator with recorder, clipboard with code record and drug calculation reference sheets	ECG leads, electrodes, conductive gel or pads; possible transcutaneous pacemaker or combination unit
Airway supply drawer or box	Oral and nasal airways, ETTs, stylet, laryngoscope handle and curved and straight blades, Magill forceps, lubricating jelly, 5-mL syringes, and tape
IV supply drawer	IV catheters of various sizes, tape, syringes, needles and needleless adaptors, IV fluids (NS, Ringer's lactate solution, and D_5W); and IV tubing
Medication drawer or box	All IV push emergency medications in prefilled syringes if available, sterile water and NS for injection, and IV infusion emergency medications (see Table 9-4)
Miscellaneous supply drawer	Sterile and nonsterile gloves, suction catheters, nasogastric tubes, chest tubes, blood pressure cuff, blood collection tubes, sutures, pacemaker magnet, extra ECG recording paper, gauze pads
Procedure trays	Cut-down, tracheostomy, and central line insertion trays

D_5W, 5% dextrose in water; *ECG*, electrocardiogram; *ETTs*, endotracheal tubes; *IV*, intravenous; *NS*, normal saline.

and blood pressure cuff. Various trays used for venous cut-down, tracheotomy, and central line insertion are also frequently kept on the crash cart.

The crash cart and defibrillator are usually checked by nursing staff at designated time intervals (every shift or every 24 hours) to ensure that all equipment and medications are present and functional. Once the cart is fully stocked, it should be kept locked, to prevent borrowing of supplies and equipment.

The nurse can become familiar with the location of items on the cart by being responsible for checking it. Management of the code is more efficient when the nurse knows where items are located on the crash cart, as well as how to use them. Many institutions require nursing staff to participate in periodic "mock" codes.

Resuscitation Efforts

The flow of events during a code is the result of a concentrated team effort. BCLS is provided until the code team arrives. Once help has arrived, CPR is continued by use of the two-person technique. Other tasks, such as connecting the patient to an ECG monitor, starting IV lines, attaching an oxygen source to the BVD, and setting up suction, are performed by available personnel as soon as possible. The activities that occur during the code are summarized in Table 9-3. Often, several activities are performed simultaneously.

The code team should be alerted to the patient's code status. The Patient Self-Determination Act of 1991 recognizes the right of an individual person to make decisions about his or her medical care, including care at the end of life. A person may have a living will documenting his or her wishes. This document provides instructions to family members, physicians, and other health care providers. An advance directive may be prepared by a physician based on the individual's living will. Frequently, critically ill patients are too ill to participate in decision making. Physicians and families should talk with the patient about preferences regarding CPR.

TABLE 9-3

Flow of Events During a Code

Priorities	Equipment from Cart	Intervention
Recognition of arrest		Assess code status, call for help, initiate CPR
Arrival of resuscitation team, emergency cart, monitor-defibrillator, AED	Cardiac board Mouth-to-mask or bag-valve-mask unit with oxygen tubing Oral airway Oxygen and regulator if not already at bedside	Place patient on cardiac board Ventilate with 100% oxygen with oral airway and mouth-to-mask or bag-valve-mask device Continue chest compressions
Identification of team leader		Assess patient Direct and supervise team members Solve problems Obtain patient history and information, events leading up to the code
Rhythm diagnosis	Cardiac monitor with quick-look paddles—defibrillator AED 12-Lead ECG machine	Apply quick-look paddles first Attach limb leads, but do not interrupt CPR
Prompt defibrillation if indicated	Defibrillator/AED	Use correct algorithm
Intubation	Suction equipment Laryngoscope Endotracheal tube and other intubation equipment Stethoscope End-tidal CO_2 or esophageal detectors	Connect suction equipment Intubate patient (interrupt CPR no more than 30 sec) Check tube position (listen over epigastrium and bilateral lung fields); confirm with secondary measure (end-tidal CO_2 detector, esophageal detector, chest x-ray) Secure tube Hyperventilate and oxygenate
Venous access	Peripheral or central IV equipment IV tubing, infusion fluid (NS)	Insert peripheral IV into antecubital sites Central line may be inserted by physician
Drug administration	Drugs as ordered (and in anticipation, based on algorithms) for bolus and continuous infusion	Use correct algorithm

Ongoing assessment of the patient's response to therapy during resuscitation		Assess frequently:
		  Pulse generated with CPR (is there a pulse?)
		  Adequacy of artificial ventilation
		  Arterial blood gases or other laboratory studies
		  Spontaneous pulse after any intervention/rhythm change (is there a pulse?)
		  Spontaneous breathing with return of pulse (is there breathing?)
		  Blood pressure, if pulse is present
		  Decision to stop, if no response to therapy

Continued

TABLE 9-3		
Flow of Events During a Code—cont'd		
Priorities	**Equipment from Cart**	**Intervention**
Drawing arterial and venous blood specimens	Arterial puncture and venipuncture equipment	Draw specimens Treat as needed, based on results
Documentation	Code record	Accurately record events while resuscitation is in progress Record rhythm strips during the code
Controlling or limiting crowd		Dismiss those not required for bedside tasks
Family notification		Keep family informed of patient's condition Notify outcome with sensitivity
Transfer of patient to critical care unit		Ensure bed assigned for patient Transfer with adequate personnel and emergency equipment
Critique		Evaluate events of code and express feelings

AED, automated external defibrillator; *CO$_2$*, carbon dioxide; *CPR*, cardiopulmonary resuscitation; *ECG*, electrocardiogram; *IV*, intravenous; *NS*, normal saline.
Source: American Heart Association (2000). Guidelines 2000 for cardiopulmonary resuscitation and emergency cardiovascular care. *Circulation (Suppl.)*, *102*(8): I1–I134; and American Heart Association. (2001). *ACLS provider manual*, Dallas, TX: Author.

Many states have implemented "no CPR" options. The patient, who usually has a terminal illness, signs a document requesting "no CPR" if there is a loss of pulse or if breathing stops. In some states, this document directs the patient to wear a "no CPR" identification bracelet. In the event of a code, the bracelet alerts the responders that CPR efforts are prohibited. The responders should respect the person's wishes.

BASIC CARDIAC LIFE SUPPORT

The purposes of BCLS are (1) to prevent respiratory and/or cardiac arrest through prompt assessment and intervention and (2) to support respiration and circulation through CPR and the use of an AED (American Heart Association, 2001b). CPR must be initiated immediately in the event of an arrest to prevent brain damage and to improve patient outcomes. Brain damage may occur after 4 to 6 minutes without adequate oxygen.

The ABCs of CPR are airway, breathing, and circulation. Assessment is a part of each step, and the steps are performed in order (Box 9-1). The following summary is adapted from the American Heart Association (AHA) standards for BCLS (AHA, 2001b).

Airway

An open airway is essential. The first intervention is to assess unresponsiveness by tapping or shaking a patient and shouting, "Are you OK?" If the patient is

---

BOX 9-1
Steps in Basic Cardiac Life Support

1. AIRWAY
Determine unresponsiveness.
Call for help.
Position patient on back.
Open airway using head-tilt/chin-lift technique.

2. BREATHING
Assess breathing (look, listen, feel).
If breathing present, maintain airway.
If breathing absent, give two slow breaths.
Activate the code team, if possible.

3. CIRCULATION
Determine pulselessness.
Activate code team, if not previously done.
If pulse present, perform rescue breathing at 12 breaths/min.
If pulse absent, perform chest compressions at rate of 100 beats/min.
Alternate compressions and breaths at a rate of 15:2.

Source: American Heart Association. (2001). *BLS for healthcare providers.* Dallas, TX: Author.

unresponsive, the nurse calls for help by shouting to fellow caregivers or by using the nurse-call system. The patient is positioned on his or her back, and the airway is opened by use of the head-tilt/chin-lift method (Figure 9-2). If the patient must be turned to the supine position, the head and body are turned as a unit to prevent possible injury.

Breathing

The second step of CPR is to assess breathing and to initiate rescue breathing if necessary. Early initiation of rescue breathing may prevent a cardiac arrest in a patient who stops breathing but still has a pulse (e.g., a patient with hypercapnia). To assess breathing, the nurse looks, listens, and feels for breathing while maintaining an open airway. The nurse looks at the chest wall to see whether it is moving up and down, listens for air movement, and feels for exhaled air. Rescue breathing, or ventilation, is initiated if the patient is not breathing.

If possible, the code team is notified of the arrest at this time. The first person who arrives to help should "call the code." Some critical care units and emergency departments have an emergency call system that can be activated from the patient's room by the pressing of a button. If this type of system is not available and the nurse is alone, he or she presses the nurse-call system and begins CPR. When the call is answered the nurse states, "Call a code!"

In mouth-to-mouth resuscitation, the open airway is maintained, and the nurse seals his or her mouth over the patient's mouth, pinches off the patient's nose, and gives two slow breaths to the patient (Figure 9-3). If the nurse experiences difficulty in ventilating the patient, the patient's head should be repositioned, because improper head position is the most common cause of inability to ventilate.

If the patient has a mouth injury or the nurse has difficulty maintaining a good seal, mouth-to-nose ventilation can be performed. Mouth-to-stoma ventilation is performed when the patient has a tracheostomy or laryngectomy.

Although health care providers should be able to provide mouth-to-mouth breathing, mouth-to-nose breathing, and mouth-to-stoma breathing, barrier devices must be available in the work place for individuals who are expected to perform CPR. In the hospital setting, these include a BVD and a face mask. Many hospitals have a pocket mask at every patient's bedside. Additionally, most critical care units have a BVD in every patient's room.

The mouth-to-mask technique involves placing a pocket mask over the patient's mouth and breathing through a mouthpiece connected to the mask (Figure 9-4). Pocket masks have a one-way valve that protects the nurse from the patient's exhalation.

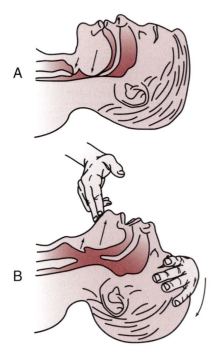

FIGURE 9-2 Head-tilt/chin-lift technique for opening the airway. **A,** Airway obstruction produced by the tongue and epiglottis. **B,** Relief by head-tilt/chin-lift. (Source: American Heart Association. [1994]. *Textbook of basic life support for healthcare providers* [pp. 4-4]. Dallas, TX: Author.)

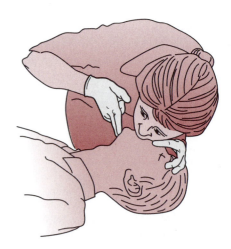

FIGURE 9-3 Mouth-to-mouth technique for rescue breathing. (Source: American Heart Association. [1997]. *Textbook of basic life support for healthcare providers* [pp. 4-7]. Dallas: Author.)

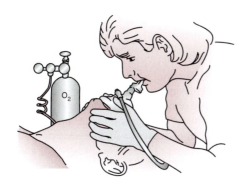

FIGURE 9-4 Mouth-to-mask technique for rescue breathing. (Source: American Heart Association. [2001]. *ACLS provider manual* [p. 25]. Dallas: Author.)

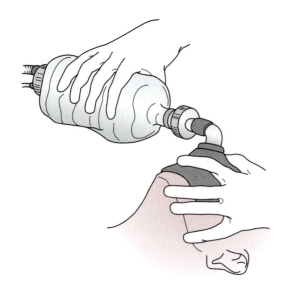

FIGURE 9-5 Rescue breathing with bag-valve device. (Modified from Kersten, L. D. [1989]. *Comprehensive respiratory nursing* [p. 629]. Philadelphia: W. B. Saunders.)

Ventilation of the patient with a BVD and face mask requires that an open airway must be maintained. Frequently, an oral airway is used to keep the airway patent and to facilitate ventilation. The BVD is connected to an oxygen source set at 15 L/min. The face mask is positioned and sealed over the patient's mouth and nose. The patient is manually ventilated with the BVD (Figure 9-5). Personnel should be properly trained to use the BVD effectively.

Circulation
The third step of CPR is to ensure adequate circulation. After the initial two breaths are given, the nurse

assesses the patient to determine the presence or absence of a pulse. (Note: The pulse check is no longer recommended for lay rescuers [AHA, 2001b].) The pulse is assessed even if the patient is attached to a cardiac monitor because artifact or a loose lead may mimic a cardiac dysrhythmia. The nurse checks the patient's carotid pulse on the side nearest the nurse. The pulse is assessed for 5 to 10 seconds to detect bradycardia.

If a pulse is present, the nurse continues to perform rescue breathing at a rate of 12 breaths per minute, or 1 breath every 5 seconds. The pulse should be assessed periodically.

If the pulse is absent, the nurse begins cardiac compressions. The patient is placed supine on a firm surface (cardiac board). Proper hand position is essential for performing compressions. The location for compressions is the lower half of the sternum above the xiphoid process. To locate the proper area, the nurse runs his or her fingers up the rib cage to the notch where the ribs and sternum meet. The heel of the second hand is placed on the lower half of the sternum. The first hand is placed on top of the second hand on the sternum so the hands are parallel. Using both hands, the nurse begins compressions by depressing the sternum 1.5 to 2.0 inches for the average adult. For the prevention of injury, care must be taken to ensure that fingers are raised off the patient's chest wall. Compressions are performed at a rate of 100 per minute at a ratio of 15 compressions to 2 breaths (15:2). The carotid pulse is checked after four cycles of compressions and ventilations. If the pulse is absent, CPR is continued until additional help arrives. With two-person CPR, one person performs compressions while the other person maintains the airway and performs rescue breathing at the same 15:2 ratio. Once the airway is secured with an endotracheal tube (ETT), a 5:1 ratio is recommended (AHA, 2001b).

ADVANCED CARDIAC LIFE SUPPORT
For cardiac or respiratory emergencies, many institutions follow the AHA standards for ACLS. The conceptual tools of management are the primary survey followed by the secondary survey (AHA, 2001a).

Primary Survey
The ABCDs of the primary survey focus on CPR and defibrillation. The ABCs of ACLS are the same as for BCLS: airway, breathing, and circulation. "D" refers to early defibrillation that can be accomplished with an AED or a conventional defibrillator. It is now a requirement that BCLS providers be trained in the use of AEDs. The AED is discussed in more detail in the electrical therapy section of this chapter.

Secondary Survey

At the time of defibrillation, the secondary survey is initiated. The ABCD (airway, breathing, circulation, differential diagnosis) in the secondary survey involves the performance of more in-depth assessments and interventions.

Airway

Airway management involves reassessment of original techniques established in BCLS. Endotracheal intubation provides definitive airway management and should be performed by properly trained personnel as soon as possible during any resuscitation effort (AHA, 2001a). Endotracheal intubation:

1. Isolates the airway and keeps it patent.
2. Facilitates the administration of a high concentration of oxygen.
3. Ensures delivery of a selected tidal volume to maintain adequate lung inflation.
4. Protects the patient from gastric distention and aspiration of stomach contents.
5. Permits effective suctioning of the trachea.
6. Provides a route for administration of certain medications.

During a cardiopulmonary arrest, CPR should not be disrupted for longer than 30 seconds while intubation is attempted. Techniques of endotracheal intubation are discussed in Chapter 8. Once intubated, the patient is manually ventilated with a BVD attached to the ETT (Figure 9-6). The BVD should have a reservoir and should be connected to an oxygen source to deliver 100% oxygen while providing a tidal volume of 10 to 15 mL/kg. Ventilation of the intubated patient should not be synchronized to chest compressions but should instead be performed asynchronously or 1 breath every 5 seconds over 1 to 2 seconds.

Breathing

Breathing assessment determines whether the ventilatory efforts are causing the chest to rise. After intubation, the nurse first auscultates the epigastrium. If stomach gurgling is heard in this area and no chest expansion is present, the ETT has mistakenly been placed in the esophagus and is removed immediately. ETT placement should be confirmed by bilateral breath sounds and observation of chest movement with ventilation. A secondary method of assessing ETT placement must be done with an end-tidal carbon dioxide detector or esophageal detector device (Figure 9-7) (AHA, 2001a). A chest x-ray study confirms placement after the code.

Circulation

Circulation focuses on IV access, attachment of monitor electrodes and leads, rhythm identification, blood pressure measurement, and medication administration. A patent IV is necessary during an arrest for the administration of fluids, medications, or both. Medications that can be administered through the ETT until an IV access is established are epinephrine, lidocaine, and atropine (AHA, 2001a).

Most critically ill patients already have IV access with an ongoing IV infusion or intermittent access device. If the patient does not have IV access, or needs additional IV access, a large-bore IV should be inserted. The antecubital vein should be the first target for

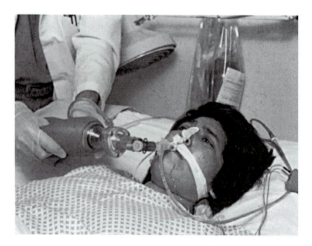

FIGURE 9-6 Ventilation with a bag-valve device connected to endotracheal tube. (From Kersten, L. D. [1989]. *Comprehensive respiratory nursing* [p. 630]. Philadelphia: W. B. Saunders.)

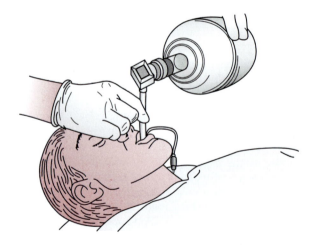

FIGURE 9-7 End-tidal carbon dioxide detector connected to an endotracheal tube. Exhaled carbon dioxide reacts with the device to create a color change indicating correct endotracheal tube placement.

IV access. Other areas for IV insertion include the dorsum of the hands and the wrist. If a peripheral IV cannot be started, the physician inserts a central line for IV access.

NS is the preferred IV fluid because it expands intravascular volume better than dextrose. When any medication is administered by the IV route, it is best followed with a 20-mL bolus of IV fluid to enhance delivery to the central circulation.

Differential Diagnosis

Differential diagnosis involves investigation into the cause of the arrest. If a reversible cause is identified, a specific therapy can be initiated. Cardiac dysrhythmias that result in cardiac arrests have many possible causes. The lethal dysrhythmias include ventricular fibrillation/ventricular tachycardia (VF/VT), asystole, and pulseless electrical activity (PEA). Other dysrhythmias that may lead to a cardiopulmonary arrest include symptomatic bradycardias and symptomatic tachycardias. Algorithms for treating these rhythm disorders have been established by the AHA (2001a). Because these algorithms periodically change, critical actions in the management of these dysrhythmias are summarized.

RECOGNITION AND TREATMENT OF DYSRHYTHMIAS

Ventricular Fibrillation and Pulseless Ventricular Tachycardia

The treatment for VF and pulseless VT is the same. If the arrest is witnessed, the patient has no pulse, and a defibrillator is not immediately available, a precordial thump may be administered.

Critical actions

- Initiate the ABCDs in the primary survey. Initiate CPR until a defibrillator is available. Defibrillate as soon as possible because early defibrillation increases the chance of survival.
- Defibrillate up to three times in rapid succession, if needed, for persistent VF/VT (200 joules [J], 200 to 300 J, 360 J, monophasic. Clinically equivalent biphasic energy doses have not yet been determined). Assess the pulse and rhythm after the third defibrillation attempt if no change has occurred in the rhythm to this point.
- If VF/VT persists, continue CPR, intubate at once, and obtain IV access. Intubation optimizes airway management and provides a route for some medication administration.
- Administer epinephrine, 1 mg IV push every 3 to 5 minutes if VF persists or vasopressin, 40 units IV push (one dose only).

- Defibrillate at 360 J, within 30 to 60 seconds of each epinephrine dose. Continue defibrillation after each dose of medication if VF persists. The pattern should be "drug-shock, drug-shock."
- Administer medications that are probably of benefit in persistent VF/VT. These medications include amiodarone, lidocaine, magnesium sulfate, and procainamide. Sodium bicarbonate is considered only if there is preexisting acidosis or tricyclic antidepressant drug overdose or if other recommended interventions within a lengthy arrest have proved ineffective. Dosages and administration are discussed in the section on pharmacological intervention.
- Reassess the patient frequently. Check for return of pulse, spontaneous respirations, and blood pressure. Resume CPR if appropriate.

Pulseless Electrical Activity

The goal in treating any rhythm without a pulse is to determine and treat the probable underlying cause of this condition. This treatment algorithm applies to any rhythm that occurs in the absence of a pulse. PEA is often associated with clinical conditions that can be reversed if they are identified early and treated appropriately (AHA, 2001a).

Critical actions

- Initiate the ABCDs of the primary and secondary survey. The patient is intubated, and IV access is obtained.
- Consider possible causes. Some of the causes of PEA include hypovolemia, hypoxia, cardiac tamponade, tension pneumothorax, drug overdose, pulmonary embolism, acidosis, massive myocardial infarction, hyperkalemia or hypokalemia, and hypothermia.
- Administer epinephrine, 1 mg IV push every 3 to 5 minutes. Additional pharmacological support includes atropine, 1 mg IV every 3 to 5 minutes up to a total of 0.04 mg/kg, if bradycardia is present.
- Continue the ABCDs of the secondary survey while identifying underlying causes and initiating related interventions.

Asystole

The absence of electrical activity in the heart continues to carry a poor prognosis. The rescuer must focus aggressively on the differential diagnosis of the secondary survey.

Critical actions

- Initiate the ABCDs of the primary and secondary survey.
- Perform CPR, intubation, and IV access.

- Confirm asystole by ensuring lead and cable connections, ensuring that the power is on, and verifying asystole in another lead. An additional lead confirms or rules out the possibility of a fine VF.
- Ensure adequate ventilation.
- Consider possible causes, including hypoxia, hypovolemia, hyperkalemia or hypokalemia, preexisting acidosis, drug overdose, cardiac tamponade, tension pneumothorax, myocardial infarction, pulmonary embolism, or hypothermia.
- Consider transcutaneous pacing. It may be effective if used early and in conjunction with medications.
- Administer medications: epinephrine, 1 mg IV push every 3 to 5 minutes, and atropine, 1 mg IV every 3 to 5 minutes up to a total dose of 0.04 mg/kg.
- Consider termination of efforts.

Symptomatic Bradycardia

This category encompasses two types: classic bradycardia (i.e., a heart rate of less than 60 beats per minute that causes symptoms) or any heart rhythm that is slow enough to cause hemodynamic compromise (Box 9-2). The cause of the bradycardia must be considered. For example, hypotension associated with bradycardia may be caused by dysfunction of the myocardium or hypovolemia, rather than by a conduction system or autonomic nervous system disturbance.

Critical actions

- Assess the ABCDs of the primary and secondary survey. Secure the airway, administer oxygen, obtain IV access, and assess vital signs. The use of a pulse oximeter is encouraged. A 12-lead ECG should be obtained.

BOX 9-2

Symptoms Associated with Bradycardia

Chest pain
Shortness of breath
Decreased level of consciousness
Weakness
Fatigue
Exercise intolerance
Dizziness
Hypotension
Diaphoresis
Pulmonary congestion
Pulmonary edema

- Administer atropine, 0.5 to 1 mg IV every 3 to 5 minutes up to a total dose of 0.04 mg/kg. It is not indicated in second-degree atrioventricular (AV) block type II or third-degree AV block.
- Identify the causative rhythm. Symptomatic bradycardias include sinus rhythm with a rate of less than 60 beats per minute, second-degree AV block types I or II, and third-degree AV block.
- Consider transcutaneous pacing for all symptomatic bradycardias. If used, analgesics or sedatives may need to be given because patients often find the pacing stimulus that is delivered with this therapy uncomfortable.
- Dopamine infusion is acceptable if low blood pressure is associated with the bradycardia. An epinephrine infusion may be administered instead if clinical symptoms are severe.
- Avoid lidocaine. Lidocaine may be lethal if the underlying bradycardia is a ventricular escape rhythm associated with a third-degree AV block. The ventricular escape rhythm indicates the failure of higher pacemakers. In this instance, lidocaine would suppress the patient's only rhythm that is providing any cardiac output, resulting in asystole.

Unstable Tachycardia

Unstable tachycardia occurs when the heart beats too fast for the patient's condition. The treatment of this group of dysrhythmias involves the rapid assessment of the patient and identification of the dysrhythmia. Synchronized cardioversion and antidysrhythmic therapy may be needed (AHA, 2001a).

Critical actions

- Initiate the primary and secondary ABCD survey. Assess the patient and recognize the signs and symptoms of cardiovascular instability including chest pain, hypotension, decreased mentation, shortness of breath, and dyspnea on exertion. Provide supplemental oxygen, establish IV access, and prepare suction and intubation equipment.
- Identify the unstable tachycardia from the monitor. This group of dysrhythmias includes atrial fibrillation and flutter, narrow complex tachycardia, wide complex tachycardia of unknown type, and VT.
- Premedicate with sedation or analgesia whenever possible. Cardioversion is an uncomfortable procedure, and a fully conscious patient is sedated before electrical intervention.
- Perform synchronized cardioversion at the appropriate energy level. Supraventricular tachycardia and atrial flutter often respond to energy levels as low as 50 J. Cardioversion for the other

tachydysrhythmias should be initiated at 100 J, increasing to 200 J, 300 J, and 360 J monophasic for subsequent attempts. Clinically equivalent biphasic energy doses have not yet been determined.

- Reassess the patient and rhythm, and consider the need for follow-up monitoring and antidysrhythmic therapy including adenosine, verapamil, diltiazem, and amiodarone.

ELECTRICAL THERAPY

The therapeutic use of electrical current has expanded over the past several years with the addition and increased use of the AED. This section addresses the use of electricity in code management for the purposes of defibrillation, cardioversion, and transcutaneous (external) pacing. Defibrillation of the patient with an implantable cardioverter-defibrillator (ICD) is also discussed.

Defibrillation

The primary treatment for VF and pulseless VT is defibrillation. VF may occur as a result of coronary artery disease, myocardial infarction, electrical shock, drug overdose, near drowning, and acid-base imbalance.

Definition. Defibrillation is the delivery of an electrical current to the heart through the use of a defibrillator (Figure 9-8); it is sometimes referred to as *countershock.* The current can be delivered through the chest wall by use of external paddles or adhesive electrode pads connected to cables. Smaller, internal paddles may be used to deliver current directly to the heart during cardiac surgery when the chest is open and the heart is visualized. Defibrillation works by completely depolarizing the heart and disrupting the impulses that are causing the dysrhythmia. Because the heart is completely depolarized, the sinoatrial node or other pacemaker can resume control of the heart's rhythm.

Defibrillation delivers energy or current in waveforms. Monophasic waveforms deliver current in one direction. More recently, defibrillators have been developed that deliver biphasic current. Biphasic waveforms deliver current that flows in a positive direction for a specified duration and then reverses and flows in a negative direction. As a result, less joules can be used for defibrillation. Biphasic defibrillation appears to work at least as effectively as monophasic defibrillation (AHA, 2001a).

Energy is delivered to the patient through a cable attached to the paddles. Newer defibrillators permit "hands-off" defibrillation. Countershocks are delivered through a cable attached to special adhesive electrode pads placed on the patient's chest.

Procedure. Two methods exist for paddle placement for external defibrillation. The standard or anterior paddle placement is used most often. In the anterior method, one paddle or adhesive electrode pad is placed at the second intercostal space to the right of the sternum, and the other paddle or adhesive electrode pad is placed at the fifth intercostal space, midaxillary line, to the left of the sternum (Figure 9-9). The alternative method is anteroposterior placement. Adhesive electrode pads are used

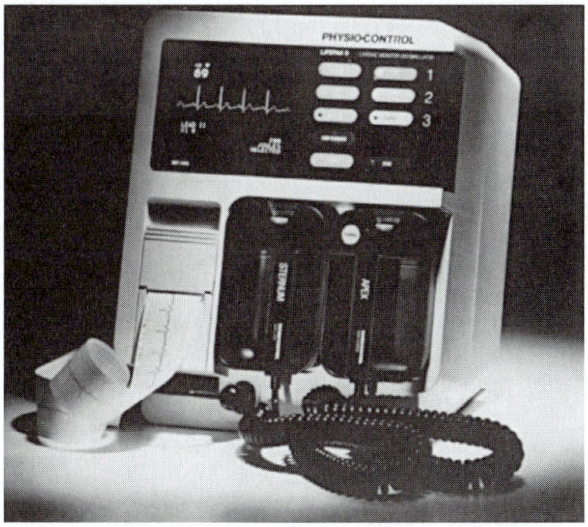

FIGURE 9-8 Defibrillator. (Courtesy of Physio-Control, Redmond, WA.)

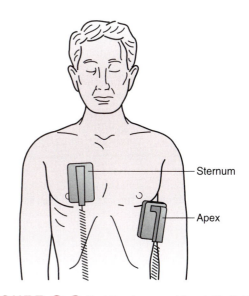

Sternum

Apex

FIGURE 9-9 Paddle placement for defibrillation.

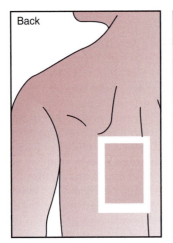
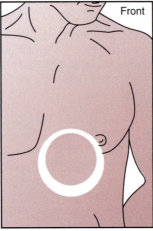
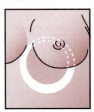

Female patients: Position electrode under breast.

FIGURE 9-10 Anteroposterior placement of adhesive electrodes for defibrillation or transcutaneous pacing.

because of the difficulty in correctly placing the paddles. The anterior adhesive electrode pad is placed at the left anterior precordial area, and the posterior electrode pad is placed at the left posterior-infrascapular area (Figure 9-10).

The amount of energy delivered is referred to as joules (J), or watt-seconds (W-s). For monophasic defibrillation, start at 200 J, then 200 to 300 J, then 360 J. For biphasic defibrillation, refer to the manufacturer's instructions for the amount of joules to deliver to the patient.

For the shock to be effective, some type of conductive medium is placed between the paddles and the skin. In the past, gel and saline pads have been used to conduct the electricity. If gel is used, it is important to cover the paddles completely with the gel. Commercially prepared defibrillator pads are also available and can be used for multiple shocks to prevent burns on the patient's skin. Newer defibrillators allow for "hands off" defibrillation. Adhesive electrode pads are attached to a cable connected to the defibrillator.

The defibrillator is charged to the desired setting. The paddles are placed firmly on the patient's chest. Firm pressure is needed to facilitate skin contact and to reduce the impedance to the flow of current.

Safety is essential during the procedure to prevent injury to the patient and the personnel assisting with the procedure. The person performing the defibrillation ensures that all personnel are standing clear of the bed and visually checks to see that no one is in contact with the patient or bed. It is important that this step not be omitted when "hands off" defibrillation is used. The countershock is then delivered. The patient's rhythm is assessed after each defibrillation.

After the initial triad of shocks for VF and pulseless VT, and after subsequent shocks, the pulse is assessed. Rhythm strips are recorded during the procedure to document response. The procedure for defibrillation is summarized in Box 9-3.

Complications of defibrillation include burns on the skin and damage to the heart muscle. Arcing of electricity can occur if the paddles are not firmly placed on the skin, excessive conductive gel is used, or the

---

BOX 9-3

Procedure for External Defibrillation

1. Apply the defibrillator pads to the patient's chest (or apply conductive gel to paddles or adhesive electrode pads).
2. Turn on the defibrillator.
3. Select the energy level.
4. Position the paddles on the patient's chest.
5. Ensure that all personnel (including yourself) are clear of the patient, the bed, and any equipment that may be connected to the patient.
6. Charge the defibrillator to the desired setting.
7. Shout "I'm clear, you're clear, everybody's clear," and look to verify.
8. Apply firm pressure on both paddles.
9. Deliver countershock by depressing buttons on each paddle simultaneously, or, if using adhesive electrode pads, press the button on the defibrillator.
10. After the defibrillation, observe the patient's heart rhythm to determine effectiveness.

skin is wet. Arcing has also been noted when patients have nitroglycerin patches or paste on the chest; therefore, topical nitroglycerin should be removed before defibrillation.

Automated External Defibrillation

The AED extends the range of personnel trained in the use of a defibrillator and shortens the time between code onset and defibrillation. The AED is considered an integral part of emergency cardiac care. Public access defibrillation programs are encouraged (AHA, 2001a).

Definition. The AED is an external defibrillator with rhythm analysis capabilities (Figure 9-11). It is used to achieve early defibrillation. Because of the ease of use, AEDs may be placed on medical-surgical patient units, emergency response vehicles, and in public places.

Indications. The AED should be used only when a patient is in cardiac arrest (unresponsive, no effective breathing, no signs of circulation including no pulse). Confirmation that the patient is in cardiac arrest must be obtained before attaching the AED (AHA, 2001a).

Procedure. The AED is attached to the patient by two adhesive pads and connecting cables. Correct placement of each adhesive pad is displayed on each adhesive pad. These pads serve a dual purpose: recording the rhythm and delivering the countershock. The AED eliminates the need for training in rhythm recognition because these microprocessor-based devices analyze the surface ECG signal. The AED "looks" at the patient's rhythm numerous times to confirm the presence of a rhythm for which defibrillation in indicated. The semiautomatic "shock advisory" AED charges the device and "advises" the operator to press a button to defibrillate. The fully automated AED requires only that the operator attach the defibrillation pads and turn on the device (Box 9-4). Both models deliver AHA-recommended energy levels for the treatment of VF/pulseless VT. They are not designed to deliver synchronous shocks and will shock VT if the rate exceeds preset values.

Cardioversion

Definition. Cardioversion is the delivery of a countershock that is synchronized with the patient's cardiac rhythm. The purpose of cardioversion is to disrupt an ectopic pacemaker that is causing a dysrhythmia and to allow the sinoatrial node to take control of the rhythm. During an emergency situation, cardioversion is used to treat patients with VT or supraventricular tachycardia who have a pulse but are developing symptoms related to a low cardiac output, such as hypotension and decreased level of consciousness. Elective cardioversion is used to treat atrial flutter and atrial fibrillation.

Cardioversion is similar to defibrillation, except the delivery of energy is synchronized to occur during

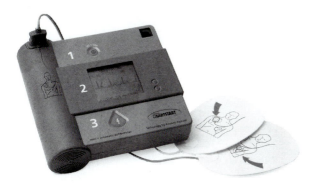

FIGURE 9-11 Automatic external defibrillator. (Courtesy of Laerdal Medical Corporation, Wappingers Falls, NY.)

> **BOX 9-4**
>
> ### Procedure for Automated External Defibrillator Operation
>
> 1. Turn the power on.
> 2. Attach the AED connecting cables to the AED "box."
> 3. Attach the AED connecting cables to the adhesive electrode pads.
> 4. Attach the adhesive electrode pads to the patient:
>   Place one electrode pad on the upper right sternal border directly below the clavicle.
>   Place the other electrode pad lateral to the left nipple with the top margin of the pad a few inches below the axilla.
>   The correct position of the electrode pads is often marked on the electrode pads.
> 5. "Clear" personnel from the patient (no one should be touching the patient), and press the "analyze" button to start rhythm analysis.
> 6. Listen or read the message "shock indicated" or "no shock indicated."
> 7. "Clear" personnel from the patient, and press the "shock" button if shock is indicated. A shock is delivered only if the AED signals that a shock is indicated and no one is touching the patient.
>
> *AED,* Automated external defibrillator.

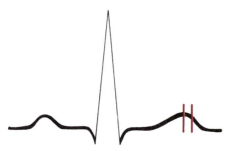

FIGURE 9-12 Approximate location of the vulnerable period. (From Conover, M. B. [2003]. *Understanding electrocardiography.* 8th ed. St. Louis: Mosby.)

ventricular depolarization (QRS complex). The rationale for delivering the shock during the QRS complex is to prevent the shock from being delivered during repolarization (T wave), often termed the *vulnerable period.* If a shock is delivered during this vulnerable period (Figure 9-12), VF may occur. Because the purpose of cardioversion is to disrupt the rhythm rather than completely depolarize the heart, less energy is usually required. Cardioversion can be performed with energy levels as low as 50 J. The amount of energy is gradually increased until the rhythm is converted.

Procedure. The procedure for cardioversion (Box 9-5) is similar to that for defibrillation. However, the defibrillator is set in the "synchronous" mode for the cardioversion. The R waves are sensed by the machine and are noted by "spikes" or other markings on the monitor of the defibrillator (Figure 9-13). It is important to assess that all R waves are properly sensed. When it is time to deliver the shock, the buttons on the paddles must remain depressed until the shock is delivered because energy is discharged only during the QRS complex. When a patient is undergoing cardioversion on a nonemergency basis, sedation is given before the procedure. Rhythm strips are recorded during cardioversion to document response.

Special Situations

When a patient with a permanent pacemaker or ICD requires defibrillation, placing the paddle near the generator is avoided. Although damage to the device rarely occurs, the generator can absorb much of the current of defibrillation from the pads or paddles and reduce the chance of success (AHA, 2001a). Patients with ICDs are at high risk for lethal dysrhythmias.

A patient may also have an ICD with dual-chamber pacing capabilities. Nurses should become familiar, whenever possible, with the type of therapy the

---

BOX 9-5

Procedure for Synchronous Cardioversion

1. Ensure that emergency equipment is readily available.
2. Explain the procedure to the patient.
3. Consider sedating the patient.
4. Attach monitor leads to the patient. Ensure that the monitor displays the patient's rhythm clearly without artifact.
5. Turn on the defibrillator to "synchronous" mode.
6. Observe the rhythm on the monitor to determine that the R wave is properly sensed and marked (usually with a spike) (see Figure 9-13).
7. Apply the defibrillator pads or adhesive electrode pads to the patient's chest (or apply conductive gel to the paddles).
8. Select the appropriate energy level.
9. Position the paddles on the patient's chest and apply firm pressure.
10. Ensure that all personnel (including yourself) are clear of the patient, the bed, and any equipment that may be connected to the patient.
11. Charge the defibrillator.
12. Shout "I'm clear, you're clear, everybody's clear," and look to verify.
13. Deliver synchronized countershock by depressing the buttons on each paddle simultaneously, or press the button on the defibrillator if you are using adhesive electrode pads. Keep the buttons depressed until the shock has been delivered.
14. After the cardioversion, observe the patient's heart rhythm to determine effectiveness.

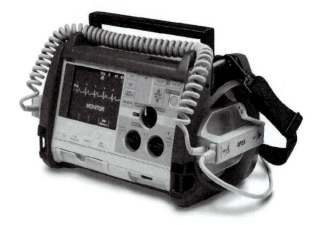

FIGURE 9-13 Monitor/defibrillator demonstrating marked R waves for cardioversion. (Courtesy of Zoll Medical, Burlington, MA.)

patient's device has been programmed to deliver. By the time VF/VT is recognized on the monitor, the rhythm should also have been recognized by the ICD. If a successful countershock by the ICD has not occurred when the rhythm is noted on the monitor, one should proceed with standard code management. If external defibrillation is unsuccessful, the location of the paddles or adhesive electrodes on the chest should be changed. Anteroposterior placement may be more effective than anterior-apex placement. External defibrillation of a patient while the ICD is firing does not harm the patient or the ICD. ICDs and permanent pacemakers are insulated from damage caused by conventional external defibrillation. There is no danger to personnel if the ICD discharges while staff members are touching the patient. However, the shock may be felt and has been compared to the sensation of contact with an electrical outlet. The pacing and sensing thresholds of the pacemaker or ICD are assessed after external defibrillation.

Transcutaneous Cardiac Pacing

Definition. Transcutaneous (external noninvasive) cardiac pacing is used during emergency situations to treat symptomatic bradycardia and asystole. In this method of pacing, the heart is stimulated with externally applied cutaneous electrodes that deliver the electrical impulse. Impulse conduction occurs across the chest wall to stimulate the cardiac contraction.

The transcutaneous pacemaker may be a freestanding unit with a monitor and a pacemaker. Some models incorporate a monitor, a defibrillator, and an external pacemaker into one system (Figure 9-14).

The advantages of transcutaneous pacemakers include the following:

- It is easy to operate.
- It requires minimal training.
- It can be initiated immediately in emergency situations.
- It eliminates the risks associated with invasive pacemakers.

Procedure. The procedure (Box 9-6) for transcutaneous pacing involves the placement of adhesive electrodes anteriorly and posteriorly on the patient (see Figure 9-10). The electrodes are connected to the external pacemaker allowing for "hands off" pacing. The pacemaker is set in either asynchronous or

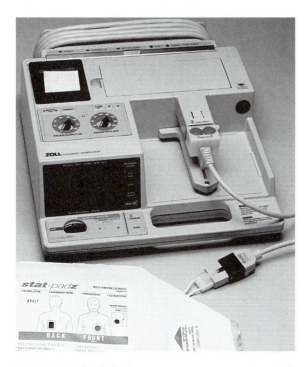

FIGURE 9-14 Transcutaneous pacemaker-defibrillator. (Courtesy of Zoll Medical, Burlington, MA.)

BOX 9-6

Procedure for Transcutaneous Pacemaker

1. Obtain the transcutaneous pacemaker, pacemaker electrodes, and emergency equipment.
2. If the patient is alert, explain the procedure.
3. Clip excess hair from the patient's chest. Do not shave hair.
4. Apply the anterior electrode to the chest. The electrode is centered at the fourth intercostal space to the left of the sternum.
5. Apply the posterior electrode on the patient's back to the left of the thoracic spine.
6. Connect the electrode to the pacemaker generator.
7. Set the pacemaker parameters for mode, heart rate, and output (mA) according to the manufacturer's instructions.
8. Turn the unit on. Choose pacing mode (if applicable).
9. Assess the adequacy of pacing:
   Pacemaker spike and QRS complex (capture)
   Heart rate and rhythm
   Blood pressure
   Level of consciousness
10. Observe for patient discomfort. The patient may need sedation and/or analgesia.
11. Anticipate follow-up treatment (e.g., insertion of a temporary transvenous pacemaker).

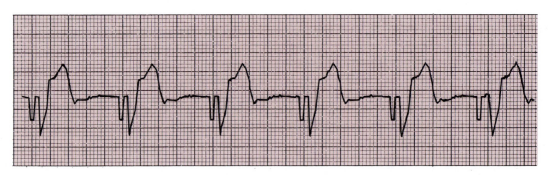

FIGURE 9-15 Electrical capture of transcutaneous pacemaker. Note the pacemaker spikes followed by a wide QRS complex and a tall T wave.

demand modes. Some devices permit only demand pacing. In the asynchronous mode, the pacemaker generates a rhythm without regard to the patient's own rhythm. In the demand mode, the pacemaker fires only if the patient's heart rate falls below a preset limit determined by the operator (e.g., 50 beats per minute). The electrical output is adjusted to stimulate a paced beat.

The electrical and mechanical effectiveness of pacing is assessed. The electrical activity is noted by a pacemaker "spike" that indicates that the pacemaker is initiating electrical activity. The spike is followed by a broad QRS complex (Figure 9-15). Mechanical activity is noted by palpating a pulse during electrical activity. Additionally, the patient has signs of improved cardiac output, including increased blood pressure and improved skin color and skin temperature. If the external pacemaker is effective, the patient may need to have a temporary transvenous pacemaker inserted, depending on the cause of the bradycardia.

The alert patient who requires transcutaneous pacing may experience some discomfort. Because the skeletal muscles are stimulated, as well as the heart muscle, the patient may experience a tingling, twitching, or thumping feeling that ranges from mildly uncomfortable to intolerable. Sedation, analgesia, or both may be indicated.

Pharmacological Intervention During a Code

Medications that are administered during a code depend on several factors: the cause of the arrest, the patient's cardiac rhythm, the physician's preference, and the patient's response. The goals of treatment are to reestablish and maintain optimal cardiac function, to correct hypoxemia and acidosis, and to suppress dangerous cardiac ectopic activity. Additionally, medications are used to achieve a balance between myocardial oxygen supply and demand, to maintain adequate blood pressure, and to relieve congestive heart failure. Because of the rapid and profound effects these drugs can have on cardiac activity and hemodynamic function, continuous ECG monitoring is essential, and hemodynamic monitoring should be instituted as soon as possible after the code. If IV push medications are given peripherally, they should be flushed with at least 20 mL of IV fluid to ensure central circulation. Additionally, because of the precise dosages and careful administration required with these medications, infusion pumps should be used when continuous infusions are given. IV infusion rates are tapered slowly, with frequent monitoring of clinical effectiveness.

The following drugs are included in ACLS guidelines (AHA, 2001a) and represent those drugs most frequently used in code management. Indications, mechanisms of action, and dosages for each drug, as well as side effects and nursing implications are discussed in this section and are summarized in Table 9-4.

OXYGEN

Oxygen is essential to resuscitation and has several pharmacological considerations. Oxygen is used to treat hypoxemia, which exists in any arrest situation as a result of lack of adequate gas exchange, inadequate cardiac output, or both. Artificial ventilation without supplemental oxygen does not correct hypoxemia.

Oxygen is used to improve tissue oxygenation. Additionally, the success of other medications and interventions, such as defibrillation, depends on adequate oxygenation and normal acid-base status.

Oxygen can be delivered via mouth to mask, BVD with mask, BVD to ETT, or other airway adjuncts. During an arrest, 100% oxygen is administered.

TABLE 9-4

DRUGS FREQUENTLY USED IN CODE MANAGEMENT

Drug	Indication	Mechanism of Action	Dosage/Route	Side Effects	Nursing Implications
Adenosine (Adenocard)	Initial drug of choice for supraventricular dysrhythmias	Slows conduction in AV node and interrupts AV nodal reentry circuits	6 mg rapid IV bolus over 1–3 sec, followed by 20-mL rapid flush; if no response in 1–2 min, give 12-mg repeat dose and flush; may repeat 12-mg dose if necessary	Headache, transient flushing, dyspnea, and chest pain; may cause asystole up to 15 sec	Half-life 10 sec; higher dose needed with theophylline, lower dose with dipyridamole or after cardiac transplantation
Amiodarone (Cordarone)	Treatment and prophylaxis of recurrent VF and hemodynamically unstable VT; rapid atrial dysrhythmias	↓ Membrane excitability, prolongs action potential to terminate VT or VF	*Cardiac arrest:* 300 mg diluted in 20–30 mL IV push followed by dose of 150 mg in 3 to 5 min (max dose of 2.2 g/24 hr) NS or D₅W *Nonarrest, rapid infusion:* 150 mg IV push over 10 min followed by 1 mg/min infusion for 6 hrs, then 0.5 mg/min for 6 hr; then 0.5 mg/min to a maximum dose of 2 g	Bradycardia, hypotension; use with caution on preexisting conduction system abnormalities	Monitor for symptomatic sinus bradycardia, PR prolongation
Atropine	Symptomatic bradycardia, asystole, bradycardic pulseless electrical activity	↑ SA node automaticity and AV node conduction activity	*Bradycardia:* 0.5–1 mg IV push every 3–5 min to max dose of 0.03–0.04 mg/kg *Asystole:* 1 mg IV push every 3–5 min to max dose of 0.04 mg/kg; 2–3 mg in 10 mL NS may be given via ETT	Tachycardia, increased myocardial oxygen consumption and ischemia	Consider transcutaneous pacing if repeated doses needed
Calcium chloride	Acute hyperkalemia, hypocalcemia, calcium channel blocker toxicity	↑ Myocardial contractility	8–16 mg/kg of 10% solution slow IV push; 10 mL of 10% solution = 10 mg/mL; repeat as needed.		Rapid administration can slow heart rate
Digitalis (Digoxin)	Atrial fibrillation or flutter with rapid ventricular response, supraventricular tachycardia	↓ Conduction through AV node	10–15 mcg/kg IV push loading dose	Dysrhythmias, changes in mental status, anorexia, nausea, vomiting	Monitor drug levels; ensure normal potassium levels; onset of action, 5–30 min; peak, 1.5–3 hr

Continued

TABLE 9-4

DRUGS FREQUENTLY USED IN CODE MANAGEMENT—cont'd

Drug	Indication	Mechanism of Action	Dosage/Route	Side Effects	Nursing Implications
Diltiazem (Cardizem)	Reentrant supraventricular tachycardias, atrial fibrillation and flutter with rapid ventricular response	Calcium channel blocker, slows conduction and prolongs refractoriness in the AV node	0.25 mg/kg IV over 2 min for rapid atrial fibrillation/flutter; repeat in 15 min at 0.35 mg/kg if needed; maintenance infusion of 5–15 mg/hr titrated to heart rate	Myocardial depression	Use with caution with left ventricular failure
Dopamine (Intropin)	Hypotension not related to hypovolemia	*Moderate doses* (5–10 mcg/kg/min): ↑ contractility and cardiac output *High doses* (10–20 mcg/kg/min): vasoconstriction and ↑ systemic vascular resistance	Continuous IV infusion, 2–5 mcg/kg/min initially and titrated as needed	Tachycardia, increased dysrhythmias	Extravasation may cause necrosis and sloughing; dilution, 400–800 mg in 250 mL D_5W = 1600–3200 mcg/mL
Epinephrine (Adrenalin)	Ventricular fibrillation, pulseless ventricular tachycardia, pulseless electrical activity, asystole	↑ Contractility, automaticity, systemic vascular resistance, and arterial blood pressure; vasoconstriction improves coronary and cerebral perfusion	1 mg IV push, or 2–2.5 mg in 10 mL via ETT; may repeat every 3–5 min		In a cardiac arrest may be used as a continuous infusion for hypotension; dilution, 1 mg/250 mL NS; infuse at 1–5 mcg/min and titrate as needed
Isoproterenol (Isuprel)	Symptomatic bradycardia in cardiac transplantation patients, or if external pacing is not available	Beta-agonist, ↑ contractility and heart rate, also greatly increases myocardial oxygen demand	Continuous IV infusion at 2 mcg/min, titrated to maintain heart rate of 60 beats/min. Dilution, 1 mg in 250 mL D_5W = 4 mcg/mL (range 2–10 mcg/min)	Myocardial ischemia, ventricular dysrhythmias	Monitor for myocardial ischemia
Lidocaine (Xylocaine)	Ventricular fibrillation, ventricular tachycardia, PVCs	Suppresses ventricular dysrhythmias, raises fibrillation threshold	*Ventricular fibrillation:* 1–1.5 mg/kg IV push, followed by 0.5–0.75 mg/kg every 5–10 min to maximum dose of 3 mg/kg; may be given by ETT at dose of 2–4 mg/kg; follow with continuous intravenous infusion at 2–4 mg/min	Neurologic toxicity if drug level excessive	Lower dose if impaired hepatic blood flow; dilution, 1 g in 250 mL or 2 g/500 mL = 4 mg/mL
Magnesium	Torsades de pointes, hypomagnesemia	Essential for enzyme reactions and sodium-potassium pump, ↓ postinfarction dysrhythmias	*Cardiac arrest:* 1–2 g in 100 mL D_5W over 1–2 min *Nonarrest:* 1–2 g in 50–100 ml of D_5W over 5–60 min, followed by infusion of 0.5 to 1 g/hr	Flushing, bradycardia, hypotension	Monitor serum levels

Drug	Action	Indications	Dosage/Administration	Adverse Effects	Nursing Considerations
Norepinephrine (Levophed)	Alpha-, beta₁-agonist, causes arterial and venous vasoconstriction, some ↑ in myocardial contractility	Hypotension uncorrected by other drugs	Continuous IV infusion at 0.5–1 mcg/min, titrated upward as needed to maximum of 30 mcg/min. Dilution: 4 mg/250 mL D₅W	Myocardial ischemia	Administer through central line, if possible; extravasation may cause necrosis and sloughing
Oxygen	↑ Arterial oxygen content and tissue oxygenation	Cardiopulmonary arrest, chest pain, hypoxemia	100% in a code via bag-valve device with mask		Monitor pulse oximetry values
Procainamide (Pronestyl)	↓ Automaticity of ectopic pacemakers; slows intraventricular conduction	PVCs, ventricular tachycardia uncontrolled by lidocaine, occasionally supraventricular dysrhythmias	Administer 20 mg/min until dysrhythmia is suppressed, hypotension occurs, or the QRS widens by >50% of original width, or 17 mg/kg has been administered, followed by a continuous infusion of 1–4 mg/min	Hypotension, heart block	Do not exceed recommended infusion rate; dilution, 1 g/250 mL = 4 mg/mL; decrease dose with cardiac or renal dysfunction
Sodium bicarbonate	Counteracts metabolic acidosis by binding with hydrogen ions to produce water and carbon dioxide	Metabolic acidosis in cardiopulmonary arrest uncorrected by defibrillation, correct CPR technique, oxygenation, and other drugs	1 mEq/kg IV push initially, may repeat 0.5 mEq/kg every 10 min as needed; administration dictated by ABG results		Ensure adequate CPR, oxygenation, and ventilation
Vasopressin	Nonadrenergic, peripheral vasoconstriction	Alternative pressor to epinephrine in ventricular fibrillation	40 units IV push (one dose only)	Cardiac ischemia	May also be useful in asystole and pulseless electrical activity, but not yet validated
Verapamil (Calan, Isoptin)	Calcium channel blocker, ↓ myocardial contractility, slows AV nodal conduction, vasodilates vascular smooth muscle	Supraventricular tachycardia unresponsive to adenosine that does not require cardioversion	Initially, 2.5–5 mg IV push over 1–2 min; repeat dose at 5–10 mg if needed in 15 to 30 min or 5 mg every 15 min, to a maximum dose of 30 mg	Hypotension, myocardial depression	Contraindicated in left ventricular failure; beta-blockers have synergistic effect; use with caution in WPW syndrome, atrial fibrillation, and flutter

ABG, Arterial blood gas; *AV*, atrioventricular; *CPR*, cardiopulmonary resuscitation; *ETT*, endotracheal tube; *NS*, normal saline; *PVC*, premature ventricular contraction; *SA*, sinoatrial; *VF*, ventricular fibrillation; *VT*, ventricular tachycardia.
Data from American Heart Association (2000). Guidelines 2000 for cardiopulmonary resuscitation and emergency cardiovascular care. *Circulation (Suppl.) 102*(8): I1-I384; and Hazinski, M. F., Cummins, R. O., and Field, J. M. (2000). *2000 handbook of emergency cardiovascular care for healthcare providers*. Dallas, TX: American Heart Association.

Effects of Adrenergic Receptor Stimulation

ALPHA
Vasoconstriction
Increased contractility

BETA$_1$
Increased heart rate
Increased contractility

BETA$_2$
Vasodilation
Relaxation of bronchial, uterine, and gastrointestinal smooth muscle

EPINEPHRINE (ADRENALINE)

Epinephrine is a potent vasoconstrictor. Because of its alpha-adrenergic and beta-adrenergic effects (Box 9-7), epinephrine increases systemic vascular resistance and arterial blood pressure, as well as heart rate, contractility, and automaticity of cardiac pacemaker cells. Because of peripheral vasoconstriction, blood is shunted to the heart and brain. Epinephrine also increases myocardial oxygen requirements.

Epinephrine is indicated for the restoration of cardiac electrical activity in an arrest. In addition, epinephrine increases automaticity and the force of contraction, an effect that makes the heart more susceptible to successful defibrillation. Epinephrine is used to treat VF or pulseless VT that is unresponsive to initial defibrillation, asystole, and PEA.

During a code, epinephrine may be given by the IV route or through an ETT. The IV dosage is 1.0 mg (10 mL of a 1:10,000 solution) and is repeated every 3 to 5 minutes as needed. When given through the ETT, 2 to 2.5 times the IV dose of epinephrine is diluted in 10 mL of NS or sterile water. (Either diluent should be preservative free to prevent injury to the lungs.)

Occasionally, epinephrine is administered by continuous infusion to increase heart rate or blood pressure. Dilution is 1 mg in 250 mL or 500 mL of 5% dextrose in water (D$_5$W) or NS. The infusion is started at 1 mcg/min and is titrated according to the patient's response in a range of 2 to 10 mcg/min. In a situation other than cardiac arrest, because epinephrine increases myocardial oxygen requirements, the nurse must monitor the patient closely for signs of myocardial ischemia.

VASOPRESSIN

Vasopressin is recommended as an alternative to epinephrine administration in VF unresponsive to shock (AHA, 2001a). At high doses, vasopressin is a potent vasoconstrictor. A single dose of 40 units IV is recommended. Repeat doses are not necessary because of its 10- to 20-minute half-life. Administration of the drug is not recommended for conscious patients with coronary artery disease because severe angina can result from the vasoconstriction.

ATROPINE

Atropine is used to increase the heart rate by decreasing the vagal tone. It is indicated for patients with symptomatic bradycardia. In an arrest, atropine may be used for asystole because it may initiate electrical activity or restore conduction through the AV node.

For symptomatic bradycardia, atropine is given in 0.5-mg doses IV and repeated every 3 to 5 minutes as needed (for a total of 0.03 to 0.04 mg/kg) to maintain a heart rate greater than 60 beats per minute or until adequate tissue perfusion is achieved (as indicated by blood pressure, level of consciousness). External pacing should be considered to maintain an adequate heart rate after the initial atropine dose in patients with myocardial ischemia to minimize the increased myocardial oxygen consumption caused by atropine. Doses lower than 0.5 mg can cause paradoxical bradycardia and may precipitate VF.

In asystole, a 1-mg dose is given and repeated every 3 to 5 minutes, if necessary, up to the maximum dose of 0.04 mg/kg. If necessary, atropine may be given via an ETT. The dose for ETT administration is 2 to 3 mg diluted in 10 mL of NS or sterile water (without preservatives).

LIDOCAINE (XYLOCAINE)

Lidocaine is an antidysrhythmic drug that suppresses ventricular ectopic activity. It depresses the ventricular conduction system and reduces automaticity. Lidocaine is the drug of choice for treating ventricular ectopy (premature ventricular contractions), VT, and VF.

During a code, a bolus dose of 1 to 1.5 mg/kg of lidocaine is administered by IV push. Additional boluses of 0.5 to 0.75 mg/kg may be administered every 5 to 10 minutes, as needed, until a total dose of 3 mg/kg has been given. If IV access is not available, 2 to 4 mg/kg of lidocaine may be given through the ETT.

If lidocaine is successful in treating the cardiac dysrhythmia, a continuous infusion should be started at 2 to 4 mg/min. Dilution is 1 g mixed in 250 mL of

D_5W, or 2 g can be mixed in 500 mL. Both solutions deliver 4 mg/mL, the standard dilution.

Dosages of lidocaine should be decreased in patients with impaired hepatic blood flow (as occurs in congestive heart failure, acute myocardial infarction, shock) and in elderly patients. Blood levels should be monitored, and the patient should be assessed for central nervous system disturbances that may indicate lidocaine toxicity. Common side effects of lidocaine include lethargy, confusion, tinnitus, muscle twitching, seizures, bradycardia, and paresthesias.

PROCAINAMIDE (PRONESTYL)

Procainamide is an antidysrhythmic drug that reduces the automaticity of ectopic pacemakers and slows intraventricular conduction. It is used to treat ventricular ectopy and VT that is uncontrolled by lidocaine. It may also be used to treat supraventricular dysrhythmias. Procainamide is not used initially in VF because of the length of time needed to achieve adequate blood levels; however, it may be used for recurrent VF.

Procainamide is given IV in 100-mg doses (diluted in 10 mL of sterile water for injection) at a rate of 20 mg/min until the dysrhythmia is controlled, the patient becomes hypotensive, the QRS widens by 50% of its original width, or a total of 17 mg/kg has been given. If procainamide successfully controls the dysrhythmia, a continuous infusion is given at a rate of 1 to 4 mg/min for maintenance. The infusion is prepared by mixing 1 g of procainamide in 250 mL of fluid, yielding 4 mg/mL. As with lidocaine, serum levels should be monitored. It should be administered in reduced dosages to patients with left ventricular dysfunction or renal failure.

Hypotension may occur after rapid injection of procainamide. Procainamide may also cause widening of the QRS interval and prolongation of PR or QT intervals, resulting in AV conduction disturbances, cardiac arrest, or both.

ADENOSINE (ADENOCARD)

Adenosine is the initial drug of choice for the diagnosis and treatment of supraventricular dysrhythmias. Adenosine slows conduction through the AV node and interrupts AV node reentrant electrical conduction, which is the cause of most supraventricular dysrhythmias. It is effective in restoring normal sinus rhythm in patients with paroxysmal supraventricular tachycardia, including that caused by Wolff-Parkinson-White syndrome. Adenosine does not convert supraventricular rhythms that do not involve the sinoatrial or AV node, such as atrial fibrillation, atrial flutter, atrial tachycardia, and VT. However, adenosine may produce a brief AV node block, thereby assisting with the diagnosis of these rhythms (Figure 9-16).

Adenosine has a half-life of less than 10 seconds; therefore, it is administered rapidly. The initial dose is a 6-mg IV push over 1 to 3 seconds, followed by a 20-mL rapid saline flush. A period of asystole lasting as long as 15 seconds may be seen after adenosine administration that reflects the suppression of AV node conduction. A second and third dose of 12 mg may be given 1 to 2 minutes later if the first dose is ineffective in converting the rhythm.

Patients receiving theophylline require higher doses of adenosine. Cardiac transplantation recipients and those receiving dipyridamole are more sensitive to adenosine and need lower doses (AHA, 2000). Common side effects include transient flushing, dyspnea, and chest pain.

VERAPAMIL (CALAN, ISOPTIN)

Verapamil is a calcium channel blocker that decreases the heart rate. Unfortunately, it also causes vasodilation and decreased cardiac contractility. Verapamil slows conduction through the AV node, thus making it effective in the treatment of most supraventricular dysrhythmias. Verapamil is useful in stable supraventricular tachycardia that does not require cardioversion.

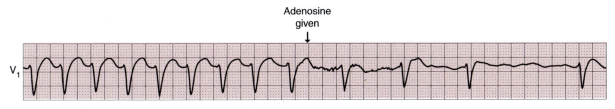

FIGURE 9-16 Atrioventricular block after intravenous administration of adenosine. (From Paul, S., & Hebra, J. D. (1998). *The nurse's guide to cardiac rhythm interpretation: Implications for patient care*. Philadelphia: W. B. Saunders.)

Verapamil is ineffective in converting paroxysmal supraventricular tachycardia caused by Wolff-Parkinson-White syndrome, because it may actually increase the ventricular rate in this syndrome and may cause VF (AHA, 2000). However, verapamil is useful in slowing rapid ventricular rates with atrial fibrillation or atrial flutter. Verapamil is not effective, and should not be used, in the treatment of VT. Severe hypotension, VF, or both, may result.

The initial dose of verapamil is 2.5 to 5 mg IV bolus given over 2 minutes. In middle-aged or older patients, verapamil should be given more slowly, at least over 3 minutes (AHA, 2000). Maximal therapeutic response occurs within 3 to 5 minutes after injection. A repeat dose of 5 to 10 mg may be given 15 to 30 minutes later if needed, up to a maximum dose of 30 mg.

Because verapamil is also a vasodilator, arterial blood pressure is monitored closely during and after administration. Verapamil is contraindicated in patients with preexisting severe heart failure because hemodynamic compromise may result.

DILTIAZEM (CARDIZEM)

Diltiazem is a calcium channel blocker that is effective in slowing heart rate but produces less myocardial depression than verapamil. Diltiazem may be as effective as verapamil in treating supraventricular tachycardias, particularly rapid atrial fibrillation or flutter (AHA, 2000).

The initial dose for supraventricular tachycardias is 0.25 mg/kg by IV bolus over 2 minutes. This regimen converts the rhythm of more than 90% of patients with supraventricular tachycardia. A second dose of 0.35 mg/kg may be given 15 minutes after the initial dose, if needed. If treating atrial fibrillation or flutter, the bolus dose is followed by a continuous infusion of 5 to 15 mg/hr. Continuous infusions at rates greater than 15 mg/hr or for longer than 24 hours are not recommended (AHA, 2000).

MAGNESIUM

Magnesium is essential for many enzyme reactions and for the function of the sodium-potassium pump. It also acts as a calcium channel blocker and slows neuromuscular transmission. Hypomagnesemia is associated with a high frequency of cardiac dysrhythmias, including refractory VF. Magnesium may also be an effective treatment for torsades de pointes. Torsades de pointes is a form of ventricular tachycardia characterized by QRS complexes that change amplitude and appearance (polymorphic) and appear to twist around the isoelectric line (Figure 9-17). The QRS complexes may deflect downward for a few beats and then upward for a few beats.

For cardiac arrest related to low magnesium or torsades de pointes, 1 to 2 g of magnesium sulfate is

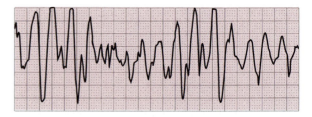

FIGURE 9-17 Torsades de pointes. The QRS complex seems to spiral around the isoelectric line. (From Paul, S., & Hebra, J. D. [1998]. *The nurse's guide to cardiac rhythm interpretation: Implications for patient care.* Philadelphia: W. B. Saunders.)

diluted in 100 mL of 5% dextrose and given via IV bolus over 1 to 2 minutes. In nonarrest situations, a loading dose of 1 to 2 g mixed in 50 to 100 mL of 5% dextrose is given over 5 to 60 minutes, followed by an infusion at 0.5 to 1 g/hr until desired effects. The side effects of rapid magnesium administration include hypotension, asystole, flushing, and sweating. Serum magnesium levels are monitored to avoid hypermagnesemia.

SODIUM BICARBONATE

A patient who has experienced an arrest quickly becomes acidotic. The acidosis results from two sources: (1) retention of carbon dioxide from inadequate ventilation and (2) buildup of acids from anaerobic metabolism induced by hypoxia. Effective ventilation with supplemental oxygen and rapid restoration of tissue perfusion (by CPR and spontaneous circulation) are the best mechanisms to correct these causes of acidosis.

Sodium bicarbonate is indicated in the treatment of metabolic acidosis only after interventions such as defibrillation, intubation, and hyperventilation with 100% oxygen, and administration of pharmacological agents have been instituted. Sodium bicarbonate buffers the increased numbers of hydrogen ions present in metabolic acidosis. It is beneficial in treating preexisting metabolic acidosis, hyperkalemia, or tricyclic antidepressant or phenobarbital overdose.

The initial dosage of sodium bicarbonate is 1 mEq/kg by IV push. Subsequent doses of half this amount may be repeated every 10 minutes, as determined by arterial blood gas results. Sodium bicarbonate should not be mixed or infused with any other medication, because it may precipitate or cause deactivation of other medications.

DOPAMINE (INTROPIN)

The indication for dopamine is symptomatic hypotension in the absence of hypovolemia. Its effects are dose related. At rates of 5 to 10 mcg/kg/min, myocardial contractility increases from alpha- and beta-adrenergic stimulation causing enhanced cardiac contractility, increased cardiac output, increased heart rate, and increased blood pressure. At rates greater than 10 mcg/kg/min, systemic vascular resistance markedly increases as a result of generalized vasoconstriction produced from alpha-adrenergic stimulation. At doses greater than 20 mcg/kg/min, marked vasoconstriction and increases in myocardial contractility occur. Myocardial workload is increased without an increase in coronary blood supply, a situation that may cause myocardial ischemia.

Dopamine is administered by continuous IV infusion starting at 5 mcg/kg/min, and the dose is titrated upward. A dilution of 400 to 800 mg of dopamine in 250 to 500 mL of D_5W delivers 1600 to 3200 mcg/mL. Box 9-8 demonstrates the steps in the calculation of an IV infusion in micrograms per kilogram per minute. The lowest dose necessary for blood pressure control should be used to minimize side effects and to ensure adequate perfusion of vital organs.

BOX 9-8

Drug Calculation Case

A 55-year-old man has been successfully defibrillated. He remains hypotensive with a blood pressure of 78/40 mm Hg despite two fluid challenges (each with 250 mL of normal saline). The decision is made to initiate a dopamine infusion at 5 mcg/kg/min. The patient weighs 165 lb. Your crash cart contains premixed dopamine with 800 mg in 250 mL of 5% dextrose in water.

Step 1. Determine the patient's weight in kilograms (2.2 lb/kg).

$$165/2.2 = 75 \text{ kg}$$

Step 2. Determine the concentration of solution: Total amount of the drug/Total amount of the solution.

  a. Convert milligrams to micrograms to determine the total amount of drug in solution.

$$800 \text{ mg} \times 1000 = 800,000 \text{ mcg}$$

  b. Divide this number by the total number of milliliters in the intravenous bag.

$$800,000/250 = 3200$$

  c. The solution contains 3200 mcg/mL dopamine.

Step 3. Determine the number of milliliters per hour that must be delivered for 5 mcg/kg/min to be provided.

Desired dose × 60 (minutes in 1 hour) ×
Body weight in kg/concentration/mL of drug:

$$(5 \times 60 \times 75)/3200 \text{ mcg/mL} =$$
$$22,500/3200 = 7.03 \text{ or } 7 \text{ mL/hr}$$

In addition to causing myocardial ischemia, dopamine may also cause cardiac dysrhythmias, such as tachycardia and premature ventricular contractions. Necrosis and sloughing of tissue may occur if the drug infiltrates; therefore, it should be infused into a central line if possible. Phentolamine, 5 to 10 mg in 10 to 15 mL of NS, can be injected into the infiltrated area to prevent necrosis.

CALCIUM CHLORIDE

Calcium increases the force of myocardial contraction. The only use of calcium chloride in a code is the treatment of underlying hypocalcemia, hyperkalemia, or calcium channel blocker toxicity that may be a cause of the arrest. Unless these conditions are present, calcium chloride should not be used in resuscitation efforts.

For hyperkalemia and calcium channel overdose in a code, 8 to 16 mg/kg of a 10% solution is administered via IV push. (A 10-mL prefilled syringe of 10% calcium chloride yields 100 mg/mL.) This dose may be repeated if necessary. Calcium must be administered slowly to prevent a decrease in the heart rate (when the heart is beating). Ventricular irritability and coronary or cerebral vasospasm may also occur after administration.

AMIODARONE (CORDARONE)

Amiodarone is a unique antidysrhythmic possessing some characteristics of all groups of antidysrhythmic drugs. It reduces membrane excitability, and by prolonging the action potential and retarding the refractory period it facilitates the termination of VT and VF. Many antidysrhythmic agents, despite their effectiveness in suppression of dysrhythmias, also have a propensity to exacerbate dysrhythmias. This property is known as prodysrhythmia. Unlike many other antidysrhythmics, amiodarone is only rarely prodysrhythmic and has not been shown to increase mortality (Kudenchuk, 2002; Dorian et al., 2002). It is less likely to produce hypotension and myocardial depression than is procainamide. Amiodarone has the added benefit of dilating coronary arteries and increasing coronary blood supply. Amiodarone also decreases systemic vascular resistance, and in patients with impaired left ventricular function it can improve cardiac pump function. A meta-analysis of studies concluded that amiodarone reduces the rate of dysrhythmic/sudden cardiac death in high-risk patients with recent myocardial infarction or congestive heart failure (Gonzalez, Kannewurf, & Ornato, 1998).

IV amiodarone is indicated for treatment and prophylaxis of recurring VF and unstable VT refractory to other treatment. It is also used in supraventricular tachycardia for rate control or conversion of atrial fibrillation or flutter, especially in patients with heart failure (Eisenberg and Mengert, 2001). Bolus and infusion rates are described in Table 9-4. During cardiac arrest, however, it may be administered as a 300 mg loading bolus. Supplemental bolus doses of 150 mg may be administered for recurrent VT/VF. A loading infusion of 360 mg amiodarone over 60 minutes may be given. A maintenance infusion is administered at a rate of 0.5 mg/min until a maximum dose of 2 g (AHA, 2000). Adverse reactions include hypotension and bradycardia, which can be prevented by slowing the infusion rate or treating the patient with fluids, vasopressors, chronotropic medications, or temporary pacing.

Special Problems During a Code

In addition to electrical and pharmacological interventions carried out in a code, immediate treatment of the underlying cause of the arrest may be necessary. Tension pneumothorax and cardiac tamponade are two such problems that require rapid invasive therapeutic techniques.

TENSION PNEUMOTHORAX

A tension pneumothorax occurs when air enters the pleural space but cannot escape (Figure 9-18). Pressure increases in the pleural space and causes the lung to collapse. Tension pneumothorax is a life-threatening emergency. It may be caused by barotrauma from mechanical ventilation, blunt or penetrating trauma,

or invasive procedures that inadvertently cause air to enter the pleural space. Symptoms of a tension pneumothorax include dyspnea, chest pain, tachypnea, tachycardia, and jugular venous distention. On assessment, breath sounds on the affected side are diminished, and the trachea may be shifted to the opposite side. If left untreated, the tension pneumothorax may progress and cause cardiovascular collapse and cardiac arrest. Because little time exists for radiographic confirmation, a needle may be inserted into the second or third anterior intercostal space on the affected side if tension pneumothorax is suspected. If air is under pressure in the pleural space, it will escape through the needle and make a hissing noise. As soon as possible after needle placement, a chest tube must be inserted to restore negative pressure in the chest and to reexpand the lung.

PERICARDIAL TAMPONADE

Pericardial tamponade is the accumulation of fluid in the pericardial sac. The fluid causes a decrease in ventricular filling and results in decreased cardiac output. PEA or cardiac arrest may follow. Cardiac tamponade can be caused by such events as trauma, pericarditis, CPR, or invasive procedures. The patient with cardiac tamponade has increased central venous pressure, hypotension with narrowing of the arterial pulse pressure, and paradoxical pulse. Paradoxical pulse is the exaggerated fluctuation of arterial pressure during the respiratory cycle. It is defined as a peak systolic blood pressure drop of greater than 10 mm Hg during normal inspiration. Further assessment may

Geriatric Assessment

- Many elderly patients in the hospital would not want their stated resuscitation preferences followed if they were to lose their decision-making capacity. They would prefer that their family and physician make resuscitation decisions for them (Puchalski et al., 2000).
- Elderly patients have an increased incidence of complications from chest compressions, including rib fractures, sternal fractures, pneumothorax, and hemothorax.
- Declines in hepatic and renal functioning occur in the elderly that may result in higher than desired serum drug concentrations and adverse drug reactions with standard therapeutic dosing regimens.
- Beta-adrenergic receptors on the myocardium in the elderly are less responsive to changes in heart rate and cardiac contractility. Heart rate responses to beta-blocker (propranolol, metoprolol) and parasympathetic (atropine) medications are less.
- A decline in heart rate and slowing of conduction through the atrioventricular node result in a narrow therapeutic range for cardiovascular medications.
- Cardiopulmonary resuscitation is less likely to be effective in patients older than 70 years of age with comorbidities, unwitnessed arrest, terminal arrhythmias (asystole, pulseless electrical activity), cardiopulmonary resuscitation duration greater than 15 minutes, metastatic cancer, sepsis, pneumonia, renal failure, trauma, and acute and sustained hypotension (Robinson, 2002).

TENSION PNEUMOTHORAX

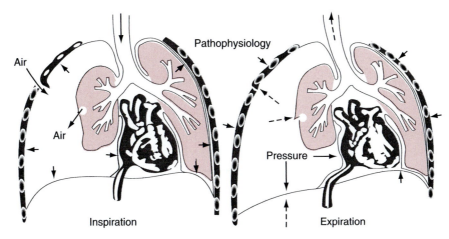

FIGURE 9-18 Tension pneumothorax. On inspiration, air enters the pleural space. On expiration, air is unable to escape the pleural space. Pressure increases, causing the lung on the affected side to collapse and the trachea to shift to the opposite side. (From Alspach, J. G. [Ed.] [2001]. *AACN instructor's resource manual for the AACN core curriculum for critical care nursing, ed. 5.* Philadelphia: W. B. Saunders.)

reveal distant or muffled heart tones. Pericardiocentesis, or needle aspiration of pericardial fluid, is performed to alleviate the pressure around the heart. Additionally, rapid administration of IV fluids (to increase preload and stroke volume) and drugs such as epinephrine or isoproterenol may be used temporarily to increase stroke volume and cardiac output.

Documentation of Code Events

A detailed chronological record of all interventions must be maintained during a code. One of the first actions of the nurse team leader or nursing supervisor is to ensure that someone is assigned to record information throughout the code.

Documentation includes the time the code is called, the time CPR is started, any actions that are taken, and the patient's response (e.g., pulse, blood pressure, cardiac rhythm). Intubation and defibrillation (and the energy used) must be documented, along with the patient's response. The time and sites of IV initiations, types and amounts of fluids administered, and medications given to the patient are all accurately recorded. Rhythm strips are recorded to document events and response to treatment. Many hospitals have standardized code records (Figure 9-19) that list actions and medications and include spaces for the time of interventions and any comments. It is best if information can be recorded directly on the code record during

the code to ensure that all information is obtained. The code record is signed by the code team and becomes part of the patient's permanent record.

Care of the Patient After Resuscitation

The survivor of a cardiac or respiratory arrest requires intensive monitoring and care. If the patient is not already in a critical care unit, he or she is transferred to one as soon as possible.

Postresuscitation goals include optimizing tissue perfusion by airway and blood pressure maintenance, oxygenation, and control of dysrhythmias. Underlying abnormalities that may have caused the arrest, such as hypokalemia and myocardial ischemia, are corrected. See the Laboratory Alerts box (p. 243) which summarizes critical electrolyte values associated with these conditions. These values are assessed and treated. Oxygenation and acid-base status must also be assessed.

Oxygen is given at a concentration of 100%. It is adjusted according to arterial blood gas and pulse oximetry values. A 12-lead ECG and chest x-ray study are done and compared to previous results. Dopamine or other pharmacological intervention may be needed for the maintenance of systolic blood pressure at or greater than 90 mm Hg. Blood pressure and heart rate are recorded at least every 30 minutes during

THE CLEVELAND CLINIC FOUNDATION
CPR DATA SHEET & EMERGENCY MEDICAL RESPONSE

DATE: ___ / ___ / ___
LOCATION OF EVENT _____
WITNESSED EVENT: ☐ Yes ☐ No

ALS INTERVENTION: CHECK IF PRESENT @ ONSET
☐ ETT ☐ VENT ☐ IV ACCESS ☐ EXTERNAL PACING
(RECORD MA AND PACER RATE UNDER SIGNIFICANT EVENTS)

CONSCIOUS @ ARREST ☐ Yes ☐ No
PULSE @ ARREST ☐ Yes ☐ No
RESPIRATION @ ARREST ☐ Yes ☐ No

RHYTHM @ ONSET ☐ NSR ☐ A FIB ☐ BRADY ☐ ASYS ☐ PEA
☐ VFIB ☐ VTACH ☐ PVC

IMMEDIATE PRECIPITATING CAUSE
☐ ARRHYTHMIA ☐ HEMORRHAGE
☐ MYOCARDIAL ISCHEMIA/INFARCT ☐ SYNCOPE
☐ HYPOTENSION ☐ SEIZURE
☐ RESPIRATORY DEPRESSION ☐ UNKNOWN
☐ METABOLIC ☐ OTHER
☐ TAMPONADE

EVENTS LEADING TO CODE:
_____
_____

RECORD (IN MILITARY TIME):
EVENT NOTED @ _____
CODE CALLED @ _____
CPR STARTED @ _____
ARRIVAL 1ST PHYSICIAN @ _____
ARRIVAL ANESTHESIA @ _____
ARRIVAL RESPIRATORY TX @ _____
PATIENT INTUBATED @ _____

RESUSCITATION EFFORTS INITIATED:
☐ CPR
☐ DEFIB/CARDIOVERTED
☐ AIRWAY/INTUBATION
☐ CVP/VENOUS ACCESS
☐ MEDS ONLY

OUTCOME:
PATIENT EXPIRED @ _____
PATIENT TRANSFERRED @ _____
PATIENT TRANSFERRED TO _____
PATIENT REMAINED @ _____
FAMILY NOTIFIED @ _____

SIGNIFICANT EVENTS
(i.e. ABG results, CT insertion, code status change, etc)

I.V. BOLUS INJECTIONS
EPINEPHRINE · ATROPINE · AMIODARONE · Ca GLUCONATE · LIDOCAINE · MAGNESIUM SULFATE · NALOXONE · PROCAINAMIDE · SODIUM BICARBONATE · VASOPRESSIN

I.V. FLUIDS

CONTINUOUS I.V. INFUSIONS
AMIODARONE · DOPAMINE · EPINEPHRINE · LIDOCAINE · PROCAINAMIDE

Vital signs columns
TIME · HEART RATE · RHYTHM · B.P. · O₂ SATURATION · RESPIRATIONS · DEFIB/CARDIO JOULES (Mono Bi) · ABG's SENT

MEDICATION NURSE _____ DRUG BOX # _____
RECORDING NURSE _____

ANESTHESIA _____ PRINT NAME   RESPIRTORY THERAPIST _____ PRINT NAME   SIGNATURE
PHYSICIAN/EMT IN CHARGE OF RESUSCITATION _____ PRINT NAME
(SIGNATURE VERIFIES SHEET REVIEWED & AGREEMENT)
WHITE= CHART COPY   YELLOW= QUALITY MGMT

FIGURE 9-19 Sample of a code sheet used for documenting activities during a code. (Courtesy of The Cleveland Clinic Foundation, Cleveland, OH.)

LABORATORY ALERTS

Laboratory Test	Critical Value	Significance	Nursing Actions
Sodium (Na)	<136 *or* >145 mEq/L	Implications for polarization of heart muscle via Na-K pump	Identify abnormal values and report to physician
Potassium (K)	<3.5 *or* >5.3 mEq/L	Affects cardiac conduction and contraction Maintains cardiac cell homeostasis *ECG:* *Hypokalemia:* depressed ST segments, flat or inverted T wave, presence of U wave *Hyperkalemia:* tall, peaked T waves, disappearance of P waves, widening of QRS; can progress to asystole	Identify abnormal values; administer replacement per protocol or physician order Recheck levels, especially with diuretic therapy, dysrhythmias
Calcium (Ca)	<8.8 *or* >10.2 mg/dl	Affects cardiac cell action potential and contraction *ECG:* *Hypocalcemia:* prolonged QT interval *Hypercalcemia:* shortened QT interval	Alert physician to abnormal values Prolonged QT interval can precipitate ventricular dysrhythmias
Magnesium (Mg)	<1.3 *or* >2.5 mEq/L	Affects contraction of cardiac muscle and promotes vasodilation that may reduce preload, alter cardiac output, and reduce systemic blood pressure *ECG:* *Hypomagnesemia:* flat or inverted T waves, ST segment depression, prolonged QT interval *Hypermagnesemia:* peaked T waves, bradycardia, signs of depressed contractility	Check levels; administer replacement per protocol or physician order Suspect hypomagnesemia with prolonged hypokalemia despite K replacement

ECG, electrocardiogram

continuous infusions of vasoactive medications. If anti-dysrhythmic drugs were used successfully during the code, additional doses may be repeated to achieve adequate blood levels, or continuous infusions may be administered for 24 hours. Other drugs may be given to improve cardiac output and myocardial oxygen supply. Arterial lines and pulmonary artery catheters are frequently inserted after a code to facilitate hemodynamic assessment and patient treatment. A Foley catheter is inserted to monitor urinary output hourly. A nasogastric tube is inserted if bowel sounds are absent and in patients with a decreased level of consciousness who are mechanically ventilated. Management of patient care continues to focus on

the differential diagnosis to identify reversible causes of the arrest and underlying pathophysiology.

Psychosocial, Legal, and Ethical Implications

PSYCHOSOCIAL CONCERNS

Emotional support is an important aspect of care after an arrest. Fear of death or of a recurrence of the arrest is common. Survivors often feel the need to discuss their experience in depth, and nurses should listen objectively and provide psychological support. In addition to the patient, many other people are affected when a code occurs. Family members, roommates and other patients, and staff members are all affected by the emergency.

In the past, family members were not given the opportunity to be present at the bedside during resuscitation. However, research now supports the benefits of family presence during a code. Families who have been present during a code describe the benefits as knowing that everything possible was being done for their loved one, feeling supportive and helpful to the patient and staff, sustaining patient-family relationships, providing a sense of closure on a life shared together, and facilitating the grief process (Meyers et al., 2000; MacLean et al., 2003; Emergency Nurses Association, 2001a and b). In a prospective study by Meyers and colleagues (2000) and Eichhorn and associates (2001), approximately one third of patients' families did not want to be present during resuscitation in the emergency department. However, 100% of those who were present said that they would choose to do it again. Many health care providers are uncomfortable with having patients' families present during a code, but they do support the practice after they have experienced it (Meyers et al., 2000).

Decisions regarding family presence should be made on an individual basis, considering individual preferences and assessment of coping mechanisms (Emergency Nurses Association, 2001a, 2001b; Tucker, 2002). If family members are not in the patient's room during resuscitation, a staff member, chaplain, volunteer, or friend should remain with them during this time and keep them informed of the patient's progress. Honesty is crucial, and it is important that they know that their family member is receiving the best possible care. If the family is not in the facility during the code, the next of kin should be called as soon as possible and informed of the patient's critical status.

If the patient is successfully resuscitated, the family should be allowed to see the patient as soon as is feasible. Communication regarding the events and status of the patient is extremely important. If the patient does not survive, the family should be encouraged to see the patient if they were not present during the code; this measure may facilitate the grief process.

All efforts should be made to remove roommates and alert patients from the scene. If this is not feasible, the curtains should be drawn. These patients may experience fear and usually want to talk about the experience. As do the survivor and family members, they require emotional support. Patient privacy must also be protected; it suffices to tell curious patients that an emergency is in progress. It is also easy to overlook other patients and their needs during a code. If staff members are not performing a specific role in the code, they should clear the area and tend to other patients.

Staff members are also affected by a code. In addition to the grief that may be felt over the loss of a patient, guilt, anger, and anxiety may also be felt. Debriefings are helpful for the staff involved in a code. In these sessions, feelings and thoughts can be discussed. This is also an opportunity to critique the code and to learn what may be useful next time (AHA, 2001a).

LEGAL AND ETHICAL CONCERNS

In the absence of a written order from a physician to withhold resuscitative measures, CPR and a code must be initiated when a patient has a cardiopulmonary arrest. The physician and family together and, if possible, the patient, generally make the decision whether to resuscitate the patient. However, it is the physician who makes the decision to terminate resuscitation efforts in progress. Decisions about resuscitation status often create ethical dilemmas for the nurse, patient, and family (see Chapter 3).

In situations of terminal or prolonged catastrophic illness, the patient may wish not to be resuscitated. A competent patient is legally and ethically allowed to make the choice concerning his or her preference. If the patient is comatose or is otherwise unable to make end-of-life decisions (e.g., from irreversible brain damage), the health care team seeks to determine whether the patient would have wanted to be resuscitated in the present situation. Previously expressed wishes may exist in written form through advance directives. The patient may have written a living will or may have assigned a health care surrogate to make decisions for him or her. In addition to discussing what their wishes are, family members may be able to express what they believe the patient would have wanted. The patient and/or family members need to voice their wishes to the physician and discuss these issues. Often, it is the nurse who must approach a physician regarding a "do not resuscitate" order and must encourage open communication with the patient and family. It is best if discussions regarding code status occur as soon as it is evident that a cardiac or respiratory arrest is possible, so the decision can be made well before a code occurs. The patient and the patient's family should understand and agree with the decision, whether it be to withhold CPR or to do everything possible to sustain life. Discussions and orders related to treatment in the event of an arrest should be clearly documented in the medical record according to hospital policy.

RESEARCH ANALYSIS

ARTICLE REFERENCE

MacLean, S. L., Guzzetta, C. E., White, C., et al. (2003). Family presence during cardiopulmonary resuscitation and invasive procedures: Practices of critical care and emergency nurses. *American Journal of Critical Care, 12*(3), 246-257.

STUDY OVERVIEW

The purpose of this study was to identify the policies, preferences, and practices of critical care and emergency nurses for having patients' families present during resuscitation and invasive procedures. A 30-item survey was mailed to a random sample of 1500 members of the American Association of Critical-Care Nurses and 1500 members of the Emergency Nurses Association.

Among the 984 respondents (33% response rate), 5% worked on units with written policies allowing family presence during both resuscitation and invasive procedures. A significantly larger percentage (45% and 51%, respectively) worked on units that allowed family presence during resuscitation and invasive procedures without written policies. Some respondents preferred written policies allowing family presence (37% for resuscitation, 35% for invasive procedures), whereas others preferred unwritten policies allowing it (39% for resuscitation, 41% for invasive procedures). Many respondents had taken family members to the bedside (36% for resuscitation, 44% for invasive procedure) or would do so in the future (21% for resuscitation, 18% for invasive procedures). Family members often asked to be present (31% for resuscitation, 61% for invasive procedures).

The authors concluded that nearly all respondents have no written policies for family presence, yet most have done (or would do) it, prefer to be allowed, and are confronted with requests from family members to be present. Written policies or guidelines for family presence during resuscitation and invasive procedures are recommended.

CRITIQUE

This is the first nursing study to determine the policies, preferences, and practices of family presence during resuscitation and invasive procedures of a large number of critical care and emergency nurses. Most critical care and emergency nurses in this study supported family presence, and those who have experienced family presence tended to support the practice. Although most units have no written policies on family presence, many respondents reported that their units allowed the option. This informal practice may reflect family-centered care and the desire to meet the holistic needs of patients and families.

One limitation of this study was lack of reliability testing and no construct validity of the survey. In addition, only one third of the sample returned the survey, thus limiting the generalizability of the findings to this group. The preferences of patients' families for being present during resuscitation and invasive procedures were not examined.

NURSING IMPLICATIONS

Family presence during resuscitation and invasive procedures is controversial. The benefits of family presence during resuscitation and invasive procedures for patients, families, and nurses have been documented in this study as well as in many others. The implication of nurses' differences about whether a written policy is needed may reflect discomfort with family presence or resistance to changing a long-standing practice. However, as a result of consumer and professional organization demands, critical care and emergency departments will need to determine whether the departments support the practice and whether formal or informal guidelines are needed.

SUMMARY

Positive patient outcomes depend on the health care team members' ability to recognize problems rapidly and to intervene effectively. When a patient suffers a cardiac or respiratory arrest, or both, in the hospital, BCLS and ACLS measures must be initiated immediately. How the code team functions and how interventions are carried out affect the patient's potential for recovery. Thus, code management is an important topic for anyone involved in the care of patients, especially those in critical care areas.

CRITICAL THINKING QUESTIONS

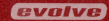

1. Discuss nursing strategies to be implemented during and after a code to provide psychosocial support to family members of patients suffering a cardiopulmonary arrest.

2. A surgical patient on a general nursing unit has just been successfully defibrillated with the use of an AED by the nursing staff. He is being manually ventilated with a BVD. Identify the current nursing priorities and their rationales.

3. You are the second nurse to respond to a code. The first nurse is administering CPR. Describe your first actions and their rationales.

4. Your patient has a permanent pacemaker or ICD. How would care and treatment of this patient differ in a code situation?

5. Some hospitals are now considering allowing family members to be present during a code.
   a. How could the presence of family members affect the management of the code?
   b. What factors should you consider before permitting family members to be present?

REFERENCES

American Heart Association. (2000). Guidelines 2000 for cardiopulmonary resuscitation and emergency cardiovascular care. *Circulation, 102*(8 suppl); I1-I384.

American Heart Association. (2001a). *ACLS provider manual.* Dallas, TX: Author.

American Heart Association. (2001b). *BLS for healthcare providers.* Dallas, TX: Author.

Dorian, P., Cass, D., Schwartz, B., Cooper, R., Gelaznikas, R., & Barr, A. (2002). Amiodarone as compared with lidocaine for shock-resistant ventricular fibrillation. *New England Journal of Medicine, 346*(12), 884-890.

Eichhorn, D. J., Meyers, T. A., Guzzetta, C. E., et al. (2001). Family presence during invasive procedures and resuscitation: Hearing the voice of the patient. *American Journal of Nursing, 101*(5), 48-55.

Eisenberg, M. S., & Mengert, T. J. (2001). Cardiac resuscitation. *New England Journal of Medicine, 344*(17), 1304-1313.

Emergency Nurses Association. (2001a). *Family presence at the bedside during invasive procedures and/or resuscitation* (ENA position statement). Des Plaines, IL: Author.

Emergency Nurses Association. (2001b). *Presenting the option for family presence.* 2nd ed. Des Plaines, IL: Author (www.ena.org).

Gonzalez, E. R., Kannewurf, B. S., & Ornato, J. P. (1998). Intravenous amiodarone for ventricluar arrythmias: Overview and clinical use. *Resuscitation 39*(1-2), 33-42.

Kudenchuk, P. J. (2002). Advanced cardiac life support antiarrhythmic drugs. *Cardiology Clinics, 20*(1), 79-87.

MacLean, S. L., Guzzetta, C. E., White, C., et al. (2003). Family presence during cardiopulmonary resuscitation and invasive procedures: Practices of critical care and emergency nurses. *American Journal of Critical Care, 12*(3), 246-257.

Meyers, T. A, Eichhorn, D. J., Guzzetta, C. E., et al. (2000). Family presence during invasive procedures and resuscitation: The experience of family members, nurses, and physicians. *American Journal of Nursing, 100*(2), 32-42.

Paul, S., & Hebra, J. D. (1998). *The nurse's guide to cardiac rhythm interpretation: Implications for patient care.* Philadelphia, PA: W. B. Saunders.

Puchalski, C. M., Zhong, Z., Jacobs, M. M., et al. (2000). Patients who want their family and physician to make resuscitation decisions for them: Observations from SUPPORT and HELP. *Journal of the American Geriatrics Society, 48*[5 suppl], S84-S90.

Robinson, E. M. (2002). Ethical analysis of cardiopulmonary resuscitation for elders in acute care. *AACN Clinical Issues, 13*(1), 132-144.

Tucker, T. L. (2002). Family presence during resuscitation. *Critical Care Clinics of North America, 14*(2), 177-185.

RECOMMENDED READINGS

Dries, D. J., & Sample, M. A. (2002). Recent advances in emergency life support. *Nursing Clinics of North America, 37*(1), 1-10.

Tsai, E. (2002). Should family members be present during cardiopulmonary resuscitation? *New England Journal of Medicine, 346*(13), 1019-1021.

Williams, J. (2002). Family presence during resuscitation: To see or not to see. *Nursing Clinics of North America, 37*(1), 211-220.

evolve *Did you remember to check out the bonus material, including free self-assessment exercises, on the Evolve Web site at http://evolve.elsevier.com/Sole/ and on the CD-ROM?*

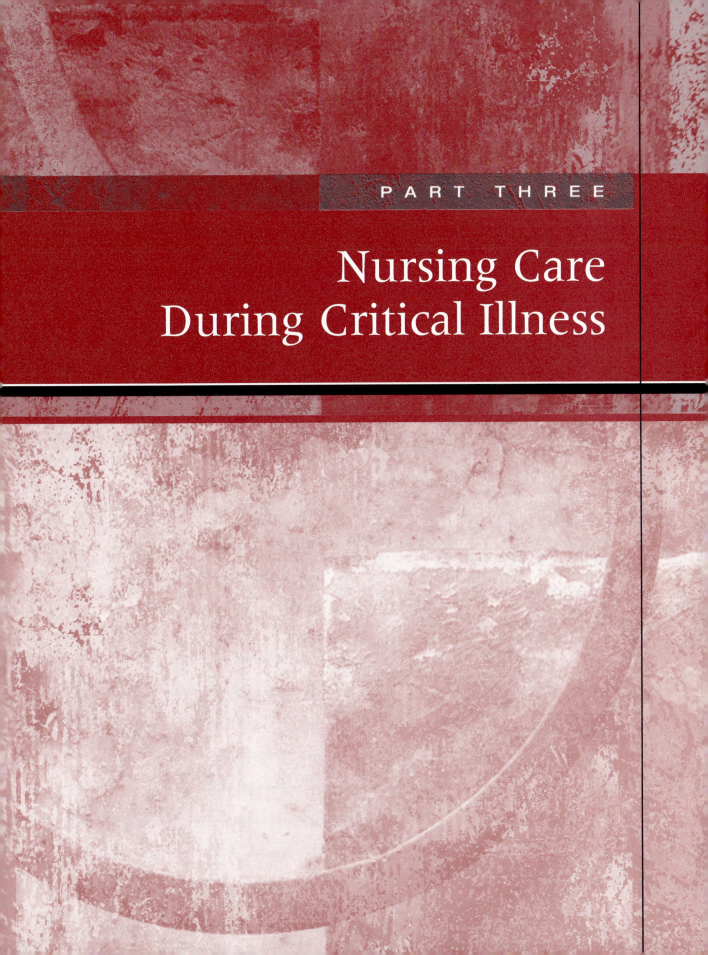

PART THREE

Nursing Care
During Critical Illness

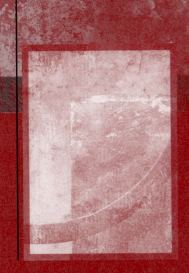

CHAPTER 10

Shock and Sepsis

Mary G. McKinley, MSN, RN, CCRN

OBJECTIVES

- Define shock.
- Describe the continuum of sepsis.
- Correlate the four classifications of shock to their pathophysiology.
- Discuss the progression of shock through three stages.
- Relate assessment findings to the classification and stage of shock.
- Describe management strategies for each type of shock.
- Develop an individualized plan of care that includes nursing diagnosis, expected outcomes, nursing interventions, and rationale.

Introduction

Shock is a clinical syndrome characterized by inadequate tissue perfusion that results in impaired cellular metabolism. This syndrome is a severe, life-threatening complication that can result from diverse patient conditions.

The effects of shock are not isolated to one organ system; instead, all body systems are affected. Shock is best described by its symptoms, the complex clinical picture that results from the underlying cause of the shock state, and the compensatory mechanisms initiated by the body in an attempt to restore homeostasis.

Athough the causes of shock differ, the end points of poor tissue perfusion and impaired cellular metabolism are common to all cases. Patient responses to the shock syndrome and its treatment vary, thus presenting a challenge to the patient and health care team. Nursing care of patients in shock requires critical thinking based on knowledge, skills, and the application of research.

The purpose of this chapter is to introduce the nurse to the complex syndrome of shock and its management. The classifications, pathophysiology, and assessment findings of shock are reviewed. Nursing diagnoses are identified to provide a plan of care. The complex management of the patient includes definitive and supportive intervention strategies related to the classification of shock. An overview of patient outcomes and a comprehensive plan of care complete the chapter.

evolve *Be sure to check out the bonus material, including free self-assessment exercises, on the Evolve Web site at http://evolve.elsevier.com/Sole/ and on the CD-ROM.*

Review of Anatomy and Physiology

The cardiovascular system is a closed, interdependent system composed of the heart, blood, and vascular bed. Arteries, arterioles, capillaries, venules, and veins make up the vascular bed. The microcirculation, the portion of the vascular bed between the arterioles and the venules, is the most significant portion of the circulatory system for cell survival (Figure 10-1). Its functions are the delivery of oxygen and nutrients to cells, the removal of waste products of cellular metabolism, and the regulation of blood volume. Additionally, the vessels of the microcirculation constrict or dilate selectively to regulate blood flow to cells in need of oxygen and nutrients.

The structure of the microcirculation differs according to the function of the tissues and organs it supplies; however, all the vascular beds have common structural characteristics (see Figure 10-1). As oxygenated blood leaves the left side of the heart and enters the aorta, it flows through progressively smaller arteries until it flows into an arteriole. Arterioles are lined with smooth muscle, which allows these small vessels to change diameter and, as a result, to direct and adjust blood flow to the capillaries. From the arteriole, blood then enters a metarteriole, a smaller vessel that branches from the arteriole at right angles. Metarterioles are partially lined with smooth muscle, which also allows them to adjust diameter size and to regulate blood flow into capillaries.

Blood next enters the capillary network by passing through a muscular precapillary sphincter. Capillaries are narrow, thin-walled vascular networks that branch off the metarterioles. This network configuration increases the surface area to allow for greater fluid and nutrient exchange. It also decreases the velocity of the blood flow to prolong transport time through the capillaries. Capillaries have no contractile ability and are not responsive to vasoactive chemicals, electrical or mechanical stimulation, or pressure across their walls. The precapillary sphincter is the only means of regulating blood flow into a capillary. When the precapillary sphincter constricts, blood flow is diverted away from a capillary bed and directed to one that supplies tissues in need of oxygen and nutrients. The capillary bed lies close to the cells of the body, a position that facilitates the delivery of oxygen and nutrients to the cells.

Once nutrients are exchanged for cellular waste products in the capillaries, blood enters a venule. These small muscular vessels are able to dilate and constrict, offering postcapillary resistance for the regulation of blood flow through capillaries. Blood then flows from the venule and enters the larger veins of the venous system.

Another component of the microcirculation consists of the arteriovenous anastomoses that connect arterioles directly to venules. These muscular vessels are able to shunt blood away from the capillary circulation and send it directly to tissues in need of oxygen and nutrients.

Changing pressures within the vessels as blood moves from an area of high pressure within the arteries and passes to the venous system, which has lower pressures, facilitate the flow of blood. The force of resistance opposes blood flow; thus, as resistance increases, blood flow decreases. Resistance is determined by three factors: (1) vessel length, (2) blood viscosity, and (3) vessel diameter (Huffstutler, 2003). Increased resistance occurs with increased vessel length, increased blood viscosity, and decreased blood vessel diameter.

Vessel diameter is the most important determinant of resistance. As the pressure of blood within the vessel decreases, the diameter of the vessel decreases, resulting in decreased blood flow. The critical closing pressure and the resultant cessation of blood flow occur when blood pressure decreases to a point at which it is no longer able to keep the vessel open. These alterations in circulation initiate the pathophysiology of shock.

PATHOPHYSIOLOGY

Shock begins when the cardiovascular system fails to function properly because of an alteration in at least one of the four essential circulatory components: blood volume, myocardial contractility, blood flow, and vascular resistance. Under healthy circumstances,

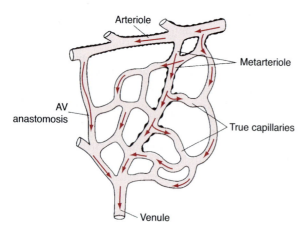

FIGURE 10-1 Microcirculation. *AV,* Arteriovenous. (Redrawn from Perry, A. G., & Potter, P. A. [1983]. *Shock: Comprehensive nursing management.* St. Louis, MO: Mosby.)

TABLE 10-1

Classification of Shock

Altered Circulation Component	Type of Shock
Blood volume	Hypovolemic shock
Myocardial contractility	Cardiogenic shock
Blood flow	Obstructive shock
Vascular resistance	Distributive shock

these components function together to maintain circulatory homeostasis. When one of these components fails, the others compensate. However, as compensatory mechanisms fail, or if more than one of the circulatory components are affected, a state of shock ensues. Shock is not a single clinical entity but a life-threatening response to alterations in circulation resulting in impaired tissue perfusion. As the delivery of adequate oxygen and nutrients decreases, impaired cellular metabolism occurs. Cells convert from aerobic to anaerobic metabolism. Less energy in the form of adenosine triphosphate (ATP) is produced. Lactic acid, a by-product of anaerobic metabolism, causes tissue acidosis. Cells in all organ systems require energy to function, and this resultant tissue acidosis causes organ dysfunction.

Diverse events can initiate the shock syndrome. These events are classified according to the affected circulatory component (Table 10-1) (Tierney & Messina, 2003).

STAGES OF SHOCK

Although the response to shock is highly individualized, a pattern of stages progresses at unpredictable rates. These stages of shock appear to occur regardless of the type of shock experienced. If these stages of shock are not recognized and treated, progression to the next stage occurs. A summary of the pathophysiological events and resultant clinical findings for each stage can be found in Table 10-2.

Stage I: Early, Reversible, and Compensatory Stage

As shock ensues, the sustained reduction in cardiac output initiates a set of neural, endocrine, and chemical compensatory mechanisms in an attempt to maintain blood flow to vital organs and to restore homeostasis. During this stage, symptoms become apparent, but shock may still be reversed with minimum morbidity if appropriate interventions are initiated (Tierney & Messina, 2003).

Neural compensation. Baroreceptors (which are sensitive to pressure changes) and chemoreceptors (which are sensitive to chemical changes) located in the carotid sinus and aortic arch detect the reduction in arterial blood pressure. Impulses are relayed to the vasomotor center in the medulla oblongata, stimulating the sympathetic branch of the autonomic nervous system to release epinephrine and norepinephrine from the adrenal medulla. In response to these catecholamines, the heart increases the rate and the force of contractions to improve cardiac output and to supply the heart muscle with more oxygen. The coronary arteries vasodilate to increase blood flow to the heart to meet the increased demands for oxygen. Systemic vasoconstriction occurs. Arterial vasoconstriction improves blood pressure, whereas venous vasoconstriction augments venous return to the heart, thus increasing cardiac output. Blood is shunted from the kidneys, gastrointestinal tract, and skin to the heart and brain. Bronchial smooth muscles are relaxed, and respiratory rate and depth are increased, thus improving oxygenation and gas exchange. Additional catecholamine effects are as follows: an increase in blood glucose level as the liver is stimulated to convert glycogen to glucose for energy production; dilation of pupils; and cool, moist skin that is caused by peripheral vasoconstriction and increased sweat gland activity.

Endocrine compensation. In response to the reduction in blood pressure, messages are also relayed to the hypothalamus, which stimulates the anterior and posterior pituitary gland. The anterior pituitary gland releases adrenocorticotropic hormone, which acts on the adrenal cortex to release glucocorticoids and mineralocorticoids (aldosterone). Glucocorticoids increase the blood glucose level by increasing the conversion of glycogen to glucose (glycogenolysis). Mineralocorticoids act on renal tubules to reabsorb sodium, chloride, and water resulting in increased intravascular volume and blood pressure. Aldosterone is also released in response to a reduction of pressure in the renal arterioles of the kidneys and/or by a decrease in sodium levels as sensed by the kidney's juxtaglomerular apparatus. In response to decreased renal perfusion, the juxtaglomerular apparatus releases renin. Renin circulates in the blood and reacts with angiotensinogen to produce angiotensin I. Angiotensin I circulates through the lungs, where it forms angiotensin II, a potent arterial and venous vasoconstrictor that increases blood pressure and improves venous return to the heart. Angiotensin II also activates the adrenal cortex to release aldosterone.

Stimulation of the posterior pituitary gland releases antidiuretic hormone, which is secreted in response

Stages of Shock

Stage of Shock	Physiological Events	Clinical Picture

Stage 1: Compensatory	Neural compensation
	Sympathetic stimulation
	  Mild to moderate vasoconstriction
	  Bronchodilation
	Endocrine compensation
	Some anaerobic metabolism
	Glycogen conversion to glucose
		↓ MAP of 5-15 mm Hg from baseline
		Normal BP with narrow pulse pressure
		Sinus tachycardia
		Rapid, deep respirations
		Initially, respiratory alkalosis with hypoxemia and mild metabolic acidosis late in compensatory stage
		↓ Urinary output
		↑ Specific gravity
		↑ Thirst
		Cool, clammy skin
		Altered level of consciousness
		Dilated pupils
		Mild hyperkalemia
		Hyperglycemia

Stage II: Progressive	Anoxia of nonvital organs Hypoxia of vital organs ↓ Production of ATP Overall anaerobic metabolism Tissue ischemia Failure of sodium-potassium pump	↓ BP with narrow pulse pressure Sinus tachycardia Rapid, deep respirations Crackles Pulmonary edema Metabolic acidosis and respiratory acidosis with hypoxemia ↓ Urinary output ↑ Urinary specific gravity and ↓ creatinine clearance ↑ BUN, creatinine, and potassium Altered level of consciousness Peripheral edema Dysrhythmias
Stage III: Irreversible	Severe tissue hypoxia with ischemia and necrosis Release of myocardial depressant factor Build-up of toxic metabolites	Severe hypotension Respiratory failure Metabolic and respiratory acidosis Peripheral edema Oliguria to anuria with acute renal failure Coagulation alterations

↑, Increased; ↓, decreased; *ATP,* adenosine triphosphate; *BP,* blood pressure; *BUN,* blood urea nitrogen; *MAP,* mean arterial pressure.

to the increased osmolarity of the blood that occurs in shock. The overall effects of endocrine compensation result in an attempt to combat shock by providing the body with glucose for energy and by increasing the intravascular blood volume.

Chemical compensation. As cardiac output decreases, pulmonary blood flow is reduced, resulting in ventilation-perfusion imbalances. The alveoli may be adequately ventilated with oxygen, but the perfusion of blood through the alveolar capillary bed is decreased. Chemoreceptors located in the aorta and carotid arteries are stimulated in response to this low oxygen tension in the blood. Consequently, the rate and depth of respirations increase. As the patient hyperventilates, carbon dioxide is excreted, and respiratory alkalosis occurs. A reduction in carbon dioxide levels and the alkalotic state cause vasoconstriction of cerebral blood vessels. This vasoconstriction, coupled with the reduced oxygen tension, may lead to cerebral hypoxia and ischemia. The overall effects of chemical compensation result in an attempt to combat shock by increasing oxygen supply; however, in doing so they cause negative effects on cerebral perfusion.

Stage II: Intermediate, or Progressive Shock

If the cause of shock is not corrected, or if compensatory mechanisms continue without reversing the shock, further patient deterioration occurs. Whereas during the compensatory stage the systemic and microcirculation worked together with vasoconstriction to increase venous return, they now begin to function independently and in opposition (Smith-Blair, 2003).

The systemic circulation continues to vasoconstrict. Although this effect shunts blood to vital organs, the decrease in cutaneous blood flow leads to ischemia in extremities, weak or absent pulses, and altered body defenses. Prolonged vasoconstriction results in decreased capillary blood flow and cellular hypoxia. The cells convert to anaerobic metabolism, producing lactic acid, which leads to metabolic acidosis. This anaerobic metabolism leads to a decrease in the production of ATP, which further reduces energy available for cellular metabolism. The lack of ATP also causes failure of the sodium-potassium pump. Sodium and water accumulate within the cell, resulting in cellular swelling and a further reduction in cellular function.

The microcirculation exerts the opposite effect and dilates to obtain the blood supply for local tissue needs. Whereas the arterioles remain constricted in an attempt to keep vital organs perfused, the precapillary sphincters relax, allowing blood to flow into the capillary bed. Meanwhile, postcapillary sphincters remain constricted. As a result, blood flows freely into the capillary bed but accumulates in the capillaries as blood flow exiting the capillary bed is impeded. Capillary hydrostatic pressure increases, and fluid is pushed from the capillaries into the interstitial space, causing edema. Fluid shift from the intravascular space is further aggravated as histamine release increases capillary permeability, and the loss of proteins through enlarged capillary pores lowers colloidal osmotic pressure. As intravascular blood volume decreases, the blood becomes more viscous, and blood flow is slowed. This situation causes capillary sludging as red blood cells, platelets, and proteins clump together. The loss of intravascular volume and capillary pooling further reduce the venous return to the heart and cardiac output. Coronary perfusion is impaired, and ischemia results when the systolic pressure is less than 60 mm Hg (Maier, 2001). Cardiac contractility, cardiac output, and blood pressure decrease,

potentiating cellular hypoxia. The vicious cycle of shock perpetuates as the body attempts to compensate with further vasoconstriction. At this point, the patient presents with classic shock signs and symptoms that affect all body systems. This phase of shock responds poorly to fluid replacement alone and requires aggressive interventions if it is to be reversed.

Stage III: Refractory, or Irreversible, Shock

Prolonged inadequate tissue perfusion that is unresponsive to therapy ultimately contributes to multiple organ dysfunction and death. A large volume of the blood remains pooled in the capillary bed, and the arterial blood pressure is too low to support perfusion of the vital organs. Poor renal function, respiratory failure, and impaired cellular function aggravate the existing state of acidosis, which, in turn, contributes to further fluid shifts, loss of vasomotor tone, and relative hypovolemia. Coronary artery perfusion and oxygen delivery to the heart muscle are reduced, causing myocardial ischemia and dysrhythmias. Myocardial depressant factor is released. These alterations in the cardiovascular system and continued acidosis cause a reduction in heart rate, impaired contractility, and a further decrease in cardiac output (Pathan, Sandford, Harding, & Levin, 2002).

Acidosis, decreased intravascular fluid volume, and sluggish blood flow through the capillaries lead to clumping of platelets and red blood cells. These aggregates form fibrin clots that occlude small vessels and further impede blood flow. This cycle depletes clotting factors and may result in alterations in coagulation. Cerebral ischemia occurs as a result of the reduction in cerebral blood flow. Consequently, the sympathetic nervous system is stimulated, an effect that aggravates the existing vasoconstriction, thereby increasing afterload and decreasing cardiac output. Prolonged cerebral ischemia eventually causes the loss of sympathetic nervous system response, and vasodilation and bradycardia result. The patient's decreasing blood pressure and heart rate cause a lethal decrease in tissue perfusion, multisystem organ failure that is unresponsive to therapy, and ultimately brain death and cardiopulmonary arrest.

CLASSIFICATIONS OF SHOCK

Hypovolemic Shock

Hypovolemic shock occurs when the circulating blood volume is inadequate to fill the vascular network. Intravascular volume deficits may be caused by external or internal losses (Box 10-1) (Tierney & Messina, 2003). In either case, the blood volume is depleted and is unavailable for the transport of oxygen and nutrients to tissues.

Causes of Hypovolemic Shock

EXTERNAL LOSSES
Blood
Plasma
Body fluid

INTERNAL LOSSES
Third-space sequestration
Fluid loss into intestinal lumen
Internal hemorrhage

External volume deficits include loss of blood, plasma, or body fluids. The most common cause of hypovolemic shock is hemorrhage. External loss of blood may occur after traumatic injury, surgery, obstetrical delivery, or with coagulation alterations (e.g., hemophilia, thrombocytopenia, disseminated intravascular coagulation, and anticoagulant medications). Hypovolemic shock resulting from hemorrhage is classified according to the volume of blood lost and the resultant effects on level of consciousness, vital signs, and urine output (Table 10-3).

External plasma losses may be seen in patients with exudative lesions or burn injuries. Excessive external loss of fluid may occur through the gastrointestinal tract (e.g., via suctioning, upper gastrointestinal bleeding, vomiting, diarrhea, reduction in oral fluid intake, fistulas), the genitourinary tract (e.g., as a result of excessive diuresis, diabetes mellitus with polyuria, diabetes insipidus, Addison's disease), or the skin (e.g., as a result of diaphoresis without fluid and electrolyte replacement).

Internal volume deficits caused by third-space sequestration, fluid leakage into the intestinal lumen, or internal hemorrhage may also result in hypovolemic shock. Third-space sequestration is seen in patients with ascites, peritonitis, and edema. Intestinal obstruction causes fluid to leak from the intestinal capillaries into the lumen of the intestine. Internal hemorrhage may be seen in patients with a ruptured spleen or liver, hemothorax, hemorrhagic pancreatitis, fractures of the femur or pelvis, and lacerations of the great vessels.

The severity of hypovolemic shock depends on the volume lost, the rate of volume loss, the patient's age, and the presence of other preexisting conditions. Hypovolemic shock results in a reduction of intravascular volume and a decrease in venous return to the right side of the heart. Ventricular filling pressures are reduced, resulting in a decrease in stroke volume and cardiac output. As the cardiac output decreases, blood pressure decreases and tissue perfusion decreases. The end result is impaired cellular metabolism as a result of the decrease in nutritional blood flow through capillaries that supply the cells with oxygen and nutrients (Figure 10-2).

TABLE 10-3

Classification of Hypovolemic Shock and Estimated Fluid and Blood Requirements*

	Class I	Class II	Class III	Class IV
Blood loss (mL)	Up to 750	750-1500	1500-2000	>2000
Blood loss (% blood volume)	Up to 15%	15%-30%	30%-40%	>40%
Pulse rate	<100	>100	>120	>140
Blood pressure	Normal	Normal	↓	↓
Pulse pressure (mm Hg)	Normal or ↓	↓	↓	↓
Respiratory rate	14-20	20-30	30-40	>35
Urine output (mL/hr)	>30	20-30	5-15	Negligible
CNS/Mental status	Slightly anxious	Mildly anxious	Anxious, confused	Confused, lethargic
Fluid replacement (3:1 rule)	Crystalloid	Crystalloid	Crystalloid and blood	Crystalloid and blood

*The guidelines are based on the "3-for-1" rule. This rule derives from the empirical observation that most patients in hemorrhagic shock require as much as 300 mL of electrolyte solution for each 100 mL of blood loss. Applied blindly, these guidelines can result in excessive or inadequate fluid administration. For example, a crush injury to the extremity may have hypotension out of proportion to blood loss and require fluids in excess of the 3:1 guidelines. In contrast, a patient whose ongoing blood loss is being replaced by blood transfusion requires less than 3:1. The use of bolus therapy with careful monitoring of the patient's response can moderate these extremes.
*For a 70-kg man.
↑, Increased; ↓, decreased; *CNS*, central nervous system.
Reproduced with permission from American College of Surgeons' Committee on Trauma. (1997). *Advanced Life Support® for Doctors*, Instructor Manual. 6th ed. Chicago: American College of Surgeons.

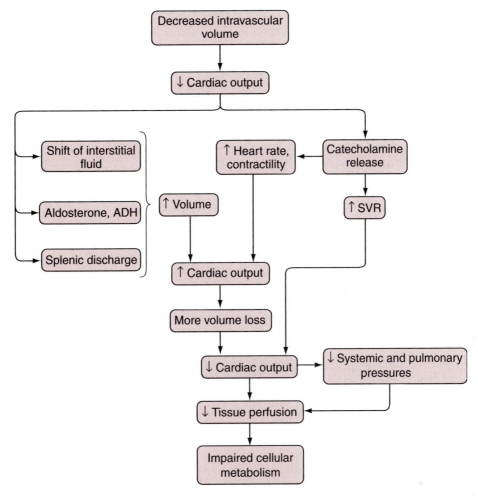

FIGURE 10-2 Hypovolemic shock. *ADH,* antidiuretic hormone; *SVR,* systemic vascular resistance. (Modified from McCance, K. L., & Huether, S. E. [eds.]. [2002]. *Pathophysiology: The biologic basis for disease in adults and children.* 4th ed. St. Louis, MO: Mosby.)

Cardiogenic Shock

Cardiogenic shock is caused when the heart fails to act as an effective pump. A decrease in myocardial contractility results in a decrease in cardiac output and impaired tissue perfusion. Cardiogenic shock is one of the most difficult types of shock to treat and carries a mortality of 50% to 80% (Hollenberg, Kavinsky, & Parillo, 1999).

Cardiogenic shock usually occurs when diseased coronary arteries are not capable of meeting the oxygen demand of the working myocardial cells, such as occurs in acute myocardial infarction. A correlation exists between the amount of myocardial damage and the likelihood of cardiogenic shock. If 40% or more of the left ventricle is damaged, the likelihood of cardiogenic shock increases (Loeb & Cohn, 2000).

Other causes of cardiogenic shock include conditions that result in ineffective myocardial cell function. These conditions include dysrhythmias, cardiomyopathy, myocarditis, metabolic derangement, valvular disease, and structural disorders.

The pathophysiology of cardiogenic shock can be understood by review of cardiac dynamics. Contractile force is responsible for the amount of blood ejected from the heart each beat, termed the *stroke volume.* Ventricular filling pressure or *preload* is the pressure in the ventricles as they fill. *Afterload* is the pressure the heart must overcome to empty the ventricles effectively. When damage to the myocardium occurs, contractile force is reduced, and stroke volume, ventricular filling pressure, and afterload are affected. Stroke volume is decreased because the heart is unable

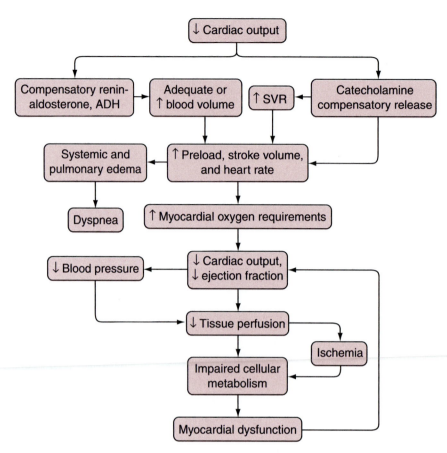

FIGURE 10-3 Cardiogenic shock. Shock becomes life threatening when compensatory mechanisms cause increased myocardial oxygen requirements. *ADH,* Antidiuretic hormone; *SVR,* systemic vascular resistance. (Modified from McCance, K. L., & Huether, S. E. [eds.]. [2002]. *Pathophysiology: The biologic basis for disease in adults and children.* 4th ed. St. Louis, MO: Mosby.)

to pump effectively and to eject adequate amounts of blood. Ventricular filling pressures begin to increase as the stroke volume decreases because blood remains in the cardiac chambers and increases pressure in the ventricles. As these two mechanisms occur, the cardiac output and ejection fraction decrease, causing hypotension. This hypotension brings about reflex compensatory peripheral vasoconstriction and increased afterload. At the same time, backup of blood into the pulmonary circulation causes decreased oxygen perfusion across alveolar membranes, thus reducing the oxygen tension in the blood and decreasing cellular metabolism (Figure 10-3).

The already failing heart is now in a crisis situation (Figure 10-4). An increased demand is placed on the myocardium as it attempts to increase perfusion to the cells. The heart rate increases as a compensatory mechanism, a phenomenon that increases the oxygen demand on an overworked myocardium, thereby compounding the problem. In patients with cardiogenic shock secondary to acute myocardial infarction, the increased demand may increase infarction size.

Obstructive Shock

Obstructive shock (also known as extracardiac obstructive shock) occurs when there is a physical impairment to adequate circulatory blood flow. The causes of obstructive shock are impaired diastolic filling, increased right ventricular afterload, and increased left ventricular afterload. Table 10-4 gives specific causes of obstructive shock.

Obstruction of the heart or great vessels either impedes venous return to the right side of the heart or prevents effective pumping action of the heart.

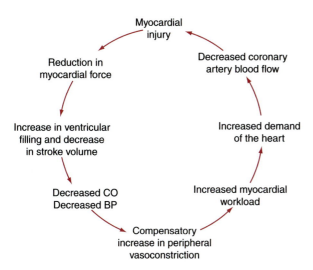

FIGURE 10-4 Cycle of cardiogenic shock. *BP,* Blood pressure; *CO,* cardiac output.

TABLE 10-4	
Causes of Obstructive Shock	

Mechanism	Examples
Impaired diastolic filling	Pericardial tamponade, tension pneumothorax, constrictive pericarditis, compression of great veins
Increased right ventricular afterload	Pulmonary emboli, pulmonary hypertension, positive end-expiratory pressure
Increased left ventricular afterload	Aortic dissection, systemic embolization, aortic stenosis, abdominal distention

This results in decreased cardiac output, a decreased blood pressure, and reduced tissue perfusion and cellular metabolism (Figure 10-5).

Distributive Shock

Distributive shock, also known as vasogenic shock, describes several different types of shock that have in common widespread vasodilation and decreased peripheral vascular resistance. Vasodilation increases the vascular capacity; however, the blood volume is unchanged, resulting in a relative hypovolemia. Neurogenic, anaphylactic, and septic are forms of distributive shock.

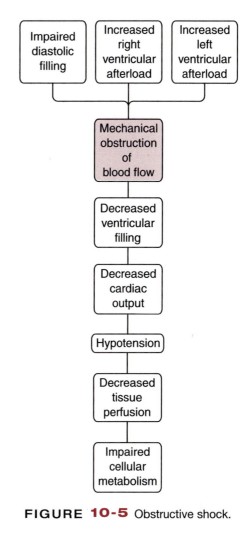

FIGURE 10-5 Obstructive shock.

Neurogenic shock. Neurogenic shock occurs when a disturbance in the nervous system affects the vasomotor center in the medulla. In healthy persons, the vasomotor center in the medulla initiates sympathetic stimulation of nerve fibers that travel down the spinal cord and out to the periphery. There, they innervate the smooth muscles of the blood vessels to cause vasoconstriction. In neurogenic shock, disturbances that interrupt sympathetic nerve impulses result in vasodilation. Consequently, these reactions create hypovolemia with decreased systemic vascular resistance, venous return, preload, and cardiac output. Bradycardia with hypotension from decreased sympathetic activity is common.

Causes of neurogenic shock include injury or disease of the upper spinal cord, spinal anesthesia, nervous system damage, ganglionic and adrenergic blocking agents, and vasomotor depression. Patients who have a cervical spinal cord injury may experience a permanent or temporary interruption in sympathetic nerve stimulation. Spinal anesthesia may extend up the spinal cord and may block sympathetic nerve impulses from the vasomotor center. Vasomotor depression may be seen with deep general anesthesia, injury to the medulla, administration of drugs, severe pain, and hypoglycemia.

Anaphylactic shock. A severe allergic reaction can precipitate a second form of distributive shock known as anaphylactic shock. Antigens, which are foreign substances to which someone is sensitive, initiate an antigen-antibody response. Table 10-5 lists some common antigens causing anaphylaxis grouped by the route in which they enter the body.

Once an antigen enters the body, antibodies are produced that attach to mast cells and basophils. The greatest concentrations of mast cells are found in the lungs, around blood vessels, in connective tissue, and in the uterus. Mast cells are also found to a lesser extent in the kidneys, heart, skin, liver, and spleen and in the omentum of the gastrointestinal tract. Basophils circulate in the blood. Both mast cells and basophils contain histamine and histamine-like substances, which are potent vasodilators.

The initial exposure to the antigen may not cause any harmful effects. However, subsequent exposures to the antigen cause an anaphylactic reaction. The antigen-antibody reaction causes cellular breakdown and the release of powerful vasoactive substances from the cells. These substances cause vasodilation, increased capillary permeability, and smooth muscle contraction. The combined effects are decreased blood pressure, relative hypovolemia caused by the vasodilation and fluid shifts, and symptoms of anaphylaxis that primarily affect the skin, respiratory, and gastrointestinal systems (see the later discussion of assessment).

Septic shock. Septic shock is one component of a continuum of progressive clinical insults including systemic inflammatory response syndrome (SIRS), sepsis, and multiple organ dysfunction syndrome (MODS). In the past, clinicians have used these terms without a common definition, and there has been much confusion about what various syndromes represent. Because of this confusion and the complexity of these syndromes, consensus definitions were identified in 1992 and were reviewed in 2001. The 2001 consensus group took the definitions a step further by identifying diagnostic criteria for sepsis. The list of signs and symptoms of sepsis reflects additional physical assessment and laboratory findings. The intent of the criteria is to provide a tool to recognize and diagnose sepsis quickly and therefore to prompt the search for an infectious source to initiate the appropriate therapy. None of the diagnostic criteria are specific for sepsis because these parameters can be altered by other findings. The definitions are presented in Box 10-2, and diagnostic criteria are presented in Box 10-3. Invasion of the host by a microorganism or an infection begins the process that progresses to sepsis, followed by severe sepsis and septic shock, which then progresses to MODS.

Once a microorganism has invaded a host, an inflammatory response is initiated to restore homeostasis. SIRS occurs, leading to a release of inflammatory mediators or cytokines, which are produced by the white blood cells. For reasons not completely understood, SIRS may progress to septic shock and MODS, as shown in Figure 10-6. Cytokines are proinflammatory or antiinflammatory. Proinflammatory cytokines (e.g., tumor necrosis factor, interleukin-1α and β) produce pyrogenic responses and initiate the hepatic response to infection. Antiinflammatory cytokines (e.g., nitric oxide, lipopolysaccharide, and interleukin 1–receptor antagonist) are compensatory, ensuring that the effect of the proinflammatory mediators does not become destructive (Sommers, 2003). In sepsis, continued activation of proinflammatory cytokines overwhelms the antiinflammatory cytokines, and excessive systemic inflammation results.

A state of enhanced coagulation occurs through stimulation of the coagulation cascade with a reduction

TABLE 10-5	
Classification of Antigens Causing Anaphylaxis	
Route	**Substance**
Medication administration	Antibiotics, analgesics, anesthetics, vaccine, hormones
Contrast media	Iodine-based radiological dye
Blood transfusions	Sensitivity to antigens in donor blood
Ingestion	Milk, egg, egg whites, oranges, mangos, bananas, beans, soybeans, sesame and sunflower seeds, seafood, shellfish, peanuts
Bites or stings	Venomous snakes, wasps, bees, hornets, yellow jackets

BOX 10-2

Definitions Relevant to Sepsis and Septic Shock

INFECTION
Inflammatory response to microorganisms

BACTEREMIA
Presence of bacteria in the blood

SYSTEMIC INFLAMMATORY RESPONSE SYNDROME (SIRS)
Systemic response to a clinical insult including infection, pancreatitis, ischemia, trauma, and hemorrhagic shock
Symptoms include fever or hypothermia, tachycardia, tachypnea, and leukocytosis or leukopenia

SEPSIS
Systemic response to infection manifested by two or more of the symptoms noted with SIRS

SEVERE SEPSIS
Sepsis associated with organ dysfunction, hypoperfusion, or hypotension
Alterations possibly including lactic acidosis, oliguria, and changes in mental status

SEPTIC SHOCK
Sepsis associated with hypotension despite adequate fluid resuscitation, along with perfusion abnormalities
Patients receiving inotropes or vasopressors may not exhibit hypotension

HYPOTENSION
Systolic blood pressure of ≤90 mm Hg or a reduction of ≥40 mm Hg from normal baseline

MULTIPLE ORGAN DYSFUNCTION SYNDROME (MODS)
Altered organ function in acutely ill patients

Modified from American College of Chest Physicians/Society of Critical Care Medicine Consensus Conference Committee. (1992). Definitions for sepsis and organ failure and guidelines for the use of innovative therapies in sepsis. *Critical Care Medicine, 20*(6), 864-874.

BOX 10-3

Diagnostic Criteria for Sepsis

Infection, documented or suspected, and some of the following:
General variables
   Fever (core temperature >38.3°C)
   Hypothermia (core temperature <36°C)
   Heart rate >90 beats/min or >2 SD above the normal value for age
   Tachypnea
   Altered mental status
   Significant edema or positive fluid balance (>20 mL/kg over 24 hr)
   Hyperglycemia (plasma glucose >120 mg/dL or 7.7 mmol/L) in the absence of diabetes
Inflammatory variables
   Leukocytosis (WBC count >12,000 μL)
   Leukopenia (WBC <4000 μL)
   Normal WBC with >10% immature forms
   Plasma C-reactive protein >2 SD above the normal value
   Plasma procalcitonin >2 SD above the normal value

Hemodynamic variables
   Arterial hypotension (SBP <90 mm Hg, MAP <70 mm Hg, or an SBP decrease >40 mm Hg in adults or <2 SD below normal for age)
   SvO_2 >70%
   Cardiac index >3.5 L/min/m^2
Organ dysfunction variables
   Arterial hypoxemia (PaO_2/FiO_2 <300)
   Acute oliguria (urine output <0.5 mL/kg/hr or 45 mmol/L for at least 2 hr)
   Creatinine increase >0.5 mg/dL
   Coagulation abnormalities (INR >1.5 or aPTT >60 sec)
   Ileus (absent bowel sounds)
   Thrombocytopenia (platelet count <100,000 μL)
   Hyperbilirubinemia (plasma total bilirubin >4 mg/dL or 70 mmol/L)
Tissue perfusion variables
   Hyperlactatemia (>1 mmol/L)
   Decreased capillary refill or mottling

aPTT, Activated partial thromboplastin time; *FiO₂,* fraction of inspired oxygen; *INR,* international normalized ratio; *MAP,* mean arterial blood pressure; *PaO₂,* partial pressure of arterial oxygen; *SBP,* systolic blood pressure; *SD,* standard deviation; *SvO₂,* mixed venous oxygen saturation; *WBC,* white blood count.
Modified from 2001 SCCM/ESICM/ACCP/ATS/SIS International Sepsis Definitions Conference. (2003). *Critical Care Medicine, 31*(4), 1250-1256.

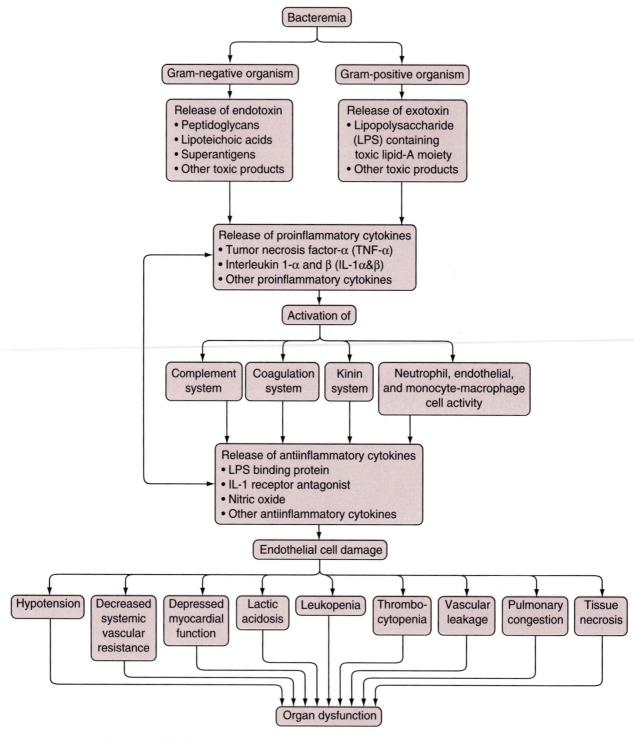

FIGURE 10-6 Septic shock cascade. (Modified from Larson, V., Barke, R. A. [1999]. Gram-negative bacterial sepsis and the sepsis syndrome. *Urology Clinics of North America, 26*[4], 687.)

in the levels of protein C and antithrombin III. This results in the generation of thrombin and the formation of microemboli that impair blood flow and organ perfusion. Fibrinolysis is activated in response to the activation of the coagulation cascade to promote clot breakdown. However, activation is followed by inhibition, further promoting coagulopathy. This imbalance among inflammation, coagulation, and fibrinolysis results in systemic inflammation, widespread coagulopathy, and microvascular thrombi that impair tissue perfusion leading to MODS.

Sepsis is present if two or more of the clinical manifestations of SIRS (temperature higher than 38°C or lower than 36°C, heart rate higher than 90 beats per minute, respiratory rate greater than 20 breaths per minute or arterial blood carbon dioxide level less than 32 mm Hg, and white blood cell count higher than 12,000 cells/µL) are identified (International Sepsis Definitions Conference, 2003). In addition to the SIRS criteria, other signs of sepsis include hypotension, chills, decreased urine output, decreased skin perfusion, poor capillary refill, skin mottling, decreased platelets, petechiae, hyperglycemia, and unexplained changes in mental status (Kleinpell, 2003). Factors that increase the risk of developing sepsis include underlying chronic disease, alteration in host defenses, long hospital stays, use of invasive catheters and devices, trauma, and surgical wounds. Additionally, the increased use of more potent and broader-spectrum antibiotics, immunosuppressive agents, and invasive technology has contributed to the increased incidence of infection in critical care. Predisposing risk factors in the development of sepsis and septic shock are summarized in Box 10-4.

Once sepsis is present, it can progress to septic shock. Septic shock is sepsis with hypotension that is unresponsive to fluid resuscitation along with signs of inadequate organ perfusion such as metabolic acidosis, acute encephalopathy, oliguria, hypoxemia or coagulation disorders, low blood pressure, low systemic vascular resistance from vasodilation, tachycardia, and fever or hypothermia. Clinical conditions, manifestations, and management in the continuum of sepsis and septic shock are summarized in Table 10-6.

Gram-negative bacteria (e.g., *Escherichia coli*, *Klebsiella* species, *Pseudomonas* species) are a common cause of infections in adults. Common sites of infection include the pulmonary system, urinary tract, gastrointestinal system, and wounds.

BOX 10-4

Predisposing Risk Factors in the Development of Sepsis and Septic Shock

COMPROMISED IMMUNITY

Chronic Debilitating Diseases

Neoplastic disease
Leukemia
Cirrhosis
Hepatitis
Diabetes mellitus
Cardiovascular disease
Pulmonary disease
Renal failure
Lupus erythematosus
Alcoholism
Human immunodeficiency virus infection

Anemia or Malnutrition

Skin Alterations

Burns
Ulcerations
Areas of tissue necrosis

Drug Therapy

Antibiotics
Immunosuppressives
Cytotoxics
Corticosteroids

Extremes of Age

<1 yr
>65 yr

SURGICAL AND INVASIVE PROCEDURES

Urological procedures
Bronchoscopy
Obstetrical-gynecological procedures
Septic abortion
Cesarean section
Hysterectomy for pelvic inflammatory disease

INVASIVE LINES AND CATHETERS

Indwelling catheters and drains
Pulmonary artery catheter
Central venous catheter
Endotracheal tube or tracheostomy

TABLE 10-6

Clinical Condition, Manifestations, and Management in the Continuum of Sepsis

Clinical Condition	Clinical Manifestations	Management
Infection	Fever	Administer antibiotics Perform surgical excision or drainage Potential future therapies: antiendotoxin/lipopolysaccharide, anti–tumor necrosis factor, or other mediator-specific therapies
Sepsis or systemic inflammatory response syndrome (SIRS)	Fever or hypothermia Tachycardia Tachypnea or $PaCO_2$ <32 mm Hg Leukocytosis, leukopenia, or >10% band forms	Administer antibiotics Remove source of infection Maintain adequate ventilation and oxygenation Replace fluid Antipyretics
Severe sepsis	As above with evidence of impaired systemic perfusion and organ function, possibly including lactic acidosis, oliguria, or acute change in mental status Possible hypotension Cardiac output typically high, systemic vascular resistance typically low	Administer antibiotics Remove source of infection Maintain adequate ventilation and oxygenation Maximize oxygen delivery, minimize oxygen demand Replace fluid Administer vasoactive medications Correct acid-base abnormalities Monitor and support organ function
Septic shock	Severe sepsis with hypotension and perfusion abnormalities despite fluid resuscitation Hypotension Lactic acidosis, oliguria, acute change in mental status Cardiac output typically high, systemic vascular resistance typically low for 24 hr	Administer antibiotics Maintain adequate ventilation and oxygenation Maximize oxygen delivery, minimize oxygen demand Replace fluid Administer vasoactive medications Correct acid-base abnormalities Monitor and support organ function
Multiple organ dysfunction syndrome (MODS)	See Table 10-12	Maintain adequate ventilation and oxygenation Maximize oxygen delivery, minimize oxygen demand Perform dialysis Monitor and support organ function Monitor clotting studies and bleeding

Gram-positive bacteria, such as *Staphylococcus aureus,* can also lead to sepsis and septic shock. These bacteria release a potent toxin that exerts its effects within hours. Gram-positive infection has been associated with the use of tampons in menstruating women (known as toxic shock syndrome); however, it is also seen after vaginal and cesarean delivery in patients with surgical wounds, deep and superficial abscesses, infected burns, abrasions, insect bites, herpes zoster, cellulitis, septic abortion, and osteomyelitis, as well as in some newborns in whom the bacteria are transmitted from the mother. Management includes antimicrobial therapy, removal of the source of infection if one is

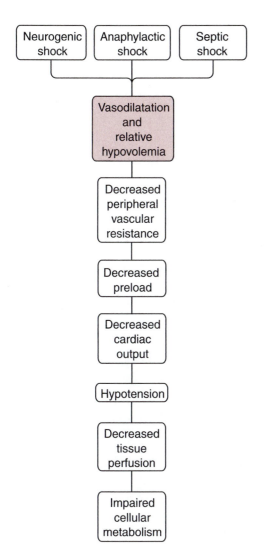

FIGURE 10-7 Distributive shock.

tissue perfusion. The end result is impaired cellular metabolism (Figure 10-7).

Assessment

Shock is a common risk to all critically ill patients. Shock is not selective in its effects—all cells, tissues, and organ systems suffer as a result of the physiological response to the stress of shock, decreased tissue perfusion, and cellular metabolism (Figure 10-8). The nurse's understanding of the pathophysiology of shock and identification of patients at risk are essential for the prevention of shock. An understanding of how cells and organ systems are affected facilitates assessment. Assessment focuses on three areas: history, clinical picture, and laboratory diagnosis. The logical approach for assessment is to examine the history of the patient and then look at the systems most sensitive to a lack of oxygen and nutrients.

HISTORY AND PREVENTION

An accurate and detailed history is essential for identifying patients with a high risk of developing shock, and it increases the likelihood that preventive steps can be taken. Information about potential causative events can assist with this identification.

Hypovolemic Shock

Hypovolemic shock may be prevented by assessment of fluid balance, hemodynamic values, and vital signs. Recognizing the need for fluid or blood product administration in those experiencing rapid or large volume losses is essential. One study demonstrated that the weekly administration of recombinant human erythropoietin (rHU-EPO or Procrit) could reduce the need for transfusion (with associated risks) and increase hemoglobin values in critically ill patients (Corwin, 2002). This may be a consideration for future prevention of hypovolemic shock in the critically ill patient. Fluid losses occur in frank or subtle ways. Assessment includes the following: weighing dressings; considering insensible losses, such as perspiration; and measuring drainage, such as from chest or nasogastric tubes. Abdominal girth is measured periodically in patients in whom hidden bleeding may be suspected or in those with ascites. Daily weights are obtained by using the same scale with the patient wearing the same clothing at approximately the same time each day.

Cardiogenic Shock

Prevention of cardiogenic shock is aimed at promoting myocardial contractile force, decreasing the myocardial oxygen demand, and increasing oxygen supply to the damaged tissue. Aggressive therapy, such as

found, fluid resuscitation, and vasoactive medication to improve cardiac performance.

All forms of distributive shock result in relative hypovolemia. Blood volume remains normal, but because of massive vasodilation and decreased peripheral vascular resistance, the blood is abnormally distributed in the resulting enlarged vascular space. This causes a decrease in venous return to the right side of the heart and a reduction in ventricular filling pressures. Anaphylactic shock and septic shock are also complicated by an increase in capillary permeability, which decreases intravascular volume, further compromising venous return. Eventually, in all forms of distributive shock, stroke volume, cardiac output, and blood pressure decrease, resulting in decreased

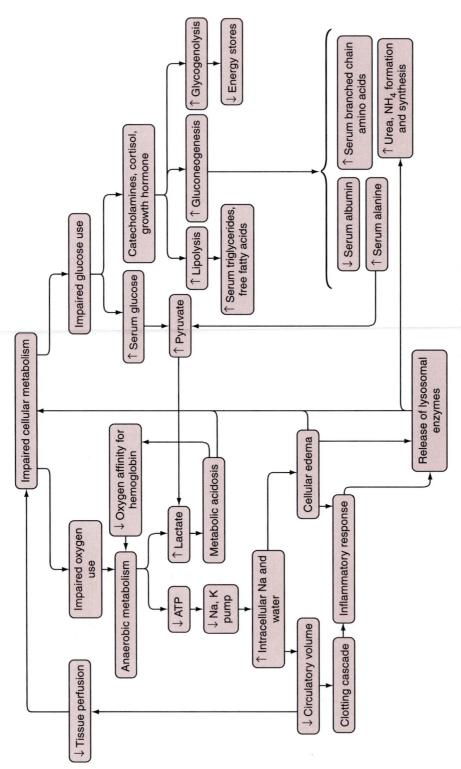

FIGURE 10-8 Impairment of cellular metabolism by shock. *ATP,* adenosine triphosphate. (From McCance, K. L., & Huether, S. E. [2002]. *Pathophysiology: The biologic basis for disease in adults and children.* 4th ed. St. Louis, MO: Mosby.)

Geriatric Assessment

- Cardiovascular changes in the elderly include the following:
  Left ventricular wall thickening, calcification and fibrosis of heart valves, less elastic and more rigid myocardium; decreased stroke volume resulting in a decreased cardiac output and decreased sensitivity of the baroreceptors (Miller, 2002). These changes create a decreased response to stress and increased oxygen demands.
  Older patients who are taking selected medications such as beta-blockers have a decreased ability to increase heart rate in the initial phase of shock.
  Arterial walls lose elasticity and vasomotor tone leading to an increase in the systemic vascular resistance and decreasing the body's ability to adapt to changing oxygen needs and response to catecholamines.
- Pulmonary changes in the elderly affect the ability of the respiratory system to assist in meeting the oxygen needs. These include: decreased elasticity in the chest wall, decreased alveolar perfusion, decreased alveolar surface area, and a thickening of the alveolar capillary membrane.
- The elderly may be more likely to suffer anaphylactic shock and transfusion reactions because of previous medication and blood administration.
- The immune system in elderly patients is less effective, so they are more susceptible to sepsis after illness or injury.
- The elderly have decreased elasticity of the skin and thinning of the epidermis, thus making assessment of skin turgor for adequate hydration difficult.
- Fluid administration in hypovolemic shock must be carefully monitored. Pulmonary artery catheterization may be needed to guide fluid resuscitation in shock.
- Older adults are more sensitive to medication dose adjustments and polypharmacy.

thrombolytic agents, glycoprotein IIb/IIIa inhibitors, beta-blockers, and percutaneous transluminal coronary angioplasty with stent placement, may help to limit the size of the infarction. Pain relief and rest are significant aids in reducing the workload of the heart and therefore infarct size. Oxygen administration increases oxygen delivery to the ischemic muscle and may help to save myocardial tissue. Close monitoring of the patient with dysrhythmias, and appropriate medical interventions, may also reduce the risk of the development of cardiogenic shock. A pulmonary artery catheter is useful in trending hemodynamic parameters. For cardiovascular changes in the elderly, see Geriatric Assessment.

Obstructive Shock

Obstructive shock may be prevented by aggressive interventions to relieve the source of the compression or obstruction. Pericardiocentesis, or the removal of fluid in the pericardial sac, is performed for the treatment of cardiac tamponade. A needle thoracentesis relieves the accumulated intrathoracic pressure associated with a tension pneumothorax that results from blunt or penetrating chest injuries. Early surgical reduction of long bone fractures, measures to enhance circulation in immobile patients (e.g., use of antiembolism hose, range-of-motion exercises), and prophylactic anticoagulant therapy reduce the risk of pulmonary emboli.

Distributive Shock

Immobilization of spinal injuries may assist in preventing severe neurogenic shock. Such measures include the use of traction devices, such as a halo brace (to maintain alignment) or surgical intervention to stabilize the injury. Frequent assessment of patients receiving spinal anesthesia can prevent the occurrence of neurogenic shock. These patients may be positioned with the head of the bed elevated to prevent the upward progression of the spinal blockade up the cord (Bernards, 2001).

The nurse can prevent anaphylactic shock by collecting detailed information about allergies and drug reactions. The nurse inquires about reactions to drugs with similar structures. For example, if patients are allergic to penicillin, they are likely to have a reaction to ampicillin (Principen), carbenicillin (Geopen), or nafcillin sodium. Response to intravenous (IV) administration of medications, particularly antibiotics, is monitored. Injecting small amounts of a drug before the entire dose is given is recommended to assist in detecting a possible reaction. Care is taken during the transfusion of blood or blood products, which can result in allergic reactions. The patient receiving any of these products is observed closely for any signs of an allergic reaction.

Prevention of septic shock is promoted through preventing infections, including proper hand washing, use of aseptic technique, and awareness of the patient at risk. The critically ill patient is debilitated and has many potential portals of entry for bacterial invasion. Meticulous technique is required during procedures (i.e., suctioning, dressings changes, and wound care) and when handling catheters or tubes. Frequent assessment of temperature, wounds, and laboratory results (e.g., white blood cell and differential counts and cultures) is important for the identification of infection. The United States Centers for Disease Control and Prevention have uniform definitions and data collection methods to collect and analyze data regarding nosocomial infections. Data are collected from patients in intensive care units and provide site-specific, risk-adjusted infection rates (Gaynes et al., 2001).

One of the greatest infection risks is the development of ventilator-associated pneumonia. Several strategies have been identified that could reduce the risk of ventilator-associated pneumonia and are easily implemented by the bedside nurse. These include maintaining the head of the bed at 30-degree elevation or greater, providing frequent oral care, ensuring that enteral feedings are initiated early, and reducing the number of ventilator circuit changes (Ahrens and Vollman, 2003). Another strategy is the use of an endotracheal tube with a dorsal lumen to allow continuous suction of secretions from the subglottic area (Centers for Disease Control and Prevention, 2004).

Clinical Picture

Multiple body systems are affected by the shock syndrome. The clinical presentation for each classification of shock is summarized in Table 10-7 (see also Clinical Alerts).

TABLE 10-7

Clinical Picture and Management of Classifications of Shock

Classification	Causes	Clinical Picture	Management
HYPOVOLEMIC	External and internal volume loss	Hypotension Tachycardia Tachypnea Oliguria Normothermia Cool, pale skin ↓ CO, CI, PAP, PAOP ↑ SVR ↓ SvO_2	Eliminate and treat cause of hypovolemia Fluid therapy
CARDIOGENIC	Myocardial ischemia End-stage cardiomyopathy Valvular disease Structural defects Dysrhythmias	Hypotension Tachycardia Tachypnea Oliguria Normothermia Cool, pale skin ↓ CO,CI ↑ PAP, PAOP ↑ SVR ↓ SvO_2	Improve CO and ↓ workload of the heart Inotropic agents Thrombolytics Afterload reducing agents Preload reducing agents Mechanical assist devices
OBSTRUCTIVE	Impaired diastolic filling ↑ Right ventricular afterload ↑ Left ventricular afterload	Hypotension Tachycardia Tachypnea Oliguria Normothermia ↓ CO, CI ↑ or normal PAP, PAOP depending on cause ↓ SVR ↑ SvO_2	Eliminate source of obstruction or compression

Continued

TABLE 10-7

Clinical Picture and Management of Classifications of Shock—cont'd

Classification	Causes	Clinical Picture	Management
DISTRIBUTIVE			
Neurogenic	Brain injury Vasomotor depression Spinal cord injury Drug overdose	Hypotension Bradycardia ↓ CO, CI ↓ PAP, PAOP ↓ SVR	Intubate and ventilate Fluid therapy Vasopressors Atropine
Anaphylactic	Repeated exposure to antigen	Hypotension Tachycardia Tachypnea and wheezing Urticaria, pruritus Edema Cyanosis ↓ CO, CI ↓ SVR ↓ SvO$_2$	Intubate and ventilate Bronchodilators Fluid therapy Steroids Antihistamines Sympathomimetics
Septic	Gram-negative bacteria Gram-positive bacteria	Hypotension Tachycardia Tachypnea ↑ Urine output, then oliguria ↑ Temperature, then ↓ Skin warm, then cool Color flushed, then pale ↑ CO, CI, then ↓ ↓ PAP, PAOP, then ↑ ↓ SVR ↑ SvO$_2$, then ↓	Find source of infection Fluid therapy Vasopressors Antibiotics based on cultures Inotropes Recombinant human activated protein C Glucose control

↑, Increased; ↓, decreased; *CI,* cardiac index; *CO,* cardiac output; *PAP,* pulmonary artery pressure; *PAOP,* pulmonary artery occlusion pressure; *SvO$_2$,* mixed venous oxygen saturation; *SVR,* systemic vascular resistance.

CLINICAL ALERTS

Assessment	Significance
Change in vital signs, hemodynamic status, sensorium	Changes occur secondary to decreased tissue perfusion associated with shock
Decreased urine output; rising blood urea nitrogen and creatinine levels	Secondary damage to kidneys related to decreased renal perfusion associated with shock
Tachypnea, worsening arterial blood gases, worsening chest radiograph	Development of acute respiratory distress syndrome secondary to shock
Bleeding from puncture sites, bruising, hematuria, occult blood in gastric aspirate or stool	Development of disseminated intravascular coagulation secondary to shock

Central Nervous System

The central nervous system is the most sensitive to changes in the supply of oxygen and nutrients. Thus, it is the first system affected by changes in cellular perfusion. Initial responses of the central nervous system to shock include agitation, anxiety, nervousness, and restlessness. As the shock state progresses, the patient becomes drowsy, confused, and lethargic because of the decreased blood flow to the brain. In stage II of shock, the patient becomes unresponsive.

Cardiovascular System

Blood pressure. A major focus of assessment is blood pressure. It is important for the nurse to know the patient's baseline blood pressure. The initial blood pressure is often normal, with a narrow pulse pressure because of the compensatory effects of the sympathetic nervous system. As the shock state progresses, the systolic blood pressure drops, whereas the diastolic pressure remains normal, resulting in a further narrowed pulse pressure. A narrowed pulse pressure is an earlier indicator of shock than is the systolic blood pressure (Mikhail, 1999). A narrowed pulse pressure denotes involvement of compensatory mechanisms and suggests significant blood loss or obstructive shock. Recommendations vary, but a drop in systolic blood pressure to less than 90 mm Hg is considered hypotensive. For hypertensive patients, a decrease in systolic pressure of 40 mm Hg from their usual systolic pressure may be considered severely hypotensive (Tierney & Messina, 2003). A point to consider is that auscultated pressures may be very inaccurate. One of the chief compensatory mechanisms occurring early in the shock state is peripheral vasoconstriction, which can lead to inaccuracies in blood pressure measurement. If blood pressure is not heard via auscultation, the approximate pressure can be assessed by palpation or ultrasound (Doppler) devices. Intraarterial lines may also be used for a direct measurement of blood pressure.

Palpable pulses can give an approximation of the blood pressure. If the brachial pulse is readily palpable, the approximate systolic pressure is 80 mm Hg. Corresponding blood pressure for the femoral and carotid pulses is 70 and 60 mm Hg, respectively.

Another measurement of the blood pressure is the tilt test, or orthostatic vital sign assessment. The patient is taken from a supine to upright (sitting or standing) position very quickly, and blood pressure and pulse before and after positioning are compared. (Patients who are volume depleted may become symptomatic in the standing position and in the interest of patient safety should be assessed going from a supine to a sitting position.) A 10-mm Hg decrease in systolic pressure is correlated with a mild degree of shock.

A decrease of 25 to 50 mm Hg approximates a moderate degree of shock, and a decrease of 50 mm Hg or greater indicates a severe state of shock. An increase in the pulse rate of 10 to 20 beats per minute is also considered to be a positive tilt, or orthostatic, sign suggesting depleted intravascular volume (Tierney & Messina, 2003). Pulsus paradoxus is assessed in patients with suspected obstructive shock caused by cardiac tamponade. Pulsus paradoxus is a decrease in systolic blood pressure of more than 10 mm Hg during inspiration.

Pulse. The rate, quality, and character of major pulses are evaluated: carotid, radial, femoral, dorsalis pedis, and posterior tibial. In shock states, the pulse is generally weak and thready. The rate is increased, usually greater than 100 beats per minute, in a compensatory response to the decreased cardiac output and demand of the cells for increased oxygen. Elderly patients may not exhibit tachycardia because of the limited response to catecholamines that occurs with the normal aging process. Normal compensatory responses to shock may be altered if the patient is taking medications such as beta-blockers. In later stages of shock, the pulse slows. The decrease in pulse rate may be related to myocardial depressant factor.

Heart sounds. Cardiac auscultation reveals abnormal heart sounds if the patient is in cardiogenic shock. A third heart sound (S_3) indicates filling of a flabby ventricle, which occurs with myocardial muscle damage. A fourth heart sound (S_4) reflects a noncompliant ventricle. Murmurs are usually present in the patient with valvular diseases.

Neck veins. Assessment of the neck veins provides information regarding the volume and pressure in the right side of the heart. It is an indirect method of evaluating the central venous pressure. Neck veins are distended in patients with obstructive or cardiogenic shock and are nondistended or flat in hypovolemic shock.

Capillary refill. Capillary refill assesses the ability of the cardiovascular system to maintain perfusion to the periphery. The normal response to pressure on the nail beds is blanching; the color returns to a normal pink hue 1 to 2 seconds after the pressure is released. A delay in the return of color indicates peripheral vasoconstriction. Capillary refill provides a quick assessment of the patient's overall cardiovascular status, but this assessment is not reliable in a patient who is hypothermic or has peripheral circulatory problems.

Right atrial pressure. A central venous catheter may be inserted to aid in the differential diagnosis of shock, to administer and monitor therapies, and to evaluate the preload of the heart. Normally, the right atrial pressure is 0 to 8 mm Hg. When blood volume decreases, such as in hypovolemic shock, the right atrial pressure decreases. In cardiogenic shock, the right atrial pressure may be increased because of the poor myocardial contractility and high filling pressure in the ventricles. In obstructive shock secondary to tamponade or tension pneumothorax, the right atrial pressure will be high.

Pulmonary artery pressure. A pulmonary artery catheter is one of the most useful tools for diagnosing and treating the patient in shock. The catheter can give information regarding cardiac dynamics, fluid balance, and effects of vasoactive agents. Table 10-8 gives hemodynamic values and alterations in shock.

Preload, which is measured by the mean right atrial pressure for the right ventricle and by the pulmonary artery occlusive pressure for the left ventricle, is used for assessing fluid balance. Vascular resistance or afterload can be measured by the systemic vascular resistance, a calculated value that offers information on the workload of the left ventricle, and the pulmonary vascular resistance, which measures right ventricular workload. Cardiac output and cardiac index give information regarding contractile force and how the heart is handling the cells' demands for nutrients.

A fiberoptic pulmonary artery catheter, which measures mixed venous oxygen saturation (SvO_2), is used to evaluate whether oxygen supply is meeting the demands of the tissues. SvO_2 reflects the amount of oxygen bound to hemoglobin in the venous circulation. SvO_2 is useful in identifying the type of shock and in evaluating the effectiveness of treatment.

Respiratory System

Respirations in the early stage of shock are rapid and deep. The respiratory center responds to shock and the resultant metabolic acidosis with an increase in respiratory rate to eliminate carbon dioxide. Direct stimulation of the medulla by chemoreceptors alters the respiratory pattern. As the shock state progresses, metabolic wastes build up and cause generalized muscle weakness resulting in shallow breathing with poor air exchange.

In anaphylactic shock, cough, runny nose, nasal congestion, hoarseness, and dysphonia are common because of upper airway obstruction from edema of the larynx, epiglottis, or vocal cords. Lower airway obstruction may result from diffuse bronchoconstriction. Patients may show signs of pulmonary edema.

Pulse oximetry is frequently used to measure arterial oxygen saturation. It must be used with caution in patients in shock because decreased peripheral circulation and low pulse pressure may result in inaccurate readings. Arterial blood gas analysis is used for more accurate assessment of oxygenation.

TABLE 10-8

Hemodynamic Alterations in Shock States

Parameter, Normal Range	Cardiogenic	Hypovolemic	Obstructive	Distributive	
				Septic	Anaphylactic/ Neurogenic
Cardiac output, 4-8 L/min	Low	Low	Low	High then low	Low
Cardiac index, 2.8-4.2 L/min/m²	Low	Low	Low	High then low	Low
Right atrial pressure, 0-8 mm Hg	High	Low	High	Low then high	Low
Pulmonary artery diastolic pressure, 4-12 mm Hg	High	Low	High	Low then high	Low
Pulmonary artery occlusion pressure, 6-12 mm Hg	High	Low	High	Low then high	Low
Systemic vascular resistance, 900-1400 dynes/sec/cm⁻⁵	High	High	Low	Low	Low
Mixed venous oxygen saturation, 60%-80%	Low	Low	High	High then low	Low

Renal System

Urine output of less than 0.5 mL/kg/hr is considered a sign of shock. Urine output decreases because of reduced renal perfusion. The kidneys compensate by reducing excreted fluids and concentrating urine. In addition, the renin-angiotensin mechanism facilitates the release of aldosterone, which promotes the retention of sodium and the reabsorption of water in the kidneys further decreasing urinary output. If decreased perfusion is prolonged, blood urea nitrogen and creatinine levels will increase and result in acute renal failure.

Gastrointestinal System

Research has demonstrated that the gastrointestinal system is affected early by the decreased tissue perfusion (Mikhail, 1999). The initial compensatory response in shock is to reduce the blood flow to nonessential organ systems, including the gastrointestinal system. This results in a slowing of intestinal activity with decreased bowel sounds, distention, nausea, and constipation. The prolonged decrease in perfusion leads to decreased motility and increased permeability of the tract lining. This results in paralytic ileus, possible ulceration, and damage to the microvilli in the lining. The damaged microvilli allow bacteria to enter the systemic circulation (Maier, 2001). This bacterial translocation increases the risk of infection and sepsis in the already compromised critically ill patient.

The liver is susceptible to the decreased perfusion that occurs with shock. The hypoperfusion leads to decreased function and may be seen as alterations in liver enzymes such as lactate dehydrogenase and aspartate aminotransferase. If decreased perfusion persists, the liver will not be able to produce compounds needed for coagulation and will not detoxify drugs or neutralize invading microorganisms. This situation results in clotting disorders, drug toxicity concerns, and increased susceptibility for infection.

Hematological System

Current research indicates an interaction between the coagulation pathway and the inflammatory process (Sommers, 2003). This interaction enhances clotting and inhibits fibrinolysis, which leads to clotting in the microcirculatory system and bleeding. Because of this, platelet counts are low, and clotting times are prolonged. Additionally, blood cells and blood flow become slow and sluggish in a state of decreased perfusion. This sluggish blood flow can also contribute to the formation of microemboli in the circulation. Leukopenia occurs secondary to the compensatory response in the early stages of shock, thus increasing the patient's susceptibility to infection. Because there is a decreased production of clotting factors by the liver, coagulation assays are abnormal, with prolonged clotting times.

Skin and Mucous Membranes

Skin color, temperature, texture, turgor, and moisture level are evaluated. Characteristic skin changes occur, depending on the type of shock. In septic shock, the skin is often dry, flushed, and warm. In hypovolemic or cardiogenic shock, the skin is pale, cool, and moist. The mucous membranes are dry and pale as a result of the decreased perfusion. In anaphylactic shock, patients may present with urticaria and pruritus. The skin may be flushed, diaphoretic, and warm because of vasodilation. In neurogenic shock, the skin is warm. In toxic shock syndrome, the patient displays a red macular rash, desquamation of the skin, and, occasionally, bright red mucous membranes. Cyanosis may be present; however, it is a late and unreliable sign. The patient may exhibit *central* cyanosis, seen in the mucous membranes of the mouth and nose, or *peripheral* cyanosis, evident in the nails and earlobes.

Musculoskeletal System

The patient in shock suffers from fatigue in all muscle systems. Generalized weakness and fatigue are major complaints with increasing lactate levels. If there is prolonged reduction in perfusion, the patient may have a breakdown of the skeletal muscle cells, with myoglobin released into the circulation. This may produce myoglobinemia and myoglobinuria. Patients with toxic shock exhibit neuromuscular symptoms, such as arthralgia, general aching, malaise, abdominal discomfort, and neck stiffness.

DIAGNOSTIC TESTS

Additional tests may assist in the differential diagnosis of the patient in shock. These include laboratory analysis and a variety of other tests (see Laboratory Alerts).

Laboratory Studies

Various laboratory tests aid in the differential diagnosis of shock (Table 10-9). A measure of the overall state of shock, regardless of the cause of inadequate perfusion, is the serum lactate level. Lactate level has been used as an indicator of decreased oxygen delivery to the cells and of the adequacy of resuscitation in shock and as an outcome predictor. Elevated levels of lactate produce an acidic environment and decrease arterial pH. The serum lactate level correlates with the degree of hypoperfusion. Elevations in lactate occur only after maximal oxygen extraction by the cells. By the time many of the laboratory test

LABORATORY ALERTS: VALUES COMMON IN SHOCK

Test	Normal Value	In Shock
Serum tests		
Blood glucose	70-105 mg/dL	Early: ↑ Late: ↓
Blood urea nitrogen	5-20 mg/dL	↑
Creatinine	0.6-1.2 mg/dL	↑
Sodium	136-145 mEq/L	↑
Chloride	97-107 mEq/L	↑
Carbon dioxide	22-30 mEq/L	Early: ↓ Late: ↑
Lactate	0.5-1.6 mEq/L	↑
AST	8-20 units/L	↑
LDH	55-102 units/L	↑
WBC	4,500-11,000 µL	↑
Arterial blood gases		
pH	7.35-7.45	Early: ↑ Late: ↓
$PaCO_2$	35-45 mm Hg	Early: ↓ Late: ↑
PaO_2	75-100 mm Hg	↓
HCO_3^-	22-26 mEq/L	Late: ↓

↑, Increased; ↓, decreased; *AST,* aspartate aminotransferase; HCO_3^-, bicarbonate, *LDH,* lactate dehydrogenase; $PaCO_2$, partial pressure of arterial carbon dioxide; PaO_2, partial pressure of arterial oxygen; *WBC,* white blood count.

results are altered, the patient is in the later stages of shock. The clinical picture is often more useful for early diagnosis and immediate treatment.

Other Diagnostic Tests

Additional diagnostic tests and assessment parameters include urine studies, chest x-ray studies, echocardiography, peritoneal lavage, ultrasonography, computed tomography (CT), and gastric tonometry (pHi).

Urine studies. Urine studies may be ordered for the examination of renal status. The urine specific gravity and osmolarity may be high because of decreased urine production, resulting from impaired renal perfusion, as well as increased release of antidiuretic hormone and aldosterone.

Chest x-ray studies. Chest x-ray studies are helpful for assessing respiratory status. They can be used to identify pulmonary edema in the patient in cardiogenic shock. Pulmonary edema can further compromise the patient's cellular oxygenation. In obstructive

shock, a chest film may help to identify a tension pneumothorax or cardiac tamponade. Chest x-ray studies are also helpful in the early recognition of acute respiratory distress syndrome, which is a common complication of the shock syndrome. In the patient admitted with chest injuries, an x-ray study assists in the diagnosis of a pneumothorax or a hemothorax.

Echocardiography. An echocardiogram is useful in the diagnosis of cardiac tamponade or other structural processes in the heart. It shows a collection of fluid in the pericardial sac.

Diagnostic peritoneal lavage. A diagnostic peritoneal lavage may be performed for the assessment of abdominal bleeding. Diagnostic peritoneal lavage is indicated in cases of severe trauma and is performed in the emergency department. Abdominal girth is also assessed. An increase in the girth may be an indicator of abdominal bleeding or fluid loss into the abdomen.

Ultrasonography. The use of ultrasonography has gained favor for the diagnosis of hypovolemic shock secondary to abdominal bleeding. In some facilities, ultrasonography has eliminated the need for diagnostic peritoneal lavage because it is less invasive and can be performed rapidly and repeatedly at the bedside.

Computed tomography. CT is useful in assisting with the differential diagnosis of shock. CT can pinpoint sources of bleeding, which can cause hypovolemic shock, or abscess formation, which can cause sepsis. A CT scan can also show spinal injuries that can precipitate neurogenic shock.

Gastric tonometry. A newer test to measure hypoperfusion is the use of gastric tonometry. Measurement of the partial pressure of carbon dioxide (PCO_2) in the gastric lumen (pHi) provides early and accurate information about tissue perfusion, the effect of various therapies, and outcomes (Mikhail, 1999). Research has shown that because of various neural and hormonal factors, the gut is extremely susceptible to hypoperfusion. These factors make it the first system affected by inadequate perfusion. Additionally, hypoperfusion in the gut itself may be a factor in contributing to the development of MODS. A pHi greater than 7.35 is normal and is an indication of normal perfusion. A drop in the pHi to less than 7.35 indicates that tissue hypoxia may be occurring (Maier, 2001). Newer technologies are making the measurement of gastric pHi easier to perform.

An alternative to gastric pHi is the measurement of sublingual PCO_2 ($PslCO_2$). This is a technically simple

TABLE 10-9

Laboratory Tests for Differential Diagnosis of Shock

Test	Normal Value	In Shock
Blood culture	No growth	Positive in septic shock
Hemoglobin (Hgb)	13.6-17.2 g/dL (men) 12-15 g/dL (women)	↓ In hypovolemic shock caused by hemorrhage
Hematocrit (Hct)	42%-52% (men) 35%-47% (women)	↓ In hypovolemic shock caused by hemorrhage
Red blood cells (RBC)	4.5-6.2 million/µL (men) 4.0-5.5 million/µL (women)	↓ In hypovolemic shock caused by hemorrhage
Cardiac enzymes		All enzymes may be ↑ in cardiogenic shock as a result of ↓ coronary artery perfusion and myocardial injury
CK	<90 units/L (men) <80 units/L (women)	
CK-MB	0-7 mcg/dL 0-6% of total CK	
Troponin	Troponin I > 2.3 mcg/L Troponin T <0.1 mcg/L	
LDH	55-102 units/L	
LDH₁	14%-26%	
LDH₂	29%-39%	

↑, Increased; ↓, decreased; *CK*, creatine kinase; *CK-MB*, creatine kinase-myocardial bound; *LDH*, lactate dehydrogenase.

and noninvasive measurement that has been shown to assess tissue hypercarbia in shock states (Marik, 2001).

Nursing Diagnosis

The primary nursing diagnosis for all patients in shock is altered tissue perfusion. This diagnosis may be related to decreased tissue perfusion, myocardial contractility, vascular resistance, obstruction, or a combination of these (see Nursing Care Plan).

Management

Management of the patient in shock consists of finding and treating the cause of the shock as rapidly as possible. Care is directed toward correcting or reversing the altered circulatory component (e.g., blood volume, cardiac contractility, obstruction, and vascular resistance) and treating clinical symptoms. A combination of fluid, pharmacological, and mechanical therapies is implemented to maintain tissue perfusion.

Nursing Care Plan for the Patient in Shock

NURSING DIAGNOSES: *Altered tissue perfusion related to:*
- *Decreased blood volume*
- *Decreased myocardial contractility*
- *Impaired circulatory blood flow*
- *Widespread vasodilatation*

Patient Outcomes	Interventions	Rationales
Tissue perfusion will be optimized as evidenced by	Monitor for early symptoms of shock (see Table 10-7)	The earlier shock is recognized, the sooner the patient can receive appropriate support reducing patient problems.

Continued

Nursing Care Plan for the Patient in Shock—cont'd

Patient Outcomes	Interventions	Rationales
Balanced fluid intake and output	Establish or maintain patent airway	The airway must be patent to provide oxygen support.
Controlled bleeding or fluid loss	Administer oxygen	Additional oxygen can increase oxygen delivery to the tissues.
Normal serum and urine laboratory values and ABG results	Prepare for intubation and mechanical ventilation as needed	Anticipating the need for advanced respiratory support ensures that oxygen delivery will be provided according to patient need.
Normal vital signs	Establish intravenous access	IV access, with large-bore IV catheters, is required for fluid administration.
Normal mentation and cognition for patient	Use large-gauge catheters (14 or 16 gauge) peripherally	Using central IV access allows for easy fluid and drug administration without the concerns of peripheral infiltration and irritation.
Normal elimination pattern	Obtain central venous access, if possible	
Normal mobility for patient	Control bleeding through the application of pressure or surgical intervention	Pressure or surgical intervention will control the blood loss.
Managed pain		
Absence of complication (e.g., ARDS, renal and hepatic failure, MODS)	Administer fluids as ordered (e.g., crystalloids, colloids, blood products)	Fluid administration provides volume to maintain tissue perfusion.
	Consider warming fluids before infusing	Warmed fluids reduce potential hypothermia and its complications.
	Type and crossmatch for blood replacement	Blood replacement is necessary if volume loss is associated with blood loss.
	Evaluate patient's response to fluid challenges and blood product administration: improvement in vital signs, level of consciousness, urinary output, hemodynamic values, and serum and urine laboratory values	Monitoring the patient's response to therapy is essential.
	Monitor cardiopulmonary status: HR, RR, BP, MAP, skin color, temperature, and moisture, capillary refill, hemodynamic values, cardiac rhythm, neck veins, lung sounds	Cardiopulmonary status is key in evaluating therapy and tissue perfusion.
	Monitor neurological status: Level of consciousness	The central nervous system is the most sensitive indicator of tissue perfusion.
	Monitor gastrointestinal status: Abdominal distention, bowel sounds, gastric pH, vomiting, large enteral feeding residual	Gastrointestinal status is evaluated for tissue perfusion and possible complications.
	Monitor fluid balance: I & O, daily weights, amount and type of drainage (e.g., chest tube, nasogastric, wounds)	Monitoring fluid balance and the response to therapy is key to evaluating need for continued support.

Continued

Nursing Care Plan for the Patient in Shock—cont'd

Patient Outcomes	Interventions	Rationales
Tissue perfusion will be optimized as evidenced by Balanced fluid intake and output	Monitor serial serum values: Hct, Hgb, PT, aPTT, fibrin degradation products, fibrinogen, platelets, ABGs, chemistry profile, lactate, cultures	Evaluation of laboratory values assists in directing care.
Controlled bleeding or fluid loss		
Normal serum and urine laboratory values and ABG results	Monitor pain level: Administer analgesics Implement comfort measures (turning, repositioning, skin care) Evaluate patient's response	Ensuring patient comfort by monitoring pain levels is necessary for comprehensive care of the patient.
Normal vital signs		
Normal mentation and cognition for patient	Administer medications as prescribed and specific for the type of shock (see Table 10-11)	Pharmacological interventions require monitoring to improve outcomes and reduce complications.
Normal elimination pattern		
Normal mobility for patient	Position in modified Trendelenburg position	Proper positioning can improve venous return and cardiac output.
Managed pain		
Absence of complication (e.g., ARDS, renal and hepatic failure, MODS)—*cont'd*	Provide wound care as indicated and evaluate healing	Providing wound care promotes healing and reduces the likelihood of introducing infection.
	Provide adequate nutritional support	Nutritional support provides for optimum cell function and healing and reduces complications.
	Early enteral feeding preferred	Enteral feeding is preferred to maintain optimal functioning of the gastrointestinal system.
	Collaborate with dietitian about patient's nutritional needs	Collaboration with a dietician assures optimal nutritional support.
	Provide psychological support for patient, family, and others	Psychological support reduces the stress response and physiological demand.
	Evaluate patient response to interventions and adjust accordingly	Continuous evaluation and adjustment of care are required for provision of quality care.
	Monitor for the development of complications	Early identification of complications assists in directing care.
	Monitor oxygenation: pulse oximetry, ABGs, mixed venous oxygen saturation	
	Monitor renal status: Hourly urine output, serum creatinine and urea nitrogen levels	

ABG, Arterial blood gas; *ARDS,* acute respiratory distress syndrome; *Hct,* hematocrit; *Hgb,* hemoglobin; *I&O,* intake and output; *MAP,* mean arterial pressure; *MODS,* multiple organ dysfunction syndrome; *PT,* prothrombin time; *HR,* heart rate; *RR,* respiratory rate; *BP,* blood pressure; *aPTT,* activated partial thromboplastin time.

Oxygen consumption increases in shock as oxygen delivery decreases, a phenomenon that has been associated with poor prognosis (Maier, 2001). Current medical management of shock includes interventions to increase oxygen delivery. These interventions include increasing cardiac output and index, increasing hemoglobin, and increasing arterial oxygen saturation. For a summary of the management for each classification of shock, see Table 10-7. Box 10-5 outlines management guidelines for severe sepsis and septic shock.

BOX 10-5

Management Guidelines for Severe Sepsis and Septic Shock

1. Early, goal-directed resuscitation during the first 6 hours after recognition of sepsis
2. Appropriate diagnostic studies (cultures) to determine causative organisms before starting antibiotics
3. Administration of broad spectrum antibiotic therapy after cultures obtained
4. Reassessment of antibiotic therapy after 48 to 72 hours with microbiology and clinical data to narrow coverage
5. Seven to ten days of antibiotic therapy guided by clinical response
6. Aggressive fluid therapy
7. Initiation of vasopressors (norepinephrine, dopamine) if fluid therapy fails to restore adequate blood pressure and organ perfusion
8. Consider initiation of an inotrope (dobutamine) in patients with low cardiac output despite adequate fluid resuscitation
9. Consider initiation of corticosteroids in patients with septic shock who, despite adequate fluid replacement, require vasopressor therapy to maintain adequate blood pressure
10. Initiation of activated protein C in patients with severe sepsis and high risk of death
11. Use of protocols for sedation (intermittent or continuous infusion) with daily interruption/lightening to assess for retitration of continuous infusion
12. Maintenance of blood glucose < 150 mg/dL after initial stabilization
13. Avoidance of neuromuscular blockage, if possible
14. Use of deep vein thrombosis and stress ulcer prophylaxis
15. Use of semirecumbent bed position unless contraindicated

Modified from Dellinger, R.P., Carlet, J.M., Masur H., et al. (2004). Surviving sepsis campaign guidelines for management of severe sepsis and septic shock. *Critical Care Medicine, 32*, 858-873

FLUID THERAPY

Regardless of the cause, shock produces profound alterations in fluid balance that affect tissue perfusion. Therefore, patients experiencing absolute hypovolemia (hypovolemic shock) or relative hypovolemia (distributive shock) require the administration of IV fluids for the restoration of intravascular volume, maintenance of oxygen-carrying capacity, and establishment of the hemodynamic stability necessary for optimal tissue perfusion. The choice of fluid and the volume and rate of infusion depend on the type of fluid lost, the patient's concurrent medical problems, and the fluid's availability.

Benefits of parenteral fluid administration include increased intravascular volume, increased venous return to the right side of the heart, optimal stretching of the ventricle, improved myocardial contractility, and increased cardiac output. The desired outcome is enhanced tissue perfusion. However, these effects may be dangerous to the patient in cardiogenic shock because large volumes of fluid overwork an already failing heart. Instead, cardiogenic shock is managed primarily with medications that reduce both preload and afterload.

Patients in severe shock may require immediate rapid volume replacement. The IV flow rate can be increased by infusion of fluids under pressure by use of a blood pump, large-bore infusion tubing, or rapid-infusion devices. Infusion pumps can be used for the accurate administration of large volumes at fast rates. One concern of administration of large volumes is hypothermia. Large volumes of room temperature fluids can rapidly drop core body temperature and can cause hypothermia. Fluid-related hypothermia causes alterations in cardiac contractility and coagulation. For this reason, fluids should be run through warming devices. Fluid administration is adjusted based on changes in blood pressure, urine output, hemodynamic values, diagnostic test results, and the clinical picture of the patient's response to treatment. Generally, volume replacement continues until an adequate mean arterial pressure (60 mm Hg or greater) is achieved and evidence of end-organ tissue perfusion is reestablished (i.e., improved level of consciousness, urinary output and peripheral perfusion) (Maier, 2001).

Intravenous Access

IV access is needed for the administration of fluids and medications. The patient in shock requires a minimum of two IV catheters, one in a peripheral vein and one in a central vein. Peripheral access via a large-gauge catheter (14- or 16-gauge) provides a route for immediate, rapid administration of fluids and medications. Establishing IV routes in a patient in shock is challenging because peripheral vasoconstriction and venous collapse make access difficult. Initially, it is usually necessary to use the large peripheral veins in the antecubital fossa (i.e., the basilic, cephalic, or accessory cephalic). In extreme emergencies, the physician may need to perform a venous cut-down.

A central venous access is established for large-volume replacement and can be used for monitoring central venous pressure or for placing a pulmonary artery catheter to guide fluid replacement. Central venous catheters are commonly inserted into the subclavian, internal jugular, or femoral veins. Multilumen catheters, which provide multiple access ports, are often used to allow the concurrent administration of fluid, medication, and blood products.

Fluid Challenge

Once IV access is established, a fluid challenge may be performed for the assessment of the patient's hemodynamic response to the rapid administration of fluid. Various methods for administering a fluid challenge exist. Typically, the physician orders a rapid infusion of 250 mL up to 2 L of a crystalloid solution. Nursing responsibilities include obtaining the baseline hemodynamic measurements, administering the fluid challenge, and assessing the patient's response.

Patient response to this initial bolus determines further treatment needs (i.e., repeat boluses, transfusion, surgical repair). Response patterns are described as rapid, transient, or minimal or no response to the initial fluid administration (American College of Surgeons, 1997). Patients in the rapid response group attain hemodynamic stability after the initial bolus and when fluids are slowed to a maintenance rate. Transient responders respond to the initial bolus, but they deteriorate as fluids are slowed to a maintenance level, indicating ongoing blood loss or inadequate resuscitation and the need for more aggressive management. Minimal or no responders do not respond to crystalloid or blood administration and require immediate surgical intervention. A description of each of these responses and treatment needs can be found in Table 10-10.

Types of Fluids

The choice of fluid or fluids depends on the cause of the volume deficit, the patient's clinical status, and the physician's preference. Although the nurse is not responsible for selecting the infusion or transfusion, an understanding of the rationale for the prescribed fluid and the expected effects is needed for the assessment of patient outcomes. The nurse carefully monitors the patient's response to fluid therapy. A return to normal laboratory and hemodynamic values, as well as the patient outcomes described in Box 10-6 are the goals of fluid therapy.

Blood, blood products, crystalloids, and colloids are used alone or in combination to restore intravascular volume. Initially, crystalloids and colloids are infused until diagnostics and blood typing and crossmatching are completed.

Blood and blood products. Whole blood, packed red blood cells, washed red blood cells, fresh frozen plasma, and platelets are given for the treatment of major blood loss. Typing and crossmatching are performed for these products, to identify the patient's blood type (A, B, AB, O), to determine the presence of the Rh factor, and to ensure compatibility with the donor blood to prevent transfusion reactions. In extreme emergencies, the patient may be transfused with O-negative blood, which is considered the universal donor blood type.

TABLE 10-10

Responses to Initial Fluid Resuscitation

	Rapid Response	Transient Response	No Response
Vital signs	Return to normal	Transient improvement; recurrence of ↓ BP and ↑ HR	Remain abnormal
Estimated blood loss	Minimal (10%-20%)	Moderate and ongoing (20%-40%)	Severe (>40%)
Need for more crystalloid	Low	High	High
Need for blood	Low	Moderate to high	Immediate
Blood preparation	Type and crossmatch	Type-specific	Emergency blood release
Need for operative intervention	Possibly	Likely	Highly likely

↑, Increased; ↓, decreased; *BP*, blood pressure; *HR*, heart rate.

Transfusions require an IV access with at least a 20-gauge, preferably an 18-gauge or larger, catheter (a 22- or 23-gauge needle or catheter may be used in neonates, children, or adults with small veins). Solutions other than 0.9% normal saline are not infused with blood because they cause red blood cells to clump, swell, and burst. In addition, IV medications are never infused in the same port with blood. Appropriate patient and blood identification is necessary before starting any transfusion.

Transfusions are administered with a blood filter to trap debris and tiny clots. Frequent patient assessment is necessary during a blood transfusion to monitor for adverse reactions. In the event of a reaction, the transfusion is stopped, the transfusion tubing is disconnected from the IV access site, and the vein is kept open with an IV of 0.9% normal saline solution. The patient is assessed, and the physician and laboratory are notified. All transfusion equipment (bag, tubing, and remaining solutions) and any blood or urine specimens obtained are sent to the laboratory according to hospital policy. The events of the reaction, interventions used, and patient response to treatment are documented.

Blood and blood products are given until the hemoglobin is 10 g/dL or greater (Tierney & Messina, 2003, Caplan & Miller, 2001). The transfusion administration time varies with the particular blood product used and the individual patient circumstances. Documentation of the transfusion includes the blood product administered, the baseline vital signs, the time the transfusion was started and completed, the volume of blood and fluid administered, the results of assessment of the patient during the transfusion, and any nursing actions taken.

Whole blood is indicated for the treatment of obvious rapid blood loss and insidious slower blood loss. It restores blood volume and oxygen-carrying capacity; however, side effects include volume overload. Acidosis, hyperkalemia, and coagulation problems are associated with transfusions of banked blood more than 24 hours old. Typing and crossmatching of whole blood are required.

Packed red blood cells increase the blood volume and oxygen-carrying capacity without causing the problems of volume overload associated with the administration of whole blood. One unit of packed red blood cells increases the hematocrit value by about 3% and the hemoglobin value by 1 g/dL (Tierney & Messina, 2003). Typing and crossmatching of packed red blood cells are required. Red blood cells tend to aggregate because of the fibrinogen coating; therefore, washed red blood cells may be given to decrease capillary sludging.

Fresh frozen plasma is administered to replace all clotting factors except platelets. When massive transfusions are infused, fresh frozen plasma is given rapidly to restore coagulation factors. One unit of fresh frozen plasma is given for every 4 to 5 units of blood transfused. Typing and crossmatching of fresh frozen plasma are required.

Platelets are given rapidly to help control bleeding caused by low platelet counts (usually less than 50,000/mm^3). Typing of platelets, but not crossmatching, is required.

Blood substitutes. Three types of red cell substitutes are currently in various stages of clinical trials: cell-free hemoglobin, perfluorocarbon emulsions, and liposome-encapsulated hemoglobin. Red cell substitutes are oxygen carriers designed to replace transfused blood temporarily. These substitutes have several advantages: potent plasma volume expanders, availability, no typing and crossmatching, no transmission of viral or bacterial infection, no immunosuppression, and long shelf life. Limitations of the substitutes include gastrointestinal side effects, fever, flulike symptoms, vasoconstriction, thrombocytopenia, dose limitations, short duration of action, and cost (Winslow, 1999; Robb, 1999). Despite these limitations, it has been suggested that the use of red blood cell substitutes may be useful in cases of shock trauma, when blood is not available (e.g., in prehospital settings) or when blood would be unlikely to remain in the intravascular space (e.g., before surgical repair of an actively bleeding site) (Robb, 1999; Winslow, 1999).

Crystalloids. Crystalloids are inexpensive and readily available commercial solutions. Lactated Ringer's solution and 0.9% normal saline are isotonic electrolyte solutions that are used to expand intravascular volume. These solutions move freely from the intravascular space into the tissues. Traditionally, 3 mL of crystalloid solution is administered to replace each 1 mL of blood loss. Current recommendations are to administer an initial rapid fluid bolus of 1 to 2 L for an adult and observe the patient's response (American College of Surgeons, 1997). Lactated Ringer's solution closely resembles plasma, rarely causes side effects, and may be the only fluid replacement required if the blood loss is less than 1500 mL (American College of Surgeons, 1997). Although 0.9% normal saline is an isotonic solution, its side effects include hypernatremia, hypokalemia, and metabolic acidosis. Solutions of 5% dextrose in water and 0.45% normal saline are hypotonic and are not used for fluid resuscitation because they rapidly leave the intravascular space, thus causing interstitial and intracellular edema.

When large volumes of crystalloids are infused, the patient is at risk of developing hemodilution of red blood cells and plasma proteins. Hemodilution of red blood cells impairs delivery of oxygen to the cells if the hematocrit value is decreased to such an extent that the cardiac output cannot increase enough to compensate. Hemodilution of plasma proteins decreases colloidal osmotic pressure and places the patient at risk of developing pulmonary edema.

Colloids. Colloids contain proteins that increase osmotic pressure. Osmotic pressure holds and attracts fluid into blood vessels, thereby expanding plasma volume. Because colloids remain in the intravascular space longer than crystalloids, smaller volumes of colloids are given.

Albumin and plasma protein fraction (Plasmanate) are naturally occurring colloid solutions that are given when the volume loss is caused by a loss of plasma rather than blood, as seen in burns, peritonitis, and bowel obstruction. Typing and crossmatching of albumin and plasma protein fraction are not required. Pulmonary edema is a potential complication of colloid administration, resulting from increased pulmonary capillary permeability seen in some stages of shock or increased capillary hydrostatic pressure in the pulmonary vasculature created by rapid plasma expansion.

Dextran is a synthetic colloid used as a plasma expander. Dextran solutions contain glucose polymers that draw water into the vascular space. Low-molecular-weight dextran (dextran 40, Rheomacrodex) has a duration of 12 hours. Its use is contraindicated in hemorrhagic shock because it causes a decrease in platelet adhesiveness and consequently increases bleeding from wounds. High-molecular-weight dextran (dextran 70, Macrodex) is effective for 24 hours, but it increases platelet aggregation and interferes with blood typing and crossmatching; therefore, these assessments should be performed before dextran 70 is infused. No more than 1 L of dextran should be given in a 24-hour period. Additional complications associated with this plasma expander include allergic reactions and renal damage. Because of the multiple concerns with blood coagulation, dextran is used very infrequently for the treatment of shock (Tierney & Messina, 2003).

Hetastarch (Hespan) is a synthetic colloid that acts as a plasma expander but carries less risk for the development of pulmonary edema. Compared with dextran, hetastarch has no apparent effect on renal function and is less likely to cause allergic reactions. Side effects of hetastarch include altered prothrombin time and partial thromboplastin time and the potential for circulatory overload. No more than 1 L should be given in a 24-hour period.

PHARMACOLOGICAL THERAPY

Pharmacological management of shock is based on the manipulation of the cardiac dynamics: contractility, preload, afterload, and heart rate. No drugs magically restore cellular nutrition, but agents are available that assist in the manipulation of the four circulatory variables, thereby making nutrients available to the cells. A list of commonly used medications is found in Box 10-7. Hemodynamic monitoring is often used to assess the effectiveness of medications.

Drugs That Affect Contractility

Positive inotropic agents, which increase the contractile force of the heart, are used in the management of cardiogenic and distributive shock. As contractility increases, two things occur: (1) ventricular emptying increases and filling pressures of the heart decrease; and (2) improved stroke volume increases cardiac output, which, in turn, increases blood pressure and improves tissue perfusion.

Positive inotropic agents increase myocardial oxygen demand, which increases the workload of the heart. Therefore, the agents must be used cautiously in patients with ischemic heart disease and in those with cardiogenic shock.

Negative inotropic agents, such as propranolol, are not used to treat shock but are discussed here because of the widespread use of these agents in the treatment of angina, hypertension, and dysrhythmias and their effect on the patient in shock. Negative inotropes work primarily by blocking the effects of the beta

---

BOX 10-7

Pharmacological Management of Shock: Manipulation of Cardiac Dynamics

Positive inotropic drugs
  Dopamine (in midrange doses: 5-10 mcg/kg/min)
  Dobutamine
  Norepinephrine
Drugs to reduce preload
  Diuretics: furosemide
  Nitroprusside
  Nitroglycerin
  Morphine sulfate
Drugs to increase afterload
  Dopamine (in high doses: 10-20 mcg/kg/min)
  Vasopressin (in low doses: 0.01-0.04 units/min)
  Norepinephrine
  Phenylephrine
Drugs to decrease afterload
  Nitroprusside
  Hydralazine

---

branch of the sympathetic nervous system and cause a decrease in heart rate and cardiac output. A patient who is taking these medications has an altered ability to respond to the stress of shock and may not exhibit the typical signs and symptoms.

Drugs that Affect Preload

Treatment aimed at increasing preload is instituted for the treatment of hypovolemic and distributive shock. The primary treatment to increase preload is the administration of fluids.

Vasopressors, such as epinephrine and norepinephrine, are also used as adjunct therapies to increase preload. These drugs cause vasoconstriction and increase the venous return to the heart. Vasopressors are used in the treatment of distributive shock. These drugs should be used with caution in patients with hypovolemic shock, because these patients need volume replacement.

In cardiogenic shock, drugs are administered to reduce preload. Drugs such as nitroprusside are given to reduce the venous return to the heart and decrease afterload through vasodilation. A serious side effect is that they reduce the preload to such an extent that hypotension ensues, thereby increasing hypoperfusion to the cells.

Drugs that Affect Afterload

Afterload is the force the heart must overcome to pump effectively. Afterload is low in distributive shock. In this situation, drugs such as epinephrine

are used to increase vascular tone, improve venous return, and consequently increase cardiac output. Vasopressin is a potent vasoconstrictor that increases blood pressure and systemic vascular resistance, and it decreases cardiac output, heart rate, left ventricular oxygen consumption, and myocardial contractility. Low-dose vasopressin is in use for cardiogenic and septic shock states (Albright, Zimmerman, & Selzman, 2002). A negative effect of drugs that increase afterload is an increase in the myocardial oxygen demand. Accurate measurement of systemic vascular resistance and pulmonary vascular resistance via a pulmonary artery catheter assists in assessment. In cardiogenic shock, nitroprusside and nitroglycerin are used to reduce afterload and consequently reduce the workload of the heart. These drugs must be carefully monitored using hemodynamic parameters to adjust the dosages.

Drugs that Alter Heart Rate

Low and high heart rates and dysrhythmias result in decreased cardiac output, which can be deleterious to the patient in shock. Chronotropic drugs and antidysrhythmic drugs are given as indicated (see Chapter 11). In neurogenic shock, sinus bradycardia secondary to cervical spinal cord injury usually does not require therapy. However, if the heart rate falls to less than 40 beats per minute, atropine, 1 mg IV, may be given in anticipation of placement of a temporary pacemaker.

Other Pharmacological Therapy

Oxygen is administered to elevate the arterial oxygen tension, thereby improving tissue oxygenation (Tierney & Messina, 2003). Oxygen is administered by methods ranging from nasal cannula to mechanical ventilation, depending on the patient's condition.

Epinephrine is the drug of choice for treating anaphylactic shock. For mild reactions, aqueous epinephrine 1:10,000 is given 0.3 to 0.5 mL, intramuscularly or subcutaneously. The dose may be repeated at 5- to 10-minute intervals. For severe reactions, 1 to 5 mL IV of the 1:10,000 aqueous solution is administered. Antihistamines and corticosteroids may be useful, but they do not replace epinephrine.

Antibiotics are used in the treatment of septic shock. The antibiotic selected is determined by culture and sensitivity tests of blood, urine, sputum, wounds, tip of a catheter, or any site that could be a source of infection. If the source of infection cannot be identified, broad-spectrum therapy is instituted to eradicate common organisms. Antibiotics do not act on the immune response to infection and do not directly improve tissue perfusion. In severe sepsis, the patient has excessive coagulation, inflammation, and impaired fibrinolysis. A newer agent recommended for use in severe sepsis is recombinant human activated protein C (drotrecogin alfa). This drug is an antiinflammatory, antithrombotic, and profibrinolytic agent that reduces the inflammatory, clotting, and bleeding responses to sepsis. It has been shown to reduce mortality significantly in septic patients (Bernard et al., 2001). It is administered at 24 mcg/kg/hr IV for 96 hours. Patients are monitored for bleeding during the infusion.

Steroids have had a controversial place in the treatment of shock, and current evidence does not support their use. The only indication for steroids is shock associated with acute adrenal insufficiency (Tierney & Messina, 2003).

Sodium bicarbonate may be given for the treatment of metabolic acidosis associated with lactic acid production. Sodium bicarbonate combines with hydrogen ions to form water and carbon dioxide to buffer metabolic acidosis. Sodium bicarbonate is administered cautiously because the carbon dioxide produced crosses rapidly into the cells and may cause a paradoxical worsening of intracellular hypercarbia and acidosis (Cummins, 2002). Other methods for treating acidosis, such as increasing ventilation, are used before sodium bicarbonate is given. Arterial blood gas analysis is used to guide treatment.

Hyperglycemia and insulin resistance may occur in the patient with sepsis. Data suggest that intensive insulin therapy to maintain blood glucose levels at or less that 110 mg/dL reduces morbidity and mortality in the septic patient (Van den Berghe et al., 2001).

Pharmacological treatment of shock includes a wide range of agents. The major medications, actions, indications, dosages, side effects, and nursing implications are found in Table 10-11.

MECHANICAL MANAGEMENT

The management of shock includes the use of mechanical devices that aid in the restoration of cellular perfusion. Mechanical devices include the intraaortic balloon pump (IABP) and ventricular assist device (VAD).

Intraaortic Balloon Pump

A common method for mechanically assisting the heart is the use of counterpulsation via the IABP (Loeb & Cohn, 2000). It is most often used in the treatment of cardiogenic shock. It is more effective if it is inserted early in the course of treatment.

The IABP is a dual-chambered balloon that is inserted into the descending thoracic aorta via the femoral artery. The tip of the balloon is positioned just distal to the left subclavian artery (Figure 10-9). The IABP is inserted percutaneously at the patient's bedside or under fluoroscopy. Correct placement is verified via chest x-ray study.

The IABP improves coronary artery perfusion, reduces afterload, and improves perfusion to vital organs. The balloon is inflated mechanically with helium. Inflation and deflation are automatically timed with the cardiac cycle. The IABP inflates during diastole when the aortic valve is closed and deflates just before systole when the aortic valve is open. The inflation cycle displaces blood backward and forward simultaneously. The backward flow increases perfusion to the coronary arteries, and the forward flow increases perfusion to vital organs.

The balloon pump also assists the heart during systole. The balloon deflates just before contraction. This sudden deflation reduces the pressure in the aorta, decreases afterload, and reduces myocardial oxygen demand.

The IABP requires a high degree of nursing skill because of the complexity of the equipment and the need for frequent monitoring. Limb ischemia and embolic phenomena are potential complications that must be assessed. Other complications include dissection of the aorta, infection, ineffective pumping, and technical problems. Use of the IABP is contraindicated in patients with aortic insufficiency and thoracic and abdominal aneurysms.

The IABP is used concurrently with pharmacological support. Long-term use can cause patients to become dependent on the pump. Weaning is performed by gradually decreasing the pump-to-cardiac cycle ratio from 1:1, in which the IABP supports every heartbeat, to 1:2 or 1:3, in which the IABP supports every second or third beat.

Ventricular Assist Device

VADs are used temporarily to support a failing ventricle that has not responded to IABP and pharmacological therapy (Loeb & Cohn, 2000). VADs are used to treat cardiogenic shock by allowing the ventricle to recover (Christensen, 2000). They can be used to support the left ventricle, the right ventricle, or both ventricles.

VADs vary in design and technology. In general, they consist of an external pump, which diverts blood from the failing ventricle or ventricles and pumps it back into the aorta (left VAD), the pulmonary artery (right VAD), or both great vessels (Bi-VAD) (Christensen, 2000). The use of VADs requires extensive training and advanced nursing care. These devices are not typically available in community hospitals.

TABLE 10-11

MEDICATIONS COMMONLY USED IN SHOCK

Drug	Action	Indications	Dosage/Route	Standard Concentration	Side Effects	Nursing Implications
Dopamine	Positive inotropic Vasopressor	↑ Myocardial contractility ↑ Afterload ↑ BP when not caused by hypovolemia	5-10 mcg/kg/min IV infusion 10-20 mcg/kg/min IV infusion	400 mg/250 mL D₅W	↑ HR, dysrhythmias ↑ Myocardial oxygen consumption Nausea/vomiting	Do not administer with alkaline solutions Monitor for myocardial ischemia Monitor BP at least every 15 min If IV infiltrates, may cause sloughing Administer via volumetric pump Should be tapered gradually Administer via central catheter, if possible Low BP associated with hypovolemia should be treated with aggressive fluid resuscitation before drug administration
Dobutamine	Positive inotropic	↑ BP in low CO states	2-20 mcg/kg/min IV infusion	500-1000 mg/ 250 mL D₅W or NS	↑ HR, dysrhythmias ↑ Myocardial oxygen consumption Headache, tremors Nausea	Monitor for myocardial ischemia Monitor BP at least every 15 min Administer via volumetric pump Should be tapered gradually Administer via central catheter, if possible
Norepinephrine	Vasopressor, some positive inotropic effects	↑ Afterload ↑ BP refractory to other drugs	2-12 mcg/min IV infusion	4 mg/250-1000 mL D₅W or NS	↑ Myocardial oxygen consumption Dysrhythmias Severe nausea	Monitor for myocardial ischemia Monitor BP at least every 15 min Administer via volumetric pump Should be tapered gradually Administer via central catheter, if possible If IV infiltrates, may cause sloughing

Continued

TABLE 10-11

MEDICATIONS COMMONLY USED IN SHOCK—cont'd

Drug	Action	Indications	Dosage/Route	Standard Concentration	Side Effects	Nursing Implications
Nitroglycerin	Venodilator	↓ Preload, pump failure	Start at 5 mcg/min and titrate to effect; 50-200 mcg/min is range for most patients An IV bolus dose of 12.5-25 mcg may be given before infusion	50-100 mg/250 mL D$_5$W	Headache Hypotension Bradycardia	Monitor BP at least every 15 min Administer via volumetric pump Should be tapered gradually Administer via central catheter, if possible Use glass or nonabsorbable container, use special IV tubing
Nitroprusside	Vasodilator	↓ Preload and afterload	0.5-10 mcg/kg/min IV infusion	50 mg/250 mL D$_5$W or NS	Myocardial ischemia Hypotension Nausea	Monitor for myocardial ischemia May cause thiocyanate intoxication in large dosages or prolonged administration Monitor BP at least every 15 min Administer via volumetric pump Should be tapered gradually Administer via central catheter, if possible Protect from light
Vasopressin	Vasoconstrictor ↑ Afterload	↑ BP ↑ SVR ↑ Myocardial contractility BP resistant to catecholemines	0.01-0.04 units/min	100 units in 100 mL D$_5$W or NS	Diaphoresis, tremors Nausea or vomiting ↓ CO Bradycardia	Monitor BP at least every 15 min Administer via central catheter and use infusion pump

↑, Increases; ↓, decreases; *BP,* blood pressure; *CO,* cardiac output; *D$_5$W,* 5% dextrose in water; *HR,* heart rate; *NS,* normal saline; *SVR,* systemic vascular resistance.

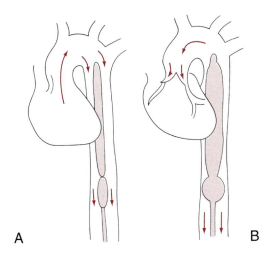

FIGURE 10-9 Intraaortic balloon pump. The balloon is deflated during systole **(A)** and inflated during diastole **(B)**.

Nursing Interventions

The nurse provides care to support tissue perfusion of the patient in shock until definitive care is under way. Supportive care is aimed at maintenance of organ function (see Nursing Care Plan).

MAXIMIZE OXYGEN DELIVERY AND REDUCE OXYGEN CONSUMPTION

Airway maintenance is the top priority. The airway is maintained by proper head position, use of oral or nasopharyngeal airways, or intubation, depending on the patient's condition (see Chapter 8). Oxygen is provided to maximize the amount of oxygen available to the cells. Suctioning and chest physical therapy facilitate secretion removal and help to maintain a patent airway. Sedation or neuromuscular blockade is considered to reduce the oxygen consumption of the patient. Arterial blood gases, pulse oximetry, and pulmonary artery hemodynamics aid in evaluation of oxygen consumption and delivery.

PATIENT POSITIONING

Proper positioning can assist in improving venous return. Traditionally, the patient in shock has been placed in the Trendelenburg position (head down and feet up). This position was thought to increase the venous return to the heart and to increase the cardiac output. However, the Trendelenburg position can actually worsen the shock state. By raising the legs, diaphragmatic movement is restricted, and this may impair ventilation. A reflex inhibition of the

baroreceptors may occur by the dramatic increase in venous return caused by the elevation of the legs. This pseudoincrease in blood volume signals the baroreceptors that blood volume is adequate, which causes the blood pressure to decrease even more. The best position for the patient in shock is one that elevates the lower extremities slightly. This elevation increases venous return without compromising the ventilatory status.

MAINTENANCE OF BODY TEMPERATURE

Care is directed toward maintaining normal body temperature. The patient's temperature is monitored frequently, and he or she is covered with light blankets. Patients should be kept warm and comfortable and yet not be overly warmed; excessive warmth increases the metabolic needs and places a larger demand on an already stressed cardiovascular system. Hypothermia depresses cardiac contractility and therefore impairs cardiac output and oxygen delivery. Hypothermia also directly impairs the coagulation pathway, which can result in significant coagulopathy (Maier, 2001). The nurse observes for hypothermia when fluids are infused rapidly and considers warming the fluids before their administration.

NUTRITIONAL SUPPORT

Establishment of nutritional support is essential for patient survival. The goals of nutritional support are to initiate enteral intake as soon as possible and to maintain sufficient caloric intake to assist in the healing process. Early enteral feeding decreases hypermetabolism, minimizes bacterial translocation, decreases diarrhea, and decreases length of stay. Nutritional requirements of the patient in shock are highly variable depending on the degree of hemodynamic stability, the cause of shock, and the patient's age, gender, and preexisting diseases. Enteral feeding is the preferred method, but the use of this mode may be limited by paralytic ileus or gastric dilation, which is commonly seen in the patient in shock. Total parenteral nutrition is used if patients are unable to tolerate enteral feeding (see Chapter 5).

MAINTENANCE OF SKIN INTEGRITY

Decreased peripheral perfusion seen in shock can precipitate injury to the skin. Meticulous skin care is required to ensure that no breaks occur in the patient's skin. The patient is turned at frequent intervals, and lotion is applied. Pressure-relieving devices, such as therapeutic beds or mattresses, may be warranted, depending on the patient's risk of skin breakdown.

RESEARCH ANALYSIS

ARTICLE REFERENCE

Boulain, T., Achard, J., Teboul, J., Richard, C., Perroting, D., & Ginies, G. (2002). Changes in blood pressure induced by passive leg raising predict response to fluid loading in critically ill patients. *Chest, 121*(4), 1245-1252.

REVIEW OF STUDY METHODS AND FINDINGS

This study was a clinical evaluation of intravascular volume status in critically ill patients with acute circulatory failure. Fluid volume replacement is often necessary to maintain adequate preload and cardiac output. Often, patients are given a fluid challenge and are monitored invasively to test preload dependence. The problem with fluid bolus is that it can sometimes result in worsening pulmonary edema. Passive leg raising was used in this study to induce change in arterial pulse pressure. It was believed that the leg raising could help to predict the response to rapid fluid loading in patients with acute circulatory failure without the potential problem of fluid overload. All the patients in the study were receiving mechanical ventilation and had a pulmonary artery catheter in place. This was a prospective clinical study of 39 patients in two medical intensive care units in university hospitals.

The measured values in this study were the pulse pressure (from the radial artery), heart rate, right atrial pressure, pulmonary artery occlusion pressure, and cardiac output. The radial artery pressure, pulmonary artery occlusive pressure, and stroke volume increased with passive leg raising. These changes rapidly reversed when the legs were lowered. The changes in pulse pressure and stroke volume were significantly correlated to the changes induced by the rapid fluid administration.

The authors concluded that the response of a patient to a rapid fluid bolus could be predicted noninvasively by observing changes in the pulse pressure during passive leg raising in patients with acute circulatory failure. The practical implications of the study were that the existence of preload-dependent problems can be detected without a pulmonary artery catheter but by using the pulse pressure. Potential harm from rapid fluid loading procedures could be avoided when unnecessary.

BRIEF CRITIQUE OF STRENGTHS AND WEAKNESSES

Strengths

The study was prospective, and the criteria for were clearly defined. Different patients in the study represented all different classifications of shock. Although the review of literature was thorough, it was somewhat dated, with references from 15 and 20 years ago. The methods and procedures used were complex but clearly explained, and the figures describing the findings contributed to the content.

Weaknesses

This is an initial study, so there is not a volume of human subjects research to support these findings. The sample size was small (39) and was limited to patients receiving mechanical ventilation. Mechanical ventilation may alter the cardiac response in patients, and the study cannot be generalized to spontaneously breathing patients without further study. The authors identified that other treatments (e.g., catecholamines) may have had effects on the study.

IMPLICATIONS OF THE STUDY FOR NURSING PRACTICE

Any time a noninvasive method of observation can be used over an invasive method, nursing and the patient will benefit. It would also be valuable to avoid unnecessary fluid overloading whenever possible. The research must be able to be generalized to be able to be used. This study should be replicated controlling for some of the factors noted in the weaknesses before it can be useful in general practice. Vasoactive and ventilatory therapy would definitely have an impact on the circulatory response of the patient. This must be identified before the findings can be generalized. The dated literature review makes it obvious that this is an area that has not been aggressively researched in the recent years and therefore is open to further study.

PSYCHOLOGICAL SUPPORT

Nursing interventions also focus on identifying the impact of the illness on the patient and the family (see Chapter 2). Nursing interventions include providing information, which is essential for the psychological well-being of the patient and the family and may help to give them a sense of understanding and control of the situation.

Patient Outcomes

The expected outcome is that the patient will have improved tissue perfusion (see Box 10-5). Specific patient outcomes include alertness and orientation, normotension, warmth, dry skin, adequate urine output, hemodynamic and laboratory values within normal limits, absence of infection, and intact skin. The patient should be relaxed and resting quietly.

COMPLICATIONS

Complications of shock are related to the metabolic and tissue changes that result. If the normal compensatory mechanisms are not supported by effective therapeutic interventions, the pathological consequences perpetuate a vicious cycle of shock. The cycle is initiated by ischemia to the cells. Ischemia results in anaerobic metabolism, which leads to an accumulation of lactic acid and metabolic acidosis. This acidosis leads to irreversible changes in the cells. Many of these complications are discussed in greater depth in other chapters.

Central Nervous System

The brain suffers as a result of anaerobic metabolism. As lactate levels begin to increase and glucose consumption decreases, the availability of energy for cells in the central nervous system declines. The cells begin to retain sodium and water, and cerebral edema ensues. This phenomenon initiates a vicious cycle in which further compromise of the tissues occurs. Neurological deficits are the end result of severe and prolonged episodes of shock.

Cardiovascular System

The major mechanisms for failure of the heart in shock include (1) a decrease in cardiac output, (2) a decrease in coronary blood flow, and (3) a marked decrease in myocardial contractility. The factors that contribute to these processes in shock are the decreased oxygen availability and the production of myocardial depressant factors.

Hematological System

Alterations in coagulation are common complications of shock. Consumption of clotting proteins leads to bleeding, so bleeding and clotting occur simultaneously. The most common occurrence is disseminated intravascular coagulation, which is a late occurrence in the shock syndrome. The shock syndrome also affects the white blood cells. Leukopenia is common and predisposes the patient to infections.

Respiratory System

The major respiratory complication is acute respiratory distress syndrome. This syndrome occurs secondary to reduced pulmonary blood flow and increased pulmonary vascular resistance. Pulmonary capillary permeability increases, resulting in noncardiogenic pulmonary edema. Surfactant production is decreased, with consequent decreased pulmonary compliance and hypoxemia that is refractory to oxygen therapy.

Renal System

Acute renal failure is a common complication of shock. Decreased renal perfusion leads to ischemic injury and acute tubular necrosis that may require renal replacement therapy (see Chapter 14).

Hepatic System

Decreased perfusion to the hepatic cells diminishes the ability to produce energy, serum proteins, and clotting factors and decreases the ability to detoxify circulating toxins. Consequences include coagulopathy, poor wound healing, and inability to detoxify drugs.

Gastrointestinal System

Ischemia to the intestines causes two distinct problems. Reduction in blood supply affects the protective mechanism of the gastrointestinal tract and leads to mucosal damage and ulceration of the intestines. Ischemia also increases the likelihood that bacteria and toxins will cross the intestinal barrier and enter the circulation, thus leading to sepsis.

Multiple Organ Dysfunction Syndrome

MODS is the progressive dysfunction of two or more organ systems as a result of the uncontrolled inflammatory response to severe illness or injury. Organ dysfunction can progress to organ failure and death. The most common causes of MODS are sepsis and septic shock; however, MODS can occur after any severe injury that activates a massive systemic inflammatory response. Precipitating conditions in the development of MODS are listed in Box 10-8.

BOX 10-8

Precipitating Conditions in the Development of Multiple Organ Dysfunction Syndrome

Sepsis or septic shock
Severe trauma
Major surgery
Burns
Hypovolemic shock
Acute pancreatitis
Acute renal failure
Acute respiratory distress syndrome (ARDS)
Necrotic tissue
Age ≥65 yr
Delayed, inadequate fluid resuscitation
Multiple blood transfusions
Persistent infection
Bowel infarction
Steroid use

The clinical presentation of MODS is caused by inflammatory mediator damage, tissue hypoxia, and hypermetabolism. Criteria used in the diagnosis of organ dysfunction and failure are described in Table 10-12.

Management focuses on prevention and early recognition so supportive therapies can be initiated as soon as possible. Potential sites of infection must be removed, including necrotic tissue and hematomas, and the number of invasive catheters and procedures must be reduced. Maintaining arterial saturation between 88% and 92% and hemoglobin at more than 10 to 12 g/dL is recommended. To promote oxygen delivery to the tissues in the presence of significant vasodilation, fluid resuscitation may be necessary. If fluid resuscitation is not effective, vasoactive and/or inotropic medications are used. Respiratory failure is treated with mechanical ventilation and high oxygen concentrations. Enteral feedings help to preserve the gut microbial barrier. Continuous renal replacement therapies may be required to maintain fluid and electrolyte balance in the presence of acute renal failure.

TABLE 10-12

Diagnostic Criteria of Organ Dysfunction and Failure

Organ or System	Dysfunction	Failure
Pulmonary	Hypoxia requiring respirator-assisted ventilation for at least 3-5 days	Progressive, ARDS requiring PEEP >10 cm H_2O and FiO_2 >0.5
Hepatic	Serum bilirubin ≥2-3 mg/dL or liver function values twice normal or higher	Clinical jaundice with bilirubin ≥ 8-10 mg/dL
Renal	Oliguria ≤479 mL/24 hr or rising creatinine (≥2-3 mg/dL)	Dialysis
Intestinal	Ileus with intolerance to enteral feeding for longer than 5 days	Stress ulcers requiring transfusion; acalculuos cholecystitis
Hematologic	PT and PTT ↑ >25% or platelets <50,000-80,000, ↑ WBC or ↓ WBC	Disseminated intravascular coagulation
Central nervous system	Confusion, mild disorientation	Progressive coma
Cardiovascular	Decreased ejection fraction, tachycardia, hypotension, Atrial or ventricular arrhythmias Elevated CVP, elevated PAOP Need for inotropic or vassopressor support	Hypodynamic (↓ CO, ↓ SVR, ↓ SvO_2) Response refractory to inotropic support

Modified from Deitch, E. A. (1992). Multiple organ failure. *Annals of Surgery, 216*(2), 117; and Balk, R. A. (2000). Pathogenesis and management of multiple organ dysfunction or failure in severe sepsis and septic shock. *Critical Care Clinics, 16*(2), 337.
ARDS, Acute respiratory distress syndrome; *PEEP,* positive end-expiratory pressure; *FiO₂,* fraction of inspired oxygen in air; *PT,* prothrombin time; *PTT,* partial thromboplastin time; *CVP,* central venous pressure; *PAOP,* pulmonary artery occlusion pressure; *CO,* cardiac output; *SVR,* systemic vascular resistance, *SvO₂,* mixed venous oxygen saturation.

Case Study

evolve

A 33-year-old man, William Rogers, was involved in a motor vehicular accident in which he sustained chest injuries. Mr. Rogers, the driver, was not wearing his seat belt, and the steering wheel was bent. At the scene, Mr. Rogers was unresponsive. Paramedics performed endotracheal intubation and assisted ventilation with 100% oxygen via a bag-valve mask device. Vital signs were a barely palpable systolic blood pressure (BP) at 60 mm Hg and a heart rate of 136 beats/min, and respirations were assisted. His skin was noted as being pale, cold, and clammy, with a delay in capillary refill. Peripheral pulses were weak and thready. Two 14-gauge peripheral intravenous lines were inserted with lactated Ringer's solution infusing wide open. The initial assessment in the emergency department (ED) noted that his palpable BP had increased to 90 mm Hg, and heart rate was 125 beats/min. He was restless in response to pain, with no other purposeful responses; pupils were equal and reacted to light. Mr. Rogers' chest expansion was unequal, and his breath sounds were markedly diminished on the right side. A chest radiograph documented a 70% hemopneumothorax on the right side, and a 36-French chest tube was inserted at the eighth intercostal space on the right midaxillary line. The immediate return was 2000 mL of blood with continuing drainage of 500 mL in 30 minutes. Initial laboratory results were as follows:

Hemoglobin: 9 g/dL
Prothrombin time: 15 sec
Hematocrit: 31%
Partial thromboplastin time: 47 sec
Platelets: 274,000/µL
Red blood cells: 2.9 million/µL
White blood cells: 5300/µL

Staff in the ED inserted a Foley catheter, and it drained 80 mL of clear, yellow urine. Fluid resuscitation was continued to maintain a systolic BP at 90 to 100 mm Hg. Mr. Rogers was taken immediately to the operating room, where a right thoracotomy was performed, with repair of the right axillary artery. In the operating room,

his vital signs remained stable with the continued fluid resuscitation of crystalloids, blood, and fresh frozen plasma.

After surgery, he was admitted to the intensive care unit, where his BP was 116/70 mm Hg, heart rate was 90 beats/min, and respirations were 24 breaths/min on the ventilator (assist/control mode with a rate setting of 20). He was responsive to commands and denied pain. He was being medicated with morphine, 4 mg intravenous push every hour, for pain. Laboratory results were as follows:

Hemoglobin: 11 g/dL
Prothrombin time: 18.7 sec
Hematocrit: 34%
Partial thromboplastin time: 71.7 sec
Platelets: 180,000/µL
Fibrinogen: 76 mg/dL
Red blood cells: 4.8 million/µL
White blood cells: 5300/µL
Arterial blood gases (on 60% assisted ventilation):
  Ph: 7.30
  $PaCO_2$: 47 mm Hg
  PaO_2: 90 mm Hg
  SaO_2: 92%
  HCO_3^-: 15 mEq/L

CASE STUDY QUESTIONS

1. What type of shock did Mr. Rogers demonstrate at the scene, and what components of his assessment supported this diagnosis?
2. In the ED, Mr. Rogers was receiving lactated Ringer's solution for fluid resuscitation. Is this the appropriate solution at this time?
3. Explain Mr. Rogers' arterial blood gas results. What treatment is indicated?
4. Describe the nursing care Mr. Rogers will receive in the first 24 hours after his surgery.
5. Describe the risk factors Mr. Rogers has for developing sepsis.

SUMMARY

The risk of shock is a common threat for all patients. Its causes are many and its treatment varied and complex. Prevention is the primary goal; it is accomplished through the identification of high-risk patient conditions and early interventions. Successful management relies on accurate nursing assessments, data analysis, implementation of definitive interventions, and evaluation of patient response to treatment. Shock is a crisis for the patient, family, nurse, and health care team. A multidisciplinary approach of clinical expertise combined with caring assists the patient in reaching a positive outcome.

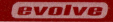
1. Several people are admitted to the critical care unit, including (1) a 79-year-old man with a small anterior myocardial infarction and no prior cardiac history, (2) a 47-year-old man admitted after surgery for an open reduction and fixation of a fractured femur, (3) a 17-year-old adolescent with cervical spine injury after a diving accident, and (4) a 23-year-old woman with sternal bruising and occasional premature ventricular contractions after a motor vehicle accident. Discuss what additional assessment information is needed in order to determine which of these patients have the potential to develop shock and why they could develop shock.

2. Differentiate hypovolemic, cardiogenic, and septic shock.

3. A patient was admitted from the emergency department after a motorcycle accident in which he sustained blunt abdominal trauma. IV access was established in the internal jugular and left antecubital veins, and lactated Ringer's solution was infused. The results of initial CT scan of the abdomen were negative. On admission to the critical care unit, you review the hematological profile for the following results:
   a. Hemoglobin: 9.1 g/dL
   b. Hematocrit: 31.1%
   c. Platelets: 274,000/μL
   d. Red blood cells: 2.9 million/μL
   e. White blood cells: 9800/μL
   f. Prothrombin time: 15 sec
   g. Activated partial thromboplastin time: 47 sec
   Explain the rationale for the alterations in these values.

4. Describe factors in the critically ill patient that increase susceptibility to the development of severe sepsis and septic shock. Describe how these can be prevented.

REFERENCES

2001 SCCM/ESICM/ACCP/ATS/SIS International Sepsis Definitions Conference. (2003). *Critical Care Medicine, 31*(4), 1250-1256.

Ahrens, T., & Vollman, K. (2003). Severe sepsis management: Are we doing enough? *Critical Care Nurse, 23* (5 suppl), 2-15.

Albright, T., Zimmerman, M., & Selzman, C. (2002). Vasopressin in the cardiac surgery intensive care unit. *American Journal of Critical Care, 11*(4), 326-332.

American College of Chest Physicians/Society of Critical Care Medicine Consensus Conference Committee. (1992). Definitions for sepsis and organ failure and guidelines for the use of innovative therapies in sepsis. *Critical Care Medicine, 20*(6), 864-874.

American College of Surgeons. (1997). *Advanced trauma life support for doctors.* Chicago: Author.

Baldwin, K., & Morris, S. (2002). Shock, multiple organ dysfunction syndrome and burns in adults. In K. L. McCance & S. E. Huether (eds.). *Pathophysiology: The biologic basis for disease in adults and children* (pp. 1483-1499). 4th ed. St. Louis: Mosby.

Bernard, G., Vincent, J., Laterre, P., et al. (2001). Efficacy and safety of recombinant human activated protein C for severe sepsis. *New England Journal of Medicine, 344* (10), 699-709.

Bernards, C. (2001). Epidural and spinal anesthesia. In P. Barash, B. Cullen, & R. Stoelting (eds.). *Clinical anesthesia* (pp. 689-710). 4th ed. Philadelphia: Lippincott Williams & Wilkins.

Boulain, T., Achard, J., Teboul, J., Richard, C., Perroting, D., & Ginies, G. (2002). Changes in blood pressure induced by passive leg raising predict response to fluid loading in critically ill patients. *Chest, 121*(4),1245-1252.

Caplan, L., & Miller, S. (2001). Shock. In P. Barash, B. Cullen, & R. Stoelting (eds.). *Clinical anesthesia* (pp. 1261-1262). 4th ed. Philadelphia: Lippincott Williams & Wilkins.

Centers for Disease Control and Prevention. (2004). Guidelines for preventing health-care associated pneumonia, 2003. *Morbidity and Mortality Weekly Report 53*(RR03):1-36.

Chambers, H. (2003). Infectious diseases. In L. Tierney, S. McPhee, & M. Papadakis (eds.). *Current medical diagnosis and treatment.* 42nd ed. (pp. 1419-1420). New York: Lange Medical Books/McGraw-Hill.

Chernecky, C., & Berger, B. (2004). *Laboratory tests and diagnostic procedures.* 4th ed. Philadelphia: Elsevier.

Christensen, D. (2000). The ventricular assist device: An overview. *Nursing Clinics of North America, 35*(2), 945-959.

Corwin, H., Gittinger, A., Pearl, R., et al. (2002). Efficacy of reombinant human erythropoietin in critically ill patients: A randomized controlled trial. *Journal of the American Medical Association, 288*, 2827-2835.

Cummins, R. (ed.). (2002). *Textbook for advanced cardiovascular life support.* Dallas, TX: American Heart Association.

Dellinger, R., Carlet, J., Masur, H., et al. (2004). Surviving sepsis campaign guidelines for management of severe sepsis and septic shock. *Critical Care Medicine, 32*, 858-873.

Gaynes, R., Richards, C., Edwards, J., et al. (2001). Feeding back surveillance data to prevent hospital-acquired infections. *Emerging Infectious Diseases, 7*(2), 295-298.

Hollenburg, S., Kavinsky C., & Parillo, J. (1999). Cardiogenic shock. *Annals of Internal Medicine, 131*(1)45-57.

Huffstutler, S. (2003). Assessment of the cardiovascular system. In W. Phipps, F. Monahan, J. Sands, J. Marek, M. Neighbors, & C. Green(eds.). *Medical-surgical nursing: Health and illness perspectives.* (pp. 611-644). 7th ed. St. Louis: Mosby.

Kleinpell, R. (2003). The role of the critical care nurse in the assessment and management of the patient with severe sepsis. *Critical Care Nursing Clinics of North America, 15,* 27-34.

Loeb, H, & Cohn, J. (2000). Shock. In J. Willerson & J. Cohn (eds.). *Cardiovascular medicine.* (pp. 1529-1536). 2nd ed. New York: Churchill-Livingstone.

Maier, R. (2001). Shock. In E. Braunwald, A. Fauci, J. Jameson, L. Kasper, S. Hauser, & D. Longo (eds.). *Harrison's principles of internal medicine.* (pp. 222-227). 15th ed. New York: McGraw-Hill.

Marik, P. (2001). Sublingual capnography: A clinical validation study. *Chest, 120*(3), 923-927.

Mikhail, J. (1999). Resuscitation endpoints in trauma. *AACN Clinical Issues, 10*(1), 10-21.

Miller, S. (2002). Acute care of the elderly units: A positive outcomes study. *AACN Clinical Issues, 13*(1), 34-42.

Pathan, N., Sandiford, C., Harding, S., & Levin, M. (2002). Characterization of myocardial depressant factor in meningococcal septicemia. *Critical Care Medicine, 30*(10), 2378-2380.

Robb, W. (1999). Massive transfusion in trauma. *AACN Clinical Issues, 10*(1), 69-84.

Seidel, H. M., Ball, J. W., Dains, J. E., & Benedict, G. W. (1999). *Mosby's guide to physical examination.* 4th ed. St. Louis: Mosby.

Smith-Blair, N. (2003). Shock. In W. Phipps, F. Monahan, J. Sands, J. Marek, M. Neighbors, & C. Green (eds.).

Medical-surgical nursing: Health and illness perspectives. (pp. 283-301). 7th ed. St. Louis: Mosby.

Sommers, M. (2003). The cellular basis of septic shock. *Critical Care Nursing Clinics of North America, 15,* 13-25.

Tierney, L., & Messina, L. (2003). Blood vessels and lymphatics. In L. Tierney, S. McPhee, & M. Papadakis (eds.). *Current medical diagnosis and treatment* (pp. 465-468). 42nd ed. New York: Lange Medical Books/McGraw-Hill.

Van den Berghe, G., Wouters, P. J., Weekers, F., et al. (2001). Intensive insulin therapy in critically ill patients. *New England Journal of Medicine, 345,* 1359-1367.

Winslow, R. (1999). New transfusion strategies: Red cell substitutes. *Annual Review of Medicine, 50,* 337-353.

RECOMMENDED READINGS

Ely, E. W., Kleinpell, R. M., & Goyette, R. E. (2003). Advances in the understanding of clinical manifestations and therapy of severe sepsis: An update for critical care nurses. *American Journal of Critical Care, 12*(2), 120-133.

Felblinger, D. (2003). Malnutrition, infection and sepsis in acute and chronic illness. *Critical Care Nursing Clinics of North America, 15,* 71-78.

Kleinpell, R. (2003). Advances in treating patients with severe sepsis. *Critical Care Nurse, 23*(3), 16-29.

Pudelek, B., (2002). Geriatric trauma: Special needs for a special population. *AACN Clinical Issues, 13*(1) 61-72.

evolve *Did you remember to check out the bonus material, including free self-assessment exercises, on the Evolve Web site at http://evolve.elsevier.com/Sole/ and on the CD-ROM?*

CHAPTER 11

Cardiovascular Alterations

Jeffrey Williams, MSN, RN, CCRN, CCNS
Virginia Oenning, MSN, RN, CNS
Beverly Tuomala, BSN, RN, CCRN

OBJECTIVES

- Contrast the pathological cause and effect mechanisms that produce acute cardiac disturbances.
- Discuss the nursing care responsibilities related to the cardiac and vascular patient.
- Compare and contrast pharmacological, operative, and electrical treatment modalities used in treatment of cardiac disease.
- Identify specific nursing interventions designed to prevent secondary occurrences or to minimize complications of cardiac and vascular patients.
- Develop a research-related care plan for the acutely ill cardiovascular patient.

Introduction

Care of the seriously ill patient with alterations in cardiac status includes those cardiac patients at risk for an uncertain prognosis. The critical care nurse needs theoretical knowledge and practice-related understanding of the common cardiac diseases to have the sound clinical judgment necessary for making rapid and accurate decisions. The purpose of this chapter is to identify and explore some of the more common cardiac alterations that are likely to be encountered by the critical care nurse caring for adult patients with compromised cardiac status and to describe the nursing care to optimize the patient's outcome.

Normal Structure and Function of the Heart

An essential component of effective nursing care is a comprehensive knowledge of the normal structure and function of the heart. The heart muscle is approximately the size of a person's closed fist and lies within the mediastinal space of the thoracic cavity between the lungs, directly under the lower half of the sternum, and above the diaphragm (Figure 11-1). It is covered by the pericardium, which has an inner visceral layer and an outer parietal layer. Certain diseases can cause this covering to become inflamed and can subsequently diminish the effectiveness of the heart as a pump. Several cubic millimeters of

evolve Be sure to check out the bonus material, including free self-assessment exercises, on the Evolve Web site at http://evolve.elsevier.com/Sole/ and on the CD-ROM.

lubricating fluid are present between these layers. Some pathological conditions can increase the amount and the consistency of this fluid, and this can also affect the pumping ability of the heart. The heart muscle itself is composed of three layers. The outer layer, or epicardium, covers the surface of the heart and extends to the great vessels; the middle, muscular layer, or myocardium, is responsible for the heart's pumping action; and the inner endothelial layer, or endocardium, covers the heart valves and the small muscles associated with the opening and closing of those valves. These layers are damaged or destroyed when a patient has a myocardial infarction (MI).

Functionally, the heart is divided into right-sided and left-sided pumps that are separated by a septum. The right side is generally considered to be a low-pressure system, whereas the left side is a high-pressure system. Each side has an atrium that receives the blood and a ventricle that pumps it out. The right atrium receives deoxygenated blood from the body through the superior and inferior venae cavae. Blood travels from the atrium to the ventricles by means of a pressure gradient between the chambers. The right ventricle pumps the deoxygenated blood to the lungs through the pulmonary artery for oxygen and carbon dioxide exchange. The left atrium receives the newly oxygenated blood by way of the pulmonary veins from the lungs, and the left ventricle pumps the oxygenated blood through the aorta to the systemic circulation (Figure 11-2).

The four cardiac valves maintain the unidirectional blood flow through the chambers of the heart. The four valves also assist in producing the pressure gradient needed between the chambers for the blood to flow through the heart. There are two types of valves: the atrioventricular (AV) valves, which separate the atria from the ventricles, and the semilunar

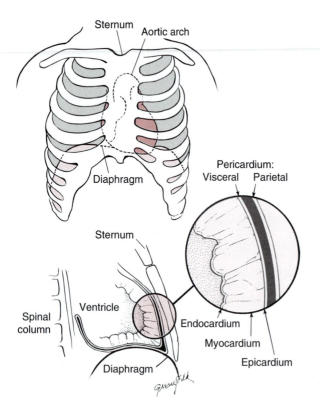

FIGURE 11-1 The heart lies in the mediastinum, between the lungs. Its apex rests on the diaphragm. The heart is covered by the pericardium. The *inset* shows the layers of the heart muscle and the pericardium. (From Price, S. A., & Wilson, L. M. [2003]. *Pathophysiology: Clinical concepts of disease processes.* 6th ed. St. Louis: Mosby.)

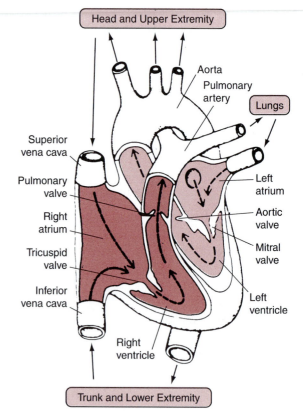

FIGURE 11-2 Structure of the heart and course of blood flow through the heart chambers. (From Guyton, A. C., & Hall, J. E. [2001]. *Textbook of medical physiology.* 10th ed. Philadelphia: W. B. Saunders.)

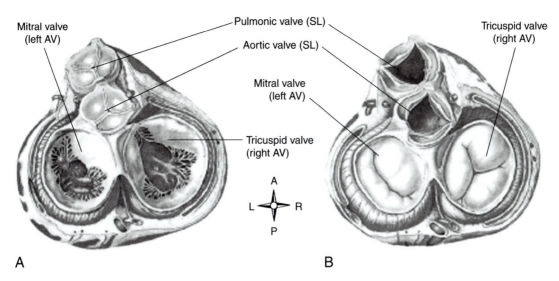

Mitral valve
(left AV)

Pulmonic valve (SL)

Aortic valve (SL)

Tricuspid valve
(right AV)

Mitral valve
(left AV)

Tricuspid valve
(right AV)

A

L — R

P

A   B

FIGURE 11-3 A, The atrioventricular (AV) valves in the open position and the semilunar (SL) valves in the closed position. **B,** The AV valves in the closed position and the SL valves in the open position. *AV,* Atrioventricular; *SL,* semilunar. (From Thibodeau, G. A. & Patton, K. T. [2003]. *Anatomy and physiology,* 5th ed. St. Louis: Mosby.)

valves, which separate the pulmonary artery from the right ventricle and the aorta from the left ventricle (Figure 11-3). The AV valves are the tricuspid valve, which lies between the right atrium and the right ventricle, and the mitral valve, located between the left atrium and the left ventricle. Each AV valve is anchored by chordae tendineae to the papillary muscles on its ventricular floor. The semilunar valves are the pulmonic valve, which lies between the right ventricle and the pulmonary artery, and the aortic valve, which is between the left ventricle and the aorta. These semilunar valves are not anchored by chordae tendineae. Instead, their closing is passive and is caused by differences in pressure between the chamber and the respective great vessel.

AUTONOMIC CONTROL

The autonomic nervous system exerts control over the cardiovascular system. The sympathetic nervous system releases norepinephrine, which has two effects. Alpha-adrenergic effects cause arterial vasoconstriction. Beta-adrenergic effects increase sinus node discharge (positive chronotropic), increase the force of contraction (positive inotropic), and accelerate the AV conduction time (positive dromotropic).

The parasympathetic nervous system releases acetylcholine through stimulation of the vagus nerve. It causes a decrease in the sinus node discharge and slows conduction through the AV node.

In addition to this innervation, receptors help to control cardiovascular function. The first receptors are the chemoreceptors, which are sensitive to changes in partial pressure of arterial oxygen (PaO_2), partial pressure of arterial carbon dioxide ($PaCO_2$), and pH blood levels. Chemoreceptors stimulate the vasomotor center in the medulla; this center controls vasoconstriction and vasodilation. Second are baroreceptors, which are sensitive to stretch and pressure. If blood pressure increases, the baroreceptors cause the heart rate to decrease. If the blood pressure decreases, the baroreceptors stimulate an increase in heart rate (Figure 11-4).

CORONARY CIRCULATION

Because many cardiac problems result from an occlusion or a partial occlusion of a coronary artery, an understanding of the coronary blood supply is necessary. The blood supply to the myocardium is derived from the coronary arteries that branch off the aorta immediately above the aortic valve (Figure 11-5). Two major branches exist: the right coronary artery and the left coronary artery, which splits into two branches, the left anterior descending and the left circumflex. Knowledge of the portion of the heart that receives its blood supply from a particular coronary artery allows the nurse to anticipate problems related to occlusion of that vessel (Box 11-1). Variations in the branching and the exact placement of the coronary arteries are common (Buja & McAllister, 2000).

Blood flow to the coronary arteries occurs during diastole, when the aortic valve is closed and the sinuses of Valsalva are filled with blood. Myocardial fibers

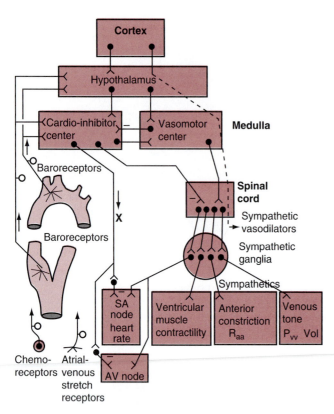

FIGURE 11-4 Autonomic control of circulation. *AV,* Atrioventricular; P_{vv}, pulmonary venules; R_{aa}, renal arterioles; *SA,* sinoatrial. (Modified from Goerke, J., & Mines, A. [1988]. *Cardiovascular physiology.* New York: Raven.)

are relaxed at this time, thus promoting blood flow through the coronary vessels. The coronary veins return blood from the coronary circulation back into the heart through the coronary sinuses to the right and left atria (Buja & McAllister, 2000).

OTHER CARDIAC FUNCTIONS

Knowledge of properties of cardiac muscle and the normal conduction system of the heart is essential since many patients have cardiac dysrhythmias (see Chapter 6). Hemodynamics of the cardiovascular system are also important in understanding pathology such as heart failure (HF).

HEART SOUNDS

The vibrations produced by vascular walls, flowing blood, heart muscle, and heart valves create sound waves known as *heart sounds.* Auscultating these sounds with a stethoscope over the heart provides valuable information about valve and cardiac function

(Figure 11-6). Ventricular systole occurs when the pulmonic and aortic valves open to allow blood to be pumped to the lungs (right ventricle-pulmonic valve) and systemic circulation (left ventricle-aortic valve). Ventricular diastole occurs when the tricuspid and mitral valves open to allow the ventricles to fill with blood.

The first heart sound is known as S_1. This sound has been described as "lubb." It is caused by closure of the mitral and tricuspid valves. It is best heard at the apex (fifth intercostal space, left midclavicular line) of the heart and represents the beginning of ventricular systole.

The second heart sound is known as S_2. It has been described as "dubb" and is caused by closure of the aortic and pulmonic valves. It is best heard at the second intercostal space at the right or left sternal border and represents the beginning of ventricular diastole. The first and second heart sounds are best heard with the diaphragm of the stethoscope with the patient lying in the supine position.

A third heart sound, S_3, can be normal in a child, but it usually represents a pathological process in the adult. The sound may be produced at the time when the heart is already overfilled or poorly compliant. The S_3 sound is low pitched and can best be heard with the bell of the stethoscope at the fifth intercostal space, at the left midclavicular line. It occurs immediately after S_2. Together with S_1 and S_2, S_3 produces a sound like "lubb-dubba" or "ken-tuk'e." S_3 is heard in patients with HF or fluid overload. A fourth heart sound, S_4, is produced from atrial contraction that is more forceful than normal. Together with S_1 and S_2, S_4 produces a sound like "te-lubb-dubb" or "ten'-ne-see." S_4 can be normal in elderly patients, but it is often heard after MI, when the atria contract more forcefully against ventricles distended with blood. In the severely failing heart, all four sounds (S_4, S_1, S_2, and S_3) may be heard, producing a "gallop" rhythm, so named because it sounds like the hoofbeats of a galloping horse. It can best be heard with the bell of the stethoscope at the fifth intercostal space, at the left midclavicular line.

HEART MURMUR

A heart murmur is a sound caused by turbulence of blood flow through the valves of the heart. In children and adults, murmurs can also be heard when a septal defect is present. In adults, murmurs can be heard when a valve, usually aortic or mitral, is narrow, inflamed, stenosed, or incompetent or when the valve leaflets fail to approximate (insufficiency). The presence of a new murmur warrants special attention, particularly in a patient with an acute MI (AMI). A papillary muscle may have ruptured, causing the valve

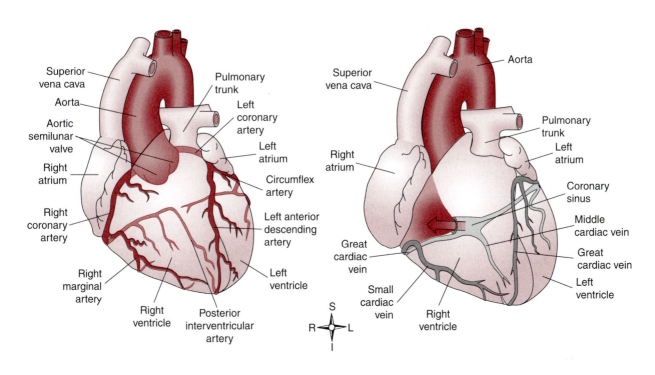

FIGURE 11-5 The coronary vessels. (From McCance, K. L., & Huether, S. E. [eds.]. [2002]. *Pathophysiology: The biologic basis for disease in adults and children.* 4th ed. St. Louis: Mosby.)

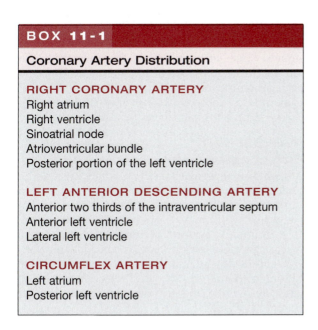

BOX 11-1

Coronary Artery Distribution

RIGHT CORONARY ARTERY
Right atrium
Right ventricle
Sinoatrial node
Atrioventricular bundle
Posterior portion of the left ventricle

LEFT ANTERIOR DESCENDING ARTERY
Anterior two thirds of the intraventricular septum
Anterior left ventricle
Lateral left ventricle

CIRCUMFLEX ARTERY
Left atrium
Posterior left ventricle

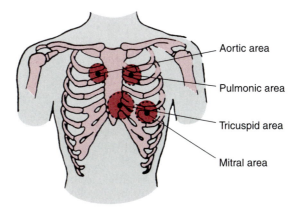

FIGURE 11-6 Chest areas from which each valve sound is best heard. (From Guyton, A. C., & Hall, J. E. [2001]. *Textbook of medical physiology.* 10th ed. Philadelphia: W. B. Saunders.)

TABLE 11-1

Grading of Heart Murmurs

Intensity of Murmur Graded from I to VI	Intensity of Murmur Graded Based on Increasing Loudness
Grade I	Lowest intensity, usually not audible by inexperienced providers
Grade II	Low intensity, usually audible by inexperienced providers
Grade III	Medium intensity without a thrill
Grade IV	Medium intensity with a thrill
Grade V	Loudest murmur audible when stethoscope is placed on the chest; associated with a thrill
Grade VI	Loudest intensity, audible when stethoscope is removed from chest; associated with a thrill

to not approximate correctly, and it can be indicative of severe damage and impending complications (e.g., HF and pulmonary edema). A murmur is usually a rumbling, blowing, harsh, or musical sound. It is important to distinguish the sound, anatomical location, loudness, and intensity of a murmur and whether extra heart sounds are heard. Table 11-1 gives a grading of heart murmurs. This skill is developed from practice in listening to many different patients' hearts and in correlating the sounds heard with the patients' pathological conditions.

Coronary Artery Disease

Coronary artery disease (CAD) is broad term used to refer to the narrowing or occlusion of the coronary arteries. Blood supply to the coronary arteries is reduced as a result of CAD. Other terms used to describe CAD include coronary heart disease and atherosclerotic heart disease.

PATHOPHYSIOLOGY

CAD is the progressive narrowing of one or more coronary arteries by atherosclerosis. CAD results in ischemia when the internal diameter of the coronary vessel is reduced by 50% to 70% (Killip, 2000) (Figure 11-7).

Atherosclerosis begins with injury to the endothelial cells in the intima of the coronary arteries (McCance & Huether, 2002). The injury results in platelet aggregation and migration of monocytes to the site. Lipoproteins enter the intima, and the result is a fatty streak. The monocytes in the fatty streak are transformed into macrophages that develop receptors for engulfing lipids, especially low-density lipoproteins (LDLs). Lipid-rich "foam cells" develop. Foam cells progress to form a fibrous plaque or atheroma. Damage to the intima liberates platelet-derived growth factor, which stimulates migration of smooth muscle cells from the media to the intima of the coronary artery and forms the atheroma. Over time, a fibrous cap is formed from connective tissue (fibroblasts and macrophages) and LDLs.

The fibrous cap often ruptures, producing a thrombus. The thrombus can occlude a coronary artery, with resulting injury and infarction. Rupture of the plaque also initiates the coagulation cascade with the initiation of thrombin production, the conversion of fibrinogen to fibrin, and platelet aggregation at the site.

Platelet changes occur in three steps. It is important to understand these steps because current therapy after an acute occlusion is targeted at altering this process. After injury to the endothelium, platelets are exposed to proteins that bind to receptors, causing adhesion of platelets at the site of injury. Next, the platelets are activated and change shape. They release thromboxane A_2 and serotonin. Each platelet has thousands of glycoprotein IIb/IIIa (Gp IIb/IIIa) receptors that are activated and bind with von Willebrand's factor and fibrinogen, which is converted to fibrin strands. At the same time, the platelets aggregate with one another. This process of adhesion, activation, and aggregation causes a rapidly growing thrombus that compromises coronary blood flow (Killip, 2000). Box 11-2 presents risk factors for CAD.

ASSESSMENT

Patient Assessment

A cardiovascular assessment is imperative to an understanding of the individual cardiac patient and is inherent to the planning of nursing care for that patient.

A thorough history includes subjective data regarding medical history, prior hospitalizations, allergies, and family medical history. A previous medical history of both pediatric and adult illnesses is of particular interest and includes a positive history for rheumatic fever, diabetes mellitus, hypertension, asthma, renal disease, or cerebrovascular accident. Knowledge of prior hospitalizations is also important so records can be obtained for review. Information regarding the patient's current medications, both

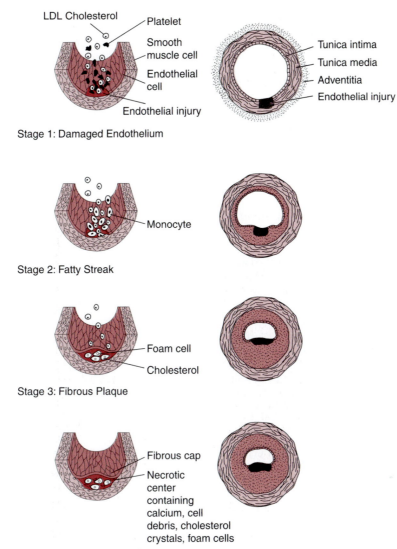

LDL Cholesterol
Platelet
Smooth muscle cell
Endothelial cell
Endothelial injury

Tunica intima
Tunica media
Adventitia
Endothelial injury

Stage 1: Damaged Endothelium

Monocyte

Stage 2: Fatty Streak

Foam cell
Cholesterol

Stage 3: Fibrous Plaque

Fibrous cap
Necrotic center containing calcium, cell debris, cholesterol crystals, foam cells

Stage 4: Complicated Lesion

FIGURE 11-7 Development of coronary atherosclerosis. (From Hansen, M. [1998]. *Pathophysiology: Foundations of disease and clinical intervention.* Philadelphia: W. B. Saunders.)

prescription and over-the-counter drugs, should include information about the patient's understanding and use of these medications. A history of the patient's use of sildenafil citrate (Viagra) and/or cialis (Levitra) is necessary to know when considering nitroglycerin (NTG) administration. These medications have been shown to potentiate the hypotensive effects of nitrates, thus concurrent use is contraindicated. It is also important to determine whether the patient has any food or drug allergies.

A psychosocial or personal history is also important for the planning of the patient's care. This history includes major stress events and everyday stressors. Additional information regarding activities for stress reduction is obtained. What, if any, is the patient's exercise routine, including the type, amount, and regularity of the activity? What is the patient's daily food pattern and intake? What is his or her sleep pattern? What are the patient's habitual social patterns in using tobacco, alcohol, drugs, coffee, tea, and caffeinated sodas?

Before beginning the physical examination, the nurse determines recent and recurrent symptoms that may be related to the patient's current problems.

BOX 11-2

Risk Factors for Coronary Artery Disease

Several risk factors predispose persons to coronary artery disease (CAD). Some risk factors cannot be changed (e.g., heredity and age). Other risk factors for CAD are modifiable (e.g., smoking, hypertension, and diabetes) and are targeted in prevention programs. Major risk factors for CAD include age, family history, high blood cholesterol, smoking, hypertension, diabetes, obesity or overweight, and physical inactivity (AHA, 2002; AHA, 2001b).

AGE
Men older than 45 years and women older than 55 years are considered at higher risk for CAD.

HEREDITY
Family history of early heart disease is an unmodifiable risk for CAD. History is defined as having a father or brother diagnosed with CAD before age 55 years or a mother or sister with CAD before age 65 years.

BLOOD CHOLESTEROL
Serum cholesterol or lipid levels play a key role in the development of atherosclerosis. Elevated total cholesterol (>200 mg/dL) is considered a risk factor for CAD (AHA, 2002). Cholesterol is insoluble in plasma and must be transported by lipoproteins that are soluble. High-density lipoproteins (HDLs) are considered the good cholesterol. HDLs assist in transporting cholesterol to the liver for removal. A high HDL level (≥60 mg/dL) may reduce the incidence of CAD, whereas a low HDL level (<40 mg/dL) is considered a risk factor for developing CAD (NIH, 2004).

Low-density lipoproteins (LDLs) are considered the bad cholesterol. LDLs transport and deposit cholesterol to the arterial vessels, thus facilitating the process of atherosclerosis. An LDL level <100 mg/dL is optimal. Other non-HDL lipoproteins also contribute to development of CAD. Very-low-density lipoproteins are largely composed of triglycerides and contribute to an increased risk of CAD (NIH 2004).

CIGARETTE AND TOBACCO SMOKE
Smokers have a higher risk of CAD. Smoking increases LDL levels and damages the endothelium of coronary vessels. These are predisposing factors for the development of atherosclerosis. Smoking also causes vasoconstriction of coronary vessels, thus decreasing blood supply.

HYPERTENSION
A blood pressure >140/90 mmHg or on antihypertensive medication is a risk for CAD (NIH, 2004). Hypertension causes direct injury to the vasculature, leading to development of CAD. Oxygen demands are also increased in patients with hypertension. The heart muscle enlarges and weakens over time, thereby increasing the workload of the heart.

DIABETES
Diabetes is associated with increased levels of LDL and triglycerides. Glycation associated with diabetes decreases uptake of LDL by the liver and increases hepatic synthesis of LDL (McCance & Huether, 2002).

OBESITY AND OVERWEIGHT
Obesity increases the atherogenic process and predisposes persons to CAD. In addition, obesity is related to hypertension and diabetes, two other major risk factors for CAD. Some research has noted that distribution of fat may also influence the risk of CAD. Persons with a greater proportion of fat through the abdomen ("apple-shaped") have been shown to have a higher incidence of CAD than those with greater fat distribution over the hips ("pear-shaped"). The waist-to-hip ratio is used to help identify this risk.

PHYSICAL INACTIVITY
Lack of physical activity is a risk factor for CAD. Regular, aerobic exercise reduces the incidence of CAD. Exercise also helps to control other risk factors such as hypertension, diabetes, and obesity.

SECONDARY RISK FACTORS
Other factors may influence the development of CAD. These factors include stress, alcohol, and the role of estrogen. Findings from recent research studies are controversial on the role of these secondary risk factors in CAD.

CLINICAL ALERT: ASSESSMENT OF THE PATIENT WITH CHEST PAIN *PQRST*

P	Provocation
Q	Quality
R	Region/Radiation
S	Severity
T	Timing (when began) and Treatment

Such information gathering should include the presence or absence of fatigue, fluid retention, dyspnea, irregular heart beat (palpitations), and chest pain (see Clinical Alert). The physical examination itself encompasses all the body systems and is not limited to the cardiovascular system, because all the body systems are interrelated and interdependent. Although it is imperative that a total evaluation is completed regarding the physical status of the patient, a patient whose primary problems are cardiovascular most commonly exhibits alterations in circulation and oxygenation. Thus, all systems should be examined from this perspective.

The examination is performed in an orderly, organized manner and should involve the techniques of inspection, palpation, percussion, and auscultation. A baseline assessment is provided in Table 11-2.

TABLE 11-2

Major Systems Assessment

System	Assessment
Neurological	Level of consciousness, orientation to person, place, time, events; presence of hallucinations, depression, withdrawal, trembling; pupils (size, equality, response); paresthesias; eye movements (nystagmus, focus, directional movement); restlessness, apprehensiveness, irritability, cooperativeness; hand grips; leg movement; response to tactile stimuli; type, location of pain; how pain is relieved; patient's complaints
Skin	Color, temperature, dryness, turgor, presence of rashes, broken areas, pressure areas, urticaria, incision site, wounds
Cardiovascular	BP; apical and radial pulses; pulse deficit; monitor leads on patient in correct placement; rhythm, frequency of ectopics; PRI, QRS, and QT intervals; heart sounds; presence of abnormalities (e.g., rubs, gallops); neck vein distention with head of bed at what angle; edema (sacral and dependent); calf pain; varicosities; presence of pulses: bilateral carotid, radial, femoral, posterior tibial, dorsalis pedis; capillary refill in extremities; hemodynamic measurements; temporary pacemaker settings; medications to maintain BP or rhythm
Respiratory	Rate, depth, and quality of respirations; oxygen; accessory muscles used; cough, sputum: type, color, suctioning frequency; symmetry of chest expansion and breath sounds, describe breath sounds; current ABGs; chest tube with description of drainage, fluctuation in water seal, bubbling, suction applied; tracheostomy or endotracheal tube; ventilator used; ventilator settings; ventilator rate versus patients's own breaths; patient's spontaneous tidal volume
Gastrointestinal	Abdominal size and softness, bowel sounds, nausea and vomiting, bowel movement, dressing and/or drainage, NG tube with description of drainage, feeding tube: type and frequency of feedings, drains
Genitourinary	Foley or voiding, urine color, quality; vaginal or urethral drainage
Intravenous	Volume of fluid, type of solution, rate; intravenous site condition
Wounds	Dry or drainage, type, color, amount, odor; hematoma, inflamed, drains, hemovac, dressing changes, cultures

ABG, Arterial blood gas; *BP*, blood pressure; *NG*, nasogastric.

Diagnostic Studies

Certain diagnostic studies are fundamental for the care and treatment of patients with CAD. The following sections contain brief descriptions of common diagnostic studies the cardiac patient may encounter.

12-Lead electrocardiography. This noninvasive test is usually preliminary to most other tests performed. It is used as a baseline for many other tests and often as a comparison of pretest and posttest changes. This test is useful in identification of rhythm disturbances, and myocardial ischemia, injury, or infarct.

Holter monitor. This noninvasive test is used to detect suspected dysrhythmias. The patient is connected to a small portable recorder (about the size of a pocket radio) by three to five electrodes; the recorder is worn for 12 to 24 hours. The patient engages in the normal daily activities, keeps an activity log, and returns to the laboratory after the designated period of time. The recording is then analyzed.

Exercise tolerance test or stress test. This is a noninvasive test in which the patient is connected to an electrocardiogram (ECG) machine while exercising for 3-minute intervals (putting stress on the heart and vascular system). Physical stress causes an increase in myocardial oxygen consumption. If oxygen demand exceeds supply, ischemia may result. The stress test is used to document exercise-induced ischemia, and it can identify those individuals prone to cardiac ischemia during activity when resting ECGs are normal (Chernecky & Berger, 2004). The exercise usually involves pedaling a stationary bike or walking on a treadmill. The patient is constantly monitored, the pulse and blood pressure are checked at intervals, and the ECG printout is analyzed at the end of the testing period. The patient usually rests in the laboratory to ensure a return to the baseline heart rate before returning to his or her room or going home.

If a patient is unable physically to perform the exercise, a pharmacological stress test can be done. For example, adenosine can be administered to mimic increased cardiac workload (Chernecky & Berger, 2004).

Chest radiography. This is a noninvasive procedure and is usually performed in the anteroposterior view. The chest x-ray study is used for detecting cardiomegaly, cardiac positioning, degree of fluid infiltrating the pulmonary space, and other structural changes that may affect the physical ability of the heart to function in a normal manner.

Echocardiography. This is a noninvasive, acoustic imaging procedure and involves the use of ultrasound to visualize the cardiac structures and the motion and function of cardiac valves and chambers. A transducer placed on the chest wall sends ultrasound waves at short intervals. The reflected sound waves, termed *echoes,* are displayed on a graph for interpretation. Echocardiography is used to assess valvular function, evaluate congenital defects, measure size of cardiac chambers, evaluate cardiac disease progression, evaluate ventricular function, diagnose myocardial tumors and effusions, and, to a lesser degree, measure cardiac output. Ventricular function is evaluated by obtaining ejection fraction. The ejection fraction is the percentage of blood ejected from the left ventricle during systole, normally 60% to 70%.

Transesophageal echocardiography. This test provides ultrasonic imaging of the heart from a view behind the heart. In transesophageal echocardiography (TEE), an ultrasound probe is fitted on the end of a flexible gastroscope, which is inserted into the posterior pharynx and advanced into the esophagus. TEE shows a clear picture because the esophagus is against the back of the heart and parallel to the aorta. TEE is indicated to visualize prosthetic heart valves, mitral valve function, aortic dissection, vegetative endocarditis, congenital heart defects in adults, cardiac masses and tumors, and embolic phenomena. It is also used intraoperatively to assess left ventricular function (Chernecky & Berger, 2004). Patients should fast (except for medications) for 6 to 8 hours before the examination. During the procedure, vital signs, cardiac rhythm, and oxygen saturation are monitored. After the procedure, the patient is unable to eat until the gag reflex returns. A rare complication of TEE is esophageal perforation, with signs of sore throat, dysphagia, stiff neck, and epigastric or substernal pain that worsens with breathing and movement or pain in the back, abdomen, or shoulder.

Diagnostic heart scans. Noninvasive scanning is often used to assess the heart. Injection of a radiopharmaceutical contrast agent assists in visualization of heart structures (Chernecky & Berger, 2004).

Technetium-99m stannous pyrophosphate. The technetium-99m stannous pyrophosphate scanning is used to assess AMI. The technetium combines with calcium in damaged myocardial cells to form spots on the scan. The spots begin within 12 hours of AMI and are prominent within 48 to 72 hours. They disappear within a week after the AMI unless myocardial damage continues.

Thallium-201. The thallium-201 scan is used to assess AMI, CAD, or effectiveness of coronary intervention such as angioplasty. The isotope is absorbed into healthy myocardium. Areas of myocardial damage are then visualized. The test may be performed as part of an exercise tolerance test. It may also be used in conjunction with dipyridamole administration because the drug causes greater uptake of thallium. The combination test is useful in individuals who cannot tolerate exercise testing with the scan.

Multigated blood pool study. The multigated blood pool study scan is used to assess left ventricular function. An isotope is injected and images of the heart are taken during systole and diastole to assess the ejection fraction of the heart. An ejection fraction of 60% to 70% and symmetrical contraction of the left ventricle are considered normal test results. This test may be done under stress.

Single-photon emission computed tomography. The single-photon emission computed tomography scan uses another form of technetium that is injected. A camera is then used to reproduce visual images taken along several planes of the heart. This nuclear medicine procedure can produce clearer, more accurate images (Chernecky & Berger, 2004).

Cardiac catheterization and arteriography. This is an invasive procedure that can be divided into two stages. Cardiac catheterization is used to confirm and evaluate the severity of lesions within the coronary arteries, to assess left ventricular function, and to measure pressures in the chambers of the heart, cardiac output, and blood gas content. Right-sided catheterization is performed by placement of a pulmonary artery catheter in the femoral or brachial vein that is carefully advanced into the right atrium, right ventricle, and pulmonary artery. The practitioner measures pressures in the right atrium, right ventricle, pulmonary artery, and pulmonary artery occlusion pressure. Oxygen saturations can be measured if indicated (i.e., valve disease or septal defect).

Left sided catheterization is performed to visualize coronary arteries, to note the area and extent of lesions within the vessel walls, to evaluate CAD and angina-related spasms, to locate areas of infarct through the use of radioisotopes, and to perform interventions such as percutaneous angioplasty or stent placement.

Left-sided catheterization is performed by cannulation of a femoral or brachial artery. The procedure entails positioning a catheter into the aorta at the proximal end of the coronary arteries. Dye is then injected into the arteries, and a radiographic picture (arteriography) is recorded as the dye progresses or fails to progress through the coronary circulation. In addition, dye is injected into the left ventricle, and the amount of dye ejected with the next systole is measured to determine the ejection fraction.

After the procedure, the catheters are removed. To prevent bleeding from the arterial site, a vascular sealing device made of collagen (e.g., AngioSeal) may be used or a stitch device (e.g., Perclose) may be used to close the puncture site in the artery. If the sealing or stitch device is not used, firm pressure is applied for 15 to 30 minutes. Commercial devices (e.g., FemoStop) (Figure 11-8) are available to assist in applying pressure to the site. Depending on the diagnostic study results, patients are usually discharged within 6 to 8 hours of completion of the test.

Nursing care for a patient undergoing cardiac catheterization and arteriography involves the pre-procedure instruction (the procedure will be performed using local anesthesia, and the patient may feel a warm or hot "flush" sensation or flutter of the catheter as it moves about) and postprocedure instruction. The postprocedure routine is noted in Box 11-3.

Magnetic resonance imaging. Magnetic resonance imaging is a noninvasive test used to detect aortic aneurysms and pericardial tumors. Magnetic resonance imaging is a technique that uses magnetic resonance to create images of hydrogen. These images are created as the ions are emitted, picked up, and fed into a computer that reconstructs the image that then can differentiate between healthy and ischemic tissue (Chernecky & Berger, 2004).

Electrophysiology study. An electrophysiology study is an invasive procedure that involves the introduction of an electrode catheter percutaneously from a peripheral vein or artery into the cardiac chamber or sinuses and the performance of programmed electrical stimulation of the heart. Use of electrophysiology studies aids in the recording of intracardiac ECGs, diagnosis of cardiac conduction defects, evaluation of effectiveness of antidysrhythmic medications, determination of proper choice of pacemaker programming, and mapping of the cardiac conduction system before ablation (Chernecky & Berger, 2004).

Laboratory Diagnostics
Other diagnostic measures include the evaluation of serum electrolyte studies and cardiac enzymes. Because many manuals are available regarding the reading and interpretation of laboratory values, this

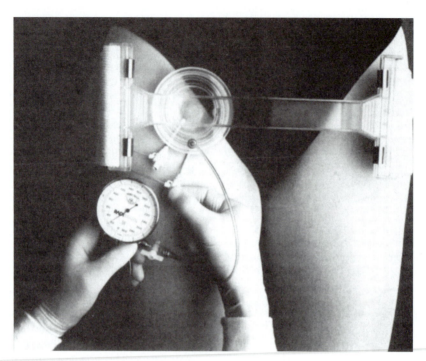

FIGURE 11-8 FemaStop in correct position. (Courtesy of RADI Medical Systems, Inc. Sweden.)

section presents a brief overview of the more important blood studies (Chernecky & Berger, 2004).

Serum electrolytes. Electrolytes are important in maintaining the function of the cardiac conduction system. Imbalances in sodium, potassium, calcium, and magnesium can result in cardiac dysrhythmias. Therefore, analysis of serum electrolytes is a routine part of assessment and treatment of the cardiac patient. Table 11-3 reviews ECG changes that may alert the nurse to possible electrolyte abnormalities.

Serum enzymes. Enzymes are proteins that are produced by all living cells and released into the bloodstream. When cells are injured or diseased, more enzymes are released. Assessments of enzyme levels released from cardiac muscle are useful in diagnosis

---

BOX 11-3

Nursing Care After Cardiac Catheterization and Arteriography

- Maintain the patient on bed rest (time varies depending on method for preventing arterial bleeding).
- Keep the extremity used for catheter insertion immobile.
- Observe the insertion site for bleeding or hematoma, especially if the patient is receiving postprocedure anticoagulant therapy.
- Mark the hematoma with a marker around outer perimeter, to aid in assessing for increased bleeding.
- Maintain head of bed elevation no higher than 30 degrees.
- Monitor peripheral pulses, color, and sensation of the extremity distal to insertion site (q15min × 4, q30min × 4, q1h × 4, then q2h). In addition, monitor the opposite extremity pulse to assess for presence of equal pulses, color, and sensation bilaterally.
- Observe cardiac rhythm.
- Encourage fluid intake.
- Monitor intake and output.
- Observe for an adverse reaction to dye (arteriography).

TABLE 11-3

ECG Changes Associated with Electrolyte Imbalances

Electrolyte Imbalance	Panic Value	Manifestations
Hypokalemia	<2.5 mEq/L	U wave, increased ventricular ectopy
Hyperkalemia	>6.6 mEq/L	Tall, peaked T waves, conduction blocks, ventricular fibrillation
Hypocalcemia	<7 mg/dL	Prolonged ST segment and QT interval
Hypercalcemia	>12 mg/dL	Shortened ST segment and QT interval
Low magnesium	<0.5 mEq/L	Prolonged PR and QT intervals, broad flat T waves, PVCs, ventricular tachycardia or fibrillation
High magnesium	>3.0 mEq/L	Prolonged PR and QT intervals, widened QRS

PVCs, Premature ventricular contractions.
Modified from Chernecky, C. C., & Berger, B. J. (2004). *Laboratory tests and diagnostic procedures.* 4th ed. Philadelphia: W. B. Saunders.

of AMI (McCance & Huether, 2002; Chernecky & Berger, 2004).

- **Creatine kinase (CK)** enzymes increase within 2 to 6 hours after onset of myocardial muscle damage. Peak levels occur within 18 to 36 hours, and levels return to baseline in 3 to 6 days. Total CK can be elevated from a variety of diseases and conditions and is nonspecific.
- **CK-MB (isoenzyme)** is a fraction of the total CK that is specific for cardiac muscle. Normal values of CK-MB are 0% to 6% of the total CK. Values are elevated after AMI, cardiac surgery, and blunt cardiac trauma. The initial rise in CK-MB levels after an AMI occurs within 4 to 8 hours after onset of damage. Peak levels occur in 18 to 24 hours, and levels return to baseline within 3 days. Total CK and CK-MB are usually ordered at initial assessment and at 8, 16, and 24 hours after onset of chest pain to assist in diagnosis of AMI.
- **Cardiac troponin I or T.** Serum troponin levels are useful in early diagnosis of AMI. Levels are normally undetectable in healthy people and elevate as early as 1 hour after myocardial cell injury. Troponin I has a greater specificity than CK-MB in the diagnosis of AMI at 7 to 14 hours after the onset of chest pain. Testing for troponin can be done quickly in the field or the emergency department and aids in the early diagnosis of AMI. The normal value of troponin I is less than 3.1 mcg/L, and that of troponin T is less than 0.2 mcg/L.
- **Myoglobin.** Serum myoglobin is released within 30 to 60 minutes after AMI. Normal values are less than 85 ng/mL. Myoglobin levels rise before CK and CK-MB and are useful in the early diagnosis of AMI. Myoglobin alone is not specific for AMI, but when used in combination with other tests, it can aid in the diagnosis. Some institutions order myoglobin levels every 2 hours. A doubling

of levels from one sample to the next sample is indicative of AMI.

NURSING DIAGNOSES

Because CAD is a very broad diagnostic area, several nursing diagnostic categories may apply. With the complications of CAD, such as angina, MI, and HF, the diagnostic categories are more specific. Nursing diagnosis of patients with CAD include the following:

- Chest pain related to decreased coronary artery tissue perfusion
- Anxiety/fear related to treatments and invasive procedures used for diagnostic testing
- Knowledge deficit related to understanding of anatomy and pathophysiology of the heart and its functions
- Health-seeking behaviors related to desire for information to decrease or alter ongoing disease process

INTERVENTIONS

Nursing Interventions

Nursing interventions are patient centered and encompass health assessment and patient education. The format and necessity of a complete health assessment are discussed in detail earlier in this chapter. The psychosocial and family support assessment, as well as the patient's history and physical examination findings, must be used. The nurse instructs the patient about risk factor modification and signs and symptoms of progression of CAD that warrant medical treatment.

Medical Management

The goals of medical management are to achieve target levels of LDL. The National Cholesterol Education Project (NIH, 2004) recommends that an optimal LDL level is less than 100 mg/dL, but the target level should be adjusted in relation to the patient's number of

LABORATORY ALERTS

Risks	Target Low-Density Lipoprotein Levels	Target High-Density Lipoprotein Levels	Target Triglyceride Levels
No CAD; 0-1 risk factors	<160 mg/dL	>40 mg/dL	<190 mg/dL
No CAD; 2 or more risk factors	<130 mg/dL	>40 mg/dL	<160 mg/dL
CAD or CAD risk equivalent (other atherosclerotic disease, diabetes, multiple risks)	<100 mg/dL	>40 mg/dL	<130 mg/dL

CAD, Coronary artery disease.

major risk factors for CAD. These include family history, age, smoking, hypertension, and diabetes. The key to lessening the burden of coronary heart disease in the United States is primary prevention, and one way this can be accomplished is through thorough management of cholesterol levels (see Laboratory Alerts for LDLs, HDLs, and triglycerides).

Strategies for risk factor modification include a low-fat, low-cholesterol diet, exercise, weight loss, smoking cessation, and control of other risks such as diabetes and hypertension. If LDL levels are not at target values after 6 months of risk factor modification, patients are started on lipid-lowering drugs.

Medications to reduce serum lipid levels.

Lipid-lowering drugs include statins, bile acid resins, and nicotinic acid (Table 11-4). The *statins* are officially classified as 3-hydroxy-3-methylglutaryl-coenzyme A (HMG-CoA) reductase inhibitors. The statins have been found to lower LDL more than other types of lipid-lowering drugs. They work by slowing the production of cholesterol and increasing the liver's ability

TABLE 11-4

MEDICATIONS FOR LOWERING CHOLESTEROL AND TRIGLYCERIDES

ANTILIPEMIC AGENTS (HMG-CoA REDUCTASE INHIBITORS)
Indications: used to lower total and LDL cholesterol and to help reduce the risk of acute myocardial infarction and stroke
Mechanism of action: competitively inhibit HMG-CoA reductase, the enzyme that catalyzes the rate-limiting step in cholesterol biosynthesis, resulting in lower total and LDL cholesterol levels with increased HDL cholesterol

Trade Name (Brand Name)	Dosage	Side Effects and Nursing Considerations
Lovastatin (Mevacor)	20-80 mg daily PO in the evening	Headache, dizziness, constipation, weakness, and increased creatine phospokinase levels Instruct patient to take with evening meal. Report severe muscle pain, weakness, or abdominal tenderness. Patient should have baseline liver function and lipid profile tests before starting therapy, then at 6 and 12 mo. Do not give in pregnancy. Patient should be instructed in a low-cholesterol diet.
Atorvastatin (Lipitor)	10-80 mg daily	Headache, peripheral edema, weakness, constipation Medicine can be taken with any meal during the day. Instruct patient to maintain fluid status every day (2 L/day) unless on fluid restriction. Do not give in pregnancy. Patient should be instructed to consume a low-cholesterol diet. Patient should have baseline liver function and lipid profile tests before starting therapy, then at 6 and 12 mo.
Pravastatin (Pravachol)	10-40 mg daily PO at bedtime	Same
Simvastatin (Zocor)	20 mg daily PO at bedtime	Same

Continued

TABLE 11-4

MEDICATIONS FOR LOWERING CHOLESTEROL AND TRIGLYCERIDES—cont'd

ANTILIPEMIC AGENTS (BILE ACID SEQUESTRANTS)
Indications: used to manage hypercholesterolemia
Mechanism of action: form a nonabsorbable complex with bile acids in the intestine, inhibiting enterohepatic reuptake of intestinal bile salts, which increases the fecal loss of bile salt–bound LDL cholesterol

Trade Name (Brand Name)	Dosage	Side Effects and Nursing Considerations
Cholestyramine (Questran)	Powder: 4-24 g 1-2 times a day Tablet: 4-16 g 1-2 times a day	Constipation, heartburn, nausea, flatulence, vomiting, abdominal pain, and headache Instruct patient to mix powder with fluid, pudding, or applesauce. Patient should take other medications at least 1 hr before taking this medication. Patient should report any stomach cramping, pain, blood in stool, and unresolved nausea or vomiting. Monitor cholesterol and triglyceride levels before and during therapy. Use during pregnancy must be cautious, weighing benefits of use against the possible risks involved.
Colestipol (Colestid)	5-30 g in divided doses 2-4 times a day	Same

ANTILIPEMIC AGENT (MISCELLANEOUS, NIACIN)
Indications: adjunctive treatment of hyperlipidemia
Mechanism of action: inhibits VLDL synthesis

Trade Name (Brand Name)	Dosage	Side Effects and Nursing Considerations
Nicotinic acid (Niacin)	1.5-6 g daily in 3 divided doses	Headache, bloating, flatulence, and nausea Instruct patient to take it as directed and not to exceed recommended dosage. Should be taken after meals. Patient should report persistent gastrointestinal disturbances or changes in color of urine or stool.

ANTILIPEMIC AGENT (FIBRIC ACID)
Indications: treatment of hypertriglyceridemia in patients who have not responded to dietary intervention
Mechanism of action: inhibits lipolysis and decreases subsequent hepatic fatty acid uptake and hepatic VLDL secretion and thus reduces serum VLDL and increases HDL

Trade Name (Brand Name)	Dosage	Side Effects and Nursing Considerations
Gemfibrozil (Lopid)	600 mg BID PO	Stomach upset, fatigue, headache, diarrhea, and nausea. Instruct patient to take before breakfast and dinner. May take with milk or meals if gastrointestinal upset occurs. Patient should report severe abdominal pain, nausea, or vomiting. Use during pregnancy must be weighed against the possible risks.

HDL, High-density lipoprotein; *HMG-CoA,* 3-hydroxy-3-methylglutaryl-coenzyme A; *LDL,* low-density lipoprotein; *VLDL,* very low-density lipoprotein.

to remove LDL from the body. Some commonly used drugs are lovastatin, atorvastatin, pravastatin, and simvastatin. The drugs are well tolerated by most patients. It is recommended that statins be given as a single dose in the evening because the body makes more cholesterol at night. LDL levels are reassessed in 4 to 6 weeks, and dosages are adjusted as needed (Skidmore-Roth, 2003). One disadvantage of the drugs is their high cost. Another disadvantage is that they can cause liver damage; therefore, it is important to ensure that the patient has liver enzymes drawn periodically to assess liver function.

The bile acid resins combine with cholestrol-containing bile acids in the intestines to form an insoluble complex that is eliminated through feces. These drugs lower LDLs by 10% to 20%. Bile acid resins include cholestyramine and colestipol. The drugs are mixed in liquid and are taken twice daily.

They are associated with side effects such as nausea and flatulence. The drugs interfere with absorption of many medications. It is recommended that other medications be given 1 hour before or 4 hours after administration of the resins to promote absorption (Skidmore-Roth, 2003).

Nicotinic acid, or niacin, reduces total cholesterol, LDLs, and triglycerides if it is given in high doses. The drug is available over the counter; however, its use in lowering cholesterol must be under the supervision of a health care provider. The drug is given three times daily; doses range from 500 mg to 2 grams daily, according to desired LDL effect. The drug should be gradually increased to the maximum effective daily dose. Common side effects include metallic taste in mouth, flushing, and increased feelings of warmth. Major side effects include hepatic dysfunction, gout, and hyperglycemia. Because nicotinic acid affects the absorption of other drugs, the nurse must give the patient information about common drug-drug interactions (Skidmore-Roth, 2003).

If triglycerides are elevated, patients may be prescribed agents that specifically lower triglycerides. One agent is gemfibrozil, a fibric acid derivative. This drug is associated with many gastrointestinal side effects.

If a patient does not respond adequately to single-drug therapy, combined-drug therapy is considered to lower LDL levels further. For example, statins may be combined with bile acid resins. Patients must be carefully monitored when two or more lipid-lowering agents are given simultaneously.

Medications to prevent platelet adhesion and aggregation. Drugs are often prescribed for the patient with CAD to reduce platelet adhesion and aggregation. They are used to provide long-term therapy for angina. Many patients with CAD take aspirin every day to prevent platelet aggregation. A single dose of 80-325 mg of an enteric-coated aspirin per day is commonly prescribed. Other agents that may be prescribed include dipyridamole (Persantine), ticlopidine (Ticlid), and clopidogrel (Plavix). Dipyridamole or clopidogrel may be given with aspirin (Skidmore-Roth, 2003).

PATIENT OUTCOMES

Expected outcomes are that the patient will
- Verbalize the absence or relief of pain.
- Experience less anxiety.
- Describe disease process, causes, and factors contributing to symptoms and the procedures for disease or symptom control and/or ask questions regarding unknown information.
- Actively adhere to health behavior modification.

Angina

Angina is chest pain or discomfort caused by myocardial ischemia that results from an imbalance between myocardial oxygen supply and demand. CAD and coronary artery spasms are common causes of angina.

PATHOPHYSIOLOGY

Angina (from the Latin word meaning "squeezing") is the chest pain associated with myocardial ischemia; it is transient and does not cause cell death, but it may be a precursor to cell death from MI. The neural pain receptors are stimulated by accelerated metabolism, chemical changes and imbalances, and/or local mechanical stress resulting from abnormal myocardial contractions. The oxygen circulating to the myocardial cells decreases, causing ischemia to the tissue and pain.

Angina occurs when oxygen demand is higher than oxygen supply. Box 11-4 shows factors influencing oxygen supply and demand that may result in angina.

TYPES OF ANGINA

Different types of angina exist: stable, unstable, and variant. *Stable angina* occurs with exertion and is relieved by rest. It is sometimes called chronic exertional angina. *Unstable angina* (along with AMI) is classified as an acute coronary syndrome. The common

---

BOX 11-4

Factors that Influence Oxygen Demand and Supply

INCREASED OXYGEN DEMAND
Increased heart rate: Exercise, tachydysrhythmias, anemia, fever, anxiety, pain, thyrotoxicosis, medications, ingestion of heavy meals, adapting to extremes in temperature
Increased preload: Volume overload, medications
Increased afterload: Hypertension, aortic stenosis, vasopressors
Increased contractility: Exercise, medications, anxiety

REDUCED OXYGEN SUPPLY
Coronary artery disease
Coronary artery spasms
Medications
Anemia
Hypoxemia

Modified from McCance, K. L., & Huether, S. E. (eds.). (2002). *Pathophysiology: The biological basis for disease in adults and children.* 4th ed. St. Louis: Mosby.

pathophysiology of these syndromes is thrombus resulting from disruption of an atherosclerotic plaque. In unstable angina, some blood continues to flow through the affected coronary artery; however, flow is diminished. The pain in unstable angina is more severe, may occur at rest, and requires more frequent NTG therapy. It is sometimes crescendo (increasing) in nature (Killip, 2000). During an unstable attack, the ECG may show ST-segment depression. The patient has an increased risk of MI within 18 months of onset of unstable angina; therefore, medical and/or surgical interventions are warranted. Patients are often hospitalized for diagnostic workup and treatment. *Variant,* or *Prinzmetal's, angina* is caused by coronary artery spasms. It often occurs at rest and without other precipitating factors. The ECG shows a marked ST-elevation (usually seen only in AMI) during the episode. The ST-segment returns to normal after the spasm subsides. AMI can occur because of prolonged coronary artery spasm, even in the absence of CAD.

ASSESSMENT

Assessment of the patient with actual or suspected angina involves continual observation of the patient and monitoring of signs, symptoms, and diagnostic findings. The patient must be monitored for the type and degree of pain (see Clinical Alert).

The precipitating factors that can be identified as bringing on an episode of anginal pain include physical or emotional stress, exposure to temperature extremes, and ingestion of a heavy meal. It is important to know what factors alleviate the anginal pain, including stopping activity or exercise and taking NTG sublingual tablets or spray.

Diagnostic Studies

Diagnostic studies for angina include the following: history and physical examination, in which patterns of pain and precipitating risk factors are sought; laboratory data, including blood studies for anemia (hemoglobin and hematocrit values), cardiac enzymes (CK-MB, cardiac troponin I, cardiac troponin T levels), and cholesterol and triglyceride levels; ECGs during resting periods, precipitating events (exercise), and anginal pain episodes; exercise tolerance or stress testing; cardiac scanning; and coronary arteriography. Complications of untreated or unstable angina include MI, HF, presence of dysrhythmias, psychological depression, and sudden death (McCance & Huether, 2002).

NURSING DIAGNOSES

Nursing diagnoses and interventions for patients with angina include the following (Ulrich, Canale, & Wendall, 2001):

- Risk of decreased cardiac output related to mechanical and electrical dysfunction of the heart associated with transient myocardial ischemia
- Chest pain related to decreased myocardial oxygenation
- Anxiety related to pain or threat of recurrent pain; lack of understanding of diagnostic tests, diagnosis, and treatment plan; unfamiliar environment; and effect of angina on lifestyle and roles
- Knowledge deficit, ineffective management of therapeutic regimen, or altered health maintenance
- Activity intolerance related to fear of recurrent angina
- Risk of self-esteem disturbance related to perceived or actual role changes
- Risk of impaired home maintenance management related to angina or fear of angina
- Risk of altered family processes related to impaired ability of person to assume role responsibilities
- Risk of sexual dysfunction related to fear of angina and altered self-esteem

CLINICAL ALERT: SYMPTOMS OF ANGINA

- Pain is frequently retrosternal, left pectoral, or epigastric. In addition, it may radiate to the jaw, left shoulder, or left arm.

- Pain can be described as burning, squeezing, heavy, or smothering.

- Pain usually lasts 1 to 5 minutes.

- Classic placing of clenched fist against chest (sternum) may be seen or may be absent if the sensation is confused with indigestion.

- Pain usually begins with exertion and subsides with rest.

INTERVENTIONS

Nursing Interventions

Nursing interventions for the patient with angina are aimed at maintaining an adequate cardiac output, relieving pain and anxiety, and providing adequate instruction to promote self-care behaviors. One key aspect within this teaching is the importance of notifying the nurse at the onset of any type of chest pain. The nurse can also aid the patient with beginning lifestyle modifications, such as weight reduction and smoking cessation. Patients who wish to stop smoking can be pointed to the World Wide Web for Internet sites that provide valuable information about smoking cessation.

Medical Interventions

Unstable angina can be treated by conservative management or early intervention with percutaneous intervention or surgical revascularization. Conservative intervention for the patient experiencing angina includes the administration of nitrates, beta-adrenergic blocking agents, and/or calcium channel blocking agents (Table 11-5). Angioplasty, stenting, and bypass surgery are approaches to revascularization.

TABLE 11-5

DRUGS FOR ACUTE CORONARY SYNDROMES

NITRATES
Indications: angina
Mechanism of action: directly relax smooth muscle, which causes vasodilation of the systemic vascular bed; decrease myocardial oxygen demands

Trade Name (Brand Name)	Dosage	Side Effects and Nursing Considerations
Nitroglycerin (Tridil, Nitro-Bid, Nitro-Dur, Nitrostat)	SL: 0.4 mg SL q5min for 3 doses Topical: 0.5-2 inches q6h IV: continuous infusion started at 5 mcg/min and titrated up to 200 mcg/min maximum	Headache, flushing, tachycardia, dizziness, and orthostatic hypotension Instruct patient to call 911 if chest pain does not subside after the third SL dose. For topical and oral doses, patient may need a nitrate-free interval (10-12 hr/day) to avoid development of tolerance. Instruct patient not to combine nitrate use keep more generic drugs for erectile dysfunction (e.g., Viagra)
Isosorbide dinitrate (Isordil)	5-40 mg TID PO, q6h except at bedtime	Same
Isosorbide mononitrate (Imdur)	5-10 mg BID PO	Same

BETA-BLOCKERS
Indications: used to treat angina, acute myocardial infarction, and heart failure
Mechanism of action: block beta-adrenergic receptors, which results in decreased sympathetic nervous system response such as decreased heart rate, blood pressure, and cardiac contractility

Trade Name (Brand Name)	Dosage	Side Effects and Nursing Considerations
Metoprolol (Lopressor, Toprol XL)	50-100 mg BID PO; 5 mg IV Toprol XL 25-200 mg daily PO	Bradycardia, hypotension, atrioventricular blocks, asthma attacks, fatigue, impotence, may mask hypoglycemic episodes Patient should be taught to take pulse and blood pressure on regular basis. Patient should not abruptly stop taking beta blockers. Close glucose monitoring if diabetic. Patient should have ECG monitoring in place for IV doses.
Propranolol (Inderal)	80-320 mg in divided doses 2-4 times a day IV: 1-3 mg SLOW IVP	Same
Labetalol (Trandate, Normodyne)	200-400 mg BID PO IV: 1-2 mg/kg slow IVP	Same Labetalol acts on both alpha and beta$_1$ and beta$_2$ receptors
Carvedilol (Coreg)	3.125-25 mg BID PO	Same

Continued

TABLE 11-5

DRUGS FOR ACUTE CORONARY SYNDROMES—cont'd

CALCIUM CHANNEL BLOCKERS

Indications: used to treat hypertension, tachydysrhythmias, vasospasms, and angina.

Mechanism of action: inhibit the flow of calcium ions across cellular membranes, with resulting increased coronary blood flow and myocardial perfusion and decreased myocardial oxygen requirements

Trade Name (Brand Name)	Dosage	Side Effects and Nursing Considerations
Verapamil (Calan, Isoptin)	80-120 mg BID PO IV: 5-10 mg slow IVP	Dizziness, flushing, headaches, bradycardia, atrioventricular blocks, and hypotension Patients should be taught to monitor pulse and blood pressure, especially if they are taking nitrates and/or beta-blockers. Tablets cannot be crushed or chewed. Instruct patient to make position changes slowly.
Nifedipine (Procardia)	10 mg TID PO	Same
Diltiazem (Cardizem, Cardizem CD)	30 mg QID PO, sustained-release 120-180 mg daily. IV: 0.25 mg/kg IV over 2 min, followed by continuous infusion at 10 mg/min	Same

ANTICOAGULANTS

Indications: unstable angina, acute myocardial infarction, and coronary interventions

Mechanism of action: inhibit clotting mechanisms within the clotting cascade or prevent platelet aggregation

Trade Name (Brand Name)	Dosage	Side Effects and Nursing Considerations
Aspirin	81-325 mg daily PO	Bleeding, epigastric discomfort, bruising, and gastric ulceration Patient should be instructed to take medication with food. Do not crush or chew the enteric-coated forms. Instruct patient to be aware of additive effects with OTC drugs containing aspirin or salicylate or other NSAIDs. Instruct patient to avoid high-risk activities that can cause injury.
Clopidogrel (Plavix)	75 mg daily PO	Same May be given before coronary intervention as loading dose of 300 mg, followed by 75 mg daily for 1-6 mo.
Dipyridamole (Persantine)	75-400 mg daily PO in divided doses	May worsen angina, dizziness, headache, and hypotension; increased risk of bleeding with aspirin use Medication should be taken 1 hr before meals with a full glass of water.
Ticlopidine (Ticlid)	250 mg BID PO	Bleeding, bruising, gastrointestinal upset, and diarrhea Instruct patient to take with food to reduce gastrointestinal upset. Instruct patient to report any unusual bleeding. Monitor CBC during therapy.

GLYCOPROTEIN IIB/IIIA INHIBITORS

Indications: acute coronary syndromes and coronary intervention patients

Mechanism of action: antiplatelet agent and glycoprotein IIb/IIIa inhibitor; act by binding to the glycoprotein IIb/IIIa receptor site on the surface of the platelet

Trade Name (Brand Name)	Dosage	Side Effects and Nursing Considerations
Abciximab (ReoPro)	0.25 mg/kg IV bolus followed by a continuous infusion at 10 mcg/min for 12-24 hr	Bleeding, bruising, hemorrhage, thrombocytopenia, and hypotension. Avoid IM injections. Avoid venipunctures. Observe and teach patient bleeding precautions and activities that may cause injury. Assess infusion insertion site for bleeding or hematoma formation. Assess femoral puncture site frequently. Abciximab is not reversible because of its binding to the platelet. For hemorrhage, give fresh frozen plasma and platelets. Monitor CBC and PTT daily.

Continued

TABLE 11-5
DRUGS FOR ACUTE CORONARY SYNDROMES—cont'd

Trade Name (Brand Name)	Dosage	Side Effects and Nursing Considerations
Tirofiban (Aggrastat)	0.4 mcg/kg/min for 30 min then continued at 0.1 mcg/kg/min for 12-24 hr	Same Tirofiban stops working when the infusion is discontinued. Platelet function is restored 4 hr after stopping the infusion.
Eptifibatide (Integrilin)	180 mcg/kg IV loading dose over 2 min, followed by continuous infusion of 2 mcg/kg/min up to 72 hr	Same Eptifibatide stops working when the infusion is discontinued. Platelet function is restored 4 hr after stopping the infusion.

ANTITHROMBIN AGENTS
Indications: prevention of or delay in thrombus formation
Mechanism of action: accelerates formation of antithrombin III–thrombin complex and deactivates thrombin, preventing conversion of fibrinogen to fibrin

Trade Name (Brand Name)	Dosage	Side Effects and Nursing Considerations
Heparin	70 units/kg IV bolus followed by initial infusion of 12-15 units/kg/hr, titrated to PTT	Bleeding, bruising, thrombocytopenia. Monitor PTT. Monitor for signs of bleeding and hematoma formation. Avoid IM injections. Do not rub the site after giving the injection.
Enoxaparin (Lovenox)	1 mg/kg subcutaneous BID, in conjunction with aspirin	Bleeding, bruising, local site hematomas, and hemorrhage. Instruct patient to report persistent chest pain, unusual bleeding or bruising. Do not rub the site after giving the injection.

ANALGESIC
Indications: pain relief and anxiety reduction during acute myocardial infarction
Mechansim of action: binds to opiate receptors in the central nervous system and causes inhibition of ascending pain pathways, altering perception and response to pain

Trade Name (Brand Name)	Dosage	Side Effects and Nursing Considerations
Morphine	2-4 mg IV push q5-10min titrated for chest pain	Hypotension, respiratory depression, apnea, bradycardia, nausea, and restlessness Monitor level of consciousness, blood pressure, respiratory rate, and oxygen saturation during therapy. Effects are reversed with naloxone (Narcan).

ANGIOTENSIN-CONVERTING ENZYME INHIBITORS
Indications: used to treat hypertension, heart failure, and patients after myocardial infarction
Mechanism of action: prevent the conversion of angiotensin I to angiotensin II resulting in lower levels of angiotensin II, which causes an increase in plasma renin activity and reduction of aldosterone secretion; also inhibit the remodeling process after myocardial injury

Trade Name (Brand Name)	Dosage	Side Effects and Nursing Considerations
Enalapril (Vasotec)	2.5-10 mg BID PO 1.25 mg slow IV over 5-6 min q6h for up to 36 hr	Hypotension, bradycardia, renal impairment, cough, and orthostatic hypotension Do not give IV enalapril to patients with unstable heart failure or in those patients having an acute myocardial infarction. Monitor urine output. Monitor potassium levels. Avoid use of NSAIDs. Instruct patient to avoid rapid change in position such as from lying to standing. Angiotensin-converting enzyme inhibitors are contraindicated in pregnancy.
Fosinopril (Monopril)	10-40 mg daily PO	Same
Captopril (Capoten)	12.5-50 mg TID	Same

CBC, Complete blood count; *ECG,* electrocardiogram; *IVP,* IV push; *NSAIDs,* nonsteroidal anti-inflammatory drugs; *OTC,* over the counter; *PTT,* partial thromboplastin time.
From Skidmore-Roth, L. (2003). *Mosby's drug guide for nurses.* 3rd ed. St. Louis: Mosby.

Nitrates are the most common medications for angina. They are direct-acting, sooth muscle relaxants that cause vasodilation of the peripheral or systemic vascular bed (Skidmore-Roth, 2003). Nitrate therapy is beneficial because it decreases myocardial oxygen demand. The vasodilating effect causes relief of pain and lowering of blood pressure. Examples of forms of or preparations of nitrates are sublingual, intravenous (IV), transdermal, spray, and ointment NTG and sublingual and oral isosorbide (Isordil). Side effects of these vasodilators include headache, flushing, tachycardia, dizziness, and orthostatic hypotension. Instructions for NTG therapy are in Box 11-5.

Beta-adrenergic blocking agents may also be used to treat angina. They block adrenergic receptors, thereby decreasing heart rate, blood pressure, and cardiac contractility (Skidmore-Roth, 2003). Examples include metoprolol, propranolol, labetalol, carvedilol, nadolol, timolol, and pindolol. The side effects of these agents include bradycardia, AV block, asthma attacks, depression, hypotension, memory loss, and masking of hypoglycemic episodes. The patient is taught to take these agents as prescribed, not to stop taking them abruptly, and to monitor heart rate and blood pressure at regular intervals.

Calcium channel blockers inhibit the flow of calcium ions across cellular membranes, an effect that causes direct increases in coronary blood flow and myocardial perfusion as well as decreases in myocardial oxygen requirements (Skidmore-Roth, 2003). These drugs are used for treating tachydysrhythmias, vasospasms, and hypertension, as well as for treating angina. Examples of calcium channel blockers include verapamil (Calan, Isoptin), nifedipine (Procardia), and diltiazem (Cardizem). The side effects of calcium channel blockers include dizziness, flushing, headaches, decreased heart rate, and hypotension. The patient is taught to monitor blood pressure for hypotension, and heart rate for bradycardia, especially if the agents are taken in combination with nitrates and beta-blockers.

Conservative treatment also includes the use of aspirin and heparin. In addition, Gp IIb/IIIa inhibitors (abciximab, tirofiban, and eptifibatide) are used in treating both unstable angina and non–Q-wave MI. Use of these drugs has shown reduction in mortality (Gylys & Gold, 2000). Low-molecular-weight heparin is now being used instead of standard heparin. Subcutaneous administration of low-molecular-weight heparin (enoxaparin) along with aspirin has been shown to be more effective than heparin in two

---

BOX 11-5

Instructions Regarding Nitroglycerin

IF THE CLIENT IS DISCHARGED ON SUBLINGUAL OR BUCCAL NITROGLYCERIN, INSTRUCT TO:
- Avoid drinking alcoholic beverages.
- Have tablets readily available.
- Take a tablet before strenuous activity and in stressful situations.
- Take one tablet when chest pain occurs and another every 5 minutes up to a total of three times if necessary; obtain emergency medical assistance if pain persists.
- Place the tablet under the tongue or in the buccal pouch and allow it to dissolve thoroughly.
- Store tablets in a tightly capped, dark glass container away from heat and moisture.
- Replace tablets every 6 months or sooner if they do not relieve discomfort.
- Avoid rising to a standing position quickly after taking nitroglycerin.
- Recognize that dizziness, flushing, and mild headache are common side effects.
- Report fainting, persistent or severe headache, blurred vision, or dry mouth.
- Caution use of drugs for erectile dysfunction (e.g. Viagra, Levitra) when taking nitrates because hypotensive effects are exaggerated.

IF NITROGLYCERIN SKIN PATCHES ARE PRESCRIBED:
- Provide instructions about correct application, skin care, the need to rotate sites and to remove the old patch, and frequency of change.
- The patch may be ordered to be left off for a period each day to prevent development of nitrate tolerance.
- Caution the client that activities that increase blood flow to the skin (e.g., hot bath or shower, sauna) can cause a sudden reduction in blood pressure.

From Ulrich, S. P. & Canale, S. W. (2001). *Nursing care plan guides for adults in acute, extended, and home care settings.* 5th ed. Philadelphia: W. B. Saunders.

trials (Massel & Cruickshank, 2002). Additional studies are under way combining low-molecular-weight heparin and the Gp IIb/IIIa inhibitors as adjunct therapy to percutaneous intervention.

OUTCOMES

The outcomes for the patient with angina are that the patient will

- Maintain adequate cardiac output.
- Have decreased or absent chest pain.
- Not experience cardiac dysrhythmias.
- Experience less anxiety.
- Actively participate in the health behaviors prescribed.
- Describe the disease process, causes, and factors contributing to symptoms and the procedure for symptom control through rest, medication, progressive activity, diet, stress control, and control of related physiological problems (McCance & Huether, 2002; Ulrich & Canale, 2001).

Acute Myocardial Infarction

AMI is ischemia with death of the myocardium that is caused by lack of blood supply from the occlusion of a coronary artery and its branches. Most cases of AMI are secondary to atherosclerosis. Other causes (less than 5%) include coronary artery spasm, coronary embolism, and blunt trauma. Cocaine use is associated with spasms (Killip, 2000).

PATHOPHYSIOLOGY

AMI is caused by an imbalance between myocardial oxygen supply and demand. This imbalance is the result of decreased coronary artery perfusion, which is usually the result of atherosclerosis, coronary artery vasospasm, coronary artery thrombus, presence of dysrhythmias, or a combination of any of these factors. Reduced blood flow to an area of the myocardium causes significant and sustained oxygen deprivation to myocardial cells. Normal functioning is disrupted as ischemia and injury lead to eventual cellular death. Myocardial dysfunction occurs as more cells become involved.

Prolonged ischemia from cessation in blood flow is called *infarction* and evolves over approximately 3 hours (McCance & Huether, 2002). It causes irreversible cellular damage and muscle death (necrosis) (Figure 11-9). Contractility in the infarcted area becomes impaired. A nonfunctional zone and a zone of mild ischemia with potentially viable tissue surrounds the infarct. The ultimate size of the infarct depends on the fate of this ischemic zone. Early interventions such as thrombolytics can restore perfusion to the ischemic zone and can reduce the area of myocardial damage.

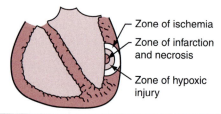

FIGURE 11-9 Three zones of myocardial infarction. (From McCance, K. L., & Huether, S. E. [eds.]. [2002]. *Pathophysiology: The biologic basis for disease in adults and children.* 4th ed. St. Louis: Mosby.)

AMI can be classified as Q-wave or non–Q-wave. It was previously believed that non–Q-wave MI was associated with damage to only a portion (subendocardial) of the cardiac muscle. Currently, both types of MI are considered to cause damage throughout the muscular layers of the ventricle. A Q-wave MI occurs as a result of total occlusion of a coronary artery secondary to a thrombus or ruptured atherosclerotic plaque. Emergency treatment with thrombolytics is recommended. ST-segment elevation and elevated cardiac enzymes are seen in Q-wave MI. The non–Q-wave MI usually results from a partially occluded coronary vessel, and it is associated with ST-segment depression in two or more leads along with elevated cardiac enzymes (Killip, 2000). Most infarcts occur in the left ventricle; however, right ventricular infarction can occur in over half of the inferior wall MIs. The treatment for RV infarcts is usually fluid therapy.

The severity of the MI is determined by the success or lack of success of the treatment and by the degree of collateral circulation that is present at that particular part of the heart muscle. The collateral circulation consists of the alternative routes, or channels, that can develop in the myocardium in response to chronic ischemia or regional hypoperfusion. Through this small network of "extra" vessels, blood flow can be improved to the threatened myocardium.

ASSESSMENT

Patient Assessment

Patient assessment includes close observation to identify the classic signs and symptoms of AMI. Chest pain is the paramount symptom. It may be severe, crushing, tight, squeezing, or simply a feeling of pressure. It can be precordial, substernal, or in the back, radiating to the arms, neck, or jaw, and/or unrelated to exertion and respirations. It does not cease with rest or nitrate administration and thus can be distinguished from the pain of an angina attack. The longer the duration and the more severe the pain, the greater the likelihood that an MI is occurring.

The skin may be cool, clammy, pale, and diaphoretic; the patient's color may be dusky or ashen; and slight hyperthermia may be present. The patient may be short of breath, dyspneic, and tachypneic; he or she may feel faint or may have intermittent loss of sensorium. Nausea and vomiting commonly occur. Hypotension may be present and is often accompanied by dysrhythmias, particularly ventricular ectopy, bradycardia, tachycardia, or heart block. The type of dysrhythmia experienced depends on the area of the MI. The patient may be anxious or restless or may exhibit certain behavioral responses, including denial, depression, and sense of impending doom.

Note: Up to 25% of patients may have ischemic episodes without knowing it (AHA, 2001b). These can occur with no presenting signs or symptoms. Asymptomatic or nontraditional symptoms are more common in elderly persons, in women, and in diabetic patients.

Assessment of a patient experiencing an MI takes all the foregoing signs and symptoms into account during the history and physical examination. Risk factors for an MI (CAD, coronary spasm, and embolism) are also considered in the determination of a diagnosis.

Diagnosis

Diagnosis of an AMI is based on symptoms, analysis of 12-lead ECG, and cardiac enzyme values. A high index of suspicion is needed for anyone older than 35 years of age who presents with chest pain lasting more than 20 minutes (Killip, 2000). The patient is assessed for other signs and symptoms indicating AMI that were previously described. The ECG is inspected for ST-segment elevation (greater than 1mm) in two or more contiguous leads. ST-segment depression (0.5 mm or greater) and bundle branch block may also suggest AMI. The type of AMI can be determined by the particular coronary artery involved and the blood supply to that area (Table 11-6).

Serum cardiac enzymes are used to confirm the diagnosis of AMI. As previously described, serum levels of total CK, CK-MB, troponin I and T, and myoglobin elevate after AMI. These tests are ordered immediately

---

TABLE 11-6

Myocardial Infarction (MI) by Site, Electrocardiographic (ECG) Changes, and Complications

Location of MI	Primary Site of Occlusion	Primary ECG Changes	Complications
Inferior MI	RCA (80%-90%) LCX (10%-20%)	Leads: II, III, aVF	First- and second-degree heart block, right ventricular infarct
Inferolateral MI	LCX	II, III, aVF, V_5, V_6	Third-degree heart block, left HF, cardiomyopathy, left ventricular rupture
Posterior MI	RCA or LCX	No lead truly looks at posterior surface Look for reciprocal changes in V_1 and V_2—tall, broad R waves; ST depression and tall T waves Posterior leads V_7, V_8, and V_9 may be recorded and evaluated	First-, second-, and third-degree heart blocks, HF, bradydysrhythmias
Anterior MI	LAD	V_2-V_4	Third-degree heart block, HF, left bundle branch block
Anterior-septal MI	LAD	V_1-V_3	Second- and third-degree heart block
Lateral MI	LAD or LCX	V_5, V_6, I, aVL	HF
Right ventricular	RCA	V_4R Right precordial leads V_1R-V_6R may be recorded and evaluated	↑ RAP, ↓ cardiac output, bradydysrhythmias, heart blocks, hypotension, cardiogenic shock

AV, Atrioventricular; *HF,* heart failure; *LAD,* left anterior descending; *LCX,* circumflex; *MI,* myocardial infarction; *RAP,* right atrial pressure; *RCA,* right coronary artery.

when a diagnosis of AMI is suspected and periodically (usually every 8 hours) during the first 24 hours to assess for increases (Killip, 2000). Emergency cardiac arteriography may be used in institutions with interventional cardiology services. Echocardiography may be useful in assessing ventricular wall motion and may assist in the diagnosis (SCCM, 2001).

NURSING DIAGNOSES

Nursing diagnoses and collaborative problems for the patient with AMI are listed here (Ulrich & Canale, 2001). Expected outcomes and interventions are specified in the Nursing Care Plan for the Patient with Acute Myocardial Infarction.

- Decreased cardiac output related to decreased contractility and altered conductivity of the heart associated with the myocardial damage that has occurred with infarction
- Pain: chest pain related to myocardial ischemia
- Activity intolerance related to tissue hypoxia associated with decreased cardiac output, difficulty resting and sleeping associated with pain, frequent assessments and treatments, fear, and anxiety
- Anxiety related to severe pain; possibility of disability or death, unfamiliar environment, and lack of understanding of diagnostic tests, the diagnosis, and treatment plan

Nursing Care Plan for the Patient with Acute Myocardial Infarction

NURSING DIAGNOSIS: *Decreased cardiac output related to decreased contractility*

Patient Outcomes	Interventions	Rationales
Improved cardiac output as evidenced by • Vital signs within normal range • Absence of fatigue and weakness • Clear breath sounds • Usual mental status • Absence of vertigo and syncope • Palpable peripheral pulses • Skin warm, dry, and usual color with capillary refill time <3, sec • Urine output at least 30 mL/hr • Absence of edema and jugular vein distention	Assess for and report diagnostic findings indicative of an MI.	Thorough assessment of patient's hemodynamic status (e.g., ECG, cardiac enzymes) allows the nurse to detect early signs of cardiac compromise.
	Prepare client for emergency interventions to restore coronary artery perfusion.	Prompt reversal of coronary occlusion helps to prevent long-term myocardial damage.
	Assist with insertion of IABP for cardiogenic shock.	IABP therapy will help decrease the workload on the heart muscle and increase coronary artery perfusion. These two actions help to preserve the patient's heart muscle.
	Perform actions to reduce cardiac workload.	Decreased cardiac workload helps the patient to tolerate activities, maintains myocardial oxygen supply and demand, and maintains stable hemodynamics.
	If PA catheter inserted, monitor CO, PAP, and PAOP on a routine basis.	PA catheters can allow for better management of the patients fluid status. Changes in pressures and CO alert the nurse to hemodynamic compromise.
	Administer medications as ordered.	Medications for MI help to prevent complications, alleviate chest pain, and also maintain hemodynamic stability.
	Consult physician if signs and symptoms of decreased CO persist or worsen.	Thorough monitoring of signs and symptoms of low CO alerts the nurse to early hemodynamic changes, and allows for prompt interventions to take place.

Nursing Care Plan for the Patient with Acute Myocardial Infarction—cont'd

NURSING DIAGNOSIS: *Pain: chest pain related to myocardial ischemia*

Patient Outcomes	Interventions	Rationales
Pain relief as evidenced by • Verbalization of same • Relaxed facial expression and body positioning • Participation in activities • Stable vital signs	Implement measures to relieve pain. Expect denial as a response. Encourage verbalization of feelings.	Adequate pain management is crucial for the patient, because untreated pain leads to hemodynamic changes having potential detrimental effects. Untreated pain increases anxiety levels. Denial is common response to chest pain related to cardiac problems. Encouraging the patient to verbalize feelings helps the patient to accept the situation better, decreases anxiety levels, and allows the nurse to facilitate learning activities for the patient.

NURSING DIAGNOSIS: *Activity intolerance, related to tissue hypoxia*

Patient Outcomes	Interventions	Rationales
Increased tolerance for activity as evidenced by • Verbalization of feeling less fatigued and weak • Ability to perform activities of daily living without exertional dyspnea, chest pain, diaphoresis, dizziness, and a significant change in vital signs	Assess for signs and symptoms of activity intolerance. Implement measures to improve activity tolerance. Instruct client to report changes in activity intolerance.	Allows for modification of activities in relation to the patient's current status and allows the nurse to prevent problems related to inadequate performance of activities. Allows the patient to tolerate activities better. Measures to increase tolerance enable the patient to see and feel actual progression toward the goal. Alerts the nurse to early signs of changes in patient's hemodynamic status and allows the nurse to modify activities as needed to prevent complications.

NURSING DIAGNOSIS: *Anxiety-related severe pain*

Patient Outcomes	Interventions	Rationales
Reduction in anxiety as evidenced by • Verbalization of feeling less anxious • Usual sleep pattern • Relaxed facial expression and body movements • Stable vital signs • Usual perceptual ability and interactions with others	Assess client for signs and symptoms of anxiety. Implement measures to reduce anxiety.	Anxiety is highly individualized, making physical and psychological changes unique to the individual patient, and is assessed routinely. Decreasing the patient's anxiety allows the patient to have greater control.

Continued

Nursing Care Plan for the Patient with Acute Myocardial Infarction—cont'd

NURSING DIAGNOSIS: *Potential complications of AMI*

Patient Outcomes	Interventions	Rationales
Absence of complications • Normal sinus rhythm • Absence of signs and symptoms of heart failure • Absence of signs and symptoms of thromboembolism • Resolution of pericarditis if it develops • No infarct extension or recurrence • No cardiogenic shock	Monitor for dysrhythmias. Assess for symptoms of heart failure. Assess for thromboembolic events.	Dysrhythmias are common during and after an MI, therefore close monitoring is warranted to detect and prevent potential life-threatening dysrhythmias. Antiarryhthmics decrease or reverse dysrhythmias. MI potentially causes heart failure; thorough assessment for signs of heart failure (crackles, JVD, and pedal edema) alerts the nurse to intervene as appropriate. Thromboembolic events (stroke, PE, and DVT) are detected and prevented or treated by thorough assessment of vascular status (peripheral and neurological).
	Implement measures to prevent the development of thromboemboli. Assess heart sounds for new murmur, muffled heart sounds, pericardial friction rub; report any abnormalities. Monitor intake and output, daily weights, and renal function tests. Monitor response to diuretics.	Measures to prevent thromboembolic events (stroke and PE) are crucial because potential complications of MI are thromboemboli formations. Changes in heart sounds signal potential hemodynamic alterations (cardiac tamponade and valve disease); therefore, thorough assessment detects these changes. Patients with heart failure frequently have impaired renal function, which can cause fluid accumulation. Decreased response to diuretics may indicate renal impairment.

NURSING DIAGNOSIS: *Knowledge deficit*

Patient Outcomes	Interventions	Rationales
Knowledge of disease process and health promotion behaviors as evidenced by • Verbalize a basic understanding of AMI • Demonstrate accuracy in counting pulse • Identify strategies for risk factor modification • Verbalize an understanding of a low-fat diet	Explain AMI in terms the client can understand; use teaching aids. Teach client how to count his or her pulse. Assess risk factors and assist in identifying strategies for risk factor modification.	Use of simple language aids in the patient's understanding of complex medical problems, and use of teaching aids (visual aids) reinforces verbal instructions. Early detection of heart rate changes allows the nurse or physician to manage the patient's situation better. Thorough assessment of the patient's risk factors allows the nurse to tailor patient education sessions including

Nursing Care Plan for the Patient with Acute Myocardial Infarction—cont'd

Patient Outcomes	Interventions	Rationales
• Verbalize an understanding of medications ordered • Verbalize an understanding of activity restrictions and progression • State signs and symptoms to report to the health care provider • Identify community resources that can assist with cardiac rehabilitation • Verbalize an understanding of and a plan for adhering to recommended follow-up care	Explain the rationale for low-fat diet; dietary consultation should be ordered for all patients with MI. Explain all medications. Reinforce instructions about activity. Reinforce instructions regarding sexual activity. Instruct client to report changes in heart rate, irregular pulse, palpitations, SOB, significant weight gain, and chest pain. Provide information and referrals for cardiac rehabilitation and community support groups.	strategies for changing modifiable risk factors (weight, diet, and smoking). A low-fat diet reduces cholesterol levels, and that, in turn, decreases the risk of heart disease. Thorough explanation of medications helps the patient to understand the disease process better and allows the patient to better communicate with health care providers. Reinforcement of activity instructions allows the patient better to understand the importance of activity modifications that help to result in decreased myocardial oxygen demands. Reinforcement of instructions regarding sexual activity helps to prevent unwanted situations (chest pain, SOB, syncope, palpitations, etc) from occurring at inopportune times. Early detection of changes leads the patient to seek medical attention and prevents potential complications. This reinforces that having an MI is an ongoing health problem for which support and assistance are available after discharge.

AMI, Acute myocardial infarction; *CO,* cardiac output; *DVT,* deep venous thrombosis; *ECG,* electrocardiogram; *IABP,* intraaortic balloon pump; *JVD,* jugular venous distention; *MI,* myocardial infarction; *PA,* pulmonary artery; *PAP,* pulmonary artery pressure; *PAOP,* pulmonary artery occlusion pressure; *PE,* pulmonary embolism; *SOB,* shortness of breath.
Modified from Ulrich, S.& Canale, S. (2001). *Nursing care planning guides for adults in acute, extended and home care settings.* 5th ed. Philadelphia: W. B. Saunders.

• Potential complications of AMI (collaborative problem)
• Knowledge deficit, ineffective management of therapeutic regimen, or altered health maintenance
• Sleep pattern disturbance related to pain, frequent assessments and treatments, fear, and anxiety
• Grieving; anticipatory grieving related to loss of normal function of the heart, possible changes in lifestyle, occupation, and roles, and uncertainty of prognosis

COMPLICATIONS

Complications include cardiac dysrhythmias, HF, thromboembolism, rupture of a portion of the heart

(e.g., ventricular wall, interventricular septum, or papillary muscle), pericarditis, infarct extension or recurrence, and cardiogenic shock (see Chapter 10) (SCCM, 2001). Dysrhythmias, HF, and pericarditis are discussed later in this chapter.

MEDICAL INTERVENTIONS

Treatment goals for AMI are to relieve symptoms, to limit the extent of myocardial damage, to reduce cardiac workload, and to manage complications (Killip, 2000). Medical treatment of AMI is aimed at relieving pain, providing adequate oxygenation to the myocardium, preventing platelet aggregation, and restoring blood flow to the myocardium through thrombolytic therapy or acute interventional therapy such as angioplasty. Hemodynamic monitoring is also used to assess cardiac function and to monitor fluid balance in some patients (AHA, 2001b). An overview of treatments is provided in the following sections (Killip, 2000).

Pain relief. The initial pain of AMI is treated with morphine sulfate administered by the IV route. The initial dose is 2 to 4 mg IV push. Patients must be observed for hypotension and respiratory depression (see Table 11-5).

NTG may be given to reduce the ischemic pain of AMI. NTG increases coronary perfusion because of its vasodilatory effects. It is usually started at titrated doses of 5 to 10 mcg/min and increased to a total of 50 to 200 mcg/min until chest pain is absent, pulmonary artery occlusion pressure decreases, and/or systolic blood pressure decreases. Caution should be used in administering NTG to patients with inferior or right ventricular infarcts.

Oxygen. Oxygen administration is important for assisting the myocardial tissue to continue its pumping activity and for repairing the damaged tissue around the site of the infarct. Treatment with oxygen via nasal cannula at 4 to 6 L/min assists in maintaining oxygenation. Rest also helps to improve oxygenation.

Antidysrhythmics. Antidysrhythmic agents are used when the heart's natural pacemaker develops an abnormal rate or rhythm (see Chapter 6).

Prevention of platelet aggregation. Alterations in platelet function contribute to occlusion of the coronary arteries. Aspirin (162.5 mg) is given immediately to all patients with suspected AMI. Aspirin blocks synthesis of thromboxane A_2, thus inhibiting aggregation of platelets. The Gp IIb/IIIa inhibitors are also being tested in combination with thrombolytics in management of AMI (Gylys & Gold, 2000). Heparin may be given, but its use is controversial. More patients are now receiving the low-molecular-weight heparins.

Thrombolytic therapy. One common treatment for AMI is thrombolytic therapy. Research has shown that occlusion of the coronary vessel does not cause immediate myocardial cell death. Injury begins within 20 minutes of the vessel occlusion. Within a period of 5 to 6 hours, irreversible damage begins at the endocardial surface and progresses to the epicardium. The extent and the progression of the injury are determined by the completeness of the occlusion and the presence of collateral circulation (AHA, 2001a). The goals are to dissolve the lesion

that is occluding the coronary artery and to increase blood flow to the myocardium. The patient must be symptomatic for less than 6 hours, have pain for 20 minutes that was unrelieved by NTG, and have an ECG with an ST segment of greater than or equal to 1 mm in two or more contiguous ECG leads or 0.5 mm depression. Table 11-7 lists some of the common thrombolytics currently available.

Many trials have been conducted on the use of thrombolytics in AMI. Results are summarized as follows (Killip, 2000):
- Fibrinolysis reduces mortality and salvages myocardium in anterior and inferior Q-wave MI.
- Fibrinolysis is not effective in treatment of unstable angina or non–Q-wave MI.
- The sooner treatment is initiated (up to 12 hours after onset of AMI), the better the outcome.
- Use of tissue plasminogen activator (t-PA) with IV heparin is slightly better than streptokinase and heparin.
- The worst possible complication of fibrinolysis is intracranial hemorrhage, although more commonly bleeding from puncture sites occurs.

More investigation is being sought to develop effective reperfusion therapy by combining thrombolytic therapy with antiplatelet therapy. Many patients do not achieve reperfusion sufficient to maintain adequate perfusion of the heart. However, with the current advances in percutaneous coronary intervention (PCI) and other new technologies, the rates of restenosis will decrease.

Nursing care of the patient includes rapid identification of suitable patients for IV thrombolytics, thus ensuring as little delay as possible before the therapy and screening for contraindications are initiated. Next, the nurse secures three vascular access lines and obtains necessary laboratory data. Initial ECG monitoring is documented before start of the infusion, at various times throughout the infusion, and at the end of the infusion. Finally, the patient is monitored for complications, including reperfusion dysrhythmias (premature ventricular contractions, sinus bradycardia, accelerated idioventricular rhythm, or ventricular tachycardia), minor oozing at venipuncture sites and gingival bleeding, reocclusion or reinfarction, and symptoms of hemorrhagic stroke.

Percutaneous coronary intervention. Emergency PCI is being used in the management of AMI with improved outcomes over thrombolytic therapy. In trials, early angioplasty led to a reduction in 30-day mortality, death, and stroke compared with the use of thrombolytics. Primary angioplasty as a treatment for AMI is most successful when it is done within 2 hours of onset of symptoms (Gylys & Gold, 2000).

TABLE 11-7

Thrombolytics

Name	Dose	Half-Life
Alteplase (tissue plasminogen activator; t-PA) Accelerated infusion	For patients weighing >67 kg, dose of 100 mg as a 15-mg bolus IV followed by 50-mg infusion over 30 min then 35-mg infusion over 60 min	4-5 min
	For patients weighing ≤67 kg, maximum dose of 100 mg as a 15-mg bolus IV followed by 0.75 mg/kg over 30 min (not to exceed 50 mg) then 0.50 mg/kg over 60 min (not to exceed 35 mg)	
Reteplase (r-PA)	10 units IV bolus, repeat in 30 min	13-16 min
Tenecteplase (TNK)	Total dose ≤50 mg, based on weight (see package insert) given over 5 sec	20-24 min
Streptokinase (SK)	1.5 million units IV infusion over 1 hr	23 min
Anistreplase (APSAC)	30 units intravenously over 4-5 min	90 min

From *Mosby's drug consult.* (2004). St. Louis: Mosby.

Facilitated percutaneous coronary intervention. Clinical trials are currently evaluating administration of thrombolytics, and combination thrombolytic therapy with Gp IIb/IIIa inhibitors, before primary angioplasty. Thrombolytic therapy promotes reperfusion to the myocardium, and the Gp IIb/IIIa inhibitors prevent platelet aggregation as the patient is prepared for arteriography and PCI (Gylys & Gold, 2000).

Medications. Several other medications may be ordered for the patient with AMI. These include nitrates, beta-blockers, angiotensin-converting enzyme (ACE) inhibitors, and magnesium (Killip, 2000).

Nitrates. Nitrates are vasodilators that reduce pain, increase venous capacitance, and reduce platelet adhesion and aggregation. Sublingual NTG is often given in the emergency department. IV NTG is effective for relieving ischemia (see Table 11-5).

Beta-blockers. Beta-blockers are used to decrease heart rate, blood pressure, and myocardial oxygen consumption. Morbidity and mortality after AMI have been reduced by the use of beta-blockers. Commonly used drugs include metoprolol, atenolol, and carvedilol. The patient is carefully assessed for hypotension and bradycardia.

Angiotensin-converting enzyme inhibitors. After an AMI (Q-wave type), the area of ventricular damage changes shape or remodels. The ventricle becomes thinner and balloons out, thus reducing contractility. ACE inhibitors should be started within 24 hours after thrombolytic therapy to reduce the incidence of ventricular remodeling. The drugs can be discontinued in 6 weeks if the patient exhibits no signs of ventricular dysfunction (see Table 11-5).

Magnesium. The use of supplemental magnesium is controversial. Results of effectiveness of supplementation have been mixed in clinical trials. In high-risk patients, an infusion of 2 g over 4 to 8 hours may be given.

OUTCOMES

Patient outcomes or goals are generalized to encompass the wide spectrum of patients who have experienced an MI, uncomplicated or complicated, that requires medical or surgical intervention. The patient will
- Verbalize an absence of chest pain concurrent with hemodynamic stability.
- Demonstrate stable or improved cardiac output.
- Demonstrate reduced anxiety levels.
- Along with family and/or support system, demonstrate increased understanding of the disease process and of health management through education, interaction, and discussion.
- Have minimized or absence of complications.

Interventional Cardiology

Several interventions are done to treat acute coronary syndromes. The goal is to treat the patient to prevent AMI. Intervention is also used after AMI to prevent further damage of the myocardium. PCIs consist of percutaneous transluminal coronary angioplasty (PTCA), percutaneous transluminal coronary rotational atherectomy, directional coronary artherectomy, laser atherectomy, and intracoronary stenting. For the purposes of this book and space, only PTCA and stenting are discussed at length. The key for nurses to know is that the postprocedure care for all patients who undergo PCI consists of the same interventions.

PERCUTANEOUS TRANSLUMINAL CORONARY ANGIOPLASTY

The purpose of PTCA is to compress intracoronary plaque to increase blood flow to the myocardium. It is usually the treatment of choice for patients with uncompromised collateral flow, noncalcified lesions, and lesions not present at bifurcations of vessels. In addition, the patient must be a candidate for coronary artery bypass graft (CABG) surgery. The PTCA is performed in the cardiac catheterization laboratory with the operating room on standby. A balloon catheter is inserted in the manner of coronary arteriography, but it is threaded into the occluded coronary artery and is advanced with the use of a guidewire across the lesion. The balloon is inflated under pressure one or several times to compress the lesion (Figure 11-10).

Single-vessel disease remains the classic indication for PTCA. This procedure best treats fixed, noncalcified lesions in the proximal two thirds of the coronary circulation that are accessible for dilation. Stenosis of the left mainstem artery is considered unacceptable for dilation. The optimal goal after PTCA is open coronary arteries (Figure 11-11).

Complications

The most common major complication of PTCA is coronary artery dissection. It is reported in approximately 1% to 3% of patients who need emergency bypass surgery; in addition, myocardial ischemia may occur from coronary artery spasm, coronary embolization, or intimal trauma. Associated complications can include bradycardia, ventricular fibrillation, hypotension, and vascular complications (AHA, 2001b).

INTRACORONARY STENT

Intracoronary stents are tubes that are implanted at the site of stenosis to widen the arterial lumen by squeezing atherosclerotic plaque against the artery's walls (as does PTCA). However, the stent can also keep the lumen open by providing structural support

(AHA, 2001a). Stent designs differ, but most are springs or slotted or mesh tubes about 15 mm long, with some resembling the spiral bindings used in notebooks. These are tightly wrapped around a balloon catheter, which is inflated to implant the stent.

The procedure for placing a stent is similar to the procedure in PTCA, in which the patient first undergoes cardiac arteriography for identification of occlusions in coronary arteries. The balloon catheter bearing the stent is inserted into the coronary artery, and the stent is positioned at the desired site. The balloon is inflated, thereby expanding the stent, which squeezes the atherosclerotic plaque and intimal flaps against the vessel wall. After the balloon is deflated and removed, the stent remains, holding the plaque and other matter in place and providing structural support that keeps the artery from collapsing (AHA, 2001a).

Aggressive anticoagulation therapy before, during, and after the procedure is necessary for the prevention of coagulation. Before sheath removal, peripheral perfusion is monitored because the sheath may cause occlusion of the femoral artery. Peripheral pulses, skin color, and temperature are monitored. The insertion site is inspected for any oozing or bleeding. After sheath removal, hemostasis is maintained with manual pressure, a femoral compression device, or an arterial puncture sealing device. Pain management and proper hydration aid in recovery. Retroperitoneal bleeding or impaired perfusion may occur after sheath removal. Restenosis can occur as a result of neointimal growth because of the body's natural defense when the inner intimal lining is injured, even slightly, as happens with stent placement. Restenosis occurs in 30% to 40% of patients who undergo this procedure (AHA, 2001b). The Gp IIb/IIIa inhibitors are being used after stent placement to prevent acute reocclusion through prevention of platelet aggregation.

After a stent procedure, a patient must take one or more antiplatelet or anticoagulant agents such as aspirin, ticlopidine, clopidogrel, and/or warfarin (AHA, 2001b). Aspirin is used indefinitely; the other drugs are used for 4 to 6 weeks. For 4 to 6 weeks after a stent procedure, it is necessary to take antibiotics for any minor surgical procedure (e.g., dental cleaning) to reduce the risk of infective endocarditis. In addition, for the next 6 to 8 weeks, a magnetic resonance imaging scan should *not* be done without a cardiologist's approval. However, metal detectors do not affect the stent.

New therapies in intracoronary stenting are being approved that use drug-eluted stents, which show promise in bringing the restenosis rate down to 0%. One such stent is coated with Sirolimus (antirejection medicine). Normal reaction from the body to vascular injury is neointimal (new intimal cell) growth. When a stent is placed, minor damage to the inner lining

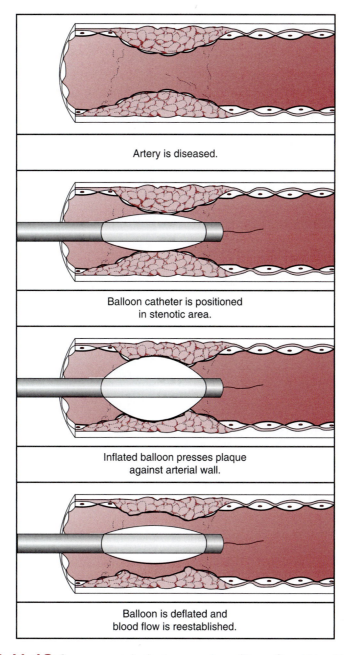

FIGURE 11-10 Coronary angioplasty procedure. (From Canobbio, M. M. [1990]. *Cardiovascular disorders: Mosby's clinical nursing series.* St. Louis: Mosby.)

of the artery occurs; thus, the body's natural defense is to grow new intimal cells to repair the damage, hence in-stent restenosis (Regar et al., 2002).

NEWER INTERVENTIONAL TECHNIQUES

Advances in interventional cardiology have led to better long-term outcomes for those patients with CAD. Two newer interventional techniques are radiation therapy and excimer laser angioplasty. Clinical

trials of both techniques have shown a decrease in restenosis rates at 6 months (Ajani, Waksman, Kim, et al., 2001; Ajani, Waksman, Sharma, et al., 2001). Radiation therapy uses either beta or gamma radiation and is delivered to the restenosis area in the same manner that the PTCA balloon is positioned within a lesion, and then the area is exposed to the radiation for varying amounts of time, usually 3 to 4 minutes. The patient is not radioactive after the

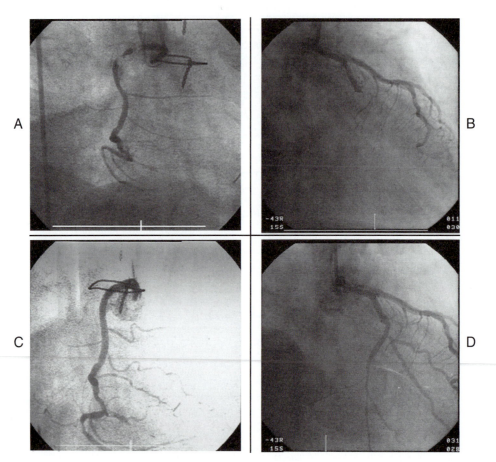

FIGURE 11-11 Radiographs of patients with triple-vessel disease with images before (**A** and **B**) and after (**C** and **D**) angioplasty. (Courtesy of University Hospital, Cardiac Catheterization Laboratory, San Antonio, TX.)

procedure, and no special precautions are needed while caring for the patient. Excimer laser coronary angioplasty uses a xenon chloride laser to photo-ablate the lesion into microscopic particles and gas. The postprocedure care for the patient who has had excimer laser coronary angioplasty is no different from that of the patient who has had PTCA.

Surgical Revascularization

Surgical approaches used for revascularization include coronary revascularization by CABG, mini-mally invasive CABG, and transmyocardial revascu-larization (TMR).

CORONARY ARTERY BYPASS GRAFT

CABG is a surgical procedure in which the ischemic area or areas of the myocardium are revascularized by implantation of the internal mammary artery or bypassing of the coronary occlusion with a saphenous

vein graft or radial artery graft. The indications for CABG are chronic stable angina that is refractory to other therapies, significant left main coronary occlusion (>50%), triple-vessel CAD, unstable angina pectoris, AMI, intractable ventricular irritability, left ventricular failure, and failure of PTCA (Eagle et al., 1999).

CABG is performed in the operating room while the patient receives general anesthesia and is intu-bated. One approach is to make a midsternal, longi-tudinal incision into the chest cavity. The patient can undergo cardiopulmonary bypass during the procedure. During cardiopulmonary bypass, blood is pumped through an oxygenator, or heart-lung machine, to receive oxygen. Cardioplegia solution is used to stop the heart so surgery can be performed.

The coronary arteries are visualized, and a segment of the saphenous vein is grafted or anastomosed to the distal end of the vessel with the proximal end of the graft vessel anastomosed to the aorta (Figure 11-12).

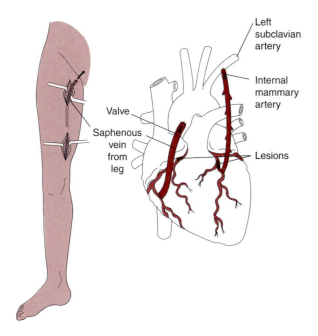

FIGURE 11-12 Coronary artery bypass graft surgery. (From Hansen, M. [1998]. *Pathophysiology: Foundations of disease and clinical intervention.* Philadelphia: W. B. Saunders.)

The internal mammary artery can also be used for creating an artery-to-artery graft. Internal mammary revascularization has been shown to have better long-term patency than saphenous vein grafts. It is the preferred graft for lesions of the left anterior descending coronary artery. The radial artery may be used as a graft. It is muscular and elastic, similar to the coronary arteries. It also has a longer duration of patency than the saphenous vein (Beghi et al., 2002). The radial artery graft is prone to spasm postoperatively; patients are given calcium channel blockers to prevent this complication.

Once grafting is done, the cardiopulmonary bypass is progressively discontinued, chest and mediastinal tubes are inserted, and the chest is closed. Box 11-6 gives information related to chest and mediastinal tubes (McHale & Carlson, 2001).

MINIMALLY INVASIVE CORONARY ARTERY SURGERY

Minimally invasive coronary artery surgery is also called limited-access coronary artery surgery (Filsoufi, Aklog, & Adams, 2001). It has been evaluated in several medical centers as an alternative to the standard methods for CABG. Two commonly used approaches

---

BOX 11-6

Key Points for Maintaining Chest and Mediastinal Tubes

DEFINITIONS

Chest tube: The tube is inserted into the pleural space to maintain the normal negative pressure and to facilitate respiration. It is inserted after cardiac surgery if the pleural space is opened. It is also inserted as treatment for pneumothorax or hemothorax.

Mediastinal tube: The tube is inserted into the mediastinal space to provide drainage after cardiac surgery.

Drainage system: A water-seal system assists in maintaining negative pressures (chest tube). Some devices are designed to function without water. Suction (up to 20 cm H_2O) is often applied to facilitate drainage.

Autotransfusion: This indicates reinfusion of autologous drainage from the system back to the patient.

BASELINE ASSESSMENT

- Make sure that all connections are tight: insertion site to the chest drainage system, suction control chamber to the suction unit.
- Assess that the dressing over insertion site is dry and intact.
- Palpate for subcutaneous emphysema around the insertion site and chest wall.
- Auscultate breath sounds.
- Observe the color and consistency of fluid in the collecting tubing (more accurate assessment than fluid in the drainage system); mark the fluid level on the drainage system.
- Assess the drainage system for proper functioning (read instructions for the device being used).
- Check the water in the water-seal level; the water level should fluctuate with respirations in chest tubes (not in mediastinal tubes).
- Check suction control and be sure that suction is on, if ordered.
- Check for intermittent bubbling in the water-seal chamber; it indicates an air leak from the pleural space (pleural tube).

Continued

include port-access coronary artery bypass (PACAB or PortCAB) and minimally invasive coronary artery bypass (MIDCAB).

In PACAB, the heart is stopped, and the patient undergoes cardiopulmonary bypass. Small incisions (ports) are made in the patient's chest. The surgical team passes instruments through the ports to perform the bypasses using the internal mammary artery, saphenous vein, or radial artery. Procedures are also being developed to replace damaged valves through limited-access ports.

The goal of MIDCAB is to avoid using cardiopulmonary bypass. It is performed while the patient's heart is still beating and is intended for use when only one or two arteries will be bypassed. MIDCAB uses a combination of small holes or ports in the chest and a small incision made directly over the coronary artery to be bypassed. The internal mammary artery is commonly used for the graft. The surgeon views and performs the attachment directly, so the artery to be bypassed must be right under the incision.

The American Heart Association's Council on Cardiothoracic and Vascular Surgery has been carefully monitoring these two procedures. MIDCAB appears to be easier on the patient and less expensive than CABG. However, complications may require an open-chest procedure. If these surgical procedures can be refined so they are no more invasive than angioplasty, they will become common.

TRANSMYOCARDIAL REVASCULARIZATION

In TMR, a high-energy laser creates channels from the epicardial surface into the left ventricular chamber (Nathan & Aranki, 2001). This procedure is also called *laser revascularization*. The purpose of TMR is to increase perfusion directly to the heart muscle. It is performed on patients who are poor candidates for CABG whose symptoms are refractory to medical treatment. To do this procedure, a surgeon makes an incision on the left side of the chest and inserts a laser into the chest cavity. With the laser, the surgeon makes channels

(1 mm) through the heart's left ventricle in between heartbeats. (The laser is fired when the chamber is full of blood so the blood can protect the inside of the heart.) Ten to 50 channels are created (Nathan & Aranki, 2001). Then the surgeon applies pressure on the outside of the heart. This seals the outer openings but lets the inner channels stay open, to allow oxygen-rich blood to flow through the heart muscle.

TMR has produced early promising results. Studies have shown that those patients who have received TMR have greater improvement in quality-of-life assessment scores at 12 months postoperatively than those patients who received only medical therapy (Nathan & Aranki, 2001). Improvement in symptoms usually occurs over time, not immediately.

TMR probably will not replace CABG or angioplasty as a common method of treating CAD. TMR may be used for people who are high-risk candidates for a second bypass or angioplasty, for example, people whose blockages are too diffuse to be treated with bypass alone, or some patients with heart transplants who develop atherosclerosis.

Management After Cardiac Surgery

Patients are usually directly admitted to the intensive care unit after cardiac surgery. The patient often has a pulmonary artery catheter, arterial catheter, peripheral IV lines, chest tubes, mediastinal tube, and a Foley catheter. The patient is usually mechanically ventilated in the immediate postoperative period. The nurse assesses the patient often and provides rapid interventions to help the patient recover from anesthesia and to prevent complications. The nurse-to-patient ratio is often 1:1 during the first few hours after surgery or until the patient is extubated. Nursing care for these patients is summarized in Box 11-7.

COMPLICATIONS OF CARDIAC SURGERY

Patients who have had cardiac surgery should be closely monitored for complications such as mediastinal bleeding, low cardiac output syndrome, atrial dysrhythmias, and hypovolemia. The critical care nurse taking care of a patient who has just undergone CABG must have quick critical thinking skills and the ability to take in the whole picture, while at the same time prioritizing interventions that need to be performed.

Cardiac Dysrhythmias

Cardiac dysrhythmias may have many causes such as CAD, AMI, electrolyte imbalances, and HF. The various dysrhythmias and patient assessment are discussed in Chapter 6. Emergency treatments of dysrhythmias,

---

BOX 11-7

Nursing Interventions After Cardiac Surgery

- Assess for hypovolemia; assess output from the chest and mediastinal tubes and urine output.
- Monitor for hypotension; administer fluids and vasopressors as ordered.
- Monitor hemodynamic pressures, cardiac output, and cardiac index; treat the patient per protocols.
- Rewarm the patient gradually (if applicable).
- Monitor fluid and electrolytes, hemoglobin, hematocrit, renal function, and coagulation studies.
- Provide pain relief.
- Monitor for complications: intraoperative acute myocardial infarction, dysrhythmias, heart failure, cardiac tamponade, thromboembolism, impaired renal function, pneumonia, pneumothorax, pleural effusion, cerebral ischemia, or stroke.
- Wean from mechanical ventilation; extubate; promote pulmonary hygiene every 1 to 2 hours while the patient is awake.
- Assess wounds and provide incisional care per hospital protocol.
- Gradually increase the patient's activity.
- Provide emotional support to the patient and family.

---

such as medications, transcutaneous pacemakers, and cardioversion and defibrillation, are discussed in Chapter 6. Other drugs that may be used in the critical care unit to manage dysrhythmias are shown in Table 11-8. Additional surgical and electrical treatments are discussed in the following sections.

RADIOFREQUENCY CATHETER ABLATION

Radiofrequency catheter ablation is a method of interrupting a supraventricular tachycardia, a dysrhythmia caused by a reentry circuit, an abnormal conduction pathway. The objective of catheter ablation is to interrupt electrical conduction or activity permanently in a region of dysrhythmogenic cardiac tissue (AHA, 2002). Indications for radiofrequency catheter ablation include the presence of two conducting pathways that are in competition with each other, causing reentrant tachycardias.

Radiofrequency ablation is performed percutaneously. The procedure begins with a diagnostic electrophysiology study. A catheter with an electrode is positioned at the accessory (abnormal) pathway, and mild, painless radiofrequency energy (similar to microwave heat) is transmitted to the pathway, causing coagulation and necrosis in the conduction fibers without destroying the surrounding tissue. This stops the area from conducting the extra impulses that caused the tachycardia. After each ablation attempt, the patient is retested until there is no recurrence of the tachycardiac rhythm (AHA, 2002).

A promising new technique that uses radio-frequency ablation to treat atrial fibrillation is called circumferential radiofrequency ablation. The lines of electrical conduction that may contribute to atrial fibrillation are located where the pulmonary veins connect to the left atrium. Radiofrequency ablation

TABLE 11-8

AGENTS USED TO TREAT DYSRHYTHMIAS

Drug	Indications	Mechanism of Action	Dosage and Route	Side Effects	Nursing Implications
Diltiazem (Cardizem)	Atrial fibrillation/ flutter SVT	Inhibits calcium ion influx into vascular smooth muscle and myocardium	IV: 20 mg over 2 min Infusion: 5-15 mg/hr × 24 hr	Hypotension, edema, dizziness, bradycardia	Often used in conjunction with digoxin for rate control Not used in heart failure Observe for dysrhythmias
Amiodarone (Cordarone)	Atrial fibrillation/ flutter SVT Ventricular dysrhythmias	Prolongs action potential phase 3	PO: 200-600 mg/day IV: 150 mg bolus in 10 min, then 1 mg/min for 6 hr, then 0.5 mg/min for 18 hr (ventricular dysrhythmias)	Bradycardia, complete atrioventricular block, hypotension Multiple side effects (thyroid, pulmonary, hepatic, neurological, dermatologic)	Long half-life Monitor rhythm closely Obtain baseline pulmonary and liver function tests
Flecainide (Tambocor)	Ventricular dysrhythmias	Decreases conduction in all parts of the heart; stabilizes cardiac membrane	PO: 50-100 mg q12h; increase as needed, not to exceed 400 mg/day	Hypotension, bradycardia, heart block, blurred vision, respiratory depression	Interacts with many other drugs; check drug guide Monitor cardiac rhythm Monitor intake and output Assess electrolytes Assess for central nervous system symptoms
Sotalol (Betapace)	Ventricular dysrhythmias	Nonselective beta-blocker	PO 80 mg BID Increase to 240-320 mg/day	Hematological disorders, bronchospasm	Monitor blood pressure and pulse rate Check baseline liver and renal function before beginning therapy Monitor hydration Watch for QT prolongation Teach patient not to decrease drug abruptly
Ibutilide (Corvert)	Atrial fibrillation/ flutter	Prolongs duration of action potential and refractory period	IV: 1 mg IV push over 10 min; may repeat after 10 min	Hypotension, bradycardia, sinus arrest	Continuous ECG monitoring to assess effectiveness Assess for central nervous system symptoms Use usually restricted to electrophysiology personnel
Propafenone (Rythmol)	Ventricular dysrhythmias	Stabilizes membranes; depresses action potential phase 0	PO: 150 mg q8h	Ventricular dysrhythmias, congestive heart failure, dizziness, nausea/ vomiting, altered taste	Monitor rhythm Use in patients without structural heart disease

ECG, Electrocardiogram; *SVT,* supraventricular tachycardia.

is done in a circular pattern around each pulmonary vein opening. This procedure has been found to be effective in treating and curing both episodic and chronic atrial fibrillation (AHA, 2002).

PERMANENT PACEMAKERS

Temporary pacemakers are used on an emergency basis to treat symptomatic bradycardia or to override tachyarrhythmias. Bradycardia often results from heart block associated with AMI, digoxin toxicity, or other cardiac abnormality. If symptomatic bradycardia continues despite treatment and resolution of the cause, a permanent pacemaker is usually indicated. Permanent pacemakers may also be used to treat recurrent tachydysrhythmias unresponsive to pharmacological treatment. Biventricular pacemakers are discussed in the section of this chapter on HF.

In the United States, most pacemakers are multiprogrammable for rate, voltage, sensitivity, stimulus duration, and refractory period. Most implanted pacemakers are of the ventricular demand type and have the ability to coincide with the patient's changing needs. Most permanent pacemakers use lithium batteries as their power source. These models have a longevity of 8 to 10 years.

Pacemaker functions are described in a code developed by the Intersociety Commission for Heart Disease (ICHD). The ICHD code has been updated to a Modified Generic Code (Table 11-9). The North American Society for Pacing and Electrophysiology (NASPE) uses a more specific code that may also be seen in the clinical setting. The code is used to denote the capabilities of the pacemaker as programmed for an individual patient. The code originally had three letters, was updated to five, but is more commonly seen with the original three letters denoting the chambers paced, the chamber sensed, and the mode of response to sensing (see Table 11-9).

Programmable pacing devices have the ability to sense as well as trigger an output; they are classified as *atrial* or *ventricular* pacemakers and are coded as such, depending on their placement and inhibiting or triggering activity. A permanent pacemaker can be inserted in a transvenous mode by use of local anesthesia, with the lead wires traversing through the subclavian vein into the right atrium and ventricle. The battery or generator is implanted into the subcutaneous tissue, usually on the left side of the chest. This procedure may be performed in the operating room, but it is commonly performed in the cardiac catheterization laboratory or special procedures area of the radiology department.

IMPLANTABLE CARDIOVERTER-DEFIBRILLATOR

Implantable defibrillators have become the dominant therapeutic modality for patients with life-threatening ventricular dysrhythmias. Implantable cardioverter-defibrillators (ICDs) were initially used for patients with one or more sudden cardiac arrests or drug-refractory sustained ventricular tachycardia or ventricular fibrillation (AHA, 2002).

Current indications for ICD therapy are listed in Box 11-8. Recent indications also include patients awaiting cardiac transplantation who sustain life-threatening dysrhythmias and prophylactic implantation in high-risk patient groups: extensive MI and low ejection fraction, history of MI with recurrent episodes of unexplained syncope, and children with congenital long-QT syndrome (Gregoratos et al., 2002).

An implantable atrial defibrillator has been introduced. In selected patients with recurrent atrial fibrillation with and without structural heart disease, a stand-alone atrial defibrillator was able to restore sinus rhythm promptly with low amounts of energy. In patients with no structural heart disease, the frequency of atrial fibrillation episodes decreased (Daoud et al., 2000).

ICDs provide high-energy shocks for ventricular fibrillation and rapid ventricular tachycardia,

TABLE 11-9

Modified Generic Code for Pacemakers

I Chamber Paced	II Chamber Sensed	III Response to Sensing	IV Programmable Functions/ Rate Modulation	V Antitachycardia Function(s)
V: Ventricle	V: Ventricle	T: Triggered	P: Programmable	P: Pace
A: Atrium	A: Atrium	I: Inhibited	M: Multiprogrammable	S: Shock
D: Dual (A + V)	D: Dual (A + V)	D: Dual (T + I)	C: Communicating	D: Dual (P + S)
O: None	O: None	O: None	R: Rate modulating	O: None
			O: None	

From Medtronic. (1998). CorePace. PowerPoint presentation package. Minneapolis, MN: Author.

BOX 11-8

Indications for an Implantable Cardioverter-Defibrillator

- Cardiac arrest resulting from ventricular fibrillation (VF) or ventricular tachycardia (VT) not produced by a transient or reversible cause
- Spontaneous sustained VT in association with structural heart disease*
- Syncope of undetermined origin with clinically relevant, hemodynamically significant sustained VT or VF induced during electrophysiological study
- Nonsustained VT in patients with coronary artery disease, prior myocardial infarction, left ventricular dysfunction, and inducible VF or sustained VT during electrophysiological study*
- Spontaneous sustained VT in patients who do not have structural heart disease that is not amenable to other treatments
- Patients with left ventricular ejection fraction of 30% or less, at least 1 month after myocardial infarction and 3 months after coronary artery bypass surgery*

*New indications or changes to an old recommendation.
From Gregoratos, G., Abrams, J., Epstein, A., et al. (2002). ACC/AHA/NASPE 2002 guideline update for implantation of cardiac pacemakers and antiarrhythmia devices. Summary article: A report of the American College of Cardiology/American Heart Association Task Force on Practice Guidelines (ACC/AHA/NASPE Committee to Update the 1998 Pacemaker Guidelines). *Circulation*, *106*, 2145-2161.

antitachycardia pacing for ventricular tachycardia, and pacing for bradycardia. Newer devices, incorporating an atrial lead, allow dual-chamber pacing with better discrimination between ventricular tachycardia (VT) and supraventricular tachycardia (SVT). ICDs can also provide resynchronization therapy for patients with HF (NASPE, 2003).

Just like the leads of a pacemaker, ICD leads are placed transvenously through the subclavian or cephalic vein and are positioned inside the heart. The defibrillator or pulse generator is placed in the pectoral region. Initially, devices were so large and cumbersome that patients found them very uncomfortable, but with each new generation of devices, they become smaller and more sophisticated. Complications associated with ICD therapy include infection, lead failure, and unnecessary shocks for SVT.

Patients and family members must be educated about the device. Teaching is highlighted in Box 11-9 (Guidant, 2002). Quarterly clinic visits are important for the monitoring of ICD function and events.

The ICD comes with an identification card that specifies the heart rate at which shocks occur, the manufacturer and model number of the ICD, and the telephone numbers of the manufacturer and the primary physician. This card is carried with the patient.

Standard emergency procedures are to be followed with patients who have these devices and suffer cardiovascular collapse. Cardiopulmonary resuscitation must not be delayed because the patient has an implanted device. Placement of paddles for external defibrillation is usually anteroposterior rather than sternum-apex.

Heart Failure

HF is a principal complication of virtually all forms of heart disease (Braunwald, Zipes, & Libby, 2001). HF is a clinical syndrome that can result from any structural or functional cardiac disorder that impairs the ability of the ventricle to fill or eject blood (Hunt et al., 2001). The cardinal manifestations of HF are dyspnea, fatigue, exercise intolerance, and fluid retention, which may lead to pulmonary and peripheral edema (Hunt et al., 2001).

Clinically, HF can be defined as the heart's inability to pump a sufficient amount of blood to meet the needs of the body tissues (Braunwald et al., 2001). HF can be acute or chronic. CAD is the underlying cause of HF in approximately two thirds of patients. The remainder have a nonischemic cause: hypertension, valvular disease, exposure to myocardial toxins, myocarditis, or unidentifiable causes such as idiopathic dilated cardiomyopathy. The classic symptoms of HF consist of progressive exertional dyspnea, paroxysmal nocturnal dyspnea, orthopnea, fatigability, loss of appetite, abdominal bloating, nausea or vomiting, and eventual organ system dysfunction, particularly the renal system as the failure advances.

PATHOPHYSIOLOGY

HF is impaired cardiac function of one or both ventricles. HF can also be classified as systolic or diastolic. Systolic HF results from impaired pumping of the ventricles. Diastolic HF results from impaired filling or relaxation of the ventricles. By far, the most common type of HF is left-sided systolic dysfunction. Right-sided dysfunction is usually a consequence of left-sided HF; however, it can be a primary cause after a right ventricular MI or secondary to pulmonary pathology. The causes of HF are noted in Box 11-10 (McCance & Huether, 2002).

In left-sided HF, the left ventricle cannot pump efficiently. The ineffective pumping action causes a decrease in cardiac output. The volume of blood

---

BOX 11-9

Patient and Family Teaching for an Implantable Cardioverter-Defibrillator

PREPROCEDURAL TEACHING
Device and how it works
Lead and generator placement
Implantation procedure
Videos and materials from the manufacturer

POSTPROCEDURAL TEACHING
Site care and symptoms of complications
Restricting activity of the arm on the side of the implant
Identification (Medic Alert jewelry and ICD card)
Diary of an event if the device fires
Response if the device fires (varies from falling, tingling, or discomfort to no awareness of the shock); family members needed to help in assessment
Safety measures:
  Avoid strong magnetic fields (no magnetic resonance imaging).
  Avoid sources of high-power electricity.
  Keep cellular phones at least 6 inches from the ICD.

Inform airline security personnel about the device; avoid the metal detector; the security wand may be used but should not be left over the device.
The defibrillator must be turned off for surgical procedures using electrocautery.
Everyday activities:
  Hairdryers, microwaves, and razors are safe.
  Sexual activity can be resumed; tachycardia associated with sexual activity may cause the device to fire; rate adjustments may be needed.
  If shock occurs during sexual activity, it will not harm the patient's partner.
  Avoid driving for 6 months if the patient has a history of sudden cardiac arrest.
Testing of the device requiring additional electrophysiological studies
Replacement of the device
Instruction of family members in cardiopulmonary resuscitation and in how to contact emergency personnel
Support groups in the local community

BOX 11-10

Causes of Heart Failure

LEFT HEART SYSTOLIC FAILURE
Myocardial infarction
Coronary artery disease
Cardiomyopathy
Hypertension
Valvular heart disease
Tachyarrhythmias
Toxins: cocaine, ethanol, chemotherapy agents
Myocarditis
Pregnancy: postpartum cardiomyopathy

LEFT HEART DIASTOLIC FAILURE
Myocardial infarction
Coronary artery disease
Hypertrophic heart disease
Pericarditis
Infiltrative disease: amyloid, sarcoid

Radiation therapy to the chest
Age
Hypertension

RIGHT HEART SYSTOLIC FAILURE
Right ventricular infarction
Left-sided heart failure
Pulmonary embolus
Pulmonary hypertension
Chronic obstructive pulmonary disease
Septal defects

RIGHT HEART DIASTOLIC FAILURE
Right ventricular hypertrophy
Infiltrative disease: amyloid, sarcoid
Radiation therapy to the chest

remaining in the left ventricle increases after each beat. As this volume builds, it backs up into the left atrium and pulmonary veins and into the lungs. Eventually, fluid accumulates in the lungs and pleural spaces, causing increased pressure in the lungs. Gas exchange (oxygen and carbon dioxide) in the pulmonary system is impaired. The backflow can continue into the right ventricle and right atrium and into the systemic circulation (right-sided HF).

When gas exchange is impaired and carbon dioxide increases, the respiratory rate increases to help eliminate the excess carbon dioxide. This phenomenon causes the heart rate to increase, pumping more blood to the lungs for gas exchange. The increased heart rate results in the pumping of more blood from the systemic circulation into the cardiopulmonary circulation, which is already dangerously overloaded, and a vicious cycle ensues.

As the heart begins to fail to meet the body's metabolic demands, several compensatory mechanisms are activated to improve cardiac output and tissue perfusion. The most noteworthy of these neurohormonal systems are the renin-angiotensin-aldosterone system and the sympathetic nervous system. These interrelated systems act in concert to redistribute blood to critical organs in the body by increasing peripheral vascular tone, heart rate, and contractility (Murray & Dugan, 2000). The activation of these diverse systems may account for many of the symptoms of HF and may contribute to the progression of the syndrome. Although these responses may be initially viewed as compensatory, many of them are or become counter-regulatory and lead to adverse effects.

The renin-angiotensin-aldosterone system plays a major role in pathogenesis and progression of HF.

Angiotensin II is a potent vasoconstrictor and promotes salt and water retention by stimulation of aldosterone release. Sodium reabsorption increases, and this, in turn, increases blood volume. In patients with impaired function, the heart is unable to handle the extra volume effectively, resulting in edema (peripheral, visceral and hepatic).

The sympathetic nervous system is activated. Although this is initially beneficial in preserving cardiac output and systemic pressure, chronic activation is deleterious. Activation (1) produces tachycardia, thereby decreasing preload and contributing to a further decrease in stroke index; (2) causes vasoconstriction, which increases afterload, further decreasing stroke index; and (3) increases contractility, which increases myocardial oxygen demand, thereby decreasing contractility and possibly decreasing stroke index.

These changes are progressive. In time, the ventricle dilates, hypertrophies, and becomes more spherical. This process of cardiac remodeling generally precedes symptoms by months or even years (Hunt et al., 2001).

ASSESSMENT

Patient assessment includes the identification of the cause of both right-sided and left-sided HF, the signs and symptoms, and precipitating factors as well as diagnostic studies. Signs and symptoms are described in Box 11-11.

Diagnosis and treatment of the patient suspected of having HF include the following:
- A complete history including precipitating factors
- Physical examination. The key aspects of the physical examination include assessment of

---

BOX 11-11

Signs and Symptoms of Heart Failure

LEFT-SIDED HEART FAILURE: POOR PUMP
Dyspnea/orthopnea
Paroxysmal nocturnal dyspnea
Cough (orthopnea equivalent)
Fatigue or activity intolerance
Diaphoresis
Slow capillary refill/cyanosis
Elevated pulmonary capillary wedge pressure
S_3 and S_4 gallop*
Increased heart rate

RIGHT-SIDED HEART FAILURE: EXCESS VOLUME
Elevated jugular venous pressure
Liver engorgement (hepatomegaly)
Edema
Elevated right atrial pressure
Loss of appetite, nausea, vomiting
Enlarged spleen

*In left-sided heart failure, the detection of an S_3, or gallop, rhythm is an important early sign. Detection of the S_3 sound and observation of other signs can precipitate early and aggressive management of impending congestive heart failure to prevent further problems and complications.

Intravascular volume with examination of neck veins and presence of hepatojugular reflux

Presence or absence of edema

Perfusion status, which includes blood pressure, quality of peripheral pulses, capillary refill, and temperature of extremities

Lung sounds, which may not be helpful; in most cases the lung fields are clear when the patient is obviously "congested," a reflection of chronicity of the disease and adaptation

- Chest x-ray study to view heart size and configuration and to check the lung fields to determine whether they are clear or opaque (fluid filled)
- Hemodynamic monitoring with pulmonary artery catheter. Mixed venous oxygen saturation (SvO_2), stroke index, cardiac index, cardiac output and pulmonary artery pressures are important parameters to assess in the most critically ill patients, especially when they do not respond to conventional therapy. Noninvasive methods of determining hemodynamics, such as bioimpedance cardiography, are gaining popularity. This technology allows stroke volume, cardiac output, thoracic fluid content, and contractility to be determined noninvasively by placing sensor pads at the root of the neck and the thorax (Ventura, Pranulis, Young, & Smart, 2000).
- Noninvasive imaging of cardiac structures. The single most useful test in evaluating patients with HF is the echocardiogram, which can evaluate ventricular enlargement, wall motion abnormalities, and valvular structures.
- Arterial blood gases to assess oxygenation and acid-base status
- Laboratory studies

Serum electrolytes. Many electrolyte derangements can be seen in patients with HF. Low serum sodium can be a sign of advanced or end-stage disease, potassium can be low (excessive diuresis) or high (renal impairment), blood urea nitrogen and creatinine can be elevated in low perfusion states or with overdiuresis.

Complete blood count to assess for anemia

B-Type natriuretic peptide (BNP), a cardiac hormone secreted by ventricular myocytes in response to wall stretch. Plasma concentrations of BNP reflect severity of HF (Hirata et al., 2001). In decompensated HF, the BNP will rise as a response to wall stress or stretch. As the HF is treated, BNP can be used to assess how well patients are responding to therapy. Less than 100 pg/mL is a normal BNP value. Patients are at risk of 30-day readmission if BNP is higher than 400 pg/mL at time of discharge. BNP is also a good marker for differentiating between pulmonary and cardiac causes of dyspnea (Morrison et al., 2002).

Liver function studies. The liver can become enlarged with tenderness because of hepatic congestion. Transaminases and bilirubin can be elevated with diminished liver function. Function usually returns once the patient is treated and euvolemic.

ECG. Intraventricular conduction delays are common. Left bundle branch blocks are often associated with structural abnormalities. Patients frequently have premature ventricular contractions, premature atrial contractions, and atrial arrhythmias such as atrial fibrillation or flutter. Resting sinus tachycardia implies substantive cardiac decompensation, and detection of this occurrence is essential.

NURSING DIAGNOSES

Priority nursing diagnoses for the patient with HF are noted here. See the Nursing Care Plan for the Patient with Heart Failure for outcomes, interventions, and rationale.

- Decreased cardiac output related to altered myocardial contractility or inotropic changes, alterations in rate, rhythm, electrical conduction, and structural changes
- Impaired gas exchange related to fluid collection or shifts into interstitial space or alveoli; weakness and anxiety
- Fluid volume excess related to reduced glomerular filtration rate (decreased cardiac output) or increased antidiuretic hormone production and sodium or water retention
- Activity intolerance related to imbalance between oxygen supply and demand, generalized weakness, and prolonged bed rest or immobility
- Impaired skin integrity related to prolonged bed rest, edema, and decreased tissue perfusion
- Potential complications of HF (collaborative problem)
- Knowledge deficit related to lack of understanding or misconceptions about cardiac function, disease, and failure

INTERVENTIONS

Medical and nursing interventions for the patient with HF consist of a threefold approach: (1) treatment of the existing symptoms of the crisis situation, (2) prevention of further or expanding complications, and (3) treatment of the underlying cause. For example, some patients with HF can be treated by controlling hypertension or by repairing or replacing abnormal heart valves.

Text continued on p. 336

Nursing Care Plan for the Patient with Heart Failure

NURSING DIAGNOSIS: *Decreased cardiac output related to impaired cardiac function*

Patient Outcomes	Interventions	Rationales
Adequate cardiac output as evidenced by • Vital signs within normal range • Resolution of gallop rhythm • Absence of fatigue and weakness • Clear breath sounds • Usual mental status • Absence of vertigo and syncope • Palpable peripheral pulses • Skin warm, dry, and usual color with capillary refill time less than 3 sec • Urine output at least 30 mL/hr • Absence of edema and jugular vein distention • Hemodynamic values WNL	Assess for signs and symptoms of HF and decreased cardiac output.	Thorough assessment of patient's hemodynamic status including diagnostic test and laboratory results (e.g., ECG, BNP level) and assessment for right-sided HF (increased JVD, hepatomegaly, peripheral edema) and left-sided HF (decreased BP, weak pulses, orthopnea) allow the nurse to detect early signs of cardiac compromise.
	Monitor ECG readings and report dysrhythmias.	Patients with heart failure frequently have atrial fibrillation and ventricular dysrhythmias.
	Monitor chest x-ray results; report findings of cardiomegaly, pleural effusion, or pulmonary edema.	Frequent evaluation of chest films assesses response to therapy and allows for early detection of problems.
	Implement measures to reduce cardiac workload and improve cardiac output.	During the decompensated phase of HF, patients can easily become fatigued and short of breath with minimal activity.
	Administer ordered medications. ACE inhibitors, diuretics, inotropic agents, vasodilators, beta-blockers, nitrates.	These drugs maintain hemodynamic stability, enhance tissue perfusion, and decrease workload on the heart.
	Prepare the patient for insertion of IABP or VAD (ventricular assist device) if indicated.	These assist devices help to maintain cardiac output in the failing heart.

NURSING DIAGNOSIS: *Impaired gas exchange related to excess fluid in lungs*

Patient Outcomes	Interventions	Rationales
Adequate gas exchange as evidenced by • Normal rate, rhythm, and depth of respirations • ↓ Dyspnea • Usual or improved breath sounds • Usual mental status • Usual skin color • Blood gases within normal range	Assess for signs and symptoms of respiratory distress.	Thorough assessment of the respiratory system allows the nurse to detect worsening HF and fluid accumulation.
	Assess lung sounds.	Crackles and wheezing may indicate pulmonary edema.
	Monitor chest x-ray studies, ABG results, and pulse oximetry values.	Frequent assessment of these diagnostic tests allows the nurse to evaluate the response to therapy.
	Elevate the head of bed, and turn and reposition patient every 2 hours.	Patients with HF often cannot tolerate being flat, and turning and repositioning allow for increased comfort and prevent skin breakdown.
	Administer oxygen; the patient may need noninvasive positive pressure ventilation (CPAP, BiPAP).	Many patients with HF have sleep apnea and Cheyne-Stokes respirations resulting in oxygen desaturation.

Nursing Care Plan for the Patient with Heart Failure—cont'd

Patient Outcomes	Interventions	Rationales
	Administer CNS depressants cautiously.	Decreasing anxiety and keeping the HF patient calm will help to lessen the work on the cardiovascular and respiratory systems.
	Administer ordered medications, diuretics, and morphine.	Morphine reduces preload and alleviates anxiety; diuretics alleviate congestion.

NURSING DIAGNOSIS: *Fluid excess related to sodium and water retention*

Patient Outcomes	Interventions	Rationales
Resolution of fluid imbalance as evidenced by • Decline in weight toward client's normal • Vital signs WNL • Balanced I&O • Usual mental status • Improved breath sounds • Hct returning toward normal range • ↓ Dyspnea and orthopnea • ↓ In edema and ascites • Resolution of neck vein distention • RAP within normal range • Serum sodium WNL	Assess for signs and symptoms of fluid volume excess. Monitor daily weight and intake and output. Monitor chest x-ray results. Restrict fluid and sodium intake as ordered. Administer diuretics as ordered. Assess for hyponatremia, nausea, vomiting, lethargy, and decreased sensorium.	Patients with HF often cannot maintain sodium and fluid balance. Evaluate the response to therapy. Weight gain and intake greater than output are signs of fluid volume excess. Frequent evaluation of chest films assesses response to therapy and allows for early detection of problems. Helps to maintain fluid balance. These drugs help to maintain fluid balance and alleviate congestion. Neurohormonal activation and excessive diuretics can cause hyponatremia.

NURSING DIAGNOSIS: *Activity intolerance, related to tissue hypoxia*

Patient Outcomes	Interventions	Rationales
↑ Tolerance for activity as evidenced by: • Verbalization of feeling less fatigued and weak • Ability to perform activities of daily living with minimal symptoms	Assess for signs and symptoms of activity intolerance. Implement measures to improve activity tolerance. Instruct client to report changes in activity intolerance	Allows for modification of activities in relation to the patient's current status and allows the nurse to prevent problems related to inadequate performance of activities. Allows the patient to tolerate activities better. Measures to increase tolerance enable the patient to see and feel actual progression toward the goal. Alerts the nurse to early signs of changes in patient's hemodynamic status and allows the nurse to modify activities as needed to prevent complications.

Continued

Nursing Care Plan for the Patient with Heart Failure

NURSING DIAGNOSIS: *Impaired skin integrity*

Patient Outcomes	Interventions	Rationales
Skin and mucous membranes will be intact as evidenced by the following indicators: skin intactness and tissue temperature in expected range.	Monitor site of skin impairment at least once a day for color changes, redness, swelling, warmth, pain, or other signs of infection.	Systematic inspection can identify impending problems early. Monitor client's continence status, and minimize exposure of skin impairment and other areas to moisture from incontinence, perspiration, or wound drainage
	For clients with limited mobility, use a risk-assessment tool to systematically assess immobility-related risk factors	A validated risk-assessment tool such as the Norton or Braden scale should be used to identify clients at risk for immobility-related skin breakdown.
	Teach skin and wound assessment and ways to monitor for signs and symptoms of infection, complications, and healing.	Early assessment and intervention help prevent serious problems from developing.
	If consistent with overall client management goals, teach how to turn and reposition at least every 2 hours.	If the goal of care is to keep a client comfortable, turning and repositioning may not be appropriate.

NURSING DIAGNOSIS: *Potential complications of HF*

Patient Outcomes	Interventions	Rationales
Absence of renal failure, cardiac dysrhythmias, thromboembolism, cardiogenic shock	Monitor for dysrhythmias.	Dysrhythmias can be common in patients with HF, and therefore close monitoring is warranted to detect and prevent potential life-threatening arrhythmias.
	Assess for thromboembolic events.	Patients with HF can have ventricular thrombi as result of low output. Thromboembolic events (stroke, PE, and DVT) are detected and prevented or treated by thorough assessment of vascular status (peripheral and neurological).
	Implement measures to prevent the development of thromboemboli.	Thromboembolic events can be a potential complication of HF; therefore, measures to prevent thromboembolic events (stroke and PE) are crucial.
	Assess heart sounds for new murmur or new S_3 and/or S_4.	Changes in heart sounds can signal worsening left ventricular functioning and fluid volume excess.

NURSING DIAGNOSIS: *Knowledge deficit, ineffective management of therapeutic regimen*

Patient Outcomes	Interventions	Rationales
Verbalizes knowledge of treatment regimen for HF	Explain HF in terms the patient can understand; use teaching aids.	Use of simple language aids in the patient's understanding of complex medical problems, and use of teaching aids (visual aids) reinforces verbal instructions.
	Teach patient how to count his or her pulse.	Use of some cardiac medications can cause bradycardia. Early detection can help to prevent complications.
	Explain the rationale for a low-sodium diet; dietary consultation should be ordered for all patients with HF.	A low-sodium diet helps to reduce fluid accumulation.
	Explain all medications.	Thorough explanation of medications helps the patient better to understand the disease process and allows the patient better to communicate with health care providers.
	Reinforce instructions about activity.	Reinforcement of activity instructions allows the patient better to understand the importance of activity modifications that help to result in decreased myocardial oxygen demands.
	Reinforce instructions regarding sexual activity.	Reinforcement of instructions regarding sexual activity helps to prevent unwanted situations (chest pain, SOB, syncope, palpitations, etc) from occurring at inopportune times.
	Instruct client to report changes in heart rate, irregular pulse, palpitations, SOB, chest pain, weight gain of more than 2 lb in 2 days, cough, or an increase in edema.	Early detection of changes leads the patient to seek medical attention and prevents potential complications.
	If patient is discharged on a diuretic, instruct to:	Diuretic instructions are important for compliance.
	Take diuretic early in the morning and second dose 6 hours later.	They improve compliance and thus avoid nocturia.
	Weigh self daily, keeping a record.	Sudden increases in weight can alert the patient of fluid accumulation.
	Change position gradually.	Diuretics can cause orthostatic hypotension.
	Monitor potassium intake.	Diuretics can alter potassium levels.
	Report the following symptoms: weight loss of more than 5 lb in a week, excessive thirst, severe dizziness, muscle weakness or cramping, nausea, vomiting, or irregular pulse.	Diuretics cause dehydration and electrolyte imbalances.

ABG, Arterial blood gas; *ACE,* angiotensin-converting enzyme; *BiPAP,* bilevel positive airway pressure; *BNP,* brain natriuretic peptide; *BP,* blood pressure; *CNS,* central nervous system; *CPAP,* continuous positive airway pressure; *DVT,* deep venous thrombosis; *ECG,* electrocardiogram; *Hct,* hematocrit; *HF,* heart failure; *IABP,* intraaortic balloon pump; *I&O,* intake and output; *JVD,* jugular venous distention; *PE,* pulmonary embolism; *RAP,* right atrial pressure; *SOB,* shortness of breath; *WNL,* within normal limits.
From Ulrich, S. & Canale, S. (2001). *Nursing care planning guide for adults in acute, extended and home care settings.* 5th ed. Philadelphia: W. B. Saunders.

Treatment of existing symptoms includes the following:

1. Improvement of pump function, fluid removal, and enhanced tissue perfusion (Table 11-10)
   a. First-line medications include ACE inhibitors and diuretics. Once symptoms and volume status are stable, a beta-blocker (metoprolol, carvedilol, bisoprolol) should be added. Once contraindicated in HF, beta-blockers have shown impressive mortality reduction and reverse remodeling of the ventricle (Hunt et al., 2001). Additional drug therapy includes digoxin, spironolactone, hydralazine, and nitrates.
   b. Inotropes (dobutamine, milrinone, amrinone) improve cardiac performance in the acute decompensated patient and aid in end-organ tissue perfusion. Prolonged or intermittent use as an outpatient has produced increased mortality rates (Peacock, Freda, Emerman, & Volturo, 2002).
   c. Nesiritide (Natrecor). During decompensated HF, endogenous BNP is produced by cardiac myocytes in an attempt to return the heart to homeostasis. In a decompensated state, not enough is produced to achieve physiological benefit. Administration of synthetic exogenous BNP (Nesiritide [Natrecor]) has shown positive effects on hemodynamics and has resulted in rapid improvement of symptoms of HF (Colucci et al., 2000).

TABLE 11-10

MEDICATIONS FOR HEART FAILURE

ANGIOTENSIN-CONVERTING ENZYME INHIBITORS (ACE-I)

Indications: used to treat hypertension, heart failure, and patients after myocardial infarction

Mechanism of action: prevent the conversion of angiotensin I to angiotensin II resulting in lower levels of angiotensin II, thus causing an increase in plasma rennin activity and reduction of aldosterone secretion; also inhibit the remodeling process after myocardial injury

Trade Name (Brand Name)	Dosage	Side Effects and Nursing Considerations
Enalapril (Vasotec)	2.5-10 mg BID PO	Hypotension, bradycardia, renal impairment, cough, and orthostatic hypotension. Do not give IV enalapril to patients with unstable heart failure or in those patients having an acute myocardial infarction. Monitor urine output. Monitor potassium levels. Avoid use of NSAIDs. Instruct patient to avoid rapid change in position such as from lying to standing. Angiotensin-converting enzyme inhibitors are contraindicated in pregnancy.
Fosinopril (Monopril)	10-40 mg daily PO	Same
Captopril (Capoten)	12.5-50 mg TID	Same

DIURETICS

Indication: for the management of edema or fluid volume overload associated with heart failure and hepatic or renal disease

Mechanism of action: inhibit reabsorbtion of sodium and chloride in the ascending loop of Henle and distal renal tubule, interfering with the chloride-binding cotransport system, causing increased excretion of water, sodium, chloride, magnesium, and calcium

Trade Name (Brand Name)	Dosage	Side Effects and Nursing Considerations
Furosemide (Lasix)	20-160 mg PO/IV BID	Orthostatic hypotension, vertigo, dizziness, gout, hypokalemia, cramping, diarrhea or constipation, hearing impairment, tinnitus (rapid IV administration). Monitor appropriate laboratory results, especially potassium levels. Monitor cardiovascular and hydration status regularly. In decompensated patients, use IV route until euvolemic status is reached. Administer first dose early in the day and second dose late in afternoon, to avoid sleep disturbance.
Bumetadine (Bumex)	0.5-2 mg daily 0.5-1 mg IV/IM q4-6h	Same
Torsemide (Demadex)	10-100 mg PO/IV BID *Max 200 mg daily	Same
Metolazone (Zaroxolyn)	2.5-10 mg 30 min before furosemide dose daily-BID	Increased diuretic effect occurs when it is given with furosemide and other loop diuretics.

TABLE 11-10

MEDICATIONS FOR HEART FAILURE—cont'd

Trade Name (Brand Name)	Dosage	Side Effects and Nursing Considerations
Ethacrynic acid (Edecrin)	50-100 mg BID	Same Used when patient has a sulfa allergy.

BETA-BLOCKERS
Indications: used to treat angina, acute myocardial infarction, and heart failure
Mechanism of action: block beta-adrenergic receptors, with resulting decreased sympathetic nervous system responses such as decreases in heart rate, blood pressure, and cardiac contractility in heart failure may improve systolic function over time

Trade Name (Brand Name)	Dosage	Side Effects and Nursing Considerations
Metoprolol (Lopressor, Toprol XL)	50-100 mg BID PO, 5 mg IV Toprol XL 25-200 mg daily PO	Bradycardia, hypotension, atrioventricular blocks, asthma attacks, fatigue, impotence, may mask hypoglycemic episodes Patient should be taught to take pulse and blood pressure on regular basis. Patient should not abruptly stop taking these drugs. Close glucose monitoring if the patient is diabetic. In heart failure, patients should be started on the lowest dose and slowly titrated to the max dose over 4-6 wk as tolerated.
Carvedilol (Coreg)	3.125-25 mg BID PO	Same This is better tolerated on a full stomach.
Bisoprolol (Concor)	2.5-20 mg daily	Same

ALDOSTERONE RECEPTOR ANTAGONIST
Indication: management of edema associated with excessive aldosterone secretion
Mechanism of action: competes with aldosterone for receptor sites in distal renal tubules, increasing sodium chloride and water excretion while conserving potassium and hydrogen ions; may block the effect of aldosterone on arterial smooth muscle

Trade Name (Brand Name)	Dosage	Side Effects and Nursing Considerations
Spironolactone (Aldactone)	25-50 mg PO daily	Monitor serum potassium and renal function. This is potassium sparing.
Eplerenone (Inspra)	50 mg PO daily, may be increased to 50 mg BID if inadequate response after 4 weeks	Monitor blood pressure closely, especially at 2 weeks. Monitor potassium and sodium levels.

INOTROPES
Indication: treatment of cardiac decompensation from heart failure, shock, or renal failure
Mechanism of action: augment cardiac output by increasing contractility and enhancing tissue perfusion; agents listed use different mechanisms

Trade Name (Brand Name)	Dosage	Side Effects and Nursing Considerations
Digoxin (Lanoxin)	0.125-0.5 mg PO/IV daily	Heart block; asystole; visual disturbances (blurred or yellow vision), confusion/mental disturbances, nausea, vomiting, diarrhea Monitor serum concentrations, digoxin possesses a narrow therapeutic range. Digoxin toxicity can be life-threatening. Maintain adequate serum potassium levels, hypokalemia increases risk of digoxin toxicity. Monitor heart rate and notify presciber if heart rate is <50/min.

Continued

TABLE 11-10

MEDICATIONS FOR HEART FAILURE—cont'd

Dopamine (Intropin)	1-5 mcg/kg/min up to 50 mcg/kg/min IV infusion titrated to desired response Always administer via infusion device; administer into large vein	Frequent ventricular ectopy, tachycardia, anginal pain, vasoconstriction, headache, nausea, or vomiting. Extravasation into surrounding tissue can cause tissue necrosis and sloughing. Monitor heart rate/rhythm and blood pressure closely. Dopamine is most frequently used for treatment of hypotension because of its peripheral vasoconstrictor action. It is often used together with dobutamine to minimize hypotension. Thus, pressure is maintained by increased cardiac output (from dobutamine) and vasoconstriction (by dopamine). Monitor the IV site frequently.
Dobutamine (Dobutrex)	2.5-20 mcg/kg/min continuous IV infusion titrated to desired response Always administer via infusion device; administer into large vein	Increased heart rate, ventricular ectopy, hypotension, angina, headache, nausea, and local inflammatory changes It has been used in outpatient settings (continuous at home or intermittent infusions in office) in patients with end-stage heart failure to stabilize symptoms, but it does increase mortality. Monitor heart rate/rhythm and blood pressure closely.
Milrinone (Primacor)	Loading dose of 50 mcg/kg administered over 10 min, followed by continuous infusion 0.375-0.75 mcg/kg/min Always administer via infusion device; administer into large vein	Same as dobutamine
Inamrinone (Inocor)	Initially, 0.75 mg/kg IV bolus over 2 to 3 minutes. Then begin maintenance infusion of 5 to 10 mcg/kg/min May give additional bolus of 0.75 mcg/kg/min 30 minutes after starting therapy. Do not exceed total daily dose of 10 mg/kg.	Same as dobutamine Because of confusion with amiodarone, the generic name amrinone was changed to inamrinone. Do not administer furosemide and inamrinone through the same IV line because precipitation occurs.

BRAIN NATRIURETIC PEPTIDE

Indication: decompensated congestive heart failure

Mechanism of action: exogenous form of hormone produced by myocardial myocytes as a result of myocardial stress and stretching; vasodilates both veins and arteries and has a positive neurohormonal effect by decreasing aldosterone and positive renal effects by increasing diuresis and natriuresis

Trade Name (Brand Name)	Dosage	Side Effects and Nursing Considerations
Nesiritide (Natrecor)	Continuous infusion: 0.01 mcg/kg/min after bolus of 2 mcg/kg	Hypotension, enhanced diuresis, electrolyte imbalances (hypokalemia) Patients will usually respond quickly to therapy. Infusions generally run for 24 hr but can continue for days in the severely decompensated patient.

NITRATES

Indications: to reduce afterload, elevated systemic vascular resistance

Mechanism of action: directly relax smooth muscle, which causes vasodilation of the peripheral vascular bed; decrease myocardial oxygen demands

Trade Name (Brand Name)	Dosage	Side Effects and Nursing Considerations
Nitroglycerin (Tridil)	IV: continuous infusion started at 5 mcg/min and titrated up to a maximum of 200 mcg/min.	Headache, dizziness, flushing, and orthostatic hypotension. Monitor blood pressure closely. Titrate to effect.

TABLE 11-1O
MEDICATIONS FOR HEART FAILURE—cont'd

ANGIOTENSION RECEPTOR BLOCKERS

Indications: hypertension, heart failure, used in patients that cannot tolerate use of angiotensin-converting enzyme inhibitors

Mechanism of action: selective and competitive angiotensin II receptor antagonists; block the vasoconstrictor and aldosterone secreting effects of angiotensin II

Trade Name (Brand Name)	Dosage	Side Effects and Nursing Considerations
Losartan (Cozaar)	25-100 mg daily	Hypotension, diarrhea, dyspepsia, upper respiratory infection Avoid use of NSAIDs, such as indomethacin or naproxen, which may cause renal impairment. Same as angiotensin-converting enzyme inhibitors.
Valsartan (Diovan)	80 mg PO daily-BID up to 320 mg total daily dose	Same
Candesartan (Atacand)	4-32 mg PO daily	Same

BID, Twice daily; *NSAIDs,* nonsteroidal antiinflammatory drugs; *TID,* three times per day.
From Skidmore-Roth, L. (2003). *Mosby's drug guide for nurses.* 3rd ed. St. Louis: Mosby.

2. Reduction of cardiac workload and oxygen consumption
   a. The intraaortic balloon pump in severe acute decompensated HF and cardiogenic shock is used to maintain systemic perfusion and to preserve end-organ function. It is no longer used as a bridge to heart transplantation. Long-term use is impractical because of immobility and the risk of infection. It is used to stabilize patients with marked hemodynamic instability to allow time for insertion of a ventricular assist device (Braunwald et al., 2001).
   b. Ventricular assist devices are capable of partial to complete circulatory support. They assist the failing heart and maintain adequate circulatory pressure. They attach to the patient's own heart and leave the patient's heart intact, with potential for removal. At present, this device is approved as a "bridge" to transplantation. Investigations are under way looking at permanent implantation of these devices (destination therapy).
   c. Biventricular pacing. Approximately 30% of patients with chronic HF have intraventricular conduction delays (Abraham, 2000), such as left bundle branch block. This results in an asynchronus contraction and places the failing heart at a significant mechanical disadvantage. Biventricular pacing involves placing a ventricular lead in the right ventricle and another lead down the coronary sinus to the left ventricle. Both ventricles are stimulated simultaneously, resulting in a synchronized contraction that improves cardiac performance, decreases wall stress, and reduces mitral regurgitation. Patients are showing improved exercise and activity tolerance and improved quality of life scores. Further studies are currently being done to determine long-term clinical effect.
   d. Nursing measures that can reduce cardiac workload and oxygen consumption are to schedule rest periods and to encourage patients to modify activities of daily living: take a break inbetween activities and to sit instead of stand to brush their teeth, shave, and comb their hair. Activity is advanced as tolerated. Many patients with HF derive tremendous benefit from formal cardiac rehabilitation to improve activity tolerance and endurance.
3. Optimization of gas exchange through supplemental oxygen and diuresis
   a. Evaluate the airway, the degree of respiratory distress, and the need for supplemental oxygenation by pulse oximetry and/or arterial blood gas measurement. Patients are more comfortable in semi-Fowler's position.
   b. Diurese aggressively. Administer IV diuretics; furosemide and bumetanide are the preferred diuretics. Ethacrynic acid is useful if the patient has a serious sulfa allergy. These agents are characterized by quick onset; diuresis can be expected 10 to 15 minutes after administration. The goal is to achieve euvolemia, which may take days. When the patient is euvolemic, oral

medications can be reinstated because they are better absorbed and the patient will be less likely to be readmitted to the acute care setting.

c. Control of sodium and fluid retention involves fluid restriction of 2 L per day and sodium restriction of 2 g per day. Daily weights are a priority in these patients. Nurses can make a tremendous impact by teaching and enforcing these concepts throughout the hospital stay. Patients may find it easier to continue these habits at discharge if their importance is stressed throughout hospitalization.

Cardiac transplantation is a therapeutic option of last resort for patients with end-stage HF. Patients who suffer severe cardiac disability refractory to expert management and who have a poor prognosis for 6-month survival are optimal candidates. For many patients with symptomatic HF and ominous objective findings (ejection fraction less than 20%, stroke volume less than 40 mL, severe ventricular arrhythmias), timing of the surgery can be somewhat difficult. A further consideration may be the quality of life, which is a judgment made by patients and the physicians caring for them. This also comes into play in patients with intractable angina and coronary vessels that cannot be bypassed (Braunwald et al., 2001).

Once the crisis stage has passed and the patient is stabilized, the precipitating factor or factors for the complications must be addressed and treated. Treatment consists of surgical or catheter-based intervention as addressed for a patient with an MI, such as CABG, PTCA or stent, and pharmacological therapy (ACE inhibitors, beta-blocker); valve replacement or repair for valvular heart disease; restoration of sinus rhythm if atrial fibrillation or flutter and tachyarrhythmias are present; and management of risk factors such as hypertension, hyperlipidemia, diabetes, and obesity (Hunt et al., 2001; AHA, 2002). Compliance with medications and sodium restriction must also be addressed.

COMPLICATIONS

Complications of HF can be devastating. Interventions must be provided to avoid extending the existing conditions or allowing the development of new, life-threatening complications. Two specific complications for which the patients are monitored are pulmonary edema and cardiogenic shock.

Pulmonary Edema

The failing heart is sensitive to increases in afterload. In some patients with HF, when systolic blood pressure is higher than the 150 mm Hg systolic range, pulmonary edema will ensue. The pulmonary vascular system becomes full and engorged. The results are increasing volume and pressure of blood in pulmonary vessels, increasing pressure in pulmonary capillaries, and leaking of fluid into the interstitial spaces of lung tissue.

Pulmonary edema greatly reduces the amount of lung tissue space available for gas exchange and results in clinical symptoms of extreme dyspnea, cyanosis, severe anxiety, diaphoresis, pallor, and blood-tinged, frothy sputum (AHA, 2002). Arterial blood gas results indicate severe respiratory acidosis and hypoxemia.

Although diuretic therapy is important, it is critical to lower the blood pressure and cardiac filling pressures. IV NTG is administered and titrated until blood pressure is controlled, resulting in a reduction in both preload and afterload. Administering IV diuretics and placing the patient in a high Fowler's position with legs dependent reduce pressures by decreasing venous return. Gas exchange is improved through the administration of 100% oxygen and aminophylline. IV morphine may be helpful to vasodilate and decrease respiratory distress and circulating catecholamine levels (Peacock, Freda, Emerman, & Volturo, 2002).

Cardiogenic Shock

Cardiogenic shock is the most acute and ominous form of pump failure. Cardiogenic shock can be seen after a severe MI, with dysrhythmias, decompensated HF, pulmonary embolus, cardiac tamponade, and ruptured abdominal aortic aneurysm. Often, the outcome of cardiogenic shock is death. Cardiogenic shock and its treatment are discussed in depth in Chapter 10.

OUTCOMES

Outcomes for the patient with HF include the following:

- Mixed venous oxygen saturation within normal limits
- Adequate stroke index, cardiac index, cardiac output
- Adequate respiratory function; absence of paroxysmal nocturnal dyspnea or orthopnea and respiratory distress
- Resolution of fluid balance; euvolemia
- Increased level of activity without symptoms
- Absence of dysrhythmias
- Knowledge and adherence to therapeutic regimen

Pericardial Disease

PERICARDITIS

Pericarditis is acute or chronic inflammation of the pericardium. It may occur as a consequence of AMI or secondary to other diseases such as renal failure (uremic pericarditis), infection, and cancer.

The pericardium has an inner and outer layer with a small amount of lubricating fluid between the layers. When the pericardium becomes inflamed, the amount of fluid between the two layers increases (pericardial effusion). This squeezes the heart and restricts its action and may result in cardiac tamponade. Chronic inflammation can result in constrictive pericarditis, which leads to scarring. The epicardium may thicken and calcify.

The patient usually presents with precordial pain; this pain frequently radiates to the shoulder, neck, back, and arm and is intensified during deep inspiration, movement, coughing, and even swallowing. Other signs and symptoms may include pericardial friction rub, dyspnea, weakness, fatigue, persistent temperature elevation, increase in white blood cell count and sedimentation rate, and increased anxiety level (AHA, 2002). Pulsus paradoxus may be noted while auscultating the blood pressure. Precordial pain must be distinguished from the pain of an AMI.

Detection of a pericardial friction rub is the most common method of diagnosing pericarditis. The friction rub is usually heard best on inspiration with the diaphragm of the stethoscope placed over the second, third, or fourth intercostal space at the sternal border. Friction rubs have been described as grating, scraping, squeaking, or scratching sounds. This rubbing sound results from an increase in fibrous exudate between the two irritated pericardial layers. Other findings of pericarditis include persistent ST-elevation on a 12-lead ECG after AMI. An echocardiogram is also useful in diagnosis to visualize the effusion.

The treatment of patients with pericarditis involves relief of pain (analgesic agents or antiinflammatory agents, such as indomethacin and ibuprofen), antibiotics if the causative agent is bacterial, and treatment of other systemic symptoms (AHA, 2002). If excess fluid is seriously affecting the heart's action, a needle can be inserted into the pericardial space to remove the fluid (pericardiocentesis). In extreme cases, surgery may be required to remove part of the pericardium (pericardial window).

Endocarditis

Infective endocarditis is an infection of microorganisms circulating in the bloodstream that attach onto an endocardial surface. It is caused by various microbes and frequently involves the heart valves. Bacteria of the genus *Streptococcus* are the organisms most commonly responsible for subacute infective endocarditis. Endocarditis can also be caused by staphylococci, gram-negative bacilli (e.g., *Escherichia coli* and *Klebsiella* species), and fungi (e.g., *Candida* and *Histoplasma* species).

Endocarditis rarely occurs in people with normal hearts. Certain preexisting heart conditions increase the risk of developing endocarditis: implantation of an artificial (prosthetic) heart valve and a history of previous endocarditis or damaged or abnormal heart valves by conditions such as rheumatic fever or congenital heart or valve defects.

Infectious lesions or vegetations form on the heart valves. These lesions have irregular edges and have been known to have a cauliflower-like appearance. The mitral valve is the most common area to be affected, followed by the aortic valve. The vegetative process can grow to involve the chordae tendineae, papillary muscles, and conduction system. Therefore, the patient may experience dysrhythmias or acute HF.

Clinical manifestations of endocarditis include fever, chills, night sweats, cough, weight loss, general malaise, weakness, fatigue, headache, musculoskeletal complaints, new murmur, right or left-sided HF, positive blood cultures, and anemia. The presenting symptoms are determined by the valve involved, the organism present, and the length of time and extent of growth of the vegetative process. Treatment involves diagnosing the infective agent, treating with the appropriate antibiotics or antifungal agents, and performing valve replacement surgery in the most serious cases (AHA, 2002).

Vascular Alterations

The aorta is the largest blood vessel in the body both in length and diameter. Shaped like a walking cane, the aorta is an artery that carries blood from the heart. Its many branches then feed all other areas of the body. The aorta is divided into the thoracic and abdominal aorta (Figure 11-13).

The thoracic aorta is divided into the ascending aorta, the aortic arch, and the descending aorta. The thoracic aorta begins at the left ventricle just beyond the aortic valve of the heart. The round segment, or cane handle is the ascending aorta and the aortic arch. Branches of the ascending aorta include the right and left coronary arteries, which feed the myocardium. The arch vessels include the innominate artery, which branches into the right subclavian artery and right common carotid artery, and the left common carotid and subclavian arteries. These branches send blood to the head and the upper extremities.

The descending thoracic aorta, the long segment of the cane, is to the left of the midline of the chest. Branches of the descending aorta are the intercostal arteries. These arteries are the major blood supply to the distal spinal cord, feeding the artery of Adamkiewicz, and they arise anywhere along the spinal cord from T8 to L2.

RESEARCH ANALYSIS

ARTICLE REFERENCE

Booker, K. J., Hom, K., Drew, B. J., et al. (2003). Frequency and outcomes of transient myocardial ischemia in critically ill adults admitted for noncardiac conditions. *American Journal of Critical Care, 12*(6), 508-517.

STUDY PURPOSE, METHODS, AND FINDINGS

The purpose of this study was to detect myocardial ischemia and injury in patients admitted for non-cardiac conditions and to examine the relationship of myocardial ischemia, injury, and acuity to cardiac events. Transient myocardial ischemia, acuity, elevations in serum troponin I, and in-hospital cardiac events were examined in 76 consecutive patients. Transient myocardial ischemia, determined by using continuous electrocardiography, was defined as a 1-mm (0.1-mV) change in ST level from baseline to event in one or more leads lasting 1 minute or more. Scores on Acute Physiology and Chronic Health Evaluation II determined acuity.

Thirty-seven ischemic events were detected in 8 patients (total n = 76 with complete electrocardiographic data): 32 were ST-segment depressions, and 35 were silent. Twelve patients had elevated levels of troponin I. Transient myocardial ischemia, elevated troponin I levels, and advanced age were significant predictors of cardiac complications. Acuity correlated only modestly with increased length of stay in the intensive care unit and with elevated troponin I levels. Patients with transient myocardial ischemia had significantly higher rates of elevations in troponin I and cardiac events than did patients without this finding.

STRENGTHS AND LIMITATIONS

One of the weaknesses of the study was the sample demographics. Most of the study participants, 90%, were white. Moreover, although this is not really a weakness in the study, the application of these findings to the practice setting will involve some expense, if an institution needs to buy technology to support continuous 12-lead monitoring.

One strength of the study was that it was conducted in consecutively admitted patients in two medical-surgical intensive care units. There was a team member on call 24 hours a day for the duration of the study, and standard protocols were used for skin preparation based on national recommendations. In addition, team members had education for correct lead placement.

IMPLICATIONS FOR PRACTICE

Continuous ST-segment monitoring is beneficial for critically ill patients in detecting transient myocardial ischemia that may indicate risk of cardiac events. There is a need for careful electrocardiographic monitoring in multiple leads. ST segment analysis remains important.

In noncardiac surgical patients, lead V_5 is primarily diagnostic of demand-related ischemia. Although lead V_5 is excellent for detecting subendocardial ischemia, ST-segment depression in this lead must be interpreted cautiously because such depression can also represent reciprocal change associated with acute myocardial infarction in nearly every major coronary occlusion. Ischemia was most frequently detected in lead V_5, but if lead V_5 had been the only lead used, only 46% of ischemic events would have been detected.

The abdominal aorta begins at the level of the diaphragm. At the umbilicus, it then forks into the iliac arteries. Abdominal branches include the celiac artery, the superior and inferior mesenteric arteries, and the renal arteries.

AORTIC ANEURYSMS

The words *aneurysm* comes from the Greek *aneurysma*, which means *widening* (Bick, 2000). An aneurysm is a diseased area of an artery causing dilatation and thinning of the wall. Pathology often reveals layered clot and mural thrombi at the aneurysm site (Faust & Cohen, 1998). Atherosclerosis and degeneration of elastin and collagen are the underlying causes in 95% of all cases. Aneurysms are frequently hereditary and are associated with hypertension in 40% of cases. The ratio of aneurysms in men compared to women is 1:1 for thoracic aneurysms and 4:1 for

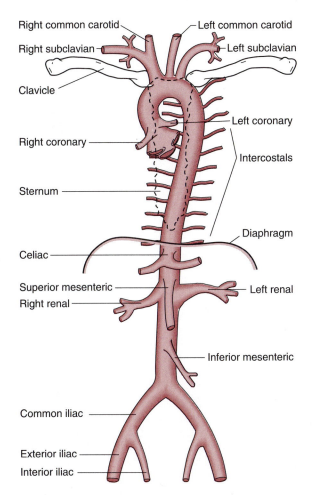

FIGURE 11-13 Anatomy of the aorta and its major branches. (From Fahey, V. A. [1999]. *Vascular nursing* [p. 213]. 3rd ed. Philadelphia, PA: W. B. Saunders.)

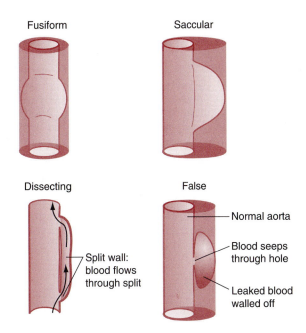

FIGURE 11-14 The fours types of aneurysms. (From Bick, C. [2000]. Abdominal aortic aneurysm repair. *Nursing Standard, 4*(15), 47-52.)

abdominal aneurysms (Cronenwett & Rutherford, 2001). In the critical care arena, abdominal aortic aneurysms are the most common. However, aneurysmal disease is systemic in 20% of patients. Other artery locations for aneurysms include the iliac, femoral, popliteal, intracranial, splenic, subclavian, and hepatic. Anastomotic aneurysms are false aneurysms found at any graft-host artery anastomosis (Faust & Cohen, 1998).

Aneurysms of the aorta are generally divided into thoracic aortic, thoracoabdominal aortic, or abdominal aortic. Most aneurysms are asymptomatic and are found on routine physical examination or when testing for another disease entity. The best intervention is to treat a patient with an aneurysm based on the symptoms of the patient and size of the aneurysm. Size is the usual determining factor for surgical repair: thoracic aortic or thoracoabdominal aortic aneurysms larger than 6 cm and abdominal aortic aneurysms 5 cm or larger. Smaller aneurysms are followed diagnostically for any change in size.

Aortic aneurysms have a usual growth rate of 10% per year. The goal of treatment is avoidance of rupture, which is dramatic and often fatal. Major risk factors for rupture include the coexisting diagnosis of hypertension or chronic obstructive pulmonary disease and larger aneurysm size (Cronenwett & Rutherford, 2001).

An aneurysm may be further classified as a false or true aneurysm (Figure 11-14). A false aneurysm results from a complete tear in the arterial wall. Blood leaks from the artery to form a clot. Connective tissue is then laid down around this cavity. One example of a false aneurysm is an arterial wall tear resulting from an arterial puncture in the groin area. This type of aneurysm is one of the more stable. True aneurysms include saccular, fusiform, and dissecting. A saccular aneurysm is a bulbous pouching of the artery usually found in the thoracic aorta. Fusiform or spindle-shaped aneurysms are generally found in the abdominal aorta and are the most common (Bick, 2000).

AORTIC DISSECTION

Second to ruptured abdominal aneurysms, aortic dissection is the next most common aortic emergency.

Dissection is a tear in the intimal layer of the vessel creating a false lumen causing blood flow diversion into a "false" lumen. Seventy-five percent of patients present with the 3 Ss: sudden, sharp, and shifting pain. Twenty-five percent of patients present with ischemic symptoms (i.e., anuria, stroke, or lower extremity ischemia), depending on which of the branch arteries are blocked by the dissection. Dissection can occur in any age group. Ascending dissections are more common in younger patients, especially those with Marfan's syndrome. Descending dissections are usually seen with advanced atherosclerotic disease and are highly associated with hypertension. These are often misdiagnosed because of the copycat pain of MI or pulmonary embolism (Cronenwett & Rutherford, 2001). Aortic dissection is a surgical emergency.

NURSING ASSESSMENT

Knowledge of anatomy is the key factor in the treatment and care of patients with aortic aneurysms. Presentation of symptoms, intraoperative risk, and postoperative care are often location dependent. Blood flow to aortic branches may be hindered by the aneurysm itself, or embolization of thrombus may cause signs and symptoms such as chest pain, transient ischemic attacks, arm paresthesia with arch location, transient paralysis with descending aorta involvement, or abdominal or flank pain with abdominal aortic aneurysm. In the presence of atherosclerosis, lower extremity and/or buttock pain or loss of peripheral pulses may occur (Fahey, 1999).

DIAGNOSTIC STUDIES

1. Physical examination is examiner dependent. A pulsatile mass may be palpated at the aneurysm site. Palpation reveals decreased or absent peripheral pulses. The patient may have a history of paresthesia, transient ischemic attacks, lower extremity or buttock claudication, and or back or abdominal pain.
2. The sonogram is widely used to diagnose aneurysm because of its availability and cost.
3. Computed tomography scan with contrast is a more accurate diagnostic test in determining the true diameter of the aneurysm.
4. Angiography should not be used as a diagnostic test for sizing an aneurysm because of the inability to detect intramural clots. However, this test is often used to evaluate the associated vascular anatomy further.

TREATMENT

Surgical repair is the treatment for aortic aneurysms. Thoracic aneurysm repair is electively done in tertiary

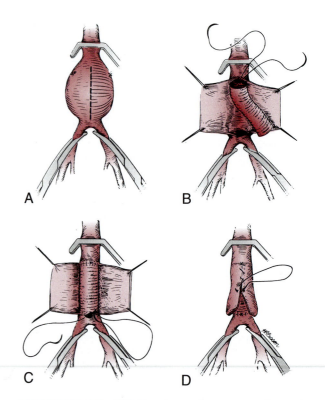

FIGURE 11-15 Classic endoaneurysmal repair of an abdominal aortic aneurysm. The aorta is controlled with vascular clamps **(A),** and opened. The prosthetic graft is sutured from within the aneurysm attaching to the proximal **(B)** and distal **(C)** aorta. **D,** The aneurysm wall is closed over the graft to assist in hemostasis and prevent contact with overlying bowel. (From Yao J. S. T., Flinn W. R., & Bergan J. J. [1984]. Technique for repairing infrarenal abdominal aortic aneurysm. In L. M. Nyhus & R. J. Baker [eds.]: *Master of surgery.* Boston: Little, Brown.)

care centers. Surgery of the ascending aorta and arch requires a mediastinal open surgical approach and cardiopulmonary bypass. Endovascular repair is not an option because of possible occlusion of major arteries leading from the aorta. Surgery of the descending aorta and the abdominal aorta may be done as an open repair or endovascularly. Both method and approach depend on the surgeon's preference and the patient's anatomy.

The open or conventional repair of aortic aneurysm is the endoaneurysmal repair (Figure 11-15). This requires a midline or transverse anterior approach or a retroperitoneal approach. The aorta is exposed and is clamped above and below the aneurysm, and a graft is sutured inside the aneurysm sac (Fahey, 1999).

Endovascular or aortic stent grafting is less invasive. Through a small opening in the exposed femoral artery, an intraluminal sheathed stent is introduced, placed, and deployed with fluoroscopic guidance. Once this is in place, the device excludes the aneurysm sac and significantly decreases the risk of rupture (Kalinowski, 2001). Patients and their families are informed during the preoperative teaching phase that a 10% to 15% chance of an intraoperative event exists and may require open repair of the aneurysm. A comparision of the endoaneurysmal, or open, repair and the endovascular stent graft repair is found in Table 11-11. Care of the vascular surgery patient is detailed in Box 11-12.

TABLE 11-11

Comparision of Open Repair and Endovascular Stent Graft Repair of Aneurysms

	Open Repair	Endovascular Stent Graft Repair
Anatomical criteria	Thoracic, thoracoabdominal, abdominal, iliac of any type	Thoracic where visceral vessels would not be covered; infrarenal AAA dependent on size and length of the neck, calcification of the neck, presence of thrombus in the neck, diameter and tortuosity of the iliac arteries
Pre-op diagnostic studies	CT scan with and without contrast in all (unless emergency); angiography not universally used	3-mm cut CT scan with and without contrast; angiogram with graduated marker needed.
Patient selection	Low to moderate cardiac or pulmonary surgical risk Consider patient preference	Severe cardiac or pulmonary surgical risk Meets anatomical requirements
Preoperative teaching	Surgical procedure; lines and catheters; pain control; pulmonary toilet; early ambulation; length of stay; physical limitations; follow-up visits	Same information; includes follow-up CT scans, possibility of endoleaks and their repair
Anesthesia	General anesthesia intraoperatively Epidural anesthesia postoperatively	Epidural with conscious sedation intraoperatively IV or PO analgesia postoperatively
Ventilation	Intubation and mechanical ventilation	No intubation
Invasive lines and catheters	Central line; A-line; peripheral IV lines; Foley catheter; nasogastric tube	Central line; A-line; peripheral IV lines; Foley catheter
Incision	Extensive	1- to 3-inch groin unilateral or bilateral incisions
Nutrition	Nasogastric tube in place until ileus resolves, then clear liquids to regular diet	May eat after PACU stay
Use of blood products	High incidence	Low incidence
Length of hospital stay and recuperation	5-10 days in hospital; 2-3 days SICU; 3-6 mo at home	1-3 days in hospital; no SICU stay necessary; 1-2 wk at home
Complications	High risk	Low risk
Follow-up	Initial postoperative, then physician discretion	CT scan at 3, 6, and 12 mo and every yr Endoleaks require further repair
Possible sexual dysfunction	25% incidence of retrograde ejaculation or impotence in men	Unlikely unless both hypogastric arteries are covered by the stent

AAA, Abdominal aortic aneurysm; *CT,* computed tomography; *PACU,* postanesthesia care unit; *SICU,* surgical intensive care unit.

BOX 11-12

Nursing Interventions After Aortic Surgery

- Monitor vital signs q1h: pulse; assess for tachycardia and irregular rhythms.
- Blood pressure: keep the patient normotensive; hypertension causes bleeding; give vasodilators per protocol. Hypotension causes organ ischemia; give fluids and vasoconstrictors.
- Monitor hemodynamic pressures: mean arterial pressure, cardiac output, and cardiac index; treat per protocols.
- Assess for hypovolemia: monitor output from chest tubes, drains, and urine output q1h.
- Assess for hypothermia: rewarm the patient gradually.
- Monitor fluid and electrolytes, hemoglobin, hematocrit, renal function, and coagulation studies.
- Monitor the radial, dorsalis pedis, and posterior tibial pulses q1h; use Doppler studies as needed. Assess the ankle-brachial index q2h or as ordered.
- Monitor for complications: intraoperative acute myocardial infarction, dysrhythmias, heart failure, cardiac tamponade, thromboembolism, impaired renal function, pneumonia, pneumothorax, pleural effusion, cerebral ischemia, or stroke.
- Wean from mechanical ventilation; extubate; promote pulmonary hygiene.
- Assess wounds and provide incisional care per protocol.
- Organize nursing care; control environmental stimuli.
- Gradually increase the patient's activity.
- Provide emotional support to the patient and family; assess the family's level of understanding; discuss the postoperative course.

 ## Case Study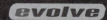

Mr. Smith was admitted to the emergency department (ED) by the emergency medical service with a complaint of sudden onset of substernal chest pain while he was mowing his lawn. The paramedics have placed Mr. Smith on oxygen at 2 L per minute by nasal cannula. They have started an 18-gauge intravenous (IV) line in his left antecubital area with normal saline to be kept open. They have given Mr. Smith aspirin and three sublingual nitroglycerin tablets en route. Mr. Smith states that his pain has gone from a 7, on a 0 to 10 scale, to a 3 now. Jane, the ED nurse, places Mr. Smith on the heart monitor and notes that he is in sinus rhythm with frequent premature ventricular contractions (PVCs). The paramedic states that Mr. Smith was diaphoretic, cool, and clammy on arrival of the emergency medical service at the scene. Mr. Smith is now warm and drier, although he still appears quite pale. Mr. Smith's blood pressure is 154/88 mm Hg, his pulse is 95 beats per minute, and respirations are 24 breaths per minute and nonlabored. While awaiting the arrival of the ED physician to examine Mr. Smith, Jane starts a second IV line, gives Mr. Smith another nitroglycerin tablet,

and then proceeds to obtain a brief history from Mr. Smith.

Mr. Smith is a 63-year-old white man, 220 lb, 6'2", and he has been married for 41 years. He is hypertensive and diabetic, and he continues to smoke 1½ packs of cigarettes per day. He is allergic to penicillin.

While Jane is obtaining the history from Mr. Smith, she looks at the monitor and notices ventricular fibrillation. She begins cardiopulmonary resuscitation. The code team arrives, and Mr. Smith is defibrillated with 200 J. His rhythm is now regular sinus with frequent PVCs. His blood pressure is 92/56 mm Hg, his pulse is thready, and he is diaphoretic. His pupils are 4 mm, equal and reactive. His respiration rate is 16 breaths per minute and shallow, and his oxygen saturation is 92%. He has developed crackles in his lower and middle lung fields bilaterally. He is not fully awake at this time, but he is moving all his extremities. A 150-mg bolus of amiodarone is given over 10 minutes, and a drip is started at 1 mg per minute. Emergency laboratory tests and arterial blood gases (ABGs) are ordered, along with a 12-lead electrocardiogram. A request for an emergency consultation is placed to the cardiologist on call.

Continued

Case Study—cont'd

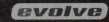

Mr. Smith's cardiac enzymes return: creatine kinase, 456 units/L; creatine kinase–myocardial band, 52% of creatine phosphokinase; and troponin T, 151 mcg/L. Electrolytes are sodium, 143 mEq/L; potassium, 3.4 mEq/L; chloride, 109 mEq/L; carbon dioxide, 34 mEq/L; glucose, 354 mg/dL; and magnesium, 1.5 mEq/L. ABGs are pH, 7.32; $PaCO_2$, 49 mm Hg; PaO_2, 77 mm Hg; and bicarbonate, 24 mEq/L. His hemoglobin is 16.9 g/dL, and his hematocrit is 47.2%. A 12-lead electrocardiogram shows ST elevation in leads V_2, V_3, and V_4. Mr. Smith is diagnosed with an acute anterior myocardial infarction. Mr. Smith's oxygen is increased to 6 L by nasal cannula. Based on these study results, tissue plasminogen activator (t-PA) is administered.

QUESTIONS

1. What do Mr. Smith's cardiac enzyme values indicate about the time and extent of his myocardial infarction?
2. What would you expect his repeat cardiac enzyme values to show at the following times after his heart attack?
   a. 8 hours
   b. 24 hours
   c. 4 days
3. What complications may be anticipated for Mr. Smith related to the infusion of t-PA? What parameters would the nurse need to monitor?
4. What assessments would indicate that the t-PA was effective?

SUMMARY

This chapter focuses on the care of the patient with alterations in cardiovascular status. Geriatric patients are increasingly having medical and surgical interventions. They have even greater needs associated with the aging process (see Geriatric Assessment). The purpose of this chapter is to acquaint the critical care nurse with the problems and pathological conditions most commonly seen in the cardiovascular patient. This chapter is intended to provide a basic understanding of the cardiovascular patient that will facilitate sound clinical judgment in the planning of care that is holistic and incorporates a cooperative, interdisciplinary approach.

Geriatric Assessment

The geriatric cardiac patient needs special considerations when planning and implementing care. Many older patients react differently and with more sensitivity to medications, procedures, and other modes of treatment. Some areas of special consideration include the following:

MEDICATIONS

Great caution must be exercised when administering any medication to a geriatric patient, especially cardiac medications. Elderly persons may have great sensitivity to these medications, they may not require the usual recommended dosage, or they may require more if they have been taking the medication in question for a period of time. Monitor the patient closely for signs of drug effectiveness, adverse reactions, and possible interactions with other medications.

PROCEDURES

The geriatric patient may need more information, support, and attendance during diagnostic or treatment procedures. Having someone always in attendance is a major consideration. It is also necessary to answer any and all questions to the extent needed for understanding and compliance.

SURGERY

Cardiac surgery is a major stress factor for anyone. The geriatric patient needs special attention to answer questions at the appropriate level of understanding and to provide the support for a very stressful, life-threatening procedure. Information and education are important, but be cautious of overwhelming the patient and causing greater stress.

Continued

Geriatric Assessment—cont'd

Postoperative
The geriatric patient has special needs in the postoperative period. The aging patient has a natural physiological process of gradually diminished circulation. Anesthesia and a major surgical procedure add to this problem area and warrant careful monitoring and continuous assessment.

FAMILY
It is imperative to have the involvement of family members or close friends. This can add a stabilizing factor that elderly patients need as they adjust to changes in treatment, activity, diet, medications, and ability to maintain activities of daily living.

REHABILITATION
Rehabilitation is a necessary part of the process for any cardiac patient, whether after a myocardial infarction or after surgery. The geriatric patient needs extra encouragement to adhere to the set regimen to progress to maximum cardiac and vascular function.

CRITICAL THINKING QUESTIONS   *evolve*

1. You are taking care of a 58-year-old post-MI patient brought back to the unit because of recurrent chest pain, shortness of breath, and the need for IV NTG.
   a. Prioritize your actions at this time.
   b. What assessment findings regarding MI would concern you?
   c. What pertinent information from the patient's history would you want to obtain ?
   d. What diagnostic tests do you anticipate?
2. Many patients now come into the hospital the same day that cardiac surgery is performed. Discuss methods for teaching patients effectively given this situation.
3. You are caring for a 63-year-old woman who has just returned to the cardiac care unit after PTCA and stent placement to the right coronary artery. Her proximal right coronary artery had a 90% occlusive lesion. She has her arterial sheath in place to the right femoral artery. She is receiving IV NTG and eptifibatide (Integrilin).
   a. What type of arrhythmia would you anticipate if her right coronary artery were to reocclude?
   b. Prioritize your actions on her arrival.
   c. What type of assessment would you perform regarding the sheath?
4. Mr. Phillips has been hospitalized three times in the past 2 months for chronic HF. What teaching and interventions can you implement to prevent rehospitalization after discharge?

REFERENCES

Abraham, W. T. (2000). Miracle trial. *Journal of Cardiac Failure, 6,* 369-380.

American Heart Association. (2002) Risk factors for coronary artery disease. Retrieved from http://www.amhrt.org/presenter.jhtml. Accessed 6/1/2003.

American Heart Association. (2001a). ACC/AHA guidelines for percutaneous coronary intervention (revision of the 1993 PTCA guidelines). Retrieved from http://www.americanheart.org/. Accessed 7/12/2004.

American Heart Association. (2001b). Heart and stroke facts. Retrieved from http://www.americanheart.org/ Accessed 7/12/2004.

Ajani, A., Waksman, R., Kim, H., et al. (2001). Excimer laser coronary angioplasty and intracoronary radiation for in-stent restenosis: Six-month angiographic and clinical outcomes. *Cardiovascular Radiation Medicine, 2,* 191-196.

Ajani, A., Waksman, R., Sharma, A., et al. (2001). Three-year follow-up after intracoronary gamma radiation therapy for in-stent restenosis: Original WRIST. *Cardiovascular Radiation Medicine, 2,* 200-204.

Beghi, C., Nicolini, F., Budillon, A., et al. (2002). Midterm clinical results in myocardial revascularization using the radial artery. *Chest, 122,* 2075-2079.

Bick, C. (2000). Abdominal aortic aneurysm repair. *Nursing Standard, 4*(15), 47-52.

Braunwald, E., Zipes, D., & Libby, P. (2001). *Heart disease: A textbook of cardiovascular medicine.* 6th ed. Philadelphia: W. B. Saunders.

Buja, L. M., & McAllister, H. A. (2000). Anatomic abnormalities and pathogenesis. In J. T. Willerson & J. N. Cohn (eds.). *Cardiovascular medicine* [p. 503-520]. New York: Churchill Livingstone.

Chernecky, C. C., & Berger, B. J. (2004). *Laboratory tests and diagnostic procedures.* 4th ed. Philadelphia: W. B. Saunders.

Colucci, W. S., Elkayam, U., Horton, D. P., et al. (2000). Intravenous nesiritide, a natriuretic peptide, in the treatment of decompensated congestive heart failure. *New England Journal of Medicine, 343,* 246-253.

Cronenwett, J. L., & Rutherford, R. B. (2001). *Decision making in vascular surgery.* Philadelphia, PA: W. B. Saunders.

Daoud, E., Timmermans, C., Fellows, C., et al. (2000). Initial clinical experience with ambulatory use of an implantable atrial defibrillator for conversion of atrial fibrillation. *Circulation, 102*(12), 1407-1413.

Eagle, K., Guyton, R., Davidoff, R., et al. (1999). ACC/AHA guidelines for coronary artery bypass graft surgery: Executive summary and recommendations. *Circulation, 100,* 1464-1480.

Fahey, V. A. (1999). *Vascular nursing.* 3rd ed. Philadelphia: W. B. Saunders.

Faust, G. R., & Cohen, J. R. (1998). *Vascular surgery for the house officer.* 3rd ed. Baltimore, MD: Williams & Wilkins.

Filsoufi, F., Aklog, L., & Adams, D. (2001). Minimally invasive CABG. *Current Opinion in Cardiology, 16,* 306-309.

Gregoratos, G., Abrams, J., Epstein, A., et al. (2002). ACC/AHA/NASPE 2002 guideline update for implantation of cardiac pacemakers and antiarrhythmia devices. Summary article: A report of the American College of Cardiology/American Heart Association Task Force on Practice Guidelines (ACC/AHA/NASPE Committee to Update the 1998 Pacemaker Guidelines). *Circulation, 106,* 2145-2161.

Guidant. (2002). *Patient guidelines before, during and after ICD implantation.* St. Paul, MN: Guidant.

Gylys, K., & Gold, M. (2000). Acute coronary syndromes: New developments in pharmacological treatment strategies. *Critical Care Nurse, 20*(Suppl), 3-14.

Hirata, Y., Matsumoto, A., Aoyagi, T., et al. (2001). Measurement of plasma brain natriuretic peptide level as a guide for cardiac overload. *Cardiovascular Research, 51,* 585-591.

Hunt, S., Baker, D., Chin, M., et al. (2001). ACC/AHA guidelines for the evaluation and management of chronic heart failure in the adult; executive summary; a report of the American College of Cardiology/American Heart Association Task Force on Practice Guidelines (Committee to Revise the 1995 Guidelines for the Evaluation and Management of Heart Failure). *Circulation, 104,* 2996-3007.

Kalinowski, H. (2001). Aortic stent grafting: A new approach to a deadly diagnosis. One hospital's findings in defining new care processes. *Lippincott's Case Management 6*(2), 79-87.

Killip, T. (2000). Treatment of myocardial infarction. In A. Grevnik, S. M. Ayres, P. R. Holbrook, & W. C. Shoemaker. *Textbook of critical care.* 4th ed. Philadelphia: W. B. Saunders.

Massel, D., & Cruickshank, M. (2002). Enoxaparin in acute coronary syndromes: Evidence for superiority over placebo or untreated control. *American Heart Journal, 143*(5), 758-752.

McCance, K. L., & Huether, S. E. (eds.) (2002). *Pathophysiology: The biologic basis for disease in adults and children.* 4th ed. St. Louis: Mosby.

McHale, D., & Carlson, K. (2001). *AACN procedure manual for critical care.* 4th ed. St. Louis: Mosby.

Morrison, L., Harrison, A., Krishnaswamy, P., et al. (2002). Utility of a rapid B-natriuretic peptide assay in differentiating congestive heart failure from lung disease in patients presenting with dyspnea. *Journal of the American College of Cardiology, 39,* 202-209.

Murray, D., & Dugan, J. (2000). Overview of recent clinical trials in heart failure: What is the current standard of care? *Cardiology in Review, 8,* 340-347.

NASPE: North American Society for Pacing and Electrophysiology (Heart Rhythm Society). (2003). http:// www.naspe.org. Retrieved June 1, 2003.

Nathan, M., & Aranki, S. (2001). Transmyocardial laser revascularization. *Current Opinion in Cardiology, 16,* 310-314.

National Institutes of Health (NIH): National Heart, Lung, and Blood Institute (NHLBI). (2001). *Third report of the National Cholesterol Education Project.* Retrieved from http://www.nhlbi.nih.gov/guidelines/cholesterol/atp3xsum.pdf. Accessed 6/1/2003.

National Institutes of Health (NIH): National Heart, Lung, and Blood Institute. (NHLBI). (2004). *Third report of the National Cholesterol Education Project: Detection, evaluation, and treatment of high blood cholesterol in adults (Adult Treatment Panel III). Executive summary.* Retrieved from http://www.nhlbi.nih.gov/guidelines/cholesterol/index.htm. Accessed 7/13/2004.

Peacock, W., Freda, B., Emerman, C., & Volturo, G. (2002). The clinical challenge of heart failure: Comprehensive, evidence-based management of the hospitalized patient with acute myocardial decompensation. *Clinical Cardiology Consensus Reports,* May 15, 2002.

Regar, E., Serruys, P., Bode, C., et al. (2002). Angiographic findings of the multicenter randomized study with the sirolimus-eluting Bx Velocity balloon-expandable stent (RAVEL trial). *Circulation, 106*(15), 1949-1960.

Seidel, H. M., Ball, J. W., Dains, J. E, & Benedict, G. W. (1999). *Mosby's guide to physical examination.* 4th ed. St. Louis: Mosby.

Skidmore-Roth, L. (2003). *Mosby's drug guide for nurses.* 3rd ed. St. Louis: Mosby.

Society of Critical Care Medicine (SCCM). (2001). *Fundamental critical care support.* 3rd ed. Anaheim, CA: Authors.

Ulrich, S., Canale, S. (2001). *Nursing care planning guides for adults in acute, extended, and home care settings.* 5th ed. Philadelphia: W. B. Saunders.

Ventura, H. O., Pranulis, M. F., Young, C., & Smart, F. W. (2000). Impedance cardiography: A bridge between research and clinical practice in the treatment of heart failure. *Congestive Heart Failure, 6*(2): 94-102.

RECOMMENDED READINGS

Albert, N. M. (2003). Cardiac resynchronization therapy through biventricular pacing in patients with heart failure and ventricular dyssynchrony. *Critical Care Nurse, 23*(3), S2-S16.

Booker, K. J., Hom, K., Drew, B. J., et al. (2003). Frequency and outcomes of transient myocardial ischemia in critically ill adults admitted for noncardiac conditions. *American Journal of Critical Care, 12*(6), 508-516.

Braunwald, E., Antman, E., Beasley, J., et al. (2002). ACC/AHA 2002 guidelines for the management of patients with ustable angina and non-ST-segment elevation myocardial infarction. *Journal of the American College of Cardiology, 40,* 1366-1374.

DeVon, H. A., & Zerwic, J. J. (2003). The symptoms of unstable angina: Do women and men differ? *Nursing Research, 52*(2), 108-118.

Scios, Inc. (2002). *Natrecor United States prescribing information.* Freemont, CA: Scios, Inc. Retreived from http://www.sciosinc.com. Accessed 6/1/2003.

evolve *Did you remember to check out the bonus material, including free self-assessment exercises, on the Evolve Web site at http://evolve.elsevier.com/Sole/ and on the CD-ROM?*

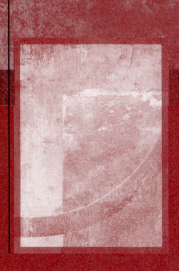

Nervous System Alterations

Janis N. Rice, MSN, RN, CS
Catherine McBride Robichaux, PhD, RN, CCRN, BSN, MSN
Anne D. Leonard, BSN, RN, MPH, FAHA

OBJECTIVES

- Review the anatomy and physiology of the central nervous system.
- Describe the pathophysiology of increased intracranial pressure.
- Describe nursing and medical management of patients with increased intracranial pressure.
- Complete an assessment on a critically ill patient with nervous system injury.
- Describe the pathophysiology of head injury.
- Describe nursing and medical management of patients with a spinal cord injury.
- Discuss the nursing assessment and care of a critically ill patient with cerebrovascular disease.
- Describe the pathophysiology and management for status epilepticus.

Introduction

Neurological illness and trauma to the central nervous system (CNS) are devastating and often life-threatening events. These patients have many unique needs during the acute phase of their illness. Critical care nurses can make a significant difference for both the patient and the family as they adjust to these events.

The brain is important in all aspects of our lives — for consciousness, thinking, problem solving, judgment, memory, language, perceptions, emotions, movements, and autonomic functions. The spinal cord is important because most sensory pathways go through the spinal cord on the way to the brain. Most motor pathways pass through the spinal cord to the rest of the body, and most reflex activity is accomplished at the spinal cord level. When these structures are damaged, a person's activities are greatly altered. In this chapter, the pathophysiology, assessment, and nursing and medical management related to increased intracranial pressure (ICP), head injury, spinal cord injury (SCI), status epilepticus (SE), and cerebrovascular diseases are discussed.

Anatomy and Physiology of the Nervous System

CELLS OF THE NERVOUS SYSTEM

The nervous system is composed of two types of cells, neurons and neuroglia. The *neuron,* or nerve cell, is the basic functioning unit of the nervous system and serves as the transmitter of nerve impulses for information (Figure 12-1). Of the estimated 12 billion neurons in the CNS, three fourths are located in the cerebral

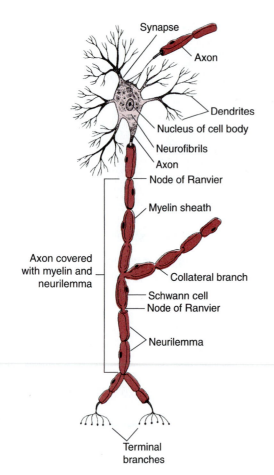

FIGURE 12-1 A neuron, the basic element of the nervous system. (From Black, J. M., & Hawks, J. A. [2005]. *Medical-surgical nursing: Clinical management for positive outcomes 7th ed.* Philadelphia: Saunders.)

Neuroglial cells (glia), which means "nerve glue," constitute the supportive tissue and form the supporting structures for the CNS. These cells are approximately 5 to 10 times as numerous as neurons, and they make up approximately one half of the total brain and spinal cord. Neuroglial cells act to control ion concentrations within the extracellular space and contribute to the transport of nutrients, gases, and waste products among neurons, the vascular system, and cerebrospinal fluid (CSF). Because neuroglial cells are capable of division, most CNS tumors originate from this cell type.

Four types of neuroglial cells exist, each with specific functions. *Microglia* act as phagocytic scavenger cells when nervous tissue is damaged. *Astrocytes,* which mean "star shaped," play a critical role in the basic structure of the blood-brain barrier. They provide nutrients for neurons and respond to brain trauma by forming scar tissue. Astrocytes also contain calcium channels essential for nerve transmission. *Oligodendrocytes* are responsible for myelin formation. *Ependymal* cells produce specialized glial tissue that forms the lining of the ventricles of the brain and the central canal of the spinal cord.

TRANSMISSION OF IMPULSES

The same principles of depolarization and repolarization that occur in the cardiac cycle apply in the conduction of an impulse in a nerve.

Various stimuli can transform the permeability of the cell membrane to certain ions, and this results in changes in the membrane potential. Sodium rapidly enters the cell and potassium exits the cell, thus creating an action potential. This positive ionic change is transmitted along the length of the neuron and is termed a *wave of depolarization;* the impulse is then conducted from one neuron to the next. The cell returns to a resting state in a process termed *repolarization.*

Along the axon at the nodes of Ranvier, the myelin sheath is noninsulated. This noninsulated feature facilitates conduction of impulses along the neuron because the action potential hops from one node to the next. This is called *saltatory conduction,* which causes rapid velocity of conduction and conserves energy. The speed of the impulse depends on both the thickness of the myelin and the distance between nodes.

SYNAPSES

The point of junction between one neuron and another neuron, a muscle cell, or a gland cell, where an impulse is transmitted is called the *synapse.* The three structures necessary for impulse transmission at the synapse are the presynaptic terminals, the

cortex. Each neuron is unique in character, and its features are determined by its specific function.

One of the functions of neurons is receiving input from other neurons via dendrites and axons. Axons normally carry nervous impulses *away* from the cell body of the neuron; dendrites conduct the impulse *toward* the cell body. Axons and dendrites are collectively referred to as nerve fibers. Each neuron possesses one axon, although it may have numerous dendrites. Some axons are surrounded by a white, protein-lipid complex (myelin) that is formed by Schwann cells in the peripheral nervous system (PNS) and by the oligodendrocytes in the CNS. Along the axons are periodic constrictions that are nonmyelinated. These areas are known as nodes of Ranvier, and they produce faster and more efficient impulse conduction (see Figure 12-1).

synaptic cleft, and the postsynaptic membrane (effector cell/neuron).

Presynaptic terminals are either inhibitory or excitatory. The neurotransmitter secretions from these terminals arise from the synaptic vesicles of the axon. Mitochondria within the axon supply the adenosine triphosphate (ATP) to form new transmitter secretions. The microscopic space between the presynaptic terminal and the receptor area of the effector cells is the synaptic cleft. The part of the effector membrane that is closest to the presynaptic terminals is the postsynaptic membrane.

As an action potential spreads through the presynaptic terminal, the membrane depolarizes. Contents from the synaptic vesicles are emptied into the cleft. The neurotransmitter that is released changes the permeability of the postsynaptic membrane, resulting in either excitation or inhibition of the neuron, depending on the type of chemical transmitter released.

NEUROTRANSMITTERS

Neurotransmitters are chemical substances that, when released from the synaptic vesicle, excite, inhibit, or modify the response of another neuron. It is generally believed that each neuron releases the same neurotransmitter at all its separate terminals. Table 12-1 provides a summary of common neurotransmitters and their actions.

TABLE 12-1

Common Neurotransmitters and Their Actions

Neurotransmitter	Action
Acetylcholine	Generally excitation; inhibitory effect on some of parasympathetic nervous system (heart by vagus)
Dopamine	Inhibitory effect
Norepinephrine	Generally excitation; inhibitory effect on postsynaptic neurons
Serotonin	Inhibitory effect
Glutamate	Generally excitation
Gamma-aminobutyric acid (GABA)	Inhibitory effect
Substance P	Excitation
Endorphin	Excitation to systems that inhibit pain

CEREBRAL CIRCULATION

The cerebral circulation must provide sufficient blood to supply oxygen, glucose, and nutrients to the cerebral tissues. The brain receives approximately 750 mL of blood per minute, or 15% to 20% of the total resting cardiac output (Hickey, 2003). The blood supply of the CNS is derived from two major sets of arteries, the vertebral arteries and the internal carotid arteries. The internal carotid arteries provide anterior circulation, whereas the vertebral arteries provide posterior circulation to the brain. These two arterial systems interconnect at the base of the brain to form the cerebral arterial circle (circle of Willis) (Figure 12-2).

The left common carotid artery originates from the aortic arch, and the right common carotid artery originates from the innominate artery. The common carotid arteries then branch to form the external and internal carotid arteries. The external carotid artery supplies the face, scalp, and other extracranial structures. Each internal carotid artery divides within the brain and supplies most of the ipsilateral cerebral hemisphere, basal ganglia, and upper two thirds of the diencephalon. Specifically, each internal carotid artery terminates by dividing into anterior cerebral, middle cerebral, and posterior communicating arteries. The anterior cerebral artery and its branches supply the medial aspects of the motor cortex and the frontal lobes. The middle cerebral artery comprises the principal blood supply of the parietal lobe. Almost 90% of all strokes involve this artery. The posterior communicating artery anastomoses with the posterior cerebral branch of the basilar artery.

The paired vertebral arteries originate from the subclavian artery and enter the skull through the foramen magnum. The vertebral arteries and their branches supply the spinal cord, medulla, and cerebellum before joining at the pons to form the basilar artery. The basilar artery sends branches to the cerebellum, medulla, pons, and internal ear. Then the basilar artery bifurcates and terminates as the posterior cerebral arteries, which serve the medial portions of the occipital and inferior temporal lobes.

Cerebral veins, which do not have a muscle layer or valves, empty blood into venous sinuses located throughout the cranium. The venous blood is emptied into the internal jugular vein and, ultimately, the superior vena cava, which returns the blood to the heart.

BRAIN METABOLISM

The continuous high activity of the brain results in large metabolic energy needs. Glucose is the brain's main source of energy for cellular function. Because the brain is unable to store glucose, it requires a continuous supply of glucose in the blood to maintain

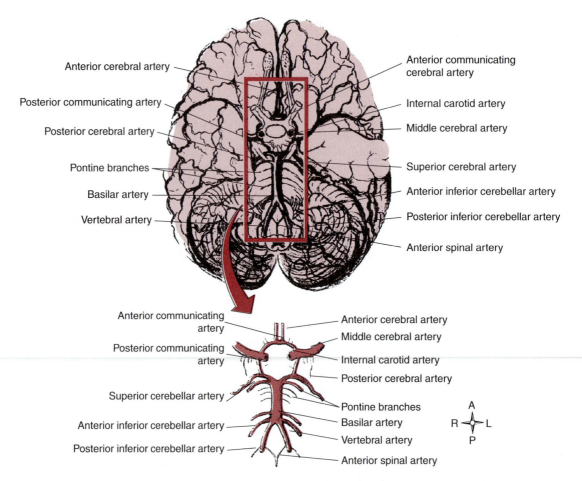

FIGURE 12-2 Arteries at the base of the brain. The arteries that compose the circle of Willis are the two anterior cerebral arteries, joined to each other by the anterior communicating two short segments of the internal carotids, off of which the posterior communicating arteries connect to the posterior cerebral arteries. (From Thibodeau, G. A., & Patton, K. I. [2003]. *Anatomy and physiology.* 5th ed. St. Louis: Mosby.)

normal brain metabolism. If the cerebral glucose level drops to less than 70 mg/100 mL, confusion will develop. Coma develops when the brain glucose level drops to less than 20 mg/100 mL. Cerebral glucose metabolism is divided into aerobic and anaerobic metabolism. Because anaerobic metabolism produces only a minimal amount of ATP, aerobic metabolism is used to meet the high cerebral energy demands. If the brain is deprived of oxygen, metabolism changes from aerobic to less efficient anaerobic cellular metabolism. The brain becomes acidotic as a result of lactic acid production. In addition, certain areas of the brain are more sensitive to lower levels of oxygen than are others (Barker, 2002).

Maintaining a constant cerebral blood flow (CBF) is essential to sustain normal cerebral metabolism.

A process called autoregulation is used by the brain to ensure continuous CBF regardless of the mean arterial pressure (MAP). Autoregulation is defined as the ability of cerebral blood vessels to adjust their diameter to arterial pressure changes within the brain. If a rapid increase in MAP occurs, the cerebral vessels constrict to prevent excessive distention of the cerebral arteries. Conversely, if the MAP drops, the cerebral blood vessels dilate to maintain normal CBF and to prevent cerebral ischemia (Barker, 2002).

CBF is determined by the cerebral perfusion pressure (CPP). CPP is the driving force that underlies CBF, and it is an estimate of the adequacy of cerebral circulation. The normal CPP in an adult is between 70 and 100 mm Hg. CPP is calculated as the difference between the MAP and the ICP or CPP = MAP – ICP.

Any factor that decreases MAP and increases ICP will decrease CPP. Ischemia develops with inadequate CPP and, if not corrected, may lead to tissue infarction. Brain hypoxia may occur with reversible injury to the cells. If an anoxic state lasts for 5 minutes or longer at normal body temperature, cerebral neurons are destroyed and cannot regenerate (Barker, 2002).

Hypercapnia ($PaCO_2$ greater than 45 mm Hg) and, to a lesser extent, hypoxia (PaO_2 less than 50 mm Hg) cause dilation of cerebral arteries and increase the blood circulation into the brain regardless of actual needs. This, in turn, causes an increase in ICP. A healthy brain can accommodate a small increase, but an injured or diseased brain is more vulnerable to the increased blood volume (Hickey, 2003).

Acidosis, an increase in hydrogen ion concentration, increases CBF. Increased CBF is a compensatory mechanism that facilitates the removal of acidic end products from cerebral tissue metabolism.

Certain vitamins are essential for normal CNS functioning. Vitamin B_1 (thiamine) is important in the Krebs cycle. Vitamin B_1 deficiency, common in patients with alcoholism, causes Wernicke-Korsakoff syndrome, which in later stages causes cerebellar degeneration. Deficiency of vitamin B_{12} results in gradual degeneration of the brain, optic nerves, and spinal cord. Pyridoxine participates in many enzymatic reactions in the CNS. Deficiencies can produce polyneuropathies.

BRAIN BARRIER SYSTEM

Two brain barrier systems exist: (1) the blood-brain barrier system, and (2) the blood-CSF barrier. The blood-brain barrier is the more extensive system.

The blood-brain barrier operates on the concept of tight junctions between adjacent cells and subsequent selective permeability that prevents the free movement of materials from the vascular bed into the brain (Minton & Hickey, 1999). The blood-brain barrier protects the brain from toxic elements and disease-causing organisms that may circulate in the blood. Water, carbon dioxide, oxygen, and glucose cross the cerebral capillaries easily. The movement of other substances into the brain is dependent on the chemical dissociation, lipid solubility, particle size, and protein-binding potential.

VENTRICULAR SYSTEM AND CEREBROSPINAL FLUID

The four ventricles of the adult brain are hollow spaces lined by ependyma. They contain specialized epithelium called the choroid plexus, a major source of CSF. CSF is continually secreted from these surfaces

at more than 400 mL per day or 18 to 24 mL per hour (Barker, 2002). The CSF provides a cushioning effect during rapid movements of the head and exerts a considerable buoyant effect on the brain (Benarroch, Westmoreland, Daube, Reagon, & Sandok, 1999). A smaller amount of CSF is secreted from the ependymal cells that line the ventricles, the blood vessels of the meninges, and the blood vessels of the brain. On average, approximately 150 mL of CSF is in the ventricles and subarachnoid space at any given time.

CSF that is produced by the choroid plexus in the lateral ventricles flows into the third ventricle through the foramen of Monro. From the third ventricle, CSF flows through the aqueduct of Sylvius into the fourth ventricle. From there, the foramina of Luschka and Magendie direct the flow of CSF into the cisterna and subarachnoid space (Figure 12-3). After circulating over the entire brain and spinal cord, most of the CSF produced is reabsorbed into the arachnoid villi, which are projections from the arachnoid space into the venous sinuses of the brain.

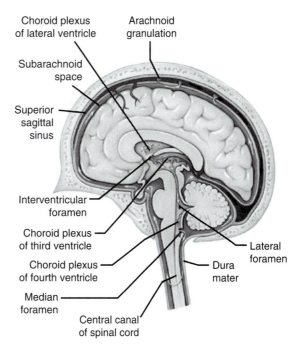

FIGURE 12-3 Cerebrospinal fluid (CSF) circulation. *Arrows* represent the route of CSF. CSF is produced in the ventricles and returns to the venous circulation in the superior sagittal sinus. (From Lewis, S. M., Collier, I. C., & Heitkemper, M. M. [2004]. *Medical-surgical nursing: Assessment and management of clinical problems.* 6th ed. St. Louis: Mosby.)

Functional and Structural Divisions of the Central Nervous System

MENINGES

Meninges cover the brain and spinal cord and consist of three layers: dura mater, arachnoid, and pia mater (Figure 12-4). Dura mater is the outermost covering and has two layers. The outer surface adheres to the skull, and the inner layer produces prominent folds (falx cerebri, tentorium cerebelli, falx cerebelli, diaphragma sellae) that subdivide the interior cranial cavity to support and protect the brain. The inner dura mater also covers the spine. The epidural space is a potential space between the skull and the outer dura mater. The subdural space is between the dura mater and arachnoid and is filled with a small amount of fluid.

The arachnoid, located between the dura and pia mater, is a delicate, avascular layer that loosely encloses the brain. It also encases the spine. The subarachnoid space, a considerable area between the arachnoid and pia, contains circulating CSF.

The pia mater closely adheres to the brain's surface, contains a network of blood vessels, and intervenes into the sulci of the brain. The pia mater surrounding the spinal cord is less vascular (Hickey, 2003).

BRAIN (ENCEPHALON)

The brain is approximately 2% of body weight. The average weight of a man's brain is approximately 1400 g. The brain of a woman weighs less, and the average brain weight of an older person is 1200 g. The brain is typically divided into three major areas: the cerebrum, the brainstem, and the cerebellum (Figure 12-5).

Cerebrum

The cerebrum (Figure 12-6) is composed of the right and left cerebral hemispheres, which are incompletely separated by a deep longitudinal fissure. The cerebral hemispheres are joined by the corpus callosum, a thick area of nerve fibers. This provides a pathway for fibers to travel from one hemisphere to the other and thus makes the two hemispheres intricately connected.

The hemispheres' surface appears wrinkled because of the numerous raised areas, or gyri, referred to as *convolutions.* The gyri fold into one another, causing the convoluted appearance and substantially increasing the surface area of the brain. The surface of the cerebral hemisphere is approximately six cells deep and is called the cerebral cortex, or gray matter. Beneath the cortex is a layer of medullary white

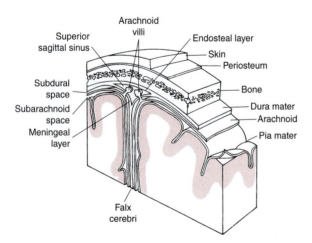

FIGURE 12-4 Coronal section of the skull and brain showing the relationships of the meninges. (From Barker, E. [2002]. *Neuroscience nursing: A spectrum of care.* 2nd ed. St. Louis: Mosby.)

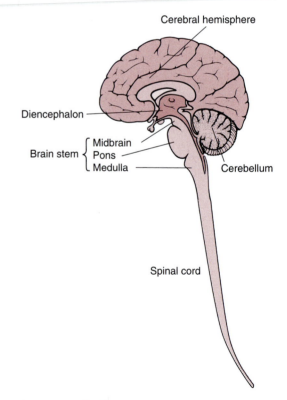

FIGURE 12-5 Major divisions of the central nervous system (CNS). (From Lewis, S. M., Collier, I. C., & Heitkemper, M. M. [2004]. *Medical-surgical nursing: Assessment and management of clinical problems.* 6th ed. St. Louis: Mosby.)

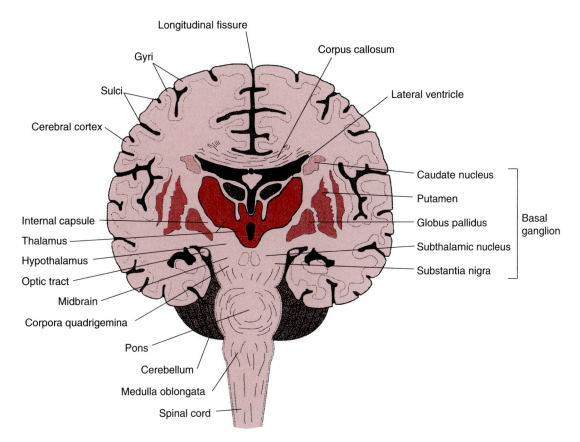

FIGURE 12-6 The structures of the brain (coronal section). (From Black, J. M., & Hawks, J. A. [2005]. *Medical-surgical nursing: Clinical management for positive outcomes of care.* 7th ed. Philadelphia: Saunders.)

matter consisting of mostly myelinated axons, which serve as association and projection pathways.

At birth, both right and left hemispheres have an equal capacity for development. Ninety percent of the population has a highly developed left hemisphere and is right-handed. Most left-handed people also have the left hemisphere as the dominant side of the brain.

A fissure, or sulcus, is a separation in the cerebral hemisphere. The fissures serve as important landmarks. The longitudinal fissure separates the cerebral hemispheres into left and right sections. The lateral fissure, or fissure of Sylvius, divides the frontal and temporal lobes. The fissure of Rolando separates the frontal and the parietal lobes. The parieto-occipital fissure separates the occipital lobe from the parietal and temporal lobes.

The cerebrum is divided into lobes (Figure 12-7). Each lobe has a specific function. The *frontal lobe*, situated anterior to the central sulcus and above the lateral fissure, has as its major functions conscious thought, abstract thinking, judgment, and initiation of motor activity. The prefontal area of this lobe is

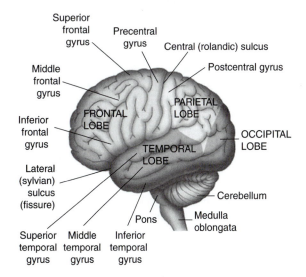

FIGURE 12-7 Cerebral hemispheres. (From McCance, K. L., & Huether, S. E. [2002]. *Pathophysiology: The biologic basis for disease in adults and children.* 4th ed. St. Louis: Mosby.)

believed to be concerned with affective reactions, memory, and concentration.

The *parietal lobes* extend from the central sulcus to the parietooccipital fissure. The primary responsibilities of this lobe are sensory functioning, sensory perception, association, and processing of general sensory modalities at a higher level.

The *temporal lobes* are located in the middle cranial fossa under the lateral fissures of Sylvius. Their major functions are localized in the primary auditory areas, which receive input from the auditory pathway and process auditory information. The auditory association area occupies a portion of the temporal gyrus and is known as Wernicke's area. The *occipital lobes* are wedge shaped and contain the primary visual cortex for visional reception and visional association.

Basal Ganglia

The basal ganglia are masses of gray matter located deep within the cerebral hemisphere. Composed of several sections, these structures influence motor control of fine body movements, particularly of the hands and lower extremities (see Figure 12-6).

Diencephalon

The diencephalon is the uppermost portion of the brainstem and is covered by the cerebrum. It is divided into four regions: thalamus, hypothalamus, subthalamus, and epithalamus. The thalamus and hypothalamus are the major areas of importance.

The *thalamus* is the largest structure within the diencephalon and integrates all bodily sensations except smell. It plays a crucial role in conscious awareness of pain, in focusing of attention, in the reticular activating system, and in the limbic system.

The right and left *hypothalamus* act as the CNS regulatory centers for the autonomic nervous system (ANS). The general functions of the hypothalamus include temperature control, water balance, control of appetite and thirst, cardiovascular regulation, sleep-wakefulness cycle, circadian rhythms, and sexual activity. The hypothalamus also controls the release of hormones from the pituitary gland.

Brainstem

The brainstem is at the central core of the brain and controls vital functions. The major divisions of the brainstem are the midbrain, pons, and medulla (Figure 12-8). The *midbrain*, also known as the mesencephalon, is a short segment of brainstem lying between the diencephalon and the pons. Cranial nerves III (oculomotor) and IV (trochlear) are associated with the midbrain. The midbrain carries impulses down from the cerebrum and controls the wakefulness of the brain via the reticular activating system.

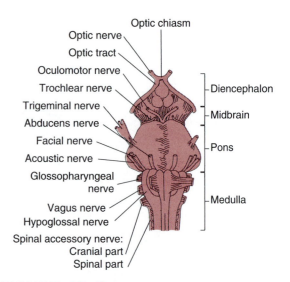

FIGURE 12-8 The brainstem (ventral view) and the cranial nerves that exit from it. (From Black, J. M., & Matassarin-Jacobs, E. [1997]. *Medical-surgical nursing: Clinical management for continuity of care*, 5th ed. Philadelphia: W. B. Saunders.)

It also serves as the center for auditory and visual reflexes.

The *pons* is seated between the midbrain and the medulla. It contains nuclei of cranial nerves V (trigeminal), VI (abducens), VII (facial), and VIII (vestibulocochlear). In conjunction with the medulla, the pons controls the rate and length of respirations.

The *medulla oblongata* is situated between the pons and the spinal cord. Cranial nerves IX (glossopharyngeal), X (vagus), XI (accessory), and XII (hypoglossal) connect to the brain within the medulla. The functions of the medulla include the regulation of the basic rhythm of respiration, rate and strength of pulse, and vasomotor activity. In addition, neurons within the medulla regulate certain reflexes including sneezing, swallowing, coughing, and vomiting.

Cerebellum

The *cerebellum* is located in the posterior fossa of the cranium (see Figures 12-5 and 12-6). It is attached to the pons, medulla, and midbrain by three paired cerebellar peduncles. The peduncles receive input from the spinal cord and brainstem and send it to the cerebellar cortex. The functions of equilibrium, fine movement, muscle tone, and coordination are mediated by the cerebellum.

SPINAL CORD

The spinal cord is a mass of nerve tissue that is located within and protected by the vertebral column and surrounded by the meninges. It is continuous with the medulla oblongata. The spinal cord usually measures 18 inches (46 cm) in the adult. The spinal canal is an extension of the fourth ventricle and contains CSF.

The spinal cord has 31 segments, each of which gives off a pair of spinal nerves. The segments include 8 cervical, 12 thoracic, 5 lumbar, 5 sacral, and 1 coccygeal (Figure 12-9). The spinal nerves carry information from the periphery to the spinal cord, and from the spinal cord to the periphery. These nerves innervate the skin and musculature of the entire body below the neck. Each spinal nerve consists of a dorsal root (posterior) and ventral root (anterior). The dorsal roots convey sensory input into the spinal cord from skin segments that represent specific areas of the body known as dermatomes. The ventral roots carry efferent impulses from the spinal cord to the body. A dermatome chart traces the spinal nerves to their point of muscle innervation and provides anatomical clues about the level of injury or dysfunction (Figure 12-10).

Two enlargements in the spinal cord provide innervation of the extremities. The cervical enlargement, located between C5 and T1, innervates the upper extremities; the lumbar enlargement, located

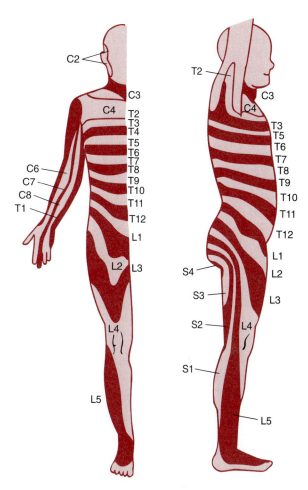

FIGURE 12-10 Cutaneous distribution of spinal nerves (dermatomes). (From Conn, P. M., [1995]. *Neuroscience in Medicine.* 5th ed. Philadelphia: J. B. Lippincott Williams & Wilkins.)

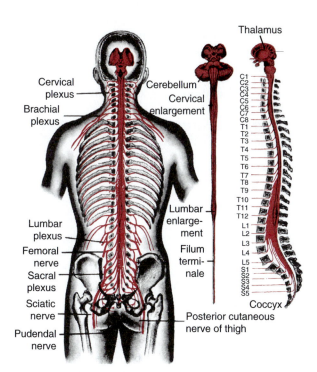

FIGURE 12-9 Spinal cord within vertebral canal and exiting spinal nerves. (From Rudy, E. B., [ed.] [1984]. *Advanced Neurological and Neurosurgical Nursing.* St. Louis: Mosby.)

between L3 and S3, innervates the lower extremities (see Figure 12-10).

Four types of nerve fibers make up the spinal nerves. *Motor fibers*, which originate in the ventral horn of the spinal cord, have efferent fibers that relay motor impulses from the CNS to skeletal muscles. *Sensory fibers*, which begin in the dorsal horn of the spinal cord, have afferent fibers that convey sensory impulses from organs and muscles to the CNS. *Meningeal fibers* relay sensory and vasomotor innervation to the spinal meninges. Autonomic fibers are discussed in the section on the ANS.

PLEXUSES

Plexuses are networks of interlacing nerves. The spinal nerves interconnect in three areas: the cervical, brachial, and lumbosacral plexuses. These plexuses innervate specific areas of the body and form the major peripheral nerves. The cervical plexus includes spinal nerves C1 to C4 and innervates the muscles of the neck and shoulders. The phrenic nerve originates at the base of the neck and supplies the diaphragm. The brachial plexus comprises spinal nerves C4 to C8 and T1 and innervates the arms via the radial and ulnar nerves. The lumbosacral plexus is formed by spinal nerves L1 to L5 and S1 to S3. The femoral nerve arises from the lumbar plexus and the sciatic nerve from the sacral plexus and innervates the legs (see Figure 12-10).

PERIPHERAL NERVOUS SYSTEM

The PNS is the portion of the nervous system that is situated outside the CNS. It is a complex web of nerves. The 12 pairs of cranial nerves and 31 pairs of spinal nerves form the PNS. Additionally, the ANS is considered a specialized part of the PNS. When the PNS nerves are damaged, loss of movement and sensation occurs in the area innervated distal to the lesion.

The 12 pairs of cranial nerves originate in the brain and brainstem and exit from the cranial cavity. Cranial nerves have either sensory or motor functions, with cranial nerves V, VII, IX, and X possessing both functions. These nerves are primarily responsible for the innervation of structures in the head and neck. A summary of the cranial nerves and functions is provided in Table 12-2. The relationship of the cranial nerves with surrounding structures is very important. Changes in cranial nerve assessment findings usually indicate intracranial disease and dysfunction.

AUTONOMIC NERVOUS SYSTEM

The ANS comprises motor nerves to visceral effectors: cardiac muscle, smooth muscle, adrenal medulla, and various glands, including salivary, gastric, and sweat glands. It controls the activities of the viscera at an unconscious level. The ANS consists of the sympathetic nervous system and the parasympathetic nervous system. These parallel systems act to regulate visceral organs in opposing ways. The purpose of the ANS is to maintain the body with a relatively stable internal environment.

One characteristic of the ANS is a two-neuron chain that relays information from the CNS to the periphery. Cell bodies and fibers are classified into preganglionic neurons and postganglionic neurons. *Preganglionic neurons* are the first neurons in the chain and are located in the brainstem or spinal cord. The axons terminate on *postganglionic cell bodies* that are located throughout the body.

The sympathetic nervous system is also known as the thoracolumbar system because the nerve fibers originate in the thoracic and lumbar regions of the spinal cord. This system contains a chain of ganglia located on both sides of the vertebrae. The sympathetic nervous system is sometimes called the fight-or-flight system because it is activated and dominates during stressful periods. Most sympathetic neurons release the chemical neurotransmitter norepinephrine at the visceral effector. Sympathetic impulses cause vasoconstriction in skin and viscera, vasodilation in skeletal muscle, elevation of heart rate and force, elevation of blood pressure, dilation of bronchioles,

TABLE 12-2		
The 12 Cranial Nerves		
Nerve	**Name**	**Major Functions**
I	Olfactory	Smell
II	Optic	Vision
III	Oculomotor	Movements of eyes; pupillary constriction and accommodation
IV	Trochlear	Movement of eyes
V	Trigeminal	Muscles of mastication and eardrum tension; general sensations from anterior half of head, including face, nose, mouth, and meninges
VI	Abducens	Movements of eyes
VII	Facial	Muscles of facial expression and tension on ear bones (stapes); lacrimation and salivation; taste
VIII	Auditory	Hearing and equilibrium reception (vestibulocochlear)
IX	Glossopharyngeal	Swallowing, salivation, taste, visceral sensory
X	Vagus	Swallowing movements and laryngeal control, parasympathetics to thoracic and abdominal viscera
XI	Spinal accessory	Movements of head and shoulders
XII	Hypoglossal	Movements of tongue

increase in sweat gland activity, dilation of pupils, decrease in peristalsis, and contraction of pilomotor muscles (gooseflesh).

The parasympathetic nervous system, the second division of the ANS, is also known as the craniosacral system because the preganglionic fibers originate at certain cranial nerves and in the sacral spinal cord. The axons are long, and ganglia are situated adjacent to or within specific organs. The parasympathetic system is dominant in nonstressful situations. It stimulates visceral activities associated with maintenance of normal functions. The effects of parasympathetic nervous system stimulation induce a return of systems to a normal state of functioning. All neurons within the parasympathetic nervous system release the neurotransmitter acetylcholine at the visceral effector.

GERIATRIC CONSIDERATIONS

Aging affects the nervous system in a variety of ways. An understanding of the changes that occur with aging is important in assessment and management of the elderly person who is critically ill (see Geriatric Assessment).

ASSESSMENT

History, along with an initial and ongoing neurological assessment, provides needed information about the patient's current condition. Ideally, the patient is the primary source of the historical data. If the patient is unable to give the history, family or friends should supply information related to symptoms, onset, progression, and chronology of the event. If headache is a presenting symptom, information must be obtained about the location, onset, type of pain, duration, presence of other symptoms, and what makes the headache better or worse. If the patient is admitted secondary to nervous system trauma, specific information concerning the mechanism of injury, immediate posttrauma care, and emergency treatments are needed.

The *Glasgow Coma Scale (GCS)* is a standardized tool used as a guide in assessing a patient with neurological injuries. It scores two aspects of the patient's level of consciousness: arousal (awareness of the environment) and cognition (demonstrating an understanding of what the observer says through an ability to perform the task). The components of this assessment tool are eye opening, verbal response, and motor response (Figure 12-11). A consistent stimulus is applied, either a verbal command or a painful stimulus. When the patient does not respond to a verbal command, a painful stimulus is applied by either a firm pressure to the patient's nailbed (use a pencil or pen), a trapezium squeeze (using thumb and two fingers, twist 2 inches of the trapezius muscle where the head

Geriatric Assessment

- Loss of myelin and altered conduction may result in a decrease in reaction time of specific nerves.
- Cellular degeneration and death of neurons may result in decreased speed and intensity of reflexes.
- Hardening of the pupil sphincter may result in decreased responsiveness to light.
- Increased rigidity of the iris may result in decreased pupil size.
- Subdural hematomas are more common in the older population because of cerebral atrophy and subsequent increase in size of the subdural space. A large amount of blood can accumulate before the patient demonstrates overt signs and symptoms. Subtle changes in mental status may indicate a substantial intracranial hemorrhage.
- Assessment of admission Glasgow Coma Scale scores may underestimate the extent of brain injury in the older patient.
- The effects of certain medications used to decrease intracranial pressure (osmotic and loop diuretics, barbiturates) should be closely monitored because of the older patient's decreased ability to absorb, metabolize, and/or excrete these drugs.
- Assessment of preexisting renal insufficiency and use of diuretics is necessary because the use of these drugs may place older patients at risk of hypokalemia or hyponatremia when they receive medications to reduce intracranial pressure.
- In the older patient, elevating the head of the bed to decrease intracranial pressure may compromise an already diminished cerebral blood flow. Continuous assessment of cerebral perfusion pressure is necessary to avoid decreasing brain blood flow.
- Central cord syndrome is more common in the older population and may result from hyperextension of an osteoarthritic spine.

Glasgow Coma Scale			
Eyes	Open	Spontaneously	4
		To verbal command	3
		To pain	2
		No Response	1
Best motor response	To verbal command	Obeys	6
	To painful stimulus	Localizes pain	5
		Flexion-withdrawal	4
		Flexion-abnormal (Decorticate rigidity)	3
		Extension (Decerebrate rigidity)	2
		No response	1
Best verbal response		Oriented and converses	5
		Disoriented and converses	4
		Inappropriate words	3
		Incomprehensible sounds	2
		No response	1
Total			3-15

FIGURE 12-11 The Glasgow Coma Scale, which is based on eye opening, verbal responses, and memory responses. Each response is given a number, and the three scores are summed. The lowest score is 3; the highest is 15. (Modified from Becker, D. P., & Gudeman, S. K. [1998]. *Textbook of head injury*. Phildelphia: W. B. Saunders.)

meets the shoulder), supraorbital pressure (place pressure on the notch felt along the bony ridge above the top of the eye), or sternal rub (grind the center of sternum using knuckles of clenched fist). The responsiveness of the patient is expressed as a number according to the listed criteria. A high number (approaching 15) indicates normal functioning, whereas a low number (approaching 3) indicates deep coma. When the score decreases over time, the level of consciousness has deteriorated. Several conditions can affect the accuracy of the GCS, including medications administered and concurrent traumatic injuries such as SCI. It remains, however, a universal, standardized approach that health care practitioners can use to monitor and look for trends in neurological assessment findings (Fischer & Mathieson, 2001). The GCS does not replace neurological assessment of the specific area of the brain.

When performing a neurological assessment, the critical care nurse focuses on mental status, level of consciousness, cranial nerve functioning, motor status, and sensory function.

Mental status. When assessing a patient's mental status, the critical care nurse tests arousal (consciousness), language, and memory.

Consciousness. The level of consciousness is evaluated by observing the patient's response to the environment. The highest level of response is the patient's acknowledgment of the nurse's presence (e.g., appropriate verbal response, gesture of greeting, eye contact). The lowest level is a lack of any response. Any change in the level of consciousness is an *early* sign of neurological deterioration and is one of the most important aspects of mental status assessment. Once consciousness is established, the nurse assesses and specifically documents the patient's orientation to person, place, and time.

Language skills. The second component is language skills. If the patient is not intubated, it is important to assess his or her ability to talk, fluency of speech, word-finding difficulty, and whether the speech is spontaneous. *Expressive dysphasia* is primarily a deficit in language output or speech production and can vary from imperfect articulation to complete loss of both verbal and written communication skills (Boss, 2002). If the patient is intubated, a similar evaluation is possible by assessing his or her writing skills. A patient with only expressive problems can comprehend language and follow commands.

The next step is to assess the patient's ability to follow verbal commands. The patient is asked to perform simple commands such as pointing to the clock, pointing to the window, or raising the right arm. On successful completion of simple commands, the patient may be presented with a complex command such as raising the right arm and folding a piece of paper. The inability to comprehend language and follow commands is called *receptive dysphasia* (Boss, 2002). A patient with only receptive problems who is not intubated can speak spontaneously, but the verbal response does not follow the context of the conversation.

Memory. The third component of mental status to be assessed is memory. Short-term memory is assessed by asking the patient to recall the names of three words or objects (e.g., chair, clock, blue) after a 3-minute interval. This simple test can be used with an intubated patient by having the patient write the words on a piece of paper. Long-term memory is tested by asking questions about the patient's distant past (e.g., birth place, year of birth, year of graduation from school, year of marriage). If intubated, the patient can write the answers.

Cranial nerve functioning. Knowledge of the function of the each of the cranial nerves (see Table 12-2) helps to localize lesions and assists the nurse in identifying patient problems related to the cranial nerve deficit. On the initial baseline neurological assessment, all cranial nerves are assessed.

Cranial nerves I and II. Cranial nerve I is responsible for the ability to smell. Tests for visual acuity and visual fields assess the function of cranial nerve II. Testing all these functions is important initially, but serial assessments can focus on direct light response and visual acuity only.

Cranial nerves III, IV, and VI. The third cranial nerve is responsible for the consensual light response, elevation of the eyelids, and eye movement. Cranial nerves III, IV, and VI affect extraocular movements of the eye. When assessing extraocular movements, the nurse assesses gaze and notes the presence of nystagmus.

In an unconscious patient, eye movements are an indication of brainstem activity and are tested by the oculocephalic response (doll's eyes maneuver). When the doll's eyes maneuver is intact, the eyes move in the opposite direction when the head is turned. Abnormal responses include movement of the eyes in the same direction as the head, or the eyes staying midline when the head is turned. An abnormal response indicates a disruption in the processing of information through the brainstem. Contraindications to performing oculocephalic testing include cervical injuries and increased ICP. This examination is performed by the physician.

An alternative test, performed only by physicians, is the oculovestibular response (ice water calorics). This test is believed to be more reliable than the oculocephalic response. To test for the oculovestibular response, the head of the patient's bed is elevated 30 degrees, and 30 to 50 mL of ice water is quickly instilled into the patient's ear. The normal response, for the eyes to move in the direction of the ice water. Any other response is considered abnormal and indicates severe brainstem injury.

Examination of the pupils includes checking for size, shape, equality, and light reflex. Normal pupil size, ranges from 1.5 to 6 mm in diameter. Exact measurement using a millimeter scale is the most reliable method of determining size and equality. Unequal pupils (anisocoria) normally occurs in approximately 10% of the general population. Otherwise, inequality of pupils (greater than 1 mm) is a sign of a pathological process.

The light reflexes are tested with a bright penlight in dim surrounding light. The direct light reflex is elicited by approaching the eye from the side with a penlight. The pupil should constrict briskly. The consensual light reflex occurs when the contralateral pupil constricts. Reaction rates are generally described as brisk, sluggish, or nonreactive. A change in pupil reaction is an important sign. These subtle changes may be an indication of increasing ICP and indicate a deterioration in neurological status.

Differences between pupils are also important. For example, pressure on the pathway of the oculomotor nerve may cause the ipsilateral pupil (same side as pressure) to be dilated and sluggish or even nonreactive to light, whereas the contralateral pupil (opposite side of pressure) remains normal in size and reactivity.

Cranial nerves V, VII, IX, and X. Cranial nerves V, IX, and X control the protective reflexes. Testing cranial nerves V and VII determines whether the corneal reflex is intact. Observing for a bilateral blink is one way to test cranial nerve V. When there is an asymmetrical blink, a wisp of cotton is used to touch the cornea. The normal response is blinking in that eye. When this reflex is absent or diminished, the patient is at risk of developing a corneal abrasion.

Testing of cranial nerves IX and X involves the cough, gag, and swallowing reflexes. The patient is instructed to cough and to swallow. To test the gag reflex, the patient is asked to open his or her mouth and say "ah." During this maneuver, observe for symmetry: the soft palate rises on both sides, and the uvula is at the midline. If the patient is unable to follow commands or is unconscious, stimulating the pharyngeal wall elicits a "retching" response. It is important to have the head of the bed elevated 30 degrees with the patient lying on his or her side before testing the gag reflex. When these reflexes are diminished or absent, the patient has difficulty handling secretions and oral intake and is at risk of aspiration.

Cranial nerves VII, VIII, XI, and XII. To test the facial nerve (cranial nerve VII), the nurse asks the patient to smile, frown, and puff out the cheeks and observes the facial expressions. The acoustic nerve (cranial nerve VIII) is tested by the patient closing his or her eyes, the nurse initiating a sound, and then asking the patient if the sound was heard. The spinal accessory (XI) enables the shoulders to move upward and allows turning the head to either side. Cranial nerve XII moves the tongue and is assessed by asking the patient to stick out the tongue and move it from side to side. The nurse observes for symmetry of movement and inspects the surface of the tongue for atrophy.

Motor status. The nurse assesses spontaneous movement of all extremities, muscle strength, muscle tone, deep tendon reflexes, Babinski's reflex, coordination, and abnormal postures. Muscle groups are assessed for symmetry.

For the conscious and alert patient, the assessment is conducted by observing responses to directions. For an unconscious patient or one who is unable to provide accurate responses, the nurse relies on neurological testing and observation skills.

Spontaneous movement. Spontaneous movement can be assessed by asking the patient to move the extremities on command or by observing while the patient moves around in bed.

Muscle strength. A grading of muscle strength is also part of the motor assessment because it offers a basis for comparative assessment throughout the course of treatment. The grading of muscle strength (5/5 scale) is based on the ability to move muscle groups, hold a position against gravity, and maintain that position against the nurse's resistance to the muscle groups. If you ask the patient to lift his or her arm and nothing occurs even when pain is inflicted, the patient is rated 0/5. If you see or feel a flicker in the biceps muscle, the patient is rated 1/5. If the patient moves the arm or wrist displaying joint movement but is unable to raise the extremity off the bed, the score is 2/5. When the patient is able to lift the extremity off the bed, but drops it as soon as you touch it, the patient is rated 3/5. This action shows the patient can overcome gravity, but has no strength. The last step is for the nurse to apply resistance to the muscles when the patient has the arm extended in front ("I am going to push your right arm/leg down, so try to prevent me from doing that"). If the patient has difficulty resisting the examiner, the rating is a 4; if the patient maintains the position with resistance, the rating is 5 (Lower, 2002). Lower extremity strength can also be tested by asking the patient to push his or her feet against the nurse's hands. Testing generalized muscle strength in a conscious patient can also be done with the drift test. The patient is asked to close the eyes and stretch out the arms with palms up for 20 to 30 seconds. A downward drift of the arm or pronation of the palm on one side indicates mild paresis of the involved extremity. This test is very sensitive to subtle changes in strength secondary to neurological deterioration. It is not possible to test strength in an unconscious patient or a patient who is receiving a paralytic agent.

Muscle tone. Muscle tone is assessed by taking each extremity through passive range of motion. Normal muscle tone shows slight resistance to the range of motion. Limp, flabby muscles are characterized by decreased or loss of tone, so there is no resistance to movement. Increased muscle tone is characterized by spasticity and rigidity, resulting in a muscle group demonstrating increased resistance to the range of motion.

Deep tendon reflexes. Deep tendon reflexes are also included in the motor assessment. Reflex testing assists in establishing the level of SCI, and the return of deep tendon reflexes below the level of injury signals the end of spinal shock. Deep tendon reflexes are obtained by a brisk tapping of a reflex hammer on the tendons of a muscle group (Figure 12-12). The response is contraction of the stimulated muscle group. Deep tendon reflexes are graded according to the response elicited (0, no reflex; 1, hypoactive; 2, normal; 3, hyperactive).

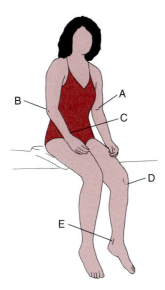

FIGURE 12-12 Deep tendon reflexes. *A,* Biceps. *B,* Triceps. *C,* Brachioradialis. *D,* Patellar. *E,* Achilles. (From Mitchell, P., Cammermeyer, M., Ozuna, J., & Woods, N. F. [1984]. *Neurological assessment for nursing practice.* Reston Publishing.)

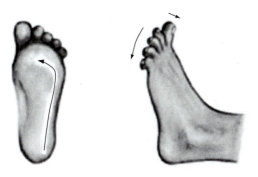

FIGURE 12-13 Babinski's reflex. With a moderately sharp object, such as a key, stroke the lateral aspect of the sole from the heel to the ball of the foot, curving medially across the ball. Use the lightest stimulus that provokes a response. Note movement of the toes, normally flexion. Dorsiflexion of the great toe with fanning of the other toes indicates upper motor neuron disease. (From Bates, B. [1991]. *Guide to physical examination.* Philadelphia: J. B. Lippincott.)

Babinski's reflex. The major pathological deep tendon reflex is Babinski's reflex (Figure 12-13). In an adult, the presence of a Babinski's reflex is a sign of an upper motor neuron lesion and damage to the corticospinal tract.

Coordination of movement. Coordination of movement is under cerebellar control. It is assessed by asking the patient to perform rapid alternating movements, placing the finger to the nose, or to running the heel down the shin bilaterally. These tests require the patient to be able to follow verbal commands.

Abnormal postures. Assessment for abnormal postures is important in neurologically injured patients.

Early *hemiplegia* exists when one side of the patient's body stops moving spontaneously. This state indicates a cortical lesion and is a sign of further neurological deterioration secondary to a mass effect. The lesion is compressing the fibers in the motor strip in the frontal lobe. Prolonged compression on motor fibers leads to paralysis.

Decorticate rigidity (Figure 12-14) can be the result of a cortical, subcortical, or diencephalon lesion.

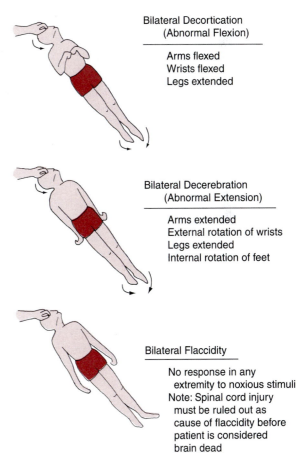

Bilateral Decortication
(Abnormal Flexion)

Arms flexed
Wrists flexed
Legs extended

Bilateral Decerebration
(Abnormal Extension)

Arms extended
External rotation of wrists
Legs extended
Internal rotation of feet

Bilateral Flaccidity

No response in any
  extremity to noxious stimuli
Note: Spinal cord injury
  must be ruled out as
  cause of flaccidity before
  patient is considered
  brain dead

FIGURE 12-14 Abnormal postures. (From Marshall, S. B., Marshall, L. F., Vos, H. R., & Chesnut, R. M. [1990]. *Neuroscience critical care.* Philadelphia: W. B. Saunders.)

Characteristics of this posture are flexion of the upper extremities and extension, with internal rotation of the lower extremities.

Decerebrate posturing is the result of a midbrain or pons lesion. In this posture, the patient's jaws are clenched, extremities are in full extension, feet are in plantar extension, forearms are pronated, and wrists and fingers are flexed (see Figure 12-14). Decerebrate and decorticate posturing can occur in response to noxious stimuli such as suctioning or pain.

In *bilateral flaccidity*, there is no response to noxious stimuli (see Figure 12-14).

Sensory assessment. Sensory assessment is performed to determine superficial response to pinprick (sharp, dull, hyperesthesia, absent), position sense, and temperature. The sensory dermatomes are the segmental distribution of sensation (see Figure 12-10; Table 12-3). The areas of sensation on the skin are supplied by one spinal segment. For example, the ability to sense a superficial pinprick on the lateral forearm, thumb, and index finger tests the innervation by dermatome C6. While undergoing sensory testing, the patient is instructed to close his or her eyes. Position sense is determined by having the nurse grasp the patient's thumb or big toe and move the digit up or down or leave it in a neutral position. The patient is asked to identify the pattern of movement. Temperature is assessed by filling up one test tube

with hot water and another test tube with cold water. The patient is asked to identify the sensation when the test tube touches the skin.

Respiratory assessment. Assessing respiratory pattern and rate is performed with each neurologically impaired patient because adequate cerebral oxygenation and carbon dioxide elimination are necessary for proper neurological function. Changes in the respiratory pattern can indicate neurological deterioration. Table 12-4 describes abnormal respiratory patterns that are a sign of neurological decline.

The assessments described in this section provide a complete neurological evaluation of a critically ill patient. The nurse reassesses the neurological parameters based on physician instructions and severity of or changes in the patient's condition. Table 12-5 contains the components of an hourly neurological assessment for patients with increased ICP, head injury, or acute stroke. Documentation of the neurological assessment findings is accomplished using a neurological flow chart and narrative charting.

Increased Intracranial Pressure

One of the most commonly encountered problems in the critical care setting is increased ICP. Brain disorders such as head injury, stroke, tumor, hydrocephalus,

TABLE 12-3

Spinal Nerve Innervation of Major Muscle Groups

Spinal Nerve	Muscle Group Movement	Assessment Technique
C4-C5	Shoulder abduction	Shrug shoulders against downward pressure of examiner's hands
C5-C6	Elbow flexion (biceps)	Arm pulled up from resting position against resistance
C7	Elbow extension (triceps)	From the flexed position, arm straightened out against resistance
C7	Thumb-index pinch	Index finger held firmly to thumb against resistance to pull apart
C8	Hand grasp	Hand grasp strength evaluated
L2-L4	Hip flexion	Leg lifted from bed against resistance
L5-S1	Knee flexion	Knee flexed against resistance
L2-L4	Knee extension	From flexed position, knee extended against resistance
L5	Foot dorsiflexion	Foot pulled up toward nose against resistance
S1	Foot plantar flexion	Foot pushed down (stepping on the gas) against resistance

TABLE 12-4

Respiratory Patterns in Neurological Disorders

Abnormal Pattern	Disorder
Cheyne-Stokes	Bilateral deep cerebral lesions or some cerebellar lesions
Central neurogenic hyperventilation	Lesions of the midbrain and upper pons
Apneustic	Lesions of the mid to lower pons
Cluster breathing	Lesions of the lower pons or upper medulla
Ataxic respirations	Lesions of the medulla

infection, cerebral edema, hematoma formation, and anoxia are often associated with life-threatening ICP.

Under normal circumstances, ICP (normal range, 0 to 15 mm Hg) fluctuates in response to changes in blood pressure, respiratory cycle, isometric contractions, coughing, and Valsalva's maneuvers (e.g., breath holding, straining). Box 12-1 lists causes of ICP fluctuations.

PATHOPHYSIOLOGY

Occurrence of increased ICP (20 mm Hg or greater persisting for 5 minutes or longer) is a life-threatening event. The rigid cranial vault contains three types of noncompressible contents: semisolid brain, intravascular blood, and CSF. When the volume of any one of these three components increases, one or both of the other components must decrease proportionally, or there will be an increase in ICP (Monro-Kellie doctrine).

BOX 12-1

Causes of Intracranial Pressure Fluctuations

INCREASES IN INTRACRANIAL PRESSURE
Defecation
Coughing
Airway obstruction
Abdominal breathing
Vomiting
Positive end-expiratory pressure
Suctioning
Muscle exertion or tension
Range-of-motion exercises
Isometric exercises
Valsalva maneuver
REM sleep
Position changes (prone, Trendelenburg's position, extreme hip flexion, neck flexion)
Hypercapnia ($PaCO_2$ greater than 42 mm Hg)
Hypoxia (PaO_2 less than 50 mm Hg)
Stress or emotional upsets
Pain and noxious stimuli
Seizure activity
Hyperthermia
Clustering of nursing activities
Discussion of the patient's condition at the bedside

DECREASES IN INTRACRANIAL PRESSURE
CNS depressant medications
Inspiration

REM, Rapid eye movement; *CNS,* central nervous system; *PaO₂,* partial pressure of oxygen; *PaCO₂,* partial pressure of carbon dioxide.
From Barker, E. (2002). *Neuroscience nursing. A spectrum of care* [p. 381]. 2nd ed. St. Louis: Mosby.

TABLE 12-5

Components of the Hourly Neurological Assessment for Patients with Increased Intracranial Pressure, Head Injury, or Acute Stroke

Mental Status	Focal Motor	Pupils	Brainstem/Cranial Nerves
Glasgow Coma Scale (GCS) Assesses level of consciousness, expressive language, ability to follow commands	Move all extremities Strength of all extremities (compares right and left sides) Motor response	Size Shape Reaction to light (direct and consensual) Extraocular movements	Corneal reflex Present: immediate blinking bilaterally Diminished: blinking asymmetrically Absent: no blinking Cough, gag, swallow reflex Observe for excessive drooling Observe for cough/swallow reflex

To compensate for an increased intracranial component, CSF is displaced into the spinal canal or absorbed into the venous system. When additional intracranial volume occurs in pathological conditions as a result of increased blood volume, increased CSF production or inability to reabsorb CSF, expanding mass lesions with cerebral edema, or cerebral hemorrhage, the compensatory mechanisms fail and the increased intracranial volume is not tolerated by the patient. At this point, the patient begins to display symptoms of increased ICP. Physiologically, the brain loses its ability to compensate, as demonstrated by an alteration in intracranial compliance (Figure 12-15).

Intracranial Compliance

Intracranial compliance is a measure of the brain's compensatory mechanisms and demonstrates the effects of volume on pressure. In Figure 12-16, the curve is flat from point *A* to point *B*. Adding volume up to this point has very little effect on pressure; the ICP remains stable. This response is known as compliance (Hickey, 2003). During normal compliance, CSF is displaced into the spinal subarachnoid space, and blood is displaced into the venous sinuses. In Figure 12-16, point *B* on the steep portion of the curve indicates the point at which small changes in volume produce large changes in pressure—when compensatory volume displacement mechanisms are exhausted (low compliance). Patients on the steep portion of this curve can experience large and dangerous increases in ICP with ordinary activities, positioning, or other nursing interventions and must be monitored closely (Le Jeune, 2002; Wojner, El-Mitwalli, & Alexandrov, 2002; Simmons, 1997).

Altered Cerebral Blood Flow

CBF brings oxygen and glucose to the brain for energy production. Waste products are then removed by the blood. When metabolism is increased, the CBF is increased to meet those demands. In pathological situations, CBF can increase to such an extent that it adds to brain bulk and, consequently, ICP. Conversely, a decrease in CBF can render an area ischemic.

CPP is an estimate of CBF. It is calculated by subtracting mean ICP from MAP. The CPP in the average adult is approximately 70 to 100 mm Hg. The CPP must be maintained near 70 to 80 mm Hg to ensure adequate blood supply to the brain. If the CPP drops below this point, ischemia may develop. When ICP approaches MAP, CPP decreases to a point at which autoregulation is impaired and CBF decreases. As CBF decreases, cellular activity is impaired, and signs and symptoms related to neurological dysfunction become apparent (Hickey, 2003).

The basis for physiological instability in critically ill patients with neurological disorders is an alteration in CBF and cerebral perfusion. These alterations lead

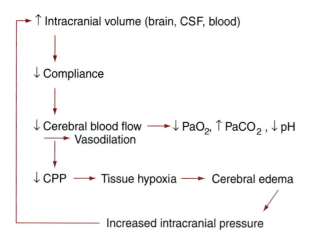

FIGURE 12-15 Pathophysiology flow diagram for increased intracranial pressure. This process contributes to decreased mentation, impaired motor function, cranial nerve dysfunction, sensory impairment, and autonomic nervous system dysfunction. (From Black, J. M., & Matassarin-Jacobs, E. [1997]. *Medical-surgical nursing: Clinical management for continuity of care.* 5th ed. Philadelphia: W. B. Saunders.)

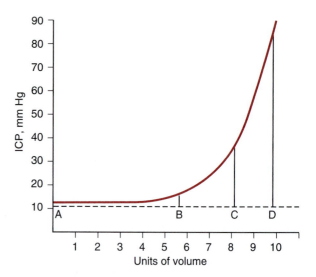

FIGURE 12-16 Pressure-volume curve. Up to point *B*, addition of volume has little effect on pressure; after point B, there is a dramatic increase in ICP in response to the addition of volume (low compliance). (From Hickey, J. V. [2003]. *The clinical practice of neurological neurosurgical nursing.* 5th ed. Philadelphia: Lippincott Williams & Wilkins.)

to hypoxia and ischemia, which can cause pathological changes to the brain. Therefore, management is focused on maintaining adequate blood flow and perfusion to the brain.

Autoregulation

Within normal limits, the cerebral vasculature exhibits pressure and chemical autoregulation. Pressure autoregulation provides a constant blood volume and CPP over a wide range of MAPs. Pathological states, such as head injury, hemorrhage, or craniotomy, lead to a loss of pressure autoregulation. When autoregulation is lost, hypertension increases CBF, and hypotension causes ischemia. Both these situations cause increased ICP.

The cerebral vessels are also sensitive to the chemical regulators carbon dioxide pressure ($PaCO_2$), oxygen pressure (PaO_2), and hydrogen ion concentration. Carbon dioxide is the most potent agent influencing CBF. When $PaCO_2$ is high, cerebral blood vessels respond by vasodilating, which increases blood flow, cerebral blood volume, and ICP. A low $PaCO_2$ causes the cerebral arteries to constrict, leading to a decreased blood flow and decreased tissue perfusion. Cerebral arteries are less sensitive to changes in PaO_2. The CBF is not affected until the PaO_2 is 40 mm Hg or less. A PaO_2 of 40 mm Hg causes hypoxia and vasodilation of the cerebral vessels, which increase CBF in an effort to raise oxygen delivery. High PaO_2 levels have not been shown to affect CBF in either direction. If PaO_2 is not raised, anaerobic metabolism begins and results in lactic acid accumulation. The increased hydrogen ion concentration causes more vasodilation (Urden, Stacy, & Lough, 2002).

Obstructed Venous Outflow

Shunting CSF into the venous system is another way to compensate for an increase in intracranial volume. In pathological states, venous outflow can become obstructed in several ways. Different neck positions (hyperflexion, hyperextension, rotation) and tightly applied tracheostomy and endotracheal ties compress the jugular vein, inhibit venous return, cause central venous engorgement, and increase ICP. A second mechanism for venous outflow obstruction is transmission of a high pressure that impairs venous return. Mechanisms that increase intrathoracic or intraabdominal pressure (e.g., coughing, vomiting, posturing, isometric exercise, Valsalva's maneuver, or positive end-expiratory pressure) produce increased pressure that impairs venous return (Figure12-17). When the jugular vein is compressed, venous return is inhibited, resulting in venous engorgement. As venous outflow decreases, an increase in ICP occurs.

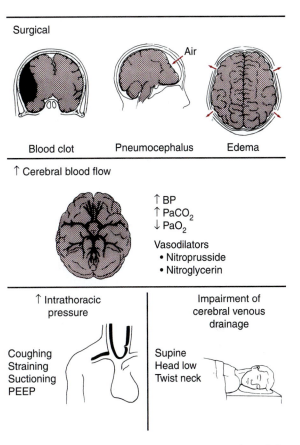

FIGURE 12-17 Schematic representation of the different causes of increased intracranial pressure. (From Frost, E. A. M. [1990] *Postanesthesia care unit*, 2nd ed., St. Louis: Mosby.)

Cerebral Edema

Cerebral edema is an increase in the water content of the brain tissue. When cerebral edema occurs, ICP increases and CBF decreases.

Cytotoxic edema and vasogenic edema are two categories of cerebral edema. Cytotoxic edema is characterized by intracellular swelling of neurons, most often the result of hypoxia and hypo-osmolality. Hypoxia causes decreased ATP production and leads to the failure of the sodium-potassium pump and causes sodium, chloride, and water to enter the cell while potassium exits. This failure leads to hypoosmolality, which causes the cells to swell and to stop functioning. Cytotoxic edema is associated with brain ischemia or hypoxic events such as stroke, cardiac arrest, and asphyxiation. It is also seen with hypoosmolar conditions including water intoxication, hyponatremia, and syndrome of inappropriate antidiuretic hormone (SIADH) secretion.

Vasogenic cerebral edema occurs as a result of a breakdown in the blood-brain barrier, leading to an increase in the extracellular fluid space. Normally, the highly selective blood-brain barrier closely regulates the internal brain environment. When this barrier is disrupted, osmotically active substances (proteins) leak into the brain interstitium and draw water from the vascular system. This results in an increase in extracellular fluid and a consequent increase in ICP. Head injuries, brain tumors, meningitis, and abscesses are common causes of vasogenic cerebral edema.

Herniation

When a mass effect occurs in the semisolid brain within a compartment, the pressure exerted by this mass is not equally divided, resulting in shifting or herniation of the brain from a compartment of high pressure to one of lower pressure. This causes pressure or traction on certain neurological structures, and an increase in neurological deficits or death can occur. Any change in intracranial compliance, CBF, autoregulation, and cerebral edema can potentially cause increased ICP and subsequent herniation.

Herniation syndromes are classified as supratentorial (cingulate, central, and uncal herniation) or infratentorial (cerebellar tonsil herniation).

Cingulate herniation. When a unilateral lesion creates a shift of brain tissue of one cerebral hemisphere under the falx cerebri to the other cerebral hemisphere, it is called cingulate herniation (Figure 12-18). This type of herniation compresses cerebral blood vessels and brain tissue and causes cerebral ischemia, cerebral edema, and increased ICP. Changes in arousal (level of consciousness) and mental status are associated with this type of herniation.

Central herniation. A downward shift of the cerebral hemispheres, basal ganglia, and diencephalon through the tentorial notch causes central herniation (Hickey, 2003). The supratentorial contents compress vital centers of the brainstem (see Figure 12-18). Early signs and symptoms include changes in arousal and mental status, increased muscle tone, motor weakness, change in the respiratory pattern (increased yawning, deep sighs, rate changes), small reactive pupils that may become dilated and fixed, and bilateral Babinski's reflexes. Late signs and symptoms include decorticate posturing and Cheyne-Stokes respirations.

Uncal herniation. When a unilateral lesion above the tentorium forces the uncus of the temporal lobe to displace through the tentorial notch, uncal herniation is the result (see Figure 12-18). The displaced uncus compresses the midbrain and causes

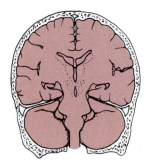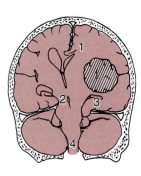

FIGURE 12-18 Types of herniation. Cross section of a normal brain *(left)* and a brain with intracranial shifts from supratentorial lesions *(right): 1,* herniation of the cingulate gyrus under the falx; *2,* central herniation causing a downward shift of the cerebral hemispheres, basal ganglia, and diencephalon through the tentorial notch; *3,* uncal herniation causing the temporal lobe to pass through the tentorial notch; *4,* tonsillar herniation causing the cerebellar tonsils to be displaced through the foramen magnum. (Modified from Plum, F., & Posner, J. [1972]. *Diagnosis of stupor and coma*. 2nd ed. Oxford University Press.)

dysfunction of the parasympathetic fibers of the ipsilateral third nerve. Signs and symptoms include unilateral pupil dilation, ipsilateral third nerve palsy, and contralateral hemiplegia. Without treatment, the patient becomes unresponsive to the environment and progresses to full coma. In addition, brainstem dysfunction (loss of oculocephalic reflex, fixed midposition pupils, and altered respirations) and decerebrate posturing are present.

Cerebellar tonsil herniation. When the cerebellar tonsils are displaced through the foramen magnum, tonsillar herniation results (see Figure 12-18). This displacement distorts the brainstem, compresses the medulla, and causes fatal damage to the respiratory and cardiac centers.

ASSESSMENT

The GCS is used in assessing the patient with increased ICP. Additionally, a thorough neurological examination must be performed with an emphasis placed on level of consciousness, motor movement, pupillary response to light, extraocular movements, and cranial nerve function testing of corneal, cough, gag, and swallow reflexes.

Vital signs. Changes in vital signs due to brain injury typically appear late in the course of neurological dysfunction. A patient may experience severe irreversible damage by the time vital sign changes occur. Respiratory changes correlate with lesions at various levels of injury; therefore, changes in respiratory rate, rhythm, and depth are important. Pulse and blood pressure changes are unreliable as part of the overall assessment. Both of these changes occur late in the course of increased ICP. Cushing's reflex is another late sign of increased ICP and consists of systolic hypertension, a widening pulse pressure (systolic pressure rises faster than does diastolic pressure) and bradycardia.

Monitoring techniques. Other assessment parameters for a patient with increased ICP include ICP, arterial, and hemodynamic monitoring.

Intracranial pressure monitoring. ICP monitoring is a common tool used to assess the balance between intracranial blood, brain tissue, and CSF. ICP monitoring provides data that add to serial neurological assessments, gauge patient progress, and allow nurses to observe patient responses to nursing interventions and medical treatments. Depending on the type of ICP catheter inserted, it may also be used to drain excessive CSF. The four sites for monitoring ICP are the intraventricular space, the subarachnoid space, the

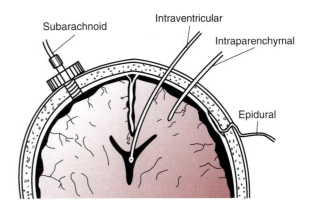

FIGURE 12-19 Intracranial pressure monitoring sites. (From Kee, K. R., Hoff, J. T. [1996] *Youman's neurological surgery*, 4th ed. Philadelphia: W. B. Saunders.)

epidural space, and the parenchyma (Figure 12-19). Each site has advantages and disadvantages for monitoring ICP (Table 12-6).

Intraventricular space. After administering local anesthesia to the patient, a small catheter is placed in the anterior horn of the lateral ventricle through a

TABLE 12-6

Intracranial Pressure (ICP) Monitoring Devices

Device	Location	Comments
Intraventricular catheter or fiberoptic transducer	Lateral ventricle of nondominant hemisphere	Therapeutic or diagnostic removal of cerebrospinal fluid Rapid CSF drainage may result in collapsed ventricle or subdural hematoma May cause intracerebral bleeding or edema Infection rate 2%-5%
Subarachnoid bolt	Subarachnoid space	Does not penetrate brain Bolt can become occluded with clots or tissue CSF drainage not possible Infection rate 1%-2%
Epidural sensor or transducer	Between the skull and the dura	Least invasive (does not penetrate dura or brain) CSF drainage not possible Infection rate <1% Head position has no effect on pressure reading Epidural pressure is slightly higher than intraventricular pressure
Intraparenchymal transducer	1 cm into brain tissue	CSF drainage not possible Catheter relatively fragile; avoid sharp kinks and pulls Head position has no effect on pressure reading Risk of intracerebral bleeding and infection

CSF, Cerebrospinal fluid.
Modified from Dennison R. (2000). *Pass CCRN®!* St. Louis: Mosby.

bur hole in a procedure known as a ventriculostomy. The side chosen for placement is usually the non-dominant hemisphere.

Subarachnoid space. A small hollow bolt or screw is inserted in the subarachnoid space through a bur hole. The bur hole is usually placed in the front of the skull behind the hairline, and local anesthesia is used.

Epidural space. After the dura is stripped from the inner table of the skull, and after local anesthesia is administered, a small fiberoptic sensor is placed in the epidural space.

Intraparenchymal space. After placing a sub-arachnoid bolt, a hole is punched in the dura, and a small fiberoptic catheter is inserted approximately 1 cm into the parenchymal tissue (Dennison, 2000; Stewart-Amidei, 1998).

Waveform monitoring. Monitoring systems allow nurses to observe an ICP waveform pattern. The normal intracranial pulse waveform has three defined peaks of decreasing height that correlate with the arterial pulse waveform and are identified as P_1, P_2, and P_3. P_1 is fairly consistent in shape and amplitude (Figure 12-20). P_1 represents the blood being ejected from the heart. Extreme hypotension or hypertension produces changes in P_1. P_2 represents intracranial brain bulk. It is more variable in shape and is most directly linked with the state of decreased compliance. Decreased compliance exists when P_2 is equal to or higher than P_1. It also is helpful in predicting the risk for increases in ICP. P_3 follows the dicrotic notch and represents closure of the aortic valve. Smaller peaks that follow the three main peaks vary among individual patients (Barker, 2002; Kirkness et al., 2000; March, 2000). The pressure is recorded as a "mean" value.

ICP waveforms can be trended over time to identify abnormal patterns: A waves, B waves, and C waves (see Figure 12-20). *A waves* (plateau waves) are waves between 50 and 100 mm Hg. These waves are associated with advanced intracranial hypertension, and immediate intervention to reduce ICP is necessary. The nurse should obtain a strip of trends to identify A waves because the waveform does not change on the actual monitor. The waveform shows a rise in ICP only for an extended period. *B waves*, less than 50 mm Hg, correspond to respirations and blood pressure. B waves may serve as a warning to the nurse of the *potential* risk of increased ICP and impairment of intracranial compliance. *C waves* are small waves (16 to 20 mm Hg) that correlate with normal changes in blood pressure and respirations. The clinical significance of C waves is not known at this time. In

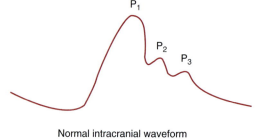

Normal intracranial waveform

A

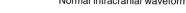
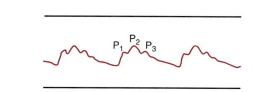

Abnormal ICP wave form

B

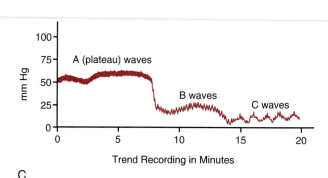

Trend Recording in Minutes

C

FIGURE 12-20 Intracranial pressure (ICP) wave-forms. **A,** Normal ICP waveform. **B,** Abnormal ICP wave-form. **C,** Intracranial pressure waves. Composite diagram of A (plateau), B (sawtooth) waves, and C (small, rhythmic) waves. (**A** and **C,** from Barker, E. (2002). *Neuroscience nursing: A spectrum of care.* 2nd ed. St. Louis, MO: Mosby; **B,** from Hickey, J. V. [2004]. *The clinical practice of neurological and neurosurgical nursing.* 5th ed. Philadelphia: Lippincott Williams & Wilkins.)

assessing ICP, the nurse uses information about wave-forms and potential changes to determine the types of interventions necessary to ensure patient safety and to promote the best patient outcome.

Hemodynamic monitoring. Hemodynamic monitoring is important for monitoring fluid management and assessing cerebral perfusion. For a detailed discussion related to this type of monitoring, refer to Chapter 7.

Monitoring cerebral oxygenation. A technique for monitoring CBF is jugular bulb oxygen saturation (S_jO_2) (Deyo, Yancy, & Prough, 2000; Kidd & Criddle, 2001). The technology is similar to mixed venous oxygen saturation (SvO_2) measured in the pulmonary artery. S_jO_2 is monitored via a fiberoptic catheter inserted through the internal jugular vein into the jugular venous bulb. Placement of the catheter is verified by skull x-ray study. S_jO_2 is a global measure of cerebral oxygenation. The normal value is 65%. Values less than 50% suggest cerebral ischemia. However, normal values do not ensure adequate perfusion to all brain areas.

Microsensor technology allows direct analysis of factors that affect brain tissue oxygenation and blood flow. The sensor is able to continuously measure brain oxygen tension, brain carbon dioxide tension, brain pH, and brain temperature. The device can be inserted with the initial ventriculostomy insertion. Another device that monitors brain tissue oxygenation is placed directly into the brain white matter. It provides information on the cellular dynamics of oxygenation and the impact of low oxygen states on the brain that may help to prevent hypoxic events, enable timely therapeutic intervention, and improve patient outcomes (Haselman & Fox, 2000; Littlejohns, Bader, & March, 2003; Bader, Littlejohns, & March, 2003).

Microdialysis is a method that measures the by-products of cellular metabolism and injury. By analyzing these neurochemicals, interventions can be developed to prevent secondary brain injury (Haselman & Fox, 2000).

Respiratory monitoring. Techniques for continuous monitoring of oxygen saturation via pulse oximetry and end-tidal carbon dioxide are useful measures to ensure adequate gas exchange in the patient. Periodic arterial blood gas samples may also be obtained.

Bedside electroencephalographic monitoring. Continuous bedside electroencephalographic (EEG) monitoring provides a recording of electrical activity in the brain. The continuous EEG allows for recording, trending, and using evoked potentials to correlate with ICP monitoring. In some cases, EEG monitoring is used to assess the effects of sedation and paralytic agents.

Cerebral blood flow monitoring. Transcutaneous Doppler is a noninvasive technology that allows for the indirect monitoring of CBF at the bedside.

Transcutaneous Doppler studies measure the velocity of arterial flow (Deyo, Yancy, & Prough, 2000). Transcutaneous Doppler measurements are correlated with ICP values to assess patient response to treatment and nursing interventions.

Evoked potential monitoring. Evoked potentials are a noninvasive way of applying sensory stimuli and recording the electrical potentials created. Each potential is recorded and stored in a computer, and an average curve is calculated. The two common types of evoked potentials are brainstem auditory evoked potentials and somatosensory evoked potentials. Brainstem auditory evoked potentials are used to evaluate brainstem function and can be conducted on a conscious or unconscious patient or even during surgery. Somatosensory evoked potentials measure peripheral nerve responses and are helpful in evaluating spinal cord function.

DIAGNOSTIC TESTING

The initial baseline laboratory tests obtained in a patient with increased ICP are the following:

- Arterial blood gases and continuous oxygen saturation
- Complete blood count, with an emphasis on red blood cells, hematocrit, and hemoglobin
- Coagulation profile (prothrombin time, partial thromboplastin time, platelet count)
- Electrolytes, blood urea nitrogen, creatinine, liver function, and serum osmolality
- Urinalysis and urine osmolality

The ongoing laboratory tests obtained in a patient with increased ICP are the following:

- Arterial blood gases and continuous pulse oximetry
- Hematocrit and hemoglobin
- Electrolytes, blood urea nitrogen, creatinine, and serum osmolality

The x-ray studies and other diagnostic tests performed on a patient with increased ICP include the following:

- Computed tomography (CT) scan (usually non-contrast)
- Magnetic resonance imaging (MRI)
- Skull x-ray studies
- EEG
- CBF studies
- Cerebral arteriography

NURSING DIAGNOSES

Refer to the Nursing Care Plan for the Patient with Traumatic Brain Injury, Increased Intracranial Pressure, or Acute Stroke for a detailed description of nursing diagnoses, specific nursing interventions, and selected rationales.

Text continued on page 378

Nursing Care Plan for the Patient with Traumatic Brain Injury, Increased Intracranial Pressure, or Acute Stroke

NURSING DIAGNOSIS: *Decreased intracranial adaptive capacity related to trauma/neurological illness*

Patient Outcomes	Interventions	Rationales
PERLA; RR, 12-20 breaths/min with normal depth and pattern; HR 60-100 beats/min; CPP 60-80 mm Hg; absence of headache, vomiting; ABG WNL; awake and exhibits appropriate responses	Assess neurological status hourly. Monitor VS. Be alert to changes in respiratory pattern, fluctuations in BP, pulse, widening pulse pressure, and decreased HR. Monitor ICP; record and report changes. Notify physician if CPP is <60 mm Hg. Maintain patent airway and monitor ABGs for evidence of hypoxemia/hypercapnia.	Decrease in LOC is early indicator of increased ICP. Change in size and reaction of pupils, decrease in motor function, and cranial nerve palsies may indicate impending herniation. Hypoxemia/hypercapnia can cause cerebral vasodilation and can increase cerebral edema and ICP.
	Maintain the patient's head in a neutral position. Ensure precise delivery of IV fluids at consistent rates. Evaluate activities that increase ICP (e.g., suctioning, bathing, dressing changes) and do not group activities together. Correct factors that may increase ICP (hypoxia, pain, anxiety, noise, abdominal/bladder distention, hip flexion). Ensure timely administration of medications prescribed to prevent sudden changes in BP, HR, or RR. Maintain head of bed elevation at level that keeps ICP <20 mm Hg and CPP >70 mm Hg.	Facilitates cerebral venous drainage and avoids increased ICP. Prevents fluid volume excess that could contribute to cerebral edema. Spacing care minimizes sustained elevations in ICP.
	If patient is hyperthermic, administer tepid baths, use a hypothermic blanket, apply ice bags to the patient's groin/axillae, administer antipyretics, and reduce ambient room temperature.	Hyperthermia increases metabolic needs.
	Assess the need for sedatives, paralytics, and antiseizure agents to decrease metabolic demand and control ICP.	Prevents excessive cerebral blood flow and/or dilation of cerebral vessels.

NURSING DIAGNOSIS: *Ineffective tissue perfusion related to increased ICP, decreased cerebral blood flow*

Patient Outcomes	Interventions	Rationales
Improved cerebral tissue perfusion as evidenced by VS, adequate hemodynamic values, NSR, improved LOC,	Assess neurological status hourly; monitor VS, assess ECG. Perform actions to prevent and treat increased ICP.	

Nursing Care Plan for the Patient with Traumatic Brain Injury, Increased Intracranial Pressure, or Acute Stroke—cont'd

Patient Outcomes	Interventions	Rationales
sensory/motor function, and adequate urine output	Implement measures to improve cerebral tissue perfusion by administering prescribed sympathomimetic agents and volume expanders and by maintaining IV fluid therapy. Monitor hemodynamic values to achieve and maintain prescribed parameters. Administer calcium channel blockers (nimodipine) if ordered, to reduce cerebral vasospasm. Assess lung sounds.	Risk of pulmonary edema is associated with vigorous fluid administration. Calcium released by injured neural cells can cause vasospasm.

NURSING DIAGNOSIS: *Impaired gas exchange related to decreased oxygen supply and increased carbon dioxide production secondary to decreased ventilatory drive occurring with pressure on respiratory center, imposed inactivity, and possible neurological pulmonary edema*

Patient Outcomes	Interventions	Rationales
PaCO$_2$ remains 35-40 mm Hg, PaO$_2$ >80 mm Hg; RR is 12-20 breaths/min with normal depth/pattern; adventitious breath sounds are absent; LOC improved	Assess patient's RR, depth, and rhythm. Auscultate breath sounds every 1-2 hr and as needed. Assess the patient for signs of hypoxia (confusion, agitation, restlessness, irritability). Ensure a patent airway and assess the need for suctioning. Hyperoxygenate the patient before and after suctioning to prevent hypoxia. Monitor ABGs and notify the physician of significant changes or findings. Be alert to levels indicative of hypoxemia and increases in PaCO$_2$. Assist with turning every 2 hr, within the limits of patient's status. Monitor I & O. Weigh the patient daily.	Prevent cerebral hypoxia. Promote lung drainage and alveolar expansion.

NURSING DIAGNOSIS: *Risk for imbalanced fluid volume related to fluids/medications administered, development of complications (diabetes insipidus; SIADH), gastrointestinal suction*

Patient Outcomes	Interventions	Rationales
Adequate VS, hemodynamic values, and I & O; appropriate weight; moist mucous membranes	Weigh the patient daily. Monitor I & O. Monitor laboratory results (electrolytes, serum and urine osmolality). Assess skin and mucous membranes. Monitor VS and hemodynamic values.	

Continued

Nursing Care Plan for the Patient with Traumatic Brain Injury, Increased Intracranial Pressure, or Acute Stroke—cont'd

NURSING DIAGNOSIS: *Imbalanced nutrition: less than body requirements related to hypermetabolic state*

Patient Outcomes	Interventions	Rationales
Weight within normal range for patient; serum proteins and albumin within normal range; positive nitrogen balance	Implement early nutritional support. Auscultate bowel sounds and monitor for abdominal distention. Weigh the patient daily. Assess gastric tube feeding residual as ordered. Monitor I & O.	Early nutritional support is associated with improved outcome. Enteral nutrition is most physiologically compatible with gut function and should be initiated as early as possible. Parenteral nutrition is indicated if enteral is contraindicated or not tolerated. Patients with neurological alterations are at increased risk of aspiration.

NURSING DIAGNOSIS: *Risk of infection related to invasive techniques and devices, compromised immune system, or bacterial invasion caused by traumatic brain injury, pneumonia, or iatrogenic causes*

Patient Outcomes	Interventions	Rationales
Free of infection as evidenced by normothermia; normal WBCs; negative culture results; HR <100 beats/min; BP within normal range for patient; absence of agitation, purulent drainage, and other clinical indicators of infection	Employ proper hand washing technique before and after patient contact. Use aseptic technique when performing invasive procedures and caring for catheters, tubes, and lines. Assess VS, body fluids, and skin for signs and symptoms of infection. Inspect cranial wounds for presence of erythema, tenderness, swelling, and drainage. Maintain a closed system for hemodynamic/ICP monitoring devices. Monitor the results of CBC and cultures. Assess and maintain adequate nutritional status. Administer antibiotics as ordered.	

NURSING DIAGNOSIS: *Risk of disuse syndrome and activity intolerance related to increased ICP, head injury, stroke, altered LOC, prolonged bed rest, and generalized weakness*

Patient Outcomes	Interventions	Rationales
Patient has baseline/optimal ROM; absence of edema or skin breakdown; absence of complications (thromboembolism, contractures, atelectasis)	Perform ROM exercises as indicated by the patient's status. Monitor ICP during exercise and be alert to elevations outside established parameters. Reposition the patient every 2 hr within restrictions of head and other injuries, using logrolling technique as indicated.	Turning the patient with increased ICP is not contraindicated but should be based on the response. If ICP remains elevated after 5 min, the patient should be returned to a position that reduces ICP and maximizes CPP.

Nursing Care Plan for the Patient with Traumatic Brain Injury, Increased Intracranial Pressure, or Acute Stroke—cont'd

Patient Outcomes	Interventions	Rationales
	Ensure proper anatomical alignment and position with use of pillows and sandbags Prevent footdrop with use of supportive devices. Perform frequent skin assessment and observe pressure point areas including the back of the head. Apply an intermittent pneumatic compression device. Assess the need for anticoagulation; monitor appropriate laboratory results. Assess breath sounds. Assess the need for PT/OT consultation.	

NURSING DIAGNOSIS: *Disturbed thought processes related to impaired cerebral functioning*

Patient Outcomes	Interventions	Rationales
Improved attention, memory, and judgment; responds appropriately with an improved level of orientation	Reorient frequently; place a clock or calendar within patient's view. Explain activities clearly and simply in a calm manner; allow adequate time for response. Instruct the family in methods to deal with patient's altered thought processes. Maintain a consistent and fairly structured routine. Allow for frequent rest periods for the patient.	

NURSING DIAGNOSIS: *Interrupted family processes related to situational crisis (patient's illness)*

Patient Outcomes	Interventions	Rationales
After interventions, family demonstrates effective adaptation to the situation as evidenced by seeking support and sharing concerns	Assess the character of family/significant others social, environmental, ethnic, and cultural relationships, role and communication patterns. Establish open, honest communication and provide information and guidance related to the patient. Assess knowledge regarding the patient's status and therapies, and allow sufficient time for questions. Acknowledge the family/significant other's involvement in patient care and promote strengths.	This assessment provides a baseline for determining interventions. This facilitates communication.

Continued

Nursing Care Plan for the Patient with Traumatic Brain Injury, Increased Intracranial Pressure, or Acute Stroke—cont'd

Patient Outcomes	Interventions	Rationales
	Provide opportunities to talk and share concerns in a private setting with nurses and other health care providers. Offer and support realistic hope. Assess for ineffective coping (depression, substance abuse, withdrawal) and the need for referral. Encourage the family/significant other to schedule periods of rest or activity outside the critical care unit and to seek support when necessary.	Assisting the family to develop realistic expectations will enable them to plan for the future.

ABG, Arterial blood gas; *BP*, blood pressure; *CBC*, complete blood count; *CPP*, cerebral perfusion pressure; *ECG*, electrocardiogram; *HR*, heart rate; *ICP*, intracranial pressure; *I & O*, intake & output; *IV*, intravenous; *LOC*, level of consciousness; *NSR*, normal sinus rhythm; *OT*, occupational therapy; P_aCO_2, partial pressure of carbon dioxide; PaO_2, partial pressure of oxygen; *PERLA*, pupils equal and reactive to light and accommodation; *PT*, physical therapy; *ROM*, range of motion; *RR*, respiratory rate; *SIADH*, syndrome of inappropriate antidiuretic hormone; *VS*, vital signs; *WBC*, white blood cell count; *WNL*, within normal limits.
Data from Swearingen, P. L., & Keen, J. H. (2001). *Manual of critical care nursing.* 4th ed. St. Louis: Mosby; and Ulrich, S. P., & Canale, S.W. (2001). *Nursing care planning guides: For adults in acute, extended, and home care settings.* Philadelphia: W. B. Saunders.

MANAGEMENT

Nursing Interventions

Nursing research has identified specific nursing activities that are associated with increases in ICP. These include endotracheal or nasal suctioning, head position, repositioning, and hygiene measures (Kerr et al., 1999; Sullivan, 2000). Elevated ICP resulting from nursing care is usually temporary, and the ICP returns to the resting baseline value within a few minutes. Sustained increases in ICP lasting longer than 5 minutes should be avoided. This is accomplished by spacing nursing care activities to prevent a continuous, detrimental increase in ICP.

Head and body positions are important factors in minimizing increased ICP and optimizing the patient's CPP. Elevating the head of the bed up to 30 degrees and keeping the head in a neutral midline position in relation to the body facilitates venous drainage and decreases the risk of venous obstruction. When the head is turned laterally 45 degrees, increases in ICP can occur as the jugular vein becomes obstructed and venous drainage is impeded. A cervical collar and excessively tight tracheostomy or endotracheal tube ties can cause the same negative effect of increased ICP. Extreme hip flexion causes an increase in intraabdominal and intrathoracic pressure and results in increased ICP. Patients with increased ICP can be turned from side to side. However, during any position change or change in elevation of the head of bed, it is imperative to monitor and document the patient's individualized cerebral and hemodynamic response carefully. If the CPP does not return to the baseline ICP within 5 minutes after the position change, the patient must return to the position that maximized CPP and minimized ICP. If the arterial oxygen saturation (SaO_2) drops because of a position change, resume the position that improves oxygenation (Sullivan, 2000; Swearingen & Keen, 2001; Yanko & Mitcho, 2001).

Endotracheal or nasal/oral suctioning may be necessary to maintain proper oxygenation. Before suctioning, the patient is preoxygenated with 100% oxygen. Each suction attempt is limited to less than 10 seconds, with no more than two passes with the suction catheter, while ensuring that the patient's head is in a neutral midline position. After suctioning, the patient is hyperventilated for 1 minute using 100% oxygen (Swearingen & Keen, 2001).

Fluid administration is provided to optimize MAP, to maintain intravascular volume without adding free water, and to normalize CPP. Normal saline solution (0.9%), an isotonic solution, is recommended for volume resuscitation. Hypotonic solutions are avoided to prevent an increase in cerebral edema and ICP.

Hypertonic saline solutions (3% normal saline) may be given to expand intravascular volume, extract water from intracellular space, decrease ICP, and increase cardiac contractility (Marik, Varon, & Trask, 2002; Yanko & Mitcho, 2001). Strict measurement of intake and output while monitoring serum sodium, potassium, and osmolarity is required. The goal is to keep serum osmolarity between 310 and 315 mOsm/L (Bullock et al., 2000). Blood products are administered to restore volume and to maintain adequate hematocrit and hemoglobin levels. Fluid restriction may be necessary when the ICP is elevated, hemodynamic values indicate excessive fluid, and other therapies are not achieving a reduced ICP. Osmotic and loop diuretics such as mannitol and furosemide (Lasix) are used to reduce cerebral brain volume by removing fluid from the brain's intracellular compartment. It is essential to evaluate fluid and electrolyte status when using diuretics. For example, hypokalemia, hyponatremia, and elevated serum osmolarity (greater than 320 mOsm/L) can occur after mannitol therapy. Hyperosmolarity can result in renal failure, neurological deterioration, and death if it is not corrected. Other factors leading to fluid and electrolyte imbalance are diabetes insipidus and SIADH secretion; either can occur with brain injury. These alterations are discussed in depth in Chapter 17. The development of diabetes insipidus and SIADH in a critically ill neurological patient presents a threat to the body's water and electrolyte balance.

Maintaining a quiet atmosphere by keeping the lighting and noise level low is usually beneficial in reducing an increased ICP. Because conversations that may emotionally stimulate the patient (e.g., discussing prognosis, condition, deficits, restraints) can cause an elevation in ICP, nurses and family members need to be cautioned to avoid unpleasant discussions (Barker, 2002). Assessing the patient's physiological response to visitors is an important nursing function. Although visitors usually have a beneficial impact on the patient physiologically, some patient-visitor interaction can be detrimental (Roland et al., 2001).

Medical (Nonsurgical) Interventions

The goal of medical management is to maintain an ICP of less than 20 mm Hg while maintaining the CPP at 70 mm Hg. The first task of the physician is to decrease ICP and then identify the cause of increased ICP. Once the cause is discovered, management is centered on permanently decreasing the high ICP, maintaining CPP, maintaining the airway, providing ventilation and oxygenation, and decreasing the metabolic demands placed on the injured brain. Management of increased ICP usually includes the following: cautious,

limited use of hyperventilation; osmotic and loop diuretics; oxygenation; euvolemic fluid administration; maintaining blood pressure; temperature control; and sedation. The use of corticosteroids for reducing ICP in patients with severe head injury is not recommended. Corticosteroids reduce cerebral edema associated with brain tumors, but more recent studies do not support the value of using corticosteroids to reduce ICP in other intracranial conditions (Littlejohns & Bader, 2001; Proctor, 2002).

Hyperventilation. Hyperventilation, which decreases $PaCO_2$, causes vasoconstriction of the cerebral arteries, reduction of CBF, and decrease in ICP. In the past, hyperventilation was commonly used to manage ICP; however, its efficacy has not been supported by research. Because hyperventilation may cause neurological damage by decreasing cerebral perfusion, it is no longer recommended as the first-line treatment to reduce ICP. Hyperventilation is only used to decrease ICP for short time periods when acute neurological deterioration is occurring (i.e., herniation) and other methods to reduce ICP have failed. During the first 24 hours after injury, it is recommended that the $PaCO_2$ be kept within a normal range, 35 to 45 mm Hg, and to avoid using hyperventilation therapy. When transporting a patient who is receiving manual ventilations via a manual resuscitation bag, it is important not to hyperventilate the patient. If the $PaCO_2$ level is purposefully lowered to less than 35 mm Hg, oxygen delivery at the cellular level should be evaluated using a jugular bulb or cerebral tissue oxygen monitor (Barker, 2002; Kidd & Criddle, 2001; Littlejohns & Bader, 2001; Oertel et al., 2002).

Diuretic therapy. Osmotic diuretics (mannitol 20%) draw water from normal brain cells to the plasma, thereby decreasing ICP. The effects of decreasing ICP and increasing CPP occur within 20 minutes of infusion. Side effects of osmotic diuretics include hypotension, electrolyte disturbance, and rebound increased ICP. If mannitol is used, the patient must have adequate intravascular volume to prevent hypotension and secondary brain injury. Osmotic diuretics are contraindicated in patients with renal disease. Osmotic diuretics are not metabolized and therefore are excreted unchanged in the urine.

Loop diuretics (furosemide, ethacrynic acid) decrease ICP by removing sodium and water from injured brain cells. These agents also decrease CSF formation.

Oxygenation. Without oxygen, the brain cannot meet metabolic demands, and the resultant hypoxia can lead to the death of neurons. For many patients with increased ICP, short-term management of the airway is accomplished by an endotracheal tube and mechanical ventilation. Long-term management entails the use of a tracheostomy tube. Additionally, adequate hematocrit and hemoglobin levels are maintained to promote oxygenation.

Blood pressure management. Blood pressure must be carefully controlled in a patient with increased ICP. Usually the MAP is kept between 70 and 90 mm Hg. However, it is critical to monitor the ICP and MAP collectively to sustain an adequate CPP. Maintaining a CPP greater than 70 mm Hg is essential to prevent cerebral ischemia. A goal for all critically ill patients is to avoid hypotension and hypertension. Hypotension decreases CBF, which leads to cerebral ischemia and therefore has a detrimental affect on patient outcome. When hypotension occurs, manipulating the systolic blood pressure with drugs and fluids may be needed to achieve an adequate CPP. This is accomplished by fluid administration and drug therapy that induces vasoconstriction. Hypertension (greater than 160 mm Hg systolic) can worsen cerebral edema by increasing microvascular pressure and leakage that lead to ischemia by compressing cerebral vessels. Systolic blood pressures greater than 160 mm Hg can be lowered using antihypertensive drugs such as labetalol. This beta-blocker decreases the response to ongoing catecholamine release from the sympathetic stimulation associated with neurological injury. Some antihypertensive agents (nitroprusside, hydralazine) and some calcium channel blockers (verapamil, nifedipine) cause cerebral vasodilation. This vasodilation increases CBF and causes increased ICP. The use of these vasodilators and calcium channel blockers is avoided in patients with poor intracranial compliance. The overall goal is to maintain an adequate MAP that will keep the CPP higher than 70 mm Hg (Hickey, 2003; Littlejohns & Bader, 2001; Yanko & Mitcho, 2001).

Reducing metabolic demands. Metabolic demands can be reduced by temperature control, sedation, analgesics, seizure prophylaxis, neuromuscular blockade, and barbiturates (Morris, Taylor, & Marshall, 2000). Aggressively managing hyperthemia is critical. The patient is kept normothermic or controlled hypothermia because fever increases oxygen demands and increases CBF, which ultimately contributes to a rise in ICP (Yanko & Mitcho, 2001). Patients are often sedated to limit and lower increased ICP related to agitation, restlessness, and resistance to mechanical ventilation. Benzodiazepines are used for sedation and do not affect CBF or ICP. Propofol is a sedative-hypnotic agent that reduces cerebral metabolism and ICP. It is a short-acting drug given by continuous infusion with a rapid onset. Morphine can be used for analgesia as a low-dose continuous infusion or given as-needed. Seizure prophylaxis may be used to prevent the increased metabolic demands associated with seizure activity. Neuromuscular blockade is considered for patients unresponsive to other treatments. Barbiturates are given selectively to reduce ICP refractory to other treatments. Pentobarbital is the most common agent used. Patients receiving neuromuscular blockade or barbiturate therapy require hemodynamic monitoring, mechanical ventilation, and intensive nursing management. Table 12-7 outlines drug therapy used in patients with increased ICP.

Surgical Interventions

Surgical intervention may be required to remove the source of a mass or lesion causing the increased ICP. This involves the removal of infarcted areas and hematomas (epidural, subdural, or intracerebral).

TABLE 12-7
DRUG THERAPY

Drug	Actions/Uses	Adult Dosage/Route	Side Effects	Nursing Implications
Mannitol	Draws water from normal brain cells into plasma; ↓ ICP; ↑ ICP	0.5 to 1 g/kg IV over 5-10 min, then 0.25-2 g/kg IVP q4-6h as needed depending on ICP, CPP, serum osmolarity	Hypotension, dehydration, electrolyte disturbances, tachycardia Rebound edema	Neurological assessment q1h; monitor ICP, CPP, serum osmolarity, electrolytes, ABG, VS, hourly I & O, daily weights; warm ampule or bottle in hot water and shake to dissolve crystals; use an in-line filter needle to administer

TABLE 12-7

DRUG THERAPY—cont'd

Drug	Actions/Uses	Adult Dosage/Route	Side Effects	Nursing Implications
Furosemide (Lasix)	Reduces cerebral edema by drawing sodium and water out of injured neurons	Edema/HF: 20-40 mg IV over 1-2 min; may repeat in 1-2 hr; if necessary, increase dosage by 20-mg increments until desired diuresis; IV dose should not exceed 1 g/day Postcardiac arrest cerebral edema: 40 mg IV over 1-2 min; if no response in 1 hr, increase to 80 mg or 0.5-1 mg/kg IV over 1-2 min; if no response, increase dose to 2 mg/kg	Ototoxicity, polyuria, electrolyte disturbances, gastric irritation, muscle cramps, hypotension, dehydration, embolism, vascular thrombosis	Monitor hourly I & O, daily weights, electrolytes, ABG, VS
Dexamethasone (Decadron)	Steroid that has a stabilizing effect on cell membrane; prevents destructive effect of O_2 free radicals; ↓ inflammation by suppressing white cells	Cerebral edema: 10-mg IV loading dose over 1 min; 4 mg q6h; reduce dose after 2-4 days; discontinue gradually over 5-7 days Cerebral edema in recurrent or inoperable brain tumor: 2 mg q8-12h (usually IM); adjust dose based on patient response	Flushing, sweating, hypertension, tachycardia, thrombocytopenia, weakness, nausea, diarrhea, gastrointestinal irritation/hemorrhage, fluid retention, poor wound healing, weight gain, hyperglycemia, peptic ulcer perforation, decreased wound healing, muscle wasting, hypokalemia	↑ or ↓ effects of anticoagulants; ↓ effects of anticonvulsants; adjust dose of antidiabetic agents; ↑ effects of digitalis; monitor glucose, potassium, daily weights, VS; causes edema; masks signs of infection; taper drug before discontinuing
Methylprednisolone (Solu-Medrol)	An adjunct to SCI management; steroids inhibit lipid peroxidation to protect the neuro-membrane from further destruction; improves blood flow to injury site facilitating tissue repair	30 mg/kg over 15 min; in 45 min, begin maintenance dose of 5.4 mg/kg/hr for 23 hr	Same as dexamethasone	Same as dexamethasone
Ranitidine (Zantac)	Inhibits histamine at the H_2-receptor sites, inhibiting gastric acid secretion; decreases gastrointestinal irritation to stress response after neurological injury and steroid use	50 mg in 50 mL 0.9% NS IVPB over 15-20 min q6-8h	Constipation or diarrhea; thrombocytopenia; dysrhythmias; burning/itching at IV site; nausea/vomiting; headache; bradycardia; confusion	May potentiate anticoagulants; monitor PT; ↑ effect of pronestyl
Pantoprazole sodium (Protonix IV)	Gastric acid pump inhibitor that suppresses gastric acid production	40 mg in 100 mL 0.9% NS IVPB over 15 min once daily for 7-10 days	Headache, abdominal pain, diarrhea, flatulence, hyperglycemia	Administer through a filter provided to remove precipitates that may form in solution

Continued

TABLE 12-7
DRUG THERAPY—cont'd

Drug	Actions/Uses	Adult Dosage/Route	Side Effects	Nursing Implications
Labetalol (Normodyne; Trandate)	Nonselective beta-blocker to decrease blood pressure	10-20 mg IVP over 2 min; may repeat with 40-80 mg IVP at 10-min intervals until desired BP is achieved; do not exceed total dose of 300 mg	Hypotension; bradycardia; HF; pulmonary edema; ventricular dysrhythmias; diaphoresis; flushing; somnolence; weakness/fatigue	Monitor BP, HR; I & O, daily weight; may ↓ glucose; may cause further hypotension with nitroglycerin; may potentiate with calcium channel blockers; adjust dosage of antidiabetic drugs
Phenytoin (Dilantin)	Inhibits the spread of seizures; status epilepticus	For status epilepticus, 10-20 mg/kg in 0.9% NS only; follow with maintenance dose of 100 mg IV over 2 min q6-8h; do not exceed a total dose of 1.5 g; if seizure not terminated, consider other anticonvulsants, barbiturates, or anesthesia	Bradycardia, hypotension, nystagmus/ataxia; gingival hyperplasia; agranulocytosis; rash; Stevens-Johnson syndrome; lymphadenopathy; nausea; cardiac arrest; heart block	Slow rate if bradycardia, hypotension, or cardiac dysrhythmias occur; monitor ECG, BP, pulse, and respiratory function; dilute with 0.9% NS only; assess oral hygiene; assess for rash; monitor renal, hepatic, and hematological status; interacts with many drugs
Fosphenytoin (Cerebyx)	Anticonvulsant; inhibits the spread of seizures; used in tonic-clonic seizures and status epilepticus	Status epilepticus loading dose 15-20 mg PE/kg IV [PE = phenytoin equivalent]; each 100-150 mg PE over a minimum of 1 min; if full effect is not immediate, may be necessary to use with benzodiazepine to control status epilepticus; maintenance dose 4-6 mg PE/kg/24 hr Nonemergency loading dose: 10-20 mg PE/kg; maintenance dose 4-6 mg PE/kg/24 hr	Transient ataxia, dizziness, headache, nystagmus, paresthesia, pruritus, somnolence, hypotension, bradycardia, heart block, respiratory arrest, ventricular fibrillation, tonic seizures, nausea/vomiting, lethargy, hypocalcemia, metabolic acidosis, rash	Slow rate or temporarily stop infusion for bradycardia, hypotension, burning, itching, numbness, or pain along injection site; assess neuro, respiratory, and cardiovascular status; assess seizure activity; monitor renal, hepatic, and hematological status; monitor for toxicity (bone marrow depression, nausea, vomiting, ataxia, diplopia, rash, cardiovascular collapse, slurred speech, confusion); interacts with many drugs
Diazepam (Valium)	Depresses subcortical areas of CNS; anticonvulsant; sedative-hypnotic; antianxiety	For status epilepticus, 5-10 mg IV; give 5 mg over 1 min. May be repeated every 10-15 min for a total dose of 30 mg; may repeat in 2-4 hr; or 0.2-0.5 mg/kg every 15-30 min for 2-3 doses; some specialists suggest 20 mg and titrate total dose over 10 min or until seizures stop; maximum dose in 24 hr is 100 mg	Respiratory depression; hypotension; drowsiness; lethargy; bradycardia; cardiac arrest	Monitor respiratory status, BP, HR; assess IV site for phlebitis and venous thrombosis
Lorazepam (Ativan)	Depresses subcortical areas of CNS; anticonvulsant; sedative-hypnotic; antianxiety	Status epilepticus: 4 mg IV over 1 min as initial dose; may repeat once in 10-15 min if seizure continues; or 0.05 mg/kg to a total of 4 mg; may repeat	Airway obstruction; apnea; blurred vision; confusion; excessive drowsiness; ↓ BP; ↓ HR; respiratory depression; somnolence	Same as diazepam

TABLE 12-7
DRUG THERAPY—cont'd

Drug	Actions/Uses	Adult Dosage/Route	Side Effects	Nursing Implications
		once in 10-15 min; do not exceed 8 mg in 12 hr Sedation: 2 mg IV over 1 min as initial dose; follow with infusion 0.5-1 mg/hr; titrate to achieve adequate sedation; increase in 1 mg/hr increments; up to 5-10 mg/hr		
Pentobarbital sodium (Nembutal sodium)	Barbiturate; sedation; hypnotic agent; anticonvulsant	100 mg IV initially; give over 2 min; additional doses in increments of 25-50 mg IV; give 50 mg over 1min; maximum dosage ranges from 200-500 mg IV Maintenance dose: 1.5-2 mg/kg IV q1-2h or an infusion of 0.5-3 mg/kg/hr; adjust to maintain pentobarbital blood level between 110 and 177 mg/L (10-50 mcg/mL) or ICP below 25	Hypotension; myocardial or respiratory depression, thrombocytopenia purpura. Overdose: apnea, coma, cough reflex depression, flat EEG, hypotension, sluggish or absent reflexes, pulmonary edema	Monitor ICP, CPP, VS, and hemodynamic responses; response of each patient is variable
Morphine	Narcotic analgesic; severe pain	IV injection: 4-10 mg IV over 4-5 min q3-4h; continuous IV infusion: 0.8-10 mg/hr; titrate to achieve pain relief with lowest dose	Confusion, sedation, respiratory depression, hypotension, bradycardia, constipation	Assess LOC, VS, level of sedation, and bowel function
Diprivan (Propofol)	Sedative (anesthetic); provides continuous sedation	Sedation of intubated mechanically ventilated: give as a continuous infusion; begin with 5 mcg/kg/min over 5 min; allow at least 5 min between adjustments to reach peak drug effect and avoid hypotension; increase slowly over 5-10 min by 5-10 mcg/kg/min to desired sedation; maintain at 5-50 mcg/kg/min	Bradycardia; cough; apnea; dyspnea; headache; hypotension; hypoventilation; burning, pain at IV site; hyperlipidemia; involuntary muscle movement	Monitor VS, ICP, CPP during infusion; assess level of sedation and response to medication; patients should awaken rapidly when the drug is discontinued; contra-indicated in patients with allergies to lipid emulsions; discard solution and IV line after 12 hr if administered directly from bottle; aseptic technique is essential; solution is capable of rapid growth of bacteria; do not use if sepa-ration of emulsion is evident
Nimodipine (Nimotop)	Calcium channel blocker; reduce neurological deficits after SAH; reduces vasospasm associated with SAH	60 mg PO q4h for 21 days; start within 96 hr of SAH	Hypotension, peripheral edema, ECG abnormalities, nausea/vomiting, diarrhea, altered liver function, HF, cough, dyspnea	Assess neurological status; monitor VS, I & O, daily weights; watch for signs of HF

↑, Increase; ↓, decrease; *ABG*, arterial blood gas; *BP*, blood pressure; *CNS*, central nervous system; *CPP*, cerebral perfusion pressure; *ECG*, electrocardiogram; *EEG*, electroencephalogram; *HF*, heart failure; *HR*, heart rate; *CVP*, central venous pressure; *I & O*, intake & output; *ICP*, intracranial pressure; *IM*, intramuscular; *IV*, intravenous; *IVPB*, intravenous piggyback; *LOC*, level of consciousness; *NS*, normal saline; *PE*, phenytoin equivalent; *PT*, prothrombin time; *SAH*, subarachnoid hemorrhage; *SCI*, spinal cord injury; *VS*, vital signs.

Data from Deglin, J.H. (2003). *Davis' drug guide for nurses.* 8th ed. Philadelphia: F.A. Davis; and Gahart, B., & Nazareno, A. (2003). *2003 Intravenous medications.* 18th ed. St. Louis: Mosby.

Another intervention used to lower ICP is drainage of CSF intermittently using an intraventricular catheter (ventriculostomy) (Figure 12-21). The decision to drain CSF from the ventriculostomy is based on the ICP exceeding a certain pressure that is individually established based on the patient's neurological condition.

Psychosocial Support

Family members of a critically ill neurological patient are different from family members of patients without neurological deficits. Neurological injury usually occurs without warning and may be severe. This places the family in a state of shock and disbelief. In addition, the patient has suffered an insult to the nervous system and may respond inappropriately or uncharacteristically or may not be able to respond at all to the family.

Neurological insults to the brain or spinal cord cause uncertainty in the patient's physical and mental outcomes. The personality and mental changes associated with brain insults can be devastating to the family. In Kosco and Warren's (2000) study, family members of the patients in the critical care unit indicated that assurance, proximity, and information ranked highest of all needs. Nurses fulfill these needs by providing information to family members and by providing psychosocial support to reduce their anxiety.

Head Injury

Head injury is a common occurrence in the United States, is the leading cause of trauma-related deaths in persons younger than 45 years, and occurs twice as often in male patients. With approximately 1.5 to 2 million traumatic brain injuries (TBIs) occurring each year, TBI is identified as a major cause of disability and death in most Western nations.

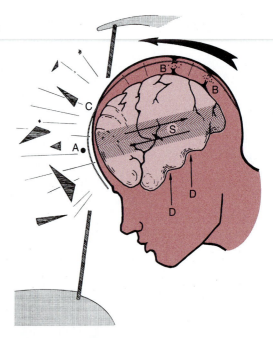

FIGURE 12-22 Closed blunt injury. Skull molding occurs at the site of impact. *A, Stippled line* indicates preinjury contour. *C, Solid line* indicates contour moments after impact, with bending inward at point *A* and bending outward at the vertex. *B,* Subdural veins torn as brain rotates forward. *S,* Shearing strains throughout the brain. *D,* Direct trauma to inferior temporal and frontal lobes over floors of the middle and anterior fossae. (From Eliasson, S. G., Prensky, A. L., & Hardin, W. B. [1978]. *Neurological pathophysiology.* 2nd ed. New York: Oxford University Press.)

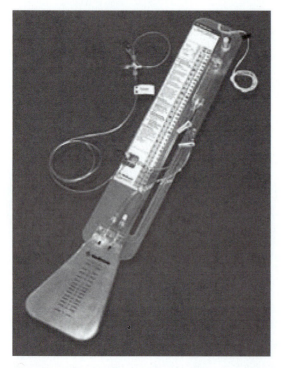

FIGURE 12-21 Becker external drainage and monitoring system. (Courtesy of Medtronic, Minneapolis, MN.)

Approximately $100 billion is spent annually in the United States on TBI. Survival is dependent on prompt emergency services and focused management of primary and secondary injuries (Davis, 2000; Littlejohns & Bader, 2001; Marik, Varon, & Trask, 2002).

PATHOPHYSIOLOGY

When head injury occurs, damage to the scalp, skull, meninges, and brain, including neuronal pathways, cranial nerves, and intracranial vessels, can occur (Figure 12-22). The head injury can be open or closed. With an open head injury, the scalp is torn or a fracture extends into the sinuses or middle ear. The meninges can also be penetrated. A closed head injury occurs when there is no break in the scalp. Acceleration-deceleration is a common mechanism for head injury. With this injury, the movement of the head follows a straight line, and the moving head (acceleration) hits a stationary object (deceleration). Rotation or a twisting of the brain within the cranial vault adds to the insult, and the extent of head injury can range from mild to severe (Figure 12-23).

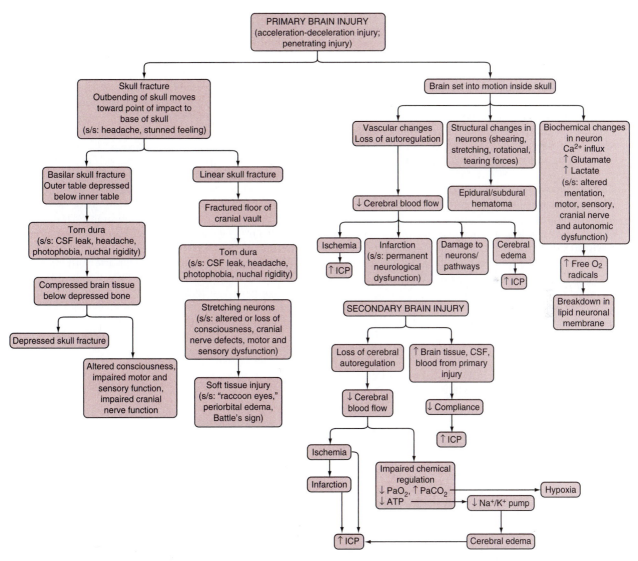

FIGURE 12-23 Pathophysiology flow diagram for head injury. *S/S*, Signs and symptoms; *CSF*, cerebral spinal fluid; *Ca²⁺*, calcium; *ICP*, intracranial pressure; *O₂*, oxygen; *PaO₂*, partial pressure of oxygen in arterial blood; *PaCO₂*, partial pressure of carbon dioxide in arterial blood; *ATP*, adenosine triphosphate; *Na⁺*, sodium; *K⁺*, potassium.

Scalp Lacerations

Scalp lacerations are common in head injury and can be associated with skull fracture. The scalp offers some resistance to compression and absorbs mild blows by distributing forces over the entire area of the scalp. The scalp is very vascular and can be the source of significant blood loss, which is difficult to stop. Once bleeding is stopped, it is important to clip the hair around the laceration. The wound is cleansed, débrided, inspected, and palpated for a depressed skull fracture. Inattention to these details can lead to infection.

Skull Fractures

The skull has high compressive strength and is somewhat elastic. After impact, the skull is compressed, and there is an in-bending of the skull at the point of impact and an out-bending at the vertex. The area of out-bending of tensile stresses creates a fracture line that moves toward the base of the skull.

There are several types of skull fractures after head injury—linear, depressed, comminuted, basilar—and various locations of the fractures (Figure 12-24). Mechanisms of closed head injury, along with associated signs and symptoms, are listed in Table 12-8.

Linear skull fracture. Linear skull fracture is the most common type. This fracture usually does not lead to significant complications unless there is an extension of the fracture to the orbit, sinus, or across a vessel. When there is extension of the fracture, the patient is admitted for observation of signs of intracranial bleeding and epidural hematoma.

Depressed skull fracture. A depressed skull fracture occurs when the outer table of the skull is depressed below the inner table of the surrounding intact skull. The dura may be intact, bruised, or torn. If the dura is torn, there is direct communication between the brain and the environment, and meningitis can occur. In addition, the compressed and bruised brain beneath the depressed bone is the source of focal neurological deficit and may become a seizure focus.

Comminuted skull fracture. Comminuted skull fracture occurs from multiple linear fractures with a depressed area at the site of impact. The fracture originates and radiates toward the impact site and base of skull. Comminuted skull fracture is referred to as an "eggshell fracture" because of the appearance of the skull.

Basilar skull fracture. A basilar skull fracture occurs at the base of the cranial vault and can extend into the anterior, middle, and posterior fossae. This type of fracture is difficult to confirm on a skull x-ray study and is diagnosed by clinical presentation of the patient (see Table 12-8). Battle's sign (bruising behind the ear) and the presence of "raccoon's eyes" (bilateral periorbital edema and bruising) may be indicative of a basilar skull fracture (Figure 12-25).

Dural tears are very common with a basilar skull fracture and may lead to meningitis. Drainage of CSF from the nose (rhinorrhea), postnasal drainage, or drainage of CSF from the ear (otorrhea) may be indicative of a dural tear. It is important to allow the CSF to flow freely. Nothing should be placed in the nose or ear, although small bandages under the nose or around the ear can be used to collect the drainage. The patient is instructed not to blow his or her nose.

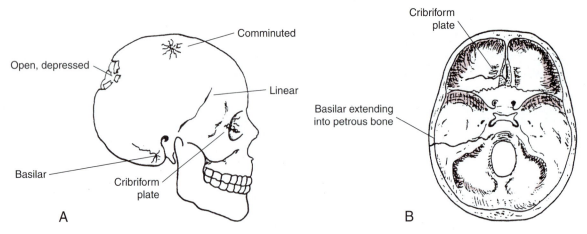

FIGURE 12-24 Skull fractures. **A,** Linear; open, depressed; basilar comminuted fractures. **B,** View of base of skull with fractures. (From Barker, E. [2002]. *Neuroscience nursing: A spectrum of care*, 2nd ed. St. Louis: Mosby.)

TABLE **12-8**

Mechanisms of Closed Head Injury with Associated Signs and Symptoms

Injury	Signs and Symptoms
SKULL FRACTURES (DEFORMATION OF SKULL, SECONDARY TO IMPACT)	
Linear: Starts at out-bent area, moves toward point of impact and to base of skull	Swelling, redness, bruising, tenderness on scalp, scalp laceration
Depressed: Outer table depressed below the inner table, associated with torn dura, and brain beneath depressed bone is bruised	Depressed area in contour of skull is palpable; CSF leak from nose, ear, postnasal; scalp bruising, tenderness, laceration
Basilar: Fracture in the anterior, middle, and/or posterior fossa along the floor of the cranial vault; dura is torn	
Anterior fossa	"Raccoon" or "panda" eyes, periorbital edema, CSF leak from nose, nasal congestion, cranial nerve deficits
Middle fossa	CSF leak ear, hemotympanum, Battle's sign, decreased hearing, cranial nerve deficits
Posterior fossa	Bruising at base of the neck, cranial nerve deficits
CELLULAR INJURIES TO BRAIN CELLS (INTERRUPTION OF NORMAL CONNECTIONS, NEURONS, PATHWAYS; BIOCHEMICAL CHANGES SECONDARY TO STRETCHING, SHEARING, ROTATIONAL, AND TEARING FORCES ASSOCIATED WITH IMPACT)	
Focal injuries: Concussion, contusion, avulsion	
Concussion: Temporary failure of impulse conduction	Altered LOC, confusion, disorientation, retrograde amnesia
Contusion: Injury can be to the area directly beneath impact (coup) or injury can be to the brain's poles (contrecoup)	Altered LOC, retrograde amnesia, motor deficits (weakness to paralysis), restlessness, combativeness, confusion, speech disturbances, cranial nerve dysfunction, decorticate and decerebrate posturing, abnormal breathing patterns, coma
Penetrating injuries: Injury is caused by deep laceration of brain tissue, damage to the ventricular system	Symptoms depend on location of injury and amount of tissue damage
Low-velocity: Stab wound: injury is caused by deep laceration of brain tissue, damage to the ventricular system	
High-velocity: Gunshot wound: extensive injury because of the entry of many bone fragments at the site; bullets spin irregularly, creating many paths and increasing the brain damage; and shock waves cause brain disruption	
Diffuse axonal injury: Tearing of axons and myelin sheaths, secondary to generalized movement of brain from impact	Prolonged coma, cranial nerve deficits, motor deficits
Secondary injury: Caused by increased ICP, cerebral edema, herniation, ischemia, hypoxia; these situations complicate intracerebral bleeds, focal and penetrating injuries	Prolonged coma, cranial nerve deficits, motor deficits
INTRACEREBRAL BLEEDING (CEREBRAL VESSELS ARE BROKEN OR SHEARED OFF SECONDARY TO IMPACT)	
Epidural: Tearing of an artery from a skull fracture; brisk bleeding and rapid accumulation in the epidural space	Short period of loss of consciousness then lucid, then confusion, irritability, headache, deterioration in LOC, motor, CN dysfunction
Subdural: Tearing of bridging cortical veins: blood accumulates in the space between the dura and arachnoid	Acute and subacute: Depressed LOC, pupil and extraocular movement changes, motor changes, headache

Continued

TABLE 12-8	
Mechanisms of Closed Head Injury with Associated Signs and Symptoms—cont'd	
Injury	**Signs and Symptoms**
	Chronic: personality changes, gait problems
Subarachnoid: Bleeding into the subarachnoid space from the rupture of a traumatic aneurysm	Altered LOC, headache, nuchal rigidity, photophobia
Intraventricular: Bleeding into the ventricles	Altered LOC, CN dysfunction, motor changes
Intracerebral: Bleeding into brain tissue, producing necrosis	Similar to focal injuries

CN, Cranial nerve; *CSF,* cerebrospinal fluid; *ICP,* intracranial pressure; *LOC,* level of consciousness.

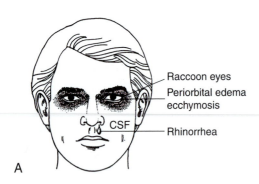

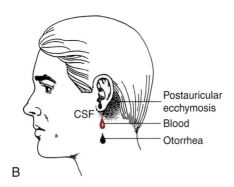

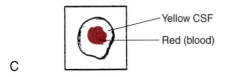

FIGURE 12-25 **A,** Raccoon eyes, rhinorrhea. **B,** Battle's sign with otorrhea. **C,** Halo or ring sign. (From Barker, E. [2002]. *Neuroscience nursing: A spectrum of care,* 2nd ed. St. Louis: Mosby.)

When blood encircled by a yellowish stain is seen on the dressing or bed linen, it is called the halo sign and usually indicates CSF (see Figure 12-25). If CSF is suspected in the drainage, a sample of the drainage is sent to the laboratory for analysis. If needed, suction catheters, nasogastric tubes, and endotracheal tubes are inserted through the mouth rather than the nose to avoid penetrating the brain as a result of the dural tear.

Brain Injury

Brain injury from head injury is classified as primary and secondary. Primary brain injury can be further divided into focal (subarachnoid hemorrhage [SAH], hematomas) and diffuse (diffuse axonal injury, contusion) lesions.

Primary brain injury. Primary brain injury is direct injury that occurs to the brain from an impact. With impact, the semisolid brain moves around inside the skull. The area under the direct impact is injured (coup injury). Injury to adjacent poles occurs from the movement of the brain inside the skull (contrecoup injury). The stretching, shearing, rotational, and tearing forces that result from impact cause an interruption of normal neuronal pathways and early vasogenic edema. This leads to cerebral edema and ischemia.

In brain injury, the initial insult causes biomechanical damage to the axonal membrane. The damaged cells trigger the inflammatory response and release of cytokines from macrophages that cause increased vascular permeability of the blood vessel wall. This allows fluid to leak from the intravascular space into the extracellular space and vasodilation, leading to vasogenic edema. The results are cerebral ischemia and impaired cerebral autoregulation. A series of biochemical events contributes to the overproduction of free oxygen radicals. Free oxygen radicals disrupt the cellular membrane and cause early neuronal deterioration. In addition, a loss of cellular calcium homeostasis inhibits cellular metabolism. Severe cellular energy failure occurs with liberation of glutamate and cellular acidosis. The decreased energy supply causes cellular ionic pumps to fail, and this leads to increased intracellular osmolality and cerebral edema. The patient shows signs or symptoms of impaired brain function and is unstable neurologically (Davis, 2000; Hickey, 2003; Lovasik, Kerr, & Alexander, 2001; Wong, 2000).

Concussion, contusion, penetrating injuries, hematomas, and intracerebral hemorrhage are all types of primary brain injury (see Table 12-8). Concussion represents a mild form of head injury, whereas contusion, penetrating injuries, hematomas, and hemorrhage constitute severe head injuries.

Concussion. Concussion occurs when there is a mechanical force of short duration applied to the skull. This injury results in the temporary failure of impulse conduction. The neurological deficits are reversible and are generally mild. Patients may lose consciousness for a few seconds at the time of injury, but lasting effects are not common.

Contusion. Contusion is the result of coup and contrecoup injuries, accompanied by bruising and generalized hemorrhage into brain tissue. Traumatic laceration of the cortical surface associated with contrecoup injuries may be greater than those seen directly under the point of impact. Signs and symptoms are variable (see Table 12-8).

Diffuse axonal injury. A more global injury is diffuse axonal involvement. With this injury, there is widespread white matter axonal damage secondary to tearing and shearing forces. This type of injury is associated with disruption of axons in the cerebral hemispheres, diencephalon, and brainstem. Clinically, these patients have no, or only minimal, signs of recovery. Signs and symptoms are variable (see Table 12-8).

Penetrating injury. Penetrating injuries are the result of low- or high-velocity forces such as gunshots, knives, or sharp objects. With this type of injury, there is a deep laceration of brain tissue and possible damage to the ventricular system. A low-velocity (stabbing) injury is limited to the tract of entry, and the greatest concern is bleeding and infection. A high-velocity (gunshot) injury causes extensive damage because of the entry of bone fragments at the site. In addition, because bullets spin irregularly, they create many paths and shock waves that cause extensive brain damage.

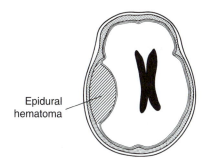

FIGURE 12-26 Epidural hematoma. (From Marshall, S. B., Marshall, L. F., Vos, H. R., & Chesnut, R. M. [1990]. *Neuroscience critical care.* Philadelphia: W. B. Saunders.)

Hematoma. Hematomas can occur as a result of injury. Acute hematomas can be life-threatening.

Epidural hematoma. Collection of blood in the space between the inner table of the skull and the dura causes an epidural hematoma (Figure 12-26). This hematoma is associated with a linear fracture of the temporal bone and results from the tearing of the middle meningeal artery. Arterial blood accumulates rapidly in this space. The patient usually experiences a lucid period before neurological deterioration. The lucid period can last for a few hours to 48 hours (Hickey, 2003). As the patient's condition deteriorates, the pupil on the side of the lesion becomes fixed and dilated.

Subdural hematoma. Collection of blood in the subdural space causes a subdural hematoma (Figure 12-27). It occurs when a surface vein is torn around the cortex. Subdural hematomas occur at all ages. In infants, they occur as a result of birth trauma; in the elderly, a subdural hematoma is most frequently

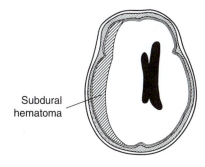

FIGURE 12-27 Subdural hematoma. (From Marshall, S. B., Marshall, L. F., Vos, H. R., & Chesnut, R. M. [1990]. *Neuroscience critical care.* Philadelphia: W. B. Saunders.)

the result of a fall. There are three kinds of subdural hematomas: acute, subacute, and chronic. *Acute* subdural hematoma occurs within 48 hours of an injury (Hickey, 2003). This type of hematoma is seen in deceleration injuries and is associated with contusions. *Subacute* hematomas occur 2 days to 2 weeks after an injury (Hickey, 2003). The onset of symptoms is much slower, and the symptoms are subtle. Prognosis is good for this kind of hematoma. *Chronic* subdural hematomas occur as a result of a low-velocity impact. They occur 2 weeks to several months after an injury. In the elderly, these hematomas usually result from a fall. Because symptoms are often subtle, diagnosis of chronic subdural hematoma may be missed in those who abuse alcohol and in the elderly population. Signs and symptoms of subdural hematomas are presented in Table 12-8.

Intracerebral hemorrhage. An intracerebral hemorrhage is a large hemorrhage into brain tissue that creates a mass lesion. This lesion can occur anywhere in the brain. Signs and symptoms vary according to the location of lesion (see Table 12-8).

Secondary brain injury. Secondary brain injury occurs after the initial trauma and causes damage to the neurons. Secondary brain injury is the result of hypoxia, hypotension, anemia, uncontrolled increased ICP, cerebral edema, hypermetabolic state, infection, and fluid and electrolyte imbalance. These insults add to the degree and extent of cellular dysfunction after head injury, can increase brain damage, and affect functional recovery. Proper management of a primary brain injury by ensuring adequate cerebral perfusion is essential to avoid secondary brain injury. These strategies include optimizing oxygenation and blood pressure; correct patient positioning; achieving normal blood glucose, normocapnia, normothermia or hypothermia; and diuretic therapy (Wong, 2000).

ASSESSMENT

The GCS is used as a guide in assessing a head-injured patient. It provides a standardized approach to assess level of consciousness objectively. In addition, the assessment of a patient is supplemented with a thorough neurological examination. Assessment should be specific to the area of the brain involved. It is best to perform a neurological assessment on the patient with the clinician who just provided care to the patient. This enables the nurse to be objective about the patient's neurological status and to identify changes in the assessment readily. All findings are documented clearly with a concise description of the patient's behavior.

Another area for assessment is respiratory status and pattern. Many severely head-injured patients arrive at the hospital hypoxic. A PaO_2 of less than 50 mm Hg causes vasodilation of cerebral vessels that increases CBF and increases ICP. This hypoxia can further compromise the patient's prognosis. Abnormal respiratory patterns must be reported and documented because pattern changes usually indicate deterioration in neurological status.

Additional assessment data include ICP, CPP, and hemodynamic monitoring. A head-injured patient requires the same laboratory and diagnostic studies as a patient with increased ICP.

NURSING DIAGNOSES

The same nursing diagnoses are applicable for a head-injured patient as for a patient with increased ICP (see Nursing Care Plan for the Patient with Increased Intracranial Pressure, Head Injury, or Acute Stroke). These diagnoses cover both primary and secondary head injuries.

MANAGEMENT
Nursing Interventions

Nursing interventions are the same as those for patients with increased ICP. Important considerations are the sequence and timing of nursing care activities. When the patient is having episodes of increased ICP, it is important to control the patient's environment and activities to minimize stimuli that contribute to the increased ICP. Monitoring the patient's response to nursing care assists the nurse in determining how to proceed with nursing care without jeopardizing the patient. For example, a patient with a severe head injury and excessively high ICP requires careful control of all activities and rest periods after each nursing intervention to allow the ICP to return to normal. Allowing frequent family visits also can aid in calming the patient. However, it is essential to observe the patient's response and to limit any interaction that has a negative physiological impact on the patient (Roland et al., 2001).

Medical (Nonsurgical) Interventions

The nonsurgical treatment of a patient with a head injury is the same as for a patient with increased ICP. The emphasis is on reducing ICP, maintaining the airway, providing oxygenation, maintaining cerebral perfusion, and preventing secondary head injury. Because the injured brain is sensitive to changes in body temperature, therapeutic hypothermia may also be implemented to protect the injured brain. Hypothermia decreases the cerebral metabolic rate and oxygen usage, lowers levels of glutamate and interleukin 1B, and decreases CBF and ICP. Protecting the brain by using hypothermia may improve outcomes in persons with TBI. Lowering the ambient room temperature, applying a cooling blanket, using antipyretics, sponging with cold water, and applying ice packs are ways to induce hypothermia. Additionally, monitoring the brain temperature to thermoregulate the patient is an optimal choice because the actual brain temperature is higher than blood temperature. The nurse should watch for adverse effects of hypothermia including dysrhythmias (atrial fibrillation), pulmonary infections, shivering, and coagulopathies (Wong, 2000).

Nutritional support after TBI is essential. Hypermetabolism, accelerated catabolism, and rampant nitrogen losses are recognized complications of TBI and SCI. They result in depletion of energy stores, loss of lean muscle mass, reduced protein synthesis, loss of gastrointestinal mucosal integrity, and immune compromise. If nutritional support is not aggressively initiated, the patient will have an increased susceptibility to infections, impaired wound healing, and difficulty in being weaned from the ventilator (Bullock et al., 2000).

Surgical Interventions

Various surgical procedures exist for head-injured patients. A patient with a depressed skull fracture may require surgery to remove bone fragments. Epidural and acute subdural hematomas are evacuated via bur holes to prevent a shift in brain tissue or herniation. Penetrating wounds to the skull and brain may necessitate a craniotomy to explore the pathway of the missile, repair laceration of intracranial vessels and brain tissue, remove bone fragments, and, in the case of a gunshot wound, retrieve the bullet.

Postoperative care is directed at the following: maintaining normal ICP, cerebral tissue perfusion, and airway; preventing fluid and electrolyte imbalance and complications of immobility; avoiding nutritional deficits; and reducing the incidence of infection. The craniotomy dressing is assessed for drainage including color, odor, and amount. Once the dressing is removed, the incision is assessed for swelling, redness, drainage, and tenderness. Persistent CSF drainage after surgery indicates a dural tear and may require a lumbar drain or intracranial CSF drain for several days to decrease pressure at the fistula site and to aid in healing. Patients with penetrating wounds to the brain are at high risk for the development of not only infections but also brain abscesses.

Acute Stroke

Stroke is a major public health problem. It is the third leading cause of death in the United States, the most frequent cause of adult disability, and the leading cause of long-term care. Although most strokes are preventable by controlling major risk factors such as hypertension, more than 700,000 new strokes occur each year in the United States, and there are more than 4 million stroke survivors (AHA, 2003). Persons who have a stroke have a 10-fold increased risk of having another stroke. The cost of hospitalization, rehabilitation, long-term care, and lost wages from stroke is estimated at $51 billion dollars annually. Stroke is a "brain attack" and as such calls for early recognition of the signs and symptoms and for rapid treatment. Strokes should be assessed and treated as a life-threatening emergency because optimal early treatment improves long-term outcome (Adams et al., 2003; Bhalla, Wolfe, & Rudd, 2001).

The hallmark of stroke is the sudden onset of focal neurological symptoms associated with changes in blood flow to the brain resulting from either a blockage of flow or hemorrhage. Stroke is also called cerebral infarction or death of a focal area of brain tissue. Stroke can present with maximal focal neurological deficits or as stroke in evolution in which symptoms evolve over several hours. Generally, the definition of stroke includes neurological deficits lasting 24 hours or longer (Hickey, 2003).

PATHOPHYSIOLOGY

Stroke occurs when the blood supply to the brain is disturbed by occlusion or hemorrhage. Brain cells survive only about 3 to 4 minutes when deprived of blood and oxygen. Normal CBF is 50 mL/100 g/min. When CBF drops to 25 mL/100 g/min, neurons become electrically silent but remain potentially viable for several hours. This region of brain is known as the ischemic penumbra (Figure 12-28). If CBF falls to less than the critical level of 10 mL/100 g/min, irreversible damage occurs. A cascade of metabolic disturbances follows, including lactic acidosis production,

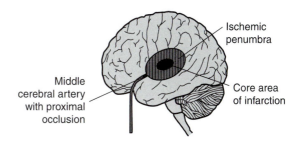

FIGURE 12-28 Proximal occlusion of left middle cerebral artery with infarction. Ischemic penumbra represents regional blood flow at about 25 mL/100 g/min. Ischemic penumbra is the area where acute therapies for stroke are targeted.

glutamate release, depletion of ATP, and the entry of sodium and calcium into the cells, leading to cytotoxic edema and mitochondrial failure (Bratina, Rapp, & Barch, 1997; Hickey, 2003). Strokes are classified as either ischemic (occlusive) or hemorrhagic (from ruptured blood vessels in the brain) (Figure 12-28).

Ischemic Stroke

Ischemic strokes are caused by large artery atherosclerosis, cardioembolic events, or by small artery occlusive disease (lacunar stroke), or the cause is unknown (cryptogenic stroke). Approximately 85% of all strokes are ischemic.

Large artery atherosclerosis. Large artery atherosclerosis is the result of stenosis caused by a cholesterol plaque, a thrombus superimposed on the plaque, or an embolus. An embolus occurs when a blood clot or plaque fractures, breaks off, and travels to the brain. This is sometimes referred to as artery-to-artery embolus. When a stenosis occurs, blood flow can be greatly reduced or occluded completely, causing ischemia and a stroke. Hypertension, diabetes, smoking, and possibly hyperlipidemia are risk factors for this type of stroke.

Cardioembolic stroke. Low-flow states or stasis of blood within the cardiac chambers may result in blood clot formation. The most common causes of cardioembolic stroke are atrial fibrillation (most common heart dysrhythmia in persons older than 65 years), rheumatic heart disease, acute myocardial infarction, endocarditis, mitral valve stenosis, and prosthetic heart valves (Figure 12-29). Because a cardiac abnormality is the source of the cerebral emboli, it is important to treat the underlying cardiac problem as well as the neurological problem. Patients commonly present with cortical features of stroke.

Lacunar stroke. Lacunar strokes (small vessel occlusive disease) are caused by chronic hypertension and diabetes. These disease states can cause a lipid material to coat the small cerebral arteries within deep structures of the brain. This process leads to a thickening of the arterial walls and ultimately a stroke. The characteristic locations of lacunar infarcts are the basal ganglia, subcortical white matter, thalamus, cerebellum, and brainstem. The recurrence rate of these strokes is about 10- to 12-fold compared with other types of stroke. This type of stroke can cause not only physical impairment, but also cognitive impairment such as vascular dementia. Patients can present with pure motor, pure sensory, or both motor and sensory features of stroke.

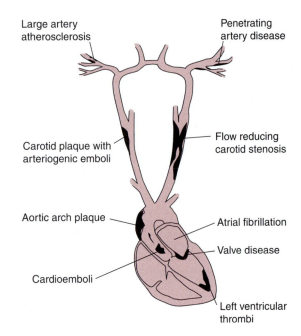

FIGURE 12-29 Common arterial and cardiac abnormalities causing ischemic stroke. (From Albers, G. W., Easton, J. D., Sacco, R. L., & Teal P. [1998]. Antithrombotic and thrombolytic therapy for ischemic stroke. *Chest, 114*[suppl 5]:683S-698S.)

Cryptogenic stroke. This subtype refers to stroke of unknown origin. This classification is used when the cause of stroke cannot be determined.

Hemorrhagic Stroke

Hemorrhagic strokes account for approximately 15% of all strokes. The most common causes of hemorrhagic stroke are primary intraparenchymal hemorrhage and ruptured cerebral aneurysm or arteriovenous malformations (AVMs). Secondary causes include overanticoagulation (warfarin, heparin, or recombinant tissue plasminogen activator [rt-PA]), vasopressor drugs, drug abuse (cocaine abuse), and coagulopathies caused by liver or renal failure or hematological disorders such as thrombocytopenia.

Intraparenchymal hemorrhage. About 10% of cerebral hemorrhages are referred to as intraparenchymal, with bleeding into the brain substance. These hemorrhages are usually caused by uncontrolled hypertension. When a blood vessel ruptures within the brain parenchyma, the escaped blood forms a mass that displaces and compresses brain tissue. The severity of the physiological symptoms depends on the location of the hemorrhage. If the bleeding is large enough, cerebral herniation may result.

Ruptured cerebral aneurysm with subarachnoid hemorrhage. Cerebral aneurysm is a localized dilation of the cerebral artery wall that causes the artery to weaken and become susceptible to rupture. The aneurysm usually occurs at the bifurcation of large arteries at the base of the brain (circle of Willis). Most patients with cerebral aneurysms are asymptomatic before the rupture unless they experience a warning "leak" or sentinel bleeding. The aneurysm commonly ruptures into the subarachnoid space of the basal cisterns and causes an SAH. Occasionally, the aneurysm ruptures into the ventricular system or into brain tissue.

Before rupturing, a cerebral aneurysm can mimic a mass lesion and compress brain tissue, cranial nerves, and blood vessels. Immediately after the rupture, bleeding into the adjacent tissue causes increased ICP, impaired cerebral autoregulation, and reduced CBF. The altered CBF causes ischemia and neurological changes. The bleeding can be stopped through the formation of a fibrin plug and platelet aggregation within the artery. Although the clot is necessary to prevent rebleeding, the clot can occlude blood flow or prevent CSF reabsorption through the arachnoid villi, thus leading to a condition called hydrocephalus.

After an aneurysm rupture, the patient can develop cardiac dysrhythmias, rebleeding, hydrocephalus, seizures, and vasospasm. Cardiac dysrhythmias can occur as a result of sympathetic nervous system stimulation. Increased sympathetic tone can cause elevated T waves, prolonged QT intervals, and ST abnormalities. Rebleeding after the initial aneurysm rupture can occur before surgical intervention is done. The mechanism causing the rebleeding is increased tension on the artery from hypertension or normal breakdown of the clot, which occurs 7 to 10 days after the initial hemorrhage. Early surgical intervention is recommended to prevent rebleeding.

SAH can impair the circulation and reabsorption of CSF. A blood clot can obstruct flow in the ventricular system, causing obstructive hydrocephalus. As blood enters the subarachnoid space, an inflammatory response is triggered that causes fibrosis and thickening of the arachnoid villi, thereby preventing reabsorption of CSF and producing hydrocephalus.

Seizures occurring within the first 12 hours after rupture are attributed to increased ICP. After the initial 12 hours and before the surgical clipping of the aneurysm, seizures are associated with rebleeding of the aneurysm. Because of the dangerous effects of seizures, most patients are given phenytoin to prevent seizure activity.

Cerebral vasospasm is a narrowing of arteries adjacent to the aneurysm that results in ischemia and infarction of brain tissue if it is not reversed. It is the leading cause of death after aneurysmal SAH. The usual period for vasospasm to occur can be anywhere between 3 and 14 days after the rupture.

The exact mechanism for vasospasm is unknown, but some factors that contribute to vasospasm are structural changes in the adjacent cerebral arteries, denervation of adjacent arteries, generation of oxygen free radicals, and release of vasoactive substances (serotonin, catecholamines, prostaglandins) that initiate vasospasm, inflammatory response, and calcium influx.

Arteriovenous malformation. AVM is a congenital abnormality: tangled, dilated vessels that form an abnormal communication network between the arterial and venous systems (Figure 12-30). Arterial blood is directly shunted into the venous system without a capillary network. This predisposes the vessels to rupture and hemorrhage into the ventricular system or subarachnoid system, thus causing SAH. Impaired perfusion of the cerebral tissue adjacent to the AVM also occurs. The size and location of the AVMs differ; however, all cause varying degrees of ischemia, scarring of brain tissue, abnormal tissue development, compression, hemorrhage, and hydrocephalus. AVMs are more prevalent in male than in female patients and are commonly diagnosed after a patient has experienced a seizure (Hickey, 2003; Ogilvy et al., 2001).

ASSESSMENT

Early identification of a stroke is imperative so rapid treatment can be initiated. The public must be educated on the symptoms of a brain attack because early intervention and treatment lead to positive patient outcomes. Patients at high risk of stroke are taught the signs and symptoms of stroke and to seek medical attention immediately (Box 12-2).

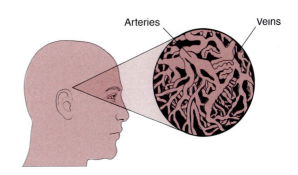

FIGURE 12-30 Arteriovenous malformation (AVM). (From Ignatavicius, D. D., & Workman, M. L. [2001]. *Medical-surgical nursing: Critical thinking for collaborative care.* 4th ed. St Louis: Mosby.)

BOX 12-2

Signs and Symptoms of Stroke

- Weakness or numbness of one side of the body (face, arm, leg, or any combination of these)
- Slurred speech
- Inability to comprehend what is being said
- Visual disturbance (transient loss of vision in one or both eyes [transient monocular blindness] or a visual field deficit)
- Dizziness, incoordination or ataxia, double vision, vertigo
- Nausea or vomiting
- Severe headache ("worst headache of my life")

Assessment in the emergency department includes an eyewitness description of symptoms, identification of exact time symptoms started, and a neurological assessment.

The neurological examination includes evaluating mental status (level of consciousness, arousal, orientation), cranial nerve function, motor strength, sensory function, neglect, coordination, and deep tendon reflexes. The National Institutes of Health Stroke Scale (NIHSS) (Table 12-9) may be used to assess severity of presenting signs and symptoms, especially if the patient is a candidate for thrombolytic therapy. Assessment of airway, breathing, and circulation is a priority to stabilize the patient who has had a stroke. Vital signs must be monitored, generally every 15 minutes. Blood pressure elevations are common in these patients. Because reducing the blood pressure can decrease blood flow and oxygenation to the ischemic brain tissue, a gradual lowering of the blood pressure is recommended to prevent enlargement of the infarcted area and worsening of the neurological deficit. The goal is to keep the MAP close to 120 mm Hg. Monitoring the respiratory pattern is important because changes can indicate that the stroke is extending and more neurological damage is occurring. Hypoxia after stroke is common as a result of concurrent medical conditions such as aspiration, pneumonia, hypoventilation, atelectasis, and pulmonary embolism (Johnston et al., 1998; Hilker et al., 2003). Baseline pulse oximetry on room air is obtained, and supplemental oxygen is added when SaO_2 is less than 95%. Cardiac assessment including the presence of cardiac dysrhythmia is important to determine whether the stroke was caused by cardiac disease. Intravenous access is obtained, and normal saline infusions are started. Hypertonic solutions are avoided. Laboratory studies include electrolytes, cardiac enzymes, blood count,

urinalysis, and coagulation studies. Serum glucose is obtained because approximately 20% to 55% of patients with stroke are initially hyperglycemic (Bhalla, Wolfe, & Rudd, 2001). In addition, 8% to 20% of patients with stroke are diabetic (Bhalla, Wolfe, & Rudd, 2001). Several studies indicate that, overall, people with hyperglycemia have poorer outcomes as compared with normoglycemic patients. The hyperglycemia seems to increase neuronal injury (Sabin-Alvarez et al., 2003).

Once the patient is transferred to the critical care unit, assessments are compared with the baseline assessments performed in the emergency department. Hemodynamic instability is common in an acute stroke because of cardiac disorders and the sympathetic response; therefore, assessment of the airway, vital signs, and fluid and electrolyte status continues to be a priority. Elderly patients with stroke often present with dehydration. Dehydration after a stroke can cause an increased hematocrit and reduced blood pressure that can worsen the ischemic process. Dehydration is caused by inadequate water intake, drowsiness, dysphagia, possible infection, diuretic use, and uncontrolled diabetes (Bhalla, Wolfe, & Rudd, 2001; Leonard, 2002). In a patient with an acute stroke, ICP, hemodynamic status, laboratory values, and cardiac function are monitored. Ongoing assessments are similar to those in patients with increased ICP.

Ruptured Cerebral Aneurysm with Subarachnoid Hemorrhage

Before the aneurysm rupture, the patient may complain of a localized headache, stiff neck (nuchal rigidity), pain above and behind the eye, and photophobia. Assessment findings may include dilated pupil, extraocular deficit, and ptosis. When arterial blood enters the subarachnoid space, its presence is irritating to the meninges. If conscious, the patient may complain of "the worst headache of my life," the patient may have photophobia and vomiting, may be unresponsive longer than an hour, and may have nuchal rigidity (Bederson et al., 2000; van Gijn & Rinkel, 2001). These patients may also experience increased ICP, alteration in CBF, hemodynamic instability, vasospasm, rebleeding, and hydrocephalus.

Neurological assessment includes level of consciousness, motor and sensory deficits, and pupillary response. Patients with SAH are usually anxious and agitated as a result of pain, altered level of consciousness, and cognitive changes.

DIAGNOSTIC TESTS

Diagnostic tests are performed to differentiate ischemic from hemorrhagic stroke and to establish baseline parameters to monitor the effects of treatment (Adams et al., 2003).

TABLE 12-9

National Institutes of Health Stroke Scale (NIHSS)

Item Tested	Title/Domain	Response/Score
1A	LOC	0 – alert 1 – drowsy 2 – obtunded 3 – coma/unresponsive
1B	Orientation	0 – answers both correctly 1 – answers one correctly 2 – answers none correctly
1C	Response/commands (two)	0 – performs both correctly 1 – performs one correctly 2 – performs none correctly
2	Gaze	0 – normal horizontal movements 1 – partial palsy 2 – complete gaze palsy
3	Visual fields	0 – no visual field defect 1 – partial hemianopia 2 – complete hemianopia 3 – bilateral hemianopia
4	Facial movement	0 – normal 1 – minor facial weakness 2 – partial facial weakness 3 – complete unilateral palsy
5	Motor function (arm) a. left b. right	0 – no drift 1 – drift before 5 seconds 2 – falls before 10 seconds 3 – no effort against gravity 4 – no movement
6	Motor function (leg) a. left b. right	0 – no drift 1 – drift before 5 seconds 2 – falls before 10 seconds 3 – no effort against gravity 4 – no movement
7	Limb ataxia	0 – no ataxia 1 – ataxia in one limb 2 – ataxia in two limbs
8	Sensory	0 – no sensory loss 1 – mild sensory loss 2 – severe sensory loss
9	Best language	0 – normal 1 – mild aphasia 2 – severe aphasia 3 – mute or global aphasia
10	Articulation dysarthria	0 – normal 1 – mild dysarthria 2 – severe dysarthria
11	Extinction or inattention	0 – absent 1 – mild (loss 1 sensory modality) 2 – severe (loss 2 modalities)

Total NIHSS Score _____ (0-42)

LOC, level of consciousness. From the National Institute of Neurological Disorders and Stroke at the National Institutes of Health. (2003). Bethesda, MD.

Initial Diagnostic Testing

- Emergency CT scan without contrast
- Twelve-lead electrocardiogram
- Chest x-ray study
- Review of time of onset and inclusion criteria for patients eligible for rt-PA, including NIHSS assessment
- Complete blood count (red blood cells, hemoglobin, hematocrit, platelet count)
- Coagulation studies: prothrombin time, activated partial prothrombin time, International Normalized Ratio (INR)
- Serum electrolytes and glucose
- Urinalysis
- Troponin and cardiac enzymes, to rule out myocardial infarction
- Cervical x-ray studies, to rule out head trauma

Additional Diagnostic Testing

The following recommendations were suggested by Adams and associates (2003):

- MRI with diffusion and perfusion images (sensitive to the presence and extent of ischemia)
- Arteriography (defines shallow ulcerated plaques, thrombus, aneurysms, dissections, multiple lesions, AVMs, collateral blood flow)
- Digital subtraction angiography (detects carotid occlusion and information about vertebral arteries)
- Doppler carotid studies (detect middle cerebral artery stenosis or occlusion)
- Transesophageal echocardiogram (identifies source of emboli from the heart)

MANAGEMENT

Nursing Diagnoses

A patient with stroke has similar nursing diagnoses as a patient with increased ICP and head injury. Refer to the Nursing Care Plan for the Patient with Increased Intracranial Pressure, Head Injury, or Stroke. Additional nursing diagnoses include Impaired Swallowing, Disturbed Sensory Perception, Hyperthermia, Acute Pain, Decreased Cardiac Output, Risk for Constipation, Risk for Imbalanced Fluid Volume, Risk for Infection, Imbalanced Nutrition, Impaired Physical Mobility, Risk for Impaired Skin Integrity, and Impaired Verbal Communication.

Ischemic Stroke

Thrombolytic candidates. Early intervention for ischemic stroke is recommended. rt-PA is the only approved therapy for acute ischemic stroke (NIH-NINDS and Stroke rt-PA Stroke Study, 1995). The medication, rt-PA, lyses the clot and restores blood flow to the ischemic penumbra, which limits secondary brain damage and improves overall neurological function. rt-PA does not affect the infarcted area but revitalizes the ischemic penumbra. Careful assessment of patients potentially eligible for thrombolytic therapy must be made. The NIH-NINDS and Stroke rt-PA Stroke Study (1995) delineated several inclusion and exclusion criteria for this drug (Box 12-3). rt-PA is recommended for acute ischemic stroke, if it is administered within 3 hours of the onset of symptoms. Stroke severity is assessed using the NIHSS (Spilker et al., 1997).

Before the administration of rt-PA, two peripheral intravenous lines are inserted, one for the administration of rt-PA and one for fluids. Any indwelling catheters that are needed (Foley, nasogastric tubes) are placed. After the administration of rt-PA, no invasive procedures are performed because of a higher risk of bleeding. rt-PA is administered within 3 hours after stroke symptom onset. Administration after 3 hours has not shown to be beneficial. The dose is 0.9 mg/kg up to a maximum of 90 mg. Initially, 10% of the total dose is administered as an intravenous bolus over 1 minute. The remaining 90% is infused over the next 60 minutes. Antithrombotics such as heparin, warfarin, and aspirin are withheld for the 24 hours after administration of rt-PA to prevent bleeding complications (Braimah et al., 1997; Hinkel & Bowman 2003).

Hemorrhage is the most common complication after rt-PA administration. Early detection of neurological changes and maintaining blood pressure less than 185 mm Hg systolic or 110 mm Hg diastolic may reduce the incidence of hemorrhage. Administration of rt-PA is contraindicated in patients with systolic blood pressure greater than 185 mm Hg or diastolic blood pressure greater than 110 mm Hg on two readings because of the increased risk of hemorrhage. Antihypertensive medication is given to these patients. The highest risk of intracerebral hemorrhage after thrombolytic therapy is within the first 36 hours. Intracerebral hemorrhage occurs as a result of secondary bleeding into the area of infarct, also known as hemorrhagic transformation. Signs and symptoms of intracerebral hemorrhage manifest as increased ICP or cerebral herniation. If intracerebral hemorrhage is suspected, the rt-PA infusion is stopped, an emergency noncontrast CT scan of the head is obtained, and fresh frozen plasma or platelets are administered (Barch et al., 1997). Internal bleeding can also occur. Signs and symptoms include hypotension, tachycardia, pallor, restlessness, or low back pain. Stool, urine, and gastric secretions are monitored for the presence of blood. Intravenous sites and gums are

BOX 12-3

Inclusion/Exclusion Criteria for the Administration of Tissue Plasminogen Activator for Acute Ischemic Stroke

ELIGIBILITY CRITERIA FOR THROMBOLYTIC THERAPY

Inclusion Criteria
1. Onset of stroke symptoms <3 hours
2. Clinical diagnosis of ischemic stroke with a measurable deficit using the National Institutes of Health Stroke Scale
3. Age >18 years
4. CT scan consistent with ischemic stroke

Exclusion Criteria
1. Stroke symptoms >3 hours of symptoms onset
2. Rapidly improving minor or major stroke (i.e., transient ischemic attack)
3. Evidence of intracerebral bleed including intraparenchymal subarachnoid hemorrhage or other pathology (neoplasm, AVM or aneurysm on CT scan)
4. Systolic blood pressure >185 mm Hg or diastolic blood pressure >110 mm Hg
5. Glucose <50 mg/dL or >400 mg/dL
6. Rapidly improving or deteriorating neurological signs or minor symptoms
7. Recent myocardial infarction
8. Seizure at the onset of stroke
9. Active internal bleeding (e.g., urinary) within 21 days
10. Arterial puncture at noncompressible site
11. Known bleeding diathesis, including but not limited to:
    a. Current use of oral anticogulants (e.g., warfarin sodium) with prothrombin time of >15 seconds
    b. Administration of heparin with 48 hours preceding the onset of stroke and have an elevated activated partial thromboplastin time at presentation
    c. Platelet count <100,000/μL
12. Lumbar puncture within 7 days, major surgery within 14 days

Dosing: 0.9 mg/kg Intravenously
Give bolus of 10% of total calculated dose intravenously over 1 minute
Give the remaining 90% over the next 60 minutes

AVM, arteriovenous malformation; *CT,* computed tomography.
Modified from the NINDS t-PA Stroke Trial Protocol Guidelines and the Activase Package insert.

monitored for signs of external bleeding. Baseline coagulation studies are compared with current studies (AANN Clinical Guideline Series, 1998).

Neurological assessment and vital signs (level of consciousness, motor and sensory testing, pupillary response, blood pressure, respiration rate, pulse and temperature) are performed every 15 minutes for the first 2 hours, every 30 minutes for the next 6 hours, and every hour for 16 hours. Accurate intake and output are maintained. Continuous cardiac monitoring is done throughout the hyperacute phase (first 24 to 72 hours). Oxygen therapy is indicated until SaO$_2$ is stable (greater than 95%). Pneumonia is a common complication after stroke; therefore, nebulizing therapy may be indicated, with frequent repositioning (Hilker et al., 2003).

Nonthrombolytic candidates. For a patient with stroke who is a not a candidate for thrombolytic therapy, interventions include neurological, respiratory, and cardiac assessments. These assessments and vital signs are performed every 1 to 2 hours during the first 24 hours after stroke: blood pressure, pulse, respiratory rate, temperature, pupillary response, motor and sensory testing, and level of consciousness. Blood pressure is controlled to prevent bleeding while maintaining an adequate CPP. For patients with uncontrolled hypertension, blood pressure is managed carefully with intravenous medications including labetalol or nicardipine. Rapid drops in blood pressure can cause further neurological deterioration by decreasing cerebral perfusion and extending the area of cerebral ischemia. Laboratory tests (complete blood count, chemistries, urinalysis, coagulations studies, cardiac enzymes) are performed, and a urinary catheter is usually indicated.

Incidence of cerebral herniation peaks at about 72 hours after the stroke. Signs and symptoms of cerebral herniation include a decrease in level of consciousness, pupillary changes (dilation on the side of herniation), respiratory pattern changes, and posturing (decerebrate or decorticate). Other interventions include the administration of medications, observation for medication side effects, and maintenance of hemodynamic stability. Anticoagulants and thrombolytics are only used for patients with an ischemic stroke. Antithrombotics such as warfarin, aspirin, and clopidogrel (Plavix), as well thrombolytics, antihypertensive agents, and anticonvulsants, may be indicated. Maintaining adequate fluid balance is crucial to achieve proper hydration. Monitoring temperature and maintaining normothermia are important. Temperature elevations exacerbate ischemia, increase the metabolic needs of the brain, and thus cause further neuronal damage. A 10% rise in oxygen consumption occurs with each centigrade degree rise in temperature. Hyperthermia may be the result of direct injury or bleeding into the hypothalamus, systemic infection, or drug-induced fever from anticonvulsant medications (Bhalla, Wolfe, & Rudd, 2001; Castillo, Davalos, Marrugat, & Noya, 1998; Ginsberg & Busto, 1998). Antipyretics such as acetaminophen, 325 to 650 mg every 4 to 6 hours as needed, may be given. Aspiration precautions are implemented including elevating the head of the bed and maintaining nothing-by-mouth status until a formal swallow study rules out dysphagia (Mann, Hankey, & Cameron, 1999).

If the patient presents for treatment longer than 3 hours after the onset of symptoms, the patient is assessed for progression of stroke symptoms. Anticoagulants, such as heparin, may be given in this situation, although clinical trials have not proved efficacy (Adams, et al., 2003). Because anticoagulants are contraindicated in hemorrhagic stroke, repeat CT scanning is necessary, to be certain that the cause of stroke progression is not hemorrhagic. Antiplatelet agents including aspirin, clopidogrel, or dipyridamole plus aspirin (Aggrenox) are recommended for secondary prevention of ischemic stroke.

Other Ischemic Events

Transient ischemic attacks. Transient ischemic attacks (TIAs) are defined as stroke symptoms that resolve within 24 hours. TIAs are important to recognize because if they are correctly diagnosed, preventive measures can be initiated to avoid stroke. TIAs are commonly caused by stenosis of the carotid arteries. TIAs can present as transient monocular blindness, a transient occlusion of the central retinal artery. Although TIA symptoms mimic those of stroke, TIA symptoms by definition, last 24 hours or less. Usually TIAs last about 5 to 10 minutes. Unfortunately, persons experiencing a TIA often ignore the symptoms because the symptoms are typically painless and short-lived. Within a year of having a TIA, many persons have a stroke and sustain permanent neurological deficits. Generally, patients presenting with symptoms of TIA should receive a complete stroke workup to determine the cause of TIA. Patients may be managed with anticoagulants such as heparin if the symptoms wax and wane or with antiplatelet therapy such as aspirin if symptoms are stable and do not recur.

People experiencing TIA with carotid stenosis may be evaluated for carotid endarterectomy or carotid stenting. If a patient has carotid stenosis greater than 69% on the symptomatic side, carotid endarterectomy is recommended (NASCET collaborators, 1995). Carotid stenting is still considered experimental; however, research trials are in progress.

Hemorrhagic Stroke

Intraparenchymal stroke. Blood pressure is carefully monitored in these patients to prevent recurrent hemorrhage. Elevations in blood pressure are not usually treated unless the blood pressure is greater than 200/110 mm Hg or the patient has a history of heart failure. If treatment is required, blood pressure is lowered cautiously to prehemorrhage levels. Maintaining blood pressure control is important to prevent continued bleeding.

Medical assessment focuses on determining the size and location of the intracranial hemorrhage and whether it is amenable to surgical intervention. Small clots usually resolve without surgery. In these instances, more aggressive blood pressure management may be indicated. If surgery is considered, it is usually for bleeding that has occurred on the non-dominant side. Surgery on the dominant side can cause severe deficits in language, speech, and motor and/or sensory function. Surgery is considered in patients with hematomas larger than 3 cm or who are deteriorating neurologically. Comatose patients with large lesions usually have poorer outcomes, regardless of treatment. (Broderick et al., 1999)

RESEARCH ANALYSIS

ARTICLE REFERENCE

Davis, A., & Gimenez, A. (2003). Cognitive-behavioral recovery in comatose patients following auditory sensory stimulation. *Journal of Neuroscience Nursing, 35*(4), 202-209.

STUDY OVERVIEW

This quasiexperimental study was conducted to determine whether an increase and improvement in arousal between the initial baseline assessment and discharge assessment occurred with the introduction of an auditory sensory stimulation program (SSP) in patients with traumatic brain injury (TBI). Additionally, the study was performed to identify the effect of sensory stimulation on the patient's cerebral and cardiopulmonary status.

The sample consisted of patients hospitalized with severe TBI. Patients suffered from various types of closed head injuries, with motor vehicle collision being the most frequent mechanism of injury. Subjects were admitted to the study a minimum of 3 days after sustaining the TBI, had a Glasgow Coma Scale (GCS) score of less than 8, a stable intracranial pressure (ICP) defined as less than 20 mm Hg for 24 hours, and a Ranchos Los Amigos Level of Cognitive Functioning Scale (RLA) indicating either unresponsive to sensory stimuli, or responding at low or inconsistent levels to sensory stimuli.

Twelve male subjects were chosen for this study, with age ranging from 17 to 55 years. Intervention participants (n = 9) were enrolled first, followed by control group participants (n = 3). At the beginning and completion of the study, arousal, cognition, behavior, and outcome measures were recorded on all participants. The intervention group received a variety of auditory stimulation that included familiar and unfamiliar voice patterns (family voices, television, radio), tone frequencies (claps, bells, music), and messages that required simple to complex interpretation. The type and duration of the stimuli stayed constant, but the sequence of delivery and number of stimulation sessions varied daily, based on visitation time of family and friends, physiological stability, and the need for procedures and diagnostic tests. Stimuli were delivered five to eight times between 8 AM and 5 PM for up to 7 days. The sessions lasted 5 to 15 minutes, with 1-hour intervals between sessions. Before and after each intervention, clinical parameters (mean arterial pressure [MAP], ICP, cerebral perfusion pressure, heart rate [HR], respiratory rate [RR]), GCS score (arousal), RLA scale (cognition), Disability Rating Scale (outcome), and Sensory Stimulation Assessment Measure (behavior) were documented. Both groups received routine nursing care and rehabilitation according to the standard of care established by the hospital for patients with TBI.

Greater improvement in GCS and RLA scores between baseline and final testing was demonstrated in those participants who received auditory sensory stimulation. However, the scores were not statistically significant between groups. When the sensory stimulation was applied, increases in ICP were not statistically or clinically significant. Significant increase in MAP, HR, and RR were isolated responses that did not change the patient's medical status or require termination or postponement of the stimulation.

CRITIQUE

Description of subject selection, auditory intervention, and standardized scales used to measure changes in arousal were well documented. The limitations of the scales to detect subtle physiological changes in arousal were stated. The sample was not statistically different between groups for age, severity of injury, and baseline GCS score. The small sample size was clearly identified as a limitation. The difference in mean time for entry into the study between the intervention group (9.4 days) and the control group (6.0 days) was discussed and may have influenced findings. The implications of undiagnosed medical problems or complications on outcomes were acknowledged.

NURSING IMPLICATION FOR PRACTICE

Although the small sample size and lack of statistical significance between groups did not provide unequivocal support for use of SSP after TBI, a progressive improvement in arousal after early implementation of a SSP was acknowledged. Using an early and repeated auditory SSP for patients with TBI deserves further research. Although no participants incurred adverse physiological effects from SSP, it is important to analyze changes in cerebral and cardiopulmonary status when any sensory stimulation is applied to patients with TBI.

Subarachnoid Hemorrhage

Management of blood pressure is an important treatment of SAH associated with a ruptured aneurysm. Medications are administered to reduce blood pressure to prehemorrhage levels without causing vasospasm. Neurological status is assessed frequently using the GCS and monitoring for focal deficits and pupillary changes. Temperature monitoring is important because persons with SAH have fever. Elevation of the head of the bed may reduce headache. A nasogastric tube is placed for nutritional support. Measures for deep vein thrombosis prevention such as compression stockings or pneumatic leg sleeves are placed. Other important interventions include providing a quiet environment, analgesia, and bed rest. Dimming the room lights and turning down the volume on the patient's monitors can be beneficial in reducing noxious stimuli. After aneurysm rupture, complications can occur including cardiac dysrhythmias, rebleeding, hydrocephalus, seizures, and vasospasm causing further neurological injury (Galley, 2000; Kirkness et al., 2002).

Monitoring for signs of vasospasm is of paramount importance, because early intervention results in better patient outcomes. Nimodipine, a neurospecific calcium channel blocker, reduces the incidence and severity of deficits associated with SAH. The recommended dosage is 60 mg every 4 hours for 21 days. Vasospasm is often treated with volume expansion to increase CPP. The three modalities used are hypervolemia, hemodilution, and hypertension, also known as "triple H therapy." Hypervolemia and hemodilution refer to increasing the blood volume by using crystalloids, colloids, albumin, plasma protein fraction, or blood. Hypertension is based on the patient's baseline blood pressure. These interventions can be used in combination or alone to prevent the release of catecholamines, thereby preventing vasoconstriction (Campbell & Edwards, 1997). If the patient's blood pressure becomes lower than prehemorrhage levels, vasoactive infusions, such as dopamine, may be administered.

More recent therapies for the treatment of symptomatic vasospasm include papaverine application and angioplasty. Papaverine increases the diameter of the vasospastic blood vessel. The effect of papaverine application lasts less than 24 hours. The frequency of clinical improvement with papaverine application is approximately 70% (Fisher & Bogousslavsky, 2001). Papaverine application is performed about 8 days after SAH when symptoms of vasospasm usually occur. Angioplasty has a longer-lasting effect than papaverine application alone, but it is associated with a risk of vessel rupture and requires anticoagulation. Recurrent vasospasm after angioplasty has been reported.

Complications of angioplasty include increased ICP, transient neurological deficits, and mydriasis (asymmetric pupils).

The CT scan helps to differentiate aneurysms from AVMs (Johnston et al., 2002; van Gijn & Rinkel, 2001). However, the definitive diagnosis is determined by cerebral angiography. Early surgical intervention (within 24 hours of admission) is recommended for patients in good neurological condition whose aneurysm is surgically accessible. The goal is to operate when there is minimal neurological dysfunction and before any episodes of rebleeding or vasospasm occur.

Surgery for a cerebral aneurysm involves occluding the neck of the aneurysm using a ligature or metal clip, reinforcing the sac by wrapping the sac with muscle, fibrin foam, or solidifying polymer, or proximal ligation of a feeding vessel. If the neck of the aneurysm is narrow, using a ligature or metal clip is desirable. When the neck of the aneurysm is too broad, reinforcing the aneurysmal sac is the goal of surgery. Proximal ligation may be preferred when the aneurysm is in the internal carotid artery. The disadvantage of this procedure is decreased CBF to certain parts of the brain.

Interventional techniques such as endovascular therapy with coils may be used to occlude the aneurysm. This therapy consists of navigating a microcatheter through the femoral artery to the aneurysm and placing platinum coils into the aneurysm sac. Thrombosis occurs, thus occluding the aneurysm from the feeder vessel. This technique can be done with ruptured or unruptured aneurysms.

Patients with severe neurological compromise after a ruptured aneurysm may benefit from emergency ventriculostomy. The ventriculostomy assists in treating the hydrocephalus associated with the bleeding.

Arteriovenous Malformation

Spontaneous bleeding from an AVM can occur into the ventricular or subarachnoid system. Blood spreads through the basal cisterns over the convexity of the brain into the spinal subarachnoid system. Arterial vasospasm may occur from irritation of blood vessels resulting from blood in CSF (Ogilvy et al., 2001). If vasospasm does occur, a decrease in local perfusion, ischemia to the area, a risk of infarction, and edema in the area may follow, causing a further decrease in perfusion. Hemorrhage from an AVM is low-pressure bleeding, and the mortality from such a hemorrhage is lower than from a ruptured aneurysm. The rebleeding rate is also much lower than that of an aneurysm.

Treatment interventions include embolization, surgical removal of the AVM, radiotherapy, or a combination of all three. Surgery for removal of an AVM is done either as a single step or in multiple stages.

Postoperatively, the major problem is breakthrough bleeding from cauterized vessels. Rapid increases in blood pressure during recovery from anesthesia are to be avoided.

POSTOPERATIVE CARE

The postoperative care of a patient who has undergone a neurosurgical procedure involves frequent and ongoing hemodynamic, respiratory, metabolic, and neurological assessments. Neurological assessments are done every 15 to 30 minutes for the first 8 to 12 hours postoperatively, then every hour while the patient is in the critical care unit. Oxygenation and tissue perfusion are monitored. Chest X-rays, CT scans, EEG scans, and other diagnostic tests may be necessary to monitor progress.

The position of the head of the bed depends on the specific surgical procedure and the physician's preference. Unconscious patients are never positioned on their backs because the tongue can slip backward and obstruct the airway. Endotracheal intubation may be necessary to protect the airway. The neck is maintained in a neutral position.

Postoperative complications include cerebral hemorrhage, increased ICP, hydrocephalus, seizures, and vasospasm (Barker, 2002). Intracerebral hemorrhage is detected by a decline in neurological status and signs of increasing ICP. It is confirmed by CT scan. Treatment depends on CT findings and may require emergency surgery.

Hydrocephalus can develop any time during the postoperative course as a result of edema or bleeding into the subarachnoid space. Blood can interfere with the normal absorption of CSF by plugging the arachnoid villi. Treatment includes placement of a ventriculostomy to drain CSF temporarily. If the hydrocephalus does not resolve, a surgical shunting procedure may be indicated to relieve the brain of excessive CSF and to prevent cerebral atrophy (Greenberg, 2001).

Seizures can occur at any time but are most common within the first 7 days after surgery. Focal seizures in the form of twitching of selected muscles, particularly of the face and hand, are seen. Because seizures are common, these patients usually receive prophylactic anticonvulsants postoperatively, most commonly phenytoin. Serum levels of phenytoin are monitored to maintain a therapeutic range.

Studies have shown that organized stroke units have better patient outcomes by decreasing the morbidity and mortality after stroke (Leonard, 2002; Sinha & Warburton, 2000). Nurses on stroke units are trained in the neurosciences, provide focused care, and can educate patients about stroke risk reduction and risk factor modification.

Seizures and Status Epilepticus

A seizure is an abnormal electrical discharge in the brain caused by a variety of neurological disorders, systemic diseases, and metabolic disorders. Seizures consist of repetitive depolarization of hyperactive, hypersensitive cells that cause an altered state of brain function. Abnormalities can occur in the motor system, sensory system, or ANS. Seizures are classified as either partial or generalized (Box 12-4). Partial seizures usually begin in one cerebral hemisphere and cause motor activity to be localized to one area of the body (e.g., arm, face). When consciousness remains intact, the seizure is classified as a simple partial seizure. If consciousness is impaired, the seizure is classified as a complex partial seizure. Generalized seizures involve both cerebral hemispheres and cause altered consciousness and motor manifestations to occur bilaterally. When seizures occur in close proximity to each other, they have the potential to lead to a life-threatening medical emergency known as status epilepticus (SE).

PATHOPHYSIOLOGY

SE can occur with any type of seizure. SE exists when seizures repeat frequently enough so brain function does not return to normal between attacks. Specifically, SE is present when seizure activity lasts for 30 minutes or when two or more sequential seizures occur without full recovery of consciousness between seizures. It has been estimated that between 100,000 and 150,000 patients experience SE each year (Smith, 2001). SE is more likely to occur with tonic-clonic seizures that have a specific causative factor than with idiopathic seizures. The most frequent precipitating factors in SE is irregular intake of anticonvulsants, withdrawal from habitual use of alcohol or sedative drugs, electrolyte imbalance, azotemia, head trauma, infection, and brain tumor.

Physiological changes that occur during SE are divided into two phases. During phase 1, when cerebral metabolism is greatly increased because of the seizure, compensatory mechanisms prevent cerebral damage from hypoxia or metabolic injury. These protective mechanisms are increased CBF and metabolism, massive autonomic activity with excessive catecholamine release, and cardiovascular changes. These changes can lead to hyperglycemia, hypertension, increased cardiac output, increased central venous pressure, tachycardia, salivation, sweating, hyperpyrexia, vomiting, and incontinence. Initial hyperglycemia is probably a result of the increased release of epinephrine and activation of hepatic gluconeogenesis. Hypertension occurs due to increased CBF to meet the metabolic demands of the neurons

BOX 12-4

Seizure Classification

Type	Symptoms
I. PARTIAL	
Simple (no loss of consciousness)	
Motor	"Jacksonian" march
	Movement of eye, head, and body on one side
	Stopping of movement or speech
Sensory or somatosensory	Tingling, numbness of body part
	Visual, auditory, olfactory, or taste sensations
	Dizzy spells
Autonomic	Pallor, sweating, flushing, piloerection, pupillary dilation
Psychic	Déjà vu(e) ("already seen"), overly familiar
	Dysphagia
	Dream states
	Distortion of time sense
	Hallucinations
	Objects appearing small, large or far away
Complex (alteration of consciousness); Automatisms	
II. GENERALIZED	
Absence	
Simple	Staring spell
	Lasting less than 15 seconds
Atypical	Starting spell with myoclonic jerks and automatisms
Myoclonic	Single jerk of one or more muscle groups
	Lasts only 1 second
Clonic	Jerking of muscle groups
Tonic	Stiffening of muscle groups
Tonic-clonic	Starts with the stiffening or tonic phase, followed by the jerking or clonic phase
	Unconsciousness
	Tongue biting
	Bowel and bladder incontinence
Atonic	Drop attack or abrupt loss of muscle tone
III. UNCLASSIFIED (INCOMPLETE DATA)	

Modified from Petit, J. M. (2001). *Primary neurologic care.* St. Louis: C. V. Mosby; and Barker, E. (2002). *Neuroscience nursing: A spectrum of care* [p. 772]. 2nd ed. St. Louis: C.V. Mosby.

for oxygen and glucose. Tachycardia occurs due to increased cardiac output. Hyperpyrexia results from excessive muscle activity and mass catecholamine release. Lactic acidosis occurs from anaerobic muscle metabolism. Elevated epinephrine and norepinephrine levels and acidosis contribute to cardiac dysrhythmias. Autonomic dysfunction causes excessive sweating and vomiting that leads to dehydration and electrolyte loss (Chapman, Smith, & Hirsch, 2001; Shorvon, 2001).

Phase 2 begins 30 to 60 minutes after phase 1. Decompensation occurs because the increased metabolic demands cannot be met. This causes decreased CBF, systemic hypotension, increased ICP, and cerebral autoregulation failure. The patient develops metabolic and respiratory acidosis from hypoxia, hypoglycemia from depleted energy stores, hyponatremia, and hypokalemia or hyperkalemia. The lack of oxygen and glucose in brain cells stimulates the production and release of glutamate. Excess glutamate changes the neuron's electrical balance and opens membrane channels, thus allowing calcium influx. The excessive intracellular calcium results in the development of oxygen free radicals; this makes brain cells electrically unstable and leads to cell injury. Pulmonary edema is common, and pulmonary aspiration can occur from decreased laryngeal reflex sensitivity. Cardiac dysrhythmia and failure result from hypoxia, hyperkalemia caused by increased muscle activity, and metabolic acidosis. Renal failure may result from rhabdomyolysis and acute myoglobinuria. This occurs because of excessive muscle activity from prolonged skeletal muscle contraction and traumatic injury. The result is disintegration of striated muscle fibers. Acute intravascular coagulation can also occur (Chapman, Smith, & Hirsch, 2001; Shorvon, 2001).

Death from SE is more likely to occur when an underlying disease is responsible for the seizure or from the acute illness that precipitated the seizure. Generalized seizures that last for 30 to 45 minutes can result in neuronal necrosis, which may result in permanent neurological deficits. Prompt diagnosis and treatment are important because seizure duration is an important prognostic factor (Bleck, 2001; Cock & Schapira, 2002).

ASSESSMENT

Assessment during SE incorporates neurological, respiratory, and cardiovascular systems. Characteristics of the seizure and the neurological state between seizures are important for the nurse to monitor. Information to collect includes precipitating factors, preceding aura, type of movement observed, automatisms, changes in size of pupils or eye deviation, responsiveness to auditory or tactile stimuli, level of consciousness throughout the seizure, urinary or bowel incontinence, patient's behavior after the seizure, weakness or paralysis of extremities after the seizure, injuries caused by the seizure, and duration of the seizure (Hickey, 2003). Assessment of respirations and monitoring of pulse oximetry values are needed to ensure the adequacy of oxygenation. Because autonomic changes can result in pulmonary edema, it is imperative to note the onset of fine basilar crackles. Suction equipment and oxygen should be readily available. Because SE may precipitate dysrhythmias, cardiac monitoring is necessary.

DIAGNOSTIC TESTS

Laboratory studies for a patient with SE include serum electrolytes, liver profile, serum medication levels, and blood and urine toxicology screens. Cardiac enzymes and arterial blood gases assist in assessing the effect of the seizure on other body systems. Patient monitoring includes ECG, EEG, noninvasive blood pressure, and pulse oximetry.

Radiological studies are performed to rule out a space-occupying lesion that may be responsible for the episode of SE. These may include CT and MRI. Additional studies may be appropriate to rule out injury.

MANAGEMENT

Nursing Diagnoses

Nursing diagnoses appropriate for a patient experiencing SE are as follows:

- Ineffective tissue perfusion (cerebral and cardiopulmonary) related to interrupted blood flow secondary to continuous seizure activity or vasodilating effects of antiepileptic medications
- Ineffective breathing pattern or impaired gas exchange related to altered oxygen supply resulting from hypoventilation and bradycardia secondary to depressant effect of seizure on respiratory center
- Ineffective airway clearance related to underlying neurological problem and seizure activity
- Risk of trauma (oral and musculoskeletal) related to underlying neurological problems and/or seizure activity
- Disturbed thought processes related to the postictal state
- Impaired verbal communication related to the postictal state
- Situational low self-esteem related to seizure activity
- Ineffective coping related to seizure activity
- Deficient knowledge related to disease process, treatment, and necessary lifestyle changes

Nursing and Medical Interventions

Management during SE incorporates maintaining a patent airway, providing adequate oxygenation, maintaining vascular access for the administration of medications and fluids, administering appropriate medications, and maintaining seizure precautions. A patent airway is facilitated by the use of an oral/nasal airway or endotracheal tube. Suctioning is often needed to remove secretions that collect in the oropharynx. Supplemental oxygen is used to improve oxygenation. Initially, oxygen is administered through nasal prongs or a face mask. Poor gas exchange during SE or as a result of respiratory depression from medications may necessitate intubation to provide adequate oxygenation. A nasogastric tube with intermittent suction may be needed to ensure that the airway is not compromised by aspiration.

Do not try to insert padded tongue blades between the clenched teeth of a patient undergoing a seizure. Patients have inadvertently been injured from aspirating teeth that were loosened during forceful attempts to insert a padded tongue blade between their teeth.

Vascular access must be maintained to provide a route for the administration of medication. If one is unable to start intravenous access, some antiseizure medications can be administered rectally. The specific medication given to arrest the seizure depends on the physician's preference and the type and duration of the seizure (see Table 12-7). It is also essential to monitor blood pressure and to administer volume replacement and vasoactive drugs if necessary. Intravenous dextrose and thiamine are given unless the patient is known to be normoglycemic or hyperglycemic.

Seizure precautions are continued during SE. This includes padding the side rails on the patient's bed and making sure that the bed has full-length side rails. The bed should remain in a low position with side rails up except when direct nursing care is being given. If patient is in a chair when a seizure begins, lower the patient to the floor and place a soft object under patient's head. It is important to remove the patient's restrictive clothing and jewelry while always maintaining the patient's privacy. Do not restrain the patient because the forceful tonic-clonic movements can traumatize the patient.

SE must be treated immediately. Initially, the nurse ensures a patent airway and maintains breathing and circulation if necessary. Significant hypoxia can occur, so protecting the cardiorespiratory function is essential. Next, medications are given using a sequential approach that progressively uses more potent medications to control the seizure. Benzodiazepines are used initially, and the drug of choice is usually intravenous lorazepam (Ativan). Diazepam may also be considered, but research shows that lorazepam has a longer duration of action, causes less cardiorespiratory depression, and reduces seizure recurrence (Cock & Schapira, 2002).

If lorazepam fails to stop seizure activity within 10 minutes or if intermittent seizures persist for longer than 20 minutes, phenytoin (Dilantin) or fosphenytoin is the next appropriate drug to administer. Phenytoin is mixed only with normal saline, and it is stable in solution for only 20 minutes, thus making it impractical for intravenous piggyback administration. It may be given as a push after clearing the line with saline or slowly pushed with normal saline infusing. Phenobarbital may be used as the third-line agent to control SE, but its utility in SE is lessened by the length of time required to achieve a therapeutic effect (Bleck, 2001).

When the patient continues in SE despite phenytoin administration, propofol (Diprivan) is given. Propofol is a general anesthetic and sedative-hypnotic agent. Patients require intubation and mechanical ventilation because of hypoxia or inefficient ventilation. General anesthesia can be also be achieved with pentobarbital therapy. With both drugs, the patient is assessed for hypotension (Shorvon, 2001). Phenobarbital can also be used. Refer to Table 12-7 for specifics regarding medication therapy for SE.

PATIENT OUTCOMES

Patient outcomes for SE are focused on protection during the life-threatening episode and prevention of recurrence. The first outcome is that the patient maintains an adequate breathing and cardiovascular pattern. Second, the patient does not experience any injury related to the seizure activity. Finally, the patient demonstrates knowledge of the disease process, including precipitating factors, medication routines, and side effects of medications.

Spinal Cord Injury

Approximately 200,000 people in the United States are living with SCI. Each year, about 11,000 additional victims sustain SCI. Fifty-five percent (55%) of SCIs occur in patients between the ages of 16 and 30 years (Barker & Saulino, 2002). The most common causes of SCI are motor vehicle accidents, falls, sports injuries, missile injuries, and diving accidents. Head injury often occurs with SCI; therefore, SCI should be considered a possibility in all unconscious patients.

Providing emergency intervention at the scene of the accident by skilled providers, decreasing transport time to the hospital, and developing specific universal SCI guidelines to standardize evidence-based care will have a profound effect on a patient's outcome.

PATHOPHYSIOLOGY

An SCI occurs when force is exerted on the vertebral column, resulting in damage to the spinal cord. A series of complex and multifaceted responses results from this injury, with altered autonomic function leading to cardiovascular instability (Figure 12-31). The loss of sympathetic input (spinal nerves T1-L1) results in bradycardia, hypotension, venous stasis, and loss of temperature control with the development of spinal shock. Spinal shock is the temporary loss of autonomic, sensory, and motor functions below the level of the lesion and occurs secondary to the loss of facilitory input from the brain and inhibitory input below the level of the injury. A sign of the termination of spinal shock is the return of reflex activity below the level of the lesion. Another response to SCI is an inflammatory reaction that creates cord edema. Cord edema compresses spinal cord tissue as well as cord blood vessels. Cord edema can ascend or descend from the level of injury.

The injury itself creates a series of biochemical changes. Potassium is lost from inside the cell to the extracellular compartment. Sodium moves into the cell causing acute cellular edema. There is also a calcium influx inside the cell that leads to the lipid membrane breakdown of neurons. The excess calcium hinders the cell's function and catalyzes neuronal death. Free oxygen radicals are released, which potentiates further breakdown of cell membranes. This results in the breakdown of free fatty acids (Dubendorf, 1999). There is a release of vasoactive substances (norepinephrine, histamine, dopamine, glutamate, endorphin, and prostaglandin) as a result of these biochemical changes. This event leads to vasoconstriction of the blood vessels, decrease in tissue oxygen, a build-up of lactic acid, and ischemia. If the ischemia is not reversed, axonal degeneration and conduction failure of the neuron occur. Eventually, there is cell death with permanent loss of function.

The final response to SCI is vascular change. Instantly after injury, there are microscopic hemorrhages in the central gray matter of the spinal cord. After several hours, these hemorrhages invade the surrounding white matter, cord blood flow is decreased, and ischemia results. If the ischemia is not reversed, neuronal cell death occurs.

SCI can result in a complete or incomplete lesion. A *complete lesion* causes total, permanent loss of motor and sensory function below the level of injury. An *incomplete lesion* results in the sparing of motor and sensory function below the level of injury. The three

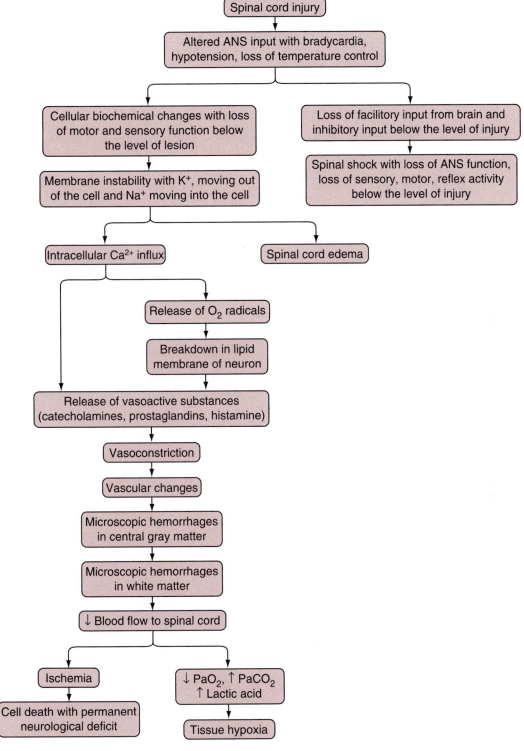

FIGURE 12-31 Pathophysiology flow diagram for spinal cord injury. *ANS,* Autonomic nervous system; *K+,* potassium; *Na+,* sodium; *Ca2+,* calcium; *O2,* oxygen; *PaO2,* partial pressure of oxygen in arterial blood; *PaCO2,* partial pressure of carbon dioxide in arterial blood.

types of incomplete lesions are central cord, anterior cord, and Brown-Séquard syndromes. The clinical presentation of each syndrome is based on damage to spinal cord organization and crossing of tracts. Most patients with an incomplete lesion show a mixed pattern of motor and sensory function rather than a classic syndrome and have a potential for some or full recovery (Figure 12-32).

ASSESSMENT
Airway and Respiratory Status

Assessment of the airway, respiratory status, and neurological status is the first assessment priority. The higher the level of SCI is, the greater is the functional impairment. Respiratory problems are frequently associated with SCI. Ineffective breathing patterns are caused by paralysis of the diaphragm or

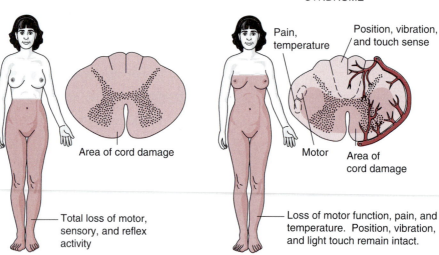

COMPLETE LESION

Area of cord damage

Total loss of motor, sensory, and reflex activity

ANTERIOR CORD SYNDROME

Pain, temperature

Position, vibration, and touch sense

Motor

Area of cord damage

Loss of motor function, pain, and temperature. Position, vibration, and light touch remain intact.

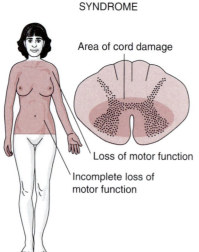

CENTRAL CORD SYNDROME

Area of cord damage

Loss of motor function

Incomplete loss of motor function

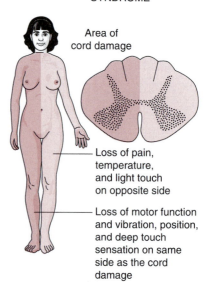

BROWN-SÉQUARD SYNDROME

Area of cord damage

Loss of pain, temperature, and light touch on opposite side

Loss of motor function and vibration, position, and deep touch sensation on same side as the cord damage

FIGURE 12-32 Common spinal cord syndromes. (Modified from Ignatavicius, D. D., & Workman, M. L. [2002]. *Medical-surgical nursing: Critical thinking for collaborative care.* 4th ed. Philadelphia: W. B. Saunders.)

BOX 12-5

Components of the Hourly Neurological Assessment for Patients with Spinal Cord Injury without Head Injury

Motor	Sensation
Respirations	Pinprick (sharp, dull)
Rate, rhythm, respiratory	All surfaces of the body
effort	Position sense
Movement/strength	Temperature
bilaterally	All surfaces of the body
Shrug shoulders	
Elbow flexion	
Elbow extension	
Bending wrists	
Touching thumb to	
index finger	
Hand grasp	
Lift leg off the bed	
Bend knee	
Extend knee	
Pull feet up	
Push feet down	

intercostal muscles and by chest trauma. Therefore, the lungs must be auscultated for the presence of breath sounds in all areas. Observing the respiratory rate and the rhythm and depth of respiration is also important. Signs of respiratory distress include excessive retraction of accessory neck muscles with respiratory effort, paradoxical expansion of the abdominal wall with inspiration, and cyanosis. Baseline arterial blood gases collected on admission and continuous monitoring of SaO_2 provide important information.

Respiratory impairment varies with the level of injury and the type of injury (complete or incomplete). Respiratory impairment results from the dysfunction or loss of the diaphragm, intercostal muscles, and abdominal muscles. Patients with complete lesions at vertebral levels C1-C3 are ventilator dependent. Patients with complete lesions at vertebral levels C4-C5 experience phrenic nerve damage and are candidates for phrenic nerve pacers. Patients with complete SCIs below vertebra C5 have intact diaphragmatic breathing without intercostal and abdominal muscle function. Patients with complete lesions from vertebral levels T1-L2 experience varying amounts of intercostal and abdominal muscle loss. Those with incomplete spinal cord lesions present with varying degrees of respiratory impairment, depending on the level of the lesion and whether the motor system is impaired; these patients may require mechanical ventilation.

Neurological Assessment

Once airway and respiratory assessment is complete, the neurological examination follows. For a patient with an SCI, all components of the neurological examination are performed, with an emphasis placed on the motor, reflex, and sensory responses. In addition, an assessment of the spinal nerve innervation of major muscle groups is completed to determine the level of injury to the motor system (see Table 12-3). Box 12-5 outlines the components of the hourly assessment for an SCI patient without a head injury, and Box 12-6 lists those for a patient with both an SCI and a head injury.

Hemodynamic Assessment

The patient requires continuous hemodynamic monitoring during the acute period after the injury to assess for hemodynamic instability. It is recommended that patients with SCI remain in a critical care unit for the first 7 to 14 days after the injury to allow early detection of hemodynamic instability (American Association of Neurological Surgeons & Congress of Neurological Surgeons, 2002). The usual hemodynamic response in injuries above the C5 level is a decrease or loss of sympathetic innervation causing vasodilation, decreased venous return, and hypotension. The patient's vasomotor response returns over the course of a couple of months. Bradycardia is common, results from the loss of sympathetic outflow, and is aggravated by hypothermia and hypoxia. The patient is therefore at risk for a vasovagal response during suctioning, which leads to hypoxia and bradycardia. This reflex is prevented by preoxygenating the patient before suctioning (Nikas, 1998).

Venous stasis occurs as a result of loss of vasomotor tone and paralysis. This stasis increases the risk of thrombosis in the legs and pelvis and pulmonary emboli.

A patient with high-level SCI (above C5) is unable to regulate body temperature. The level of injury interrupts the pathway between the hypothalamus and the blood vessels and causes body temperature to rise and fall according to the environmental temperature.

BOX 12-6

Components of the Hourly Neurological Assessment for Patients with Spinal Cord and Head Injury

Mental Status	Motor	Pupils	Brainstem/Cranial Nerves	Sensation
Glasgow Coma Scale	Respirations	Size	Corneal reflex	Pinprick (sharp, dull)
Assesses level of consciousness, expressive language, ability to follow commands	Rate, rhythm, respiratory effort	Shape	Present	All surfaces of the body
	Assess movement/strength bilaterally	Reaction to light (direct and consensual)	Diminished	Position sense
	Shrug shoulders	Extraocular movements	Absent	Temperature
	Elbow flexion		Cough, gag, swallow reflex	All surfaces of the body
	Elbow extension		Observe for excessive drooling	
	Bending wrists		Observe for cough/swallow reflex	
	Touching thumb to index finger			
	Hand grasp			
	Lift leg off the bed			
	Bend knee			
	Extend knee			
	Pull feet up			
	Push feet down			

Gastrointestinal Tract Assessment

The loss of autonomic tone causes abdominal distention and paralytic ileus. During the first 72 hours after SCI, a nasogastric tube for decompression is inserted until bowel sounds return. This also helps to prevent vomiting and possible aspiration. Abdominal decompression may help to improve pulmonary function by decreasing abdominal distention. Stress ulcers can occur as a result of vagus-stimulated gastric acid production. Histamine (H_2)-antagonists are used to prevent stress ulcers. Steroid therapy may be part of acute management, but it also irritates the gastric mucosa. A thorough nutritional assessment is necessary because the SCI leads to a hypermetabolic state.

Bowel and bladder assessment. Bowel and bladder atony occurs during spinal shock. The bladder does not contract, and the detrusor muscle does not open because of the paralysis. Urinary retention is a common problem, and a Foley catheter is used during spinal shock. The bowel does not have peristaltic movement secondary to SCI. This loss of peristaltic movement places the patient at risk of paralytic ileus. The patient is assessed for return of bowel sounds, flatus, and bowel movement. A bowel care program should be started within the first 72 hours after injury (Guin, 2001; Prendergast & Sullivan, 2000).

Autonomic Dysreflexia

Autonomic dysreflexia is a medical emergency. It occurs after spinal shock has ceased and can be an ongoing problem for a patient with an SCI lesion above T6. Autonomic dysreflexia is characterized by an exaggerated response of the sympathetic nervous system to a variety of stimuli. Causes of autonomic dysreflexia include the following: stimuli to the bladder by a kinked Foley catheter, bladder distention, infection, calculi or cystoscopy; stimuli to the bowel by fecal impaction, rectal examination, or suppository insertion; and stimuli to the skin by tight clothing and bed linens, temperature extremes, or broken skin. This exaggerated response by the sympathetic nervous system results from the lack of input from the brain because of blockage from the SCI. Common signs and symptoms are as follows: sudden, severe, pounding headache; elevated, uncontrolled blood pressure; bradycardia; nasal congestion; blurred vision; profuse sweating above the level of the lesion; flushing of the face and neck; pallor, chills, vasoconstriction, and pilomotor erection below the level of the injury; and/or anxiety. Blood pressure can rise to a dangerous level, making autonomic dysreflexia an emergency situation. Treatment is directed at finding and removing the cause. Once the cause has been located and removed, the symptoms quickly disappear. If symptoms persist, treatment with vasodilating drugs including nitroglycerin, nifedipine, hydralazine, or nitroprusside are instituted to decrease blood pressure. If autonomic dysreflexia is not identified and treated promptly, seizures, SAH, cerebrovascular accident, and myocardial infarction can occur (Swearingen & Keen, 2001).

Skin Assessment

Because of impaired circulation and immobility, the patient with SCI is at risk of skin breakdown. Preventive skin care is essential. All skin surfaces are routinely inspected. The skin around the halo or tong pins is inspected, and pin care is performed every 8 hours. Assessment includes observing the site for redness, swelling, drainage, and pain. Inspecting areas under the halo brace for signs of skin breakdown is also important. The skin surrounding the cervical collar is assessed for skin integrity with an emphasis on pressure points (occipital, chin, and sternal region).

Psychological Assessment

A psychological assessment is important during the acute period of injury. Initially, the patient is concerned with surviving the injury and does not realize the extent of injury or disability. The patient's perceptions are also impaired by medications and the physiological effects of injury. As the patient gains insight into the situation, it is important for the nurse to include the patient in planning his or her care and to give the patient choices, because feelings of powerlessness are common (Mitcho & Yanko, 1999).

Family members also go through a similar experience. First they experience shock related to the injury itself and the seriousness of the patient's condition. During this time, the family needs support and answers to their questions. Consultation with a psychiatric or mental health nurse or a psychiatrist may be indicated (Gill, 1999).

DIAGNOSTIC STUDIES

Baseline laboratory studies include electrolytes, complete blood count, prothrombin time, partial thromboplastin time, platelet count, and arterial blood gases. Common diagnostic studies to confirm the extent of vertebral injury and SCI include anteroposterior and lateral spine x-ray studies, chest x-ray studies, CT scan, MRI, myelography, and somatosensory-cortical evoked potentials. This last test is performed to see whether sensory pathways between the site of stimulation and the site of recording are intact. This test requires tactile stimulation to elicit a response.

MANAGEMENT

Nursing Interventions

Nursing interventions are focused on maintaining stabilization of the spinal alignment, preserving the airway and respiratory status, and preventing complications associated with immobility and the SCI (see Nursing Care Plan for the Patient with Spinal Cord Injury).

Text continued on page 414

Nursing Care Plan for the Patient with Spinal Cord Injury

NURSING DIAGNOSIS: *Risk for injury related to displacement of fracture, spinal shock, or ascending cord edema*

Patient Outcomes	Interventions	Rationales
Maintenance of vertebral alignment Absence of progressive neurological dysfunction Improved sensory, motor, and reflex function	Perform neurological assessments (motor, reflex, and sensory). Report progression of deficits from baseline (↑ difficulty with swallowing secretions or coughing, presence of respiratory stridor with retraction of accessory muscles of respiration, bradycardia, fluctuating BP, and ↑ motor and sensory loss at a higher level than the initial findings). Explain immobilization. Maintain halo or tong traction for immobilization. Perform pin care every 8 hr. If skeletal traction slips or is accidentally removed, maintain the patient's head in a neutral position.	Subtle changes in neurological signs indicate deterioration or improvement in neurological status. Spinal injury may be getting progressively worse. Prevents infection at the pin insertion site.

Continued

Nursing Care Plan for the Patient with Spinal Cord Injury—cont'd

Patient Outcomes	Interventions	Rationales
	Turn, lift, and transfer the patient with at least three people with one at head to stabilize neck and to coordinate the move.	Proper turning keeps the spinal cord in alignment and prevents further trauma to the spinal cord.

NURSING DIAGNOSIS: *Impaired gas exchange related to altered oxygen supply associated with hypoventilation secondary to paresis or paralysis of respiratory muscles (diaphragm, intercostals)*

Patient Outcomes	Interventions	Rationales
Adequate gas exchange as evidenced by full orientation; PaO_2 ≥80 mm Hg; $PaCO_2$ ≤45 mm Hg; RR 12-20 breaths/min with normal depth and pattern; HR 60-100 beats/min; BP stable Motor and sensory losses remaining at the same spinal cord level as initial findings	Assess for signs of respiratory dysfunction (shallow, slow, or rapid respirations; vital capacity ≤1 L; changes in sensorium; anxiety; restlessness; tachycardia; pallor; inability to move secretions). Monitor ABG studies. Monitor chest x-ray studies. Monitor for evidence of ascending cord edema (↑ difficulty with swallowing secretions or coughing, presence of respiratory stridor with retraction of accessory muscles of respiration, bradycardia, fluctuating BP, and ↑ motor and sensory loss at a higher level than the initial findings). Monitor respiratory status, especially in a patient with cranial tongs or traction with a halo vest. Assess for absent or adventitious breath sounds and inspect chest movement.	Indicates the need for assisted ventilation caused by atelectasis or respiratory fatigue. Spinal injury may be getting progressively worse. Ensures that the vest is not restricting diaphragmatic movement.

NURSING DIAGNOSIS: *Ineffective airway clearance related to decreased or absent cough reflex secondary to cervical or high thoracic spine injury or depressant effect of some medications*

Patient Outcomes	Interventions	Rationales
Within 24-48 hr, airway clear as evidenced by absence of adventitious breath sounds	Monitor respiratory status, be alert to adventitious breath sounds, ↓ or absence breath sounds, ↑ HR >100 beats/min, BP >10 mm Hg over normal, ↓ tidal volume, shallow or rapid respirations, use of intercostal or abdominal muscles, pallor, cyanosis, increased restlessness, and anxiety. Monitor oxygen saturation, ABG, chest x-ray study, and temperature. Administer oxygen as needed. Suction secretions according to auscultated findings. Hyperoxygenate before and after suctioning. Perform incentive spirometry every hour the patient is awake.	Indicates the need for assisted ventilation caused by atelectasis or respiratory fatigue. Provides adequate oxygenation before suctioning.

Nursing Care Plan for the Patient with Spinal Cord Injury—cont'd

NURSING DIAGNOSIS: *Ineffective thermoregulation related to inability of body to adapt to environmental temperature changes secondary to loss of sympathetic innervation*

Patient Outcomes	Interventions	Rationales
Within 2-4 hr of diagnosis, patient normothermic	Monitor temperature at least every 4 hr. Assess for signs of ineffective thermoregulation (complaints of being too warm, excessive diaphoresis, skin warmth above level of injury; complaints of being too cold, pilomotor erection, or cool skin below level of injury. Implement measures to attain normothermia (regulate room temperature, provide extra blankets, protect patient from drafts, use fans, provide tepid bath or cooling blanket; ice packs at neck, axillae, groin). Provide antipyretics.	The patient may be developing autonomic dysreflexia.

NURSING DIAGNOSIS: *Risk for autonomic dysreflexia related to abnormal response of the autonomic nervous system to a stimulus*

Patient Outcomes	Interventions	Rationales
No symptoms of autonomic dysreflexia as evidenced by dry skin about level of injury; BP within patient's normal range; HR >60 beats/min; absence of headache; ECG NSR	Assess for throbbing headache, cutaneous vasodilation above injury level (skin warmth above level of injury), cool skin below level of injury; grossly elevated BP, nasal stuffiness, nausea, chest pain, or blurred vision. Determine and remove the offending stimulus (check for bladder distention; urinary catheter draining freely; check for fecal impaction; check for sensory stimuli and loosen clothing, bed covers, or any constricting factor). Administer an antihypertensive agent. Raise the head of the bed. Remain calm and supportive of the patient.	Removes the agent causing autonomic dysreflexia. Reduce severe hypertension associated with autonomic dysreflexia. Promote venous pooling and subsequent ↓BP.

NURSING DIAGNOSIS: *Decreased CO related to relative hypovolemia secondary to enlarged vascular space occurring during neurogenic/spinal shock*

Patient Outcomes	Interventions	Rationales
Adequate CO as evidenced by orientation to name, place, time SBP >90 mm Hg; urine output ≥0.5 mL/kg/hr; ECG NSR	Monitor decrease SBP >20 mm Hg; SBP <90 mm Hg, HR >100 beats/min; lightheadedness, confusion, flushed skin, diminished peripheral pulses.	Identifies changes associated with ↓CO.

Continued

Nursing Care Plan for the Patient with Spinal Cord Injury—cont'd

Patient Outcomes	Interventions	Rationales
Normal peripheral pulses	Monitor hemodynamic measurements. Continuously assess the ECG. Monitor the patient's mental status, and report changes. Implement measures to prevent orthostatic hypotension: Change the patient's position slowly. Use antiembolic hose. Administer fluids. Administer and monitor the effects of vasopressor drugs.	Indicates fluid status. Increases SVR to increase BP.

NURSING DIAGNOSIS: *Imbalanced nutrition: less than body requirements related to hypermetabolic state; decreased oral intake secondary to anorexia; difficulty eating in prone position; fear of choking and aspiration; inability to feed self; decreased gastroinestinal motility resulting from autonomic nervous system dysfunction*

Patient Outcomes	Interventions	Rationales
Adequate nutrition evidenced by balanced nitrogen state; serum albumin 3.5-5.5 g/dL	Weigh the patient daily. Use an NGT on low suction to prevent abdominal distention or aspiration. The patient remains NPO until bowel sounds are present. Assess readiness for oral intake (bowel sounds present, passing flatus, or bowel movement). Perform a nutrition assessment. Give parenteral or enteral nutrition if ordered. Progress slowly from liquids to solids. Give small, frequent feedings.	Decompresses the patient's stomach, to prevent aspiration of gastric contents and to decrease the risk of paralytic ileus. This approach causes less abdominal distention, which can compromise respiratory effort, and it is less tiring.

NURSING DIAGNOSIS: *Ineffective tissue perfusion related to interrupted blood flow associated with thrombophlebitis, DVT, and PE secondary to venous stasis, vascular intimal injury, and hypercoagulability from decreased vasomotor tone and immobility*

Patient Outcomes	Interventions	Rationales
No symptoms of thrombophlebitis, DVT, and PE as evidenced by absence of heat, swelling, discomfort, and erythema in calves and thighs; HR <100 beats/min, RR <20 breaths/min with normal respiratory pattern and depth PaO$_2$ >80 mm Hg; absence of chest or shoulder pain	Assess for sudden chest or shoulder pain, tachycardia, dyspnea, tachypnea, hypotension, pallor, cyanosis, cough with hemoptysis, restlessness, increasing anxiety, or low PaO$_2$. Change the patient's position every 2 hr. Perform ROM exercises on all the patient's extremities every 1-2 hr. Avoid knee gatch or pillows under the knees. Apply sequential compression devices or antiembolic hose.	These are indicators of PE. This promotes venous return and prevents venous stasis. These positions compromise circulation

Nursing Care Plan for the Patient with Spinal Cord Injury—cont'd

Patient Outcomes	Interventions	Rationales
	Maintain adequate hydration of the patient.	Prevents dehydration and increased blood viscosity, which can promote thrombus formation.
	Administer prophylactic low-dose, low-molecular-weight heparin.	An anticoagulant prevents or decreases thrombus formation.
	If the patient develops signs of thrombophlebitis or DVT, notify the physician, maintain the patient at bed rest, and keep the extremity in a neutral or elevated position.	Prevents a clot from dislodging.
	If the patient develops evidence of PE, elevate the head of the bed, administer oxygen, administer vasopressors for hypotension and analgesics for pain as ordered, and prepare the patient for a diagnostic procedure.	

NURSING DIAGNOSIS: *Risk for infection related to inadequate primary defenses (broken skin) secondary to immobilization and presence of invasive devices*

Patient Outcomes	Interventions	Rationales
Free of infection at insertion site for tongs, IV, Foley catheter, ETT Negative culture results Absence of erythema, swelling, warmth, purulent drainage, tenderness, normal WBCs	Perform pin, IV, and Foley catheter care. Monitor WBCs. Use sterile technique to change the central IV dressing. Use proper hand-washing techniques.	Prevents infection.

NURSING DIAGNOSIS: *Risk for impaired skin integrity related to prolonged immobility*

Patient Outcomes	Interventions	Rationales
Skin remains intact	Assess the patient's skin every 4 hr, especially over bony prominences, dependent or edematous areas, and the area under the halo vest and the cervical collar. Ensure that the patient's skin is clean and dry. Pad the halo vest to decrease irritation and friction. Turn the patient every 2 hr.	

NURSING DIAGNOSIS: *Constipation related to neuromuscular impairment secondary to spinal shock, SCI*

Patient Outcomes	Interventions	Rationales
Soft, formed bowel movement within 48 hr of admission	Monitor for nausea, vomiting, abdominal distention, malaise, and the presence of a hard fecal mass on digital examination Monitor the patient's bowel sounds.	Indicates constipation and fecal impaction.

Continued

Nursing Care Plan for the Patient with Spinal Cord Injury—cont'd

Soft, formed bowel movement within 48 hr of admission—*cont'd*	Keep the patient NPO with an NGT until bowel sounds return. Administer stool softeners. Document the patient's bowel movements.

NURSING DIAGNOSIS: *Fear/anxiety related to loss of motor and sensory function; immobilizing device to stabilize and align spine; lack of understanding of diagnostic tests and treatment; unfamiliar environment; financial concerns; anticipated effect of SCI on lifestyle and roles*

Patient Outcomes	Interventions	Rationales
Experiencing reduced fear and anxiety as evidenced by: verbalization of feeling less anxious; usual sleep pattern; relaxed facial expression; healthy interaction with others	Assess for signs and symptoms of fear and anxiety (tense, insomnia). Implement measures to reduce fear and anxiety. Explain the need for frequent neurological checks. Provide information concerning all nursing care. Assure the patient that staff members are nearby; provide a call signal that is adapted to meet the patient's needs. Answer the call signal as soon as possible. Include the patient in planning care. Provide an environment conducive to rest and expressions of fear or questions. Listen and clarify perceptions.	Decreases stimuli that cause stress; expressing fears assists in coping with changes and reduces anxiety. Promotes successful resolution of the crisis and establishes a positive coping mechanism.

NURSING DIAGNOSIS: *Powerlessness related to SCI*

Patient Outcomes	Interventions	Rationales
Verbalizing of increased control over activities	Encourage talk. Include the patient in planning. Allow the patient to make choices. Display sensitivity toward events that could cause powerlessness. Encourage asking questions.	Facilitates communication.

↑, Increase; ↓, decrease; *ABG,* arterial blood gas; *BP,* blood pressure; *CO,* cardiac output; *DVT,* deep vein thrombus; *ECG,* electrocardiogram; *ETT,* endotracheal tube; *HR,* heart rate; *IV,* intravenous; *NGT,* nasogastric tube; *NPO,* nothing by mouth; *NSR,* normal sinus rhythm; *PaCO$_2$,* partial pressure of carbon dioxide; *PaO$_2$,* partial pressure of oxygen; *PE,* pulmonary embolus; *RR,* respiratory rate; *SCI,* spinal cord injury; *SBP,* systolic blood pressure; *SVR,* systemic vascular resistance; *WBC,* white blood cell count.
Data from Swearingen, P. L., & Keen, J. H. (2001). *Manual of critical care nursing.* 4th ed. St Louis: Mosby; and Ulrich, S. P., & Canale, S. W. (2001). *Nursing care planning guides: For adults in acute, extended, and home care settings.* Philadelphia: W. B. Saunders.

Medical Interventions

Maintaining a patent airway and respiratory function is a priority. If the patient is having difficulty sustaining respiration, endotracheal intubation and mechanical ventilation are the treatments of choice.

Initial stabilization of the spinal cord must occur at the scene of the accident to prevent or reduce untoward movement of the spine. A rigid cervical collar with supporting blocks on a rigid backboard is recommended (American Association of Neurological Surgeons & Congress of Neurological Surgeons, 2002). Stabilization of the fracture or dislocation to create spinal alignment and to prevent further neurological deterioration is accomplished by skeletal traction—a halo vest or tongs (Figure 12-33). The halo vest offers many advantages, such as easy access to the neck for

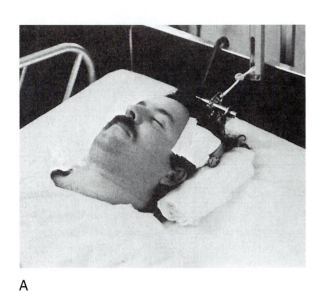

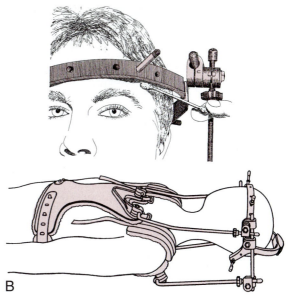

A   B

FIGURE 12-33 A, Skeletal traction with Crutchfield tongs. **B,** Halo fixator. (**A,** from Hickey, J. V. [1992]. *Clinical practice of neurological and neurosurgical nursing.* 3rd ed. Philadelphia: J. B. Lippincott; **B,** courtesy of DePuy Acromed, Raynham, MA.)

diagnostic procedures and surgery, early mobilization, and ambulation.

Maintaining perfusion to the spinal cord is crucial and therefore monitoring blood pressure is a priority. Systolic blood pressure lower than 90 mm Hg must be avoided, and the MAP should be maintained at 85 to 90 mm Hg for the first 7 days after the SCI. Hypotension contributes to secondary injury by decreasing spinal cord blood flow and perfusion leading to ischemia, which may be one of the most important causes of neuronal injury and neurological deficit. Fluid volume and vasopressor drugs may be needed to maintain the MAP at 85 to 90 mm Hg (American Association of Neurological Surgeons & Congress of Neurological Surgeons, 2002). A pulmonary artery catheter may be used to determine the need for fluids accurately.

Although controversial, glucocorticoids have been used in the treatment of SCI for many years. The guidelines of the American Association of Neurological Surgeons and the Congress of Neurological Surgeons (2002) for the management of acute cervical spine and spinal cord injuries state that treatment with high-dose methylprednisolone (Solu-Medrol) within the first 8 hours of injury is an option for the patient with SCI. The dosing regimen is initiated with a bolus of 30 mg/kg over 15 minutes, followed in 45 minutes by a continuous intravenous infusion of 5.4 mg/kg/hr for 23 hours. Potential adverse effects of glucocorticoids include hyperglycemia, infection, insulin resistance, gastrointestinal hemorrhage, poor wound healing, edema, and thrombocytopenia. These side effects can adversely affect the patient with SCI (Hurlbert, 2000; American Association of Neurological Surgeons & Congress of Neurological Surgeons, 2002).

Because of limited mobility, measures to prevent the formation of deep vein thrombosis and pulmonary embolism are started immediately on admission. Intermittent pneumatic compression devices are used. If there is not a risk of intramedullary or epidural hemorrhage into the spine, use of low-dose or low-molecular-weight heparin may be initiated. If the patient does not respond to anticoagulation, a vena cava filter may be inserted. Because deep vein thrombosis and pulmonary embolism are common complications of acute SCI, nurses need to assess for the development of these conditions (Barker, 2002; Prendergast & Sullivan, 2000). See SCI Nursing Care Plan.

Surgical Intervention

SCI may require surgical intervention to gain greater neurological recovery, to restore spinal stability, and to protect the patient from further neurological deterioration. Surgery is recommended when neurological deterioration occurs, for intraspinal compression, and for surgically correctable problems. The issue of when surgery should be performed remains controversial (Barker, 2002).

Case Study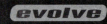

Ms. Jones is a 45-year-old patient who had a clipping of an aneurysm 5 days ago. At present, she is receiving mechanical ventilation and has a pulmonary artery catheter, arterial line, and ventriculostomy in place. Cerebral angiography performed today indicates that she is experiencing cerebral vasospasm. To reverse or overcome the vasospasm, she is started on oral nimodipine and "triple H" therapy (hypervolemia, hemodilution, and hypertension).

QUESTIONS
1. When is the patient at greatest risk of developing vasospasm?
2. What effects does vasospasm have on cerebral function?
3. Discuss the benefits of administering nimodipine and "triple H" therapy.
4. Explain the purpose of the ventriculostomy in this patient.

SUMMARY

Care of the patient with a neurological problem is challenging and complex. Knowledge of normal structure and function of the nervous system is essential to understand common disorders and injuries. Nurses must carefully consider how interventions affect patients. Skills in neurological assessment are important to learn, because changes are often subtle. Nursing assessments and interventions that are tailored to each patient are essential to promote positive patient outcomes.

CRITICAL THINKING QUESTIONS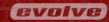

1. You are caring for Tim Smith, who has suffered a closed head injury from a motor vehicle accident. He has an intraventricular catheter for continuous measurement of ICP. His ICP has been stable at 13 mm Hg for the past 4 hours. The alarm on the monitor sounds because his ICP is now 20 mm Hg. What are your priority assessments and interventions at this time?

2. Many nurses believe that visiting should be restricted for neurological patients, especially those with head injuries. What assessments can you make to determine whether family visits are helpful or harmful to your patient?

3. What interventions can you teach families to assist in the care and rehabilitation of patients with prolonged unconsciousness after a head injury or cranial surgery?

4. Barry Brown is an 18-year-old patient who was admitted in generalized convulsive SE. Describe the appropriate nursing and medical interventions.

REFERENCES

Adams, H. P., Goldstein, L. B., Grubb, R. L., et al. (2003). Guidelines for the early management of patients with ischemic stroke: A scientific statement from the Stroke Council of the American Heart Association. *Stroke, 34,* 1056-1083.

American Association of Neurological Surgeons & Congress of Neurological Surgeons (2002). Guidelines for the management of acute cervical spine and spinal cord injuries. *Neurosurgery, 50*(3), S1.

American Association of Neuroscience Nurses, & Schooley, Y. (1998). *Recommendations for the nursing management of the hyperacute ischemic stroke patients* [pp. 1-20]. Clinical Guidelines Series. Glenview, IL: American Association of Neuroscience Nurses.

American Heart Association. (2003). *Stroke facts.* Dallas: Author.

Bader, M., Littlejohns, L., & March, K. (2003). Brain tissue oxygen monitoring in severe brain injury. II. Implications for critical care teams and case study. *Journal of Neuroscience Nursing, 23*(4), 29-44.

Barch, C., Spilker, J., Bratina, P., et al. (1997). Nursing management of acute complications following rt-PA in acute ischemic stroke. *Journal of Neuroscience Nursing, 29*(6), 367-372.

Barker, E. (2002). *Neuroscience nursing: A spectrum of care.* 2nd ed. St. Louis: Mosby.

Barker, E., & Saulino, M. (2002). First-ever guidelines for spinal injuries. *RN, 65*(10), 32-37.

Bederson, J. B., Awad, I. A., Wiebers, D. O., et al. (2000). Recommendations for the management of patients with unruptured intracranial aneurysms: A statement for healthcare professionals from the Stroke Council of the American Heart Association. *Circulation, 102,* 2300-2308.

Benarroch, E. E., Westmoreland, B. F., Daube, J. R., Reagan, T. J., & Sandok, B. A. (1999). *Medical neurosciences: An approach to anatomy, pathology and physiology by systems and levels.* New York: Lippincott Williams & Wilkins.

Bhalla, A., Wolfe, C. D. A., & Rudd, A. G. (2001). Management of acute physiological parameters after stroke. *QJM, 94,* 167-172.

Bleck, T. (2001). Seizures in the critically ill. In J. Parrillo & R. Dellinger (eds.). *Critical care medicine: Principles of diagnosis and management in the adult.* 2nd ed. St. Louis: Mosby.

Braimah, J., Kongable, G., Rapp, K., et al. (1997). Nursing care of acute stroke patients after receiving rt-PA therapy. *Journal of Neuroscience Nursing, 29*(6), 373-383.

Bratina, P., Rapp, K., & Barch, C. (1997). Pathophysiology and mechanisms of acute ischemic stroke. *Journal of Neuroscience Nursing, 29*(6), 356-359.

Broderick, J. P., Adams, H. P., Barsan, W., et al. (1999). Guidelines for the management of spontaneous intracerebral hemorrhage: A statement for health care professionals from a special writing group of the Stroke Council, *30*(4), 905-915. American Heart Association,

Bullock, R., Chestnut, R. M., Clifton, G., et al. (2000). *Management and prognosis of severe traumatic brain injury.* New York: Brain Trauma Foundation and American Association of Neurological Surgeons.

Campbell, P. J., & Edwards, S. M. (1997). Hyperdynamic therapy: The nurse's role in the treatment of cerebral vasospasm. *Journal of Neuroscience Nursing, 29*(5), 318-324.

Castillo, J., Davalos, A., Marrugat, J., & Noya, M. (1998). Timing for fever related brain damage in acute ischemic stroke. *Stroke, 29,* 2455-2460.

Chapman, M., Smith, M., & Hirsch, N. (2001). Status epilepticus. *Anaesthesia, 56,* 648-659.

Cock, H. R., & Schapira, A. H. V. (2002). A comparison of lorazepam and diazepam as initial therapy in convulsive status epilepticus. *QJM, 95*(4), 225-231.

Davis, A. (2000). Cognitive impairments following traumatic brain injury. *Critical Care Nursing Clinics of North America, 12*(4), 447-456.

Deglin J. H. (2003). *Davis' drug guide for nurses.* 8th ed. Philadelphia: F. A. Davis.

Dennison, R. (2000). *Pass CCRN.* 2nd ed. St. Louis: Mosby.

Deyo, D. J., Yancy, V., & Prough, D. S. (2000). Brain function monitoring. In A. Grenvik, S. M. Ayers, P. R. Holbrook, & W. C. Shoemaker (eds.). *Textbook of critical care.* 4th ed. Philadelphia: W. B. Saunders.

Dubendorf, P. (1999). Spinal cord injury pathophysiology. *Critical Care Nursing Quarterly, 22*(2), 31-35.

Fischer, J., & Mathieson, C. (2001). The history of the Glasgow Coma Scale: Implications for practice. *Critical Care Nursing Quarterly, 23*(4), 52-58.

Fisher, M., & Bogousslavsky, J. (2001). *Current review of cerebral vascular disease.* 4th ed. Philadelphia: Current Medicine.

Galley, H. (2000). *Neurologic injury: Critical care focus 3.* London: BMJ Books, BMJ Publishing Group.

Gill, M. (1999). Psychosocial implications of spinal cord injury. *Critical Care Nursing Quarterly, 22*(2), 1-7.

Ginsberg, M. D., & Busto R. (1998). Combating hyperthermia in acute stroke. *Stroke, 29,* 529-534.

Greenberg, M.S. (2001). Handbook of neurosurgery, 5th ed. Lakeland FL: Greenberg Graphics.

Guin, P. (2001). Advances in spinal cord injury care. *Critical Care Nursing Clinics of North America, 13*(3), 399-409.

Haselman, M., & Fox, S. (2000). Microsensor and microdialysis technology. *Critical Care Nursing Clinics of North America, 12*(4), 437-446.

Hickey, J. V. (2003). *The clinical practice of neurological and neurosurgical nursing.* 5th ed. Philadelphia: Lippincott Williams & Wilkins.

Hilker, R., Poetter, C. Findeisen, N., Sobesky, J., Jacobs, A., Neveling, M., & Heiss, W-D. (2003). Nosocomial pneumonia after acute stroke: Implications for neurological intensive care medicine. *Stroke, 34,* 975.

Hinkel, J. L., & Bowman, L. (2003). Pharmacology update: neuroprotection for ischemic stroke. *J Neuroscience Nursing, 35*(2), 114-118.

Hurlbert, R. (2000). Methylprednisolone for acute spinal cord injury: An inappropriate standard of care. *Journal of Neurosurgery, 93,* 1-7.

Johnston, K.C., Li, J. Y., Lynden, P.D., et al. (1998). Medical and neurological complications of ischemic stroke. *Stroke, 29,* 447-453.

Johnston, S. C., Higashida, R. T., Barrow, D. L., et al. (2002). A statement for healthcare professionals from the Committee on Cerebrovascular Imaging of the American Heart Association Council on Cardiovascular Radiology. *Stroke, 33,* 2536-2544.

Kerr, M., Weber, B. B., Sereika, S. M., et al. (1999). Effect of endotracheal suctioning on cerebral oxygenation in traumatic brain-injured patients. *Critical Care Medicine, 27*(12), 2776-2781.

Kidd, K., & Criddle, L. (2001). Using jugular venous catheters in patients with traumatic brain injury. *Critical Care Nurse, 21*(6), 16-22.

Kirkness, C., Mitchell, P. H., Barr, R. L., et al. (2000). Intracranial pressure waveform analysis: clinical and research implications. *Journal of Neuroscience Nursing, 32*(5), 271-277.

Kirkness, C. J., Thompson, J. M., Ricker, B. A., Buzaitis, A., Newell, D. W., Dikmen, S., & Mitchell, P.H. (2002). The impact of aneurysmal subarachnoid hemorrhage on functional outcome. *Journal of Neuroscience Nursing, 34*(3), 134-141.

Kosco, M. & Warren, N.A. (2000). Critical care nurses' perspective of family needs as met. *Critical Care Nursing Quarterly, 23(2),* 60-72.

Le Jeune, G. (2002). Nursing assessment and management of patients with head injury. *Dimensions of Critical Care Nursing, 21* (6), 54-62.

Leonard, A. (2002). *Acute stroke principles of modern management: General care after stroke, including stroke units and prevention and treatment of complications of stroke.* St. Paul, MN: American Academy of Neurology.

Lewis, S., Collier, I., & Heitkemper, M. (2003). *Medical-surgical nursing: Assessment and management of clinical problems.* 6th ed. St. Louis: Mosby.

Littlejohns, L., Bader, M., & March, K. (2003). Brain tissue oxygen monitoring in severe brain injury. *Critical Care Nurse, 23*(4), 17-25.

Littlejohns, L., & Bader, M. (2001). Guidelines for the management of severe head injury: Clinical application and changes in practice. *Critical Care Nurse, 21*(6), 48-65.

Lovasik, D., Kerr, M., & Alexander, S. (2001). Traumatic brain injury research: A review of clinical studies. *Critical Care Nursing Quarterly, 23*(4), 24-41.

Lower, J. (2002). Facing neuro assessment fearlessly. *RN, 32*(2), 58-62.

Mann G., Hankey, G. J., Cameron, D. (1999). Swallowing function after stroke. *Stroke, 30*(4), 744-748.

March, K. (2000). Application of technology in the treatment of traumatic brain injury. *Critical Care Nursing Quarterly, 23*(3), 26-37.

Marik, P., Varon, J., & Trask, T. (2002). Management of head trauma. *Chest, 122*, 699-711.

Minton, M., & Hickey, J. (1999). A primer of neuroanatomy and neurophysiology. *Nursing Clinics of North America, 34*(3), 555-572.

Mitcho, K., & Yanko, J. (1999). Acute care management of spinal cord injuries. *Critical Care Nursing Quarterly, 22*(2), 60-79.

Morris, G. F., Taylor, W. R., & Marshall, L. F. (2000). Management of traumatic brain injury in the intensive care unit. In A. Grenvik, S. M. Ayers, P. R. Holbrook, & W. C. Shoemaker (eds.). *Textbook of critical care.* 4th ed. Philadelphia: W. B. Saunders.

NIH-NINDS and Stroke rt-PA Stroke Study Group. (1995). Tissue plasminogen activator for acute ischemic stroke. *New England Journal of Medicine, 333*, 1581-1587.

Nikas, D. L. (1998). The neurologic system. In J. G. Alspach (ed.). *AACN core curriculum for critical care nursing.* 4th ed. Philadelphia: W. B. Saunders.

North American Symptomatic Carotid Endarterectomy Trial (NASCET) collaborators. (1995). Beneficial effect of carotid endarterectomy in symptomatic patients with high-grade carotid stenosis. *New England Journal of Medicine, 325*(7), 445-453.

Oertel, M., Kelly, D. F., Lee, J. H., et al. (2002). Efficacy of hyperventilation, blood pressure elevation, and metabolic suppression therapy in controlling intracranial pressure after head injury. *Journal of Neurosurgery, 95*, 1045-1053.

Ogilvy, C. S., Stieg, P. E., Awad, I., et al. (2001). Recommendations for the management of intracranial arteriovenous malformations: A statement of healthcare professionals from a special writing group of the Stroke Council, American Heart Association. *Circulation, 103*, 2644-2657.

Prendergast, V., & Sullivan, C. (2000). Acute spinal cord injury. *Critical Care Nursing Clinics of North America, 12*(4), 499-508.

Proctor, M. (2002). Spinal cord injury. *Critical Care Medicine, 30*(11), S489-S499.

Roland, R., Russel, J., Richards, K. C., et al. (2001). Visitation in critical care: Processes and outcomes of a performance improvement initiative. *Journal of Nursing Care Quality, 15*(2), 18-26.

Sabin-Alverez, J., Molina, C. A., Montaner, J., et al. (2003). Effects of admission hyperglycemia on stroke outcome in reperfused tissue plasminogen activator treated patients. *Stroke, 34*, 1235.

Shorvon, S. (2001). The management of status epilepticus. *Journal of Neurology, Neurosurgery, & Psychiatry, 70*[suppl II], ii22-ii27.

Simmons, B. J. (1997). Management of intracranial hemodynamics in the adult: A research analysis of head positioning and recommendations for clinical practice and future research. *Journal of Neuroscience Nursing, 29*(1), 44-49.

Sinha, S., & Warburton, E. A. (2000). The evolution of stroke units: towards a more intensive approach. *QJM, 93*, 633-638.

Smith, B. (2001). Treatment of status epilepticus. *Neurologic Clinics, 19*(2), 347-367.

Spilker, J., Kongable, G., Barch, C., et al. (1997). Using the NIH stroke scale to assess stroke patients. *J Neuroscience Nursing, 29*(6), 384-391.

Stewart-Amidei, C. (1998). Neurologic monitoring in the ICU. *Critical Care Nursing Quarterly, 21*(3), 47-54.

Sullivan, J. (2000). Positioning of patients with severe traumatic brain injury: Research-based practice. *Journal of Neuroscience Nursing, 32*(4), 204-209.

Swearingen, P., & Keen, J. (2001). *Manual of critical care nursing.* 4th ed. St. Louis: C. V. Mosby.

Urden, L., Stacy, K., & Lough, M. (2002). *Critical care nursing: Diagnosis and management.* St. Louis: Mosby.

van Gijn, J., & Rinkel, G. J. E. (2001). Subarachnoid haemorrage: Diagnosis, causes and management. *Brain, 124*, 249-278.

Wojner, A., El-Mitwalli, A., & Alexandrov, A. (2002). Effect of head positioning on intracranial blood flow velocities in acute ischemic stroke. *Critical Care Nursing Quarterly, 24* (4), 57-66.

Wong, F. (2000). Prevention of secondary brain injury. *Critical Care Nurse, 20*(5), 18-27.

Yanko, J., & Mitcho, K. (2001). Acute care management of severe traumatic brain injury. *Critical Care Nursing Quarterly, 23*(4), 1-23.

RECOMMENDED READINGS

Neatherlin, J. (2000). Head trauma in the older adult population. *Critical Care Nursing Quarterly, 22*(4), 49-58.

Pudelek, B. (2002). Geriatric trauma: Special needs for a special population. *AACN Clinical Issues: Advanced Practice in Acute and Critical Care, 13*(1), 61-72.

Stewart-Amidei, C. (2002). Pharmacology advances in the neuroscience intensive care unit. *Critical Care Nursing Clinics of North America, 14*(1), 31-38.

evolve *Did you remember to check out the bonus material, including free self-assessment exercises, on the Evolve Web site at http://evolve.elsevier.com/Sole/ and on the CD-ROM?*

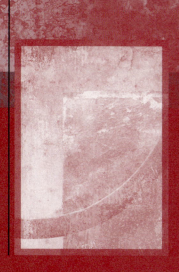

CHAPTER 13

Acute Respiratory Failure

Linda M. Tamburri, MS, RN, CNS, C, CCRN
Carolyn D. Hix, ASN, BSN, MSN, CNAA

OBJECTIVES

- Describe the pathophysiology of acute respiratory failure.
- Examine the etiology, pathophysiology, assessment, nursing diagnoses, interventions, and outcomes for acute respiratory failure in the patient with adult respiratory distress syndrome, chronic obstructive pulmonary disease, asthma, pneumonia, and pulmonary embolus.
- Formulate a plan of care for the patient with acute respiratory failure.

Introduction

Acute respiratory failure (ARF) may occur in many disease states. It may be the patient's primary problem, or it may be a complicating factor in other conditions. This chapter reviews the pathophysiology of ARF, several common causes, and the nursing care involved in the treatment of these patients.

Acute Respiratory Failure

DEFINITION

ARF is defined as a state of altered gas exchange resulting in abnormal arterial blood gas (ABG) values, a partial pressure of oxygen (O_2) in arterial blood (PaO_2) value of less than 60 mm Hg, and a partial pressure of carbon dioxide (CO_2) in arterial blood ($PaCO_2$) value of greater than 50 mm Hg with a pH of less than 7.30 when the patient is breathing room air. Patients with ARF are placed into one of three categories: failure of respiration or oxygenation, failure of ventilation, or a combination of respiratory and ventilatory failure. ARF differs from chronic respiratory failure in the length of time necessary for it to develop. It occurs rapidly, with little time for bodily compensation. Chronic respiratory failure develops over time and allows the body's compensatory defenses to activate. ARF and chronic respiratory failure are not mutually exclusive. ARF may occur when a person who has chronic respiratory failure develops a sudden respiratory infection or is exposed to other types of stressors.

PATHOPHYSIOLOGY
Failure of Oxygenation

Failure of oxygenation is present when the PaO_2 cannot be adequately maintained. Five generally accepted mechanisms that reduce arterial O_2 concentrations and create a state of hypoxemia are (1) hypoventilation,

evolve **Be sure to check out the bonus material, including free self-assessment exercises, on the Evolve Web site at http://evolve.elsevier.com/Sole/ and on the CD-ROM.**

(2) intrapulmonary shunting, (3) ventilation/perfusion mismatching, (4) diffusion defects, and (5) decreased barometric pressure (Figure 13-1). All these mechanisms may contribute to the failure of oxygenation associated with ARF. The least common mechanism, decreased barometric pressure, which occurs at high altitudes, is not addressed in this text. In addition, other conditions, such as decreased cardiac output (CO) and low hemoglobin level, may result in tissue hypoxia.

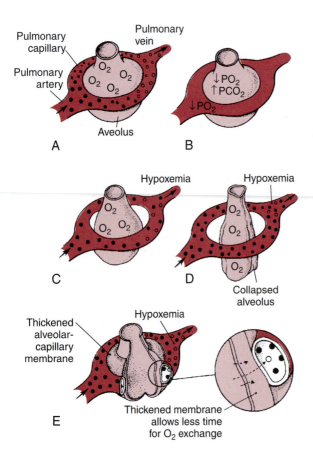

A

B

Hypoxemia   Hypoxemia

C

D

Collapsed alveolus

Hypoxemia

E

Thickened membrane allows less time for O_2 exchange

FIGURE 13-1 Physiological causes of hypoxemia. **A,** A normal alveolar-capillary unit. Unoxygenated blood *(filled circles)* in the pulmonary capillary obtains O_2 from the alveolus. Oxygenated blood *(open circles)* leaves via the pulmonary veins. **B,** Hypoventilation results in an increased PCO_2 and decreased PO_2. **C,** Ventilation/perfusion mismatch resulting from poor alveolar ventilation; hypoxemia results. **D,** Right-to-left shunt. Hypoxemia results from many disorders, all of which lead to collapsed alveoli. **E,** Diffusion defect. The diffusion of O_2 across the alveolar-capillary membrane is decreased when the membrane is thickened or filled with fluid. (From Yee, B. H., & Zorb, S. L. [1985]. *Cardiac critical care nursing* [p. 109]. Boston: Little, Brown).

Hypoventilation. In the normal lung, the partial pressure of alveolar O_2 (PAO_2) is approximately equal to the PaO_2. Alveolar ventilation refers to the amount of gas that enters the alveoli per minute. If the alveolar ventilation is reduced because of hypoventilation, the PAO_2 and the PaO_2 are reduced. Factors that may lead to hypoventilation include drug overdose that causes central nervous system (CNS) depression, neurological disorders that cause a decrease in the rate or depth of respirations, and abdominal or thoracic surgery leading to shallow breathing patterns secondary to pain on inspiration. Hypoventilation also produces an increase in the alveolar CO_2 level because the CO_2 that is produced in the tissues is delivered to the lungs but is not released from the body. This buildup of CO_2 in the alveoli displaces O_2 and contributes to reduced PaO_2 (Schumann, 2000).

Intrapulmonary shunting. In a normally functioning lung, a small amount of blood returns to the left side of the heart without engaging in alveolar gas exchange. This blood is referred to as the *physiological shunt*. If, in addition to the normal shunt, more blood returns to the left side of the heart without being oxygenated, a decrease in the PaO_2 occurs. This condition exists when areas of the lung that are inadequately ventilated are adequately perfused (see Figure 13-1). The blood therefore is shunted past the lung and returns unoxygenated to the left side of the heart. Causes of shunting include atrial or ventricular septal defects, atelectasis, pneumonia, and pulmonary edema.

As the shunt increases, the PaO_2 continues to decrease. This cause of hypoxemia cannot be effectively treated by increasing the fraction of inspired O_2 (FiO_2), because the unventilated alveolar units do not receive any of the enriched air.

Ventilation/perfusion mismatching. The rate of ventilation ($\dot{V}$) usually equals the rate of perfusion ($\dot{Q}$), resulting in a ventilation/perfusion ($\dot{V}/\dot{Q}$) ratio of 1. If ventilation exceeds blood flow, the $\dot{V}/\dot{Q}$ ratio is greater than 1; if ventilation is less than blood flow, the $\dot{V}/\dot{Q}$ ratio is less than 1. In respiratory failure, $\dot{V}/\dot{Q}$ mismatching is the most common cause of hypoxemia. At any given moment, the lung has various $\dot{V}/\dot{Q}$ ratios; one region may be better ventilated and another better perfused. One compensatory mechanism for $\dot{V}/\dot{Q}$ mismatch is hypoxic pulmonary vasoconstriction. When a decrease in $\dot{V}/\dot{Q}$ causes alveolar hypoxia, blood flow to the affected area decreases. This mechanism can partially correct $\dot{V}/\dot{Q}$ mismatch.

In the failing lung, a reduction in the ventilation to a region may occur as a result of increased secretions that obstruct the airway or as a result of bronchospasms. If partial ventilation of the alveoli is involved, the hypoxemia caused by this $\dot{V}/\dot{Q}$ mismatch responds somewhat to an increase in FiO_2. If perfusion is reduced to an area that has normal ventilation, as in pulmonary embolus (PE), the dead space increases in relation to the tidal volume (V_T). The effect of this $\dot{V}/\dot{Q}$ mismatch is discussed later, in the section on failure of ventilation.

Diffusion defects. Diffusion is the movement of gas from an area of high concentration to an area of low concentration. The alveolar-capillary membrane consists of six barriers for diffusion of O_2 and CO_2: surfactant, the alveolar membrane, interstitial fluid, the capillary membrane, plasma, and the red blood cell membrane. Under normal circumstances, O_2 and CO_2 diffuse across the alveolar-capillary membrane in 0.25 second. The distance between the alveoli and the pulmonary capillaries is usually only one or two cells thick. This narrowness of space facilitates efficient diffusion of O_2 and CO_2 across the cell membrane. In respiratory failure, the distance between the alveoli and the capillaries may be increased by the addition of fluid into the interstitial space (see Figure 13-1). Changes in capillary perfusion pressure, leaking of plasma proteins into the interstitial space, and destruction of the capillary membrane contribute to the build-up of fluids around the alveolus. Fibrotic changes in the lung tissue itself may also contribute to a reduction in the diffusion capacity of the lung. As this capacity is reduced, PaO_2 is the first parameter affected, and hypoxemia results. Because CO_2 is more readily diffusible than O_2, hypercapnia is a late sign of diffusion defect.

Low cardiac output. Adequate tissue oxygenation depends on a balance between O_2 supply and demand. CO is the mechanism for delivering O_2 to the tissues, and normal O_2 transport is between 600 and 1000 mL/min.

CO is the product of heart rate times stroke volume. If the CO decreases, less blood is delivered to the tissues. To maintain normal aerobic metabolism, the tissues must extract increasing amounts of O_2 from the blood. When this increase in extraction can no longer compensate for the decreased CO, anaerobic metabolism occurs. This results in a build-up of lactic acid, which further depresses the myocardium and results in an even lower CO. The patient exhibits a low PaO_2 and a low mixed venous O_2 saturation. This reduction in mixed venous O_2 saturation reflects the increased extraction of O_2 at the tissue level. This reduction in oxygenation is seen in patients with reduced CO with or without concomitant pulmonary disease.

Low hemoglobin level. Approximately 95% of the body's O_2 is transported to the tissues bound to hemoglobin. Each gram of hemoglobin can carry 1.34 mL of O_2 when all of its O_2 binding sites are completely filled. The term *oxygen saturation* (SaO_2) refers to the percentage of O_2 binding sites on each hemoglobin molecule that is filled with O_2. For example, a hemoglobin molecule with half of its binding sites filled is said to be 50% saturated. The hemoglobin of a healthy person breathing room air is about 95% saturate. If a patient's hemoglobin level is less than normal, O_2 supply to the tissues may be impaired, and tissue hypoxia may occur. An alteration in hemoglobin function (i.e., carbon monoxide poisoning) can also decrease O_2 delivery to the tissues (Pierson, 2002).

Tissue hypoxia. Anaerobic metabolism occurs when the tissues can no longer obtain adequate O_2 to meet their metabolic needs. In addition, some conditions such as cyanide poisoning may leave the tissues unable to use O_2 despite normal O_2 delivery (Pierson, 2002). Anaerobic metabolism is inefficient and results in the build-up of lactic acid. The point at which anaerobic metabolism begins to occur is not known and may vary with different organ systems. The effects of tissue hypoxia vary with the severity of the hypoxia.

Failure of Ventilation

$PaCO_2$ is the index used in the evaluation of ventilation. When ventilation is reduced, $PaCO_2$ is increased (hypercapnia). When ventilation is increased, $PaCO_2$ is reduced (hypocapnia). Hypoventilation and $\dot{V}/\dot{Q}$ mismatching are the two mechanisms responsible for hypercapnia. Hypercapnia greatly increases cerebral blood flow and may result in headache, increased cerebrospinal fluid pressure, and papilledema. The patient may appear restless and anxious and may demonstrate slurred speech and a depressed level of consciousness.

Hypoventilation. Hypoventilation is the cause of respiratory failure that occurs in patients with neuromuscular disorders, drug overdoses, and chest wall abnormalities (see Figure 13-1). In hypoventilation, CO_2 accumulates in the alveoli and is not blown off. Respiratory acidosis occurs rapidly before renal compensation can occur. Mechanical ventilation may be necessary to support the patient until the initial cause of the hypoventilation can be corrected.

Ventilation/perfusion mismatching. Because the upper and lower airways do not play a part in gas exchange, the volume of inspired gas that fills these structures is referred to as dead space. This dead space is normally 25% to 30% of the inspired volume.

A major mechanism for changes in $PaCO_2$ is an alteration in the volume of dead space (V_D) in relation to the entire V_T (V_D/V_T). The V_D in the lung increases when perfusion is reduced to an area that is ventilated, because that area no longer participates in gas exchange. A change in the V_D/V_T ratio must be accompanied by an increase in minute ventilation for the $PaCO_2$ to remain normal. If the V_D/V_T increases without an accompanying change in minute ventilation, then the $PaCO_2$ increases.

ASSESSMENT

Assessment of gas exchange is discussed in depth in Chapter 8. Assessment of the patient with ARF begins with the neurological system. Changes in mental status resulting from hypoxia and hypercapnia include anxiety, restlessness, confusion, and lethargy, and they may progress to severe somnolence and coma.

The respiratory assessment continues with inspection. The critical care nurse observes the rate, depth, and pattern of respiration. The presence of a cough and the amount and characteristics of any sputum production are noted. Diaphoresis, use of accessory muscles, and retractions indicate respiratory muscle fatigue. The chest is palpated for bilaterally equal respiratory excursion and tactile fremitus. Auscultation assesses the adequacy of airflow and the presence of adventitious breath sounds. For concerns regarding the older adult, see Geriatric Assessment.

A thorough cardiac assessment provides information about the heart's ability to deliver O_2 to the tissues. The patient must be closely monitored for changes in blood pressure, heart rate, and dysrhythmias. Peripheral pulses are assessed for strength and bilateral equality. The skin is assessed for a decrease in temperature, and cyanosis or pallor in color, possibly indicating poor perfusion.

The patient's nutritional status must be evaluated because this is an important factor in maintaining respiratory muscle strength. The nurse looks for recent weight loss, muscle wasting, nausea, vomiting, abdominal distention, and skin turgor quality.

It is important to assess the patient's psychosocial status. This includes identifying the patient's significant others and their role in the family structure. An understanding of the patient's educational level, socioeconomic background, spiritual beliefs, and cultural or ethnic practices will be key in determining an educational plan for discharge and future self-care.

Serial chest x-rays and pulmonary function tests provide important information. Laboratory studies that are essential for the patient with respiratory failure include the following: electrolytes, which determine adequate muscle function; hemoglobin and hematocrit to evaluate the blood's O_2 carrying capacity; and

Geriatric Assessment

- Visual inspection of the elderly patient's chest will reveal diminished chest wall mobility and an increase in anteroposterior diameter. This results from calcification of costal and sternal cartilage and from skeletal changes such as osteoporosis, spinal degeneration, and kyphosis.
- The impact of physiological changes associated with aging is evident in pulmonary function tests, which show increases in functional residual capacity and residual volume, and decreases in tidal volume, vital capacity, and forced expiratory volume.
- Because of age-related decreases in chemoreceptor and central nervous system function, older adults may be less likely to perceive the sensation of dyspnea despite the presence of bronchospasm.
- Older patients have a lower ventilatory response to hypoxia and hypercapnia.
- Hypoxia in the elderly may not produce the same compensatory increases in heart rate, stroke volume, and cardiac output that are seen in younger adults.
- PaO_2 decreases by approximately 4 mm Hg for every decade of life after the 30s. Aging does not, however, produce alterations in $PaCO_2$. For this reason, hypercapnia and a falling pH are causes for concern.
- Increasing age leads to a slower response to oxygen therapy.
- The geriatric patient is more at risk of developing atelectasis and pneumonia as a result of a diminished cough reflex, fewer cilia, a decline in surfactant, thickening of the alveolar-capillary membrane, and a decrease in the effectiveness of the immune system.

Data from Phelan, B. B., Cooper, D. A., & Sangkachand, P. (2002). Prolonged mechanical ventilation and tracheostomy in the elderly. *AACN Clinical Issues, 13*, 84-93; and Zelzenik, J. (2003). Normative aging of the respiratory system. *Clinics in Geriatric Medicine, 19*, 1-18.

ABG measurements. Noninvasive monitoring of the patient's oxygenation and ventilation, such as pulse oximetry and end-tidal CO_2 monitoring, is helpful.

INTERVENTIONS

The goals of treating patients with ARF are five-fold and include (1) maintaining a patent airway, (2) optimizing O_2 delivery, (3) minimizing O_2 demand, (4) treating the cause of ARF, and (5) preventing complications.

If a patient is unable to *maintain a patent airway*, it is the responsibility of the critical care team to protect the airway. This usually involves insertion of an endotracheal tube (ETT) or tracheostomy tube. Safeguarding the position of the tube to prevent inadvertent extubation resulting from patient-related factors requires interventions that range from adequately securing the tube and reassuring or reorienting the patient, to providing sedation or applying restraints. As a last resort, therapeutic paralysis may be required. (Refer to Chapter 8 for nursing care interventions.)

Optimizing O_2 delivery can be achieved in many ways, depending on the needs of the patient. The first is to provide supplemental O_2 via nasal cannula, face mask, or mechanical ventilation. Position the patient for comfort and to enhance $\dot{V}/\dot{Q}$ matching. Some patients who are alert and are very dyspneic oxygenate more effectively in the semi-Fowler's to high-Fowler's position. Patients with unilateral lung disease should be positioned with the better-functioning lung down to perfuse the side that has the best ventilation. Other components of O_2 delivery include adequate hemoglobin levels to carry O_2 and sufficient CO to deliver O_2 to the tissues.

Decreasing O_2 demand begins with providing opportunities for rest. Unnecessary physical activity is avoided in the patient with ARF. Agitation, restlessness, fever, sepsis, and patient-ventilatory dyssynchrony must be addressed because they all contribute to increased O_2 demand and consumption.

While the patient's hypoxia is being treated, efforts must be made to *identify and reverse the cause* of the ARF. Specific interventions for acute respiratory distress syndrome (ARDS), chronic obstructive pulmonary disease (COPD), asthma, pneumonia, and PE are detailed later in this chapter.

Finally, the critical care nurse must be alert to the potential complications that the patient with ARF may encounter in the critical care unit. Preventive measures must be taken to *avoid the complications* of immobility, adverse effects from medications, fluid and electrolyte imbalances, and the hazards of mechanical ventilation, including aspiration, volutrauma, O_2 toxicity, and ventilator-associated pneumonia (VAP).

NURSING DIAGNOSES

Several nursing diagnoses must be considered in the care of a patient with ARF. Establishing appropriate nursing diagnoses assists the critical care nurse in meeting the major goals of therapy. To meet these goals, the critical care nurse devises a plan of care that includes some or all of the following nursing diagnoses:

- Ineffective breathing pattern related to hypoventilation secondary to bronchospasms, infection, inflammation, or CNS depression as indicated by dyspnea, cough, tachypnea, use of accessory muscles, and abnormal ABG results
- Impaired gas exchange related to increased pulmonary edema, secretions, bronchospasms, alteration in amount of dead space, fluid in the interstitial capillaries, or fibrotic changes in the lung tissue, as indicated by hypoxemia, restlessness, and increased $\dot{V}/\dot{Q}$ mismatch
- Risk for infection related to illness and invasive procedures, as indicated by fever; warm, flushed skin; and increased white blood cell count
- Altered nutrition (less than body requirements) related to increased metabolic demands and decreased ability to take in food as a result of infection, trauma, and/or mechanical ventilation, as indicated by calorie counts that do not meet metabolic demands
- Risk for impaired skin integrity related to bed rest and inadequate nutrition
- Risk for anxiety related to inability to speak, situational crisis, uncertainty, and lack of control, as indicated by increased heart rate, blood pressure, respiratory rate; increased muscle tension; and inappropriate behaviors
- Risk for ineffective family coping related to knowledge deficits of family members that result from inadequate information and uncertain outcomes, as indicated by verbalization of fears

OUTCOMES

Therapies and interventions for ARF are chosen based on the individual patient's clinical data. The critical care nurse must continuously reassess the patient's responses to interventions to determine whether therapies can be altered or discontinued. In each situation, health care team members must work with patients and their families to reach common goals. The expected patient outcomes for a patient with ARF include the following:

- Effective breathing pattern and adequate gas exchange without mechanical ventilation
- Adequate oxygenation to the organs and peripheral tissues

- Decreased O_2 consumption
- Minimal damage to lung tissues
- Normothermia
- Absence of infection
- Adequate nutrition to meet metabolic demands
- Intact skin
- Stable blood pressure and CO
- Reduction or elimination of anxiety, fears, and social isolation
- Gradual increase in activity back to baseline without signs of tachypnea, dyspnea, or abnormal ABG results

A review of the care of the patient with ARF can be found in the Nursing Care Plan for a Patient with Acute Respiratory Failure.

Respiratory Failure in Acute Respiratory Distress Syndrome

DEFINITION

ARDS was originally described in 1967 by Ashbaugh, Bigelow, Petty, and Levine as an acute illness manifested by dyspnea, tachypnea, decreased lung compliance, and diffuse alveolar infiltrates on chest x-ray studies. The syndrome was observed in young adult patients after trauma in a clinical setting of shock and/or the need for excessive fluid administration. Autopsy of the initial patients revealed that pathological heart and lung findings were similar to those described in infant respiratory distress syndrome.

 Nursing Care Plan for a Patient with Acute Respiratory Failure

NURSING DIAGNOSIS: *Ineffective breathing pattern related to increased hypoventilation secondary to bronchospasm, infection, inflammation, central nervous system depression*

Patient Outcomes	Interventions	Rationales
Respiratory distress will be absent. Respirations will be unlabored at a rate of 12-16 breaths/min. Arterial blood gases will be WNL.	Assess and document respiratory status every 1 to 2 hr, including breathing pattern, rate, depth, and rhythm.	A normal respiratory rate for an adult is 12-16 unlabored breaths/min. With secretions in airway the respiratory rate will increase.
	Monitor for dyspnea and signs of increasing respiratory distress. Assist with activities designed to conserve energy.	Breath sounds are normally clear or have scattered fine crackles at bases which clear with deep breathing. The presence of coarse crackles during late inspiration indicates fluid in the airway; wheezing indicates an airway obstruction. Signs of increasing distress and dyspnea indicate worsening of condition.
	Position patient in semi-Fowier's position or that in which breathing pattern is most comfortable.	An upright position allows for maximal air exchange and lung expansion.
	Administer medications to increase airflow as ordered; evaluate their effectiveness; may include such drugs as albuterol (Ventolin) and metaproterenol sulfate (Alupent).	Decrease airway resistance secondary to bronchoconstriction.
	Give oxygen therapy or maintain mechanical ventilation as indicated.	To correct hypoxemia.
	Monitor arterial blood gases.	Monitor for hypoxemia. Hypoxemia can result from ventilation/perfusion mismatches secondary to respiratory secretions.
	Provide patient with adequate periods of rest	Patients with dyspnea are easily exhausted and need additional rest.

Nursing Care Plan for a Patient with Acute Respiratory Failure—cont'd

NURSING DIAGNOSIS: *Impaired gas exchange related to pulmonary edema, secretions, bronchospasms, amount of dead space, fluid in interstitial capillaries, or fibrotic changes*

Patient Outcomes	Interventions	Rationales
Gas exchange will be adequate.		Monitor for oxygenation problems and alteration in acid-base balance.
	Monitor arterial blood gases; assess for hypoxemia and hypercapnia.	
	Assess for restlessness or change in the level of consciousness. Position for maximal gas exchange; place the "good" lung down.	Change in behavior and mental status can be early signs of impaired gas exchange.
	Encourage coughing and deep breathing.	Controlled coughing uses the diaphragmatic muscles, which makes the cough more forceful and effective.
	If patient is mechanically ventilated, use paralysis and sedation as ordered to maintain optimal gas exchange.	Medications can decrease sympathetic nervous system discharge that accompanies hypoxia.

NURSING DIAGNOSIS: *Altered nutrition (less than body requirements) related to increased metabolic demands and decreased ability to take food related to infection, trauma, and/or mechanical ventilation, as indicated by calorie counts that do not meet the metabolic demands*

Patient Outcomes	Interventions	Rationales
Decrease in metabolic demands will occur as condition improves. Calorie counts are indicative of nutritional requirements being met. No weight loss will occur. Laboratory results will be WNL.	If patient is able to take food by mouth, provide frequent small meals that are high in calories.	Eating small frequent meals reduces the sensation of fullness and reduces the amount of energy expended.
	Increase usual caloric intake by 1.5-2 times normal.	Caloric requirements are increased by enhanced metabolic demands in critical illness. Inadequate nutritional intake compromises healing.
	If patient is mechanically ventilated, provide enteral or parenteral nutrition.	Mechanisms to provide needed nutrition are used.
	If enteral feedings are used, elevate the head of the bed and monitor gastric residual volumes every 2 hr. Monitor weight and caloric counts.	Decreases the risk of aspiration of gastric contents.

NURSING DIAGNOSIS: *Risk for infection related to illness and invasive procedures, as indicated by elevated temperatures; warm, flushed skin; and increased white blood cell count*

Patient Outcomes	Interventions	Rationales
Temperature will be normothermic. White blood cell count will be WNL. Infection will be absent.	Monitor temperature every 4 hr, more frequently if elevated.	Fever may be first sign of infection.
	Monitor white blood cell count; notify physician if it is elevated. Provide good	Laboratory values are correlated with physical examination to provide a

Continued

Nursing Care Plan for a Patient with Acute Respiratory Failure—cont'd

Patient Outcomes	Interventions	Rationales
Temperature will be normothermic. White blood cell count will be WNL. Infection will be absent.—*cont'd*	pulmonary hygiene. Assess central line and intravenous site for signs of infection: redness, swelling, and drainage. Use aseptic technique with all invasive procedures and dressing changes. Change dressings per protocol and as needed if they become soiled.	global view of the immune system and develop a plan of care. Aseptic technique decreases risk of complications from invasive sites.

NURSING DIAGNOSIS: *Risk for impaired skin integrity related to bed rest and altered metabolic state*

Patient Outcomes	Interventions	Rationales
Skin will remain intact. Perfusion to all areas of the body will be maximized.	Assess every shift for areas of skin breakdown. Keep patient's skin clean and dry. Reposition every 1-2 hr. If unable to turn patient because of hemodynamic instability, place on specialized bed or mattress.	Inspection can identify impending problems early. Decreases the risk of skin breakdown. Repositioning reduces pressure on bony prominences for extended periods of time.

NURSING DIAGNOSIS: *Risk for anxiety related to inability to speak, situational crises, uncertainty, and lack of control, as indicated by an elevated heart rate, blood pressure, and respiratory rate; increased muscle tension; and inappropriate behaviors*

Patient Outcomes	Interventions	Rationales
Vital signs will be WNL. Muscle tension will be reduced; patient will remain relaxed. Anxiety will be reduced, and patient will not exhibit inappropriate behaviors, e.g., anger, fear, withdrawal, or regression.	Monitor for signs of anxiety: increased heart rate, blood pressure, respiratory rate, muscle tension; inappropriate behaviors. Develop trusting relationship with the patient by using calm, consistent, and reliable behaviors. Always introduce yourself and all unfamiliar persons to the patient and explain why they are there. Provide nurturing environment and increase attention to the patient as indicated. Allow the patient some control over decision making. Do not reinforce inappropriate behaviors. Attempt to structure environment by providing consistent caregivers and decreased stimulation. Teach relaxation techniques, e.g., the use of slow rhythmic breathing during stressful periods. Administer sedatives as ordered if indicated. Allow frequent family visits to decrease isolation.	Anxiety is highly individualized response to life events. Signs must be recognized to provide interventions. Being supportive and approachable encourages communication and enhances feeling of safety. Uncertainty and lack of predictability contribute to feelings of anxiety. Relaxation techniques enhance coping.

Nursing Care Plan for a Patient with Acute Respiratory Failure—cont'd

NURSING DIAGNOSIS: *Risk for ineffective family coping related to knowledge deficits of family members due to inadequate information and uncertain outcomes, as indicated by verbalization of fears*

Patient Outcomes	Interventions	Rationales
Family integrity will be maintained. Family members will verbalize educational needs. Family members will verbalize fears and feel comfortable asking questions related to patient's prognosis. Family members will be together in making decisions for their loved one when necessary.	Assess family unit and coping behaviors.	Assessment allows for anticipatory care and guidance to help family unit maintain support and coping strategies.
	Assist family to identify roles to maintain family integrity.	Positive feedback from one family member can reinforce a behavior of another member.
	Assist family members to verbalize distress.	Sharing feelings allows family an opportunity to communicate in an effective way.
	Explain procedures, equipment, changes in patient's condition, and outcomes to family members in a sensitive manner.	Establishes a trusting relationship.
	Always allow time for family members to ask questions and to verbalize fears.	Encourages compliance with treatment and enhances feelings of control.
	Inform family of resources available to them, such as chaplain and psychiatric liaison.	Enhances the use of services that could assist family during time of crisis.
	Provide conferences with family and health care providers to supply information, be supportive, and allow family members to see that all members of health care team are working together to provide the best quality and continuity of care of their loved one.	Establishes trust with health care team and encourages compliance with treatments.

WNL, within normal limits.
From Ackley, B. J., & Ladwig, G. B. (2002). *Nursing diagnosis handbook: A guide to planning care.* St. Louis: Mosby.

The definition of ARDS has been expanded and refined over the years. Murray, Matthay, Luce, & Fick (1988) were the first to suggest a three-part definition. The first component reflects the condition. The second component designates the causes or risk factors. The third is a scoring mechanism determining the degree of injury to the lung. The lung injury score consists of four aspects of pulmonary assessment: the amount of infiltrates on chest x-ray, the degree of hypoxemia (PaO_2/FiO_2), the amount of positive end-expiratory pressure (PEEP), and the static lung compliance. The scoring system quantifies the severity of the acute lung injury. ARDS is the most severe degree of lung injury as shown in Table 13-1. In 1994, the American-European Consensus Conference recommended that the definition of ARDS consist of three criteria in the presence of a risk factor. The three criteria are PaO_2/FiO_2 less than 200, bilateral infiltrates, and pulmonary

TABLE 13-1

Expanded Definition of ARDS: Severity of Acute Lung Injury

Component	Score
CHEST X-RAY SCORE (ALVEOLAR CONSOLIDATION)	
None	0
Confined to one quadrant	1
Confined to two quadrants	2
Confined to three quadrants	3
In all four quadrants	4
HYPOXEMIA SCORE(PaO_2/FiO_2)	
≥300	0
225-299	1
175-224	2
100-174	3
<100	4
PEEP SCORE (WHEN VENTILATED)	
≤5 cm H_2O	0
6-8 cm H_2O	1
9-11 cm H_2O	2
12-14 cm H_2O	3
≥15 cm H_2O	4
COMPLIANCE SCORE (WHEN AVAILABLE)	
≥80 mL/cm H_2O	0
60-79 mL/cm H_2O	1
40-59 mL/cm H_2O	2
20-39 mL/cm H_2O	3
≤19 mL/cm H_2O	4
LUNG INJURY	
The final value is obtained by dividing the aggregate sum by the number of components that were used:	
No lung injury	0
Mild to moderate lung injury	0.1-2.5
Severe lung injury (ARDS)	> 2.5

From Murray, J. F., Matthay, M. A., Luce, J. M., & Fick, M. R. (1988). An expanded definition of the adult respiratory distress syndrome. *American Review of Respiratory Disease, 138*(3), 720-723.

artery occlusion pressure less than 18 mm Hg or no clinical evidence of left atrial hypertension (Bernard et al., 1994).

ETIOLOGY

Although the signs, symptoms, and pathophysiology are the same, many potential causes have been implicated in the development or worsening of ARDS. Some possible causes of ARDS are listed in Box 13-1, and are categorized into direct and indirect factors (Bernard et al., 1994). Certain risk factors have a higher associated frequency of ARDS, and the presence of two or more factors increases the risk. The most common risk factors or disease processes associated with ARDS are sepsis, pneumonia, multiple transfusions, aspiration of gastric contents, trauma, and ischemia reperfusion (Brower, Ware, Berthiaume, & Matthay, 2001).

BOX 13-1

Possible Causes for Acute Respiratory Distress Syndrome

DIRECT CAUSES
Aspiration of gastric contents
Diffuse pneumonia
Fat embolism
Near-drowning
Neurogenic pulmonary edema
Oxygen toxicity
Prolonged mechanical ventilation
Pulmonary contusion
Multisystem trauma (chest and/or lung injury)
Radiation (chest)

INDIRECT CAUSES
Cardiopulmonary bypass
Anaphylaxis
Disseminated intravascular coagulation
Drug overdose
Eclampsia
Fractures, especially of the pelvis or long bones
Increased intracranial pressure
Leukemia
Multiple transfusions
Pancreatitis
Sepsis
Thrombotic thrombocytopenic purpura
Hypotension
Multisystem trauma
Radiation

The mortality rate for patients diagnosed with ARDS is 43% to 70% (Schumann, 2000). A study of 109 patients who survived ARDS revealed that lung volume and spirometric measurements were normal by 6 months, but functional disability persisted 1 year after discharge. Most of these patients had extrapulmonary conditions, with muscle wasting and weakness being prominent (Herridge et al., 2003).

The cause of ARDS is an important factor in the planning of collaborative interventions to attain successful patient outcomes. Although treatment plans may be similar because of the overall problems with oxygenation and fluid balance, all the possible underlying causes must be considered. This careful consideration guides the therapy and can improve the patient's chances for a successful outcome.

PATHOPHYSIOLOGY

ARDS is characterized by acute and diffuse injury to the lung, leading to respiratory failure. The initial response is a systemic inflammatory reaction secondary to the direct or indirect lung injury. Several cell types and inflammatory mediators have key roles in the pathological changes that occur at the cellular level after the injury. The most significant of these are neutrophils, complement, endotoxins, and arachidonic acid metabolites. Initial injury causes damage to the pulmonary capillary endothelium, which activates massive aggregation of platelets and formation of intravascular thrombus. The platelets release serotonin and a substance that activates neutrophils. Neutrophil activation causes release of several chemotactic mediators (i.e., tumor necrosis factor, interleukin 1, cytokines, and hydroxyl radicals). The release of the chemotactic mediators damages lipid membranes, lung fibroblasts, parenchymal cells, and endothelial cells. Neutrophils also release platelet-activating factor causing additional agglutination of platelets and neutrophils. Microembolization occurs, leading to pulmonary vasoconstriction and hypertension (Schlicher, 2001).

Endothelial damage initiates the complement cascade including the anaphylatoxins C3a and C5a. The complement components promote release of histamine by mast cells causing large gaps to develop in the capillary membrane. Additional destructive complement components including proteolytic enzymes, O_2 free radicals, prostaglandins, thromboxanes and leukotrienes are activated. All of these complement components combine to cause damage to the alveolar-capillary membrane increasing capillary permeability.

Increased capillary permeability allows fluids, protein, and blood cells to leak from the capillary beds into the alveoli and results in pulmonary edema. Pulmonary edema worsens $\dot{V}/\dot{Q}$ mismatch.

The production of surfactant is stopped, and the surfactant present is inactivated.

The lungs become less compliant, and ventilation decreases. A right-to-left shunt of pulmonary blood develops, and hypoxemia refractory to O_2 supplementation becomes profound. This entire process leads to fibrosis destroying the alveoli, bronchioles, and interstitium.

The neutrophils and inflammatory mediators may also cause generalized endothelial damage and capillary permeability throughout the entire body. This damage can lead to the development of multiorgan dysfunction. The development of multiorgan dysfunction increases ARDS mortality to 90% (Schlicher, 2001). The pathophysiology of ARDS is outlined in Figure 13-2.

ASSESSMENT

Early assessment and diagnosis of ARDS guide the caregivers to institute appropriate therapies. One of the initial signs of ARDS is restlessness, change in the patient's personality, disorientation, and change in levels of consciousness. Other early warning signs are dyspnea and hyperventilation with normal breath sounds. Patients may also exhibit a cough accompanied by respiratory alkalosis. If the patient is mechanically ventilated, the critical care nurse may observe an increase in peak inspiratory pressures. This finding is an indication of a decrease in compliance. Pulse and temperature may be increased, and chest x-ray studies are usually normal in the initial stage.

As the process progresses and the PaO_2 decreases, dyspnea becomes severe, and the patient may grunt with respirations. The $PaCO_2$ continues to decrease, resulting in respiratory alkalosis without an improvement in oxygenation. Intercostal and suprasternal retractions are present on physical examination. Hypocapnia and hypoxemia do not respond to increasing levels of O_2. Tachycardia and pallor are present, and central cyanosis may be evident.

The respiratory alkalosis is accompanied by metabolic acidosis that is caused by lactic acid buildup. The presence of this condition can be confirmed by serum lactate level determinations. As the ARDS progresses, the nurse auscultates crackles, rhonchi, and bronchial breath sounds. A chest x-ray study shows bilateral patchy infiltrates, which progress to complete opacity, often referred to as a "whiteout" (see Acute Respiratory Failure Clinical Alerts).

Pulmonary mechanics show a decrease in lung volume, especially functional residual capacity, and a decrease in static and dynamic compliance. As the patient's condition deteriorates, peak inspiratory pressures continue to rise.

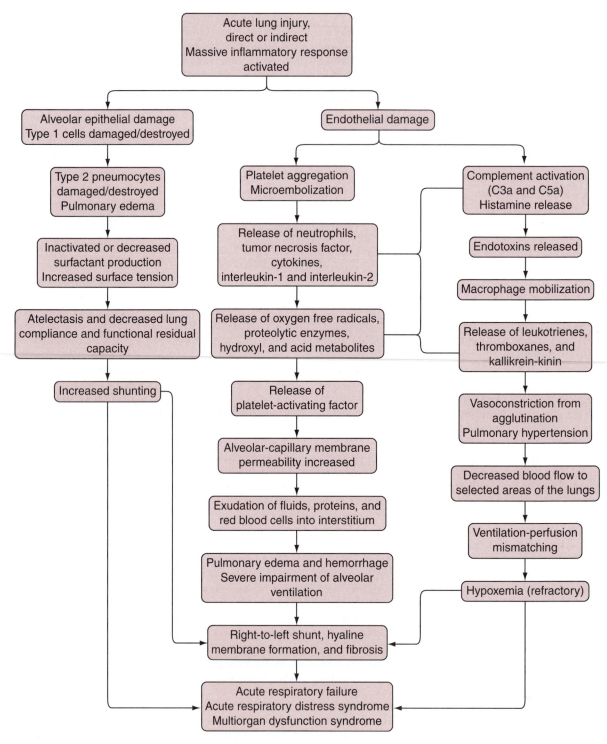

FIGURE 13-2 Pathophysiology of acute respiratory distress syndrome. (From Schlicher, M. [2001]. Using liquid ventilation to treat patients with acute respiratory distress syndrome: A guide to a breath of fresh liquid. *Critical Care Nurse, 21*(5), 55-65.)

ACUTE RESPIRATORY FAILURE CLINICAL ALERTS

Concern	Symptoms	Nursing Actions

Respiratory muscle fatigue	Diaphoresis
	Nasal flaring
	Tachypnea
	Abdominal paradox
	Muscle retractions
	  Intercostal
	  Suprasternal
	  Supraclavicular
	Tachycardia
	Central cyanosis
		Improve oxygen delivery
		  Administer oxygen
		  Ensure adequate cardiac output
		  Correct low hemoglobin
		Decrease oxygen demand
		  Provide rest
		  Decrease pain and anxiety
		  Decrease work of breathing
		  Administer bronchodilators

Cerebral hypoxia and carbon dioxide narcosis from increased carbon dioxide retention	Lethargy Somnolence Coma Respiratory acidosis	Position patient for optimum gas exchange and perfusion Maintain airway patency Prepare for intubation and mechanical ventilation

Assessment of a patient with ARDS is collaborative. A key clinical finding that is often diagnostic of ARDS is a lung insult followed by respiratory distress with profound dyspnea, tachypnea, and hypoxemia that does not respond to O_2 therapy. Once the condition is diagnosed, important assessment data that are used to guide treatment include hemodynamic measurements, ABGs, mixed venous blood gases, breath sounds, serial chest x-ray studies, fluid and electrolyte values, metabolic and nutritional needs, and psychosocial needs of the patient and family.

INTERVENTIONS

The treatment of ARDS demands that the health care team focus on the goals outlined in the section on ARF. Although current research has provided a clearer understanding of the pathophysiology of ARDS, treatment of the illness remains largely supportive.

Oxygenation

Patients with ARDS usually require intubation and mechanical ventilation (see Chapter 8). Selection of ventilator settings is based on lung-protective strategies that attempt to achieve adequate oxygenation while minimizing the risks of ventilator-associated complications. Until recent years, high levels of V_T were routinely used in the treatment of ARDS. Studies conducted since the mid-1990s demonstrated reduced mortality and complications with the use of lower V_T. The target V_T recommended is 6 mL/kg of ideal

body weight. It may be reduced to 4 to 5 mL/kg to maintain the end-inspiratory plateau pressure at 30 cm H_2O or less. These lower volumes prevent the alveoli from overdistending and minimize shearing (Davies, 2002). The respiratory acidosis that occurs secondary to the hypercapnia can be controlled with a sodium bicarbonate infusion and/or by increasing the ventilator respiratory rate. The total CO_2 should be kept within a permissive hypercapnia range of 50 to 70 mm Hg (Brower, Ware, Berthiaume, & Matthay, 2001).

Patients with ARDS require significant support to achieve and/or maintain arterial oxygenation. To prevent O_2 toxicity, the lowest FiO_2 is used to maintain the PaO_2 above 60 mm Hg. Research has shown no detectable O_2 toxicity when the FiO_2 is less than 0.50. Impaired gas exchange has been noted after breathing 100% O_2 at sea level for approximately 40 hours (Brower, Ware, Berthiaume, & Matthay, 2001).

Ventilatory support typically includes PEEP to improve arterial oxygenation by ventilating collapsed alveoli. The appropriate amount of PEEP to use is controversial. A research trial conducted in the late 1990s to examine the role of higher PEEP to keep the lungs open between breaths and to improve lung healing and repair was inconclusive. Additional studies are ongoing to assist in answering the question whether high PEEP levels are beneficial as an open lung approach (Thompson, Hayden, Matthay, Brower, & Parson, 2001). The amount of PEEP used in critical care settings varies considerably. High levels of PEEP carry two major risks. First, excessive pressure in stiff lungs increases peak inspiratory and plateau pressures which may result in barotrauma and pneumothorax. Treatment of a pneumothorax requires prompt insertion of a chest tube. Second, high levels of PEEP can decrease venous return to the heart and result in lower CO and blood pressure.

A few unconventional modes of mechanical ventilation have been used in the treatment of ARDS when patients are unable to be oxygenated with standard modes of ventilation (i.e., high-frequency ventilation; pressure-controlled, inverse-ratio ventilation; airway pressure release ventilation). These modes have been developed to improve alveolar ventilation and arterial oxygenation while decreasing the risk of lung injury. None have been successful enough to be considered standard therapy. (See Chapter 8 for additional information on advanced modes of mechanical ventilation.)

Comfort

Sedation and pain relief are essential for promoting comfort and decreased O_2 consumption in the patient with ARDS. Clinical indications of pain or anxiety include tachycardia, hypertension, restlessness, and diaphoresis. When using continuous sedation, the patient's sedation level should be monitored carefully using a clinical observation scale (e.g., Ramsay Sedation Scale) or objective technique (e.g., bispectral index monitoring) to prevent oversedation. In some patients, therapeutic paralysis with a neuromuscular blocking agent is required to control ventilation completely and to oxygenate the patient adequately. Administration of neuromuscular blockade is required when using unconventional modes of ventilation because these modes are uncomfortable for the patient and are an unnatural means of respiration. The critical care nurse should use a peripheral nerve stimulator to monitor the degree of paralysis achieved by the blocking agent. This will guide drug titration and decrease the risk of prolonged muscle weakness that has been associated with the use of paralytic agents. Because of the intense fear and anxiety that a patient may experience while undergoing neuromuscular blockade, it is vital that the patient receives intravenous anxiolytic medication to maintain an appropriate level of deep sedation (Davies, 2002; Luer, 2002).

Positioning

Patient positioning has had a long-standing role in promoting comfort and preventing skin breakdown. It has also been used as a treatment for ARDS. Some studies have been conducted on turning patients to the prone position to improve oxygenation. In 2001,

Gattinoni and colleagues found that prone positioning improved oxygenation in more than 70% of the patients studied. CT studies demonstrated that pulmonary infiltrates, atelectasis, and collapsed lung regions were primarily located in the dorsal regions when patients were supine. After turning to the prone position, the pulmonary infiltrates were redistributed toward the ventral region, thus reducing intrapulmonary shunting and increasing pulmonary perfusion (Murray & Patterson, 2002). A small study of 51 patients resulted in a statistically significant decrease in VAP when patients with ARDS were turned to the prone position. The incidence of VAP was 20% in the group of patients turned to the prone position daily versus 38.4% in the group left in the supine position. Although results of studies on placing these patients in the prone position have been encouraging, they have not clearly outlined the optimal timing, frequency, and duration of this positioning. Two multi-institutional studies are occurring in Europe to determine whether prolonged use of the prone position will reduce mortality (Krieger, 2002). Some research is suggesting that placing patients in the prone position early in the course of treatment may be optimal (Brower, Ware, Berthiaume, & Matthay, 2001; Ward, 2002).

Turning patients to the prone position is a cumbersome procedure with safety concerns. Care must be taken during the turning procedure to prevent dislodging the multiple tubes and lines connected to the severely ill patient. During the turning procedure, several health care professionals are needed to ensure the patient's safety. In 1996, the Vollman Prone Positioner was introduced by the Hill-Rom Services Corporation to assist with the turning procedure (Figure 13-3).

Other potential complications from the prone position are peripheral nerve injury, skin necrosis, corneal

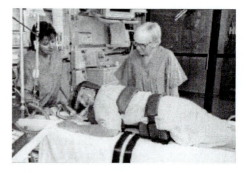

FIGURE 13-3 Patient in the prone position using the Vollman Prone Positioner. (© 2003 Hill-Rom Services, Inc. Reprinted with permission. All rights reserved).

ulceration, and facial edema (Murray & Patterson, 2002). Before the turning procedure, the critical care nurse develops a plan to prevent these complications. A moisture barrier is applied to the patient's entire face to protect the skin from the massive amount of drainage from the mouth and nose. Protective pads are used at the shoulders, iliac crest, and knees to decrease alteration in skin integrity and peripheral nerve damage. The prone position usually results in massive facial edema. The eyes must be protected to prevent direct ocular pressure. The eyes are either taped shut or have lubricant applied to prevent corneal drying and abrasions. To avoid peripheral nerve injury and contractures of the shoulders, the arms are positioned carefully and repositioned often (Balas, 2000).

Fluid and Electrolytes

Optimal fluid management in patients with ARDS is a controversial issue. The ARDS Network is currently conducting a clinical trial to examine two strategies for managing fluid balance in these patients. The study is testing a liberal fluid strategy aimed at improving the overall circulation volume versus a fluid conservative strategy that potentially avoids excess lung fluid accumulation. Until the outcome of these studies is known, the International Consensus Committee recommends timely fluid resuscitation and achievement of normal hemodynamics (Brower, Ware, Berthiaume, & Matthay, 2001).

Nutrition

Nutritional support for critically ill patients including those with ARDS is a standard of care. The goals of the therapy are to provide adequate nutrition to meet the patient's level of metabolism, to prevent and treat deficiencies of macronutrients and micronutrients, and to prevent complications related to the route of administration (Brower, Ware, Berthiaume, & Matthay, 2001). Enteral nutrition is preferred in patients with functioning gastrointestinal tracts. If the gastrointestinal tract is not functioning, parenteral nutrition may be used. Enteral formulas lower in carbohydrates than normal may be used to decrease CO_2 formation if the patient is retaining CO_2. A research study is currently under way to determine whether nutritional products containing antioxidants that promote cell regeneration may decrease production of inflammatory mediators (Davies, 2002).

Psychosocial Support

The onset of ARDS and its long recovery phase result in stress and anxiety for both the patient and the family. The patient may also experience feelings of isolation and dependence because of the length of the recovery phase. Health care team members must always remember to provide a warm, nurturing environment in which the patient and family can feel safe.

All health care team members should take the time to explain procedures, equipment, changes in the patient's condition, and outcomes to patients and families. The patient should be allowed to participate in the planning of care as much as possible, and be encouraged to verbalize fears and questions. In the intubated patient, communication is impaired, which may increase the patient's sense of isolation. The isolation and accompanying depression can be minimized by encouraging frequent visits from family and friends and displaying personal items from home, such as photographs of loved ones.

Other Therapies

Because there is no definitive treatment for ARDS, significant efforts have been ongoing to test the efficacy of a variety of therapies. The following therapies are still under investigation, and there are no clinical trials that support routine use in patients with ARDS. Most of them are considered rescue therapy for refractory hypoxemia in ARDS.

Inhaled nitric oxide is a short-acting, potent vasodilator that selectively works on the vascular endothelium to increase pulmonary blood flow to ventilated alveoli. This lessens shunting and improves oxygenation. Potential complications associated with nitric oxide therapy are methemoglobinemia, increased nitrogen dioxide levels, pulmonary edema, acidosis, and hypotension. In addition, because nitric oxide is a pollutant, precautions must be taken to limit the amount of nitric oxide released into the patient care environment. The Occupational Safety and Health Administration set the threshold at 25 ppm averaged over an 8-hour work shift for workplace exposure to this substance (Qureshi, Shah, Hemmen, Thill, & Kruse, 2003).

Another potential therapy is liquid ventilation. This process involves filling the functional residual capacity of the lungs with perfluorocarbon liquid to enhance gas exchange. The liquid prevents alveolar collapse, increases lung compliance, and promotes gas exchange in previously unventilated alveoli (Brower, Ware, Berthiaume, & Matthay 2001; Schlicher, 2001).

Extracorporeal membrane oxygenation (ECMO) is a process where the patient's blood is circulated through a membrane oxygenator to exchange gases and partially perform the work of the lungs. This therapy provides the patient's lungs with an opportunity to rest and recover from the injury (Dirkes, 2002). ECMO is only performed in a few hospitals because of the specialized equipment and staff skills the therapy requires.

Various clinical trials are under way looking at single therapies and therapies in combination. Several pharmacological agents are being studied and show promise. Corticosteroids, inhaled nitric oxide, alveolar surfactant, and vasodilators are being evaluated. Replacements of anticoagulation mediators may have beneficial effects (Tasaka, Hasegawa, & Ishizaka, 2002). Combination albumin and furosemide therapy is being researched for hypoproteinemic patients with ARDS (Martin et al., 2002). Combination therapies such as high-frequency oscillatory ventilation and nitric oxide, use of sigh in supine and prone position, and inhaled nitric oxide and prone position are being investigated (Mehta et al., 2003; Pelosi et al., 2003; Rialp, Betbese, Perez-Marquez, & Mancebo, 2001).

Acute Respiratory Failure in Chronic Obstructive Pulmonary Disease

PATHOPHYSIOLOGY

COPD is characterized by progressive and often irreversible airflow limitations, associated with an abnormal inflammatory response to noxious particles or gases (Pauwels, Buist, Calverley, Jenkins, & Hurd, 2001). COPD is the fourth leading cause of death in the United States after cardiac disease, cancer, and stroke. Whereas the mortality rates for heart disease and stroke have declined significantly in the past few decades, the death rate for COPD has increased by 71% (Hurd, 2000). The primary cause of COPD is tobacco smoke. Smoking cessation has been described as "the single most effective—and cost effective—way to reduce the risk of developing COPD and to stop its progression" (Pauwels et al., 2001). Other contributing factors to the development of COPD include air pollution, occupational exposure to dust or chemicals, and the genetic abnormality α_1-antitrypsin deficiency (Pauwels et al., 2001).

The primary pathogenic mechanism in COPD is chronic inflammation. Exposure to inhaled particles leads to airway inflammation and injury. The body repairs this injury through the process of airway remodeling, which causes scarring, narrowing, and obstruction of the airways. Destruction of alveolar walls and connective tissue results in permanent enlargement of air spaces. Also present are an enlargement of mucus-secreting glands and an increase in the number of goblet cells, both of which lead to increased mucus production. Areas of cilia are destroyed, contributing to the patient's inability to clear thick, tenacious mucus that blocks the airways. Structural changes in the pulmonary capillaries thicken the vascular walls and inhibit gas exchange. Table 13-2 outlines the physiological changes that result from this pathological process.

Although COPD is marked by a gradual decline in lung function, ARF can occur at any time in the patient with COPD. These patients normally have little respiratory reserve, and any condition that increases the work of breathing worsens $\dot{V}/\dot{Q}$ mismatching. Common causes of ARF in patients with COPD are acute exacerbations, heart failure, dysrhythmias, pulmonary edema, pneumonia, dehydration, and electrolyte imbalances.

ASSESSMENT

The hallmark symptoms of COPD are dyspnea, chronic cough, and sputum production. The diagnosis

---

TABLE 13-2

Pathological and Physiological Changes in Chronic Obstructive Pulmonary Disease

Pathological Changes	Physiological Changes
Mucus hypersecretion	Sputum production
Ciliary dysfunction	Retained secretions
	Chronic cough
Chronic airway inflammation	Expiratory airflow limitation
Airway remodeling	Terminal airway collapse
	Lung hyperinflation
	Poor gas exchange with hypoxemia and hypercapnia
Thickening of pulmonary vessels	Poor gas exchange with hypoxemia and hypercapnia
	Pulmonary hypertension
	Cor pulmonale (right ventricular enlargement and heart failure)

Data from Pauwels, R. A., Buist, A. S., Calverley, P. M., Jenkins, C. R., & Hurd, S. S. (2001). Global strategy for the diagnosis, management, and prevention of chronic obstructive pulmonary disease: NHLBI/WHO Global Initiative for Chronic Obstructive Lung Disease (GOLD) workshop summary. *American Journal of Respiratory and Critical Care Medicine*, *163*, 1256-1276; and Brashers, V. L., & Davey, S. S. (2002). Structure and function of the pulmonary system. In M. McCance & S. E. Huether (eds.). *Pathophysiology: The biologic basis for disease in adults and children* [pp. 1082-1104]. 4th ed. St. Louis: Mosby.

is confirmed by postbronchodilator spirometry that documents irreversible airflow limitations (Pauwels et al., 2001). These pulmonary function tests show an increase in total lung capacity and a reduction in forced expiratory volume over 1 second (FEV_1). Functional residual capacity is increased as a result of air trapping. On physical examination, the chest is overexpanded, or barrel-shaped, because the antero-posterior diameter increases in size. Respiration may include the use of accessory muscles and pursed-lip breathing. Clubbing of the fingers indicates long-term hypoxemia. Lung auscultation usually reveals diminished breath sounds, prolonged exhalation, wheezing, and crackles. ABG results may show mild hypoxemia in the early stages of the disease. With disease progression, ABGs reveal worsening hypoxemia and hypercapnia. Over time, as a compensatory mechanism, the kidney increases bicarbonate production and retention in an attempt to keep the pH within normal limits.

Exacerbations of COPD may result from infection, cardiac disease, inhalation of irritants, or illnesses that contribute to respiratory muscle fatigue. The patient usually reports worsening dyspnea and an increase in sputum production. Changes in the character of the sputum may signal the development of a respiratory infection that could produce profound respiratory failure. Additional symptoms may include anxiety, chest tightness, weakness, malaise, weight loss, fever, and sleeping difficulties. Wheezing indicates narrowing of the airways, and the patient is generally more comfortable in the upright position. Retraction of the intercostal muscles may occur with inspiration, and exhalation is prolonged through pursed lips. Tachycardia and hypotension may result from reduced CO.

ABG monitoring is a sensitive indicator of the patient's respiratory status. It is extremely important for the critical care nurse to know the COPD patient's baseline ABGs to detect changes that indicate ARF. The patient with COPD who chronically retains CO_2 may have baseline ABG results that show a normal pH, a moderately low PaO_2 in the range of 60 to 65 mm Hg, and $PaCO_2$ in the range of 50 to 60 mm Hg. When ARF ensues, the $PaCO_2$ increases, and the PaO_2 may decrease further, resulting in acidosis and tissue hypoxia (see Chronic Obstructive Pulmonary Disease Clinical Alert).

INTERVENTIONS

Box 13-2 outlines the care of patients with stable COPD. When a patient experiences acute exacerbation, the goals of therapy are to provide support during the episode of acute failure, to treat the triggering

CHRONIC OBSTRUCTIVE PULMONARY DISEASE CLINICAL ALERT

The risk of relapse, acute respiratory failure, and death are highest in patients with chronic obstructive pulmonary disease who have an acute exacerbation with a low PaO_2, respiratory acidosis, and significant comorbidities, and in those who require frequent bronchodilator therapy (Snow, Lascher, & Moltur-Pilson, 2001; Pauwels et al., 2001).

event, and to return the patient to his or her previous level of functioning.

Oxygen

The most important intervention for acute exacerbation is to correct hypoxemia. O_2 should be administered to achieve a PaO_2 greater than 60 mm Hg or SaO_2 greater than 90% (Pauwels et al., 2001). Delivering high concentrations of O_2 in an attempt to raise the PaO_2 to more than 60 mm Hg will not significantly raise the SaO_2. (This is illustrated by the upper plateau of the oxyhemoglobin dissociation curve seen in Chapter 8.) Administering high concentrations

BOX 13-2

Treatment of Stable Chronic Obstructive Pulmonary Disease

- Reduce exposure to airway irritants
- Counseling/treatment for smoking cessation
- Remain in air-conditioned environment during times of high air pollution
- Pulmonary rehabilitation program with exercise training
- Annual influenza vaccine
- Inhaled bronchodilators (short-acting, long-acting, or combination)
- Inhaled corticosteroids (for moderate or severe disease)
- Long-term administration of oxygen more than 15 hours/day (for severe disease)

Data from Pauwels, R. A., Buist, A. S., Calverley, P. M., Jenkins, C. R., & Hurd, S. S. (2001). Global strategy for the diagnosis, management, and prevention of chronic obstructive pulmonary disease: NHLBI/WHO Global Initiative for Chronic Obstructive Lung Disease (GOLD) workshop summary. *American Journal of Respiratory and Critical Care Medicine*, 163, 1256-1276.

of O_2 may also blunt the patient's hypoxic drive, which can diminish respiratory efforts and increase the risk of CO_2 retention. Signs of worsening failure are a rising $PaCO_2$ accompanied by acidosis.

Bronchodilator Therapy

Table 13-3 lists commonly administered bronchodilator agents. Short-acting inhaled beta$_2$-agonists cause bronchial smooth muscle relaxation and reverse bronchoconstriction. They are administered via nebulizer or a metered-dose inhaler with a spacer. The dosage and frequency vary, depending on the delivery method and the severity of bronchoconstriction. Adverse effects are dose related and most commonly include tachycardia, dysrhythmias, tremors, hypokalemia, anxiety, bronchospasm, and dyspnea. Beta$_2$-agonists should be administered cautiously in patients with cardiac disease. Long-acting beta$_2$-agonists are useful in controlling stable COPD, but their onset of action is too long to be useful in the treatment of acute exacerbation.

Anticholinergics such as ipratropium bromide may also be administered to treat bronchoconstriction. They are indicated for patients who can not tolerate beta$_2$-agonists, or they may be used in combination with beta$_2$-agonists (Adkinson & Konzem, 2001). Side effects include palpitations, dry mouth, and drying of respiratory secretions. The use of methylxanthines for acute exacerbation is controversial and requires the monitoring of trough blood levels to maintain therapeutic concentrations (Adkinson & Konzem, 2001). Cardiac side effects may be seen in addition to CNS stimulation that may lead to headache, restlessness, and seizures. The use of expectorants, mucolytic agents, and chest physical therapy have not been found to be effective in the management of COPD exacerbations and therefore should be avoided.

Corticosteroids

The use of systemic corticosteroids for a period of 10 to 14 days to decrease airway inflammation has been shown to be beneficial in the management of an acute exacerbation of COPD. Studies show a reduction in hospital length of stay and improved FEV_1, with no significant difference seen between oral and parenteral steroids (Singh, Palda, Stanbrook, & Chapman, 2002). Common adverse effects of steroid therapy include hyperglycemia and increased risk of infection. There is also an unexplained association between steroid use in the critically ill and the development of skeletal muscle myopathy.

Antibiotics

Antibiotic therapy is most effective in severe exacerbations when increased dyspnea is also accompanied by increased sputum volume and purulence (Adkinson & Konzem, 2001; Pauwels et al., 2001). The most common organisms are *Haemophilus influenzae*, *Streptococcus pneumoniae*, and *Moraxella catarrhalis* (Adkinson & Konzem, 2001; Pauwels et al., 2001).

TABLE 13-3

Bronchodilators

Medication	Mechanism of Action	Adverse Effects/Nursing Implications
Beta$_2$-agonists (short-acting) Albuterol Bitolterol Pirbuterol Terbutaline	Bronchial smooth muscle relaxation; relief of acute symptoms	Tremor, anxiety, bronchospasm, dyspnea, tachycardia, dysrhythmias, palpitations, hypertension, hypokalemia
Beta$_2$-agonists (long-acting) Salmeterol	Bronchial smooth muscle relaxation; long-term prevention of symptoms	Same as above; do not use to treat acute exacerbations
Anticholinergics Ipratropium bromide	Inhibit action of acetylcholine causing bronchial smooth muscle relaxation	Drying of mouth and respiratory secretions, dizziness, bronchodilation, palpitations; lower incidence of tachycardia than beta$_2$-agonists; avoid contact with eyes
Methylxanthines Theophylline Aminophylline	Phosphodiesterase inhibitor	Tremor, tachycardia, dysrhythmias, CNS stimulation (headache, seizures, restlessness), nausea, vomiting; do not crush sustained-release capsules; monitor trough levels

Because of the growing problem of antimicrobial resistance, antibiotic selection should be based on sensitivity reports from sputum cultures.

Ventilatory Assistance

Patients with ARF from COPD exacerbation may benefit from early treatment with noninvasive positive pressure ventilation (NPPV). Unlike invasive mechanical ventilation, which requires an ETT or insertion of a tracheostomy tube, NPPV assists the patient's respiratory efforts by delivering positive airway pressure through a nasal or face mask. Candidates for NPPV should be hemodynamically stable, have a patent airway and minimal secretions, and be free of mental status changes (Hill, 2001). Studies on the use of NPPV in COPD exacerbation have shown a decrease in the need for intubation and mechanical ventilation and less-serious complications than invasive ventilation (American Thoracic Society et al., 2001; Peter, Moran, Phillips-Hughes, & Warn, 2002).

Intubation and mechanical ventilation are indicated in those patients who, despite aggressive therapy, develop mental status changes, respiratory muscle fatigue, respiratory acidosis, or significant hypoxemia. Because of the progressive nature of COPD, ethical dilemmas may arise when the patient with COPD and ARF requires mechanical ventilation. There are no accurate objective predictors of the likelihood of survival after mechanical ventilation in these patients. Because many patients with COPD do survive mechanical ventilation and hospitalization, mechanical ventilation should not be foregone solely on the basis of a history of COPD (Breen, Churches, Hawker, & Torzillo, 2002).

In the late stages of severe COPD, patients often report that their quality of life deteriorates because of severe activity limitations and comorbid conditions. Decisions regarding the use or avoidance of intubation, mechanical ventilation, cardiopulmonary resuscitation, and other forms of life support should be made by the patient in conjunction with his or her family before ARF occurs. Critical care nurses are in an ideal position to facilitate discussions about advance directives and to answer questions for the patient and significant others.

Acute Respiratory Failure in Asthma

PATHOPHYSIOLOGY

Asthma is a chronic inflammatory disorder of the airways, which is becoming more prevalent, particularly in children. The chronic inflammation of asthma causes the airways to be hyperresponsive when the patient inhales allergens, viruses, or other irritants (Box 13-3). Airflow obstruction occurs in patients with asthma because these irritants cause bronchoconstriction, airway edema, mucus plugging, and airway remodeling (National Heart, Lung and Blood Institute, 1997). The airway obstruction results in air trapping, prolonged exhalation, and $\dot{V}/\dot{Q}$ mismatching, with an increased intrapulmonary shunt. Unlike in COPD, however, the airflow limitations in asthma are largely reversible.

ASSESSMENT

Early symptoms of asthma exacerbation are wheezing, dyspnea, chest tightness, and cough. The patient initially hyperventilates, producing respiratory alkalosis. As the airways continue to narrow, it becomes more difficult for the patient to exhale. The lungs become overinflated and stiff, which further increases the work of breathing. Nursing assessment will reveal tachypnea, tachycardia, pulsus paradoxus greater than 25 mm Hg, agitation, possible use of accessory muscles, and evidence of suprasternal retractions. Peak expiratory flow readings will be less than 50% of the

---

BOX 13-3

Asthma Triggers

INHALANT ALLERGENS
- Animals
- House-dust mites
- Cockroaches
- Indoor fungi
- Outdoor allergens

OCCUPATIONAL EXPOSURE

IRRITANTS
- Tobacco smoke
- Indoor/outdoor pollution
- Fumes: perfumes, cleaning agents, sprays

OTHER FACTORS INFLUENCING ASTHMA SEVERITY
- Viral respiratory infections
- Rhinitis/sinusitis
- Gastroesophageal reflux
- Sensitivity: aspirin, other nonsteroidal anti-inflammatory drugs, sulfites
- Topical and systemic beta-blockers

National Heart, Lung and Blood Institute. (1997). *Guidelines for the diagnosis and management of asthma.* Publication No. 97-4051. Bethesda, MD: National Institutes of Health.

ASTHMA CLINICAL ALERT

Signs of impending acute respiratory failure in a patient with severe asthma may include:
- Breathlessness at rest and the need to sit upright
- Speaking in single words; unable to speak in sentences or phrases
- Lethargy or confusion
- Paradoxical thoracoabdominal movement
- Absence of wheezing ("silent chest") indicating no air movement and respiratory muscle fatigue
- Bradycardia
- Respiratory acidosis with $PaCO_2 \geq 42$ mm Hg and $PaO_2 < 60$ mm Hg

From National Heart, Lung and Blood Institute, National Asthma Education and Prevention Program Expert Panel Report. (2002). *Guidelines for the diagnosis and management of asthma: Update on selected topics.* Publication No. 02-5075. Bethesda, MD: National Institutes of Health.

patient's normal values. Severe asthma exacerbation, often referred to as status asthmaticus, occurs when the bronchoconstriction does not respond to bronchodilator therapy, and ARF ensues. The patient experiences fatigue from the severe dyspnea, cough, and increased work of breathing. Hypercapnia, hypoxia, and respiratory acidosis develop, and CO decreases as a result of a decreased venous return that is related to increased intrathoracic pressures (see Asthma Clinical Alert).

INTERVENTIONS

Mild exacerbations of asthma can be managed by the patient at home with the use of short-acting beta$_2$-agonists (see Table 13-3) to treat bronchoconstriction. Treatment of moderate to severe exacerbations of asthma requires O_2 therapy, systemic steroid administration, and inhaled bronchodilator therapy (Table 13-4). Patients must be monitored closely for signs of response to this therapy. Most patients respond well to treatment, but some may need intubation

TABLE 13-4

Emergency Treatment of Severe Asthma

Therapy	Purpose	Goals
Oygen via nasal cannula or face mask	Correct hypoxemia	Maintain $SaO_2 \geq 90\%$ (or $\geq 95\%$ in pregnant women and patients with cardiac disease)
Inhaled short-acting beta$_2$-agonists by MDI or nebulizer every 20 minutes or continuously in the first hour, then every 1-4 hr (systemic beta$_2$-agonists can also be given by injection; however, no proven advantage over aerosol has been shown)	Relieve airway obstruction caused by bronchoconstriction	Achieve PEF >70% of predicted or personal best Normalizing/improved arterial blood gases Respiratory rate <30 breaths/minute without use of accessory muscles
Inhaled anticholinergics (added to beta$_2$-agonist therapy)	Relieve bronchoconstriction	Relief of sensation of dyspnea; able to complete full sentences without breathlessness
Systemic corticosteroids administered orally or intravenously	Reverse airway inflammation	Improved lung sounds Prevent intubation

MDI, metered-dose inhaler; *PEF,* peak expiratory flow.
National Heart, Lung and Blood Institute. National Asthma Education and Prevention Program Expert Panel Report. (2002). *Guidelines for the diagnosis and management of asthma: Update on selected topics.* Publication No. 02-5075. Bethesda, MD: National Institutes of Health.

and mechanical ventilation. These patients are at increased risk of lung injury from barotrauma, volutrauma, or hyperinflation (auto-PEEP) (Burns & Lawson, 1999).

In a patient with severe, refractory status asthmaticus, oxygenation may be improved by delivering a mixture of helium and O_2 (heliox) to the lungs. Because helium is lighter than O_2, it allows for enhanced gas flow through the constricted airways and improves oxygenation. Another treatment option is the use of permissive hypercapnia (Burns & Lawson, 1999).

During a patient's recovery from a severe asthmatic event, the critical care nurse should focus efforts on teaching the patient asthma management techniques, because patient and family education is essential for asthma control. It can significantly reduce future emergency department visits and hospitalizations. Persons with asthma are taught how to monitor their symptoms, implement environmental controls, properly take their medications with a metered-dose inhaler and spacer, and measure their lung function daily with a hand-held peak flow meter. A written action plan from the health care provider will guide patients in their daily asthma management and will help with early identification and treatment of exacerbations.

Acute Respiratory Failure Resulting From Ventilator-Associated Pneumonia (Nosocomial Pneumonia)

DEFINITION AND ETIOLOGY

Nosocomial pneumonia is defined as pneumonia occurring more than 48 hours after hospital admission excluding any infection incubating at the time of admission. Because it is not a reportable illness, it is difficult to know the exact incidence. Pneumonia accounts for 31% of infections in medical/surgical critical care units in the United States. Critically ill patients who are mechanically ventilated are especially vulnerable to development of a nosocomial pneumonia known as ventilator-associated pneumonia (VAP) (Figure 13-4). VAP accounts for 83% of the cases of nosocomial pneumonia occurring in critical care units. Epidemiological investigations have shown the incidence of VAP to be 10% to 25% for intubated patients, with crude mortality varying from 10% to 40% and reaching as high as 76% if the disease is caused by high-risk pathogens. One episode of VAP is estimated to extend patient hospitalization as much as 13 days (Chastre & Fagon, 2002; Collard, Saint, & Matthay,

2003; Kennedy, O'Heron, Jaloway, & Steinfeld, 2002). One study of 9080 patients demonstrated that VAP was associated with an increase of $40,000 in mean hospital charges per patient (Rello et al., 2002).

PATHOPHYSIOLOGY

The pathogens responsible for nosocomial pneumonia may be inherent in the patient's endogenous flora or in the hospital environment. VAP typically occurs from aspiration of bacteria colonizing the oropharynx or gastrointestinal tract. VAP is categorized into two stages based on the time of onset from intubation. Early-onset VAP occurs in less than 4 days from intubation and is commonly associated with community-acquired organisms. The community-acquired organisms are typically *S. pneumoniae*, methicillin-susceptible *Staphylococcus aureus*, and *H. influenzae*. Late-onset VAP is usually associated with enteric gram-negative rods and antibiotic-resistant nosocomial organisms. The pathogens associated with

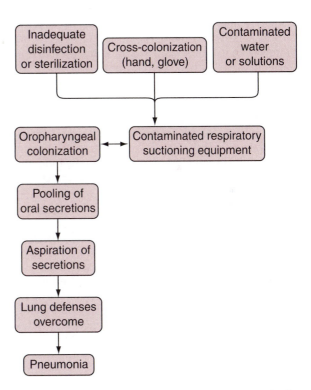

FIGURE 13-4 Role of airway management in the pathogenesis of nosocomial pneumonia. Based on the model proposed by the Centers for Disease Control and Prevention. (From Sole, M. L., Poalillo, F. E., Byers, J. F., & Ludy, J. E. [2002]. Bacterial growth in secretions and on suctioning equipment of orally intubated patients: A pilot study. *American Journal of Critical Care, 11*(2), 141-144.)

late-onset VAP include *Pseudomonas aeruginosa, Enterobacter, Acinetobacter* species, and methicillin-resistant *S. aureus* (Collard, Saint, & Matthay, 2003; Kennedy, O'Heron, Jaloway, & Steinfeld, 2002; Rello et al., 2001).

ASSESSMENT

The diagnosis of VAP is complicated by a lack of sensitive and specific criteria. It is problematic because many other conditions can produce new lung infiltrates in critically ill patients. There is no "gold standard." A protected-specimen brush culture with at least 10^3 cfu/mL, a positive result of a bronchoalveolar lavage fluid smear, or a bronchoalveolar lavage fluid culture is considered specific for VAP in patients without recent changes in antimicrobial therapy. These techniques are not standardized, nor do they have consensus from physicians of their benefit versus risk value. Some clinicians diagnose VAP by the presence of a new or persistent lung density seen on chest radiography with one or more of the following: temperature of more than 38.5°C or less than 36.5°C, leukocyte count of more than 11,000 cells/μL or fewer than 5000 cells/μL, and the presence of purulent endotracheal secretions (Lambotte et al., 2002).

INTERVENTIONS

The interventions for VAP are aimed at prevention and treatment. If the patient develops VAP, therapy is required to treat the infection. Strategies for prevention of VAP, as well as unresolved issues, are summarized in Box 13-4.

Prevention

The most effective method to prevent VAP caused by the hospital environment is hand hygiene. Health care workers should decontaminate hands with soap and water or with a waterless alcohol-based antiseptic agent before and after every patient contact even if gloves are worn (CDC Recommendation on Hand-Hygiene, 2002). Microorganisms can permeate latex and vinyl gloves, and bacteria can be transferred from hand to gloves. Hand hygiene should also be performed before and after touching any patient's respiratory equipment (CDC Healthcare Infection Control Practices Advisory Committee, 2004; Kennedy, O'Heron, Jaloway, & Steinfeld, 2002).

Universal precautions must be observed. Gloves are required when suctioning the patient both orally and through the ETT tube including the closed-suction technique. A gown, mask, and protective eye wear should be worn if the caregiver's clothing may be contaminated or if splashing of any patient fluid could occur.

The presence of the ETT contributes to the development of VAP. The ETT causes injury to the tracheal mucosa, which reduces mucociliary function. It impairs the gag and cough reflexes that help to keep organisms out of the lower respiratory tract. It prevents the upper respiratory system from heating and humidifying inspired air, leading to thickening of secretions. The ETT can create binding sites for bacteria in the bronchial tree and can increase mucus secretion. It serves as a reservoir where bacteria remain inaccessible to antibiotics. Bacteria that colonize the ETT form a bacterial biofilm. Suctioning, coughing, or movement of the tube may dislodge this biofilm. Instillation of normal saline occasionally used during suctioning may facilitate entry of bacteria into the respiratory tract by dislodging bacteria adhered to the ETT and should not routinely be done (CDC Healthcare Infection Control Practices Advisory Committee, 2004; Kennedy, O'Heron, Jaloway, & Steinfeld, 2002; Pfeifer, Orser, Gefen, McGuinness, & Hannon, 2001).

Maintaining aseptic technique during ETT suctioning and meticulous care of the respiratory equipment are needed to decrease the incidence of VAP. Minimizing ventilator tubing manipulation can help to prevent aspiration. Aspiration can occur when condensation forms in the ventilator tubing. The health care team members should prevent accidental lavage of the condensation down the ETT into the patient. The ventilator tubing should be periodically drained and condensation directed away from the patient. Limiting the number of times the ventilator circuit is opened reduces the likelihood of cross-contamination among patients. The ventilator circuit is changed only if it is visibly soiled or mechanically malfunctioning. (CDC Healthcare Infection Control Practices Advisory Committee, 2004). A study by Sole, Poalillo, Byers, and Ludy (2002) found that oral and endotracheal suctioning equipment became colonized with potential pathogens for VAP within 24 hours of use. They recommend using separate suction tubings for oral and closed suction, rinsing tonsil (Yankauer) oral suction devices with sterile water and drying on a paper towel, and considering disposable suction swabs and/or tonsil suction devices. Additional research is needed to determine effectiveness in preventing VAP (Sole et al., 2002). A clean manual resuscitation bag must be used for each patient and changed if it becomes visibly soiled. (CDC Healthcare Infection Control Practices Advisory Committee, 2004; Pfeifer et al., 2001).

Aspiration of oropharyngeal secretions is a primary route for mechanically ventilated patients to acquire VAP. Oropharyngeal secretions accumulate above the endotracheal cuff and may result in miniaspirations. The critical care nurse should implement strategies to reduce the risk of aspiration. The ETT cuff pressure

BOX 13-4

Prevention of Ventilator-Associated Bacterial Pneumonia

1. Educate staff on preventing infection.
2. Conduct surveillance for pneumonia in high-risk patients.
3. Prevent transmission of microorganisms.
   a. Use sterile water for rinsing reusable semicritical respiratory equipment, including nebulizer equipment.
   b. Change the ventilator circuit only when visibly soiled.
   c. Drain condensate in ventilator circuits periodically; do not drain toward the patient.
   d. Use sterile water in humidifiers.
   e. Change heat moisture exchanger (HME) when malfunctions or visibly soiled; do not change more often than every 48 hours.
4. Prevent person-to-person transmission.
   a. Ensure hand hygiene with antimicrobial soap and water, or alcohol-based waterless soap.
   b. Wear gloves for handling secretions or objects contaminated with secretions.
   c. Wear gown if needed.
   d. Use sterile, single-use catheters for open suctioning; rinse with sterile water in between suction attempts.
5. Modify host risk for infections: prevent aspiration.
   a. Use noninvasive ventilation if possible.
   b. Remove tubes and devices as soon as clinically indicated.
   c. Avoid reintubation.
   d. Intubate patients orally rather than nasally.
   e. If feasible, use endotracheal tube that allows continuous aspiration of subglottic secretions.
   f. Suction secretions from above the cuff before deflating endotracheal tube cuff or repositioning tube.
   g. Elevate the head of bed 30 to 45 degrees unless contraindicated.
   h. Verify feeding tube placement.
   i. Develop and implement a comprehensive oral-hygiene program.
   j. Use oral chlorhexidine rinse during perioperative period for cardiac surgery patients.
6. Unresolved issues in prevention of ventilator-associated pneumonia.
   a. Placing filters at distal end of ventilator circuit to collect condensate.
   b. Effectiveness of heat moist exchangers versus heated humidifiers.
   c. Closed versus open suctioning.
   d. Clean versus sterile gloves for endotracheal suctioning.
   e. Frequency of changing closed suction catheters.
   f. Enteral administration of glutamine.
   g. Routine adminstration of granulocyte-colony stimulating factor (GCSF) or intravenous gamma globulin.
   h. Routine oral chlorhexidine rinse for all high-risk patients.
   i. Routine administration of topical antimicrobial agents for oral decontamination .
   j. Preferential adminstration of sucralfate, H_2-antagonists, and/or antacids for stress-bleeding prophylaxis.
   k. Routine selective decontamination of the digestive tract of all high-risk patients.
   l. Use of small-bore tubes for enteral feeding.
   m. Continuous versus intermittent enteral feedings.
   n. Placing feeding tubes distal to the pylorus.
   o. Acidification of gastric feedings.
   p. Turning or rotational therapy, either by "kinetic" therapy or by continuous lateral rotational therapy.

Modified from Centers for Disease Control and Prevention Healthcare Infection Control Practices Advisory Committee. (2004). *Guidelines for Prevention of Health-care–Associated Pneumonia*, 2003 *MMWR*, 53(RR03);1-36. (Available at www.cdc.gov/mmwr.)

should be kept at 20 cm H_2O. Cuff pressures less than 20 cm H_2O increase the risk of VAP, and higher cuff pressures may cause tracheal damage. The pressure should be checked routinely and recorded in the medical record. Repositioning and retaping the ETT are routine procedures typically performed according to hospital protocol. The rationale for repositioning the ETT is to prevent breakdown of oral mucosa. Secretions tend to pool above the cuff on the ETT; therefore, before repositioning the tube, it is essential to suction the pooled secretions. The mouth and the area above the ETT cuff should also be suctioned periodically because coughing or any movement of the ETT can cause these secretions to enter into the lungs (Pfeifer et al., 2001). A special dual-lumen ETT that has a suction port in the subglottic area above the cuff is now commercially available (see Chapter 8). The suction port is used to suction secretions continuously in the subglottic region. Some randomized, controlled studies have found a decrease in VAP with continuous aspiration of subglottic secretions (CDC Healthcare Infection Control Practices Advisory Committee, 2004; Collard, Saint, & Matthay, 2003; Kennedy, O'Heron, Jaloway, & Steinfeld, 2002; Pfeifer et al., 2001).

Strategies to reduce aspiration of gastric secretions are also important in reducing VAP. A nasal or orogastric tube impairs swallowing, produces stagnation of oropharyngeal secretions, increases reflux, and acts as a conduit for bacteria to migrate from the stomach to the oropharynx. Enteral feedings increase the risk of VAP by promoting overgrowth of gram-negative organisms secondary to an increased pH of stomach content, increased gastric volume, and an increased reflux. Even with these risks, enteral feeding is preferred over parenteral nutrition if the gastrointestinal system is functioning. Enteral feedings should be started as soon as possible to prevent breakdown of the gut mucosa and to minimize the effect of malnutrition on the immune system. Malnutrition increases the risk of many complications, including pneumonia (Harris & Miller, 2000). Placing the patient in a semiupright position can be extremely beneficial in reducing aspiration. The head of the bed should be continuously elevated to an angle of 30 to 45 degrees. If the patient cannot tolerate the head of the bed elevated secondary to hemodynamic instability, the enteral feedings may need to be discontinued. Placement of the feeding tube should be verified routinely, before feedings are started and before medications are instilled, by aspiration of gastric content and/or pH testing. Intestinal motility should be routinely assessed by auscultation of bowel sounds, measurement of residual gastric volumes, and abdominal girth measurements. Gastric reflux and aspiration can occur if enteral feedings increase intragastric volume and pressure. The feeding should be adjusted to prevent gastric distention (Harris & Miller, 2000; Kennedy, O'Heron, Jaloway, & Steinfeld, 2002; Pfeifer et al., 2001).

Oral and nasal hygiene are important nursing interventions that may be overlooked. Oral care was once considered to be a comfort measure and not a high priority. New research has found that it is a primary intervention in prevention of VAP. Within 48 hours of hospitalization, the oropharyngeal flora of critically ill patients changes to predominately gram-negative organisms. These gram-negative organisms are frequently the same organisms causing VAP. These microorganisms are concentrated in dental plaque. Reducing the pool of organisms in the oral cavity reduces the amount of organisms available to translocate or be aspirated into the lungs. The right tools are necessary to perform effective oral care. Box 13-5 gives an example of an oral care policy and procedure designed to reduce respiratory pathogens. The antiseptic chlorhexidine gluconate was used successfully as a perioperative oral rinse to decrease the incidence of nosocomial respiratory tract infections in patients who underwent cardiac surgery (Houston, et al., 2002). Additional studies are needed to determine if it would be useful in preventing VAP in other types of patients. The CDC recommends the use of orotracheal or orogastric tubes instead of nasally inserted tubes. The use of nasal tubes increases the occurrence of nosocomial maxillary sinusitis (CDC Healthcare Infection Control Practices Advisory Committee, 2004; Grap, Munro, Ashtiani, & Bryant, 2002).

Many critically ill patients receive prophylaxis for gastrointestinal bleeding, but this treatment has been implicated as a factor contributing to VAP. A gastric pH higher than 3.5 is associated with increased gastric colonization. Research comparing stress ulcer prophylaxis with sucralfate and histamine (H_2)-antagonists suggests a decreased incidence of VAP with sucralfate. The use of sucralfate versus H_2-antagonists must be weighed against the risk of gastrointestinal bleeding. The CDC recommends the use of sucralfate, H_2-antagonists, and/or antacids interchangeably for stress bleeding prophylaxis in mechanically ventilated patients (CDC Healthcare Infection Control Practices Advisory Committee, 2004; Collard, Saint, & Matthay, 2003).

Turning and positioning of patients may reduce the incidence of VAP. The supine position places unconscious and mechanically ventilated patients at risk for aspiration of gastric contents. Studies have shown that placing patients in the semirecumbent position (45-degree angle) was statistically significant in reducing the risk of VAP. Routine turning and repositioning assist in mobilization of secretions. There is some evidence that the incidence of VAP may be reduced with the use of continuously laterally rotating beds in surgical patients and in patients with neurological problems; however, further study is warranted (CDC Healthcare Infection Control Practices Advisory Committee, 2004; Collard, Saint, & Matthay, 2003; Kennedy, O'Heron, Jaloway, & Steinfeld, 2002).

Treatment

VAP is considered a potentially severe infection with a high risk of mortality if an appropriate antibiotic

---

BOX 13-5

Policy and Procedure for Oral Care to Prevent Ventilator-Associated Pneumonia

POLICY
1. Assess the oral cavity on admission and daily.
2. Administer oral care to unconscious or intubated patients every 2 to 4 hours and as needed.
3. Assess intubated patients every 2 hours and before repositioning or deflating the endotracheal tube, and as needed to determine the need for removal of oropharyngeal secretions. Suction as the need is identified.

EQUIPMENT
1. Soft-tipped, covered Yankauer for nontraumatic suctioning
2. Soft-suction toothbrush with a compact head that can maneuver around the endotracheal tube
3. Suction oral swab for stimulation of mucosal tissue
4. 1.5% hydrogen peroxide mouth rinse for oral cleansing and reduction of respiratory pathogens
5. Water-based mouth moisturizer with vitamin E to improve the healing of lesions
6. Deep suction catheter for suctioning subglottal secretions
7. Dedicated tubing for oral suctioning equipment for infection control

PROCEDURE
1. Set up the suction equipment.
2. Position the patient's head to the side or place in semi-Fowler's position.
3. Provide deep oropharyngeal suction as needed to remove secretions that may migrate down the tube and settle on top of the cuff.
4. Brush the patient's teeth using a suction toothbrush, small amounts of water, and a 1.5% hydrogen peroxide oral rinse.
5. Brush for approximately 1 to 2 minutes.
6. Exert gentle pressure while moving in short horizontal or circular strokes.
7. Gently brush the surface of the patient's tongue.
8. Use a suction swab to clean the teeth and tongue between brushing, or if brushing causes discomfort or bleeding.
9. Place the swab perpendicular to the gum line, and apply gentle mechanical action for 1 to 2 minutes.
10. Turn the swab in clockwise rotation to remove mucus and debris.
11. Apply mouth moisturizer.

Data from Schleder, B. J. (2003). Taking charge of ventilator-associated pneumonia. *Nursing Management, 8,* 29-33; and Schleder, B. J., Stott, K., & Lloyd, R. C. (2003). The effect of a comprehensive oral care protocol on patients at risk for ventilator-associated pneumonia. *Journal of Advocate Health Care, 4*(1) 27-30.

---

regimen is not started in a timely manner. Research has shown a trend for decreased mortality if antibiotic therapy is started within 48 hours of suspected diagnosis with a known pathogen. The lack of a gold standard for diagnosis is problematic. The use of monotherapy, combination therapy, and duration of treatment are all areas of controversy. The following recommendations are based on a consensus of experts. Pathogens that are likely to cause early-onset VAP in patients who have received antibiotic therapy previously are adequately treated with monotherapy. Some experts recommend combination therapy for early-onset VAP in patients with a history of COPD, prolonged use of corticosteroid therapy, or malnutrition.

The bacteria causing late-onset VAP usually require combination therapy. (Rello et al., 2001).

Acute Respiratory Failure Resulting From a Pulmonary Embolism

DEFINITION

An embolus is a clot or plug of material that travels from one blood vessel to another smaller vessel. The clot or plug lodges in the smaller vessel and obstructs blood flow. An embolus that lodges in the pulmonary vasculature is called a pulmonary embolism (PE).

RESEARCH ANALYSIS

ARTICLE REFERENCE

Grap, M. J., Munro, C. L., Ashtiani, B., Bryant, S. (2003). Oral care interventions in critical care: Frequency and documentation. *American Journal of Critical Care, 12*(2), 113-119.

PURPOSES AND METHODS

Bacterial colonization of the orpharynx is a risk factor for the development of ventilator-associated pneumonia (VAP) in patients receiving mechanical ventilation. Oral hygiene to remove plaque and microbes may decrease the incidence of VAP. The purpose of this study was to describe the frequency and type of oral care interventions reported by nurses in the medical respiratory, surgical trauma, and neuroscience critical care units of a large academic medical center.

Surveys of oral care practices were sent to all nursing care providers in the three critical care units and 77 surveys (45%) were completed. Respondents were asked to report how frequently they performed oral care for intubated and non-intubated patients. Using a visual analog scale, the survey asked how frequently a variety of oral care products were used. Additionally, nurses were asked to rate the priority they gave to oral care interventions. On 5 randomly selected dates during a 1-month period, medical record reviews were conducted to determine how often oral care practices were documented on the critical care unit flowsheets.

STUDY FINDINGS

The reported frequency of oral care practices was notably different for intubated versus non-intubated patients. Seventy-five percent of respondents reported providing oral care 2 or 3 times per day for non-intubated patients, and 72% reported providing care 5 times per day for those who were intubated. The reported use of a toothbrush and toothpaste was significantly greater in non-intubated patients ($P < .001$), and use of a sponge swab was greater in intubated patients ($P < .001$). There were no significant differences in the reported use of mouthwash, isotonic sodium chloride solution, hydrogen peroxide mixture, or chlorhexidine between the two groups of patients. On an analog scale of 1-100, nurses rated the priority of oral care at 53.9. In the review of 170 medical records, oral care was documented 205 times in the previous 24 hours, for a mean of 1.2 times per patient.

STUDY STRENGTHS

This was a descriptive study conducted at one institution to examine oral care practices. The literature review outlines the problem of VAP, the risks of oral colonization, and the associated nursing interventions for prevention. When conducting the survey, all nursing staff employed in the 3 critical care units at the time of the study had an opportunity to complete the survey. The detailed description of the survey facilitates future replication of this study. Dates for medical record reviews were randomly selected, and all adult patients from medical and surgical critical care units were included in the sample.

STUDY LIMITATIONS

The frequency of oral care provided to patients in this study is self-reported by the nursing staff, which may not be an accurate accounting of actual interventions. In addition, the comparatively lower number of oral care interventions recorded in the medical record may reflect omissions in documentation rather than the actual frequency of oral care. This study was conducted in one hospital and findings may not be reflective of practice in other institutions or with other patient populations.

IMPLICATIONS FOR PRACTICE

Providing good oral hygiene is one nursing intervention that can decrease oropharyngeal colonization and help prevent VAP. Education to help nurses understand this causal relationship may increase the priority nurses place on providing oral care. While there are a variety of oral care products available, previous research has found toothbrushes to be more effective than foam swabs in removing plaque. Further research is needed to determine the optimal method and frequency of oral care, and to measure the quantitative impact it has on the incidence of VAP.

The embolus may be a clot that has broken off from a deep vein thrombosis, a globule of fat from a long bone fracture, a septic vegetation, or an iatrogenic catheter fragment. Most PEs originate from thrombosis in the legs or pelvis (Kroegel & Reissig, 2003; Wood, 2001a).

PEs are classified as massive, submassive, or minor, depending on the amount of pulmonary vascular occlusion. Minor emboli are considered insignificant because one of the functions of the pulmonary capillary bed is to act as a "filter." Massive and submassive emboli are clinically significant. A massive embolus obstructs 50% or more of the pulmonary vasculature. Anatomically massive PE is not associated with a high mortality rate unless the patient is hemodynamically unstable and in shock. The presence of shock is associated with a three- to sevenfold increase in mortality. Major PE is a combination of embolism size and underlying cardiopulmonary status. When either the size or the combination of PE and underlying cardiovascular status results in hemodynamic instability, it is considered a medical emergency. Most patients presenting with hemodynamic instability and shock die within the first hour and require rapid, accurate assessment and treatment (Wood, 2001a; Wood, 2002).

ETIOLOGY

The three main mechanisms that favor the development of venous thrombi, often referred to as Virchow's triad, are (1) venous stasis, or a reduction in blood flow; (2) altered coagulability of blood; and (3) damage to the vessel walls. Specific causes of PE that fall under these three categories are listed in Box 13-6. Both a hypercoagulable state and venous wall damage contribute to the development of a thrombus, but may not alone cause a thromboembolism. They are seen in conjunction with other factors that result in stasis.

Acute PE remains a cardiovascular emergency with an estimated annual incidence of 200,000 cases in the United States (Aquila, 2001). Without treatment, PE has a mortality rate of approximately 30%, causing more than 50,000 deaths per year (Kroegel & Reissig, 2003).

PATHOPHYSIOLOGY

The pulmonary circulation has an enormous capacity to compensate for PE. This compensatory mechanism results from lung vasculature necessary to accommodate increased blood flow during exercise. After an embolus lodges in the pulmonary vasculature, blood flow to the alveoli beyond the occlusion is eliminated. The result is a lack of perfusion to ventilated alveoli, an increase in dead space, a $\dot{V}/\dot{Q}$ mismatch, and a decrease in CO_2 tension in the embolized lung zone. Gas exchange cannot occur, and hypocarbia results. The hypocarbia affects the bronchial smooth muscle by causing bronchoconstriction, increased pulmonary resistance, and decreased compliance.

Constriction in the terminal airways of the non-perfused lung zones results in alveolar shrinking and

---

BOX 13-6

Risk Factors Associated with Deep Venous Thrombosis/Pulmonary Embolism

VENOUS STASIS
Heart disease
  Heart failure
  Myocardial infarction
  Cardiomyopathy
  Constrictive pericarditis
Dehydration
Immobility (bed rest >72 hours, long travel)
Paralysis
Incompetent venous valves
Obesity (>20% ideal body weight)
Pregnancy
Surgery lasting more than 45 minutes
Age >40 years

VESSEL WALL INJURY
Trauma
  Fracture
  Extensive burns
Infection
Venipuncture
Intravenous infusion of irritant solutions
Previous history of deep venous thrombosis
History of previous major surgery

HYPERCOAGULABILITY
Alterations in hemostatic mechanisms
  Protein C resistance or deficiency
  Antithrombin III deficiency or resistance
  Protein S deficiency
  Factor V R506Q (Leiden) mutation
  Polycythemia vera
  Anemias
Trauma/surgery
Malignancy
Oral contraceptive use
Systemic infection

From Aquila, A. M. (2001). Deep venous thrombosis. *Journal of Cardiovascular Nursing, 15*(4), 28.

decreased wasted ventilation. The result is an increase in the work of breathing for the critically ill patient. The reduction in blood flow to the alveoli also results in hypoxia for the type II pneumocytes, which are responsible for the production of surfactant. Although the effects are not seen for 24 to 48 hours, the decrease in surfactant results in an unequal gas distribution, an increase in the work of breathing, and a stiffening and collapse of the alveoli. Ventilation is then shifted away from these units, thus worsening the $\dot{V}/\dot{Q}$ mismatch.

Atelectasis and shunting may also occur as a result of the release of serotonin from the platelets that surround the clot. The result is peripheral airway constriction, which often involves functioning alveoli. In this situation, perfusion with inadequate ventilation occurs. Pulmonary hypertension may also occur if greater than 50% of the functional cross-sectional area of the pulmonary vascular bed is occluded.

The overall prognosis after a PE depends on two main factors. The first is whether any underlying cardiopulmonary problem preceded the PE, and the second is the extent of the pulmonary vascular circulation that is occluded by the thrombus. The PE is considered major if circulatory shock occurs. The embolus material blocking the pulmonary outflow tract causes a mechanical obstruction and mediates neurohumoral factors. The embolus causes pulmonary outflow impedance and creates a pressure load on the right ventricle resulting in multiple effects on right and left ventricular function (Wood, 2001a).

ASSESSMENT

Because many PEs originate from deep vein thrombosis in the lower extremities, the critical care nurse assesses for leg pain, localized tenderness, swelling, erythema, and pain on palpating the calf or along a vein (Aquila, 2001). The most common symptom of PE is sudden onset of dyspnea. The patient may also be especially apprehensive or anxious, with a feeling of impending doom. Other common signs and symptoms of PE are chest pain aggravated by deep inspiration, decreased SaO_2, tachycardia, cough, crackles, wheezing, and hemoptysis. Other signs and symptoms that may occur are accentuated pulmonic component of the second heart sound, fever, phlebitis, cyanosis, diaphoresis, and syncope.

ABGs typically show a PaO_2 of less than 80 mm Hg and a $PaCO_2$ of less than 36 mm Hg on room air. The electrocardiogram may be normal but may show the following: nonspecific ST-segment and T-wave changes; peaked P waves in leads II, III, and aVF; or right bundle branch block. The pattern of anterior T-wave inversions in the precordial leads correlates best with PE severity. Chest radiograph abnormalities

are often seen in PE. The typical findings are elevated hemidiaphragm, consolidation, pleural effusion, atelectasis, decreased pulmonary vascularity, and/or a prominent central pulmonary artery (Wood, 2001a). The echocardiogram may show signs of enlarged right-sided chambers or tricuspid regurgitation. Right-ventricular dilation is reported in 50% to 100% of patients with a PE. Transthoracic echocardiography and tranesophageal echocardiography may detect emboli in transit. Spiral CT is an excellent diagnostic tool for diagnosing central or proximal embolus. In acute PE associated with right ventricular dilation, CT sensitivity and specificity are almost 100%. Magnetic resonance imaging has sensitivity and specificity comparable to that of spiral CT, but it is rarely used to diagnosis a PE in critically ill patients. A $\dot{V}/\dot{Q}$ scan may detect dead space from impaired perfusion of ventilated alveoli. Results of $\dot{V}/\dot{Q}$ scans are reported as low, medium, or high probability (Kearon, 2003; Olin, 2002; Wood, 2001b).

A pulmonary angiogram is considered the gold standard for detecting PE. It provides direct anatomical visualization of the pulmonary vasculature. Pulmonary angiography is an invasive procedure consisting of a right-heart catheterization with contrast medium injected through the catheter into the pulmonary vasculature system. CT may be replacing pulmonary angiography as the standard because it is noninvasive and has a high level of sensitivity and specificity.

INTERVENTIONS

In the case of a PE, the best therapy is prevention. Several prophylactic nursing interventions can be instituted in the hospitalized patient that may decrease the chance of PE development. Early postoperative ambulation or, when such ambulation is not possible, use of pneumatic boots that provide intermittent compression of the lower extremities increases venous flow. Walking schedules along with active and passive range-of-motion exercises also increase circulation.

Other nursing interventions that may reduce the risk of deep vein thrombosis and PE include not adjusting the knee section of the patient's bed and avoiding the use of pillows below the knees. Proper application of elastic stockings is also essential. The patient should be instructed not to cross his or her legs and to make frequent position changes to promote circulation when sitting for long periods. Box 13-7 gives nursing interventions to prevent deep vein thrombosis.

Most critically ill patients fall into a high-risk category for PE and are often treated prophylactically. Treatment includes the use of low-dose heparin, low-molecular-weight heparin, graduated

---

BOX 13-7

Nursing Measures to Prevent Deep Venous Thrombosis

- Identify risk factors predisposing patient to deep venous thrombosis; reevaluate status frequently.
- Implement ordered prophylactic regimen:
  - Nonpharmacological (mechanical)
    Graduated compression stockings
    Intermittent (external) pneumatic compression
    Venous foot pump
  - Pharmacologic
    Subcutaneous low-dose unfractionated heparin
    Subcutaneous low-molecular-weight heparin
    Oral anticoagulants
  - Document patient tolerance to ordered prophylactic regimens.
- Assess all of the patient's extremities on a regular basis.
  - Pain/tenderness
  - Unilateral edema
  - Erythema
  - Warmth
- Encourage early ambulation and active leg exercises every hour the patient is awake.
- Perform passive range-of-motion exercises every shift if the patient is immobile.
- Monitor for low-grade fever to detect thrombophlebitis.
- Encourage fluid intake to avoid dehydration; maintain accurate intake and output measurements.
- Avoid the use of knee gatch or pillows under the knees.
- Patient education:
  - What deep venous thrombosis is and why it develops
  - Risk factor awareness; highlight any risk factors the patient possesses (see Box 13-6).
  - Describe the signs and symptoms.
  - Discuss prevention methods:
    Perform regular activity to promote venous return (i.e., walking, swimming, cycling).
    Avoid prolonged sitting or standing.
    Elevate legs with prolonged sitting.
    Avoid constrictive garments: girdles, tight-fitting stockings, garters.

Modified from Aquila, A. M. (2001). Deep venous thrombosis. *Journal of Cardiovascular Nursing, 15*(4), 41.

---

compression stockings, and/or intermittent pneumatic compression.

Thrombolytic therapy is the standard of care for patients with PE who are in shock or hemodynamically unstable. Evaluations by angiogram, perfusion scans, and echocardiograms have shown that thrombolytic therapy produces clot lysis faster than heparin alone. The research has not shown one thrombolytic agent to be superior if they are given in equivalent doses. After thrombolytic agents are given, a heparin infusion is started.

A heparin infusion is often the treatment of choice with or without thrombolytic therapy. The heparin does not dissolve the existing clot, but it prevents the clot from enlarging and prevents more thrombi from forming by inhibiting the conversion of prothrombin to thrombin. Heparin may also stimulate the intrinsic fibrinolytic system, thereby enhancing the degradation of the PE (Schumann, 2000). An initial bolus is given followed by a continuous infusion to achieve an activated partial thromboplastin time 1.5 to 2.5 times greater than control value (2.0 to 4.0 International Normalized Ratio [INR]). Studies have demonstrated that using a dose-adjusted nomogram based on weight is more likely to achieve the desired INR within the first 24 hours. The heparin infusion is continued for 5 to 7 days. Oral anticoagulation with warfarin should overlap with the heparin for at least 4 to 5 days (Hyers et al., 2001). It is essential that the critical care nurse regularly monitor the laboratory values to titrate the heparin to a therapeutic level and to monitor the patient for any signs or symptoms of bleeding or heparin-induced thrombocytopenia. The nurse must be attuned to major bleeding such as intracranial or retroperitoneal hemorrhage, and minor bleeding. Heparin-induced thrombocytopenia is a well known complication of heparin therapy. It is caused by antibodies that activate platelets and leads to thrombocytopenia (Aquila, 2001).

Other treatments should be focused on maintaining airway, breathing, and circulation. Supplemental O_2 may be administered to maintain SaO_2 at more than 90%. If the location of the PE is known, place the "good" lung in the dependent position. Administer analgesics to the patient to alleviate pain and anxiety. If the patient is hemodynamically unstable, inotropic support may be required. Drugs that dilate the pulmonary vessels may be needed if pulmonary hypertension and heart failure are present (Wood, 2001c; Aquila, 2001).

Surgical intervention may be necessary for some patients, including those in whom anticoagulants and thrombolytics are contraindicated, those who do not respond to medical treatment, those who are having life-threatening complications, and often those who have greater than 50% obstruction. Surgical procedures include an embolectomy, ligation of the inferior vena cava, and transvenous placement of a vena cava umbrella, a device placed in the inferior vena cava to trap emboli as they migrate toward the pulmonary vasculature.

Case Study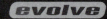

Mrs. P. is a 57-year-old woman admitted to the trauma intensive care unit after an automobile accident. She has multiple long bone fractures, a chest contusion, and an episode of hypotension in the emergency department (ED). She received 3 units of blood and 2 L of intravenous fluid in the ED. Within 12 hours she became short of breath with an increase in respiratory rate requiring high levels of supplemental oxygen. She was electively intubated and placed on volume-control mechanical ventilation with positive end-expiratory pressure (PEEP) of 5 cm H_2O. Over the next 8 hours, her oxygen saturation (SaO_2) steadily deteriorated, and the high-pressure alarms on the ventilator activated frequently. The nurse noted steadily rising peak airway pressures. The fraction of inspired oxygen (FiO_2) had to be increased to 0.80 to maintain her PaO_2 at 65 mm Hg. Her chest x-ray study showed bilateral infiltrates, and her lung injury score was 2.5. A pulmonary artery catheter was inserted with an initial pulmonary capillary wedge pressure of 14 mm Hg. The diagnosis of acute respiratory distress syndrome (ARDS) was made.

Over the next 6 hours, she steadily became more hypoxemic. She was changed to pressure-controlled ventilation with a PEEP of 18 cm H_2O. The FiO_2 had to be increased to 1.0 (100%) to maintain a PaO_2 of greater than 60 mm Hg. She was extremely restless, with tachycardia, diaphoresis, and a labile SaO_2. The decision was made to start a neuromuscular blocking agent with sedation. Over the next few hours her general condition continued to deteriorate. Her SaO_2 ranged from 85% to 89%. Her chest x-ray findings looked worse, and the nurses and physicians decided to turn her to the prone position. An hour after turning her to the prone position, her SaO_2 began to slowly rise. After 2 hours in the prone position, her SaO_2 had stabilized at 95%. Slowly, the FiO_2 was decreased to 50%, with a stable SaO_2 of 95%. After 12 hours, she was returned to the supine position. Her SaO_2 slowly decreased until it reached 90%. It remained stable at 90%.

Mrs. P. slowly improved over the next week. She was weaned off the PEEP and changed from pressure-controlled to assist-control ventilation. The neuromuscular blocking agent and sedation were discontinued without any negative outcomes. Within 2 weeks, she was extubated and transferred to the general orthopedic nursing unit.

QUESTIONS

1. Identify the risk factors Mrs. P. had for developing ARDS.
2. The American-European Consensus Conference recommended three criteria for diagnosing ARDS in the presence of a risk factor. List the criteria.
3. Explain the use of PEEP and the pressure-controlled ventilation mode. What other unconventional modes of mechanical ventilation have been used in the treatment of ARDS? What is the rationale for each mode?
4. Explain the rationale for the use of neuromuscular blocking agents and what nursing interventions should occur when using these agents.
5. Explain the rationale for placing the patient in the prone position and what nursing interventions should occur before turning a patient to the prone position.

Severe Acute Respiratory Syndrome

Severe acute respiratory syndrome (SARS), an emerging illness, is a highly contagious and potentially fatal syndrome. Between the winter of 2002 through the summer of 2003, it infected more than 8400 people and caused more than 800 deaths worldwide (Marthaler, Keresztes, & Tazbir, 2003).

ETIOLOGY

SARS is caused by a new variety of coronavirus. It is spread by person-to-person contact, and possibly by contact with objects that are contaminated with infectious droplets. It is also possible that SARS can be spread through the air. The incubation period for SARS is generally between 2 to 10 days. It usually begins with an elevated temperature of greater than 100.4°F. The fever may be associated with chills, headache, malaise, and body pain. Some patients may experience mild respiratory symptoms. After 3 to 7 days, patients typically develop lower respiratory symptoms. The symptoms may include a dry, nonproductive cough and dyspnea. In some patients, the symptoms progress to severe respiratory distress requiring intubation and mechanical ventilation. The death rate from SARS ranges from 13% for patients younger than 60 years to 47% for those 60 years old and older (Donnelly et al., 2003; Marthaler, Keresztes, & Tazbir, 2003). Case definition

and assessment criteria are being revised frequently by the CDC, and readers should refer to the CDC's Web site for the most current information (CDC, 2004).

PRECAUTIONS

If a patient suspected of having SARS is admitted to the hospital, infection control personnel should be notified immediately. Infection control measures must include the following:
- Routine standard precautions (e.g., careful hand hygiene). In addition, eye protection for all patient contact should be included.
- Contact precautions including the use of gown and gloves for all patient contact or contact with their environment.
- Airborne precautions (e.g., an isolation room with negative pressure and use of an N-95 filtering disposable respirator for persons entering the room).
- Emergency department, outpatient laboratory staff, and other personnel should carefully triage all patients entering the hospital to identify those with any respiratory symptoms, give those patients a mask to wear, and isolate them when appropriate until a diagnosis can be made.

SUMMARY

ARF is a disorder that can affect all segments of the population from young trauma victims to elderly

---

| CRITICAL THINKING QUESTIONS | 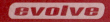 |

1. Mr. R. is a 66-year-old man who has smoked 1.5 packs of cigarettes a day for 40 years (60 pack-years). He is admitted with acute exacerbation of COPD. His baseline ABGs drawn in the clinic 2 weeks ago showed: pH, 7.36; $PaCO_2$, 55 mm Hg; PaO_2, 69 mm Hg; bicarbonate, 30 mEq/L; SaO_2, 92%. In the critical care unit, Mr. R. has coarse crackles in his left lower lung base and a mild expiratory wheeze bilaterally. His cough is productive of thick yellow sputum. His skin turgor is poor; he is febrile, tachycardic, and tachypneic. Currently, Mr. R.'s ABGs on O_2 at 2 L/min via nasal cannula are: pH, 7.32; $PaCO_2$, 64 mm Hg; PaO_2, 50 mm Hg; bicarbonate, 30 mEq/L; SaO_2, 86%.
   a. What is your interpretation of Mr. R.'s baseline ABGs from the clinic?
   b. What is the probable cause of Mr. R.'s COPD exacerbation, and what treatment is indicated at this time?
   c. What ABG changes would indicate that Mr. R.'s respiratory status is deteriorating?

2. Ms. T. is a 41-year-old woman admitted to the critical care unit and mechanically ventilated for acute asthma. She was extubated yesterday and will be transferred out of the critical care unit tomorrow. What are the important points you must cover in your teaching with Ms. T.?

3. Mr. B. has just been intubated for ARF. Currently, he is agitated and very restless. What risks are associated with Mr. B.'s agitation? What nursing actions are indicated in this situation?

4. Mr. C., age 27 years, was hospitalized 3 days ago after fracturing his femur in a snow-skiing accident. He has just been admitted to the critical care unit with a PE and is orally intubated and receiving mechanical ventilation. What actions would you take to decrease Mr. C.'s risk of developing nosocomial pneumonia?

persons with long-standing pulmonary disease. Patients in the critical care areas are at high risk of ARF. The critical care nurse must be constantly alert to signs of impending respiratory failure. Changes in respiratory rate and character, breath sounds, and blood gases must be closely evaluated. Frequent position changes, good pulmonary hygiene, and careful attention to the nutritional status all contribute to maintaining a patient's respiratory system and to the prevention of ARF.

REFERENCES

Adkinson, J. D., & Konzem, S. L. (2001). Management of acute exacerbations of chronic obstructive pulmonary disease. *Pharmacotherapy, 21*(8), 929-939.

American Thoracic Society, European Respiratory Society, European Society of Intensive Care Medicine, and Société de Réanimation de Langue Française. (2001). International consensus conference in intensive care medicine: Noninvasive positive pressure ventilation in acute respiratory failure. *American Journal of Respiratory and Critical Care Medicine, 163*, 283-291.

Aquila, A. M. (2001). Deep venous thrombosis. *Journal of Cardiovascular Nursing, 15*(4), 25-44.

Ashbaugh, D. G., Bigelow, D. B., Petty, T. L., & Levine, B. E. (1967). Acute respiratory distress in adults. *Lancet, 2*(3), 319-323.

Balas, M. C. (2000). Prone positioning of patients with acute respiratory distress syndrome: Applying research to practice. *Critical Care Nurse, 20*(1), 24-36.

Bernard, G. R., Aritgas, A., Brigham, K. L., et al., and the Consensus Committee. (1994). The American European consensus conference on ARDS: Definitions, mechanisms, relevant outcomes and clinical trial coordination. *American Journal of Critical Care Medicine, 149*[suppl], 818-824.

Brashers, V. L. (2002). Structure and function of the pulmonary system. In M. McCance & S. E. Huether. *Pathophysiology: The biologic basis for disease in adults and children* [pp. 1082-1104]. 4th ed. St Louis: Mosby.

Breen, D. Churches, T., Hawker, F., & Torzillo, P. J. (2002). Acute respiratory failure secondary to chronic obstructive pulmonary disease treated in the intensive care unit: A long term follow up study. *Thorax, 59*, 29-33.

Brower, R. G., Ware, L. B., Berthiaume, Y., & Matthay, M. A. (2001). Treatments of ARDS. *Chest, 120*(4), 1347-1367.

Burns, S. M., & Lawson, C. (1999). Pharmacological and ventilatory management of acute asthma exacerbations. *Critical Care Nurse, 19*(4), 39-54.

Centers for Disease Control and Prevention Healthcare Infection Control Practices Advisory Committee (2004). Guidelines for Prevention of Health-care–Associated Pneumonia, 2003 *MMWR,* 53(RR03);1-36 (Available at www.cdc.gov/mmwr)

Centers for Disease Control and Prevention. (September 15, 2003). Hand hygiene guidelines fact sheet. Retrieved from http://www.cdc.gov. Accessed 3/15/2004 .

Centers for Disease Control and Prevention. (January 8, 2004). Severe acute respiratory syndrome (SARS). www.cdc.gov/ncidod/sars.htm. (March 15 2004).

Collard, H. R., Saint, S., & Matthay, M. A. (2003). Prevention of ventilator-associated pneumonia: An evidence-based systematic review. *Annals of Internal Medicine, 138*(6), 494-506.

Chastre, J., & Fagon J. Y. (2002). Ventilator-associated pneumonia. *American Journal of Respiratory and Critical Care Medicine, 165*(7), 867-903.

Davies, P. (2002). Guarding your patient against ARDS. *Nursing, 32*(5), 38-41.

Dirkes, S. (2002). Help for ARDS patients. *RN, 65*(8), 52-58.

Donnelly C. A., Ghani, A. C., Leung, G. M., et al. (2003). Epidemiological determinants of spread of causal agent of severe acute respiratory syndrome in Hong Kong. *Lancet, 361*(9371), 1761-1766.

Gattinoni, L., Tognoni, G., Pesenti, A., et al. (2001). Effect of prone positioning on the survival of patients with acute respiratory failure. *New England Journal of Medicine, 345*(8), 568-573.

Grap, M. J., Munro, C. L., Ashtiani, B., & Bryant, S. (2003). Oral care interventions in critical care: Frequency and documentation. *American Journal of Critical Care, 12*(2), 113-119.

Harris, J. R., & Miller, T. H. (2000). Preventing nosocomial pneumonia: Evidence-based practice. *Critical Care Nurse, 20*(1), 56-65.

Herridge, M. S., Cheung, A. M., Tansey, M. S., et al. (2003). One-year outcomes in survivors of the acute respiratory distress syndrome. *New England Journal of Medicine, 348*(8), 683-693.

Hill, N. S., (2001). Using NPPV to optimal benefit in acute respiratory failure. *Journal of Critical Illness, 16(8)*, 361-366.

Houston, S., Hougland, P., Anderson, J. J., LaRocco, M., Kennedy, V., & Gentry, L. O. (2002). Effectiveness of 0.12% chlorhexidine gluconate oral rinse in reducing prevalence of nosocomial pneumonia in patients undergoing heart surgery. *American Journal of Critical Care, 11*(6), 567-570.

Hurd, S. (2000). The impact of COPD on lung health worldwide: Epidemiology and incidence. *Chest, 117*(2), 1S-4S.

Hyers, T. M., Agnelli, G., Hull, R. D., Morris, T. A., Samama, M., Tapson, V., & Weg, J. G. (2001). Antithrombotic therapy for venous thromboembolic disease. *Chest, 119*[suppl 1], 176S-193S.

Kearon, C. (2003). Diagnosis of pulmonary embolism. *Canadian Medical Association Journal, 168*(2), 183-201.

Kennedy, V., O'Heron, S., Jaloway, J., & Steinfeld, C. (2002). Nosocomial infections in intensive care patients. *Critical Care Nursing Clinics of North America, 14,* 417-426.

Krieger, B. P. (2002). Top ten list in mechanical ventilation. *Chest, 122*(5), 1797-1800.

Kroegel, C., & Reissig, A. (2003). Principle mechanisms underlying venous thromboembolism: Epidemiology, risk factors, pathophysiology and pathogenesis. *Respiration, 70*(1), 7-30.

Lambotte, O., Timsit, J., Garrouste-Orgeas, M., Misset, B., Benali, A., & Carlet, J. (2002). The significance of distal bronchial samples with commensals in ventilator-associated pneumonia: Colonizer or pathogen? *Chest, 122*(4), 1389-1399.

Luer, J. M. (2002). Sedation and neuromuscular blockage in patients with acute respiratory failure. *Critical Care Nurse, 22*(5), 70-75.

Martin, G. S., Mangialardi, R. J., Wheeler, A. P., Dupont, W. D., Morris, J. A., & Bernard, G. R. (2002). Albumin and furosemide therapy in hypoproteinemic patients with acute lung injury. *Critical Care Medicine, 30*(10), 2376-2367.

Marthaler, M., Keresztes, P., & Tazbir, J. (2003). SARS What have we learned? *RN, 66*(8), 58-62.

Mehta, S., MacDonald, R., Hallett, D. C., Lapinsky, S. E., Aubin, M., & Stewart, T. E. (2003). Acute oxygenation response to inhaled nitric oxide when combined with high-frequency oscillatory ventilation in adults with acute respiratory distress syndrome. *Critical Care Medicine, 31*(2), 383-389.

Murray, J. F., Matthay, M. A., Luce, J. M., & Fick, M. R. (1988). An expanded definition of the adult respiratory distress syndrome. *American Review of Respiratory Disease, 138*(3), 720-723.

Murray, T.A. & Patterson, L. A. (2002). Prone positioning of trauma patients with acute respiratory distress syndrome and open abdominal incisions. *Critical Care Nurse, 22*(30), 52-56.

National Heart, Lung and Blood Institute. (1997). *Guidelines for the diagnosis and management of asthma.* Publication No. 97-4051. Bethesda, MD: National Institutes of Health.

Olin, J. W. (2002). Pulmonary embolism. *Review of Cardiovascular Medicine, 3*[suppl 2], S68-S75.

Pauwels, R. A., Buist, A. S., Calverley, P. M., Jenkins, C. R., & Hurd, S. S. (2001). Global strategy for the diagnosis, management, and prevention of chronic obstructive pulmonary disease: NHLBI/WHO Global Initiative for Chronic Obstructive Lung Disease (GOLD) workshop summary. *American Journal of Respiratory and Critical Care Medicine, 163*, 1256-1276.

Pelosi, P., Bottino, N., Chiumello, D., et al. (2003). Sigh in supine and prone position during acute respiratory distress syndrome. *American Journal of Respiratory and Critical Care Medicine, 167*(4), 521-527.

Peter, J. V., Moran, J. L., Phillips-Hughes, J., & Warn, D. (2002). Noninvasive ventilation in acute respiratory failure: A meta-analysis update. *Critical Care Med, 30*(3), 555-562.

Pfeifer, L. T., Orser, L., Gefen, C., McGuinness, R., & Hannon, C. V. (2001). Preventing ventilator-associated pneumonia. *American Journal of Nursing, 101*(8), 24AA-24GG.

Pierson, D. J. (2002). Indications for mechanical ventilation in adults with acute respiratory failure. *Respiratory Care, 47*, 249-262.

Qureshi, M. A., Shah, N. J., Hemmen, C.W., Thill, M. C., Kruse, J. A. (2003). Exposure of intensive care unit nurses to nitric oxide and nitrogen dioxide during therapeutic use of inhaled nitric oxide in adults with acute respiratory distress syndrome. *American Journal of Critical Care, 12*(2), 147-153.

Rello, J., Paiva, J. A., Baraibar, J., et al. (2001). International conference for the development of consensus on the diagnosis and treatment of ventilator-associated pneumonia. *Chest, 120*(3), 955-967.

Rello, J., Ollendorf, D. A., Oster, G., Vera-Llonch, M., Bellm, L., Redman, R., & Kollef, M. H. (2002). Epidemiology and outcomes of ventilator-associated pneumonia in a large US database. *Chest, 122*(6), 2115-2121.

Rialp, G., Betbese, A. J., Perez-Marquez, M., & Mancebo, J. (2001). Short-term effects of inhaled nitric oxide and prone position in pulmonary and extrapulmonary acute respiratory distress syndrome. *American Journal Respiratory and Critical Care Medicine, 164*(20), 243-249.

Schlicher, M. (2001). Using liquid ventilation to treat patients with acute respiratory distress syndrome: A guide to a breath of fresh liquid. *Critical Care Nurse, 21*(5), 55-65.

Schleder, B., Stott, K., & Lloyd, R. C. (2003). The effect of a comprehensive oral care protocol on patients at risk for ventilator-associated pneumonia. *Journal of Advocate Health Care, 4*(1), 27-30.

Schumann, L. (2000). Respiratory function and alteration in gas exchange: Obstructive pulmonary disorders and restrictive pulmonary disorders. In L. C. Copstead. & J. L. Banasik *Pathophysiology: Biological and behavioral perspectives* [pp. 504-586]. 2nd ed. Philadelphia: W. B. Saunders.

Singh, J. M., Palda, V. A., Stanbrook, M. B., & Chapman, K. R. (2002). Corticosteroid therapy for patients with acute exacerbations of chronic obstructive pulmonary disease: A systematic review. *Archives of Internal Medicine, 162*(22), 2527-2536.

Sole, M. L., Poalillo, F. E., Byers, J. F., & Ludy, J. E. (2002). Bacterial growth in secretions and on suctioning equipment of orally intubated patients: A pilot study. *American Journal of Critical Care, 11*(2), 141-144.

Tasaka, S., Hasegawa, N., & Ishizaka, A. (2002). Pharmacology of acute lung injury. *Pulmonary Pharmacology Therapy, 15*(2), 83-95.

Thompson, B. T., Hayden, D., Matthay, M. A., Brower, R., & Parsons, P.E. (2001). Clinicians' approaches to mechanical ventilation in acute lung injury and ARDS. *Chest, 120*(5), 1622-1627.

Ward, N. S. (2002). Effects of prone position ventilation in ARDS: An evidence-based review of the literature. *Critical Care Clinics, 18*(1), 35-44.

Wood, K. E. (2001a). Major pulmonary embolism. Part 1: Presentation and basic diagnostic studies. *Journal of Critical Illness, 16*(9), 395-405.

Wood, K. E. (2001b). Major pulmonary embolism. Part 2: Diagnostic confirmation. *Journal of Critical Illness, 16*(11), 476-484.

Wood, K. E. (2001c). Major pulmonary embolism. Part 3: Treatment strategy. *Journal of Critical Illness, 16*(12), 524-528.

Wood, K. E. (2002). Major pulmonary embolism: Review of a pathophysiologic approach to the golden hour of hemodynamically significant pulmonary embolism. *Chest, 122*(6), 2264-2265.

RECOMMENDED READINGS

Berry, B. E., & Pinard, A. E. (2002). Assessing tissue oxygenation. *Critical Care Nurse, 22*(3), 22-42.

Fiore, M. C., Bailey, W. C., Cohne, S. J., et al. (2000). *Treating tobacco use and dependence: Quick reference guide for clinicians.* Rockville, MD: U.S. Department of Health and Human Services. Public Health Service. Retrieved from http://www.ahrq.gov/path/tobacco.htm. Accessed 3/15/2004.

Moore, M. J., & Schmidt, G. A. (2001a). Keys to effective noninvasive ventilation. Part 1: Initial steps. *Journal of Critical Illness, 16*(2), 64-70.

Moore, M. J., & Schmidt, G.A. (2001b). Keys to effective noninvasive ventilation. Part 2: Technique tips. *Journal of Critical Illness, 16*(3), 118-124.

Munro, C. L. & Grap, M. J. (2004). Oral health and care in the intensive care unit: State of the science. *American Journal of Critical Care, 13(1),* 25-34.

Schleder, B. (2003). Taking charge of ventilator-associated pneumonia. *Nursing Management, 8,* 29-33.

Togger, D. A. & Brenner, P. S. (2001). Metered dose inhalers. *American Journal of Nursing, 101*(10), 26-32.

evolve *Did you remember to check out the bonus material, including free self-assessment exercises, on the Evolve Web site at http://evolve.elsevier.com/Sole/ and on the CD-ROM?*

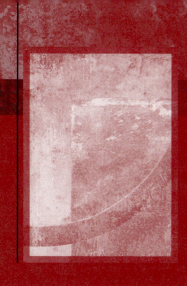

CHAPTER 14

Acute Renal Failure

Janet Goshorn, MSN, ARNP, BC

OBJECTIVES

- Review the anatomy and physiology of the renal system.
- Describe the pathophysiology of the three categories of acute renal failure.
- Identify the systemic manifestations of acute renal failure.
- Describe the methods for assessing the renal system, including physical assessment, interpretation of serum and urine laboratory values, and radiological diagnostic tests.
- Develop a patient-centered plan of care for the patient with acute renal failure including nursing management and anticipated patient outcomes.
- Describe the medical management of the patient with acute renal failure.
- Discuss the nursing assessment and care of the patient receiving dialysis or continuous renal replacement therapy.

Introduction

The renal system is the primary regulator of the body's internal environment and is thus essential to the maintenance of life. With sudden cessation of renal function, the body is incapable of maintaining a stable internal environment, and all body systems are thereby disrupted. Acute renal failure occurs in about 1% of hospitalized patients and in up to 20% of critical care patients. Community-acquired acute renal failure occurs at a rate of 209 patients per 1 million population. Renal replacement therapies are necessary in about 30% of patients who develop acute renal failure (Albright, 2001).

Despite the advanced treatments available, acute renal failure is still associated with significant morbidity and 50% mortality, depending on the type of acute renal failure and other patient comorbidities (Nally, 2002). Mortality rates have not improved much since the mid-1970s, thus making prevention of acute renal failure a high priority for all health care professionals. Nursing can play a pivotal role in promoting positive outcomes in patients with acute renal failure. Recognition of high-risk patients, preventive measures, sharp assessment skills, and supportive nursing care are fundamental to ensuring delivery of high-quality care to these challenging and complex patients. In this chapter, the pathophysiology,

evolve *Be sure to check out the bonus material, including free self-assessment exercises, on the Evolve Web site at http://evolve.elsevier.com/Sole/ and on the CD-ROM.*

assessment, and collaborative management of acute renal failure are discussed.

Review of Anatomy and Physiology

The kidneys are a pair of highly vascularized, bean-shaped organs that are located retroperitoneally on each side of the vertebral column, adjacent to the first and second lumbar vertebrae. The right kidney sits slightly lower than the left kidney because the liver lies above it. An adrenal gland sits on top of each kidney and is responsible for the production of aldosterone, a hormone that influences sodium and water balance. Each kidney is divided into two regions: an outer region, called the *cortex*, and an inner region, called the *medulla*.

The nephron is the basic functional unit of the kidney. A nephron is composed of a renal corpuscle (glomerulus and Bowman's capsule) and a tubular structure, as depicted in Figure 14-1. Approximately 1 to 3 million nephrons exist in each kidney. About 85% of these nephrons are found in the cortex of the

kidney and have short loops of Henle. The remaining 15% of nephrons are called *juxtamedullary nephrons* because of their location just outside the medulla. Juxtamedullary nephrons have long loops of Henle and, along with the vasa recta (long capillary loops), are primarily responsible for concentration of urine.

The kidneys receive approximately 20% to 25% of the cardiac output, which computes to 1200 mL of blood per minute. Blood enters the kidneys through the renal artery, travels through a series of arterial branches, and reaches the glomerulus by way of the afferent arteriole (*afferent* meaning to carry toward). Blood leaves the glomerulus through the efferent arteriole (*efferent* meaning to carry away from), which then divides into two extensive capillary networks called the *peritubular capillaries* and the *vasa recta.* The capillaries then rejoin to form venous branches by which blood eventually exits the kidney via the renal vein. The glomerulus is a cluster of minute blood vessels that filter blood. The glomerular walls are composed of three layers: the endothelium, the basement membrane, and the epithelium. The epithelium of the glomerulus is continuous with the inner

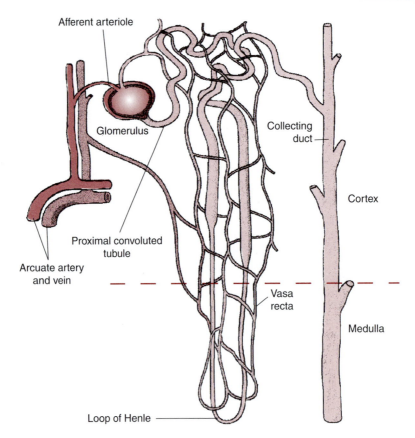

FIGURE 14-1 Anatomy of the nephron, the functional unit of the kidney.

layer of Bowman's capsule, the sac that surrounds the glomerulus. Bowman's capsule is the entry site for filtrate leaving the glomerulus (Briggs, Kriz, & Schnermann, 2001).

The kidneys perform numerous functions that are essential for the maintenance of a stable internal environment. The following text provides a brief overview of key roles the kidneys perform in maintaining homeostasis. Box 14-1 provides a listing of kidney functions.

REGULATION OF FLUID AND ELECTROLYTES AND EXCRETION OF WASTE PRODUCTS

As blood flows through each glomerulus, water, electrolytes, and waste products are filtered out of the blood across the glomerular membrane and into Bowman's capsule, to form what is known as filtrate. The glomerular capillary membrane is approximately 100 times more permeable than other capillaries. It acts as a high-efficiency sieve and normally allows only substances with a certain molecular weight to cross. Red blood cells, albumin, and globulin are too large to pass through the healthy glomerular membrane. Normal glomerular filtrate is basically protein free and contains electrolytes, including sodium, chloride, and phosphate, and nitrogenous waste products, such as creatinine, urea, and uric acid, in amounts similar to those in plasma (Unwin & Capasso, 2000).

Glomerular filtration occurs as a result of a pressure gradient, which is the difference between the forces that favor filtration and the pressures that oppose filtration. Generally, the capillary hydrostatic pressure favors glomerular filtration, whereas the colloid osmotic pressure and the hydrostatic pressure in Bowman's capsule oppose filtration (Figure 14-2). Under normal conditions, the capillary hydrostatic pressure is greater than the two opposing forces, and glomerular filtration occurs.

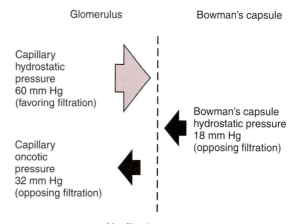

FIGURE 14-2 Average pressures involved in filtration from the glomerular capillaries.

At a normal glomerular filtration rate (GFR) of 80 to 125 mL per minute, the kidneys produce 180 L of filtrate a day. As the filtrate passes through the various components of the nephron's tubules, 99% is reabsorbed into the peritubular capillaries or vasa recta. *Reabsorption* is the movement of substances from the filtrate back into the capillaries. A second process that occurs in the tubules is *secretion,* or the movement of substances from the peritubular capillaries into the tubular network. Various electrolytes are reabsorbed or secreted at numerous points along the tubules, thus helping to regulate the electrolyte composition of the internal environment (Figure 14-3). Aldosterone and antidiuretic hormone play a role in water reabsorption in the distal convoluted tubule and collecting duct. Aldosterone also plays a role in sodium reabsorption. Eventually, the remaining filtrate (1% of the original 180 L per day) is excreted as urine, for an average urine output of 1 to 2 L per day.

REGULATION OF ACID-BASE BALANCE

The kidneys help to maintain acid-base equilibrium in three ways: reabsorption of filtered bicarbonate, production of new bicarbonate, and excretion of small amounts of hydrogen ions (acid) buffered by phosphates and ammonia (Batlle, 2001). The tubular cells are capable of generating ammonia to help with excretion of hydrogen ions. This ability of the kidney to assist with ammonia production and excretion of hydrogen ions (in exchange for sodium) is the predominant adaptive response by the kidney when the patient is acidotic. When alkalosis is present, increased

---

BOX 14-1
Functions of the Kidney

- Regulation of fluid volume
- Regulation of electrolyte balance
- Regulation of acid-base balance
- Regulation of blood pressure
- Excretion of nitrogenous waste products
- Regulation of erythropoiesis
- Metabolism of vitamin D
- Synthesis of prostaglandin

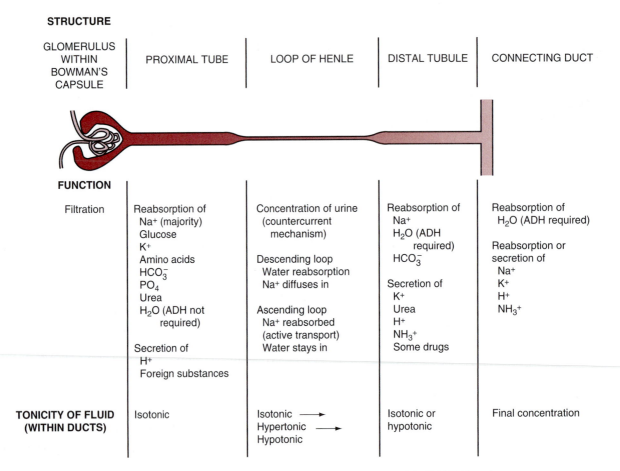

FIGURE 14-3 Major functions of the nephron. (From Noland, L. [2002]. Renal system. In J. Thompson, G. McFarland, J. Hirsch, & S. Tucker [eds.]. *Mosby's clinical nursing* [p. 862]. 5th ed. St. Louis: Mosby).

amounts of bicarbonate are excreted in the urine and cause the serum pH to return toward normal.

REGULATION OF BLOOD PRESSURE

Specialized cells in the afferent and efferent arterioles and the distal tubule are collectively known as the juxtaglomerular apparatus. These cells are responsible for the production of a hormone called *renin*, which plays a role in blood pressure regulation. Renin is released whenever blood flow through the afferent and efferent arterioles decreases. A decrease in the sodium ion concentration of the blood flowing past the specialized cells (e.g., in hypovolemia) also stimulates the release of renin. Renin activates the renin-angiotensin-aldosterone cascade, as depicted in Figure 14-4, which ultimately results in angiotensin II production. Angiotensin II causes vasoconstriction and release of aldosterone from the adrenal glands, thereby raising blood pressure and flow and increasing sodium and water reabsorption in the distal tubule

and collecting ducts. In addition, aldosterone promotes the excretion of potassium.

Pathophysiology of Acute Renal Failure

DEFINITION

Acute renal failure is the sudden deterioration of renal function, resulting in retention of nitrogenous waste products (azotemia). It is usually accompanied by oliguria (urine output less than 400 mL in 24 hours), although many patients are nonoliguric and have a urine output of greater than 400 mL every 24 hours (Holley, 2001). Patients with nonoliguric acute renal failure may even excrete 2 to 4 L of fluid in 24 hours, but the fluid is deficient in the solutes and waste products that compose normal urine. Anuria (urine output less than 100 mL in 24 hours) is less commonly seen in acute renal failure.

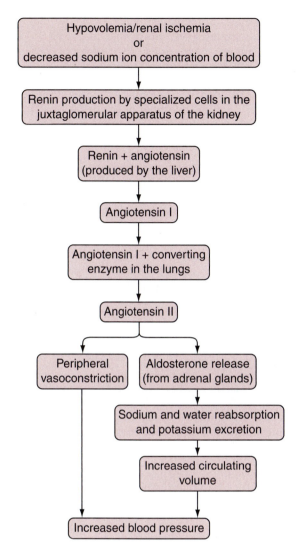

FIGURE 14-4 Renin-angiotensin mechanism.

BOX 14-2

Prerenal Causes of Acute Renal Failure

VOLUME DEPLETION
Hemorrhage
Trauma
Surgery
Postpartum period
Gastrointestinal loss
Diarrhea
Nasogastric suction
Vomiting
Renal loss
Diuretics
Osmotic diuresis
Diabetes insipidus
Volume shifts
Burns
Ileus
Pancreatitis
Peritonitis
Hypoalbuminemia

VASODILATION
Sepsis
Anaphylaxis
Drugs
Antihypertensives
Afterload reducers
Anesthesia

IMPAIRED CARDIAC PERFORMANCE
Heart failure
Myocardial infarction
Cardiogenic shock
Dysrhythmias
Pulmonary embolism
Pulmonary hypertension
Positive-pressure ventilation
Pericardial tamponade

MISCELLANEOUS
Angiotensin-converting enzyme inhibitors in renal artery stenosis
Inhibition of prostaglandins by nonsteroidal antiinflammatory drug use during renal hypoperfusion
Renal vasoconstriction
Norepinephrine
Ergotamine
Hypercalcemia

ETIOLOGY

Numerous conditions can precipitate acute renal failure. In general, the causes of acute renal failure are classified into three categories: prerenal, postrenal, and intrarenal, depending on where the precipitating factor exerts its pathophysiological effect on the kidney.

Prerenal Causes of Acute Renal Failure

Conditions that produce acute renal failure by interfering with renal perfusion are classified as *prerenal*. Most prerenal causes of renal failure are fluid volume loss, extracellular fluid volume sequestration (third spacing), inadequate cardiac output, or vasoconstriction of the renal blood vessels. Common prerenal causes of acute renal failure are listed in Box 14-2.

All these conditions reduce the glomerular perfusion and the GFR and hence hypoperfuse the kidney. For example, major abdominal surgery can cause hypoperfusion of the kidney as a result of blood loss during surgery or as a result of excess vomiting or nasogastric suction during the postoperative period. The body attempts to normalize renal perfusion by reabsorbing sodium and water. If adequate blood flow is restored to the kidney, normal renal function resumes. However, if the prerenal situation is prolonged or severe, it can progress to intrarenal damage, acute tubular necrosis (ATN), or acute cortical necrosis (Pruchnicki & Dasta, 2002a, 2002b; Iglesias & Lieberthal, 2000). Therefore, implementation of preventive measures, recognition of the condition, and prompt treatment of prerenal conditions are extremely important.

Postrenal Causes of Acute Renal Failure

Acute renal failure resulting from obstruction of the flow of urine is classified as *postrenal,* or obstructive renal failure. Obstruction can occur at any point along the urinary system (Box 14-3). With postrenal conditions, increased intratubular pressure results in a decrease in the GFR and in abnormal nephron function. Acute renal failure caused by postrenal conditions usually reverses rapidly once the obstruction is removed (Palmieri, 2002).

Intrarenal Causes of Acute Renal Failure

Conditions that produce acute renal failure by directly acting on functioning kidney tissue (either the glomerulus or the renal tubules) are classified as *intrarenal.* The most common intrarenal condition is ATN. This condition may occur after prolonged ischemia (prerenal), exposure to nephrotoxic substances, or a combination of these. Ischemic ATN usually occurs when perfusion to the kidney is considerably reduced. The renal ischemia overwhelms

the normal autoregulatory defenses of the kidneys and thus initiates cell injury that may lead to cell death. Some patients have ATN after only several minutes of hypotension or hypovolemia, whereas others can tolerate hours of renal ischemia without having any apparent tubular damage. The most commonly injured portions of the renal tubule are the proximal tubule and the ascending limb of the loop of Henle. (Esson & Schrier, 2002; Woroniecki & Devarajan, 2002).

Nephrotoxic agents (particularly aminoglycosides and radiographic contrast materials) can also damage the tubular epithelium as a result of direct drug toxicity, intrarenal vasoconstriction, and intratubular obstruction. Acute renal failure does not occur in all patients who receive nephrotoxic agents; however, predisposing factors, such as advanced age, diabetes mellitus, and dehydration, enhance susceptibility to intrinsic damage (Albright, 2001). Patients with nephrotoxic ATN often have a good chance of complete recovery from renal failure. Other intrarenal causes of acute renal failure are listed in Box 14-4.

ACUTE TUBULAR NECROSIS PATHOPHYSIOLOGY

Dramatic advances have been made in our understanding the of pathophysiology of ATN (Lieberthal & Nigam, 2000; Woolfson & Hillman, 2000; Woroniecki & Devarajan, 2002). Multiple studies with renal biopsies have shown the following typical cellular findings in ATN:

- Patchy loss of epithelial cells that causes gaps and exposed basement membrane
- Diffuse loss of brush cell border in the proximal tubule
- Patchy necrosis most often in the outer medulla region
- Dilatation of tubules with tubular cast formation and sloughing
- Evidence of cellular regeneration along with freshly damaged cells that suggests multiple cycles of injury and repair

Extensive research has identified multiple mechanisms involved in the pathophysiology of ATN. Figure 14-5 is a detailed schematic of some of the mechanisms that play a role in the ATN cascade resulting in a reduced GFR. Some of the mechanisms involved are as follows:

1. *Alterations in renal hemodynamics:* Decreases in cardiac output, intravascular volume, or renal blood flow activate the renin-angiotensin system. Angiotensin II causes further renal vasoconstriction and decreased glomerular capillary pressure, resulting in a decreased GFR. The decreased GFR and renal blood flow lead to tubular dysfunction.

BOX 14-3

Postrenal Causes of Acute Renal Failure

- Benign prostatic hypertrophy
- Blood clots
- Renal stones or crystals
- Tumors
- Postoperative edema
- Drugs
  Tricyclic antidepressants
  Ganglionic blocking agents
- Foley catheter obstruction
- Ligation of ureter during surgery

BOX 14-4

Intrarenal Causes of Acute Renal Failure

GLOMERULAR, VASCULAR, OR HEMATOLOGICAL PROBLEMS
Glomerulonephritis (poststreptococcal)
Vasculitis
Malignant hypertension
Systemic lupus erythematosus
Hemolytic uremic syndrome
Disseminated intravascular coagulation
Scleroderma
Bacterial endocarditis
Preeclampsia of pregnancy
Thrombosis of renal artery or vein

TUBULAR PROBLEM (ACUTE TUBULAR NECROSIS OR ACUTE INTERSTITIAL NEPHRITIS)
Ischemia
Any of the causes of prerenal azotemia (see Box 14-2)
Hypotension from any cause
Hypovolemia from any cause
Obstetric complications (hemorrhage, abruptio placentae, placenta previa)
Nephrotoxic agents
  Drugs: aminoglycosides, amphotericin B, penicillins, acyclovir, vancomycin, pentamidine, rifampin, cisplatin, cyclosporine, methotrexate, nonsteroidal antiinflammatory drugs, cephalosporins
  Radiocontrast dyes
  Endogenous substances: transfusion reaction causing hemoglobinuria, tumor lysis syndrome, rhabdomyolysis (caused by trauma, crush injuries, alcohol or drug abuse, heat stroke, status epilepticus, thyroid storm, strenuous exercise beyond usual capabilities)
  Miscellaneous: heavy metals (mercury, arsenic), paraquat, snake bites, organic solvents (ethylene glycol, toluene, carbon tetrachloride), pesticides, fungicides

---

In addition, administration of medications that cause vasoconstriction of the renal vessels can precipitate ATN, including nonsteroidal antiinflammatory drugs, angiotensin-converting enzyme inhibitors, angiotensin receptor blockers, cyclosporine, and tacrolimus. Endogenous substances that have been implicated in both causing and maintaining renal vessel vasoconstriction include endothelium 1, prostaglandins, adenosine, angiotensin II, and nitric oxide. A deficiency of renal vasodilators (prostaglandins, atrial natriuretic peptide, and endothelium-derived nitric oxide) has also been implicated (Thompson & King, 2003; Woroniecki & Devarajan, 2002).

2. *Alterations in tubular function:* The renal tubules in the medulla are very susceptible to ischemia (the medulla receives only 20% of the renal blood flow and is very sensitive to any reduction in blood flow). When the tubules are damaged, necrotic endothelial cells and other cellular debris accumulate and can obstruct the lumen of the tubule.

This intratubular obstruction increases the intratubular pressure, which decreases the GFR and leads to tubular dysfunction. In addition, the tubular damage often produces alterations in the tubular structure that permit the glomerular filtrate to leak out of the tubular lumen and back into the plasma. This backleak of filtrate results in oliguria (Kelly & Agraharkar, 2002).

3. *Alterations in tubular cell metabolism:* Ischemic episodes result in decreased energy supplies, such as adenosine triphosphate (ATP). Oxygen deprivation results in a rapid breakdown of ATP. The proximal tubule is very dependent on ATP, a feature that explains why it is often the most commonly injured portion of the renal tubule. Without ATP, the sodium-potassium ATPase of the cell membrane can no longer effectively transport electrolytes across the membrane. This leads to an increase of intracellular calcium, free radical formation (which produces toxic effects), and breakdown of phospholipids. Cellular edema occurs and

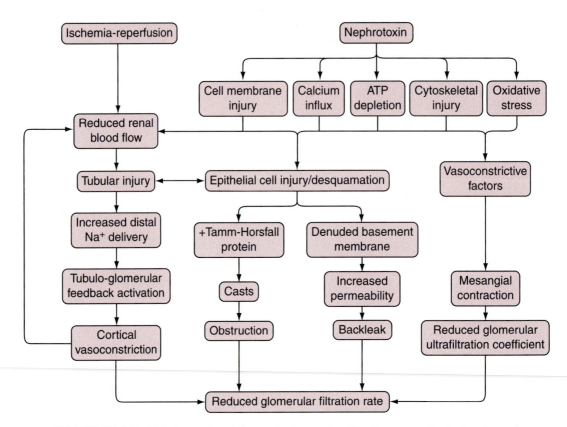

FIGURE 14-5 Schematic of loss of glomerular filtration seen in ischemic and nephrotoxic acute tubular necrosis. (From Woolfson, R., & Hillman, K. [2003]. Causes of acute renal failure. In R. Johnson & J. Feehally [eds.]. *Comprehensive clinical nephrology* [pp.16.1-16.16]. London: Mosby.)

further decreases renal blood flow, damages the tubules, and ultimately leads to tubular dysfunction and oliguria (Woolfson & Hillman, 2000).

Course of Acute Renal Failure

The patient with acute renal failure progresses through three phases of the disease process: the initiation phase, the maintenance phase, and the recovery phase (Finn, 2001).

Initiation (onset) phase. The initiation phase is the period that elapses from the occurrence of the precipitating event to the beginning of the change in urine output. This phase usually spans several hours to 2 days, during which time the normal renal processes begin to deteriorate, but actual intrinsic renal damage is not yet established. The patient cannot compensate for the diminished renal function and exhibits substantial clinical signs and symptoms that reflect the chemical imbalances in the internal environment. Acute renal failure is potentially reversible during the initiation phase.

Maintenance (oliguric/anuric) phase. During the maintenance phase, intrinsic renal damage is well established, and the GFR stabilizes at approximately 5 to 10 mL per minute. Urine volume is usually at its lowest point during the maintenance phase; however, patients may be nonoliguric, with urine outputs greater than 400 mL in 24 hours. This phase usually lasts 8 to 14 days, but it may last as long as 1 to 11 months. The longer a patient remains in this stage, the slower the recovery will be and the greater the chance of permanent renal damage is. Complications resulting from uremia, including hyperkalemia and infection, usually arise during this phase.

Recovery (diuretic) phase. This phase is the period during which the renal tissue recovers and repairs itself. A gradual increase in urine output and an improvement in laboratory values occur. Some patients may have a large diuresis during this phase that is caused by (1) salt and water accumulation in extracellular spaces that results from inability of the renal tubules to regulate sodium and water,

(2) osmotic diuresis that results from retained waste products, or (3) diuretics given to speed up salt and water excretion. However, with early and aggressive use of dialytic therapy, many patients are maintained in a relatively "dry" or volume-depleted state and do not experience a large post-ATN diuresis. Recovery may take as long as 4 to 6 months.

Assessment

PATIENT HISTORY

Several aspects of the patient's history are important to keep in mind in discussions of the renal system. Many patients do not volunteer essential parts of the history unless they are asked specific questions. Renal-related symptoms provide valuable clues to assist the clinician in focusing the assessment to obtain essential data. For example, dysuria, frequency, incontinence, nocturia, pyuria, and hematuria can be indicative of urinary tract infection.

The history provides clues about medical conditions that predispose the patient to acute renal failure, including diabetes mellitus, hypertension, immunological diseases, and any hereditary disorders, such as polycystic disease. The medical record should be carefully examined to elicit additional risk factors, such as hypotensive episodes or any surgical or radiographic procedures performed.

Information regarding exposure to potential nephrotoxins is extremely important. The most common nephrotoxins are antibiotics, such as aminoglycosides, penicillins, amphotericin B, cephalosporins, tetracyclines, and sulfonamides. Nephrotoxicity occurs in 10% to 30% of patients receiving aminoglycosides. Risk factors for development of aminoglycoside nephrotoxicity include volume depletion, prolonged use of the drug (more than 10 days), hypokalemia, sepsis, preexisting renal disease, high trough concentrations, concurrent use of other nephrotoxic drugs, and older age. Symptoms of acute renal failure are usually seen about 1 to 2 weeks after exposure. Because of this delay, the patient must be questioned about any recent medical therapy (clinic or emergency room visits) for which an aminoglycoside may have been prescribed. Nephrotoxicity is also common in patients receiving amphotericin B and nonsteroidal antiinflammatory agents (Guo & Nzerue, 2002).

VITAL SIGNS

Changes in blood pressure are common in acute renal failure. Patients with renal failure from prerenal causes may be hypotensive and tachycardic as a result of volume deficits. ATN, particularly if associated with oliguria, often causes hypertension. Patients may hyperventilate as the lungs attempt to compensate for the metabolic acidosis often seen in acute renal failure. Body temperature may be decreased (as a result of the antipyretic effect of the uremic toxins), normal, or increased (as a result of infection) (Lentino & Leehey, 2001).

PHYSICAL ASSESSMENT

The patient's general appearance is assessed for signs of uremia, such as malaise, fatigue, disorientation, and drowsiness. The skin is assessed for color, texture, bruising, petechiae, or edema. The patient's hydration status is also carefully assessed. Current and admission body weight and intake and output information are evaluated. Skin turgor, mucous membranes, breath sounds, presence of edema, neck vein distention, and vital signs (blood pressure and heart rate) are all key indicators of fluid balance. An oliguric patient with weight loss, tachycardia, hypotension, dry mucous membranes, flat neck veins, and poor skin turgor may be volume depleted (prerenal cause). Weight gain, edema, distended neck veins, and hypertension in the presence of oliguria suggest an intrarenal cause. Table 14-1 summarizes the systemic manifestations of acute renal failure according to body system and also lists the pathophysiological mechanisms that underlie a specific manifestation.

EVALUATION OF LABORATORY VALUES

Because the renal system is the primary regulator of the internal environment of the body, any alteration in its function is rapidly evident in the serum and urine laboratory values. Serum laboratory values of a patient with acute renal failure are usually monitored at least daily, whereas urinary laboratory values are checked much less frequently. The clinician assesses the laboratory values for deviations from normal and expected changes for a patient with acute renal failure. Tables 14-2 and 14-3 list normal values and the anticipated values for a patient with acute renal failure.

Assessment of the urine is extremely valuable in the evaluation of acute renal failure. The best measure of renal function is urinary creatinine clearance. Creatinine is a metabolic by-product of creatine and phosphocreatine in the muscles. Because persons do not usually alter muscle mass rapidly, the levels of creatinine produced by the body remain relatively stable. Because of this stability, creatinine levels rapidly reflect changes in renal function.

For accurate determinations of creatinine clearance, the nurse and patient must rigidly adhere to the following procedure:

1. The patient empties his or her bladder, the exact time is recorded, and the specimen is discarded.
2. All urine for the next 24 hours is saved.
3. Exactly 24 hours after the start of the procedure, the patient voids again, and the specimen is saved.

TABLE 14-1

Systemic Manifestations of Acute Renal Failure

System	Manifestation	Pathophysiological Mechanism
Cardiovascular	Fluid overload	↓ Excretion of fluids
	Heart failure	Fluid overload and hypertension
	Pulmonary edema	Fluid overload
		↑ Pulmonary capillary permeability
		Left ventricular dysfunction
	Dysrhythmias	Electrolyte imbalances (especially hyperkalemia, hypocalcemia, and variations in sodium)
	Peripheral or systemic edema	Right ventricular dysfunction
	Hypertension	Fluid overload
		↑ Sodium retention
		Inappropriate activation of the renin-angiotensin system
Hematological	Anemia	↓ Erythropoietin secretion
		Loss of RBCs through GI tract, mucous membranes, or dialysis
		↓ RBC survival time from uremic toxins
		Uremic toxins' interference with folic acid secretion
	Alterations in coagulation	Platelet dysfunction from uremic toxins
	↑ Susceptibility to infection	↓ Neutrophil phagocytosis and chemotaxis from uremic toxins
	Electrolyte imbalances	↓ Excretion
	Metabolic acidosis	↓ Hydrogen ion excretion
		↓ Sodium ion reabsorption
		↓ Bicarbonate ion reabsorption and generation
		↓ Excretion of phosphate salts or titratable acids
		↓ Ammonia synthesis and ammonium excretion
Respiratory	Pneumonia	Thick tenacious sputum from ↓ oral intake
		Weak, lethargic with depressed cough reflex
		↓ Pulmonary macrophage activity
	Pulmonary edema	Fluid overload
		Left ventricular dysfunction
		↑ Pulmonary capillary permeability
Gastrointestinal	Anorexia, nausea, vomiting	Uremic toxins
		Decomposition of urea in GI tract, releasing ammonia that irritates mucosa
	Stomatitis and uremic halitosis	Uremic toxins
		Decomposition of urea in oral cavity, releasing ammonia
	Gastritis and bleeding	Uremic toxins
		Decomposition of urea in GI tract, releasing ammonia that irritates mucosa, causing ulcerations
		Increased capillary fragility
Neuromuscular	Drowsiness, confusion, irritability, and coma	Uremic toxins produce encephalopathy
		Metabolic acidosis
		Electrolyte imbalances
	Tremors, twitching, and convulsions	Uremic toxins produce encephalopathy
		↓ Nerve conduction from uremic toxins

Continued

TABLE **14-1**

Systemic Manifestations of Acute Renal Failure—cont'd

System	Manifestation	Pathophysiological Mechanism
Psychosocial	Decreased mentation, decreased concentration, and altered perceptions (even to point of psychosis)	Uremic toxins produce encephalopathy Electrolyte imbalances Metabolic acidosis Tendency to develop cerebral edema
Integumentary	Pallor Yellowness Dryness Pruritus Purpura Uremic frost (seen only in terminal or critically ill patients)	Uremic anemia Retained urochrome pigment excretion through skin ↓ Secretions from oil and sweat glands from uremic toxins Dry skin Calcium and/or phosphate deposits in skin Uremic toxins' effect on nerve endings ↑ Capillary fragility Platelet dysfunction Urea or urate crystal excretion
Endocrine	Glucose intolerance (usually not clinically significant)	Peripheral insensitivity to insulin from uremia Prolonged insulin half-life from ↓ renal metabolism
Skeletal	Hypocalcemia	Hyperphosphatemia from ↓ excretion of phosphates ↓ GI absorption from ↓ renal conversion of vitamin D Deposition of calcium phosphate crystals in soft tissues

↑, Increased; ↓, decreased; *GI*, gastrointestinal; *RBC*, red blood cell.

4. The serum creatinine level is assessed at the end of 24 hours.
5. All the urine that was saved is sent to laboratory for testing. (Urine can also be obtained from a Foley catheter.)

Urinary creatinine clearance is calculated by use of the following formula:

$$U_c \times V/P_c = C_{cr}$$

where U_c = concentration of creatinine in the urine, V = volume of urine per unit of time, P_c = concentration of creatinine in the plasma, and C_{cr} = creatinine clearance.

Creatinine clearance is an estimate of GFR and is measured in milliliters per minute. Thus, given the following set of patient data,

U_c = 175 mg/100 mL
V = 288 mL/1440 min (24 hr = 1440 min)
P_c = 17.5 mg/100 mL

the patient's creatinine clearance would be calculated as follows:

$$\frac{175 \text{ mg}/100 \text{ mL} \times 288 \text{ mL}/1440 \text{ min}}{17.5 \text{ mg/mL}} = 2 \text{ mL/min}$$

Because a normal creatinine clearance is about 84 to 138 mL per minute, the clinician would recognize this patient's creatinine clearance as being consistent with severe renal dysfunction. Creatinine clearance decreases by 10% each decade of life after age 40 years. If no urine is available for a creatinine clearance determination, the following formula may be used to determine the creatinine clearance from a serum creatinine value:

$$C_{cr} = \frac{(140 - \text{Age in years}) \times (\text{Lean body weight [kg]})}{72 \times \text{Serum creatinine (mg/dL)}}$$

For female patients, the aforementioned calculated result is then multiplied by 0.85 (Swan & Keane, 2001).

In lieu of using creatinine clearance for the evaluation of renal function, the next best measure is serum creatinine level, followed by serum blood urea nitrogen (BUN) level. Of these two values, BUN level is the least reflective of renal function because the rate of protein metabolism is not constant. The relationship between BUN and creatinine, known as the BUN/creatinine ratio, provides useful information. The normal BUN/creatinine ratio is 10:1 to 20:1 (e.g., BUN

TABLE 14-2

Normal Serum Laboratory Values and Variations Seen in Acute Renal Failure

Parameter	Normal Values	Variation In Acute Renal Failure
Sodium	136-145 mEq/L	Varies with free water load
Potassium	3.5-5.3 mEq/L	↑
Chloride	97-107 mEq/L	Varies
Blood urea nitrogen	Age <40 yr: 5-18 mg/dL Age 40-60 yr: 5-20 mg/dL Age >60 yr: 8-21 mg/dL	↑
Creatinine	Female: 0.5-1.1 mg/dL Male: 0.6-1.2 mg/dL Elderly may be lower	↑
Calcium	Age 18-60 yr: 8.6-10 mg/dL Age 60-90 yr: 8.8-10.2 mg/dL Age >90 yr: 8.2-9.6 mg/dL	↓
Phosphorus	Age <60 yr: 2.7-4.5 mg/dL Age >60 yr/female: 2.8-4.1 mg/dL Age >60/male: 2.3-3.7 mg/dL	↑
Uric acid	Adult female: 2.4-6 mg/dL Adult male: 3.4-7.0 mg/dL	↑
Carbon dioxide total content	22-30 mEq/L	↓
Magnesium	1.8-3 mg/dL	↑ or normal
Hematocrit	Female: 35%-47% Male: 42%-52%	↓
Hemoglobin	Female: 12-15 g/dL Male: 13.6-17.2 g/dL	↓

↑, Increased; ↓, decreased.

level, 20 mg, and creatinine level, 1.0 mg). If this ratio is greater than 20:1 (e.g., BUN level, 60 mg, and creatinine level, 1.0 mg), problems other than renal failure are probably the cause. Extrarenal factors, including dehydration, high-protein diet, starvation, blood in the gastrointestinal tract, corticosteroids, and fever, all can elevate the BUN. For example, when a patient has gastrointestinal bleeding, the blood in the gut breaks down and results in increased protein load and hence an elevated BUN. In prerenal conditions, an increased BUN/creatinine ratio is typically noted. With prerenal conditions, there is a decrease in the GFR and hence a drop in urine flow through the renal tubules. This allows more time for urea to be reabsorbed from the renal tubules back into the blood. Creatinine is not readily reabsorbed; therefore, the serum BUN rises out of proportion to the serum creatinine level. A normal BUN/creatinine ratio is present in ATN. With ATN, there is actual injury to the renal tubules and a rapid decline in the GFR; hence urea and creatinine levels both rise proportionally as a result of increased reabsorption and decreased clearance (Anderson, 2000).

Analysis of urinary sediment and electrolyte levels is extremely helpful in distinguishing among the various causes of acute renal failure. Urine should be inspected for the presence of cells, casts, and crystals. In prerenal conditions, the urine typically has no cells but may contain hyaline casts (Woroniecki & Devarajan, 2002). Casts are cylindrical bodies that form when proteins precipitate in the distal tubules and collecting ducts. Postrenal conditions may present with stones, crystals, sediment, bacteria, and clots from the obstruction. Coarse, muddy brown granular casts

TABLE 14-3

Normal Urine Laboratory Values and Variations Seen in Acute Renal Failure

Parameter	Normal Values	Variation in Acute Renal Failure
Amount	0.6-1.5 L/24 hr	↓
Specific gravity	1.003-1.030	Fixed at 1.010 or less
pH	4.5-8.0	↑
Glucose	Negative	Normal
Protein	Negative	Normal (can vary)
Creatinine	0.8-2.0 g/24 hr	↓
Osmolarity	200-1200 mOsm/kg H_2O	↓
Sodium	75-200 mEq/24 hr	↑ In oliguria; can vary in nonoliguria
Potassium	25-123 mEq/24 hr; intake dependent	↓
Chloride	110-250 mEq/24 hr	↓
	Age >60 yr: 95-195 mEq/24 hr	
Calcium	110-250 mg/24 hr; diet dependent	↓
Phosphorus	0.4-1.3 g/24 hr	↓
Magnesium	12-199 mg/24 hr	↓

↑, Increased; ↓, decreased.

are classic findings in ATN (Holley, 2001). Microscopic hematuria and a small amount of protein (less than 1 g/dL) may also be seen.

Urine electrolyte levels help one to discriminate between prerenal causes and ATN. The nurse must obtain urine samples for electrolyte determinations before diuretics are administered because these drugs alter the urine results for up to 24 hours. Urinary sodium concentrations of less than 10 mEq/L are seen in prerenal conditions as the kidneys attempt to conserve sodium and water to compensate for the hypoperfusion state. Urine sodium concentrations are greater than 40 mEq/L in ATN as a result of impaired reabsorption in the diseased tubules (Nally, 2002).

The fractional excretion of sodium (FE_{Na}) is a useful test for assessing how well the kidney can concentrate urine and conserve sodium. To determine the FE_{Na} the following formula is used:

$$FE_{Na} = \frac{(Urine\ sodium)\ (Serum\ creatinine) \times 100}{(Urine\ creatinine)\ (Serum\ sodium)}$$

In prerenal conditions, the FE_{Na} will be less than 1%, although ATN presents with an FE_{Na} of greater than 1% (Albright, 2001). Table 14-4 summarizes laboratory data useful in differentiating among the three categories of acute renal failure.

Urine specific gravity and osmolality have a limited role in the diagnosis of acute renal failure, especially in older adults, because the body's ability to concentrate urine decreases with age (Pahnu & Halloran, 2001). In general, prerenal conditions cause concentrated urine (high specific gravity and osmolality), whereas intrinsic azotemia causes dilute urine (low specific gravity and osmolality). The volume of urine output is also not a good indicator of renal function. Patients with nonoliguric acute renal failure excrete large volumes of fluid with little solute. These patients still have renal dysfunction and azotemia, even though they excrete large volumes of fluid. In an older adult, assessment parameters are modified when assessing for acute renal failure (see Geriatric Assessment).

DIAGNOSTIC PROCEDURES

Various diagnostic procedures are used to evaluate renal function. Noninvasive diagnostic procedures are often performed before any invasive diagnostic procedures are conducted.

Noninvasive diagnostic procedures that assess the renal system are radiography of the kidneys, ureters, and bladder (KUB) and renal ultrasonography. The KUB study delineates the size, shape, and position of the kidneys. It may also demonstrate abnormalities, such as calculi, hydronephrosis (enlargement of the

TABLE 14-4

Laboratory Findings Useful in Differentiating Causes of Acute Renal Failure

Type of Acute Renal Failure	Specific Gravity	Urine Osmolality	Urine Sodium	Microscopic Examination	Bun/ Creatinine Ratio	FE$_{Na}$
Prerenal	>1.020	>500 mOsm/L	<10 mEq/L	Few hyaline casts possible	Elevated	<1%
Intrarenal	1.010	<350 mOsm/L	>20 mEq/L	Epithelial casts Red blood cell casts Pigmented granular casts	Normal	>1%
Postrenal	Normal to 1.010		Normal to 40 mEq/L	May have stones, crystals, sediment, clots, or bacteria	Normal	>1%

FE$_{Na}$, fractional excretion of sodium.

renal pelvis), cysts, or tumors. Renal ultrasound is helpful in evaluating the urinary collecting system for obstruction, which is manifest by dilation of the collecting system and ureters (Palmieri, 2002).

Invasive diagnostic procedures for assessing the renal system include intravenous pyelography, computed tomography, renal angiography, renal scanning, and renal biopsy. These procedures are summarized in Table 14-5.

For all diagnostic procedures, the clinician implements the following general interventions:

- Explain the procedure to the patient, reinforce previous explanations provided by other health care personnel, and emphasize the patient's responsibilities during the procedure.
- Determine whether the patient has any allergies to contrast media and notify the physician if an allergy is present.
- Carry out any preparatory activities for the procedure, such as administration of special diet, bowel preparations, laboratory testing, insertion of intravenous access, and completion of consent forms.
- Provide appropriate fluids to assist the patient in maintaining adequate hydration before and after the procedure.

Geriatric Assessment

- The typical signs and symptoms of acute renal failure may be attributed to other disorders associated with aging, thus delaying prompt diagnosis and treatment.
- Volume status is difficult to assess in older adults because of altered skin turgor and decreased skin elasticity, decreased baroreceptor reflexes, and mouth dryness caused by mouth breathing.
- Urinary indices are of limited value in assessment of older adults because of impaired ability to concentrate urine.
- Serum creatinine may remain the same in older adults even with deteriorating renal function because of decreased muscle mass and hence decreased creatinine production.
- Glomerular filtration rate decreases beginning about age 40 with a yearly decline of approximately 1 mL per minute.
- Older patients tend to exhibit uremic symptoms at lower levels of serum blood urea nitrogen and creatinine than do younger patients.
- Older patients may exhibit atypical signs and symptoms of uremia, such as an unexplained exacerbation of well-controlled heart failure, unexplained mental status changes, or personality changes.

TABLE 14-5

Invasive Diagnostic Procedures for Assessing the Renal System

Procedure	Purpose	Potential Problems
Intravenous pyelography	To visualize the renal parenchyma, calyces, renal pelvis, ureters, and bladder to obtain information regarding size, shape, position, and function of the kidneys	Hypersensitivity reaction to contrast medium Acute renal failure
Computed tomography	To visualize the renal parenchyma to obtain data regarding the size, shape, and presence of lesions, cysts, masses, calculi, obstructions, congenital anomalies, and abnormal accumulations of fluid	Hypersensitivity reaction to contrast medium (if used)
Renal angiography	To visualize the arterial tree, capillaries, and venous drainage of the kidneys to obtain data regarding the presence of tumors, cysts, stenosis, infarction, aneurysms, hematomas, lacerations, abscesses	Hypersensitivity reaction to contrast medium Hemorrhage or hematoma at the catheter insertion site Acute renal failure
Renal scanning	To determine renal function by visualizing the appearance and disappearance of the radioisotopes within the kidney; also provides some anatomical information	Hypersensitivity reaction from contrast medium
Renal biopsy	To obtain data for making a histological diagnosis to determine the extent of the pathology, the appropriate therapy, and the possible prognosis	Hemorrhage Postbiopsy hematoma

- Provide emotional support to the patient before, during, and after the procedure.
- Assist with the procedure as necessary.
- Monitor the patient for any complications after the procedure, particularly for signs of infection after any invasive diagnostic procedure.
- Document the patient's response to the procedure.

Nursing Diagnoses

Nursing care of the patient with acute renal failure is complex. Multiple nursing diagnoses must be dealt with in these often critically ill patients. The nurse formulates a plan of care that addresses the following nursing diagnoses (see Nursing Care Plan):

- Excess fluid volume related to sodium and water retention and excess intake
- Risk for infection related to depressed immune response secondary to uremia and impaired skin integrity
- Imbalanced nutrition: less than body requirements related to uremia, altered oral mucous membranes, and dietary restrictions
- Anxiety related to diagnosis, treatment plan, prognosis, and unfamiliar environment

- Deficient knowledge related to disease process and therapeutic regimen

Nursing Interventions

Measurement of intake and output, and determination of daily weights are two vital procedures performed by the nurse who is caring for patients with acute renal failure. Accuracy is extremely important. Appropriate measuring devices rather than clinician "guesstimations" must be used for the measurement of urine. For example, a urine meter or some other type of accurate measuring device is used if the patient has an indwelling catheter. Normal urine output is 0.5 to 1 mL per kg of body weight each hour. Oral fluid intake must also be carefully monitored. Fluid intake levels are often restricted to the amount of urine output in a 24-hour period plus insensible losses (approximately 600 to 1000 mL per day) (Hutchinson, 2001).

Daily weights are one of the most useful noninvasive diagnostic tools available for clinicians (Esson & Schrier, 2002). Daily weights are used to validate intake and output measurements. One kilogram of body weight gain is equal to 1000 mL of fluid gain.

Nursing Care Plan for the Patient with Acute Renal Failure

NURSING DIAGNOSIS: *Excess fluid volume related to sodium and water retention and excess intake*

Patient Outcomes	Interventions	Rationales
I & O will be balanced. Body weight will be within 2 lb of dry weight. Vital signs will be stable. RAP will be 0 to 8 mm Hg. Skin turgor, moisture, and elasticity will be normal. Oral mucosa will be normal, hydrated. Bilateral breath sounds will be clear.	Maintain accurate I & O records. Obtain daily weights. Assess vital signs every 2 to 4 hr. Conduct a head-to-toe assessment every 8 hr. Monitor respiratory status, including rate and breath sounds. Administer all fluids and medications precisely. Administer blood products before or during dialysis. Prepare the patient for dialysis or CRRT.	Early recognition of signs and symptoms of fluid volume excess allow for prompt intervention. Careful monitoring of all fluids helps to reduce accumulation of excess fluid. Restricting sodium intake causes less sodium and subsequently less water reabsorption by the kidneys.

NURSING DIAGNOSIS: *Risk for infection related to depressed immune response secondary to uremia and impaired skin integrity*

Patient Outcomes	Interventions	Rationales
Infection will be absent. The patient will be afebrile. Breath sounds, chest x-ray will be normal. Cultures will be negative for all body fluids and wounds. WBC count and differential will be normal.	Monitor environment, visitors, and personnel caring for patient for possible contamination. Assess all abrasions, cuts, incisions every 8 hr. Inspect all intravenous sites every 2 to 4 hr. Monitor temperature every 4 hr. Avoid invasive equipment whenever possible. Monitor laboratory values and diagnostic tests frequently (WBC count, cultures). Perform pulmonary preventive program (turn, cough, deep breathing).	Infection is a leading cause of morbidity and mortality in patients with acute renal failure. These measures will help prevent infection and allow early detection of any infection so appropriate interventions may be taken.

NURSING DIAGNOSIS: *Imbalanced nutrition: less than body requirements related to uremia, altered oral mucous membranes, and dietary restrictions*

Patient Outcomes	Interventions	Rationales
Nutritional and caloric intake will be adequate. Body weight will be consistent with the patient. Energy level will be appropriate. The patient will verbalize comfort of the oral cavity. The patient will verbalize the ability to taste food appropriately.	Monitor body weight and caloric intake daily. Provide diet with essential nutrients but within restrictions. Provide small frequent feedings. Remove noxious stimuli from the environment. Promote dietary goals with the patient.	An awareness of the amount of foods and fluids the patient consumes alerts the nurse to deficits in nutritional intake. Early recognition of signs and symptoms of malnutrition allows for prompt intervention.

Nursing Care Plan for the Patient with Acute Renal Failure—cont'd

Patient Outcomes	Interventions	Rationales
	Administer vitamins, medications, and nutritional supplements as prescribed. Instruct the patient to suck on hard candy or chew gum to alleviate mouth dryness. Assess oral cavity every 4 hr. Assist with oral care every 2 hr, before meals, and at bedtime.	

NURSING DIAGNOSIS: *Anxiety related to diagnosis, treatment plan, prognosis, and unfamiliar environment*

Patient Outcomes	Interventions	Rationales
The patient will have a relaxed facial expression and body posture. The patient will demonstrate a reduced anxiety level. The patient will demonstrate effective coping mechanisms. The patient will participate in the treatment plan.	Monitor for signs of anxiety: tachycardia, hypertension, muscle tension, inappropriate behaviors. Use a calm, trusting approach with the patient and family. Explain all procedures. Provide a calm, relaxed environment; attempt to decrease stimulation. Allow the patient to make decisions as appropriate. Administer sedatives as prescribed.	Early recognition of signs and symptoms of anxiety allows for prompt intervention. A sense of calm conveys to the patient that the nurse is in control of the situation and this helps reduce anxiety. Factual information and an awareness of what to expect help to decrease anxiety. A calm, restful environment facilitates relaxation.

NURSING DIAGNOSIS: *Deficient knowledge related to disease process and therapeutic regimen*

Patient Outcomes	Interventions	Rationales
The patient will have sufficient, accurate information to be an informed participant in his or her own care. The patient will verbalize information known and ask questions about the disease process and health care regimen. The patient will cooperate and participate in his or her own care.	Assess content of patient's verbalizations and questions daily. Provide specific and factual information about the disease process, its impact on the patient, and its effect on care. Reinforce information and update daily. Include the family in the process.	Knowledge will enhance the patient's and family's understanding of the disease and therapeutic regimen. Factual information and an awareness of what to expect help the patient and family to make better-informed decisions. Clear explanations will help with patient compliance with the treatment plan.

CRRT, Continuous renal replacement therapy; *I & O,* intake and output; *RAP,* right atrial pressure; *WBC,* white blood cell count.

Weights should be obtained at the same time each day by use of the same scale. Many critical care beds have built-in scales, which have simplified the procedure. When the patient is weighed, the nurse ensures that the scale is properly calibrated and that the same number of bed linens and pillows is weighed with the patient each time.

The nurse plays a key role in prevention of infection in patients with acute renal failure. Infection accounts for about 75% of deaths in patients with acute renal failure (Agrawal & Swartz, 2000). Indwelling urinary catheters should not automatically be placed, because they increase the risk of infection, and many patients remain oliguric for 8 to 14 days. Strict aseptic technique with all intravenous lines (central and peripheral), including temporary access devices used for dialysis, is also of extreme importance, both at the time of insertion and during daily maintenance.

Another important role of the nurse in prevention and progression of acute renal failure is monitoring of peak and trough drug levels. Nurses are responsible for scheduling and obtaining the peak and trough blood levels at the appropriate times to ensure accurate results. Drug dosage adjustments must be made to avoid accumulation of the drug and toxic side effects. For example, aminoglycoside doses are based on drug levels and the patient's estimated creatinine clearance. Based on the results of the drug levels, either the dose of the aminoglycoside can be kept constant and the interval between doses increased or the interval can be kept constant and the dose can be decreased if the drug level is too high. A *peak level* is usually drawn 1 to 2 hours after the drug is administered and reflects the highest level achieved after the drug has been rapidly distributed and before any substantial elimination has occurred. A *trough level* is drawn just before the next dose is given and is an indicator of how the body has cleared the drug.

When caring for the patient with acute renal failure, the nurse is alert for signs and symptoms indicative of clinical deterioration. The Clinical Alerts describe common clinical scenarios that may occur when caring for a patient with acute renal failure and that warrant prompt recognition, notification of the physician, and intervention.

MEDICAL MANAGEMENT OF ACUTE RENAL FAILURE (PRERENAL CAUSES)

Acute renal failure from prerenal conditions is usually reversible if renal perfusion is quickly restored; therefore, early recognition and prompt treatment are essential. However, prevention of prerenal conditions is just as important as early recognition and aggressive management. Prompt replacement of extracellular fluids and aggressive treatment of shock may help to prevent acute renal failure.

Hypovolemia is treated in various ways, depending on the cause. Blood loss necessitates blood transfusions, whereas patients with burns, pancreatitis, and peritonitis are usually treated with isotonic solutions, such as normal saline. Hypovolemia resulting from large urine or gastrointestinal losses often requires the administration of a hypotonic solution, such as 0.45% saline. Patients suffering from cardiac instability usually require positive inotropic agents, antidysrhythmic agents, preload or afterload reducers, or intraaortic balloon pumping. Hypovolemia from intense vasodilation may require vasoconstrictor medications, isotonic fluid replacement, pharmacological blood pressure support, and antibiotics (if the patient is septic) until the underlying problem has been resolved. Invasive hemodynamic monitoring with a pulmonary artery catheter is extremely valuable in the management of fluid balance.

MEDICAL MANAGEMENT OF ACUTE RENAL FAILURE (POSTRENAL CAUSES)

Postrenal obstruction should be suspected whenever a patient has an unexpected decrease in urine volume. Postrenal conditions are usually resolved with the insertion of an indwelling bladder catheter, either transurethral or suprapubic. Occasionally, a ureteral stent may have to be placed if the obstruction is caused by calculi or carcinoma.

MEDICAL MANAGEMENT OF ACUTE TUBULAR NECROSIS

Common interventions for the patient with ATN include the following: drug therapy, such as diuretics and dopamine; dietary management, such as protein and electrolyte restrictions; management of fluid and electrolyte imbalances; and dialysis or continuous renal replacement therapies (CRRTs).

Considering the detrimental impact of acute renal failure, nurses should implement measures to prevent this disorder. The most important preventive strategy includes identification of patients at risk and elimination of potential contributing factors. Aggressive treatment must begin at the earliest sign of renal dysfunction.

In general, maintenance of cardiovascular function and adequate intravascular volume are the two key goals in the prevention of ATN. Primary measures include the following:

1. Maintaining an adequate hydration state for the patient, especially before surgery or invasive procedures and before excretion urography studies

CLINICAL ALERTS RENAL FAILURE

Clinical Concern	Significance	Nursing Actions*
Hypertension, edema, crackles, neck vein distention, ↑ PA pressures, ↓ urine output, ↓ hematocrit, weight gain, S_3 heart sound	Indicative of fluid volume overload; may lead to pulmonary edema	Prepare to administer diuretics. Assess IV fluid rates and maintain fluid restriction as prescribed. Prepare the patient for dialysis. Monitor respiratory status and have emergency equipment available for endotracheal intubation and mechanical ventilation.
ECG changes: tall tented T waves, prolonged PR interval and wide QRS, serum K^+ >6.6 mEq/L	Indicative of hyperkalemia; may lead to ventricular fibrillation and cardiac arrest	Check IV solutions, medications, and diet for potassium. Prepare to administer IV glucose, insulin, sodium bicarbonate, and 10% calcium gluconate. Prepare to administer sodium polystyrene sulfonate (Kayexalate). Prepare the patient for dialysis. Continuous cardiac monitoring
Paresthesias, muscle cramps, weakness, fatigue, hypotension, prolonged QT interval, laryngeal stridor, serum Ca^{++} <7 mg/dL	Indicative of hypocalcemia that may precipitate seizures, heart blocks, and cardiac arrest	Continuous cardiac monitoring. Implement seizure precautions. Monitor respiratory status. Prepare to administer 10% calcium gluconate.
Altered level of consciousness, confusion, serum Na^+ <136 mEq/L, anorexia, weakness	Indicative of hyponatremia that may precipitate seizures and coma	Monitor neurological status closely. Prepare to administer oral and IV sodium replacement. Maintain fluid restrictions as prescribed. Implement seizure precautions.
Pale skin, tachycardia, ↓ hemoglobin and hematocrit, fatigue, angina	Indicative of anemia	Prepare to administer blood transfusions as prescribed. Prepare to administer erythropoietin as prescribed. Monitor for blood loss.
Hyperventilation, headache, lethargy, low serum pH, low serum bicarbonate, low $PaCO_2$	Indicative of metabolic acidosis that may cause hypotension, ↓ myocardial contractility, ↓ level of consciousness, and seizures	Prepare to administer IV $NaHCO_3$. If repeated IV $NaHCO_3$ is necessary, be alert for sodium overload, which can precipitate pulmonary edema.

*The physician is notified for all alerts.
Ca^{++}, Calcium; *ECG*, electrocardiogram; *IV*, intravenous; K^+, potassium; $NaHCO_3$, sodium bicarbonate; *PA*, pulmonary artery; $PaCO_2$, partial pressure of carbon dioxide in arterial blood.

2. Maintaining renal perfusion by administering vasoactive agents that may increase renal blood flow, such as low doses of dopamine, acetylcholine, isoproterenol, kinins, prostaglandins, and calcium antagonists

3. Monitoring the duration, dosage, and combinations of all nephrotoxic agents (radiocontrast agents, antibiotics, chemotherapy and nonsteroidal drugs) administered to the patient, weighing the risk-to-benefit ratio carefully, and considering nontoxic alternatives (Guo & Nzerue, 2002)

PHARMACOLOGIC MANAGEMENT
Diuretics

Diuretic therapy in the treatment of patients with acute renal failure is controversial. Diuretics are commonly used to convert oliguria to a nonoliguric state (urine output greater than 400 mL per day). This conversion has been found to be beneficial for several reasons. In general, nonoliguric patients are easier to treat because they require less hemodialysis, have a shorter hospital stay, and have fewer complications and a lower mortality rate (Lameire, Vanholder, & Van Biesen, 2002). It is believed that diuretics increase renal blood flow, GFR, and intratubular pressure while decreasing tubular obstruction and dysfunction. However, the problem with using diuretics is that they only increase urine flow without affecting GFR or tubular function and may thus compromise an already insulted renal system (Pruchnicki & Dasta, 2002a, 2002b). Diuretics may increase the risk of acute renal failure (from volume depletion) when they are given before procedures requiring radiological contrast agents. Even though diuretics are commonly given, there is little evidence that they are of any benefit to patients with acute renal failure, and their widespread use should be discouraged (Mehta, Pascual, Soroko, & Chertow, 2002).

Hypovolemia should be corrected before any diuretics are administered. If diuretic therapy is implemented, a loop diuretic is commonly ordered. Furosemide has the dual effect of creating a solute diuresis (increased flow of tubular cellular debris) and augmenting renal blood flow (Agraharkar & Gupta, 2003). Large doses of furosemide are often needed in acute renal failure to induce diuresis. This may lead to excessive diuresis and volume depletion. High doses of furosemide have been associated with deafness, which may become permanent. Patients who are also receiving aminoglycosides are at increased risk of ototoxicity (Lameire, Vanholder, & Van Biesen, 2002).

Mannitol, an osmotic diuretic often used in acute renal failure, increases plasma volume and is believed to protect the kidney by minimizing post ischemic swelling. However, it may cause volume depletion and may inhibit oxygen perfusion and increase oxygen demand in the renal medulla (Pruchnicki & Dasta, 2002a, 2002b).

Dopamine

The role of dopamine, like that of diuretics, is controversial in the treatment of acute renal failure. Low-dose dopamine is often used in acute renal failure despite numerous studies that have failed to show any benefit. Dopamine in low doses (1 to 3 mcg/kg per minute) may increase renal blood flow and GFR by stimulating the dopaminergic receptors in the kidney. Sodium excretion is increased as a result of the enhanced blood flow (Pierce, Morris, & Clancy, 2002). The administration of dopamine immediately at the onset of acute renal failure (particularly if the patient is hypotensive) is believed to avert further damage and to help maintain urine output (Saxena, 2002). However, there has been growing concern regarding potential adverse effects of dopamine even at low doses. Dopamine causes a decrease in T-cell function and thereby increases susceptibility to infection. It has been found to suppress circulating concentrations of most anterior pituitary–dependent hormones such as prolactin, growth hormone, and thyrotropin, which alters normal endocrine responses in critical illness. Dopamine has also been shown to reduce respiratory drive, increase intrapulmonary shunting, decrease splanchnic perfusion, and cause tachyarrhythmias (O'Leary & Bihari, 2001). The use of low-dose dopamine as a renal protective agent remains controversial. The routine administration of dopamine most likely will diminish because of growing evidence that it has no role in prevention of acute renal failure and may actually be detrimental (Bellomo, Chapman, Finfer, Hickling, & Myburgh, 2000).

Acetylcysteine

Studies have been conducted using prophylactic acetylcysteine (mucomyst) in patients at risk of contrast-induced acute renal failure. Important risk factors for contrast-induced renal failure include preexisting renal dysfunction, diabetic nephropathy, dehydration, and administration of angiotension-converting enzyme inhibitors. Contrast agents are believed to reduce renal function by altering renal hemodynamics and through direct toxic effects on the tubular cells by reactive oxygen species (Tepel et al., 2000). Acetylcysteine, an antioxidant, is thought to protect these patients by interfering with these mechanisms. Studies have demonstrated that prophylactic administration of acetylcysteine (600 mg orally twice a day on the day before and on the day of the contrast), along with hydration ($\frac{1}{2}$ normal saline at 1 mL/kg per hour overnight before procedure) decreases the amount of acute renal damage in high-risk patients undergoing procedures requiring contrast agents (Shyu, Cheng, & Kuan, 2002; Thompson & King, 2003).

Fenoldopam

Another promising agent that is postulated to protect against contrast-induced acute renal failure is fenoldopam, a dopamine A1 receptor agonist. Fenoldopam (Corlopam) acts predominately as a vasodilator of peripheral arteries (reducing blood pressure) and as a potent renal vasodilator (increasing renal blood flow) (Murphy, Murray, & Shorten, 2001). It is six times more potent than dopamine in increasing renal blood flow, especially to critical regions in the renal medulla. Fenoldopam is given via intravenous infusion several hours before the contrast agent is given and is continued for a minimum of 4 hours after the procedure (Chamsuddin et al., 2002). Studies are ongoing with the use of fenoldopam in the prevention of contrast-induced acute renal failure.

Miscellaneous Agents

Multiple miscellaneous agents have been administered in an attempt to attenuate the course of acute renal failure and to hasten recovery. None, however, has consistently proved effective. Many of these drugs attempt to improve renal blood flow through vasodilation (atrial natriuretic peptide [ANP], endothelium-1 receptor antagonists, prostaglandin E_1), prevent accumulation of intracellular calcium, as occurs in ischemic azotemia (calcium channel blockers), protect renal tubule cells during ischemia (glycine, magnesium adenosine triphosphate dichloride), or stimulate renal cell regeneration (epidermal growth factor, growth hormone, insulin-like growth factor). Many of these agents and numerous others have shown beneficial results in experimental models but have had inconsistent results in the clinical setting. Studies are currently being conducted using many of the previously mentioned agents in the prevention and treatment of acute renal failure (Lennon, Coleman, & Brady, 2000; Pruchnicki & Dasta, 2002a, 2002b). Prostaglandin E_1 has a vasodilatory effect and has been shown in small studies to counteract the vasoconstriction from radiocontrast media that may cause acute renal failure in high-risk patients (Koch et al., 2000).

Epogen (Epoetin Alfa)

Patients with acute renal failure may develop anemia from a variety of causes (see Table 14-1). Epoetin alfa is an agent commonly used to treat the anemia of chronic renal failure, but it is occasionally used in acute renal failure. Patients should have adequate iron stores (serum ferritin must be at least 300 ng/mL) before epoetin alfa is administered. If iron levels are low, oral or intravenous iron therapy is indicated. The most prominent side effect of epoetin alfa is hypertension. Blood pressure must be adequately controlled before starting epoetin alfa and closely monitored thereafter. Various dosing patterns may be used; however, starting doses in the range of 50 to 100 units per kg three times weekly are commonly used.

Pharmacologic Management Considerations

Drug therapy for the patient with acute renal failure poses a challenge because about two thirds of all drugs or their metabolites are eliminated from the body by the kidneys (Guo & Nzerue, 2002). In acute renal failure, substantial alterations in drug dosages are often necessary to prevent toxic levels and adverse reactions. Assessment of renal function by creatinine clearance is often used to assist with drug dosing. The pharmacokinetic characteristics of the drug to be given, the route of elimination, and the extent of protein binding are also considered.

Many drugs are removed by dialysis, and extra doses are often required to avoid suboptimal drug levels. In general, drugs that are primarily water soluble, such as vitamins, cimetidine, and phenobarbital, are removed by dialysis and should be administered after dialysis. Drugs that are protein bound, lipid bound, or metabolized by the liver, such as phenytoin, lidocaine, and vancomycin, are not removed by dialysis and can be given at any time (Johnson & Simmons, 2002). Box 14-5 is a partial list of drugs that are removed by dialysis.

DIETARY MANAGEMENT

Dietary management in patients with acute renal failure continues to be a major component of the therapeutic regimen. Energy expenditure in catabolic patients with acute renal failure is much higher than normal basal requirements. Dialysis also contributes to protein catabolism. The loss of amino acids and water-soluble vitamins in the dialysate solution constitutes another drain on the patient's nutritional stores.

The overall goal of dietary management for acute renal failure is provision of adequate energy, protein, and micronutrients to maintain homeostasis in patients who may be extremely catabolic. Nutritional recommendations include (Charney & Charney, 2002; Druml, 2002) the following:

- Caloric intake of 25 to 35 kcal per kg of ideal body weight per day

BOX 14-5

Common Drugs Removed by Hemodialysis*

- Aminoglycosides (gentamicin, tobramycin)
- Cephalosporins (including cefoxitin and ceftazidime)
- Penicillins (piperacillin, penicillin G)
- Erythromycin
- Isoniazid
- Sulfonamides (sulfamethoxazole, sulfisoxazole)
- Trimethoprim-sulfamethoxazole
- Procainamide
- Quinidine
- Nitroprusside
- Lithium carbonate
- Water-soluble vitamins
- Folic acid
- Phenobarbital
- Cimetidine
- Ranitidine

*If possible, hold daily doses until after dialysis; supplemental doses may be required for many of these agents.

- Protein intake of no less than 0.8 g/kg body weight. Patients who are extremely catabolic should receive 1.5 to 2 g per kg of ideal body weight per day, 75% to 80% of which contains all the required essential amino acids.
- Sodium intake of 0.5 to 1.0 g per day
- Potassium intake of 20 to 50 mEq per day
- Calcium intake of 800 to 1200 mg per day
- Fluid intake equal to the volume of the patient's urine output plus an additional 600 to 1000 mL per day

In addition, patients undergoing dialysis usually receive multivitamins, folic acid, and occasionally an iron supplement to replace the water-soluble vitamins and other essential elements lost during dialysis.

If the patient is unable to ingest or tolerate an adequate oral nutritional intake, total parenteral nutrition is prescribed. Total parenteral nutrition therapy supplies the patient with sufficient nonprotein glucose calories, essential amino acids, fluids, electrolytes, and essential vitamins to create a more stable internal environment. Such an internal environment not only prevents further catabolism, negative nitrogen balance, muscle wasting, and other uremic complications, but also enhances the patient's tubular regenerating capacity, resistance to infection, and ability to combat other multisystem dysfunctions. To facilitate the administration of total parenteral nutrition, the physician must also prescribe early dialysis therapy to handle the increased fluid volume requirements.

MANAGEMENT OF FLUID, ELECTROLYTE, AND ACID-BASE IMBALANCES

Fluid Imbalance

Volume overload is generally managed by dietary restriction of salt and water and administration of diuretics. In addition, dialysis or other renal replacement therapies may be indicated for fluid control. These modalities are discussed later in this chapter.

Electrolyte Imbalance

Common electrolyte imbalances in acute renal failure are listed in the Laboratory Alerts, along with their "critical" values, signs and symptoms, and nursing actions. Hyperkalemia occurs when potassium excretion is reduced as a result of the decrease in GFR. Hyperkalemia is common in acute renal failure, especially if the patient is hypercatabolic. Sudden changes in the serum potassium level can be fatal. In general, three primary approaches are used for the treatment of hyperkalemia: (1) reducing the body potassium content, (2) shifting the potassium intracellularly, and (3) antagonizing the membrane effect of the hyperkalemia. These approaches, which may be used simultaneously or separately, are summarized in Table 14-6. Only two methods are effective in reducing plasma potassium and total body potassium content in a patient with acute renal failure: (1) dialysis and (2) the use of cation exchange resins (sodium polystyrene sulfonate [Kayexalate]) with sorbitol. The other methods listed "protect" the patient for a short time until dialysis or cation exchange resins can be instituted.

A commonly prescribed regimen for hyperkalemia consists of the following orders (Weiner & Wingo, 2002):

- Calcium gluconate, 10 mL of a 10% solution given intravenously over 5 minutes
- Glucose (50 mL of 50% dextrose) given intravenously
- Regular insulin, 10 units given intravenously.
- Sodium bicarbonate, 50 to 100 mEq/L given intravenously
- Sodium polystyrene sulfonate (Kayexalate), 15 to 30 g every 3 to 4 hours with 50 to 100 mL of a 20% sorbital solution given by mouth or as a retention enema

Hyponatremia is generally the result of water overload. However, as nephrons are progressively damaged, the ability to conserve sodium is lost, and major salt-wasting states can develop, causing hyponatremia. This condition is usually treated with fluid restriction,

TABLE 14-6

Treatment Approaches for Hyperkalemia

Approach	Methods	Efficacy
Reduce the body potassium content	Decrease potassium intake Increase the fecal excretion of potassium by using cation-exchange resins, such as sodium polystyrene sulfonate (Kayexalate) Increase the renal excretion of potassium by using mineralocorticoid agents, increasing salt intake, or using diuretic agents	May ↓ plasma and total body potassium content over time Takes hours to be effective but eventually ↓ both plasma and total body potassium content Any of these would be effective in ↓ both plasma and total body potassium content if the patient has normal renal function ↓ Both plasma and total body potassium content within a 4- to 6-hr time frame
Shift the potassium intracellularly	Administer glucose and insulin intravenously Administer an alkali (e.g., sodium bicarbonate)	↓ Plasma potassium level for about 2 hr but has no effect on total body potassium content ↓ Plasma potassium level for a short time but has no effect on total body potassium content
Antagonize the cellular membrane effect	Administer calcium salts Administer hypertonic sodium salts	Has no effect on either plasma or total body potassium content Has no effect on either plasma or total body potassium content

↓, Decrease.

specifically restriction of free water intake. Alterations in the serum calcium and phosphorus levels occur frequently in acute renal failure as a result of abnormalities in excretion, absorption, and metabolism of the electrolytes. Mild degrees of hypermagnesemia are common in acute renal failure as a result of decreased renal excretion.

Acid-Base Imbalance

Metabolic acidosis is the primary acid-base imbalance seen in acute renal failure. Box 14-6 summarizes the causes and the signs and symptoms of metabolic acidosis in acute renal failure. Treatment of metabolic acidosis depends on its severity. In mild metabolic acidosis, the lungs are able to compensate by excreting carbon dioxide. Patients with a serum bicarbonate level of less than 15 mEq/L (normal, 24 to 28 mEq/L) and a pH of less than 7.20 are usually treated with intravenous sodium bicarbonate. The goal of treatment is to raise the pH to a value greater than 7.20. Rapid correction of the acidosis should be avoided, however, because tetany may occur as a result of hypocalcemia. The pH determines how much ionized calcium is present in the serum: the more acidic the serum is, the more ionized calcium is present. If the metabolic

acidosis is rapidly corrected, the serum ionized calcium level decreases as the calcium binds with albumin and other substances, such as phosphate and sulfate. For this reason, intravenous calcium gluconate may be prescribed. Dialysis also corrects the metabolic acidosis because it removes excess hydrogen ions and because bicarbonate is added to the dialysate cleansing solution (Whitney & Szerlip, 2002).

RENAL REPLACEMENT THERAPY

Renal replacement therapy is the primary treatment for the patient with acute renal failure. Without some form of renal replacement therapy, the patient is unable to sustain life during the acute renal failure episode. Therapy may include hemodialysis, CRRT, or peritoneal dialysis.

Definition

Dialysis is defined as the separation of solutes by differential diffusion through a porous or semipermeable membrane that is placed between two solutions. This general definition permits the clinician to distinguish among the various types of dialyses merely by identifying the semipermeable membrane and describing the two solutions that are involved.

LABORATORY ALERTS IN ACUTE RENAL FAILURE

Laboratory Test	Critical Value	Significance	Nursing Actions
Potassium (K+)	>6.6 mEq/L	Hyperkalemia: Electrocardiographic changes: tall tented T waves, increased PR interval, widening QRS (sine wave), complete heart block, asystole, ventricular fibrillation, muscle weakness, abdominal cramps, diarrhea	Continuous cardiac monitoring. Prepare to administer IV glucose, insulin, sodium bicarbonate and 10% calcium gluconate and sodium polystyrene sulfonate (Kayexelate). Prepare the patient for dialysis.
Sodium (Na+)	≤110 mEq/L	Hyponatremia: Nausea, vomiting, headache, fatigue, lethargy, confusion, coma, seizures, diarrhea	Restrict fluid intake as ordered. Monitor neurological status. Administer diuretics as prescribed. Prepare the patient for dialysis if volume overloaded.
Total calcium (Ca++)	<7 mg/dL	Hypocalcemia: Paresthesias, tetany, seizures, cramps, laryngospasm, positive Chvostek's sign, positive Trousseau's sign	Continuous cardiac monitoring. Implement seizure precautions. Monitor respiratory status. Prepare to administer 10% calcium gluconate slowly IV (1 mL/min).
Magnesium (Mg+)	>3mg/dL	Hypermagnesemia: Lethargy, coma, hypotension, hypoventilation, flaccid muscles, weak to absent deep tendon reflexes, prolonged PR interval and QT interval, bradycardia, heart blocks	Monitor respiratory and neurological status. Continuous cardiac monitoring. Prepare to administer diuretics or normal saline to encourage magnesium loss. Prepare patient for dialysis. Prepare to administer 10% calcium gluconate to minimize symptoms.

Indications for Dialysis

Dialysis is used in acute renal failure for many reasons. Fluid overload with pulmonary edema, hypertension, heart failure, electrolyte imbalances, and acid-base imbalances are the most common reasons for instituting dialysis. Dialysis therapy is usually initiated early in the course of the renal failure before uremic complications can occur, such as nausea and vomiting, pericarditis, and hematological abnormalities (Schiffl, Lang, & Fischer, 2002). In addition, dialysis is often started for fluid control when total parenteral nutrition is administered.

Principles and Mechanisms

Dialysis therapy is based on two physical principles that operate simultaneously: diffusion and ultrafiltration

(Murray & Hall, 2000). *Diffusion* (or clearance) is the movement of solutes, such as urea, from the patient's blood to the dialysate cleansing fluid, across a semipermeable membrane (the artificial kidney). Substances such as bicarbonate may also cross in the opposite direction, from the dialysate across the semipermeable membrane into the patient's blood. Movement of solutes across the semipermeable membrane is dependent on the following:

- The amount of solutes on each side of the semipermeable membrane; typically, the patient's blood has larger amounts of solutes, such as urea, creatinine, and potassium
- The surface area of the semipermeable membrane, in other words, the size of the artificial kidney
- The permeability of the semipermeable membrane

BOX 14-6

Metabolic Acidosis in Acute Renal Failure

ETIOLOGY

Inability of kidney to excrete hydrogen ions produced by body; decreased production of ammonia by the kidney (normally assists with hydrogen ion excretion)

Retention of acid end-products of metabolism, which use available buffers in the body; inability of kidney to synthesize bicarbonate

SIGNS AND SYMPTOMS

Low pH of arterial blood (pH <7.35)

Low serum bicarbonate, carbon dioxide combining power, $PaCO_2$

Increased rate and depth of respirations to excrete carbon dioxide from the lungs (compensatory mechanism); known as Kussmaul's respiration

Lethargy and coma if severe

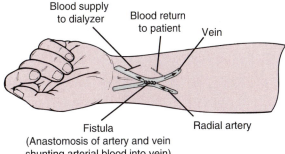

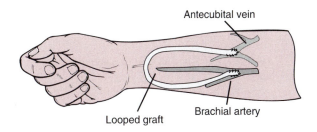

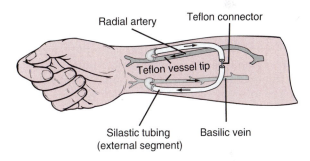

FIGURE 14-6 Hemodialysis access devices. (From Lewis, S. L., Heitkemper, M. M., & Dirksen, S. R. [2004]. *Medical-surgical nursing: Assessment and management of clinical problems.* 6th ed. St. Louis: Mosby).

- The size and charge of the solutes
- The rate of blood flowing through the artificial kidney
- The rate of dialysate cleansing fluid flowing through the artificial kidney

Ultrafiltration is the removal of plasma water and some low-molecular-weight particles by use of a pressure or osmotic gradient. Ultrafiltration is primarily aimed at controlling fluid volume, whereas dialysis is aimed at decreasing waste products and treating fluid and electrolyte imbalances.

Vascular Access

An essential component of all the renal replacement therapies is adequate, easy access to the patient's bloodstream. Various types of vascular access devices (Figures 14-6 and 14-7) are used for hemodialysis: percutaneous venous catheters, arteriovenous fistulas, arteriovenous grafts, and external arteriovenous shunts. The nurse will find that the terms *fistula, graft,* and *shunt* are often used interchangeably. Temporary *percutaneous catheters* are most commonly used in patients with acute renal failure because they can be used immediately. They are inserted into the subclavian, jugular, or femoral vein. The typical catheter has a single or double lumen and is designed only for short-term renal replacement therapy during acute situations. One example of such a device is the Vas-Cath catheter.

An *arteriovenous fistula* is an internal, surgically created communication between an artery and a vein.

The most frequently created fistula is the Brescio-Cimino fistula, which involves anastomosing the radial artery and cephalic vein in a side-to-side or end-to-side manner. The anastomosis permits blood to bypass the capillaries and to flow directly from the artery into the vein. As a result, the vein is forced to dilate to accommodate the increased pressure that accompanies the arterial blood. This method produces a vessel that is easy to cannulate for the renal replacement therapies.

Arteriovenous grafts are created by use of different types of prosthetic material, most commonly polytetrafluoroethylene and Gore-Tex (Hakaim & Oldenburg, 2001). Anastomoses are made with the graft ends connected to an artery and a vein.

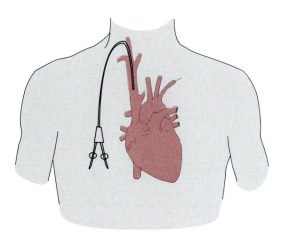

FIGURE 14-7 Central venous catheter used for hemodialysis.

An external *arteriovenous* shunt (Quinton-Scribner) consists of a surgically implanted extracorporeal apparatus that connects an artery and a vein. This type of device has become less popular since the advent of percutaneous catheters but may occasionally be used in the critical care unit. The external shunt poses a risk of infection and clotting problems.

Nursing care of arteriovenous fistula or graft.

The nurse is always protective of the vascular access site. An arteriovenous fistula or graft should be auscultated for a bruit and palpated for the presence of a thrill or buzz every 8 hours. The extremity that has a fistula or graft must never be used for drawing blood specimens, obtaining blood pressure measurements, intravenous therapy, or intramuscular injections. Such activities produce pressure changes within the altered vessels that could result in clotting or rupture. The nurse can alert other health care personnel of the presence of the fistula or graft by posting a large sign at the head of the patient's bed that indicates which arm should be used. Constrictive clothing and jewelry must be avoided on the affected arm. Patients should be cautioned against sleeping on the affected arm. All these situations may decrease blood flow through the fistula or graft and may cause clotting. The presence and strength of the distal pulse past the fistula or graft are evaluated at least every 8 hours. Inadequate collateral circulation past the fistula or graft may result in loss of this pulse. The physician is notified immediately if no bruit is auscultated, no thrill is palpated, or the distal pulse is absent (Emery, 2001).

Nursing care of percutaneous catheters.

Strict aseptic technique must be applied to any percutaneous catheter placed for dialysis. Exit sites should be inspected daily for signs of infection, such as redness, drainage, and swelling. Dressing changes are performed using sterile technique. To avoid accidental dislodging, there is minimal manipulation of the catheter. The catheter is not used for the administration of fluids or medications or for the sampling of blood unless a specific order is obtained to do so. Dialysis personnel place heparin in the catheter to maintain patency, and the catheter is clamped.

Hemodialysis

Hemodialysis is the most frequently used renal replacement therapy for treating acute renal failure. Hemodialysis consists of simply cleansing the patient's blood through an artificial kidney or dialyzer by use of diffusion and ultrafiltration. Water and waste products of metabolism are easily removed. Hemodialysis is efficient and corrects biochemical disturbances quickly. Treatments are typically 3 to 4 hours long and are performed in the critical care unit at the patient's bedside. Patients with acute renal failure may be hemodynamically unstable and unable to tolerate conventional hemodialysis. In those instances, other methods of renal replacement therapy, such as peritoneal dialysis or CRRT, are considered.

Complications.

An assortment of complications may occur in the patient undergoing hemodialysis. Hypotension occurs in approximately 10% to 50% of patients and is usually the result of preexisting hypovolemia, excessive amount of fluid removal, or excessively rapid removal of fluid (Bregman, Daugirdas, & Ing, 2001). Other factors that may contribute to hypotension during hemodialysis include left ventricular dysfunction from preexisting heart disease or medications, autonomic dysfunction resulting from medication or diabetes, and inappropriate vasodilation resulting from sepsis or antihypertensive drug therapy. Dialyzer membrane incompatibility may also cause hypotension.

Dysrhythmias may occur during dialysis and are often caused by a rapid shift in the serum potassium level, clearance of antidysrhythmic medications, preexisting coronary artery disease, hypoxemia, or hypercalcemia from rapid influx of calcium from the dialysate solution.

Muscle cramps may occur during dialysis, but they occur more commonly in chronic renal failure. Cramping is thought to be caused by ischemia of the skeletal muscles that results from aggressive fluid removal. The cramps typically involve the legs, feet, and hands and occur most often during the last half of the dialysis treatment.

A decrease in the arterial oxygen content of the blood can occur in patients undergoing hemodialysis. Usually, the decrease ranges from 5 to 35 mm Hg (mean, 15 mm Hg) and is not clinically significant except in the critically ill patient. Several theories have been offered to explain the hypoxemia, including leukocyte interactions with the artificial kidney and a decrease in carbon dioxide levels, resulting from either an acetate dialysate solution or a loss of carbon dioxide across the semipermeable membrane (Bregman, Daugirdas, & Ing, 2001).

Dialysis disequilibrium syndrome is most likely to occur after the first or second dialysis treatment or in patients who have had sudden large decreases in BUN and creatinine levels as a result of the hemodialysis. Because of the blood-brain barrier, dialysis does not deplete the concentrations of BUN, creatinine, and other uremic toxins in the brain as rapidly as it does those substances in the extracellular fluid. An osmotic concentration gradient established in the brain allows fluid to enter until the concentration levels equal those of the extracellular fluid. The extra fluid in the brain tissue creates a state of cerebral edema for the patient, which results in severe headaches, nausea and vomiting, twitching, mental confusion, and occasionally seizures. The incidence of dialysis disequilibrium syndrome may be decreased by the use of shorter, more frequent, dialysis treatments. It is also safest to use a dialysis solution sodium value close to the patient's serum sodium value to avoid fluid shifts into the brain (Bregman, Daugirdas, & Ing, 2001).

Infectious complications associated with hemodialysis include vascular access infections and hepatitis C. Vascular access infections are usually caused by a break in sterile technique, whereas hepatitis C is usually acquired through transfusion.

Hemolysis, air embolism, and hyperthermia are rare complications of hemodialysis. Hemolysis can occur when the patient's blood is exposed to incorrectly mixed dialysate solution or hypotonic chemicals (formaldehyde and bleach). An air embolism can occur when air is introduced into the bloodstream through a break in the dialysis circuit. Hyperthermia may result if the temperature control devices on the dialysis machine malfunction. Complications of hemodialysis are summarized in Box 14-7.

Nursing Care of the Patient.

The critical care nurse is responsible for the following tasks in regard to hemodialysis:
- Monitor laboratory values as ordered and report abnormal results to nephrologist and dialysis staff.

BOX 14-7

Complications of Dialysis

- Hypotension
- Cramps
- Bleeding/clotting
- Dialyzer reaction
- Hemolysis
- Dysrhythmias
- Infections
- Hypoxemia
- Pyrogen reactions
- Dialysis disequilibrium syndrome
- Vascular access dysfunction
- Technical mishaps (incorrect dialysate mixture, contaminated dialysate, or air embolism)

- Weigh patient daily; 1 kg of body weight gain is equal to 1000 mL of retained fluid.
- On the day of dialysis, withhold any dialyzable (water-soluble) medications until after treatment; check with the dialysis nurse or pharmacist to determine which medications to withhold; administer supplemental doses as ordered after treatment.
- Avoid administering antihypertensive agents for 4 to 6 hours before treatment, if possible. Reduce other medications that lower blood pressure (narcotics, sedatives), if possible.
- Assess the percutaneous catheter, fistula, or graft frequently; report any unusual findings, such as loss of bruit, redness, or drainage at site.
- Assess the patient frequently after treatment for signs of bleeding, hypovolemia, and dialysis disequilibrium syndrome.

Continuous Renal Replacement Therapy

CRRT is frequently used in patients with acute renal failure because of its ability to provide continuous ultrafiltration of fluids and clearance of uremic toxins. CRRT is particularly useful for patients in the critical care unit whose cardiovascular status is too unstable for rapid fluid removal. Table 14-7 outlines the various CRRT modalities.

Indications. The clinical indications for CRRT are similar to those for dialysis, such as hypervolemia, cardiac failure, and electrolyte and acid-base imbalances. CRRT modalities have also been thought to absorb specific proinflammatory substances such as tumor necrosis factor in patients with septic shock (Ronco, Bellomo, & Kellum, 2002).

TABLE 14-7

Continuous Renal Replacement Therapies (CRRTs)

Abbreviation	Name	Purpose	Vascular Access Required	Brief Description
CAVH	Continuous arteriovenous hemofiltration	Fluid removal	Arterial and large venous catheter	Arterial blood is circulated through a hemofilter and returned to the patient through a venous catheter; ultrafiltrate (fluid removed) is collected in a drainage bag as it exits the hemofilter
CAVHD	Continuous arteriovenous hemodialysis	Fluid and uremic waste product removal	Arterial and large venous catheter	Arterial blood is circulated through a hemofilter (surrounded by a dialysis solution) and returned to the patient through a venous catheter; ultrafiltrate (fluid and waste products removed) is collected in a drainage bag as it exits the hemofilter
CVVH	Continuous venovenous hemofiltration	Fluid removal	Dual-lumen venous catheter or two large venous catheters	Venous blood is circulated through a hemofilter and returned to the patient through a venous catheter; ultrafiltrate (fluid removed) is collected in a drainage bag as it exits the hemofilter
CVVHD	Continuous venovenous hemodialysis	Fluid and uremic waste product removal	Dual-lumen venous catheter or two large venous catheters	Venous blood is circulated through a hemofilter (surrounded by a dialysis solution) and returned to the patient through a venous catheter; ultrafiltrate (fluid and waste products removed) is collected in a drainage bag as it exits the hemofilter

Advantages of CRRT over hemodialysis include the following:
- CRRT is a continuous, 24-hour-a-day process.
- CRRT has more gradual solute removal.
- The risk of hemodynamic instability is less with CRRT.
- CRRT allows increased flexibility in fluid administration.
- CRRT requires only minimal heparinization.
- CRRT requires minimal staff education for implementation of the therapy.
- CRRT is ideal for physiologically unstable patients.

Disadvantages of CRRT include the following:
- The patient must remain in bed during the entire therapy.
- Vascular access and anticoagulation are necessary with CRRT.

- One-to-one nursing care may be needed for the patient undergoing CRRT.

Principles. CRRT is extracorporeal circulation of blood through a hemofilter for the removal of fluid and small solutes via the process of hemofiltration. Hemofiltration occurs when blood under pressure passes down one side of a highly permeable membrane allowing both water and other substances to pass across the membrane. Several different types of hemofilters are available, but all have highly porous membranes that permit the clearance of molecules less than 50,000 daltons, such as urea, creatinine, sodium, and potassium (Kaplow & Barry, 2002). Substances such as albumin and red blood cells are too large to pass through the hemofilter. Solute clearance can be enhanced with the addition of a dialysate solution, either a standard commercially prepared peritoneal solution (1.5% dextrose most commonly used) or specially prepared dialysate solutions formulated to meet individual patient's electrolyte needs. Automated devices are currently marketed to facilitate the procedure.

Depending on the method of CRRT, vascular access is gained via arterial or venous cannulation. In continuous arteriovenous hemofiltration (CAVH), an arterial and a venous catheter are inserted; the patient's own blood pressure pumps the blood through the hemofilter system and returns the blood via the venous catheter. However, because of complications with arterial vascular access, most clinicians now recommend the use of two venous accesses or a dual-lumen venous catheter. For example, in continuous venovenous hemofiltration (CVVH), venous blood from the patient is circulated through the hemofilter system by a blood pump and is then returned to the patient through the venous catheter (Figure 14-8). A constant heparin infusion is usually necessary to keep the filter from clotting with either

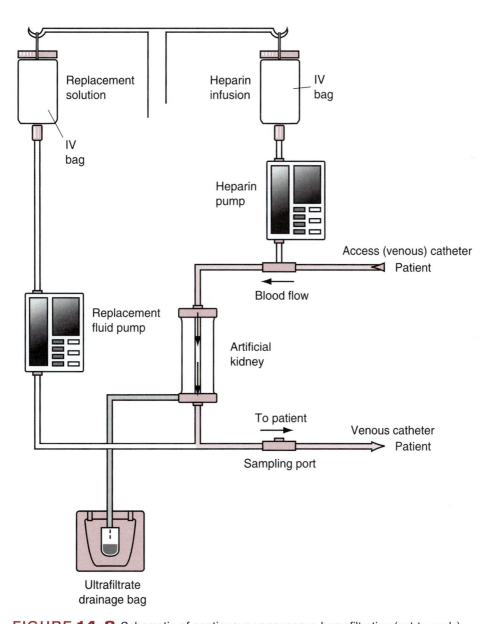

FIGURE 14-8 Schematic of continuous venovenous hemofiltration (not to scale).

method. Another option to continuous heparin therapy is sodium citrate, which anticoagulates blood by binding with calcium ions.

In CAVH or continuous arteriovenous hemodialysis (CAVHD), ultrafiltration (rate of fluid removal) occurs as a result of the difference between the patient's hydrostatic pressure and oncotic pressure. In CVVH or continuous venovenous hemodialysis (CVVHD), the clinician has the ability to control blood flow and ultrafiltration rates by adjusting the blood pump speed and ultrafiltration pump rate (Dirkes, 2000).

Fluid replacement therapy is occasionally used with CRRT to achieve optimal fluid balance. The most commonly administered solutions are normal saline, lactated Ringer's, or a physiological solution prepared by the pharmacy containing a bicarbonate base (Kaplow & Barry, 2002). Replacement fluid can be administered before the hemofilter (known as predilution) or after the hemofilter (postdilution).

Complications. Numerous complications are associated with CRRT, including the following:
- Electrolyte and acid-base imbalances
- Fluid imbalances
- Depletion of vitamins, amino acids, and other substances
- Hemorrhage and exsanguination resulting from anticoagulation or disruption of the filter or tubing
- Infection
- Hypothermia because of the extracorporeal nature of the hemofilter circuit
- Rupture or leakage of the filter
- Clotting of the filter
- Air embolism
- Vascular access failure

Responsibilities of the critical care nurse.
The critical care nurse is responsible for the following tasks in regard to CRRT:
- Monitor hemodynamic status hourly.
- Assess ultrafiltration rate hourly (volume of fluid removed) and administer appropriate replacement fluid.
- Assess hemofilter every 2 to 4 hours for clotting (as evidenced by dark fibers or rapid decrease in amount of ultrafiltration without a change in patient's hemodynamic status). If clotting is suspected, flush system with 50 mL of normal saline and observe for dark streaks or clots; the system may have to be changed.
- Monitor results of serum chemistries, clotting studies, and other tests as ordered.
- Frequently assess the CRRT system: keep filter and lines visible at all times, avoid kinks, and keep tubing warm to the touch (Figure 14-9).

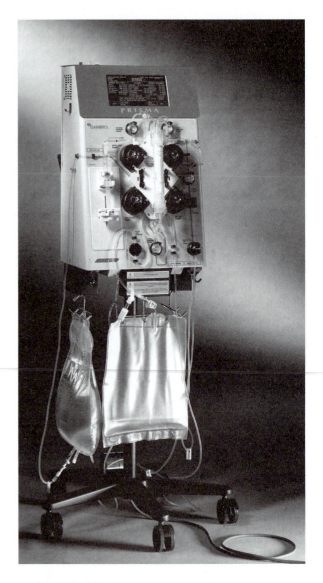

FIGURE 14-9 Prisma continuous renal replacement therapy system. (Courtesy of Gambro, Lakewood, CO.)

- Assess the ultrafiltrate for blood (pink-tinged to frank blood), which is indicative of membrane rupture.
- Maintain the heparin infusion per hospital protocol.
- Collaborate with the nephrologist and dialysis nurse for system or patient problems.
- Maintain sterile technique: swab ports with povidone-iodine (Betadine) before any blood is removed for samples, during dressing changes, or when the system is changed.

Peritoneal Dialysis

Peritoneal dialysis is the removal of solutes and fluid by diffusion through a patient's own semipermeable membrane (the peritoneal membrane) with a dialysate solution that has been instilled into the peritoneal cavity. The peritoneal membrane surrounds the abdominal cavity and lines the organs inside the abdominal cavity. This renal replacement therapy is not commonly used for the treatment of acute renal failure because of its comparatively slow ability to alter biochemical imbalances.

Indications. Clinical indications for peritoneal dialysis include acute and chronic renal failure, severe water intoxication, electrolyte disorders, and drug overdose. It offers several *advantages:*

- The equipment is easily and rapidly assembled and relatively inexpensive.
- Minimal physical preparation of the patient is required.
- The danger of acute electrolyte imbalances or hemorrhage is minimal.
- The dialysate solution can be easily individualized.
- The process can be implemented in either general care or specialty care areas.

Peritoneal dialysis also has several *disadvantages:*

- It is time-intensive, usually requiring at least 36 hours for a therapeutic effect to be achieved.
- Biochemical disturbances are corrected slowly.
- Protein loss is about 30 g per a 36-hour dialysis session.
- Access to the peritoneal cavity is sometimes difficult.
- The risk of peritonitis is high.

Complications. Although rare, many complications can result from peritoneal dialysis. Complications can be divided into three categories: mechanical problems, metabolic difficulties, and inflammatory reactions. The potential complications resulting from *mechanical problems* include the following:

- The abdominal viscera may be perforated during insertion of the catheter.
- Hemorrhage may result from the catheter insertion.
- The catheter may be improperly placed.
- Poor drainage may occur as a result of catheter blockage.
- Fluid may leak around the catheter.
- The patient may experience pain during the catheter insertion.
- The patient may experience discomfort as a result of the pressure of the fluid within the peritoneal cavity.
- Pulmonary complications may occur as a result of the pressure of the fluid in the peritoneal cavity.

Complications that may result from *metabolic difficulties* are as follows:

- Hypovolemia and hypernatremia may result from excessively rapid removal of fluid.
- Hypervolemia may result from impaired drainage of fluid.
- Hypokalemia may result from the use of potassium-free dialysate.
- Alkalosis may result from the use of an alkaline dialysate.
- Disequilibrium syndrome may result from excessively rapid removal of fluid and waste products.
- Hyperglycemia may result from the high glucose concentration of the dialysate.

These complications may result from *inflammatory reactions:*

- Peritoneal irritation may be produced by the catheter.
- Peritonitis may result from bacterial infection.

Peritonitis is the most common complication encountered in peritoneal dialysis therapy and is usually caused by contamination in the system. It is manifested by abdominal pain, cloudy peritoneal fluid, fever and chills, nausea and vomiting, and difficulty in draining fluid from the peritoneal cavity. Appropriate antibiotic treatment is indicated for peritonitis.

Contraindications. Although conflicting opinions exist, the following conditions are considered contraindications for peritoneal dialysis: acute active peritonitis, recent or extensive abdominal surgery, peritoneal adhesions, severe abdominal trauma or burns, massive intraperitoneal hematoma, and any major vascular anastomosis in the abdomen (Dirkes, 2000).

Geriatric Assessment in the Management of Acute Renal Failure

Older adults are at increased risk of developing acute renal failure as a result of the normal decline in renal function associated with aging, because of multiple comorbidities such as diabetes mellitus and hypertension, and from the multitudes of medications older adults may take. Two commonly prescribed classes of agents are nonsteroidal antiinflammatory agents and angiotensin-converting enzyme inhibitors, both of which have adverse effects on renal autoregulatory mechanisms (Albright, 2001). In addition, older adults are more prone to develop volume depletion (prerenal conditions) than are younger patients because of a decreased ability to concentrate urine and conserve sodium. Important issues in the management of acute renal failure in the patient who is an older adult are

RESEARCH ANALYSIS

ARTICLE REFERENCE
Kay, J., Chow, W., Chan, T., et al. (2003). Acetylcysteine for prevention of acute deterioration of renal function following elective coronary angiography and intervention: A randomized controlled trial. *Journal of the American Medical Association, 289*(5), 553-558.

STUDY OVERVIEW
Radiocontrast-induced nephropathy has long been a significant cause of acute renal failure, resulting in prolonged hospitalization and increased morbidity and mortality. The purpose of this study was to determine whether acute renal failure could be prevented by administering oral acetylcysteine to patients with moderate renal insufficiency who were undergoing elective coronary angiography. Acute renal failure was defined as a greater than 25% increase in serum creatinine from the admission serum creatinine.

The researchers randomly assigned 200 patients with stable moderate renal insufficiency (glomerular filtration rate of less than 60 mL or serum creatinine greater than 1.2 mg/dL) to one of two groups. The two groups were similar in age, weight, serum creatinine, and diabetic status. One group received oral acetylcysteine (600 mg twice per day), and the other group received a placebo on the day before and the day of the procedure. All patients received normal saline intravenously at 1 mL/kg body weight for the 12 hours before the procedure and for 6 hours after the contrast. Serum creatinine levels were measured at admission, then at 24 and 48 hours, and again at 7 days after the procedure. Twenty-four hour urine collections were also done at admission, at 48 hours, and at 7 days after the procedure. All patients received a nonionic, low-osmolality contrast agent (mean volume 139 mL).

Results of the study revealed that 12 placebo-treated patients (12%) and 4 acetylcysteine-treated (4%) patients developed acute renal failure within 48 hours of the procedure. Serum creatinine levels in the acetylcysteine group during the first 48 hours after the procedure decreased significantly from 1.35 to 1.22 mg/dL. In the placebo group, there was no significant change in serum creatinine during the first 48 hours after the procedure. Creatinine clearance also increased significantly in the acetylcysteine group during the same time frame. Again, the placebo group did not have any significant change in creatinine clearance. Patients who received acetylcysteine had a shorter length of hospitalization by an average of one-half day. No patients in the study required dialysis as a result of the administration of the contrast agent. No major adverse events were reported in either group directly related to acetylcysteine. The researchers concluded that acetylcysteine protects patients with moderate chronic renal insufficiency from contrast-induced worsening of renal function without any adverse effects and at a low cost.

STUDY STRENGTHS AND WEAKNESSES
One strength of this study is that the researchers measured varying renal end points and defined acute renal failure in a similar manner as prior studies, so data could be compared. One limitation of the study is the small sample size of 200 patients. All patients received intravenous hydration before the procedure and for several hours after contrast administration; however, the researchers did not study or comment on the role hydration may have played in prevention of acute renal failure. Prior studies have demonstrated hydration as playing a key role in prevention of acute renal failure in this population.

IMPLICATIONS FOR NURSING PRACTICE
In this study, the researchers concluded that there was a protective benefit against contrast-induced renal failure from acetylcysteine. Therefore, nurses need to be alert to patients who are at risk of developing acute renal failure and to administer acetylcysteine as prescribed. Prevention is key to avoid morbidity, the need for dialysis, and poor outcomes.

Geriatric Considerations in the Management of Acute Renal Failure

1. The aging kidney is more susceptible to nephrotoxic and ischemic injury:
   - Monitor drug dosages carefully.
   - Adjust drug dosages for underlying renal insufficiency.
   - Use nephrotoxic agents judiciously.
   - Monitor radiographic contrast media usage closely using only as necessary.
   - Maintain adequate hydration if radiographic contrast media must be used.
2. Older adults are more prone to volume depletion:
   - Be sure fluids are easily within reach of older adults not on fluid restriction.
   - Offer fluids frequently if not on fluid restriction (diminished in the thirst response and may not feel thirsty).
   - Provide intravenous fluids to maintain adequate hydration as prescribed.
3. Older adults often have poor nutritional status before acute renal failure and require early and adequate nutrition.
4. Older adults have special needs in regard to renal replacement therapies:
   - They may need dialysis or continuous renal replacement therapy earlier than younger patients, because they tend to become symptomatic with lower serum creatinine and blood urea nitrogen levels than younger patients.
   - Monitor for increased vascular access problems from comorbidities such as diabetes mellitus and peripheral vascular disease.
   - Keep ultrafiltration rate less than 1 L per hour because decreased cardiac reserve and autonomic dysfunction make ultrafiltration difficult.
   - Supply supplemental oxygen if needed to offset the hypoxemia that often develops at the start of dialysis.
   - Monitor for increased risk of complications associated with systemic heparinization, including subdural hematomas from falls and gastritis.
5. Older adults are more prone to infection because of a compromised immune system:
   - Use meticulous technique for all procedures.
   - Avoid indwelling catheterization especially if the patient is anuric; use intermittent catheterization as necessary.

 ## Case Study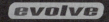

Mr. K. G. is an thin, 60-year-old man admitted to the hospital for cardiac catheterization for recurrent angina. Past medical history includes hypertension, type 2 diabetes mellitus, and a previous myocardial infarction 2 years ago. Current medications are metformin (Glucophage), glipizide (Glucotrol), enteric-coated aspirin (Ecotrin), and lisinopril (Zestril). Laboratory tests on admission revealed the following: normal electrolytes; blood urea nitrogen (BUN), 40 mg/dL; and serum creatinine, 2.0 mg/dL. A complete blood cell count and urinalysis were unremarkable. Mr. K. G. receives intravenous fluids at a KVO (keep vein open) rate (20 mL/hour) on the morning of the procedure. He successfully undergoes the catheterization and returns to the telemetry unit. The day after the procedure, Mr. K. G.'s urine output decreases to less than 10 mL per hour. Mr. K. G. is given a fluid bolus of normal saline without any increase in urine output. Furosemide is administered intravenously, with a slight increase in urine output to 15 mL per hour for several hours. Laboratory studies reveal the following: potassium, 5.9 mEq/L; BUN, 70 mg/dL; serum creatinine, 7.1 mg/dL; and carbon dioxide total content, 16 mEq/L. The next day Mr. K. G. has 2+ edema and basilar crackles, and he complains of feeling short of breath. A preliminary diagnosis of acute renal failure is made.

QUESTIONS

1. What are possible factors predisposing Mr. K. G. for acute renal failure?
2. What laboratory studies would be useful to assist in the diagnosis of acute renal failure? Describe expected results for a patient with acute tubular necrosis.
3. What medical interventions do you anticipate for Mr. K. G.?
4. What interventions could have been taken before Mr. K. G.'s cardiac catheterization to possibly prevent his acute renal failure?
5. Discuss the advantages and disadvantages of using diuretic therapy in patients with acute renal failure.

described in the Geriatric Considerations. Assessment considerations for the geriatric patient with acute renal failure were previously discussed in this chapter.

OUTCOMES

With appropriate interventions, expected outcomes for the patient with acute renal failure include the following:

- Fluid balance and hemodynamic status are stable.
- Body weight is within 2 lb of dry weight.
- Vital signs are stable and are consistent with baseline.
- Skin turgor is normal, and oral mucosa is intact and well hydrated.
- Serum laboratory values and arterial blood gas results are within normal limits.

- Infection is absent.
- Nutritional intake is adequate for the maintenance of the desired weight.
- The patient and family members are able to participate in the patient's care and are able to make informed decisions.

SUMMARY

The patient with acute renal failure poses many clinical challenges for health care personnel. Many of these patients have multisystem failure and require intensive and aggressive care. In addition, the development of acute renal failure is an event that often catches the patient and family unprepared. Nurses play a pivotal role in promoting positive patient outcomes through prevention, sharp assessment skills, and supportive nursing care.

CRITICAL THINKING QUESTIONS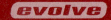

1. Identify strategies that the critical care nurse can use to help prevent acute renal failure.
2. Describe physical examination findings that may be seen in patients with prerenal acute renal failure.
3. What are three basic principles used in managing patients with acute renal failure?
4. You are caring for a patient with acute renal failure postoperatively. The cardiac monitor

demonstrates tall, tented T waves and a PR interval of 0.26 second.
   a. What electrolyte imbalance do you suspect?
   b. What medical interventions do you anticipate?
   c. Describe the mechanism of action for each medical intervention.
5. What are common indications for initiating dialysis in patients with acute renal failure?

REFERENCES

Agraharkar, M., & Gupta, R. (2003). Acute renal failure. *Emedicine,* topic 1595. Retrieved January 8, 2003, from http://www.emedicine.com/med/topic1595.htm.

Agrawal, M., & Swartz, R. (2000). Acute renal failure. *American Family Physician, 61*(7), 2077-2088.

Albright, R. (2001). Acute renal failure: A practical update. *Mayo Clinic Proceedings, 76*(1), 67-74.

Anderson, R. (2000). Clinical and laboratory diagnosis of acute renal failure. In B. Molitoris & W. Finn (eds.). *Acute renal failure: A companion to Brenner & Rector's the kidney* [pp. 157-168]. Philadelphia: W.B. Saunders.

Batlle, D. (2001). Metabolic acidosis. In A. Greenberg (ed.). *Primer on kidney diseases* [pp. 71-81]. 3rd ed. San Diego, CA: Academic Press.

Bellomo, R., Chapman, M., Finfer, S., Hickling, K., & Myburgh, J. (2000). Low-dose dopamine in patients with early renal dysfunction: A placebo-controlled randomized trial. Australian and New Zealand Intensive Care Society (ANZICS) clinical trials group. *Lancet, 356*(9248), 2139-2143.

Bregman, H., Daugirdas, J., & Ing, T. (2001). Complications during hemodialysis. In J. Daugirdas, P. Blake, & T. Ing

(eds.). *Handbook of dialysis* [pp. 148-168]. 3rd ed. Philadelphia: Lippincott Williams & Wilkins.

Briggs, J., Kriz, W., & Schnermann, J. (2001). Overview of renal function and structure. In A. Greenberg (ed.). *Primer on kidney diseases* [pp. 3-19]. 3rd ed. San Diego, CA: Academic Press.

Chamsuddin, A., Kowalik, K., Bjarnason, H., et al. (2002). Using a dopamine type 1A receptor agonist in high-risk patients to ameliorate contrast-associated nephropathy. *American Journal of Roentgenology, 179*(6), 591-596.

Charney, P., & Charney D. (2002). Nutrition support in renal failure. *Nutrition in Clinical Practice, 17*(4), 226-236.

Dirkes, S. (2000). Continuous renal replacement therapy: Dialytic therapy for acute renal failure in intensive care. *Nephrology Nursing Journal, 27*(6), 581-592.

Druml, W. (2002). Nutritional support in acute renal failure. In W. Mitch & S. Klahr (eds.). *Handbook of nutrition and the kidney* [pp. 191-213]. Philadelphia: Lippincott Williams & Wilkins.

Emery, J. (2001). Nursing care of patients with dialysis access. In J. Akoh & N. Hakim (eds.). *Dialysis access: Current practice* [pp. 371-395]. London: Imperial College Press.

Esson, M., & Schrier, R. (2002). Diagnosis and treatment of acute tubular necrosis. *Annals of Internal Medicine, 137*(9), 744-752.

Finn, W. (2001). Recovery from acute renal failure. In B. Molitoris & W. Finn (eds.). *Acute renal failure: A companion to Brenner & Rector's the kidney* [pp. 425-250]. Philadelphia: W. B. Saunders.

Guo, X., & Nzerue, C. (2002). How to prevent, recognize, and treat drug-induced nephrotoxicity. *Cleveland Clinic Journal of Medicine, 69*(4), 289-312.

Hakaim, A., & Oldenburg, W. (2001). Use of autogenous vein or synthetic grafts. In J. Akoh & N. Hakim (eds.). *Dialysis access: Current practice* [pp. 181-210]. London: Imperial College Press.

Holley, J. (2001). Clinical approach to the diagnosis of acute renal failure. In A. Greenberg (ed.). *Primer on kidney diseases* [pp. 245-250]. 3rd ed. San Diego, CA: Academic Press.

Hutchinson, F. (2001). Management of acute renal failure. In A. Greenberg (ed.). *Primer on kidney diseases* [pp. 275-280]. 3rd ed. San Diego, CA: Academic Press.

Iglesias, J., & Lieberthal, W. (2000). Clinical evaluation of acute renal failure. In R. Johnson & J. Feehally (eds.). *Comprehensive clinical nephrology* (pp.15.1-15.16). London: Mosby.

Johnson, C., & Simmons, W. (2002). *2002 Dialysis of drugs.* Verona, WI: Nephrology Pharmacy Associates.

Kaplow, R., & Barry, R. (2002). Continuous renal replacement therapies. *American Journal of Nursing, 102*(11), 26-33.

Kelly, B., & Agraharkar, M. (2002). Acute tubular necrosis. *Emedicine,* topic 39. Retrieved January 1, 2003, from http://www.emedicine.com/med/topic39.htm.

Koch, J., Plum, J., Grabensee, U., Modder, M., & PGE₁ Study Group. (2000). Prostaglandin E₁: A new agent for the prevention of renal dysfunction in high risk patients caused by radiocontrast media? *Nephrology, Dialysis, Transplantation, 15*(1), 43-49.

Lameire, N., Vanholder, R., & Van Biesen, W. (2002). Loop diuretics for patients with acute renal failure: Helpful or harmful? *Journal of the American Medical Association, 288*(20), 2599-2601.

Lennon, A., Coleman, P., & Brady, H. (2000). Management and outcome of acute renal failure. In R. Johnson & J. Feehally (eds.). *Comprehensive clinical nephrology* [pp.19.1-19.14]. London: Mosby.

Lentino, J., & Leehey, D. (2001). Infections. In J. Daugirdas, P. Blake., & T. Ing (eds.). *Handbook of dialysis* [pp. 495-521]. 3rd ed. Philadelphia: Lippincott Williams & Wilkins.

Lieberthal, W., & Nigam, S. (2000). Acute renal failure. II. Experimental models of acute renal failure: Imperfect but indispensable. *American Journal of Physiology Renal Physiology, 278*(1), F1-F12.

Mehta, R., Pascual, M., Soroko, S., & Chertow, G. (2002). Diuretics, mortality, and nonrecovery of renal function in acute renal failure. *Journal of the American Medical Association, 288*(20), 2547-2553.

Murphy, M., Murray, C., & Shorten, G. (2001). Fenoldopam: A selective peripheral dopamine-receptor agonist for the treatment of severe hypertension. *New England Journal of Medicine, 345*(21), 1548-1557.

Murray, P., & Hall, J. (2000). Renal replacement therapy for acute renal failure. *American Journal of Respiratory Care Medicine, 162*(3), 776-781.

Nally, J. (2002). Acute renal failure in hospitalized patients. *Cleveland Clinic Journal of Medicine, 69*(7), 569-574.

O'Leary, M., & Bihari, D. (2001). Preventing acute renal failure in the critically ill. *British Medical Journal, 322*(7003), 1437-1439.

Pahnu, N., & Halloran, P. (2001). The kidney in aging. In A. Greenberg (ed.). *Primer on kidney diseases* [pp.377-381]. 3rd ed. San Diego, CA: Academic Press.

Palmieri, P. (2002). Obstructive nephropathy: Pathophysiology, diagnosis, and collaborative management. *Nephrology Nursing Journal, 29*(1), 15-23.

Pierce, J., Morris, D., & Clancy, R. (2002). Understanding renal dose dopamine. *Journal of Infusion Nursing, 25*(6), 365-371.

Pruchnicki, M., & Dasta, J. (2002a). Acute renal failure in hospitalized patients: Part I. *Annals of Pharmacotherapy, 36*(7-8), 1261-1267.

Pruchnicki, M., & Dasta, J. (2002b). Acute renal failure in hospitalized patients: Part II. *Annals of Pharmacotherapy, 36*(9), 1430-1442.

Ronco, C., Bellomo, R., & Kellum, J. (2002). Continuous renal replacement therapy: Opinions and evidence. *Advances in Renal Replacement Therapy, 9*(4), 229-244.

Saxena, A. (2002). Dopamine "renal-dose": An appraisal of current concepts, controversies and concerns. *Dialysis and Transplantation, 31*(9), 615-624.

Schiffl, H., Lang, S., & Fischer, R. (2002). Daily hemodialysis and the outcome of acute renal failure. *New England Journal of Medicine, 346*(5), 305-310.

Shyu K., Cheng, J., & Kuan P. (2002). Acetylcysteine protects against acute renal damage in patients with abnormal renal function undergoing a coronary procedure. *Journal of the American College of Cardiology, 40*(8), 1383-1388.

Swan, S., & Keane, W. (2001). Clinical evaluation of renal function. In A. Greenberg (ed.). *Primer on kidney diseases* [pp. 25-28]. 3rd ed. San Diego, CA: Academic Press.

Tepel, M., van der Giet, M., Schwarzfeld, C., Laufer, U., Liermann, D., & Zidek W. (2000). Prevention of radiographic-contrast-agent-induced reductions in renal function by acetylcysteine. *New England Journal of Medicine, 343*(3), 180-184.

Thompson, E., & King, S. (2003). Acetylcysteine and fenoldopam: Promising new approaches for preventing effects of contrast nephrotoxicity. *Critical Care Nurse, 23*(3), 39-46.

Unwin, R., & Capasso, G. (2000). Renal physiology. In R. Johnson & J. Feehally (eds.). *Comprehensive clinical nephrology* [pp. 2.1-2.12]. London: Mosby.

Weiner, D., & Wingo, C. (2002). Hyperkalemia. In T. Dubose & L. Hamm (eds.). *Acid-base and electrolyte disorders: A companion to Brenner & Rector's the kidney* [pp. 395-412]. Philadelphia: W. B. Saunders.

Whitney, G., & Szerlip, H. (2002). Acid-base disorders in the critical care setting. In T. Dubose & L. Hamm (eds.). *Acid-base and electrolyte disorders: A companion to Brenner & Rector's the kidney* [pp. 165-187]. Philadelphia: W. B. Saunders.

Woolfson, R., & Hillman, K. (2003). Causes of acute renal failure. In R. Johnson & J. Feehally (eds.). *Comprehensive clinical nephrology* [pp.16.1-16.16]. London: Mosby.

Woroniecki, R., & Devarajan, P. (2002). Acute tubular necrosis. *Emedicine,* Topic 28. Retrieved January 1, 2003, from http://www.emedicine.com/med/topic28.htm.

RECOMMENDED READINGS

Daugirdas, J. (2002). Peritoneal dialysis in acute renal failure: Why the bad outcome? *New England Journal of Medicine,* 347(12), 933-935.

Haney, S. (2002). Drug use in renal failure. *Critical Care Nursing Clinics of North America, 14*(1), 77-80.

Reddy, V. (2002). Prevention of postoperative acute renal failure. *Journal of Postgraduate Medicine, 48*(1), 64-70.

Sauret, J., & Marinides, G. (2002). Rhabdomyolysis. *American Family Physician, 65*(5), 907-912.

Thorsen, M., & Poole, J. (2002). Renal disease in pregnancy. *Journal of Perinatal and Neonatal Nursing, 15*(4), 13-26.

Van de Noortgate, N., Verbeke, F., Dhondt, A., et al. (2002). The dialytic management of acute renal failure in the elderly. *Seminars in Dialysis, 15*(2), 127-132.

evolve *Did you remember to check out the bonus material, including free self-assessment exercises, on the Evolve Web site at http://evolve.elsevier.com/Sole/ and on the CD-ROM?*

CHAPTER **15**

Hematological and Immune Disorders

Gaye B. Padayao, BSN, RN, CCRN, OCN
Patricia B. Wolff, MSN, APRN, BC
Carol J. Thompson, MSN, RN, AOCN, CS

OBJECTIVES

- Explain the normal anatomy and physiology of the hematological and immune systems.
- Describe pathophysiological changes that affect hematological and immunological structure and function.
- Discuss the risk factors, pathophysiological process, clinical findings, nursing care, and medical management of anemia, neutropenia, malignant white blood cell disorders, human immunodeficiency virus, thrombocytopenia, and disseminated intravascular coagulation.
- Develop plans of care for the immunocompromised host and the patient who has a bleeding disorder.

Introduction

Hematological and immunological functions are necessary for gas exchange, tissue perfusion, nutrition, acid-base balance, protection against infection, and hemostasis. These complex, integrated responses are easily disrupted, and most critically ill patients experience some abnormalities in hematological and immune function. This chapter provides a general overview of the pertinent anatomy and physiology of these organ systems and the typical alterations in red blood cells (RBCs), immune activity, and coagulation function. Table 15-1 defines key terms used in this chapter in describing hematological and immunological disorders. The text provides guidelines for general assessment and nursing care strategies needed by beginning critical care nurses caring for patients at risk of these disorders.

Review of Anatomy and Physiology

HEMATOPOIESIS

Hematopoiesis is defined as the formation and maturation of blood cells. The primary site of hematopoietic cell production is the bone marrow; however, secondary hematopoietic organs that participate in this process include the spleen, liver, thymus, lymphatic system, and lymphoid tissues. Negative feedback mechanisms within the body induce the bone marrow's pluripotent hematopoietic stem cells to differentiate into one of the three blood cells: erythrocytes (RBCs), leukocytes (white blood cells [WBCs]), or thrombocytes (platelets) (McCance, 2002) (Figure 15-1).

In infancy, most bones are filled with blood-forming red marrow; later in childhood, productive

evolve *Be sure to check out the bonus material, including free self-assessment exercises, on the Evolve Web site at http://evolve.elsevier.com/Sole/ and on the CD-ROM.*

TABLE 15-1

Hematology-Immunology Key Terms

Term	Definition
Active immunity	A term used when the body actively produces cells and mediators that result in the destruction of the antigen
Anemia	A reduction in the number of circulating red blood cells or hemoglobin that leads to inadequate oxygenation of tissues. Subtypes named by etiology (e.g., aplastic anemia means "without cells") or by cell appearance (e.g., macrocytic anemia has large cells)
Antibody	Immune globulin, created by specific lymphocytes, and designed to immunologically destroy a specific foreign antigen
Anticoagulants	Factors inhibiting the clotting process
Antigen	Any substance that is capable of stimulating an immune response in the host
Autoimmunity	Situation in which the body abnormally sees self as nonself, and an immune response is activated against those tissues
Bone marrow transplant	Replacement of a defective bone marrow with one that is functional; described in terms of the source (e.g., autologous comes from self, and allogeneic comes from another person)
Cellular immunity	Production of cytokines in response to foreign antigen
Coagulation pathway	A predetermined cascade of coagulation proteins that are stimulated by production of the platelet plug, and occurs progressively, producing a fibrin clot; there are two pathways (intrinsic and extrinsic) triggered by different events that merge into a single list of events leading to a fibrin clot; clotting may be initiated by either or both pathways
Coagulopathy	Disorder of normal clotting mechanisms; usually used to describe inappropriate bleeding more often than excess clotting, but can refer to either one
Cytokines	Cell killer substances, or mediators secreted by white blood cells; when secreted by a lymphocyte, may also be called *lymphokine*, and secretions from monocytes are called *monokines*
Disseminated intravascular coagulation	Disorder of hemostasis characterized be exaggerated microvascular coagulation and depletion of clotting factors, with subsequent bleeding, also called *consumption coagulopathy*
Ecchymosis	Blue or purplish hemorrhagic spot on skin or mucous membrane, round or irregular, nonelevated
Epistaxis	Bleeding from the nose
Erythrocyte	Red blood cell
Fibrinolysis	Breakdown of fibrin clots that naturally occurs 1-3 days after clot development
Hemarthrosis	Blood in a joint cavity
Hematemesis	Bloody emesis
Hematochezia	Blood in stool; bright red
Hematoma	Raised, hardened mass indicative of blood vessel rupture and clotting beneath the skin surface; if subcutaneous, will appear as a blue-purple or purple-black area, but may occur in spaces such as pleural or retroperitoneal area
Hematopoiesis	Development of the early blood cells (erythrocytes, leukocytes, thrombocytes), encompassing their maturation in the bone marrow or lymphoreticular organs
Hematuria	Blood in the urine
Hemoglobinuria	Hemoglobin in the urine
Hemoptysis	Coughing up blood from the airways or lungs
Hemorrhage	Copious, active bleeding
Hemostasis	A physiological process involving hematological and nonhematological factors to form a platelet or fibrin clot to control the loss of blood

Continued

TABLE 15-1	
Hematology-Immunology Key Terms—cont'd	
Term	**Definition**
Human immunodeficiency virus	A retrovirus that transcribes its RNA-containing genetic material into DNA of the host cell nucleus; this virus has a propensity for the immune cells, replacing the RNA of lymphocytes and macrophages, causing an immunodeficient state
Humoral immunity	Production of antibodies in response to foreign proteins
Immunocompromised	Quantitative or qualitative defects in white blood cells or immune physiology; defect may be congenital or acquired and involve a single element or multiple processes; immune incompetence leads to lack of normal inflammatory, phagocytic, antibody, or cytokine responses
Immunoglobulin	A specific type of antibody named by its molecular structure (e.g., immunoglobulin A or immunoglobulin against cytomegalovirus)
Leukocyte	General word encompassing white blood cells; made up of three major subtypes: granulocytes (neutrophils, basophils, eosinophils), lymphocytes, and monocytes
Lymphoreticular system	Cells and organs containing immunologically active cells
Macrophage	Differentiated monocyte that migrates to lymphoreticular tissues of the body
Melena	Blood pigments in stool; dark or black
Menorrhagia	Excessive bleeding during menstruation
Neutropenia	Serum neutrophil count lower than normal; predisposes patients to infection
Passive immunity	A situation in which antibodies against a specific disease are transferred from another person
Petechiae	Small, red or purple, nonelevated dots indicative of capillary rupture, often located in areas of increased pressure (e.g., feet or back), or on the chest and trunk
Primary immunodeficiency	Congenital disorders in which some part of the immune system fails to develop
Procoagulants	Factors enhancing clotting mechanisms
Purpura	Large, mottled bruises
Reticulocytes	Slightly immature erythrocytes able to continue some essential functions of red blood cells
Secondary or acquired immunodeficiency	Immune disorder resulting from factors outside the immune system and involving the loss of a previously functional immune defense
Thrombocyte	Platelet
Thrombocytopenia	Serum platelet count less than normal. Predisposes individuals to bleeding as a result of inadequate platelet plugs
Thrombosis	Creation of clots; usually refers to excess clotting
Tissue anergy	Absence of a "wheal" tissue response to antigens and evidence of altered antibody capabilities
Tolerance	The body's ability to recognize self as self and therefore mount a rejection response against nonself, but not itself
Transfusion	Intravenous infusion of blood or blood products

bone marrow is found in the vertebrae, skull, thoracic cage, shoulder and pelvis, and femora and humeri (parts of long bones) (Hutchison & Davey, 2001). The hematopoietic and immunological organs and their key functions are summarized in Figure 15-2.

Changes in the immune and hematological systems occur in the elderly. These changes and implications are described in the Geriatric Assessment.

COMPONENTS AND CHARACTERISTICS OF BLOOD

Blood was recognized as being essential to life as early as the 1600s, but the specific composition and characteristics of blood were not defined until the twentieth century. Blood has four major components: (1) a fluid component called plasma, (2) circulating solutes such as ions, (3) serum proteins, and (4) cells.

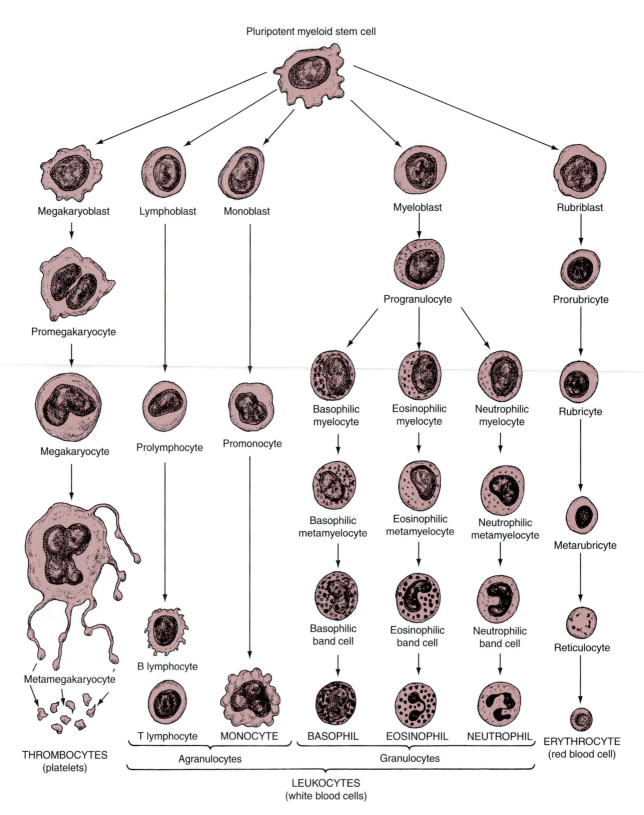

Pluripotent myeloid stem cell

Megakaryoblast   Lymphoblast   Monoblast   Myeloblast   Rubriblast

Promegakaryocyte   Progranulocyte   Prorubricyte

Megakaryocyte   Prolymphocyte   Promonocyte   Basophilic myelocyte   Eosinophilic myelocyte   Neutrophilic myelocyte   Rubricyte

Basophilic metamyelocyte   Eosinophilic metamyelocyte   Neutrophilic metamyelocyte   Metarubricyte

B lymphocyte   Basophilic band cell   Eosinophilic band cell   Neutrophilic band cell   Reticulocyte

Metamegakaryocyte   T lymphocyte   MONOCYTE   BASOPHIL   EOSINOPHIL   NEUTROPHIL   ERYTHROCYTE (red blood cell)

THROMBOCYTES (platelets)

Agranulocytes   Granulocytes

LEUKOCYTES (white blood cells)

FIGURE 15-1 Hematopoietic stem cell and lineage.

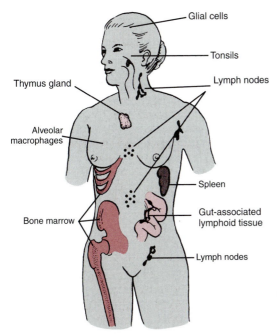

Organ	Key Functions
Spleen	The spleen is a highly vascular organ involved in the production of lymphocytes; the filtering and destruction of erythrocytes; the filtering and trapping of foreign matter, including bacteria and viruses; and the storage of blood. Although it is not necessary for survival, the spleen plays an important role in hemostasis and protection against infection.
Liver	The liver produces clotting factors, produces bile from RBC breakdown, and detoxifies many substances in the blood; its proper functioning is essential for normal hemostasis and metabolism. The liver filters and stores blood in addition to its many other metabolic functions.
Thymus gland	The thymus gland and lymph nodes are also part of the hematopoietic system; they are primarily involved in immunological functions.
Bone marrow	Site of production for all hematopoietic cells.
Tonsils, glial cells, alveolar macrophages, gut-associated lymphoid tissue	Lymphoid tissue responsive to antigens passing the initial barrier defenses, and possessing some inflammatory properties.
Lymph nodes	Storage site for lymphocytes. Part of the continuous lymphatic system that filters foreign matter.

FIGURE 15-2 Hematopoietic organs and their function. (Figure modified from Black, J. M. & Hawks, J. H. [2005]. [eds.]. *Medical-surgical nursing: Clinical management for positive outcomes.* 7th ed. Philadelphia: W. B. Saunders.)

Geriatric Assessment

Age-Related Change	Implications
Decreased percentage of marrow space occupied by hematopoietic tissue	Ineffective erythropoiesis, especially after blood loss
Decreased number of T cells produced	Delayed hypersensitivity
Decreased T-cell function	Increased incidence of infection
Appearance of autoimmune antibodies	Increased risk of autoimmune disorders
Increased immunoglobulin A and decreased immunoglobulin G levels	Increased prevalence of infection

Plasma comprises about 55% of blood volume and is the transportation medium for important serum proteins such as albumin, globulin, fibrinogen, prothrombin, and plasminogen. The hematopoietic cells comprise the remaining 45% of blood volume. Characteristics of blood and potential alterations that may be encountered in critically ill patients are shown in Table 15-2 (McCance, 2002).

HEMATOPOIETIC CELLS

Erythrocytes

Erythrocytes (RBCs) are flexible biconcave discs without nuclei whose primary component is an oxygen-carrying molecule called hemoglobin. This physiological configuration permits RBCs to travel at high speeds and to perfuse small blood vessels, exposing more surface area for gas exchange. In each milliliter of blood, there are approximately 5 million RBCs (McCance, 2002).

RBCs are generated from precursor stem cells under the influence of a growth factor called *erythropoietin*. Erythropoietin is secreted by the kidney in response to a perceived decrease in perfusion or tissue hypoxia. Maturation of RBCs takes 4 to 5 days, and their life span is about 120 days. *Reticulocytes* are immature RBCs that may be released when there is a demand for RBCs that exceeds the number of available mature cells. Reticulocytes are active but less effective than mature cells and circulate about 24 hours before maturing. The spleen and liver are important for removal and clearance of senescent RBCs (McCance, 2002).

The RBC transports hemoglobin, whose function is the transport of oxygen and carbon dioxide.

TABLE 15-2

Characteristics of Blood

Characteristic	Normal	Alterations
Color	Arterial: bright red Venous: dark red or crimson	Hypochromic (light color) in anemia Lighter color in dilution
pH	Arterial: 7.35-7.45 Venous: 7.31-7.41	↓ In systemic acidosis such as renal failure, diabetic crisis, infection ↑ In alkalosis such as vomiting, diuretic use, or hyperventilation
Specific gravity	Plasma: 1.026 Red blood cells: 1.093	— —
Viscosity	3.5-4.5 times that of water	Loss of plasma volume such as dehydration ↑ Cell production such as polycythemia Abnormal immunoglobulin such as multiple myeloma increases viscosity
Volume	Plasma volume 45 mL/kg Cell volume 30 mL/kg Average male is about 5000 mL	Fat tissue contains little water, so total blood volume best correlates to lean body mass Women have more fat, and therefore blood volume is usually lower than in men
		Plasma volume rises with progression of pregnancy Volume ↑ with immobility and ↓ with prolonged standing. May be result of changes in pressure in glomerulus and glomerular filtration rate Blood volume highest in neonate and lowest in elderly Lack of nutrients causes ↓ red blood cell and plasma formation ↑ Environmental temperature ↑ blood volume

↑, Increased; ↓, decreased.

Hemoglobin binds with oxygen in the lungs and transports it to the tissues. The rate of erythrocyte production increases when oxygen transport to tissues is impaired, and it decreases when tissues are hypertransfused or exposed to high oxygen tension. The oxygen affinity for hemoglobin is modulated primarily by the concentration of 2,3-diphosphoglycerate (2,3-DPG) and depends on the blood pH and body temperature. Erythrocytes are also vital in the maintenance of acid-base balance, because they transport carbon dioxide away from the tissues (Hutchison & Davey, 2001; Shelton, 2000).

Platelets (Thrombocytes)

Platelets, or *thrombocytes,* are the smallest of the formed elements of the blood. A normal platelet count ranges from 150,000 to 400,000/μL of blood. Platelets are created by hematopoietic stem cells in response to hormonal stimulation. Platelets have a life span of 8 to 11 days, but they may be used more rapidly if there are many vascular injuries or clotting stimuli. Two thirds of the platelets circulate in the blood. The spleen stores the remaining third, and may become enlarged if excess or rapid platelet removal occurs. In patients who have had a splenectomy, 100% of the platelets remain in circulation (Hutchison & Davey, 2001).

Platelets are the first responder in the clotting response, and they form a platelet plug that temporarily repairs an injured vessel. During circulation they detect and adhere to roughened, or sheared surfaces, such as blood vessel walls or indwelling catheters. Platelets also release mediators necessary for completion of clotting. Mediators include histamine and serotonin, which contribute to vasospasm; adenosine diphosphate, which assists platelet adhesion and aggregation; and calcium and phospholipids, which are necessary for clotting (McCance, 2002).

Leukocytes

WBCs (commonly called leukocytes) are classified according to their structure (granulocytes or agranulocytes) and function (phagocytes or immunocytes). The granulocytes include neutrophils, basophils, and eosinophils, and all function in phagocytosis. The agranulocytes consist of monocytes (phagocytes) and lymphocytes (immunocytes) (McCance, 2002).

Leukocytes (WBCs) are larger and less numerous than RBCs and have nuclei. The three types of leukocytes are classified by their structure, function, and affinity for certain dyes. The average number of WBCs ranges from 5000 to 10,000/μL of blood in the adult (Chernecky & Berger, 2001). Leukocytes are released into the bloodstream for transport to the tissues, where they perform specific functions (McCance, 2002).

Leukocytes are derived from hematopoietic stem cells that are stimulated by a triggering mechanism within the integrated immunological response. Leukocytes vary in appearance, function, storage site, and life span. Specific characteristics of cell development and life cycle are shown in Table 15-3.

WBCs play a key role in the defense against infectious organisms and foreign antigens. They produce and transport factors such as antibodies that are vital in maintaining immunity. Although they possess a variety of unique and specialized functions, WBCs work in an integrated fashion to protect the body. Numbers of WBCs are increased in circumstances of inflammation, tissue injury, allergy, or invasion with pathogenic organisms. Their numbers are diminished in malnutrition, advancing age, and immune diseases (Pagana & Pagana, 2002).

WBCs are classified into two categories: granulocytes (polymorphonuclear leukocytes) and nongranular leukocytes. These delineations are based on the appearance and staining characteristics of the cells. Polymorphonuclear leukocytes include neutrophils, eosinophils, and basophils. Nongranular leukocytes include monocytes and lymphocytes.

Granular leukocytes

Neutrophils. Neutrophils are the most numerous of the granulocytes, constituting 55% to 70% of the WBC differential count (Pagana & Pagana, 2002). The differential count measures the percentage of each type of WBC present in the venous blood sample. These cells are further broken down into segmented neutrophils, in which filaments in the cell give the nuclei an appearance of having lobes, and band neutrophils, which are immature and have a thicker or U-shaped nucleus. Normally, segmented neutrophils make up the majority of WBCs, whereas band neutrophils constitute only about 5% (Chernecky & Berger, 2004). The phrase "a shift to the left" refers to an increased number of "bands," or band neutrophils, compared with mature neutrophils on a complete blood count (CBC) report. This finding generally indicates an acute bacterial infectious process that draws on the WBC reserves in the bone marrow and causes less mature forms to be released. Likewise, a "shift to the right" indicates an increased number of circulating mature cells and may be associated with liver disease, Down syndrome, and megaloblastic and pernicious anemia (Chernecky & Berger, 2004).

The survival time of neutrophils is short. Once released from the bone marrow, they circulate in the blood less than 24 hours before migrating to the tissues, where they live another few days. When serious infection is present, neutrophils may live only hours while they phagocytize infectious organisms (Hutchison & Davey, 2001; McCance, 2002; Pagana & Pagana, 2002). Because of this short life span, drugs that affect rapidly multiplying cells (e.g., chemotherapeutic agents) quickly decrease the neutrophil count and thus alter the patient's ability to fight infection.

Eosinophils. Eosinophils are larger than neutrophils and make up 1% to 4% of the WBC count (McCance, 2002; Pagana & Pagana, 2002). They are important in the defense against allergens and parasites and are thought to be involved in the detoxification of foreign proteins. Eosinophils are found largely in the tissues of the skin, lung, and gastrointestinal tract. Eosinophils respond to chemotactic mechanisms triggering them to participate in phagocytosis, but they also contain bactericidal substances and lysosomal enzymes that aid in the destruction of invading organisms (Hutchison & Davey, 2001).

Basophils. The third type of granulocyte is the basophil, which has large granules that contain heparin, serotonin, and histamine. Basophils participate in the body's inflammatory and allergic responses by releasing these substances. Basophils, which constitute 0.5% to 1.0% of the WBC differential, play an important role in acute systemic allergic reactions and inflammatory responses (Pagana & Pagana, 2002).

Nongranular leukocytes (agranulocytes)

Monocytes. Monocytes are the largest of the leukocytes and constitute only 3% to 7% of the WBC differential (Chernecky & Berger, 2004; McCance, 2002). Once they migrate from the bloodstream into the tissues, monocytes mature into tissue macrophages, which are powerful phagocytes. In the lung, these tissue macrophages are known as alveolar macrophages; in the liver, they are Kupffer's cells; in connective tissue, they are histiocytes. In addition to "eating" large foreign particles and cell fragments,

TABLE 15-3

Overview of Leukocytes

Cell Type	Characteristics	Development and Migration	Life Span
GRANULOCYTES (polymorphonuclear leukocytes, polys)	Large granules and horseshoe-shaped nuclei that differentiate and become multilobed	Mature in the bone marrow Maturing granulocytes that are no longer dividing, accumulate as a reserve in the bone marrow Normally about a 5-day supply in the bone marrow	Average of 12 hr in the circulation About 2 to 3 days in the tissues
Neutrophils	Have small, fine, light pink or lilac acidophilic granules stained and a segmented, irregularly lobed, purple nucleus		
Band neutrophils	Bands less well defined, because they are slightly immature forms of the same cell		
Eosinophils	Have large, round granules that contain red-staining basic mucopolysaccharides and multilobed purple-blue nuclei		
Basophils	Coarse blue granules conceal the segmented nucleus Granules contain histamine, heparin, and acid mucopolysaccharides		
AGRANULOCYTES			
Lymphocytes	Small cell with a large, round, deep-staining, single-lobed nucleus and very little cytoplasm Cytoplasm slightly basophilic and stains pale blue	T lymphocytes constantly circulating, following a path from the blood to the lymphatic tissue, through the lymphatic channels, and back to the blood through the thoracic duct B lymphocytes largely noncirculating; remain mainly in the lymphoid tissue and may differentiate into plasma cells	Life span varies Small populations of memory lympho-cytes survive for many years Most T lymphocytes of the peripheral lymphatic tissue recirculate about every 10 hr Mature plasma cells have a survival rate of about 2 to 3 days
Monocytes	Large cell with a prominent, multishaped nucleus that is sometimes kidney shaped Chromatin in the nucleus looks like lace, with small particles linked together like strands Blue-gray cytoplasm filled with many fine lysozymes that stain pink with Wright's stain	Monocytes spend less time in the bone marrow pool than granulocytes	Circulation about 36 hr After the monocyte is transformed into macrophage in the tissues, life span ranges from months to years

macrophages are vital in the phagocytosis of necrotic tissue and debris. Like eosinophils, macrophages contain lysosomal enzymes and bactericidal substances. When activated by antigens, macrophages secrete substances called *monokines,* which act as chemical communicators between the cells involved in the immune response. Although monocytes may circulate for only 36 hours, they can survive for months or even years as tissue macrophages (McCance, 2002).

Lymphocytes. In the adult, approximately 25% to 33% of the total WBCs are lymphocytes (Chernecky & Berger, 2004; McCance, 2002). They contribute to the body's defense against microorganisms, but they are also essential for tumor immunity (surveillance for abnormal cells), delayed hypersensitivity reactions, autoimmune diseases, and foreign tissue rejection. Lymphocytes are responsible for specific immune responses and participate in two types of immunity: humoral immunity, which is mediated by B lymphocytes; and cellular immunity, which is mediated by T lymphocytes. B lymphocytes, or B cells, originate in the bone marrow and are also thought to mature there. B cells perform in antibody production. T lymphocytes, or T cells, comprise 60% to 70% of the circulating lymphocytes (McPherson, 2001). They live longer than B cells and participate in long-term immunity. T cells are produced in the bone marrow, but they migrate to the thymus for maturation; then most travel and reside in lymphoid tissues throughout the body. The natural killer cell is a third type of lymphocyte thought to be a differentiated form of the T lymphocyte. It is responsible for surveillance and destruction of virus-infected and malignant cells. T-cell functions include delayed hypersensitivity, graft rejection, graft versus host reaction, defense against intracellular organisms, and defense against neoplasms. Lymphocytes circulate in and out of tissues and may live days or years, depending on the type of lymphocyte (Hutchison & Davey, 2001).

IMMUNE ANATOMY

Immune activity involves an integrated, multilevel response against invading pathogens. It requires both WBCs of the hematopoietic system and the secondary hematopoietic organs, also termed the *lymphoreticular system.* The lymphoreticular system consists of lymphoid tissue, lymphatic channels and nodes, and phagocytic cells, which engulf and process foreign materials (see Figure 15-2).

The body's ability to resist and fight infection is termed *immunity.* Our bodies are constantly exposed to normal and unusual microorganisms that are capable of causing disease. The healthy person's immune system recognizes potential pathogens and destroys them before tissue invasion can occur; however, the person with a dysfunctional immune system is at risk of overwhelming, life-threatening infection.

IMMUNE PHYSIOLOGY

The immune response protects the body from disease by recognizing, processing, and destroying foreign invaders. It aids in the removal of damaged cells and defends the body against the proliferation of abnormal or malignant cells. To understand immune physiology, the critical care nurse should have a working knowledge of the key terms included in Table 15-1.

The recognition and destruction of nonself molecules called *antigens* are the key triggering activities of the immune system. Microorganisms (e.g., bacteria, viruses, fungi, and parasites), abnormal or mutated cells, transplanted cells, nonself protein molecules (e.g., vaccines), and nonhuman molecules (e.g., penicillin) can act as antigens. These antigens are detected by the body as foreign, or nonself, and are destroyed by immunological processes. The body's response to an antigen is determined by factors such as genetics, amount of antigen, and route of exposure (Rote, 2002a). In autoimmunity, the body abnormally sees self as nonself (i.e., it has no tolerance), and an immune response is activated against those tissues. Autoimmunity can result from injury to tissues, infection, or malignancy, although in many cases the cause is not known. An example of an autoimmune disease is systemic lupus erythematosus.

An intact and healthy immune system consists of both natural, or nonspecific, defenses and acquired, or specific, defenses. The nonspecific defenses are the first line of protection and include the processes of phagocytosis and inflammation. When nonspecific mechanisms fail to protect the body from invasion, the specific defenses of humoral and cellular immunity are put into action. *Active immunity* is a term used when the body actively produces cells and mediators that result in the destruction of the antigen. *Passive immunity* is that which is transferred from another person (e.g., maternal antibodies transferred to the newborn through the placenta and breast milk) (Rote, 2002a).

Nonspecific Defenses

The body's nonspecific defenses consist of the physical and chemical barriers to invasion, the protective and repairing processes of inflammation and phagocytosis, and other substances that stimulate the body to fight back. The body's first line of defense against infection consists of physical and chemical barriers.

Epithelial surfaces. The epithelial surfaces are those that are exposed to the environment. Intact skin and mucous membranes provide a protective covering; they also secrete substances that have antimicrobial effects. For example, sweat glands produce an antimicrobial enzyme, lysozyme, and sebaceous glands secrete sebum, which has antimicrobial and antifungal properties. The skin is also constantly exfoliating, a process that sloughs off bacterial and chemical hazards. These same epithelial surfaces are colonized by "normal" bacterial flora. These normal flora help to protect the body from microorganisms by occupying space on the epithelium, which prevents pathogen attachment.

Epithelial surfaces also have unique physical and chemical properties protecting them from pathogen invasion. For example, mucus and cilia work together to trap and remove harmful substances in the respiratory tract. The motility of the intestines maintains an even distribution of bacterial flora, thereby preventing overgrowth or invasion of pathogens, and promotes evacuation of harmful microbes. Chemical barriers to pathogenic entry include the unique pH of the skin and mucosa of the gastrointestinal and urinary tracts. This pH inhibits the growth of many microorganisms. Immunoglobulin A (IgA, also called *secretory IgA*) and phagocytic cells are biological factors present in respiratory and gastrointestinal secretions. They are essential for destruction of particular pyogenic bacteria (Rote, 2002a).

Inflammation and phagocytosis. The second line of defense involves the processes of inflammation and phagocytosis. Inflammation is initiated by cellular injury, is necessary for tissue repair, and is harmful when uncontrolled. When cellular injury occurs, a process called *chemotaxis* generates both a mediator and a neutrophil response. Mediator substances (histamine, serotonin, kinins, lysosomal enzymes, prostaglandin, platelet-activating factor, clotting factors, and complement proteins) are released at the site of injury. These mediators cause vasodilation, increase blood flow, induce capillary permeability, and promote chemotaxis and phagocytosis by neutrophils. Inflammatory symptoms such as redness, heat, pain, and swelling are sequelae of these responses. Complement proteins enhance the antibody activity, phagocytosis, and inflammation (Rote, 2002b).

Neutrophils are attracted to and migrate to areas of inflammation or bacterial invasion, where they ingest and kill invading microorganisms by phagocytosis. The inflammatory response is a rapid process initiated by granulocytes and macrophages, with granulocytes arriving within minutes of cellular injury (Casey, 2002). Once phagocytes have been attracted to an area by the release of mediators, a process called opsonization occurs, in which antibody and complement proteins attach to the target cell and enhance the phagocyte's ability to engulf the target cell. Once the bacteria have been engulfed, they are killed and digested within the cell by lysosomal enzymes. Exudate formation at the inflammatory site has three functions: to dilute toxins produced, to deliver proteins and leukocytes to the site, and to carry away toxins and debris (Rote, 2002b).

When infectious organisms escape the local phagocytic responses, they may be engulfed and destroyed in a similar fashion by the tissue macrophages within the lymphoreticular organs. The portal circulation of the spleen and liver filters the majority of blood, where infectious organisms can be removed before infecting the tissues. In the lymphatic system, pathogenic substances are filtered by the lymph nodes and are phagocytized by tissue macrophages. Here they may also stimulate immune responses by the lymphoid cells.

Other nonspecific defenses. Another nonspecific defensive activity is the release of cytokines from WBCs. Cytokines secreted by macrophages are known as monokines, whereas those secreted by lymphocytes are known as lymphokines. These substances, which include interleukins, tumor necrosis factor, colony-stimulating factors, and interferons, mediate various interactions between immune system cells (Rote, 2002a). Interleukin-1 is a monokine that increases body temperature in infection, thereby inhibiting the growth of temperature-sensitive pathogens. Interferons have antitumor and antiviral activity (Lewis & Weiner, 2003). Through recombinant DNA technology, interferons and other naturally occurring substances can be produced synthetically for the treatment of many disorders. Interferons and monoclonal antibodies are two biological therapies currently approved by the United States Food and Drug Administration for the treatment of certain malignant disorders (Lewis & Weiner, 2003).

Specific Defenses

Specificity refers to the finding that an immune response stimulates cells to develop immunity for a specific antigen. Two types of specific immune response exist: humoral immunity and cell-mediated immunity. They are not mutually exclusive but act together to provide immunity.

Humoral immunity. Humoral immunity is mediated by B lymphocytes and involves the formation of antibodies (immunoglobulins) in response to specific antigens that bind to their receptor sites. Antigen binding activates B-lymphocyte differentiation into plasma cells that produce specific antibodies in response to those antigens. Five classes of immunoglobulins exist: IgG, IgM, IgA, IgE, and IgD. For more detail about the clinical features and abnormalities associated with immunoglobulins, see Table 15-4 (Rote, 2002a).

Once antibodies have been synthesized and released, they bind to their specific antigen and form an antigen-antibody complex that activates phagocytosis and complement proteins. This humoral response is regulated by the activity of T lymphocytes. Helper T cells promote B-lymphocyte activity and the production of antibodies, whereas suppressor T cells downgrade the humoral response.

The body generates both primary and secondary humoral responses. In the primary response, antigens that have evaded the nonspecific defenses are engulfed and processed by macrophages. The macrophages then present the processed antigens to the lymphocytes, which proliferate, differentiate, and produce antibodies. In this first exposure, antibodies of the IgM subtype appear in the serum after 7 to 10 days, but by the peak of antibody levels at about 21 days, IgG is predominant. During this primary response, the cells develop an immunological memory for antigens that provides the basis for the secondary response on subsequent exposure.

When any subsequent exposure to the antigen occurs, a quicker, stronger, and longer-lasting IgG-mediated secondary response occurs. IgG antibodies peak within 7 to 10 days and may be detectable in the serum for years (Rote, 2002a).

Cell-mediated immunity. Cellular immunity is mediated by the T lymphocyte. Cell-mediated immunity is a more delayed reaction than the humoral

TABLE 15-4

Immunoglobulins

Antibody	Description	Normal Value
IgG	Most abundant immunoglobulin Major influence with bacterial disease Crosses the placenta Coats microorganisms to enhance phagocytosis Activates complement	75% of total 500-1600 mg/dL
IgM	Primary Ig response to antigen, with levels increased within 7 days of exposure Presents mostly in intravascular space Causes antigenic agglutination and cell lysis via complement activation	10% of total 60-280 mg/dL
IgA	Found on mucosal surfaces of respiratory, GI, and GU systems preventing antigen adherence Influential with bacteria and some viral organisms First antibody formed with exposure to antigen but rapidly diminishes as IgG increases Does not cross the placenta, but passes to newborn through colostrum and breast milk Deficiency caused by congenital autosomal dominant or recessive disease or related to anticonvulsant use Deficiency (< 5 mg/dL) manifests as chronic sinopulmonary infection	15% of total 90-450 mg/dL
IgD	Activates B lymphocytes to plasma cells, which are the key immunoglobulin-producing cells	1% of total 0.5-3 mg/dL
IgE	Attaches to mast cells and basophils on epithelial surfaces and enhances release of histamine and other vasoactive mediators responsible for the "wheal flare" reaction Important for allergic responses, inflammatory reactions, and parasitic infections	0.002% of total 0.01-0.04 mg/dL

GI, Gastrointestinal; *GU,* genitourinary.

response and can occur only when in direct contact with sensitized lymphocytes. It is important in viral, fungal, and intracellular infections and is the mechanism involved in transplant rejection and recognition of neoplastic cells.

Cell-mediated immunity is initiated by macrophage recognition of nonself foreign materials. The macrophages trap, process, and present such materials to T lymphocytes, which then migrate to the site of the antigen, where they complete antigen destruction. Once contact is made with a specific antigen, the T lymphocyte differentiates into helper/inducer T cells, suppressor T cells, and cytotoxic killer cells. Although these T cells are microscopically identical, they can be distinguished by proteins present on the cell surface called cluster of differentiation (CD) (Rote, 2002a). Helper T cells (also known as T4 cells because they carry a CD4 marker) enhance the humoral immune response by stimulating B cells to differentiate and produce antibodies. Suppressor T cells downgrade and suppress the humoral and cell-mediated responses. The ratio of helper to suppressor T cells is normally 2:1, and an alteration in this ratio may cause disease (Chernecky & Berger, 2004). For example, a depressed ratio (a decrease of helper T cells in relation to suppressor T cells) is found in acquired immunodeficiency syndrome (AIDS), whereas a higher ratio (a decrease in suppressor T cells in relation to helper T cells) is a feature of an autoimmune disease. Cytotoxic or killer T cells participate directly in the destruction of antigens by binding to and altering the intracellular environment, which ultimately destroys the cell. Killer cells also release cytotoxic substances into the antigen cell that cause cell lysis.

T cells additionally provide the body with immunosurveillance capabilities that monitor for abnormal cells or tissue. This mechanism is responsible for the rejection of transplanted tissue and the destruction of single malignant cells.

HEMOSTASIS

Hemostasis is a physiological process involving platelets, blood proteins (clotting factors), and the vasculature. This process involves the formation of blood clots to stop bleeding from injured vessels and natural anticoagulant and fibrinolytic systems to limit clot formation. Many substances are released during tissue destruction, including collagen, proteases, and bacterial endotoxins that may activate the clotting system. The three physiological mechanisms known to trigger clotting in the body are tissue injury, vessel injury, and the presence of a foreign body in the bloodstream. When one of these trigger factors is present, a series of physical events occurs that results in a fibrin clot. Although the events of hemostasis are sequential,

they require integration of components from the hematopoietic and coagulation systems. Within seconds after injury, platelets are attracted to the site and adhere to the site of injury. The activated platelets then undergo changes in shape to expose receptors on their surfaces. RBCs increase the rate of platelet adherence by facilitating migration of platelets to the site and by liberating adenosine diphosphate, which enables platelets to stick to the exposed tissue (collagen) (McCance, 2002). The exposed receptors on the activated platelet surfaces are capable of binding fibrinogen, an essential component underlying platelet aggregation (Miller, 2001). Serotonin and histamine are released by the adhered platelets and cause immediate constriction of the injured vessel to lessen bleeding. Vasoconstriction is followed by vasodilation, bringing the necessary cellular products of the inflammatory response to the site. With minor vessel injury, hemostasis is temporarily achieved with platelet plugs, usually within 3 to 5 minutes (McCance, 2002). The platelet plug is solidified with fibrin, an end product of the coagulation pathways. This process is shown in Figure 15-3.

Coagulation Pathway

The cascade theory of coagulation has been modified (Kroll, 2001; McCance, 2002; VanCott &

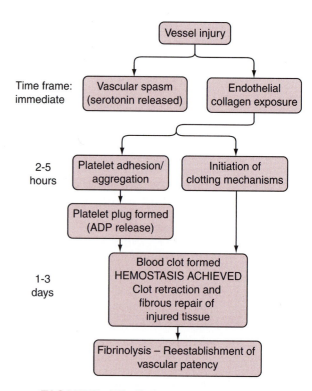

FIGURE 15-3 Coagulation physiology.

Laposata, 2001). The original theory described coagulation as occurring through two distinct pathways, intrinsic and extrinsic, which share a common "final" pathway, blood clot formation (Figure 15-4).

The cascade theory describes how both pathways begin with an initiating event and have a cascade sequence of clotting factor activation precipitated by a preceding reaction. The soluble clotting factors become insoluble fibrin. When blood is exposed to subendothelial collagen or is "injured," factor XII is activated, which initiates coagulation via the *intrinsic pathway*. In the *extrinsic pathway*, tissue injury

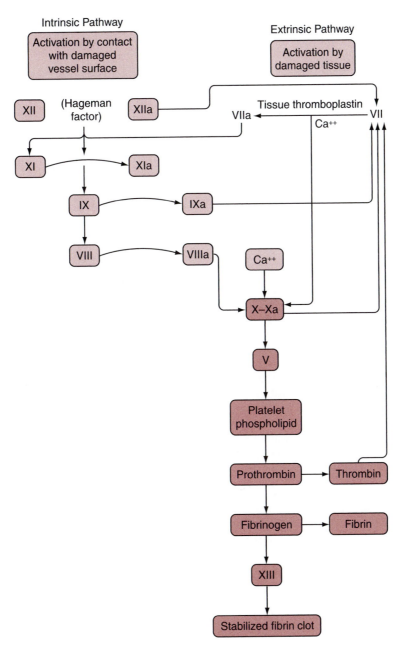

FIGURE 15-4 Coagulation cascade. (From McCance, K. L. [2002]. Structure and function of the hematological system. In K. L. McCance & S. E. Huether [eds.]. *Pathophysiology: The biologic basis for disease in adults and children. 4th ed.* [p. 834]. St. Louis: Mosby.)

precipitates release of a substance known as *tissue factor,* which activates factor VII. Factor VII is key in initiating blood coagulation. It is theorized that factor XI (activated by thrombin, generated in the extrinsic pathway) is what actually initiates the intrinsic pathway (Kroll, 2001; VanCott & Laposata, 2001). The coagulation factors are mostly plasma proteins that circulate as inactive enzymes.

Both theories (the original and the newly evolving) of coagulation pathways illustrate a final common pathway of clot formation, retraction, and fibrinolysis. Most coagulation factors are synthesized in the liver; therefore, liver disease can lead to problems with coagulation and bleeding. Vitamin K is necessary for synthesis of factors II, VII, IX, X, protein C, and protein S (anticoagulation factors); thus, a vitamin K deficiency can also lead to bleeding problems (Mansen & McCance, 2002b).

Coagulation Antagonists and Clot Lysis

Activation of the clotting factors, inhibition of these activated clotting factors, and production of circulating anticoagulant proteins maintain the balance of the coagulation processes. Normal vascular endothelium is smooth and intact, thereby preventing the collagen exposure that initiates the intrinsic clotting pathway. In addition, negatively charged proteins on the endothelium repel positively charged clotting factors. Rapid blood flow serves to dilute and disperse clotting factors. Clotting factors that are not contained within a formed clot are filtered and removed from circulation by the liver. Several plasma proteins, including antiplasmin and antithrombin III, are present to localize clotting at the site of injury. When coagulation protein levels are deficient, clotting may become inappropriately widespread, such as in disseminated intravascular coagulation (DIC). The most potent anticoagulant forces are the fibrin threads, which absorb 85% to 90% of thrombin during clot formation; and antithrombin III, which inactivates thrombin that is not contained within the clot. Heparin, which is produced in small quantities by basophils and tissue mast cells, acts as a potent anticoagulant. Heparin combines with antithrombin III to increase the effectiveness of the latter greatly. This complex removes several of the activated coagulation factors from the blood (McCance, 2002).

Once blood vessel integrity has been restored via hemostasis, blood flow must be reestablished. This goal is accomplished by the fibrinolytic system, by which clots are broken down (lysed) and removed. Fibrinolysis occurs 1 to 3 days after clot formation and is mediated by plasmin, an enzyme that digests fibrinogen and fibrin (Figure 15-5). The plasma protein, plasminogen, is the inactive form of plasmin. It is incorporated into the blood clot as the clot forms,

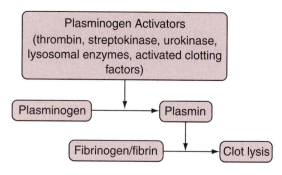

FIGURE 15-5 Fibrinolysis.

and it cannot initiate clot lysis until it is activated. Substances capable of activating plasminogen include thrombin, factor XII, lysosomal enzymes, urokinase (found in urine), and streptokinase (released from streptococcal bacteria).

Thrombin and plasmin are key for the balance between coagulation and lysis. Fibrinolysis is active within the microcirculation, where it maintains the patency of the capillary beds. Larger vessels contain less plasminogen activator, a characteristic that may predispose them to clot formation.

When plasmin digests fibrinogen, fragments known as fibrin split products, or fibrin degradation products, are produced and function as potent anticoagulants. In cases of excessive clotting and clot lysis, these fibrin split products contribute to the coagulopathy. Fibrin split products are not normally present in the circulation but are seen in some hematological disorders as well as with thrombolytic therapy.

Nursing Assessment of Hematological and Immunological Function

Critical care nurses' understanding of both normal and disrupted hematological and immunological system activities is paramount to good assessment skills and use of therapeutic interventions. Nursing assessment involves evaluation of risk factors for hematological and immunological alterations, assessment of the patient's complaints, performance of a focused physical examination, and interpretation of pertinent laboratory tests. Changes in the elderly are noted in the Geriatric Considerations (McCance, 2002).

PAST MEDICAL HISTORY

A complete health history includes a record of prior medical and surgical problems, allergies, medication or homeopathic remedies use, and family history. Important risk factors for hematological and immunological disorders are noted in Box 15-1.

Geriatric Considerations

Age-Related Changes	Implications
Decreased percentage of marrow space occupied by hematopoietic tissue	Ineffective erythropoiesis, especially after blood loss
Decreased number of T cells produced	Delayed hypersensitivity
Decreased T cell function	Increased incidence of infection
Appearance of autoimmune antibodies	Increased risk for autoimmune disorders
Increased IgA and decreased IgG levels	Increased prevalence of infection

EVALUATION OF PATIENT COMPLAINTS AND PHYSICAL EXAMINATION

During the physical examination, the nurse notes the patient's general appearance and assesses for signs of fatigue, acute illness, or chronic disease. The most common manifestations of either hematological or immunological disease include indicators of altered oxygenation, bleeding or clotting tendencies, and infection or accentuated immunological activity. The most important assessment parameters for detection of anemia, bleeding, and infection are shown in Table 15-5.

DIAGNOSTIC TESTS

Patients with hematological or immunological abnormalities can usually be diagnosed using the clinical profile in conjunction with a few key laboratory tests.

BOX 15-1

Risk Factors for Hematological and Immunological Problems*

HEMATOLOGICAL DISORDERS
Alcohol consumption, excess
Allergies
Anemia of any kind
Benzene exposure (gasoline, dry cleaning chemicals)
Blood clots
Delayed wound healing
Excess bleeding
Jaundice
Liver disease
Medications: allopurinol, antibiotics, anticoagulants, anticonvulsants, antidiabetics, antidysrhythmics, antiinflammatory agents, aspirin derivatives, chemotherapy, histamine blockers
Neoplastic disease
Pertinent surgical procedures: hepatic resection, partial or total gastric resection, splenectomy, tumor removal, valve replacement
Pesticide exposures
Previous blood or blood product transfusions
Poor nutrition
Radiation: occupational, environmental
Recurrent infection
Renal disease
Substance abuse

IMMUNOLOGICAL DISORDERS
Alcohol consumption, excess
Allergies
Anorexia
Bone tenderness
Delayed wound healing
Diabetes mellitus
Diarrhea
Fever
Joint pain
Liver disease
Lymphadenopathy
Medications: antibiotics, antiinflammatory agents, corticosteroids, chemotherapy, immunosuppressives
Nausea and vomiting
Neoplastic disease
Night sweats
Pertinent surgeries: hepatic resection, lung resection, partial or total small bowel resection, splenectomy, tumor removal
Pesticide exposure
Poor nutrition
Previous blood or blood product transfusions
Radiation: occupational, environmental
Recurrent infections
Renal disease
Sexual practices
Substance abuse
Weight loss

*A thorough history assessing for the foregoing clinical conditions may provide information suggesting predisposition to hematological or immunological disorders. This chart does not correlate specific risks with particular disease conditions, because many overlap or are not confirmed risk factors. History information should be supplemented with physical examination and laboratory test information.

TABLE 15-5

Physical Assessment for Heme-Immune Disorders

Body System	Anemia	Bleeding	Infection*
Neurological	Difficulty concentrating Dizziness Fatigue Somnolence Vertigo	*Bleeding into brain* (cerebrum, cerebellum): alteration in level of consciousness, focal deficits such as unequal pupils or motor movement, headache *Bleeding into potential spaces*	*Encephalitis:* confusion, lethargy, difficulty arousing, headache, visual difficulty/photosensitivity, nausea, hypertension *Meningitis:* lethargy and somnolence, confusion nuchal rigidity
Head/Neck	Headache Tinnitus	*Bleeding into eye:* visual disturbances, frank hemorrhagic conjunctiva, bloody tears *Bleeding into nasopharyngeal area:* nasal stuffiness, epistaxis *Oral bleeding:* petechiae of buccal mucosa or gums, hemorrhagic oral lesions *Bleeding into subcutaneous tissue of head or neck:* enlarged, bruised areas, racoon's eyes, bruising	*Conjunctivitis:* reddened conjunctiva, excess tearing of eye, puslike exudate from eye, blurred vision, swelling of eyelid, eye itching *Otitis media:* earache, difficulty hearing, itching inner ear, ear drainage *Sinusitis:* discolored nasal mucus, nasal congestion, face pain, eye pain, blurred vision *Oropharyngeal:* oral ulcerations or plaques, halitosis, reddened gums, abnormal papillae of the tongue, sore throat, difficulty swallowing *Lymphadenitis:* Swollen neck lymph glands, tender lymph glands, a lump left when patient swallows
Pulmonary	Air hunger Anxiety Dyspnea Tachypnea	*Alveolar bleeding:* crackles on breath sound assessment, alveolar fluid on x-ray, low oxygen saturation *Upper airway bleeding* (e.g., trachea or bronchi): hemoptysis *Pleural space bleeding:* decreased breath sounds, unequal chest excursion	*Bronchitis:* persistent cough, sputum production, gurgles in upper airways, wheezes in upper airways, hypoxemia and/or hypercapnia *Pneumonia:* chest discomfort pronounced with inspiration, persistent cough, sputum production, diminished breath sounds, crackles or gurgles, asymmetrical chest wall movement, labored breathing, nasal flaring with breathing, hypoxemia *Pleurisy:* chest discomfort pronounced with inspiration, sides of chest more painful, usually unilateral discomfort, splinting with deep breaths
Cardiovascular	Clubbing of digits Heart murmur Hypotension Nailbeds pale and slow capillary refill Peripheral pulses weak and thready Tachycardia	*Pericardial bleeding:* dyspnea, chest discomfort, hypotension, narrow pulse pressure, muffled heart sounds, increased jugular venous distention *Vascular bleeding:* visible blood, hematoma, or bruising of subcutaneous tissue	*Myocarditis:* dysrhythmias, murmurs or gallops, elevated jugular venous pulsations, weak thready pulses, hypotension, point of maximal impulse shifted laterally *Pericarditis:* constant, aching, discomfort in the chest unrelieved by rest or nitrates; pericardial rub; muffled heart sounds

Continued

TABLE 15-5

Physical Assessment for Heme-Immune Disorders—cont'd

Body System	Anemia	Bleeding	Infection*
Gastrointestinal	Abdominal pain Constipation Splenic enlargement, tenderness	*Upper GI bleeding:* hematemesis, vomiting (coffee ground appearance) *Lower GI bleeding:* melena *Hepatic or splenic rupture:* acute abdominal pain; abdominal distention, rapid onset hypotension with ↓ hematocrit and hemoglobin *Hemorrhagic pancreatitis:* acute abdominal pain, abdominal distention, hypotension with ↓ hematocrit and hemoglobin	*Gastritis:* nausea, vomiting within 30 min of eating, heme-positive emesis, gastric pain that is initially improved by eating *Infectious diarrhea:* greater than six loose stools per day, clay-colored stools, foul-smelling stools, abdominal cramping, or distention *Cholelithiasis/pancreatitis:* epigastric discomfort, intolerance to high-fat meal, clay-colored stools, nausea and vomiting, hyperglycemia, hypocalcemia, hypoalbuminemia, ↑ lipase and amylase *Hepatitis:* jaundice, right upper quadrant discomfort, hepatomegaly, elevated transaminases and bilirubin, fatty food intolerances, nausea and vomiting, diarrhea
Genitourinary		Bladder spasms with distended bladder Hematuria	*Urethritis:* painful urination, difficulty urinating, genitourinary itching *Cystitis:* small frequent urination, feeling of bladder fullness *Nephritis:* flank discomfort, oliguria, protein in urine *Vaginitis:* itching of vaginal area, vaginal discharge
Musculoskeletal	Muscle fatigue Muscle weakness	Altered joint mobility Painful joints Swollen joints; warm, painful, swollen muscles	*Arthritis:* joint discomfort, swollen and warm joints *Myositis:* aching muscles, weakness
Dermatological	Cyanosis Jaundice (hemolytic anemia) Pallor Poor skin turgor Skin cool to touch	Bleeding from line insertion sites, puncture wounds, skin tears Ecchymoses Petechiae	*Superficial skin infection:* rashes; itching; raised and/or discolored skin lesions; open-draining skin lesions; patterns are unique to specific microorganism *Cellulitis:* redness, warmth and swelling of subcutaneous tissue area, radiating pain from area toward middle of body
Hematological/ Immunological			*Bacteremia:* low diastolic blood pressure, headache, confusion, oliguria, ↓ bowel sounds, warmth, flushing, positive blood cultures

*Signs and symptoms presented in this chart are unique features of each process and do not include the common constitutional signs and symptoms seen with all infections such as fever, chills, malaise, leukocytosis, positive tissue culture for microorganisms, or increased erythrocyte sedimentation rate.
↑, Increased; ↓, decreased.

The most invasive microscopic examinations of the bone marrow or lymph nodes are reserved for circumstances when laboratory tests are inconclusive or when an abnormality in cellular maturation is suspected (e.g., aplastic anemia, leukemia, or lymphoma). The first screening diagnostic tests performed on patients who are at risk or exhibiting signs or symptoms of hematological or immunological dysfunction are a CBC with differential and a coagulation profile.

The CBC reveals the total RBC count and RBC indices, hematocrit, hemoglobin, WBC count and differential, platelet count, and cell morphologies. Depending on these findings and the patient's clinical presentation, further studies may be performed. A summary of common hematological diagnostic laboratory tests, with their normal values, and general implications of abnormal findings, is shown in Table 15-6 (RBCs and WBCs), and Table 15-7 (coagulation).

TABLE 15-6

Functions and Normal Values of Blood Cells

Test	Reason Evaluated	Normal Value	Alterations
RBCs			
Erythrocyte (red blood cell [RBC])	Respiration Oxygen transport Acid-base balance	5 million/µL	↑ Polycythemia, dehydration ↓ Anemia, fluid overload, hemorrhage
Mean corpuscular volume (MCV)	Average size of each RBC reflects maturity	82-98 μm^3	Immature cells such as in nutrition deficiency cause ↑; ↓ with iron deficiency
Mean corpuscular hemoglobin (MCH)	Average amount of hemoglobin in each RBC	26-34 pg	↓ With disorders of hemoglobin production
Mean corpuscular hemoglobin concentration (MCHC)	Average concentration of hemoglobin within a single RBC	31%-38%	↓ When cell has hemoglobin deficiency
Reticulocyte count	Immature RBCs released when sudden ↑ demand	1%-2% of total RBC count	↑ After recent blood loss or with chronic hemolysis
Serum folate	Amount of available vitamin for RBC development	95-500 mcg/mL	↓ In malnutrition or folic acid deficiency
Serum iron level	Iron stores within the body	40-160 mcg/dL	↓ When normal iron intake is inadequate or when there is inadequate absorption (e.g., gastric resection)
Total iron binding capacity (TIBC)	Reflection of liver function and nutrition	250-400 mcg/dL	↓ In chronic illness (infection, neoplasia, cirrhosis)
Ferritin level	Precursor to iron reflective of body's ability to create new iron stores	15-200 ng/mL	↓ Levels demonstrate inability to regenerate iron stores and hemoglobin
Transferrin level	Protein that binds to iron for removal or recirculation after RBCs are hemolyzed	200-400 mg/dL	↓ With excess hemolysis
Haptoglobin level	Protein that binds with heme for removal or recirculation after RBCs are hemolyzed	40-240 mg/dL	↓ With excess hemolysis

Continued

TABLE 15-6

Functions and Normal Values of Blood Cells—cont'd

Test	Reason Evaluated	Normal Value	Alterations
WBCs			
Leukocyte (WBC)	Inflammatory and immune responses Defend against infection, foreign tissue	4500-11,000/µL	↑ Inflammation, tissue necrosis, infection, hematologic malignancy ↓ Bone marrow depression (radiation, immune disorders), chronic disease
GRANULAR LEUKOCYTES			
Neutrophils	Polymorphonuclear neutrophils Phagocytosis of invading organisms	50%-70% of WBCs	↑ Inflammation, infection, surgery, myocardial infarction ↓ Aplastic anemia, hepatitis, some pharmacological agents
Eosinophils	Defend against parasites; detoxification of foreign proteins Phagocytosis	1%-5% of WBCs	↑ Allergic attacks, autoimmune diseases, parasitic infections, dermatologic conditions ↓ Stress reactions, severe infection
Basophils	Release heparin, serotonin, and histamine in allergic reactions; inflammatory response	0%-1% of WBCs	↑ Postsplenectomy, hemolytic anemia, radiation, hypothyroidism, leukemia, chronic hypersensitivity ↓ Stress reactions
NONGRANULAR LEUKOCYTES			
Monocytes	Mature into macrophages; phagocytosis of necrotic tissue, debris, foreign particles	1%-8% of WBCs	↑ Bacterial, parasitic, and some viral infections, chronic inflammation ↓ Stress reactions
Lymphocytes	Defend against microorganisms	20%-40% of WBCs	↑ Bacterial and viral infections, lymphocytic leukemia
B lymphocytes	Humoral immunity and production of antibodies		↓ Chemotherapy, immunodeficiencies, HIV disease, end-stage renal disease, immunosuppressive drugs
T Lymphocytes	Cell-mediated immunity		
PLATELETS			
Thrombocytes (platelets)	Blood clotting; hemostasis	150,000-400,000/µL	↑ Polycythemia vera, postsplenectomy, certain cancers ↓ Leukemia, bone marrow failure, disseminated intravascular coagulation, hemorrhage, hypersplenism, radiation exposure, large foreign bodies in blood (e.g., aortic balloon pump), hypothermia, hyperthermia, severe infection

↑, Increased; ↓, decreased; *HIV,* human immunodeficiency virus; *RBC,* red blood cell; *WBC,* white blood cell.

TABLE 15-7

Coagulation Profile Studies

Test	Normal Value	Comments
Lee-White clotting time	6-12 min	Nonspecific for clotting abnormalities
Activated partial thromboplastin time (APTT)	<35 sec	Used to monitor heparin therapy and detect bleeding tendencies, hemorrhagic disorders ↑ In anticoagulation therapy, liver disease, vitamin K deficiency, DIC
Prothrombin time (PT)	10-15 sec 1-1.2 INR	Evaluates extrinsic pathway; used to monitor oral anticoagulant therapy ↑ In warfarin sodium therapy, liver disease, vitamin K deficiency, obstructive jaundice
Thrombin time (TT)	9-13 sec	Used to detect fibrinogen abnormalities, monitor heparin therapy ↑ In fibrinogen abnormalities, multiple myeloma, cirrhosis of liver, heparin therapy
Fibrinogen level	150-400 mg/dL	↓ In DIC and fibrinogen disorders ↑ With acute infection, hepatitis or with oral contraceptive use
Fibrin degradation products (FDPs)	<10 mcg/mL	Evaluates hematologic disorders ↑ In DIC, fibrinolysis, thrombolytic therapy
Fibrin D-dimer	0-0.5 mcg/mL	Presence of D-dimer fragment of fibrinogen diagnostic for disseminated intravascular coagulation
Platelet count	150,000-400,000/µL	Measures number of circulating platelets ↓ In thrombocytopenia
Platelet aggregation test	3-5 min	Measures platelet adherence ability Prolonged in von Willebrand's disease, acute leukemia, idiopathic thrombocytopenic purpura, liver cirrhosis, aspirin use
Bleeding time	1-4 min	Evaluates platelet function ↑ In thrombocytopenia and aspirin therapy
Calcium	9-11 mg/dL	↓ With massive transfusions of stored blood

DIC, Disseminated intravascular coagulation; *Hgb*, hemoglobin; *INR*, international normalized ratio.

Selected Erythrocyte Disorders

Many pathological conditions affect the erythrocytes, ranging from mild anemias to life-threatening RBC lysis. A decrease in functional RBCs with a resulting oxygenation deficit is termed *anemia* and is a common problem experienced by critically ill patients. Polycythemia, a disorder in which the number of circulating RBCs is increased, is seen less often but can affect hypoxic patients (e.g., chronic obstructive pulmonary disease). It leads to increased blood viscosity and thrombotic complications.

ANEMIA
Pathophysiology

The term *anemia* refers to a reduction in the number of circulating RBCs or hemoglobin, which leads to inadequate oxygenation of tissues. Although symptoms may vary depending on the type, cause, or severity of anemia, the basic clinical findings are the same. As oxygenation delivery is decreased, tissues become hypoxic, and 2,3-DPG increases to cause hemoglobin to release oxygen. Blood flow is redistributed to areas where oxygenation is most vital, such as the brain, heart, and lungs. Anemia is described as mild, moderate, or severe, based on symptoms, irrespective of actual RBC serum values. Patients are able to adjust and compensate to lower RBC levels when the condition is chronic or slow in onset.

Anemia may be classified by its origin or by the microscopic appearance of the RBCs. Hematologists generally use the microscopic classifications (e.g., microcytic, hypochromic), but critical care nurses can best plan their nursing care by using the etiological classifications. Anemia may be caused by (1) blood loss (acute or chronic), (2) impaired production, (3) increased RBC destruction, or (4) combination of these. Iron deficiency anemia is the most common type of anemia. Symptoms begin gradually and initially may include fatigue, weakness, and shortness of breath (Mansen & McCance, 2002a). The types of anemia are described in Table 15-8.

Assessment and Clinical Manifestations

Symptoms of anemia are related to three physiological effects of reduced RBCs: (1) decreased circulating volume caused by loss of RBC mass, (2) decreased oxygenation of tissues resulting from reduced hemoglobin binding sites, and (3) compensatory mechanisms implemented by the body in its attempt to improve tissue oxygenation. Decreased circulating volume may be manifested by clinical findings reflective of low blood volume (e.g., low right atrial pressure) and the effects of gravity on the lack of volume (e.g., orthostasis). Inadequate oxygenation of the tissues will lead to organ dysfunction. Tissue hypoxia from inadequate oxygen delivery results in compensatory activities; the body shunts blood away from nonvital organs to perfuse the vital organs.

In addition to the general symptoms of anemia, unique disorders have their own classic clinical features. The patient with *aplastic anemia* may experience bruising, nosebleeds, petechiae, and decreased ability to fight infections. These effects result from thrombocytopenia and decreased WBC counts, which occur when the bone marrow fails to produce blood cells. Assessment of the patient with *hemolytic anemia* may reveal jaundice, abdominal pain, and enlargement of the spleen or liver. These findings result from the increased destruction of RBCs, their sequestration (abnormal distribution in the spleen and liver), and the accumulation of breakdown products. Patients with *sickle cell anemia* may have joint swelling or pain and delayed physical and sexual development. In crisis, the sickle cell patient often has decreased urine output, peripheral edema and signs of uremia because the renal tissue perfusion is impaired as a result of sluggish blood flow.

Laboratory findings in anemia include decreased RBC count, hemoglobin, and hematocrit levels. The reticulocyte count is usually increased, indicating a compensatory increased RBC production with release of immature cells. Patients with hemolytic anemia also have an increased bilirubin level. In sickle cell disease, a stained blood smear reveals sickled cells. In aplastic anemia, the reticulocyte, platelet, and RBC and WBC counts are decreased because the marrow fails to produce any cells.

Nursing Diagnoses

Nursing diagnoses of the anemic patient may include the following:

- Decreased cardiac output related to decreased circulating blood volume
- Altered tissue perfusion related to decreased or dysfunctional RBCs or hemoglobin
- Impaired gas exchange related to decreased or dysfunctional RBCs or hemoglobin
- Risk for fluid volume excess or deficit related to fluid replacement or hemorrhage
- Impaired skin integrity related to inadequate perfusion and tissue hypoxia
- Pain related to tissue ischemia and microvascular occlusion
- Risk for infection related to bone marrow failure and low WBC count
- Risk for injury related to transfusions
- Activity intolerance related to tissue hypoxia

Medical Interventions

Medical treatment of anemia includes identification and removal of causative agents or conditions, supplemental oxygen, blood component therapy, and cardiovascular system support. In blood loss anemia, initial treatment is restoration of blood volume with intravenous administration of volume expanders (colloid and crystalloid substances). Dextrans, mannitol, and albumin are examples of colloids, whereas normal saline, Ringer's solution, and lactated Ringer's solution are examples of crystalloid solutions. Erythropoietin products are available for use for stimulation of RBC production (Gillespie, 2003; Rudnicke, 2003). For certain types of anemia, cause-specific interventions may be indicated. Splenectomy may be performed for hemolytic anemia, and bone marrow transplantation may be preferred for refractory aplastic anemia. In sickle cell disease, oxygenation and correction of dehydration are important for the prevention or reversal of erythrocyte sickling. Therapies currently being researched include the use of several different hemoglobin and platelet alternatives (Rudnicke, 2003).

Text continued on page 514

TABLE 15-8

Anemias

	Marrow Failure to Produce RBCs / Aplastic Anemia	Hemolytic Anemia	Sickle Cell Anemia (Hemolytic Subtype)	Vitamin B_{12} Deficiency	Folic Acid Deficiency	Iron Deficiency
Pathophysiology	Disorder or bone marrow toxin damages the erythrocyte precursors, leading to ↓ RBC production	Stimulus causes extrasplenic destruction of the RBC, leading to hemolyzed RBC fragments in the circulating bloodstream; cell fragments ↑ blood viscosity and slow blood flow, leading to ischemia and/or infarction Extrasplenic hemolysis also leads to ↑ levels of circulating bilirubin, and unbound iron	Presence of abnormal hemoglobin causes RBCs to assume a sickle or crescent shape if ↓ oxygen, ↓ pH, or ↑ 2,3-DPG level Sickling alters the blood viscosity, leading to microvascular occlusion; sickling crisis can be life-threatening because vascular occlusion leads to continued hypoxia, exacerbation of sickling, thrombosis, and infarction in tissues and organs	Pernicious anemia is caused by decreased gastric production of HCl and intrinsic factor that play a role in vitamin B_{12} absorption	Malabsorption of dietary folic acid resulting from the lack of intake or absorption	Body's iron stores inadequate for RBC development; Hgb-deficient RBCs result
Etiology	*Disorders:* Bone metastases *Drugs:* Chemotherapy agents Antiretrovirals: reverse transcriptase inhibitors	*Disorders:* Immune suppression Postorthotopic liver transplant status Pregnancy Vitamin B_{12} deficiency Viral infection: EBV, CMV	*Abnormal RBC membrane or hemoglobin:* Anemia of liver or renal disease Hereditary RBC shape disorders Paroxysmal nocturnal hemoglobinuria Hereditary hemolytic anemia caused by abnormal amount of hemoglobin S in relation to hemoglobin A	Familial incidence related to autoimmune response with gastric mucosal atrophy Higher incidence in autoimmune disorders; SLE,	Common in infants, adolescents, pregnant and lactating women, alcoholic patients, older adults, cancer, intestinal disease	10%-30% of all American adults; primarily from dietary deficiency Also in pregnant and lactating women, infants,

Toxic Exposures: Radiation to long bones	Drugs: Anticonvulsants Antidysrhythmics Antiinflammatory agents Chloramphenicol Quinines Toxic exposures: Benzene Arsenic Herbicides/ Insecticides Lacquers Paint thinners Radiation exposure Toluene (glue)	Porphyria Sickle cell disease G6PD deficiency Thalassemias Immune reaction: Autoimmune hemolytic syndrome: BMT Hemolytic transfusion reaction Autoimmune diseases Physical damage to RBC: Blunt trauma Extracorporeal circulation Prosthetic heart valves Thermal injury Unknown: Diabetes mellitus IgA deficiency Illicit drug stimulants: cocaine Ovarian cyst Snake or spider bite	myxedema, Graves' disease Common in Northern Europeans; rare in children, black and Asian populations Occurs postoperatively with gastric surgery	(jejunitis, small bowel resection), prolonged anticonvulsants and estrogens, excessive cooking of foods	adolescents Malabsorption such as diarrhea, gastric resection, blood loss, or intravascular hemolysis
Clinical Presentation ↓ Production of cells in the earliest phase: bone marrow resulting in low RBC count	Symptoms of infection, bleeding, and anemia occur simultaneously, although earliest	Rapid hemolysis of RBCs leads to spleen uptake with enlarged and tender spleen; metabolism of RBCs often	Hyperviscosity and poor perfusion (e.g., altered mentation, hypoxemia, abdominal cramping); sickled	Inhibited growth of all cells: anemia, leukopenia, thrombocytopenia	Similar to vitamin B_{12} deficiency but without neurological symptoms

Classic: "pica" (desire to eat nonfood items), ice or dirt cravings Symptoms of

Continued

TABLE 15-8

Anemias—cont'd

	Marrow Failure to Produce RBCs	Aplastic Anemia	Hemolytic Anemia	Sickle Cell Anemia (Hemolytic Subtype)	Vitamin B₁₂ Deficiency	Folic Acid Deficiency	Iron Deficiency
	Signs and symptoms are those common in profound anemia	symptoms are usually the result of early WBC dysfunction Platelet production abnormalities lead to bleeding symptoms within 7-10 days followed by symptoms of anemia	leads to excess bilirubin with jaundice and itching	cells removed from circulation, causing enlarged and tender spleen; long-term sickling and thrombosis causes ↓ joint mobility, gut dysfunction, cardiac failure, and potentially stroke	Demyelination of peripheral nerves to spinal cord Triad: weakness, sore tongue, paresthesias	Signs: poor oxygenation, dizziness, irritability, dyspnea, pallor, headache, oral ulcers, tachycardia	cardiovascular/respiratory compromise: hypoxia, fatigue, headache, cracks in mouth corners, smooth tongue, paresthesias, neuralgias
Diagnostic Tests	CBC used as screening test Bone marrow aspiration and biopsy can confirm maturation failure	CBC used as screening test Bone marrow aspiration and biopsy reflect absence of precursor or stem cells	Reticulocytes usually ≥4% total RBC count ↑ Total bilirubin ↑ Direct bilirubin ↓ Transferrin ↓ Haptoglobin	Hemoglobin electrophoresis abnormality	Schilling test ↓ Hgb and RBC ↑ MCV ↓ MCHC ↓ WBC ↓ platelets ↑ LDH	Macrocytosis Serum folate <4 mg/dL Abnormal platelet appearance ↑ Reticulocyte count	↓ Hct and Hgb ↓ Iron level with ↑ binding capacity ↓ Ferritin level ↓ RBC with hypochromia and microcytes ↓MCHC
Management	Erythropoietin per dosing guidelines (Procrit, Aranesp)	Eliminate cause Bone marrow stimulants may be tried early Corticosteroids	Staphylococcal protein A is capable of trapping IgG complexes that are	Administer large volumes of IV fluids to dilute viscous blood Oxygen therapy	Vitamin B₁₂ 30 mcg IM or deep subcutan for 5-10 days then 100-	Folic acid 0.25-1 mg/day PO	Ferrous sulfate 325 mg PO tid and ascorbic acid

Nursing Implications	Monitor diet and medications that may interfere with marrow production of cells	Immunosuppressive agents if suspected autoimmune process Chelating (iron binding) agents Limit transfusions when possible to ↓ risk of rejection if later perform transplant Allogenic BMT	thought to cause RBC autoantibodies If autoantibodies are present, give immunosuppressive agents Administer antiplatelet medications (e.g., salicylic acid)	reduces sickling Treat infections early with fluids and antibiotics Sickling causes extreme pain (result of ischemia) and most acute episodes require narcotics Gene transplants used experimentally	200 mcg IM or deep subcutan q mo	to aid absorption Iron replacement
	High risk of infection and bleeding: implement preventive strategies and aggressively manage early problems Administer transfusions cautiously, because they ↑ exposure to antigens that may enhance rejection if BMT is required later	*Administration guidelines:* Begin plasma reinfusion at a rate of 25 mL/hr for 15 minutes, then ↑ to 100 mL/hr *Nursing care:* Assess for hypersensitivity Assess for fluid shifts into the interstitial spaces during infusion or within 6-12 hr after infusion Monitor for vomiting, pain at infusion site, diarrhea	Disorder currently incurable, although severity seems to remain consistent throughout lifetime Children who do not have pain managed effectively can develop maladaptive coping Life expectancy has been prolonged as a result of more effective supportive care Common cause of death for these patients is intracranial thrombosis or hemorrhage	Lifetime treatment requires ongoing patient teaching Heart failure prevention Special oral hygiene Monitor for persistent neurological deficits	Foods high in folic acid: beef, liver, peanut butter, red beans, oatmeal, asparagus, broccoli	Monitor for allergic reactions to iron, give oral supplements with straw so not to stain teeth; causes skin irritation and iron deposits

↑, Increased; ↓, decreased; *BMT*, bone marrow transplant; *CMV*, cytomegalovirus; *2,3-DPG*, 2-3, diphosphoglyerate; *EBV*, Epstein-Barr virus; *G6PD*, glucose-6-phosphate dehydrogenase; *Hct*, Hematocrit; *Hgb*, hemoglobin; *LDH*, lactate dehydrogenase; *MCHC*, mean corpuscular hemoglobin concentration; *MCV*, mean corpuscular volume; *RBC*, red blood cell; *SLE*, systemic lupus erythematosus.

Nursing Interventions

Nursing management of anemia is based on a continuous, thorough nursing assessment and the prescribed medical treatment. Physical assessment is vital; monitoring of vital signs, the electrocardiogram, hemodynamics, heart and lung sounds, and peripheral pulses assists the nurse in the assessment of tissue perfusion and gas exchange. Tachycardia and orthostatic hypotension are important signs that indicate that the patient's cardiovascular system is not adequately compensating for the anemia. Mental status, urine output, and skin color or temperature are important general indicators of tissue perfusion. Pain management and comfort measures are instituted as needed. Scrupulous skin care is given to prevent tissue breakdown, and the patient is monitored closely for signs of infection. For patients at risk of further blood loss, bleeding precautions are instituted. Interventions for patients at risk of bleeding or infection are listed later in this chapter.

Laboratory results, such as the CBC, are carefully monitored. Other vital nursing interventions include the following: promotion of rest and oxygen conservation; careful administration of blood components, drug therapy, and intravenous fluids; and monitoring of the patient's responses to the therapy.

Patient Outcomes

The following are the goals of care for the patient with anemia:
- Optimal tissue perfusion, oxygenation, and gas exchange will be maintained, as evidenced by the patient's response to treatment (e.g., normal vital signs, hemodynamics, mental status, organ function, and ability to tolerate activity).
- The CBC will reflect an adequate RBC and hemoglobin count.
- The patient will have adequate hydration and absence of transfusion reaction, pain, and infection.

White Blood Cell and Immune Disorders

Many pathological conditions can be classified as WBC or immune disorders. They may involve the WBCs themselves or other complementary immune processes. The immune system can fail to develop properly, can lose its previous ability to react to invasion by pathogens, can overreact to otherwise harmless antigens, or can turn immune functions against self. Regardless of the cause, WBC and immune disorders or their treatments suppress the mechanisms needed for inflammation and combating infection. Because the clinical features and complications are similar among a variety of disorders, this first section addresses general causes, signs and symptoms, and management of immunological suppression. This is followed by in-depth descriptions of specific WBC and immune disorders.

THE IMMUNOCOMPROMISED PATIENT
Pathophysiology

The immunocompromised patient is one with defined quantitative or qualitative defects in WBCs or immune physiology. The defect may be congenital or acquired and may involve a single element or multiple processes. Regardless of the cause, the physiological outcome is immune incompetence, with lack of normal inflammatory, phagocytic, antibody, or cytokine responses. Immune incompetence is often asymptomatic until pathogenic organisms invade the body and create infection. Infection is the leading cause of death in the immunocompromised patient.

Assessment and Clinical Manifestations

The nursing diagnosis "risk for infection" is frequently documented in critically ill patients, and is the primary clinical problem for those with immune compromise. A detailed database containing the patient's history, physical examination findings, and laboratory studies is paramount for rapid detection of infection.

Immunocompromise in the critically ill is caused by many factors. In addition to existing immunodeficiency diseases and life-threatening illness, immune defenses are altered by invasive procedures, inadequate nutrition, and the presence of opportunistic pathogens. Many of the drugs and treatments administered in critical care can also depress the patient's immune system. The patient's medical and social history, current medications, and risk factors for infection are evaluated. Risk factors for immune compromise are described in Table 15-9. Immunosuppressed patients do not respond to infection with typical signs and symptoms of inflammation (see Clinical Alert).

Laboratory diagnostic tests such as leukopenia, low CD4 counts, and decreased immunoglobulin levels may demonstrate disorders of immune components. A common test of the humoral (antibody) response to antigens is a skin test with intradermal injection of typical pathogens capable of initiating an antibody response. Absence of a "wheal" tissue response to the antigens (called tissue anergy) is evidence of altered antibody capabilities.

Nursing Diagnoses

The patient with compromised immune system function is most likely to have one of the following nursing diagnoses:
- Risk for infection
- Hyperthermia
- Altered protection

TABLE 15-9

Risk Factors for Infections in the Immunocompromised Patient

Patient Characteristics	Physiological Mechanism of Risk of Infection
HOST CHARACTERISTICS	
Alcoholism	↓ Neutrophil activity
	Hepatic/splenic congestion also slows phagocytic response
Abuse of intravenous drugs	Chronic altered barrier defense leads to reduced WBCs and slowed phagocytic responses
	Constant viral exposure may also alter T-cell function
Older adults	Slowed phagocytosis: ↑ bacterial infection, more rapid dissemination of infection
	Slowed macrophage activity—more fungal infection, more visceral infection
	Atrophy of thymus: ↑ risk of viral illness
	↓ Antigen-specific immunoglobins: diminished immune memory
Frequent hospitalizations	Frequent exposure to environmental organisms other than own normal flora
	Potential exposure to resistant organisms
	Potential exposure to other people's organisms via equipment, supplies, transport, person-to-person exposure
Malnutrition	Inadequate WBC count: infection
	↓ Neutrophil activity: bacterial infection, at risk of infection dissemination
	Impaired phagocytic function: bacterial infection
	Impaired integumentary/mucosal barrier: general infection risk
	↓ Macrophage mobilization: ↑ risk of fungal or rapidly disseminating infection
	↓ Lymphocyte function: ↑ risk of viral and opportunistic infection
	Thymus and lymph node atrophy with iron deficiency
Stress	Induces ↑ release of adrenal hormones (cortisol), which causes ↓ circulating eosinophils and lymphocytes
IMMUNE DEFECTS AND DISORDERS	
Lymphopenia	↓ Antibody response to previous exposed antigens
	↓ Recognition and destruction of viral and opportunistic organisms
Macrophage dysfunction/destruction	Altered response to fungi
	Inadequate antigen-antibody response
	Greater potential for visceral infection
Neutropenia	Inadequate neutrophils to combat pathogens (especially bacterial)
Splenectomy	Inability to recognize and remove encapsulated bacteria (e.g., streptococcus)
	Compromised reticuloendothelial system and ↓ antibodies lead to frequent and early bacteremia
DISEASE PROCESSES	
Burns	Altered barrier defenses allowing pathogen entry
	Physiological stressor thought to ↓ phagocytic responses
	Protein loss through skin leads to malnutrition-related immunocompromise
Cancer	Structural disruption may lead to bone marrow or lymphatic abnormalities
	Certain cancers have specific immune defects (e.g., diminished phagocytic activity or T-cell defects)
	Radiation therapy destroys lymphocytes and causes shrinkage of lymphoid tissue
	Chemotherapy causes ↓ lymphocytes and alters the proliferation and differentiation of stem cells
Cardiovascular disease	Inadequate tissue perfusion slows WBC response to tissue with pathogenic organism

Continued

TABLE 15-9

Risk Factors for Infections in the Immunocompromised Patient—cont'd

Patient Characteristics	Physiological Mechanism of Risk of Infection
Diabetes mellitus	↓ Numbers of neutrophils
	Hyperglycemia causes ↓ phagocytic activity and immunoglobin defects
	Vascular insufficiency leads to slowed phagocytic response to pathogens
	Neuropathy and glycosuria predisposes person to ↓ bladder emptying and urinary tract infections
Gastrointestinal disease	↓ Bowel motility allows normal flora to translocate across the gastrointestinal wall to the bloodstream
Hepatic disease	↓ Neutrophil count
Infectious diseases	↓ Phagocytic activity
	Hypermetabolism with infection accelerates phagocytic cell use and death
	Certain viral and opportunistic infections ↓ bone marrow production of WBCs
Pulmonary disease	Inadequate oxygenation suppresses neutrophil activity
Renal disease	↓ Neutrophil activity caused by uremic toxins
	↓ Immunoglobulin activity
Traumatic injuries	Altered barrier defenses allowing pathogen entry
	Type of infection dependent on source and severity of injury (e.g., soil contamination, water contamination, skin flora)
MEDICATION/TREATMENT	
Antibiotics	Normal flora destroyed and enhanced resistant organism growth, fungal superinfection
Immunosuppressive agents and corticosteroids	↓ Phagocytic activity
	Altered T-cell recognition of pathogens, especially viral
	↓ Interleukin-2 production leads to increased risk of malignancy
	↓ IgG production
	Lack of immune memory to recall antibodies to previously encountered pathogens
Invasive devices	Altered barrier defenses allowing pathogen entry, especially skin organisms
Surgical procedures/wounds	Normal flora may be translocated by surgical procedure
	Altered barrier defenses caused by surgical entry
	Stress of surgery and anesthetic agents reduce neutrophil activity
Transfusion of blood products	Risk of transfusion-transmitted infections undetected by donor screening: cytomegalovirus, hepatitis, human immunodeficiency virus
	Exposure to foreign antigens in blood products causes T-lymphocytic immune suppression and increases risk of infection

↑, Increased; ↓, decreased; *WBC,* white blood cell.

CLINICAL ALERT: INFECTION IN IMMUNOCOMPROMISED PATIENTS

Immunocompromised patients do not have typical signs and symptoms of infection.
- Erythema, swelling, and exudate formation are usually not evident.
- Symptoms of infection may be absent, masked, or present atypically.
- Fever is considered the cardinal and sometimes only symptom of infection.
- Patients are also more likely to describe pain at the site of infection, although physical inflammatory signs may be absent.

Medical Interventions

Primary medical therapy is directed at reversing the cause of the immune dysfunction and preventing infectious complications. In primary immunodeficiencies, B-cell and T-cell defects are treated with specific replacement therapy or bone marrow transplantation. IgG blood levels of less than 300 mg/dL warrant immunoglobin infusion. Gene replacement therapy may soon be a realistic curative treatment option for some disorders. In secondary immunodeficiencies, the underlying causative condition is treated. For example, malnutrition is corrected, doses of immunosuppressive medications are reduced or stopped, and infections are treated.

Additional risk factors for infection are carefully monitored and avoided when possible. Invasive lines pose the most common risk for iatrogenic infection; lines should be kept to a minimum and managed with meticulous sterile technique. Studies of catheters impregnated with antimicrobials or heavy metals have shown mixed success at reducing infection rates. Invasive device factors known to increase the risk of infection include (1) large lumen size, (2) multiple lumina, (3) placement after onset of immune compromise, and (4) inconsistent management techniques.

Administration of prophylactic antimicrobial agents during the period of highest risk of infection is also a common practice. For example, patients receiving bone marrow–suppressing cancer chemotherapy can receive broad-spectrum antimicrobials during the time of their lowest WBC count. Patients who have human immunodeficiency virus (HIV) infection or are recovering from organ transplantation have defined CD4 or immune suppression levels that place them at risk of specific infections. Depending on predetermined criteria, these patients can receive antimicrobial prophylaxis against infections with herpes simplex, *Candida albicans, Pneumocystis carinii, Mycobacterium avium-intracellulare, Mycobacterium tuberculosis,* and cytomegalovirus.

Nursing Interventions

Nursing interventions focus on protecting the patient from infection. It has been proposed that a protective environment could reduce risk of infection. Research studies support the use of high-efficiency particulate air (HEPA) filtration of air and laminar air flow in single-patient rooms for prevention of infection with airborne microorganisms. Comparative studies of isolation precautions and careful infection control practices, such as hand-washing with an antimicrobial soap, do not demonstrate any added advantage to isolation techniques.

Nurses should diligently ensure adequate hygiene measures that include general bathing with antimicrobial soaps, oral care, and perineal care. Nursing staff members play an important role in limiting breaks in skin integrity and ensuring sterile technique when procedures are unavoidable.

The patient's diet should not include raw fruits or vegetables because they harbor bacteria. Fresh plants and flowers are not allowed in the patient's room because the standing water or soil also contains harmful bacteria. General health promotion of adequate fluid, nutrition, and sleep are also important in bolstering the patient's defenses against infection. For a more comprehensive list of nursing interventions, consult the Nursing Care Plan for the Immunocompromised Patient.

Patient Outcomes

Patients with compromised immune function will experience optimal outcomes when the following objectives are achieved:

- Fever is absent.
- Wound, orifice, blood, and exudate cultures are negative.
- Laboratory tests show normalized WBC count, immunoglobulin levels, and tissue anergy.
- The patient and family members verbalize methods of controlling infection risks within the environment and their personal care routines.

NEUTROPENIA

Pathophysiology

Neutropenia is generally defined as an absolute neutrophil count (ANC) less than 1500 cells/μL of blood. Neutropenia is further classified into mild (1000-1500 cells/μL), moderate (500-1000 cells/μL), and severe (fewer than 500 cells/μL); predictive of the patient's infection risk (Shelton & Soloman, 2000). Neutropenia may occur as a result of inadequate production or excess destruction. Patients with low neutrophil counts are predisposed to infections because of the body's reduced phagocytic ability. In studies of infections in neutropenic versus nonneutropenic patients with cancer, those with neutropenia had double the incidence of sepsis and a higher mortality rate.

Assessment and Clinical Manifestations

The nurse must obtain a thorough medical and social history to identify risk factors for neutropenia. Common causes include acute or overwhelming infections, radiation, exposure to chemicals and drugs, or other disease states (Box 15-2).

Nursing Care Plan for the Immunocompromised Patient

NURSING DIAGNOSIS: *Risk for infection related to immunocompromise or immunosuppression, invasive procedures, presence of opportunistic pathogens*

Patient Outcomes	Interventions	Rationales
Patient will remain free of infection, as evidenced by absence of fever, redness, swelling, pain, and heat; WBC and differential, urinalysis, and cultures within normal limits; chest x-ray study without infiltrates, absence of adventitious breath sounds	Establish baseline assessment with documented history, physical examination, and laboratory study results.	Baseline enables one to determine trends.
	Follow universal precautions.	
	Plan nurses' assignments to reduce the possibility of infection spread between patients.	Prevent spread of infection.
	Be particularly careful handling secretions/excretions that are known to be infected (e.g., use different washcloth for rectal and urinary areas).	Prevent cross-contamination.
	Monitor visitors for any recent history of communicable diseases.	Prevent infection.
	Clean all multipurpose equipment (e.g., oximeter probes, noninvasive BP cuffs, bed scale slings, electronic thermometers) between patient use.	Prevent cross-contamination.
	Assess patient for signs/symptoms of infection.	
	Monitor vital signs with temperature at least every 4 hr; any elevation in temperature is reported and investigated.	Rectal temperatures are not recommended.
	Monitor laboratory results: WBC and differential, blood, urine, sputum, wound, and throat cultures; report abnormal results.	Assess for infection.
	Note the presence of chills, tachycardia, oliguria, or altered mentation that may indicate sepsis; report subtle changes to physician	Assess for infection.
	Use strict hand-washing procedure before, during, and after each patient contact.	Prevent spread of infection.
	Promote optimal hydration and nutrition.	
	Encourage incentive spirometry, changes of position every 1-2 hr.	Prevent atelectasis.
	Avoid breaks in the skin and mucous membrane integrity, change position every 2 hr, avoid wetness, provide skin lubricants, provide meticulous oral and bathing hygiene.	Maintain intact skin—the first line of defense.
	Use strict aseptic technique for dressing changes, performing with frequency defined by institutional standards for immunocompromised patients.	
	Change IV tubings every 96 hr.	
	Avoid stopcocks in IV systems, used closed injection site systems.	Stopcocks can harbor bacteria and are a source of entry for any infectious agent.
	Limit invasive devices/procedures when possible.	
	Use private room, limit visitors, limit fresh flowers and standing water, provide cooked or well-washed fruits or vegetables, avoid food cooked in uncontrolled environment.	Fresh flowers and raw fruits or vegetables have a potential to introduce pathogenic organisms.

Nursing Care Plan for the Immunocompromised Patient—cont'd

Patient Outcomes	Interventions	Rationales
	Ensure that sleep needs are being met.	To enhance resistance to infection and aid in healing.
	Control glucose levels, so that unintentional hyperglycemia does not occur	Hyperglycemia compromises phagocytic activities that fight infection).
	If construction is occurring, consider applying a mask on the patient during intrahospital transport; if HEPA filtration or other airflow protection is provided to the patient while in the unit and building air systems are old, masks may be considered for transport of these patients.	Prevent patient exposure.
	Consider closed endotracheal tube suction systems.	
	Change oxygen setups with humidification (e.g., nasal cannula) every 24 hr.	Prevent bacterial growth.
	For first fever (38.0°C two times 4 hr apart or any three consecutive times) or new fever (38.3°C after 72 hr on an antimicrobial regimen), perform cultures:	To determine site of infections and pathogens.
	Blood cultures from two different sites	
	Blood cultures from existing venous/arterial access devices	
	Urine culture	
	Sputum culture if obtainable	
	Stool culture if obtainable	
	Culture any open lesions or wounds: also consider any oral lesions.	
	Administer antimicrobial therapy as ordered.	
	Perform antimicrobial peak and trough levels as ordered; be certain that the exact time of last medication is listed in order to calculate levels accurately.	To determine effectiveness of antibiotics.
	Be alert to superinfection with fungal flora any time 7-10 days after initiation of broad-spectrum antibiotics; prophylaxis (e.g., oral nystatin or topical nystatin powder) may be started in some patients.	

NURSING DIAGNOSIS: *Risk for impaired skin integrity and altered oral mucous membranes related to immobility, invasive devices and procedures, dehydration, malnutrition, immunosuppression*

Patient Outcomes	Interventions	Rationales
Patient's skin and mucous membranes will remain intact; will be absent of signs of pressure areas, breakdown, lesions, excoriation; skin turgor and moisture of	Assess skin and mucous membranes every shift for signs of pressure, breakdown, lesions, and excoriation.	
	Monitor incisions, IV and venipuncture sites, axillae, perineal areas for redness, swelling, pain, heat.	These signs of infection may not be obvious.

Continued

Nursing Care Plan for the Immunocompromised Patient—cont'd

mucous membranes will remain adequate; patient will remain free of signs of infection	Provide meticulous skin care; keep skin clean, dry, and lubricated.	Prevent infection.
	Provide frequent mouth care with nonirritating solutions and soft-bristled brush.	Maintain moisture of mucous membranes.
	Turn/reposition the patient at least every 2 hr; evaluate need for therapeutic beds/mattresses.	Prevent skin breakdown.
	Treat any pressure ulcers or areas of breakdown promptly; provide protection from further damage.	
	Consider consultation to skin care specialist if the patient is at high risk of skin breakdown.	
	Maintain adequate hydration and optimal nutritional status.	

NURSING DIAGNOSIS: *Altered nutrition (less than body requirements) related to NPO status, anorexia, nausea/vomiting, painful oral mucosa*

Patient Outcomes	Interventions	Rationales
Patient will maintain optimal nutritional status, as evidenced by adequate caloric and protein intake; ideal/stable body weight; laboratory values will remain within normal limits (total protein, serum albumin, electrolytes, hemoglobin, and hematocrit)	Assess baseline nutritional status: height and weight, laboratory values; presence of weakness, fatigue, infection, or other signs of malnutrition.	To obtain baseline assessment.
	Obtain dietary consult to determine nutrients/intake required. Assess need for enteral/parenteral nutritional therapy; administer as ordered and observe response.	To optimize therapy especially if the patient is at high risk of complications.
	Establish food preferences.	
	Determine deterrents to adequate intake: fasting (NPO) status, presence of anorexia, nausea, vomiting, stomatitis.	
	Monitor daily weight, laboratory values, protein and caloric intake, I & O. Schedule weights for the same time every day.	Monitor status.
	Encourage small, frequent, high-calorie and high-protein meals.	
	Provide meticulous mouth care before and after meals.	
	Encourage meals from home/significant others and relaxed atmosphere/socialization during meals.	
	Administer antiemetics as needed, 30 min before meals.	

BP, Blood pressure; *HEPA,* high-efficiency particulate air; *I & O,* intake and output; *NPO,* nothing by mouth; *WBC,* white blood cell.

There are no specific signs or symptoms of a low neutrophil count, although many patients describe fatigue or malaise that coincides with the drop in counts and precedes infectious signs and symptoms. This lack of a clear pattern of symptoms makes it essential to evaluate the patient carefully for risk factors for neutropenia. In addition to risk factor analysis, the patient is monitored for clinical findings consistent with infection.

Every body system is examined for physical findings of infection. Typical signs may not be evident. Pain such as sore throat or urethral discomfort may

BOX 15-2

Causes of Neutropenia

MALNUTRITION
Vitamin B deficiency
Calorie deficiency
Iron deficiency
Protein deficiency

HEALTH STATES
Addison's disease
Anaphylactic shock
Anorexia nervosa
Brucellosis
Chronic fever
Chronic illness
Cirrhosis
Diabetes mellitus
Elderly status
Hypothermia
Infectious diseases (any severe bacterial or viral): mononucleosis, measles, mumps, influenza
Renal trauma

MEDICATIONS
Alcohol
Alkylating agents (antineoplastic and immunosuppressive; e.g., cyclophosphamide)
Anticonvulsants (e.g., phenytoin)
Antidysrhythmics (e.g., procainamide, quinidine)
Antimicrobials (e.g., aminoglycosides, chloramphenicol, sulfonamides, trimethoprim-sulfamethoxazole)
Antiretroviral agents (e.g., zidovudine)
Antitumor antibiotics (e.g., bleomycin, doxorubicin [Adriamycin])
Arsenic
Phenothiazines (e.g., prochlorperazine)
Allopurinol (Zyloprim)

be indicative of an infected site. Areas of heavy bacterial colonization (e.g., oral mucosa, perineal area, and venipuncture and catheter sites) have the highest risk of infection; however, the most common clinical infections are septicemia and pneumonia. Additional signs or symptoms of systemic infection include a rise in temperature from its normal set point, chills, and accompanying tachycardia.

The diagnostic test indicated when neutropenia is suspected is the WBC count with differential. The differential demonstrates the percentage of each type of WBC circulating in the bloodstream. The ANC is calculated by multiplying the total WBC count times the percentages of polymorphonuclear leukocytes (polys; also called *segs* or *neutrophils*) and bands (immature neutrophils). This gives an actual number that is translated into the categories of mild, moderate, or severe neutropenia.

Nursing Diagnoses
The specific nursing diagnosis related to all patients with neutropenia is as follows:
• Risk for infection

Medical Interventions
Medical treatment of neutropenia is aimed at preventing and treating infection while reversing the cause of neutropenia. Patients with anticipated neutropenia, such as those receiving antineoplastic or antiretroviral therapy, may be administered bone marrow growth factors. Also known as colony-stimulating factors (CSF), these agents enhance bone marrow regeneration of the granulocyte (G-CSF), macrophage (M-CSF) or both cell lines (GM-CSF) (McCance, 2002; Ozer et al., 2000).

Prophylactic antiinfective agents may be ordered to prevent infection, and potent broad-spectrum bactericidal antimicrobial agents are ordered when there is evidence of infection. In unresolvable sepsis accompanying neutropenia, granulocyte transfusions are occasionally used to supplement phagocytosis.

Nursing Interventions
Nursing care of patients with neutropenia are the same as for all immunocompromised patients (see Nursing Care Plan for the Immunocompromised Patient).

Patient Outcomes
The following are the goals of care for the patient with neutropenia:
• The patient will remain free of infectious symptoms.
• The absolute neutrophil count will be greater than 1500 cells/µL.
• Body site and fluid cultures will remain negative for pathogenic organisms.

MALIGNANT WHITE BLOOD CELL DISORDERS: LEUKEMIA, LYMPHOMA, AND MULTIPLE MYELOMA

Pathophysiology
Malignant diseases involving WBCs are termed leukemia, lymphoma, and plasma cell neoplasm (multiple myeloma). They are differentiated by the cell affected and by the stage of cell development when malignancy occurs. Regardless of the specific neoplastic disorder, a deficiency of functional WBCs is a common problem. The unique pathophysiological and clinical characteristics of these disorders are described in Table 15-10. Despite what may appear

TABLE 15-10

Malignant White Blood Cell Disorders

Characteristic	Leukemia	Lymphoma	Multiple Myeloma
Pathophysiology	Cancer involving any of the WBCs during the early phase of maturation within the bone marrow	Cancer affects the lymphocytes after their bone marrow maturation, when they reside within the lymph node	Cancer involves the mature and differentiated immunoglobulin-producing macrophage called a plasma cell; the malignancy is primarily manifested by excess abnormal immunoglobulin
Classification	Excess proliferation of immature cells is termed *acute* leukemia Excess proliferation of mature cells is termed *chronic* leukemia Leukemias are further classified according to whether they originate in the lymphocyte cell line or are nonlymphocytic	Hodgkin's and non-Hodgkin's subtypes have more subclassifications denoting the maturity of the cell involved and aggressiveness of the malignancy	Disease is classified as limited or extensive depending on the plasma viscosity, bone manifestations, presence of hypercalcemia, and renal involvement
Risk factors	Chromosomal abnormalities Viral infection Radiation Herbicides/pesticides Benzene/toluene Immunosuppressive therapy (e.g., high-dose steroids or posttransplant immunosuppressives) Alkylating agents	Chromosomal abnormalities Viral infection Radiation Herbicides/pesticides Benzene/toluene Immunosuppressive therapy (e.g., high-dose steroids or posttransplant immunosuppressives) Alkylating agents Autoimmune disease	Older age Male gender African-American descent Chronic hypersensitivity reactions Autoimmune diseases
Clinical manifestations	Fever Constitutional symptoms: fatigue, malaise, weakness, night sweats Easy bruising and bleeding from mucous membranes such as gums Bone pain	Enlarged >2 cm, nontender lymph node Usually immovable, and irregularly shaped Masses in body cavities or other organs (e.g., peritoneal cavity, lungs)	Thrombotic events: deep vein thrombosis, pulmonary embolism, cerebral infarction Bone pain Renal failure
Acute complications	Leukostasis Disseminated intravascular coagulation Tumor lysis syndrome	Airway obstruction Superior vena cava syndrome Bowel obstruction Neoplastic tamponade Pleural effusion	Hyperviscosity Renal failure Hypercalcemia

Continued

TABLE 15-10

Malignant White Blood Cell Disorders—cont'd

Characteristic	Leukemia	Lymphoma	Multiple Myeloma
Staging	All patients are viewed as having systemic disease, or late-stage disease	Classified by the number of lymph nodes involved, the number of lymph node groups, whether involved nodes are only above the diaphragm or on both sides of the diaphragm, and how many extranodal sites are involved	Disease is classified as limited when there are only elevated abnormal immunoglobin levels It is described as extensive when there are bone lesions, evidence of hypercalcemia, or accompanying renal dysfunction
Diagnostic tests	CBC will show either ↓ WBC or large number of immature WBCs called blasts, ↓ RBCs, ↓ platelets Bone marrow aspiration and biopsy	Lymph node biopsy CT scans Chemistry: alkaline phosphatase	Bence Jones protein in urine Immunoglobulin electrophoresis Plasma viscosity
Medical management	Systemic chemotherapy BMT	Radiation therapy for single node or node group if above diaphragm for control or remission Radiation also used if palliation of tumor is goal of therapy Systemic chemotherapy for multinode involvement, aggressive tumor subtypes Autologous BMT for patients with high risk of relapse Allogeneic BMT for patients with residual disease, especially involving bone marrow	Systemic chemotherapy still only provides average of 14-36 mo BMT or "double" BMT used Radiation therapy used to palliatively treat bone lesions
Nursing care issues	Infection control practices Bleeding precautions	Infection control practices Edema management Monitoring for lymphoma masses compressing body organs	Infection control practices Safe mobility Thrombosis precautions Aspiration precautions if hypercalemic

↓, Decreased; *BMT,* bone marrow transplant; *CBC,* complete blood count; *CT,* computed tomography; *RBC,* red blood cells; *WBC,* white blood cells.

to be normal serum cell counts, WBC activity is always impaired, and infection is the most common complication of all these disorders.

Assessment and Clinical Manifestations

Malignant hematological diseases have common risk factors such as genetic mutations, viral infection (especially retroviral), radiation, carcinogens, benzene derivatives, pesticides, and T-lymphocyte immune suppression (e.g., high-dose steroids, immunosuppressives after transplantation) (Shelton & Soloman, 2000). Other risk factors that are unique to the specific malignancy are included in Table 15-10.

Assessment findings common to all malignant WBC disorders involve alterations in the immunological response to injury or microbes. As in other disorders affecting WBC function, minimized inflammatory reactions and response to pathogens are typical. Fever is particularly difficult to interpret, because it may be a manifestation of the disease process or may accompany an infectious complication. General symptoms such as fatigue, malaise, myalgias, activity intolerance, and night sweats are nonspecific indicators of immune disease in which malignancy is one of the differential diagnoses. Each malignant WBC disorder is also associated with signs and symptoms representative of the cell line and location of the malignancy. For example, bone pain is common in multiple myeloma while lymph node enlargement is more representative of lymphoma (Shelton & Soloman, 2000). When symptoms overlap into more than one component of the immune system, it may be difficult to differentiate between these disorders.

The critical care nurse must be aware of unique oncological emergencies associated with these malignant diseases. Oncological emergencies may be the consequence of the cancer itself, a specific treatment plan, or tumor lysis. These complications are more likely to precipitate admission to the intensive care unit and are associated with significant morbidity and mortality. Nursing texts provide detailed information about complications identified in Table 15-10.

Nursing Diagnoses

The nursing diagnoses associated with hematological malignancies have some variation with each disorder, but the common issues are as follows:
* Risk for infection
* Altered tissue perfusion related to anemia
* Risk for injury (bleeding)
* Ineffective individual or family coping
* Anxiety related to fear of dying, procedures, and the unknown
* Anticipatory grieving

Medical Interventions

Each major subtype of hematological malignancy denotes an additional list of further classification subdivisions, each with slightly differing presenting symptoms, prognostic variables, and treatment implications. The treatment plan is based on the stage of the disease and commonly includes chemotherapy, biotherapy, and bone marrow transplantation. Lymphoma is the only one of these malignant diseases that may be radiosensitive when the disease is limited to single nodes or node groups; however, many patients with lymphoma have metastatic disease. Surgical interventions may be used with lymphoma, but not as a primary treatment. Surgery is performed to establish a pathological diagnosis or to debulk large tumor masses interfering with other body functions. Localized disease cannot exist in leukemia; it is considered "systemic" at diagnosis and requires an intense and usually toxic chemotherapy treatment plan. Some types of leukemia are also followed with bone marrow transplantation because of the high risk of relapse and subsequent death. Multiple myeloma is less clear because the disease is systemic, but severity is gauged as limited or extensive according to the degree of end-organ damage by the malignant immunoglobulin. Chemotherapy is used as primary treatment, and radiation therapy is used palliatively to control the pain associated with bone lesions. Bone marrow transplantation is also indicated in patients with lymphoma and multiple myeloma who are at high risk of early relapse, although the impetus to find a matched donor is less pressing, and autologous hematopoietic stem cells are often used because the cancer itself does not usually involve the bone marrow. With the exception of patients with Hodgkin's lymphoma involving a single node group, few current therapies for hematological malignancies are considered curative. Carefully selected candidates for bone marrow transplantation may achieve this objective in certain subtypes of leukemia. More realistically, selected therapies for most cases of hematopoietic cancers are hoping to achieve a long-term remission of 5 to 10 years.

Nursing Interventions

The care of patients with hematological malignancies is similar to all patients with a compromised immune system; however, specialized management of cancer therapies must be incorporated into the individual care plan. Refer to oncology nursing references for chemotherapy administration guidelines, management of acute therapy-related nausea and vomiting, and oncological treatment modalities.

Selected Immunological Disorders

PRIMARY IMMUNODEFICIENCY

Primary immunodeficiencies are those in which the primary dysfunction exists in the immune system. Most primary immunodeficiencies are congenital disorders in which some part of the immune system fails to develop. Disorders are grouped by the immunological disruption.

SECONDARY IMMUNODEFICIENCY

In secondary, or acquired, immunodeficiency, the immune disorder is the result of factors outside the immune system and involves the loss of a previously functional immune defense. HIV disease is a common secondary immunodeficiency disorders experienced by critically ill patients and is discussed in more detail in the next section. Other secondary immuno-deficiency syndromes are described in Table 15-9.

Acquired Immunodeficiency Syndrome

Pathophysiology. HIV is a retrovirus, which transcribes its RNA-containing genetic material into DNA of the host cell nucleus by using an enzyme called reverse transcriptase. HIV causes AIDS by depleting helper T cells, CD4 cells, and macrophages. Seroconversion is manifested by the presence of HIV antibodies and is likely to occur within 4 to 7 weeks after infection through blood products, or it may take several months when a patient is infected through sexual exposure (Rote, 2002c). This seroconversion is followed by a decrease in the HIV antibody titer as infected cells are sequestered in the lymph nodes. The earlier stages of HIV may last as long as 10 years and may produce few or no symptoms, although viral particles are actively replacing normal cells. This phenomenon is evident through the decreasing CD4 cell counts as the disease progresses. As the CD4 count decreases, the patient becomes more susceptible to opportunistic infections, malignancies, and neurological disease. AIDS is the final stage of HIV infection. Figure 15-6 shows the progression of disease and common clinical manifestations. A few HIV-infected patients are termed "long-term nonprogressors;" these patients fail to develop AIDS 7 years or more after seroconversion. These patients are able to maintain immune function with CD4$^+$ cell counts of greater than 600/μL. The predominant theory for this phenomenon is that disease progression is dependent on viral load, and persons with minimal viral innoculation will take longer to progress to AIDS than those with high viral antigen exposure.

HIV is transmitted through exposure to infected body fluids, blood, or blood products. Common modes of transmission include rectal or vaginal intercourse with an infected person, intravenous drug use with contaminated equipment, transfusion with contaminated blood or blood products, and accidental exposure through needle sticks, breaks in the skin, gestation, or childbirth (from mother to fetus). Risk of transmission is more likely when the infected person has advanced disease, although transmission of HIV can occur at any time or stage of infection. Since the 1980s, all blood products have been screened for HIV, hepatitis virus, and human T-cell lymphotrophic virus (Rudnicke, 2003). The risk of transmission to health care workers is small and can be further diminished through consistent observance of universal precautions.

Assessment and clinical manifestations. The initial phase of HIV disease may be asymptomatic, or it may manifest as an acute seroconversion syndrome with symptoms similar to those of mononucleosis. This is followed by asymptomatic disease as HIV progressively destroys immune cells. The United States Centers for Disease Control and Prevention differentiate HIV infection from actual AIDS by the presence of a CD4 count less than 200/μL and presence of an indicator condition (see Figure 15-6). The signs and symptoms of AIDS vary with the CD4 count and the particular indicator disease manifested.

Diagnosis of HIV infection is made by the presence of one of the core antigens of HIV or the presence of antibodies to HIV. Core antigens are tested through protein electrophoresis. HIV antibodies are detected by enzyme-linked immunosorbent assay and are confirmed by the Western blot test and polymerase chain reaction (Chernecky & Berger, 2001; Stillwell, 2002). Positive antibody test results are accurate for the presence of HIV infection, although a negative test result does not rule out HIV infection. Additional laboratory findings in AIDS may include an abnormal helper-to-suppressor ratio (less than 1.0), leukopenia, and thrombocytopenia.

Nursing diagnoses. Nursing care of the patient with AIDS is complex, and nursing diagnoses depend on the particular clinical manifestations of the disease. Universal nursing diagnoses for these patients may include the following:
- Risk for infection
- Impaired tissue integrity
- Altered nutrition
- Activity intolerance
- Altered thought processes
- Pain
- Knowledge deficit regarding disease transmission, course of disease, treatments, or medications
- Anxiety
- Anticipatory grieving

Medical interventions. Antiretroviral therapy has had dramatic effects on morbidity and mortality of HIV-infected persons. These people are living longer, and their quality of life has improved (Janssen, 2001). Medical treatment consists of primary control of HIV invasion of CD4 cells. Antiretroviral medications are categorized as nucleoside reverse transcriptase inhibitors, nonnucleoside reverse transcriptase inhibitors, and protease inhibitors. The specific agents used and the strategies of combination therapy are a rapidly changing science that would be quickly outdated if included in this text.

Equally important to quality of life are prevention and management of opportunistic infections.

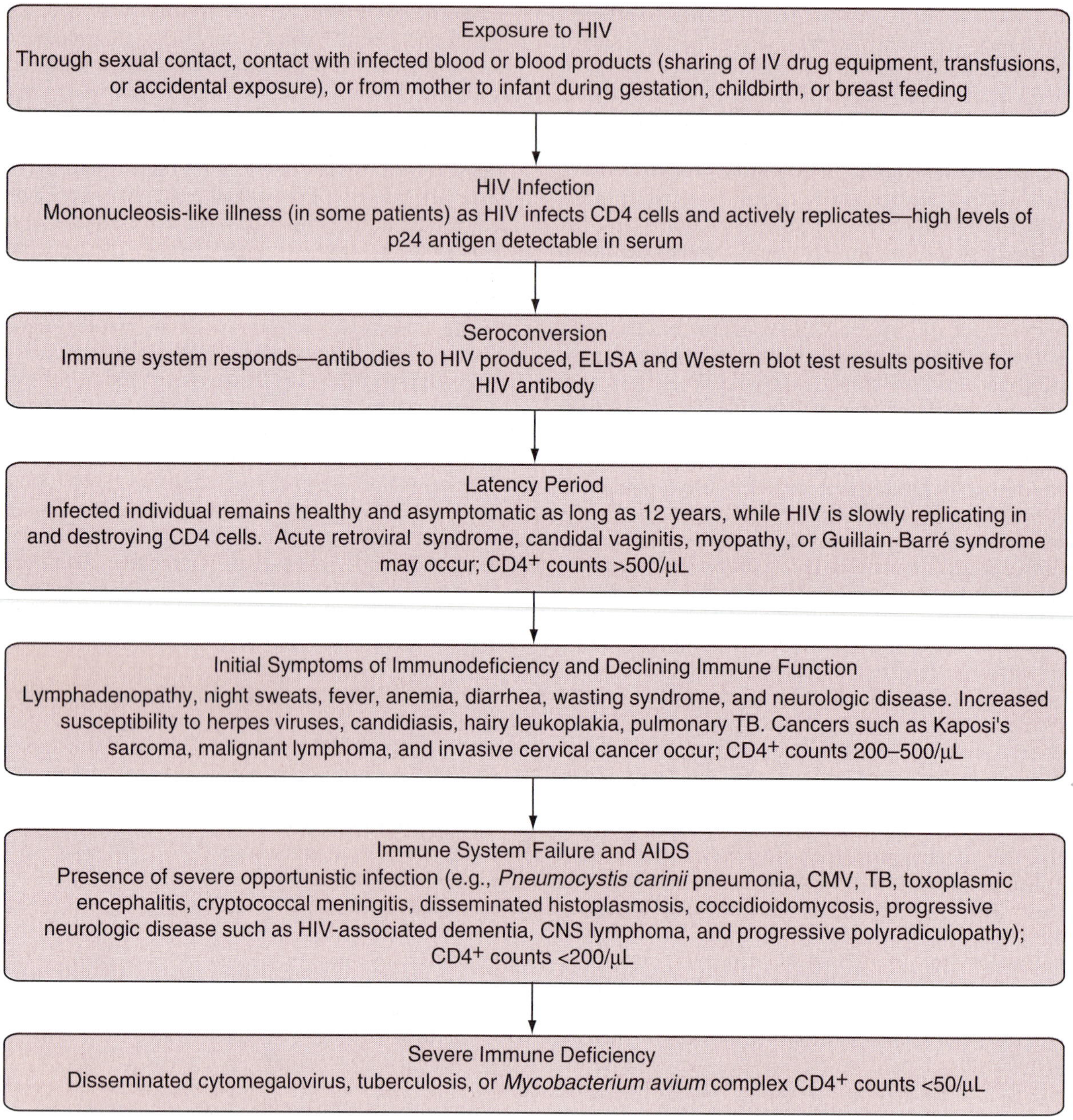

Exposure to HIV
Through sexual contact, contact with infected blood or blood products (sharing of IV drug equipment, transfusions, or accidental exposure), or from mother to infant during gestation, childbirth, or breast feeding

↓

HIV Infection
Mononucleosis-like illness (in some patients) as HIV infects CD4 cells and actively replicates—high levels of p24 antigen detectable in serum

↓

Seroconversion
Immune system responds—antibodies to HIV produced, ELISA and Western blot test results positive for HIV antibody

↓

Latency Period
Infected individual remains healthy and asymptomatic as long as 12 years, while HIV is slowly replicating in and destroying CD4 cells. Acute retroviral syndrome, candidal vaginitis, myopathy, or Guillain-Barré syndrome may occur; CD4$^+$ counts >500/μL

↓

Initial Symptoms of Immunodeficiency and Declining Immune Function
Lymphadenopathy, night sweats, fever, anemia, diarrhea, wasting syndrome, and neurologic disease. Increased susceptibility to herpes viruses, candidiasis, hairy leukoplakia, pulmonary TB. Cancers such as Kaposi's sarcoma, malignant lymphoma, and invasive cervical cancer occur; CD4$^+$ counts 200–500/μL

↓

Immune System Failure and AIDS
Presence of severe opportunistic infection (e.g., *Pneumocystis carinii* pneumonia, CMV, TB, toxoplasmic encephalitis, cryptococcal meningitis, disseminated histoplasmosis, coccidioidomycosis, progressive neurologic disease such as HIV-associated dementia, CNS lymphoma, and progressive polyradiculopathy); CD4$^+$ counts <200/μL

↓

Severe Immune Deficiency
Disseminated cytomegalovirus, tuberculosis, or *Mycobacterium avium* complex CD4$^+$ counts <50/μL

FIGURE 15-6 Human immunodeficiency virus (HIV) pathophysiology. *CMV,* Cytomegalovirus; *CNS,* central nervous system; *ELISA,* enzyme-linked immunosorbent assay; *TB,* tuberculosis.

Antimicrobials are administered to prevent high-risk opportunistic infections when predefined CD4 levels are reached. Additional treatment may include respiratory support, nutritional support, administration of blood products or intravenous fluids, administration of analgesics, and physical therapy.

Nursing interventions. Nursing care of patients with HIV infection requires complex assessment and intervention skills. As with all immunosuppressed patients, those with HIV infection must be protected from infection. Precautions outlined in the Nursing Care Plan for the Immunocompromised Patient should be followed. These patients provide additional clinical challenges because of their multisystemic clinical complications.

Nursing assessment must be comprehensive and include evaluation of the neurological status, mouth, respiratory status, abdominal symptoms, and peripheral sensation. For unclear reasons, persons with HIV infection have a higher propensity for adverse reactions than other patient groups and require careful monitoring of all medication regimens.

Staff members are encouraged to consult with support personnel and psychosocial health professionals to assist with the physical and emotional demands of caring for this population. The potential risk of exposure, although small, places an additional emotional stressor on nurses. Prevention of transmission of HIV in the clinical setting is accomplished by practicing universal precautions at all times. Continuing education must be available to address prevention of HIV transmission, current research, and treatments.

Patient Outcomes. The following are the goals of care for the patient with AIDS:
- Infection will be absent.
- Oxygenation and ventilation will be adequate.
- Hydration and optimal nutritional status will be adequate.
- Skin and mucous membrane integrity will be maintained.
- The patient will have manageable discomfort.
- The patient will be alert and oriented, demonstrating behavior appropriate to developmental stage.
- Diarrhea will be controlled adequately to regulate fluid and electrolyte balance.
- The patient will be free of injury related to seizures; seizures will be controlled.
- The patient will understand disease transmission, course of disease, symptoms of opportunistic infections, treatments, and medications.

Bleeding Disorders

Patients with abnormal hemostasis often require critical care. A general approach to assessing and managing the bleeding patient is addressed before a more thorough discussion of thrombocytopenia and DIC.

THE BLEEDING PATIENT
Pathophysiology
Bleeding disorders, also referred to as coagulopathies, are caused by abnormalities in one of the stages of clotting: (1) vasoconstriction, (2) creation of a platelet plug, (3) development of the fibrin clot, or (4) fibrinolysis. Disorders are considered inherited (e.g., hemophilia, von Willebrand's disease) or acquired (e.g., vitamin K deficiency, DIC). Coagulopathies induce bleeding manifestations, and many care principles are universal. This section addresses the universal care of patients with disorders of coagulation.

Assessment and Clinical Manifestations
A patient with abnormal bleeding requires a careful medical and social history. It is important to assess for medical disorders and medications known to interfere with platelets, coagulation proteins, or fibrinolysis. Disruptions in hemostasis commonly occur in conjunction with renal disease, hepatic or gastrointestinal disorders, and malnutrition. Medications that may alter hemostasis include aminoglycosides, anticoagulants, antiplatelets, cephalosporins, histamine blockers, nitrates, sulfonamides, sympathomimetics, and vasodilators (Box 15-3). Recognition of these risk factors, and modification when possible, may reduce the severity of bleeding.

The physical examination is extremely important. Although many patients with bleeding disorders demonstrate active bleeding from body orifices, mucous membranes, and open lesions or intravenous line sites, equal numbers of patients have less immediately obvious bleeding. The most susceptible sites for bleeding are existing openings in the epithelial surfaces. Mucous membranes have a low threshold for bleeding because the capillaries lie close to the membrane surface, and minor injury may damage and expose vessels. A general overview of assessment findings that may be indicative of bleeding is included in Table 15-5.

Substantial blood loss can occur in any coagulopathy. The physical consequences of blood loss are apparent in all body systems, most prominently the cardiac and pulmonary systems. Guidelines for assessment of bleeding and blood loss are described in the Nursing Care Plan for the Patient with a Bleeding Disorder.

Diagnostic tests are performed to evaluate the cause of the bleeding disorder and the extent of blood loss. The CBC provides quantitative values for RBCs and platelets. When the disorder arises from coagulation protein or clot lysis abnormalities, screening coagulation tests of fibrinogen level, prothrombin time, and partial thromboplastin time are usually ordered. Bedside rapid response tests for hemoglobin, hematocrit, and partial thromboplastin time are important resources to obtain rapid feedback regarding the patient's response to interventions in a bleeding disorder. In certain disease states, additional specialized

---

BOX 15-3

Heparin-induced Thrombocytopenia (HIT)

DEFINITION

Two types of HIT have been identified. Type I HIT is a non-immunologic response to heparin treatment. Type I HIT is thought to occur from an interaction between heparin and circulating platelets. It is usually self-limiting. Type II HIT is a severe immune-mediated drug reaction that can occur in any patient who has received heparin. Heparin binds to platelet factor 4, forming an antigenic complex on the surface of the platelets. Some patients develop an antibody to this complex. The antibody stimulates removal of platelets by splenic macrophages, and thrombocytopenia develops. Thrombosis also occurs secondary to platelet activation and generation of pro-coagulants.

RISKS

Up to 50% of patients who receive heparin will develop antibodies. About 3% will develop Type II HIT. All patients who have been exposed to heparin are at risk for Type II HIT.

COMPLICATIONS

Complications of Type I HIT are those associated with a low platelet count. Type II HIT is more severe, and its major complications are thromboembolic in nature. These include deep vein thrombosis, pulmonary embolism, myocardial infarction, arterial occlusion in limbs, occlusive stroke, and end-organ damage.

DIAGNOSIS

HIT is often under-diagnosed. Type I HIT occurs within 2-3 days after initiation of heparin therapy, and the platelet count does not usually fall below 100,000 μL; no laboratory tests are required. Type II HIT is suspected if the platelet count drops below 100,000 μL or more than 50% from baseline values. Antibody testing assists in confirmation of Type II HIT; however, treatment should start if HIT is suspected.

TREATMENT

Type I HIT is usually self-limiting. Type II HIT is treated by discontinuing all heparin products, including heparin flushes and heparin-coated infusion catheters. Treatment focuses on administration of drugs that inhibit thrombin formation, or cause direct thrombin inhibition. These drugs include lepirudin (Refludan), bivalirudin (Angiomax), or argatroban (Argatroban).

From Mansen, T. J., & McCance, K. L. (2002). Alteration of leukocytes, lymphoid and hemostatis function. In K. L. McCance and S. E. Huether (eds.). *Pathophysiology: The biologic basis for disease in adults and children* (pp. 865-899). St. Louis: Mosby; Retrieved from http://www.argatroban.com/hit_02.htm (accessed 7/1/2004); retrieved from http://www.refludan.com/hit (accessed 7/1/2004).

---

tests such as bleeding time and fibrin degradation products are monitored.

Nursing Diagnoses

The actively bleeding patient or one with a hemostatic disorder can experience bleeding into any body system. The major diagnoses include the following:

- Risk for bleeding
- Altered protection caused by inadequate clotting
- Fluid volume deficit resulting from blood loss
- Pain resulting from bleeding into body organs
- Potential for decreased tissue perfusion because of inadequately circulating blood volume, decreased cardiac output, or bleeding into tissue
- Altered self-image because of active bleeding, ecchymoses, mottling

Medical Interventions

Medical treatment for bleeding patients depends on the suspected cause. Component-specific replacement transfusions are preferred over whole blood because they provide more specific treatment of the bleeding disorder. Transfusion thresholds are established based on laboratory values and patient-specific variables. In general, a threshold for RBC transfusion is considered a hematocrit of 28% to 31%, based on the patient's cardiovascular tolerance. If angina or orthostasis is present, a higher threshold may be maintained. The platelet count may drop as low as 5000 to 10,000/μL before spontaneous bleeding is likely to occur. This transfusion threshold may be too low for patients with preexisting conditions such as recent surgical procedures or peptic ulcer disease. A more

Nursing Care Plan for the Patient with a Bleeding Disorder

NURSING DIAGNOSIS: *Altered tissue perfusion related to abnormal clotting, hypotension, and/or anemia*

Patient Outcomes	Interventions	Rationales

Adequate perfusion will be maintained and damage to vital organs will be prevented, as evidenced by:
  Vital signs and
    hemodynamics stable
    and within normal limits
  Normal mental status
  ABG results within normal
    limits
  Urine output >30 mL/hr
  Adequate peripheral pulses,
    skin warm with normal
    color
	Monitor hemodynamics, vital signs, electrocardiogram,
	  ABGs, I & O, and laboratory results.
	Assess for and report signs of altered perfusion.
	
	Provide good skin and oral care.
	Evaluate vital signs or orthostatic changes
	
	Recognize signs and symptoms of subcutaneous
	  bleeding (e.g., ecchymoses, hematomas).
	Note increased girth of limbs or abdomen. Make
	  anatomical area for consistency of measurement
	Elevate any limb that is bleeding to reduce blood
	  flow to the area (Table 15-12).
	Administer blood components as ordered and monitor
	  for adverse effects (Table 15-12).
	Administer selective vasoconstrictor agents (e.g.,
	  vasopressin) as ordered.
	Administer procoagulants (e.g., somatostatin, estrogen)
	  as ordered.
		Symptoms of decreased
		  tissue perfusion occur
		  with blood loss.
		To promote circulation.
		Change in vital signs
		  and/or orthostasis occur
		  with blood loss.
		
		Assess for bleeding into
		  limbs and/or abdomen.

NURSING DIAGNOSIS: *Fluid volume deficit related to hemorrhage*

Patient Outcomes	Interventions	Rationales

Patient will be free of bleeding and will be normovolemic, as evidenced by:
  Absence of oozing/bleeding
  Laboratory study results within
    normal limits
  Vital signs and hemodynamics
    stable and within normal limits
	Monitor hemodynamics, vital signs, I & O, and
	  laboratory study results.
	Weigh dressings/linens to estimate blood loss.
	Check body fluids for occult blood.
	
	Assess and report signs of bleeding, such as oozing
	  or bleeding from venipunctures, IV access sites,
	  incisions, wounds, mucous membranes, and
	  body orifices.
	Control bleeding using ice packs, pressure dressings,
	  or direct pressure.
	Leave existing clots undisturbed.
	Administer topical hemostatic agents as ordered.
	Severe bleeding requires administration of fluid to
	  replenish volume even as blood components are
	  administered (normal saline or Ringer's lactate).
		Assesses for changes in
		  volume status.
		
		To assess for hidden
		  sources of blood loss.
		To assess sources of blood
		  loss.
		
		Ringer's lactate aids in
		  maintaining the acid-base
		  balance.

ABGs, Arterial blood gases; *I & O,* intake and output; *RBC,* red blood cells; *WBC,* white blood cells.

conservative transfusion marker used in many critical care units is between 20,000 and 50,000/μL. Cryoprecipitate is usually infused if the fibrinogen level is less than 100 mg/dL(Geiter, 2003). Fresh frozen plasma is used to correct a prolonged prothrombin time and partial thromboplastin time or a specific factor deficiency (Lapointe & Von Rueden, 2002). A summary of blood product components, clinical indications, and nursing implications is included in Table 15-11.

When the cause of bleeding is unknown or multifactorial, nonspecific interventions aimed at stopping bleeding are used. These include local and systemic procoagulant medications and therapies.

Local therapies to stop bleeding are also used when systemic anticoagulation is necessary for treatment of another health condition (e.g., myocardial infarction, ischemic stroke, or pulmonary embolism). Local procoagulants usually act by direct tissue contact and initiation of a surface clot.

Systemic procoagulant medications may be used to enhance vasoconstriction (e.g., vasopressin), enhance clot formation (e.g., somatostatin), or prevent clot breakdown (e.g., aminocaproic acid) (Kroll, 2001). These agents are used judiciously in clinical situations when it is believed that inadequate clot formation and premature clot dissolution are the causes of excess bleeding. Each agent has significant adverse effects that must be considered before implementation. All may enhance clot production and induce thrombotic vascular or neurological events. They may be contraindicated when the patient has simultaneous procoagulant risk factors.

Nursing Interventions

Patients with bleeding disorders often have multisystemic manifestations. Prioritization of administration of fluids and blood products is an important nursing activity that requires careful consideration of the patient's specific coagulation defect. When the patient's blood does not clot because of thrombocytopenia, administration of RBCs before platelets will result in RBC loss from disrupted vascular structures.

Precautions such as limiting invasive procedures, including Foley catheters or rectal temperatures, are important. A comprehensive listing of bleeding precautions are included in the Nursing Care Plan for the Patient with a Bleeding Disorder.

THROMBOCYTOPENIA
Pathophysiology

A quantitative deficiency of platelets is termed *thrombocytopenia*. By definition, this is a platelet count of less than 100,000/μL; however, levels greater than 50,000/μL rarely cause significant complications.

This condition can cause severe hemorrhage if it is not corrected. The pathophysiology may be related to decreased production of platelets by the bone marrow, increased destruction of platelets, or sequestration of platelets (abnormal distribution) (Mansen & McCance, 2002b).

Assessment and Clinical Manifestations

Many critical care therapies and medications interfere with platelet production or life span and cause thrombocytopenia. A thorough medical, social, and medication history can help to identify factors that may cause thrombocytopenia. A comprehensive listing of causes is included in Box 15-4

Clinically, the patient with thrombocytopenia presents with petechiae, purpura, and ecchymoses, with oozing from mucous membranes. Laboratory findings reveal a platelet count of less than 150,000/μL, predisposing the patient to an increased risk of bleeding. When the count drops to less than 20,000 to 30,000/μL, spontaneous bleeding may occur. Fatal hemorrhage is a great risk when the count is less than 10,000/μL (Mansen & McCance, 2002b).

Nursing Diagnoses

In addition to many of the nursing diagnoses listed in care of the bleeding patient, those with thrombocytopenia may have the following:
- Potential for bleeding resulting from inadequate platelet activity
- Altered body image resulting from petichiae and ecchymoses

Medical Interventions

Medical treatment of thrombocytopenia includes infusions of platelets. Patients who require multiple platelet transfusions should be evaluated for single-donor platelet products. A single-donor product permits administration of 6 to 10 units of platelets with exposure to the antigens of only one person. For every 1 unit of single-donor platelets, the platelet count should increase 30,000-36,000 cells/μL (Meehan et al., 2000). Patients who receive many platelet transfusions can become refractory, or alloimmunized, to the many different platelet antigens and may fail to obtain benefit from non–human leukocyte antigen (HLA)-matched platelets (tissue typed to match the patient). After multiple platelet transfusions, febrile and allergic transfusion reactions are common but can be reduced by administration of acetaminopen and diphenhydramine before transfusion.

When thrombocytopenia results from inadequate production, a bone marrow growth factor called oprelvekin (Neumega) can be administered to enhance platelet production and differentiation

TABLE 15-11

Summary of Blood Products and Administration

Blood Component	Description	Actions	Indications	Administration	Complications
Whole blood	RBCs, plasma, and stable clotting factors	Restores oxygen-carrying capacity and intravascular volume	Symptomatic anemia with major circulating volume deficit Massive hemorrhaging with shock	Donor and recipient must be ABO compatible and Rh compatible Use microaggregate filter Rate of infusion: usually 2-4 unit/hr but more rapid in cases of shock	Hemolytic reaction Allergic reaction Hypothermia Electrolyte disturbances Citrate intoxication Infectious diseases
Red blood cells (RBCs)	RBCs centrifuged from whole blood	Restores oxygen-carrying capacity and intravascular volume	Symptomatic anemia when patient is at risk for fluid overload Acute hemorrhage	Donor and recipient must be ABO compatible and Rh compatible Use microaggregate filter Rate of infusion: 2-4 unit/hr but more rapid in cases of shock	Infectious diseases Hemolytic reaction Allergic reaction Hypothermia Electrolyte disturbances Citrate intoxication
Leukocyte-poor cells or washed red blood cells	RBCs from which leukocytes and plasma proteins have been reduced	Restores oxygen-carrying capacity and intravascular volume	Symptomatic anemia when patient has history of repeated febrile nonhemolytic transfusion reactions Acute hemorrhage	Donor and recipient must be ABO compatible and Rh compatible Use microaggregate filter Rate of infusion: 2-4 unit/hr but more rapid in cases of shock	Allergic reaction Hemolytic reaction Hypothermia Electrolyte disturbances Citrate intoxication Infectious diseases
Fresh frozen plasma	Plasma rich in clotting factors with platelets removed	Replaces clotting factors	Deficit of coagulation factors as in DIC, liver disease, and massive transfusions Major trauma victims with signs/symptoms of hemorrhage	Donor and recipient must be ABO compatible, but not necessary to be Rh compatible Rate of infusion: 10 mL/min	Allergic reaction Febrile reactions Circulatory overload Infectious diseases

Continued

TABLE 15-12

Summary of Blood Products and Administration—cont'd

Blood Component	Description	Actions	Indications	Administration	Complications
Platelets	Removed from whole blood	Increases platelet count and improves hemostasis	Thrombocytopenia Platelet dysfunction (prophylactically for platelet counts 10,000-20,000/μL), evidence of bleeding with platelet count <50,000/μL	Do not use microaggregate filter; component filter obtained from blood bank ABO testing not necessary unless contaminated with RBCs but is usually done Usually give 6 units at one time	Infectious diseases Allergic reactions Febrile reactions
Cryoprecipitate antihemophilic factor	Primarily coagulation factor VIII with 250 mg of fibrinogen and 20%-30% of factor XIII	Replace selected clotting factors	Hemophilia A, von Willebrand's disease Hypofibrinogenemia Factor XIII deficiency Massive transfusions	Repeat doses may be necessary to attain satisfactory serum level Rate of infusion: approximately 10 mL of diluted component per minute	Allergic reactions Infectious diseases (e.g., hepatitis)
Albumin	Prepared from plasma	Intravascular volume expansion by increasing oncotic pressure	Hypovolemic shock Liver failure	Special administration set Rate of infusion: over 30-60 min	Circulatory overload Febrile reaction
Granulocytes	Prepared by centrifugation or filtration leukopheresis, which removes granulocytes from whole blood	Increase the leukocyte level	Decreased WBCs usually from chemotherapy or radiation	Must be ABO compatible and Rh compatible Rate of infusion: 1 unit over 2-4 hr; closely observe for reaction	Rash Febrile reaction Hepatitis
Plasma proteins	Pooled from human plasma	Intravascular volume expander by increasing oncotic pressure	Hypovolemic shock	ABO compatibility not necessary Rate of infusion: over 30-60 min	Circulatory overload Febrile reaction

DIC, Disseminated intravascular coagulopathy; *RBC*, red blood cell; *WBC*, white blood cell.

BOX 15-4

Causes of Thrombocytopenia

BONE MARROW SUPPRESSION
Aplastic anemia
Burns
Cancer chemotherapy
Exposure to ionizing radiation
Nutritional deficiency (vitamin B_{12}, folate)

INTERFERENCE WITH PLATELET PRODUCTION (OTHER THAN NONSPECIFIC MARROW SUPPRESSION)
Alcohol
Histamine$_2$-blocking agents
Histoplasmosis
Hormones
Thiazide diuretics

PLATELET DESTRUCTION OUTSIDE THE BONE MARROW
Artificial heart valves
Cardiac bypass machine
Heat stroke
Heparin
Infections: severe or sepsis
Large-bore intravenous lines
Intraaortic balloon pump
Splenic sequestration of platelets
Sulfonamides
Transfusions
Trimethoprim-sulfamethoxazole

IMMUNE RESPONSE AGAINST PLATELETS
Idiopathic thrombocytopenic purpura
Mononucleosis
Thrombotic thrombocytopenic purpura
Vaccinations
Viral illness

INTERFERENCE WITH PLATELET FUNCTION
Aminoglycosides
Catecholamines: epinephrine, dopamine
Cirrhosis
Dextran
Diabetes mellitus
Diazepam
Digitoxin
Hypothermia
Loop diuretics (e.g., furosemide)
Malignant lymphomas
Nonsteroidal antiinflammatory agents
Phenothiazines
Phenytoin
Salicylate derivatives
Sarcoidosis
Scleroderma
Systemic lupus erythematosus
Thyrotoxicosis
Tricyclic antidepressants
Uremia
Vitamin E

(Ferrari et al., 2002). Other less research-supported medications used to enhance platelet production include corticosteroids and lithium carbonate. Some thrombocytopenias are autoimmune induced and may respond to filtration of antibodies via plasmapheresis or immune suppression with corticosteroids. When the spleen is enlarged and tender and these other supportive therapies are unsuccessful, splenectomy can alleviate the autoimmune reaction (see Clinical Alert: Bleeding Disorders).

Nursing Interventions

Nursing interventions for the patient with thrombocytopenia are similar to those listed for the bleeding patient. The nurse must also recognize and limit complications or interventions that can deplete or shorten the life span of platelets. For example, high fevers and high metabolic activity (e.g., seizures) prematurely destroy platelets.

Patient Outcomes

The following are the goals of care for the patient with thrombocytopenia:
- The patient will maintain adequate tissue perfusion.
- Tissue integrity will be maintained.
- Bleeding will be promptly recognized and treated.
- Pain will be managed.

CLINICAL ALERT: BLEEDING DISORDERS

All body surfaces should be inspected for overt bleeding or bruising and petechiae indicative of subcutaneous bleeding. Subtle symptoms indicative of internal bleeding may occur even without a known injury and are more challenging for clinicians to readily recognize.

DISSEMINATED INTRAVASCULAR COAGULATION

Pathophysiology

DIC is a serious disorder of hemostasis characterized by exaggerated microvascular coagulation, depletion of clotting factors, and subsequent bleeding. Because clotting factors are used up in the abnormal coagulation process, this disorder is also termed consumption coagulopathy. The disorder often manifests with acute and severe symptoms and is associated with a high mortality rate.

The clinical course of DIC can range from an acute, life-threatening process to a chronic, low-grade condition. Sepsis is the most common cause of acute DIC (Mansen & McCance, 2002b). Acute DIC develops rapidly and is the most serious form of acquired coagulopathy. With chronic DIC, the patient may have more subtle clinical and laboratory findings.

Whatever the initiating event in DIC, procoagulants that cause diffuse uncontrolled clotting are released. The intrinsic or extrinsic pathways can be activated. Large amounts of thrombin are produced, and this

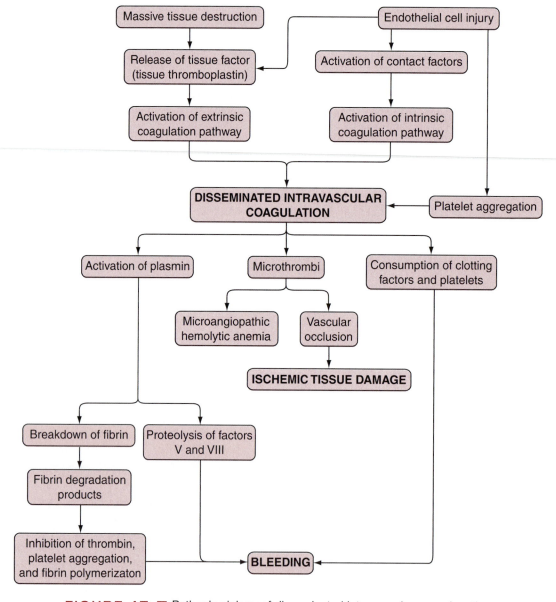

FIGURE 15-7 Pathophysiology of disseminated intravascular coagulopathy.

results in the deposition of fibrin in the microvasculature, the consumption of available clotting factors, and the stimulation of fibrinolysis.

Clotting in the microvasculature of the patient with DIC causes organ ischemia and necrosis. The skin, lungs, and kidneys are most often damaged. Thrombophlebitis, pulmonary embolism, cerebrovascular accident, gastrointestinal bleeding, and renal failure may result from thrombosis. Additionally, microvasculature thrombosis may result in cyanosis of the fingers and toes, purpura fulminans, or infarction and gangrene of the digits or tip of the nose (Mansen & McCance, 2002b).

The fibrinolysis that ensues results in the release of fibrin degradation products, which are potent anticoagulants that interfere with thrombin, fibrin, and platelet activity. RBCs are damaged as they try to pass through the blocked capillary beds; the damage to RBCs causes excess hemolysis. The lack of available clotting factors coupled with the anticoagulant forces result in an inability to form clots when needed and predisposes the patient with DIC to hemorrhage (Figure 15-7).

Assessment and Clinical Manifestations

DIC is always a secondary complication of excessive clotting stimuli and may be triggered by vessel injury caused by disease states, tissue injury, or a foreign body in the bloodstream. The greater the clotting stimulus, the higher is the risk of developing the disorder. Sepsis, multitrauma, and burns are the largest risk factors for this complication and also provide the most significant stimuli for the clotting cascade. Recognition of potential risk factors and conscientious monitoring of the high-risk patient can permit early intervention. A summary of common risk factors for DIC is included in Table 15-12.

Clinically, the patient with DIC first develops microvascular thrombosis. Thrombosis leads to organ ischemia and necrosis that may be manifested as changes in mental status, angina, hypoxemia, oliguria, or nonspecific hepatitis. Cyanosis of the fingers and toes and infarction of the same as well as the tip of the nose may occur if the DIC is severe. After a thrombotic phase of hours to a few days, depletion of clotting factors and clot lysis cause excessive bleeding. Early signs may include occult blood in the stool, emesis, and urine. Capillary fragility and depleted clotting factors often appear early as mucosal or subcutaneous tissue bleeding seen as gingival bleeding, petechiae, or ecchymoses. Overt bleeding ranges from mild oozing from venipuncture sites to massive hemorrhage from all body orifices. Occult bleeding into body cavities, such as the peritoneal and

TABLE 15-12	
Causes of Disseminated Intravascular Coagulation	
Infection	**Examples**
Infections	Bacterial (especially gram-negative), fungal, viral, mycobacterial, protozoan, rickettsial
Trauma	Burns; head, crush, or multiple injuries; snakebite
Obstetrical	Abruptio placentae, placenta previa, amniotic fluid embolism, retained dead fetus, missed abortion, eclampsia, hydatidiform mole
Hematological/ immunological disorders	Transfusion reaction, transplant rejections, anaphylaxis, autoimmune disorders, sickle cell crisis
Oncological disorders	Carcinomas, leukemias
Miscellaneous	Extracorporeal circulation, pulmonary or fat embolism, anoxia, acidosis, hyperthermia or hypothermia, hypovolemic hemorrhagic shock, ARDS, sustained hypotension

ARDS, Acute respiratory distress syndrome.

retroperitoneal spaces, may be detected by vital sign changes or other classic signs of blood loss.

Diagnosis of DIC is made based on recognition of pertinent risk factors, clinical symptoms, and the results of laboratory studies. Evidence of factor depletion in the form of thrombocytopenia and hypofibrinoginemia is seen in the early phase; however, definitive diagnosis is made by evidence of excess fibrinolysis detectable by elevated fibrin degradation products, an increased D-dimer level, or a decreased antithrombin III level (Mansen & McCance, 2002b). Altered laboratory values in DIC are noted in Laboratory Findings in Disseminated Intravascular Coagulation.

Nursing Diagnoses

The patient with DIC is likely to have multiple system involvement that encompasses thrombotic and hemorrhagic manifestations. Nursing diagnoses may include the following:

- Altered tissue perfusion related to abnormal clotting and thrombosis

LABORATORY FINDINGS IN DISSEMINATED INTRAVASCULAR COAGULATION

Test	Normal Value	Alteration
Platelet count	150,000-400,000/μL	↓
Prothrombin time	11-16 sec	Prolonged
Activated partial thromboplastin time	30-45 sec	Prolonged
Thrombin time	10-15 sec	Prolonged
Fibrinogen	150-400 mg/dL	↓
Fibrin degradation products	<10 mcg/mL	↑
Antithrombin III	>50% of control (plasma)	↓
D-Dimer assay	<100 mcg/L	↑
Protein C	71%-142% of normal activity	↓
Protein S	61%-130% of normal activity	↓

- Fluid volume deficit related to hemorrhage
- Impaired skin integrity
- Anxiety related to the fear of dying, the procedures being performed, and the unknown
- Pain related to tissue ischemia, bleeding into tissues, and therapeutic/diagnostic interventions

Medical Interventions

Medical treatment of DIC is aimed at identifying and treating the underlying cause, stopping the abnormal coagulation, and controlling the bleeding. Correction of hypotension, hypoxemia, and acidosis is vital, as is treatment of infection if it is the triggering factor. If the cause is obstetrical, evacuation of the uterus for retained fetal or other tissue must be performed. Blood volume expanders and crystalloid intravenous fluids, such as lactated Ringer's solution or normal saline, are given to counteract hypovolemia caused by blood loss.

Blood component therapy is used in DIC to replace deficient platelets and clotting factors and to treat hemorrhage. Platelet infusions are usually necessary because of consumptive thrombocytopenia. They are viewed as the highest priority for transfusion, because they will provide the clotting factors needed to establish an initial platelet plug from any bleeding sites.

Fresh frozen plasma is administered for fibrinogen replacement. It contains all clotting factors and antithrombin III; however, factor VIII is often inactivated by the freezing process, thus necessitating administration of concentrated factor VIII in the form of cryoprecipitate. Transfusions of packed RBCs are given to replace cells lost in hemorrhage.

Heparin is a potent thrombin inhibitor and may be administered to block the clotting process that initiates DIC. Heparin is given to prevent further clotting and thrombosis that may lead to organ ischemia and necrosis. Although heparin's antithrombin activity prevents further clotting, it may increase the risk of bleeding and may cause further problems. Its use is controversial when it is administered to patients with DIC who are experiencing more hemorrhage than thrombosis.

Other pharmacological therapy in DIC includes the administration of synthetic antithrombin III, which also inhibits thrombin (Geiter, 2003). Antithrombin III concentrates may shorten the course of the disease and may increase the survival rate. Administration of aminocaproic acid (Amicar) inhibits fibrinolysis by interfering with plasmin activity. It may be given in combination with heparin to prevent the lysis of existing clots, thereby preventing the release of fibrin degradation products that contribute to hemorrhage. Other treatments being investigated for use in DIC include administration of other thrombin inhibitors such as protein S and protein C directed at the microbes that trigger sepsis and DIC (Mulroy & DeJong, 2003).

Nursing Interventions

Nursing care of the patient with DIC is aimed at the prevention and recognition of thrombotic and hemorrhagic events. Continuous assessment for complications facilitates prompt and aggressive interventions that may improve outcomes. Psychosocial support of the patient and family is very important. Few patients who survive DIC are without some functional deficits caused by ischemia or hemorrhage. The patient with DIC and his or her family are assessed for the level of anxiety and coping mechanisms available. Communication is encouraged, and feelings are acknowledged. Maintenance of an open, honest, and supportive environment may lessen stress and anxiety.

Pain relief and promotion of comfort are important nursing priorities. The location, intensity, and quality of the patient's pain are assessed, along with the patient's response to discomfort. The nurse is conscientious not to enhance vasoconstriction, because it will contribute to tissue ischemia and its associated discomfort. Relief of discomfort also reduces oxygen

RESEARCH ANALYSIS

ARTICLE REFERENCE
Smith, M. C., Kemp, J., Hemphill, L., Vojir, C. P., & Smith, M. C. (2002). Outcomes of therapeutic massage for hospitalized cancer patients. *Journal of Nursing Scholarship, 34*(3), 257-262.

REVIEW OF STUDY METHODS AND FINDINGS
The purpose of this study was to examine the effects of therapeutic massage on perception of pain, subjective sleep quality, symptom distress, and anxiety in patients hospitalized for treatment of cancer. The sample consisted of 41 patients admitted to the oncology unit at a large urban medical center for chemotherapy or radiation therapy. Twenty participants received therapeutic massage, and 21 received the control therapy, nurse interaction. The outcome variables were measured on admission and at the end of 1 week. Mean scores for pain, sleep quality, symptom distress, and anxiety improved from baseline for the subjects who received therapeutic massage; only anxiety improved from baseline for participants in the comparison group. Statistically significant interactions were found for pain, symptom distress, and sleep. Sleep improved only slightly for the participants receiving massage, but it deteriorated significantly for those in the control group. The findings support the potential for massage as a nursing therapeutic for patients with cancer who are receiving chemotherapy or radiation therapy.

CRITIQUE OF STUDY STRENGTHS AND WEAKNESSES
The study did not have random assignment to the groups; however, the staff of the study unit believed that patients would perceive care inequities if some received massage and others did not. So for this reason the patients were recruited to one group in the first 8 months of the study, and the patients were recruited for the second group in the last 8 months of the study. The study was done in a sample that was 95% male; thus, the generalizability is questioned. One of the strengths of this study was that the nurse who administered the massage was the same nurse who interacted with the study participants during the deliberate focused communication. This use of the same person was intentional, to limit the bias. Another strength of the study was the use of a theoretical framework in the design of the study that was partially supported in the findings.

IMPLICATIONS OF THE STUDY FOR NURSING PRACTICE
Therapeutic massage may be an integral and important part of the nursing care plan to alleviate pain and symptoms in patients with cancer. The massage in this study was defined as 15 to 30 minutes of light Swedish techniques of effleurage and petrissage in the patient's own bed, for a total of three massages during the 1-week hospitalization. Each of the massages was at least 24 hours apart. Although immediate comfort and relaxation follow any massage, a longer-lasting effect on these outcomes seems more likely with two to three massages per week. Massage and interaction with a nurse may decrease anxiety, which is consistent with the assumption that presence can be calming and reassuring to patients during times of crisis and uncertainty. Quality of sleep often deteriorates in a hospital setting; massage may prevent this deterioration and may promote more natural sleep in patients with cancer.

consumption, which is important for these patients with limited circulatory flow. Pain medication is offered as ordered and before painful procedures. Positioning, with support and proper body alignment and frequent changes, also enhances the patient's level of comfort.

Laboratory coagulation studies are carefully monitored for evidence of disease resolution. As fewer clots are created, the platelet count and fibrinogen level are among the first laboratory tests to return to normal. The fibrin degradation products and D-dimer levels will fall and antithrombin III levels will rise as fibrinolysis slows. Other coagulation tests are less sensitive and are not usually assessed.

Patient Outcomes
The following are the goals of care for the patient with DIC:
- Adequate tissue perfusion will be maintained as abnormal clotting and thrombosis are controlled.
- Cardiac output and gas exchange will be sufficient to provide adequate tissue oxygenation.
- Bleeding or thrombotic events will be prevented.
- Skin integrity will be maintained and healing promoted.
- The patient will be able to verbalize fears and will have sufficient emotional support. Effective coping patterns will be fostered.
- The patient will remain as comfortable as possible.

Case Study

evolve

Mr. Garcia is a 70-year-old man who is admitted to the hospital because of generalized ecchymoses, with multiple large bruises primarily involving the flanks and lower extremities. He has a previous diagnosis of prostate cancer with metastasis to the bone for which he received radiation therapy 5 years earlier. There is no evidence of mucosal bleeding. His current platelet count is 62,000/μL, his prothrombin time is 14.8 seconds (international normalized ratio = 1.21), the activated partial thromboplastin time is 32.6 seconds, the serum fibrinogen is 87 mg/dL, and the D-dimer level is increased to 8 mcg/mL. Mr. Garcia's coagulation factors improved with the administration of

low-dose heparin by continuous infusion, cryoprecipitate, and platelets, in addition to estramustine phosphate (Kampel, 2003). He was discharged after 6 days with a platelet count of 83,000/μL, normal prothrombin and activated partial thromboplastin times, a serum fibrinogen level of 195 mg/dL, and a D-dimer level of 1 mcg/mL.

1. What conditions may be associated with DIC?
2. What are possible signs and symptoms of DIC?
3. What is the priority of care for the patient with DIC?
4. What are key nursing interventions for the patient with DIC?

SUMMARY

All patients in critical care have the potential for hematological and immunological dysfunction. A thorough understanding of normal anatomy and physiology provides the critical care nurse with a basis on which a comprehensive assessment and treatment approach can be built. Because nurses play a key role in the outcome of patients with serious alterations in the hematological and immune systems, this knowledge is critical and has great impact on the well-being of their patients.

CRITICAL THINKING QUESTIONS

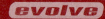

1. What disorders in critical care are associated with anemia?
2. Why is the critical care unit often a dangerous place for the immunosuppressed patient?
3. How can therapeutic choices such as interventions and medications worsen the hematological or immunological compromise of critically ill patients?
4. What criteria should be used for prioritization of nursing and medical interventions for the bleeding patient?
5. Why does the treatment of DIC (blood products, heparin) often exacerbate the problem?

REFERENCES

Casey, G. (2002). Wound repair: Advanced dressing materials. *Nursing Standard, 17*(4), 49-53.

Chernecky, C. C., & Berger, B. J. (2004). *Laboratory tests and diagnostic procedures.* 4th ed. Philadelphia: W. B. Saunders.

Cunningham-Rundles, C. (2001). Immunodeficiency disorders. In J. B. Henry (ed.). *Clinical diagnosis and management by laboratory methods* [pp. 963-973]. 12th ed. Philadelphia: W. B. Saunders.

Ferrari, S., Danova, M., Porta, C., Brugnatelli, S., Pugliese, P., Bertolini, A., & Riccardi, A. (2002). Recombinant human interleukin-11 (Neumega, rhIL-11) reduces thrombocytopenia in breast cancer patients receiving tandem autologous circulating progenitor cell transplantation. *Annals of Hematology, 81*, 354-356.

Geiter, H. (2003). Disseminated intravascular coagulopathy. *Dimensions of Critical Care Nursing, 22*(3), 108-114.

Gillespie, T. W. (2003). Anemia in cancer: Therapeutic implications and interventions. *Cancer Nursing, 26*(2), 119-128.

Hutchison, R. E., & Davey, F. R. (2001). Leukocytic disorders. In J. B. Henry (ed.). *Clinical diagnosis and management by laboratory methods* [pp. 586-622]. 12th ed. Philadelphia: W. B. Saunders.

Janssen, R. S., Holtgrave, D. R., Valdiserri, R. O., Shepherd, M., Gayle, H. D., & DeCock, K. M. (2001). The serostatus approach to fighting the HIV epidemic: Prevention strategies for infected individuals. *American Journal of Public Health, 91*(7), 1019-1024.

Kampel, L. J. (2003). Challenging problems in advanced malignancy: Disseminated intravascular coagulation in metastatic hormone-refractory prostate cancer. *Journal of Clinical Oncology, 21*(16), 3170-3171.

Karon, J. M., Fleming, P. L., Steketee, R. W., & De Cock, K. M. (2001). HIV in the United States at the turn of the century: An epidemic in transition. *American Journal of Public Health, 91*(7), 1060-1068.

Kroll, M. H. (2001). *Manual of coagulation disorders.* Williston, VT: Blackwell Science.

Lapointe, L. A., & Von Rueden, K. T. (2002). Coagulopathies in trauma patients. *AACN Clinical Issues, 13(2), 192-203.*

Lewis, N. L,. & Weiner, L. M. (2003). Biologic therapy. In B. Furie, P. A. Cassileth, M. B. Atkins, & R. J. Mayer (eds.). *Clinical hematology and oncology: Presentation, diagnosis, and treatment* [pp. 376-390]. Philadelphia: Churchill Livingstone.

Mansen, T. J., & McCance, K. L. (2002a). Alteration of erythrocyte functions. In K. L. McCance & S. E. Huether (eds.). *Pathophysiology: The biologic basis for disease in adults and children* [pp. 843-864]. St. Louis: Mosby.

Mansen, T. J., & McCance, K. L. (2002b). Alteration of leukocytes, lymphoid and hemostatic function. In K. L. McCance & S. E. Huether (eds.). *Pathophysiology: The biologic basis for disease in adults and children* [pp. 865-899]. St. Louis: Mosby.

McCance, K. L. (2002). Structure and function of the hematological system. In K. L. McCance & S. E. Huether (eds.). *Pathophysiology: The biologic basis for disease in adults and children* [pp. 811-842]. St. Louis: Mosby.

McPherson, R. A. (2001). Overview of the immune system and immunologic disorders. In J. B. Henry (ed.). Clinical diagnosis and management by laboratory methods [pp. 817-820]. 12th ed. Philadelphia: W. B. Saunders.

Meehan, K. R., Matias, C. O., Rathore, S. S., Sandler, S. G., Kallich, J., LaBrecque, J., Erder, H., & Schulman, K. A. (2000). Platelet transfusions: Utilization and associated costs in a tertiary care hospital. *American Journal of Hematology, 64,* 251-256.

Miller, J. (2001). Blood platelets. In J. B. Henry (ed.). *Clinical diagnosis and management by laboratory methods* [pp. 623-641]. 12th ed. Philadelphia: W. B. Saunders.

Mulroy, J. F., & DeJong, M. J. (2003). Syndromes of hypercoagulability: Protein C and protein S deficiencies in acutely ill adults. *American Journal of Nursing, 103*(5), 64KK-64SS.

Needle, R. H., Trotter, R. T., Singer, M., Bates, C., Page, J. B., Metzger, D., & Marcelin, L H. (2003). Rapid assessment of the HIV/AIDS crisis in racial and ethnic minority communities: An approach for timely community interventions. *American Journal of Public Health, 93*(6), 970-979.

Ozer, H., Armitage, J. O., Bennett, C. L., Crawford, J., Demetri, G. D., Pizzo, P. A., Schiffer, C. A., Smith, T. J., Somlo, G., Wade, J. C., Wade, J. L., Winn, R. J., Wozniak, A. J., & Somerfield, M. R. (2000). 2000 Update of recommendations for the use of hematopoietic colony-stimulating factors: Evidence-based, clinical practice guidelines. *Journal of Clinical Oncology, 18*(20), 3558-3585.

Pagana, K. C., & Pagana, T. J. (2002). *Mosby's manual of diagnostic and laboratory tests* [pp. 477-483]. 2nd ed. St. Louis: Mosby.

Rote, N. S. (2002a). Immunity. In K. L. McCance & S. E. Huether (eds.). *Pathophysiology: The biologic basis for disease in adults and children* [pp. 168-196]. St. Louis: Mosby.

Rote, N. S. (2002b). Inflammation. In K. L. McCance & S. E. Huether (eds.). *Pathophysiology: The biologic basis for disease in adults and children* [pp. 197-226]. St. Louis: Mosby.

Rote, N.S. (2002c). Infection and alteration in immunity and inflammation. In K. L. McCance & S. E. Huether (eds.). *Pathophysiology: The biologic basis for disease in adults and children* [pp. 227-271]. St. Louis: Mosby.

Rudnicke, C. (2003). Transfusion alternatives. *Journal of Infusion Nursing, 26*(1), 29-33.

Shelton, B. K. (2000). Normal and altered erythrocyte function. In B. Bullock & R. L. Henze (eds.). *Focus on pathophysiology* [pp. 337-357]. Philadelphia: Lippincott-Raven.

Shelton, B. K. & Soloman, A. B. (2000). Normal and altered leukocyte function. In B. Bullock & R. L. Henze (eds.), Focus on pathophysiology [pp. 358-374]. Philadelphia: Lippincott-Raven.

Stillwell, S. B. (2002). *Mosby's critical care nursing reference.* 3rd ed. St. Louis: Mosby.

VanCott, E. N. & Laposata, M. (2001). Coagulation, fibrinolysis, and hypercoagulation. In J. B. Henry (ed.). *Clinical diagnosis and management by laboratory methods* [pp. 642-658]. 12th ed. Philadelphia: W. B. Saunders.

RECOMMENDED READINGS

Aird, W. C. (2003). The hematologic system as a marker of organ dysfunction in sepsis. *Mayo Clinic Proceedings, 78,* 869-881.

Angerio, A. D., & Fink, D. A. (2002). Thromboembolic disease and cancer: Possible new treatments. *Critical Care Nursing Quarterly, 25*(2), 67-73.

Egger, M., May, M., Chene, G., et al. (2002). Prognosis of HIV-1 infected patients starting highly active antiretroviral therapy: A collaborative analysis of prospective studies. *Lancet, 360,* 119-129.

Furie, B., Cassileth, P. A., Atkins, M. B., & Mayer, R. J. (eds.). *Clinical hematology and oncology: Presentation, diagnosis, and treatment.* Philadelphia: Churchill Livingstone.

Otto, S. E. (2003). Understanding the immune system: Overview for infusion assessment. *Journal of Infusion Nursing, 26*(2), pp. 79-85.

Schulman, C. S., & Hare, K. (2003). New thoughts on sepsis: The unifier of critical care. *Dimensions of Critical Care Nursing, 22*(1), 20-30.

Tan, S. J. (2002). Recognition and treatment of oncologic emergencies. *Journal of Infusion Nursing, 25*(3), 182-188.

evolve *Did you remember to check out the bonus material, including free self-assessment exercises, on the Evolve Web site at http://evolve.elsevier.com/Sole/ and on the CD-ROM?*

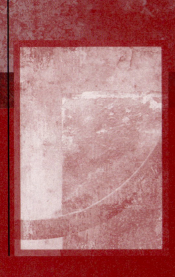

CHAPTER **16**

Gastrointestinal Alterations

Lisa Robinson, MSN, RN, CCRN

OBJECTIVES

- Review the anatomy and physiology of the gastrointestinal system.
- Describe general assessment of the gastrointestinal system.
- Compare the pathophysiology, assessment, nursing diagnoses, outcomes, and interventions for acute upper gastrointestinal bleeding, acute pancreatitis, and hepatic failure.
- Formulate a plan of care for the patient with acute upper gastrointestinal bleeding, acute pancreatitis, or hepatic failure.

Introduction

Body cells require water, electrolytes, and nutrients (carbohydrates, fats, and proteins) to obtain the energy necessary to fuel body functions. The primary function of the alimentary tract (oropharyngeal cavity, esophagus, stomach, and small and large intestine) and accessory organs (pancreas, liver, and gallbladder) is to provide the body with a continual supply of nutrients. Additionally, food must move through the system at a rate slow enough for digestive and absorptive functions to occur but also fast enough to meet body needs. Meeting these goals requires the appropriate and timely movement of nutrients through the gastrointestinal (GI) tract (motility), the presence of specific enzymes to break down nutrients (digestion), and the existence of transport mechanisms to move the nutrients into the bloodstream (absorption). Each part is adapted for specific functions, including food passage, storage, digestion, and absorption. This chapter provides a brief physiological review of each section of the GI system and a general assessment of the GI system. This provides the foundation for the discussion of the GI disorders most commonly encountered in the critical care setting: acute upper GI bleeding, acute pancreatitis, and liver failure. The remainder of the chapter reviews the pathophysiology of each disorder, nursing and medical assessments, nursing diagnoses, nursing and medical interventions, and patient outcomes. Complete nursing plans of care for select nursing diagnoses are provided; these serve as valuable summaries of the most common patient care problems and collaborative interventions.

evolve *Be sure to check out the bonus material, including free self-assessment exercises, on the Evolve Web site at http://evolve.elsevier.com/Sole/ and on the CD-ROM.*

Review of Anatomy and Physiology

GASTROINTESTINAL TRACT

The anatomical structure of the GI system is shown in Figure 16-1. It comprises the alimentary canal (beginning at the oropharynx and ending at the anus) and the accessory organs (liver, pancreas, and gallbladder) that empty their products into the canal at certain points. A review of the anatomy of the gut wall is provided as an introduction to this section because it is the foundation for the understanding of absorption of nutrients and GI protective mechanisms.

Gut Wall

The GI tract begins in the esophagus and extends to the rectum. It is composed of multiple tissue layers.

Mucosa. The innermost layer, the mucosa, is the most important physiologically. This layer is exposed to food substances, and it therefore plays a role in nutrient metabolism. The mucosa is also protective. The cells in this layer are connected by tight junctions that produce an effective barrier against large molecules and bacteria and protect the GI tract from bacterial colonization. The goblet cells in the mucosa secrete mucus, which provides lubrication for food substances and protects the mucosa from excoriation.

Gastric mucosal barrier. In the stomach, the special architecture of cells of the mucosa and the mucus that is secreted are known as the *gastric mucosal barrier*. This physiological barrier is impermeable to hydrochloric acid, which is normally secreted in the stomach, but it can be permeable to other substances, such as salicylates, alcohol, steroids, and bile salts. The disruption of this barrier by these types of substances is thought to play a role in ulcer development. Additionally, these cells have a special feature—they regenerate rapidly—that explains how disruptions in the mucosa can be quickly healed.

Submucosa. The second layer of the gut wall, the submucosa, is composed of connective tissue, blood vessels, and nerve fibers. The muscular layer is the major layer of the wall. The serosa is the outermost layer.

Beneath the mucosa, submucosa, and muscular layer are various nerve plexuses that are innervated by the autonomic nervous system. Disturbances in these neurons in a given segment of the GI tract cause a lack of motility.

Oropharyngeal Cavity

Mouth. Food substances are ingested into the oral cavity primarily according to the intrinsic desire for food called *hunger*. Food in the mouth is initially subject to mechanical breakdown by the act of chewing (mastication). Chewing of food is important for digestion of all foods, but particularly for digestion of fruits and raw vegetables, because they require the cellulose membranes around their nutrients to be broken down. The muscles used for chewing are innervated by the motor branch of the fifth cranial nerve.

Salivary glands. Saliva is the major secretion of the oropharynx and is produced by three pairs of salivary glands: submaxillary, sublingual, and parotid. Saliva is rich in mucus, which lubricates food. Salivary amylase, a starch-digesting enzyme, is also secreted. Stimuli such as sight, smell, thoughts, and taste of food stimulate salivary gland secretion. Parasympathetic stimulation promotes a copious secretion of watery saliva. Conversely, sympathetic stimulation produces a scant output of thick saliva. The normal daily secretion of saliva is 1200 mL.

Pharynx. Swallowing is a complex mechanism involving oral (voluntary), pharyngeal, and esophageal stages. It is made more complex because the pharynx serves several other functions, the most important of which is respiration. The pharynx participates in the function of swallowing for only a few seconds

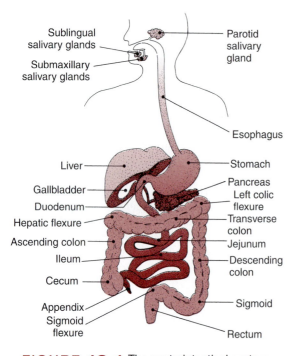

Sublingual salivary glands
Submaxillary salivary glands
Parotid salivary gland
Esophagus
Liver
Stomach
Gallbladder
Pancreas
Duodenum
Left colic flexure
Hepatic flexure
Transverse colon
Ascending colon
Jejunum
Ileum
Descending colon
Cecum
Appendix
Sigmoid flexure
Sigmoid
Rectum

FIGURE 16-1 The gastrointestinal system.

Swallowing Stages

ORAL: VOLUNTARY
Initiation of the swallowing process, usually stimulated by a bolus of food in the mouth near the pharynx

PHARYNGEAL: INVOLUNTARY
Passage of food through the pharynx to the esophagus

ESOPHAGEAL: INVOLUNTARY
Promotes passage of food from the pharynx to the stomach

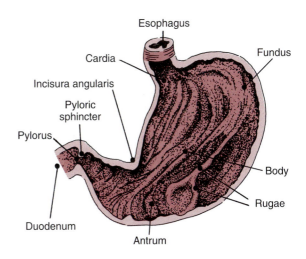

FIGURE 16-2 The stomach.

at a time to aid in the propulsion of food, which is triggered by the presence of fluid or food in the pharynx. Box 16-1 outlines the three broad stages of swallowing.

Esophagus

Once fluid or food enters the esophagus, it is propelled through the lumen by the process of peristalsis, which involves the relaxation and contraction of esophageal muscles that are stimulated by the bolus of food. This process occurs repeatedly until the food reaches the lower esophageal sphincter, which is the last centimeter of the esophagus. This area is normally contracted and thus prevents reflux of gastric contents into the esophagus, a phenomenon that would damage the lining by gastric acid and enzymes. Waves of peristalsis cause this sphincter to relax and allow food to enter the stomach. Mucosal layers in the esophagus secrete mucus, which protects the lining from damage by gastric secretions or food and also serves as a lubricant.

Stomach

The stomach is located at the distal end of the esophagus. It is divided into four regions: the cardia, the fundus, the body, and the *antrum* (Figure 16-2). The muscular walls form multiple folds that allow for greater expansion of the stomach. The opening at the distal end of the stomach opens into the small intestine and is surrounded by the pyloric sphincter. The motor functions of the stomach include storage of food until it can be accommodated by the lower GI tract, mixing of food with gastric secretions until it forms a semifluid mixture called chyme, and slow emptying of the chyme into the small intestine at a rate that allows for proper digestion and absorption. Motility is accomplished through peristalsis. The pyloric sphincter at the distal end of the stomach prevents duodenal reflux.

Gastric secretions are produced by mucus-secreting cells that line the inner surface of the stomach and by two types of tubular glands: oxyntic (gastric) glands and pyloric glands. Table 16-1 summarizes the major gastric secretions.

An oxyntic gland is composed of three types of cells: mucous neck cells; peptic, or chief, cells; and oxyntic, or parietal, cells. Mucous cells secrete a viscid and alkaline mucus that coats the stomach mucosa, thereby providing protection and lubrication for food transport. Parietal cells secrete hydrochloric acid solution, which begins the digestion of food in the stomach. Hydrochloric acid is very acidic (pH, 0.8). Stimulants of hydrochloric acid secretion include vagal stimulation, gastrin, and the chemical properties of chyme. Histamine, which stimulates the release of gastrin, also stimulates the secretion of hydrochloric acid. Current drug therapies for ulcer disease use

TABLE 16-1

Gastric Secretions

Gland/cells	Secretion
Cardiac gland	Mucus
Pyloric gland	Mucus
Fundic (gastric) gland	Mucus
Mucous neck cells	Mucus
Parietal cells	Water
	Hydrochloric acid
	Intrinsic factor
Chief cells	Pepsinogen
	Mucus

H_2-histamine receptor blockers that block the effects of histamine and therefore hydrochloric acid stimulation. The acidic environment of the stomach promotes the conversion of pepsinogen, a proteolytic enzyme secreted by gastric chief cells, to pepsin. Pepsin begins the initial breakdown of proteins. Pepsin is active only in a highly acidic environment (pH less than 5); therefore, hydrochloric acid secretion is essential for protein digestion.

An essential protein secreted only by the stomach's parietal cells is intrinsic factor. Intrinsic factor is necessary for the absorption of vitamin B_{12} in the ileum. Vitamin B_{12} is critical for the formation of red blood cells (RBCs), and a deficiency in this vitamin causes anemia.

The stomach also secretes fluid that is rich in sodium, potassium, and other electrolytes. Therefore, loss of these fluids via vomiting or gastric suction places the patient at risk for fluid and electrolyte imbalances and acid-base disturbances (Table 16-2).

Small Intestine

The segment spanning the first 10 to 12 inches of the small intestine is called the duodenum. This anatomical area is physiologically important because pancreatic juices and bile from the liver empty into this structure. The duodenum also contains an extensive network of mucus-secreting glands called Brunner's glands. The function of this mucus is to protect the duodenal wall from digestion by gastric juice. Secretion of mucus by Brunner's glands is inhibited by sympathetic stimulation, which leaves the duodenum unprotected from gastric juice. This inhibition is thought to be one of the reasons why

this area of the GI tract is the site for more than 50% of peptic ulcers.

The segment spanning the next 7 to 8 feet of the small intestine is called the jejunum, and the remaining 10 to 12 feet comprise the ileum. The opening into the first part of the large intestine is protected by the ileocecal valve, which prevents reflux of colonic contents back into the ileum.

The movements of the small intestine include mixing contractions and propulsive contractions. The chyme in the small intestine takes 3 to 5 hours to move from the pylorus to the ileocecal valve, although this activity is greatly increased after meals. Digestion and absorption of foodstuffs occur primarily in the small intestine. The anatomical arrangement of villi and microvilli in the small intestine greatly increases the surface area in this part of the intestine and accounts for its highly digestive and absorptive capabilities. Located on the entire surface of the small intestine are small pits called crypts of Lieberkühn, which produce intestinal secretions at a rate of 2000 mL per day. These secretions are neutral in pH and supply the watery vehicle necessary for absorption.

In the small intestine, digestion of carbohydrates, fats, and proteins begins with degradation by pancreatic enzymes that are secreted into the duodenum. Pancreatic juice contains enzymes necessary for digesting all three major types of food: proteins, carbohydrates, and fats (Table 16-3). It also contains large quantities of bicarbonate ions, which play an important role in neutralizing acidic chyme that is emptied from the stomach into the duodenum. Pancreatic juice is primarily secreted in response to the presence of chyme in the duodenum.

The small intestine also handles water, electrolyte, and vitamin absorption. Up to 10 L of fluid enters the GI tract daily, and fluid composition of stool is only

---

TABLE 16-2

Electrolyte and Acid-Base Disturbances Associated with the Gastrointestinal Tract

Fluid Loss	Imbalances
Gastric juice	Metabolic alkalosis
	Potassium deficit
	Sodium deficit
	Fluid volume deficit
Small intestine juice/large intestine juice (recent ileostomy)	Metabolic acidosis
	Potassium deficit
	Sodium deficit
	Fluid volume deficit
Biliary or pancreatic fistula	Metabolic acidosis
	Sodium deficit
	Fluid volume deficit

TABLE 16-3

Pancreatic Enzymes and Their Actions

Enzyme	Action
Trypsin*	Digests proteins
Chymotrypsin*	Digests proteins
Carboxypolypeptidase*	Digests proteins
Ribonuclease	Digests proteins
Deoxyribonuclease	Digests proteins
Pancreatic amylase	Digests carbohydrates
Pancreatic lipase	Digests fats
Cholesterol esterase	Digests fats

*Becomes activated only after it is secreted into the intestinal tract.

about 200 mL. Sodium is actively reabsorbed in the small intestine. In the ileum, chloride is absorbed and sodium bicarbonate is secreted. Potassium is absorbed and secreted in the GI tract. Vitamins, with the exception of B_{12}, and iron are absorbed in the upper part of the small bowel. As mentioned earlier, vitamin B_{12} is absorbed in the terminal ileum in the presence of intrinsic factor.

Large Intestine

The large intestine, or colon, is anatomically divided into the ascending colon, transverse colon, descending colon, and rectum (Figure 16-3). The functions of the colon are absorption of the water and electrolytes from the chyme and storage of fecal material until it can be expelled. The proximal half of the colon performs primarily absorptive activities, whereas the distal half performs storage activities. The characteristic contractile activity in the colon is called *haustration;* it propels fecal material through the tract. A mass movement moves feces into the rectal vault, and then the urge to defecate is elicited. The mucosa of the large intestine is lined with crypts of Lieberkühn, but the cells contain very few enzymes. Rather, mucus is secreted, and this protects the colon wall against excoriation and serves as a medium for holding fecal matter together.

ACCESSORY ORGANS

Pancreas

The pancreas is located in both upper quadrants of the abdomen, with the head in the upper right quadrant and the tail in the upper left quadrant. The head and tail are separated by a midsection called the body of the pancreas (Figure 16-4). Because the pancreas lies retroperitoneally, it cannot be palpated; this characteristic explains why diseases of the pancreas can cause pain that radiates to the back. Additionally, a well-developed pancreatic capsule does not exist, and this may explain why inflammatory processes of the pancreas can freely spread and affect the surrounding organs (stomach and duodenum).

The pancreas has both exocrine (production of digestive enzymes) and endocrine (production of insulin and glucagon) functions. The cells of the pancreas, called *acini,* secrete the major pancreatic enzymes essential for normal digestion (see Table 16-3). Trypsinogen and chymotrypsinogen are secreted in an inactive form so autodigestion of the gland does not occur. Bicarbonate is also secreted by the pancreas and plays an important role in enabling the pancreatic enzymes to work to break down foodstuffs. After breakdown by pancreatic enzymes, food is further digested by enzymes in the small intestine and is absorbed into the bloodstream. The presence of acid in the stomach stimulates the duodenum to produce the hormone secretin, which stimulates pancreatic secretions. Protein substances in the duodenum stimulate the production of cholecystokinin.

The endocrine functions of the pancreas are accomplished by groups of alpha and beta cells that compose the islets of Langerhans. Beta cells secrete insulin, and alpha cells secrete glucagon. Both are essential to carbohydrate metabolism. When beta cells are affected by disease, blood glucose levels can increase.

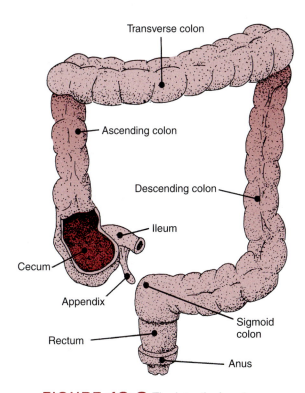

FIGURE 16-3 The intestinal system.

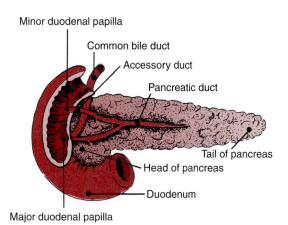

FIGURE 16-4 The pancreas.

The exocrine and endocrine functions of the pancreas are essential to digestion and carbohydrate metabolism, respectively. Therefore, pancreatic dysfunction can predispose the patient to malnutrition and accounts for many clinical problems.

The pancreatic response to low-flow states (decreased cardiac output), or hypotension, is often ischemia of the pancreatic cells. This ischemia is thought to play a role in the release of cardiotoxic factors (myocardial depressant factor), which are known to decrease cardiac output. Pancreatic ischemia can also result in acute pancreatitis, which is discussed later in the chapter.

Liver

The liver is the largest internal organ of the body; it is located in the right upper abdominal quadrant. The basic functional unit of the liver is the liver lobule (Figure 16-5). Hepatic cells are arranged in cords that radiate from the central vein into the periphery. Blood from portal arterioles and venules empties into channels called sinusoids. Lining the walls of the sinusoids are specialized phagocytic cells called Kupffer's cells. These cells remove bacteria and other foreign material from the blood.

The liver has a rich blood supply. It receives blood from both the hepatic artery and the portal vein, which drains structures of the GI tract. The blood supplied to the liver by these two vessels accounts for approximately 25% of the cardiac output.

The liver performs more than 400 functions. The following discussion of hepatic functions is based on the classification by Guyton (2001) and includes vascular, secretory, and metabolic functions. These actions are summarized in Box 16-2.

Vascular Functions

Blood storage. Resistance to blood flow (hepatic vascular resistance) in the liver is normally low. Any increase in pressure in the veins that drain the liver

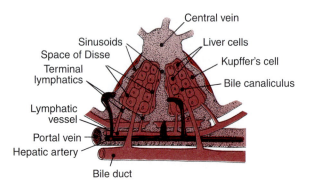

Central vein	
Sinusoids	Liver cells
Space of Disse	
Terminal lymphatics	Kupffer's cell
	Bile canaliculus
Lymphatic vessel	
Portal vein	
Hepatic artery	
Bile duct	

FIGURE 16-5 The normal liver lobule.

BOX 16-2

Functions of the Liver

VASCULAR FUNCTIONS
Blood storage
Blood filtration

SECRETORY FUNCTIONS
Production of bile salts
Secretion of bilirubin
Conjugation of bilirubin

METABOLIC FUNCTIONS
Carbohydrate metabolism
Fat metabolism
Protein metabolism
Synthesis of prothrombin (factor I), fibrinogen (factor II), and factors VII, IX, and X
Removal of activated clotting factors
Detoxification of drugs, hormones, and other substances

STORAGE FUNCTIONS
Blood
Glucose
Vitamins (A, B_{12}, D, E, K)
Fat

---

causes blood to accumulate in the sinusoids. The liver sinusoids can store up to 400 mL of blood. This blood volume can serve as a compensatory mechanism in cases of hypovolemic shock; blood from the liver can be shunted into the circulation to increase blood volume.

Filtration. As mentioned earlier, Kupffer's cells that line the sinusoids cleanse the blood of bacteria and foreign material that have been absorbed through the GI tract. These cells are extremely phagocytic and thus normally prevent almost all bacteria from reaching the systemic circulation.

Secretory Functions

Bile production. The secretion of bile is a major function of the liver. Bile is composed of water, electrolytes, bile salts, phospholipids, cholesterol, and bilirubin. Approximately 500 to 1000 mL of bile is produced daily. Bile salts emulsify fats and foster their absorption. The bile salts are reabsorbed in the terminal portion of the ileum and are then transported back to the liver, where they can be used again. Bile travels to the gallbladder via the common bile duct, where it is stored and concentrated.

Bilirubin metabolism. Bilirubin, a physiologically inactive pigment, is a metabolic end product of the degradation of hemoglobin (Hgb). Bilirubin enters the circulation bound to albumin and is "free," or unconjugated. This portion of the bilirubin is reflected in the "indirect" serum bilirubin level. Accumulation of unconjugated bilirubin is toxic to cells. In the liver, bilirubin is conjugated with glucuronic acid. Conjugated bilirubin is soluble and excreted in bile. Some conjugated bilirubin returns to the blood and is reflected in the "direct" serum bilirubin level.

Excess bilirubin accumulation in the blood results in *jaundice*. Jaundice has several categories including hepatocellular, hemolytic, and obstructive. Hemolytic jaundice results from increased RBC destruction, such as that resulting from blood incompatibilities and sickle cell disease. Viral hepatitis is the most common cause of hepatocellular jaundice (jaundice caused by hepatic cell damage). Cirrhosis and liver cancer can also decrease the liver's ability to conjugate bilirubin. Obstructive jaundice is usually caused by gallbladder disease, such as gallstones.

Metabolic Functions

Carbohydrate metabolism. The liver plays an important role in the maintenance of normal blood glucose concentration. When the concentration of glucose increases to greater than normal levels, it is stored as glycogen (glycogenesis). When blood glucose levels decrease, glycogen stored in the liver is split to form glucose (glycogenolysis). If blood glucose levels decrease to less than normal and glycogen stores are depleted, the liver can make glucose from proteins and fats (gluconeogenesis).

Fat metabolism. Almost all cells in the body are capable of lipid metabolism; however, the liver metabolizes fats so rapidly that it is the primary site for these functions. The liver is also the primary site for the conversion of excess carbohydrates and proteins to triglycerides.

Protein metabolism. All nonessential amino acids are produced in the liver. Amino acids must be deaminated (cleared of ammonia) to be used for energy by cells, or converted into carbohydrates or fats. Ammonia is released and removed from the blood by conversion to urea in the liver. The urea that is secreted by the liver into the bloodstream is excreted by the kidneys.

With the exception of gamma globulins, the liver also produces all plasma proteins in the blood. The major types of plasma proteins are albumins, globulins, and fibrinogen. Albumin maintains blood oncotic pressure and prevents plasma loss from the capillaries.

Globulins are essential for cellular enzymatic reactions. Fibrinogen helps to form blood clots.

Production and removal of blood clotting factors. The liver synthesizes prothrombin (factor I), fibrogen (factor II), and factors VII, IX and X. Vitamin K is essential for synthesis of other clotting factors. The liver also removes active clotting factors from the circulation and therefore prevents clotting in the macrovasculature and microvasculature.

Detoxification. Drugs, hormones, and other toxic substances are metabolized by the liver into inactive forms for excretion. This process is usually accomplished by conversion of the fat-soluble compounds to water-soluble compounds. They can then be excreted via the bile or the urine.

Vitamin and mineral storage. In addition to magnesium, excess amounts of vitamins A, B_{12}, D, E, and K are stored in the liver. The liver also contains up to 30% of the total body iron supply.

Gallbladder

The gallbladder is a saclike structure that lies beneath the right lobe of the liver. Its primary function is the storage and concentration of bile. The gallbladder can hold approximately 70 mL of bile. Bile salts are secreted into the duodenum when nutrients are ingested. The gallbladder is connected to the duodenum via the common bile duct. Bile flow is controlled by contraction of the gallbladder and relaxation of the sphincter of Oddi, which is located at the junction of the common bile duct and the duodenum. Contraction of the gallbladder is controlled by hormonal (cholecystokinin) and central nervous system (CNS) signals and is initiated by the presence of food in the duodenum. Bile salts emulsify fats and also assist in the absorption of fatty acids.

NEURAL INNERVATION OF THE GASTROINTESTINAL SYSTEM

Functions of the GI system are influenced by neural and hormonal factors. The autonomic nervous system exerts multiple effects. Parasympathetic cholinergic fibers, or drugs that mimic parasympathetic effects, are stimulatory to GI secretion and motility. Sympathetic stimulation, or drugs with adrenergic effects, tend to be inhibitory. Parasympathetic and sympathetic fibers also innervate the gallbladder and the pancreas. Other neural regulators of gastric secretions are stimulated by sight, smell, and thoughts of food and by the presence of food in the mouth. In this phase (cephalic), the brain centers reflexively cause parasympathetic stimulation of gastric secretions by chief and parietal cells.

HORMONAL CONTROL OF THE GASTROINTESTINAL SYSTEM

The GI tract is considered to be the largest endocrine organ in the body. Hormones that influence GI function include those produced by specialized cells in the GI tract and those produced by other endocrine organs (pancreas and gallbladder). GI hormones modulate motility, secretion, absorption, and maturation of GI tissues. Table 16-4 summarizes the common GI hormones and their actions.

BLOOD SUPPLY OF THE GASTROINTESTINAL SYSTEM

Blood supply to organs within the abdomen is referred to as the *splanchnic circulation.* The GI system receives the largest single percentage of the cardiac output. Approximately one third of the cardiac output supplies these tissues. The superior and inferior mesenteric and celiac arteries supply the stomach, small and large intestines, pancreas, and gallbladder. The liver has a dual blood supply and receives part of its blood supply from the hepatic artery. Circulation to the GI system is unique in that venous blood draining the system empties into the portal vein, which then perfuses the liver. The portal vein supplies approximately 70% to 75% of liver blood flow.

Because of the large percentage of cardiac output that perfuses the GI tract, the GI tract is a major source of blood flow during times of increased need, such as during exercise or as a compensatory mechanism in hemorrhage. Conversely, prolonged occlusion or hypoperfusion of a major artery supplying the GI tract can lead to mucosal ischemia and eventually necrosis.

Necrosis of intestinal villi can destroy the GI tract's barrier to harmful toxins and bacteria. These bacteria can then enter the blood supply and cause septic shock.

Geriatric Considerations

Several changes occur in the GI system as a result of the aging process. The Geriatric Assessment highlights these changes and related nursing implications (Jarvis, 2004).

General Assessment of the Gastrointestinal System

A comprehensive assessment of the abdomen includes a history, inspection, auscultation, percussion, and palpation. Mapping of the abdomen for descriptive purposes is usually performed by use of the four-quadrant method by drawing imaginary lines crossing at the umbilicus: right upper, right lower, left upper, and left lower. Symptoms such as pain may also be described by the use of these landmarks.

HISTORY

An assessment of the GI system begins with a history, unless an emergency situation exists that requires immediate physiological assessment and intervention. The patient is questioned about any past problems with indigestion, difficulty swallowing (dysphagia), pain on swallowing, nausea and vomiting, heartburn, belching, abdominal distention or bloating, diarrhea, constipation, or bleeding. Problems such as anorexia, fatigue, and headache also point to specific GI ailments and should be noted. All symptoms should be explored in terms of when the symptoms became apparent, any

TABLE 16-4

Actions of Gastrointestinal Hormones

Action	Gastrin	Cholecystokinin	Secretin	Gastric Inhibitory Peptide
Acid secretion	Stimulates	Stimulates	Inhibits	Inhibits
Gastric motility	Stimulates	Stimulates	Inhibits	—
Gastric emptying	Inhibits	Inhibits	Inhibits	Inhibits
Intestinal motility	Stimulates	Stimulates	Inhibits	—
Mucosal growth	Stimulates	Stimulates	Inhibits	—
Pancreatic HCO_3^- secretion	Stimulates	Stimulates	Stimulates	0
Pancreatic enzyme secretion	Stimulates	Stimulates	Stimulates	0
Pancreatic growth	Stimulates	Stimulates	Stimulates	—
Bile HCO_3^- secretion	Stimulates	Stimulates	Stimulates	0
Gallbladder contraction	Stimulates	Stimulates	Stimulates	—

0, No effect; —, not yet tested; HCO_3^-, bicarbonate.

Geriatric Assessment

Physiological Changes	Nursing Implications
Salivation decreased, resulting in dry mouth	Mouth care is essential to keep mucous membranes moist.
Decreased sense of taste	Providing adequate nutrition to those taking oral feedings may be more difficult because food may not be as appealing.
Esophageal emptying delayed	The risk of aspiration is higher; elevate the head of the bed for feedings.
Gastric acid secretion decreased	This may result in anemia; anemia can lead to hypoxemia. Assess complete blood count, arterial blood gases, and pulse oximetry values.
Incidence of gallstones increased	Assess for signs and symptoms of cholecystitis; the patients may be at higher risk for complications of gallbladder disease such as pancreatitis.
Drug metabolism by liver impaired as blood flow decreases by almost half by age 85	Assess for drug toxicity; drug dosages may need to be reduced.
Delayed bowel emptying resulting in higher incidence of constipation	Assess bowel function; patients may need extra fluids, fiber, stool softeners, or laxatives to facilitate bowel function. Provide assistance to facilitate toileting.

precipitating factors, what treatment was sought, factors that relieved or made the symptoms worse, and whether the symptom is current. A weight history is also important and includes usual and ideal body weight along with a history of fluctuations, acute weight loss, and interventions used for weight loss.

Careful pain assessment is a challenging aspect of the history. Pain receptors in the abdomen are less likely to be localized and are mediated by common sensory structures projected to the skin. Therefore, distinguishing the pain of a peptic ulcer or cholecystitis from that of a myocardial infarction is often difficult. Abdominal pain is most often caused by engorged mucosa, pressure in the mucosa, distention, or spasm. Visceral pain is more likely to cause pallor, perspiration, bradycardia, nausea and vomiting, weakness, and hypotension and should also be assessed. Increasing intensity of pain, especially after a therapeutic regimen, is always significant and usually signifies complicating factors, such as increasing inflammation, gastric distention, hemorrhage into tissue or the peritoneal space, or peritonitis from perforation or anastomosis leakage. The nurse obtains a description of the location and the type of pain in the patient's own words.

A history of any GI surgical procedures, including the specific types and dates, should be discussed. A current list of medications is also important, especially because many drugs have GI side effects.

INSPECTION

General inspection of the abdomen focuses on the following characteristics: skin color and texture, symmetry and contour of the abdomen, masses and pulsations, and peristalsis and movement.

Skin Color and Texture

The nurse observes for pigmentation of skin (jaundice), lesions, discolorations, old or new scars, and vascular and hair patterns. General nutrition and hydration status may also be discerned.

Symmetry and Contour of Abdomen

The nurse notes the size and shape of the abdomen and visible protrusions and adipose distribution. Abdominal distention, particularly in the presence of pain, should always be investigated because it usually indicates trapped air or fluid within the abdominal cavity.

Masses and Pulsations

The nurse looks for any obvious abdominal masses, which are best seen on deep inspiration. Pulsations, if they are seen, usually originate from the aorta.

Peristalsis and Movement

Motility of the stomach may be reflected in movement of the abdomen in lean patients and therefore is a normal sign. However, strong contractions are abnormal and indicate the presence of disease.

AUSCULTATION

Bowel sounds are high-pitched, gurgling sounds caused by air and fluid as they move through the GI tract. Auscultation of bowel sounds is performed before the abdomen is manipulated so the frequency of bowel sounds is not altered. Optimal positioning of the patient to relax the abdomen is performed before auscultation is begun. A supine position with the patient's arms at the sides or folded at the chest is usually the recommended position. Placing a pillow under the patient's knees also helps to relax the abdominal wall.

Bowel sounds are best heard with the diaphragm of the stethoscope and are systematically assessed in all four quadrants of the abdomen. The frequency and character of the sounds are noted. The frequency of bowel sounds has been estimated at 4 to 34 per minute, and the sounds are usually irregular. Therefore, the abdomen must be auscultated for at least 5 minutes before an assessment of absence of bowel sounds can be made. Box 16-3 reviews common causes of increased and decreased bowel sounds as they relate to acute illness.

Vascular sounds, such as bruits, may also be heard and indicate dilated, tortuous, or constricted vessels. Venous hums are also normally heard from the inferior vena cava. A hum in the periumbilical region in a patient with cirrhosis indicates obstructed portal circulation. Peritoneal friction rubs may also be heard and may indicate infection, abscess, or tumor.

PERCUSSION

Percussion is aimed at detecting fluid, gaseous distention, or masses. Because of the presence of gas within the GI tract, percussed tympany predominates. Solid masses are dull on percussion. Organ borders of the liver, spleen, and stomach may also be ascertained.

PALPATION

Palpation is used to evaluate the major organs with respect to shape, size, position, mobility, consistency, and tension. Palpation is performed last because it often elicits pain or muscle spasm. Deep abdominal tenderness and rebound tenderness must be differentiated. Rebound tenderness occurs when pain is elicited after the examiner's hand is quickly released after deep palpation. Rigidity or guarding of the abdomen is also noted. Masses in the liver, spleen, kidneys, gallbladder, and descending colon can also be palpated.

Acute Upper Gastrointestinal Bleeding

PATHOPHYSIOLOGY

Many causes of acute upper GI bleeding necessitate admission of a patient to the critical care unit. Box 16-4 reviews the most common causes of this GI emergency.

Peptic Ulcer Disease

Duodenal and gastric ulcers are the most common cause of upper GI bleeding. Duodenal and gastric ulcers are characterized by a break in the mucosa that extends through the muscularis mucosae. The ulcer crater is usually surrounded by either acutely or chronically inflamed cells. Over time, the inflamed tissue is replaced by necrotic tissue, then by granulation tissue, and finally by scar tissue.

The role of gastrin, which stimulates excess secretion of acid, is important in the pathogenesis of duodenal ulcer disease. Parietal cell mass in this patient population is 1.5 to 2 times greater than in persons with no ulcer disease. In patients with normal acid secretion, impaired mucosal resistance to acids is being studied as a cause of duodenal ulcer disease. Duodenal ulcer disease is also associated with several chronic diseases, including chronic pulmonary disease, cirrhosis, renal failure and transplantation, renal stones, and coronary artery disease.

Risk factors for the development of this disease have also been widely studied. Although certain foods, beverages, and spices may cause dyspepsia (Box 16-5), no supportive data indicate that diet causes or reactivates duodenal ulcers. Furthermore, a cause-and-effect relationship between a bland diet or milk consumption and duodenal ulcer disease has not been substantiated.

BOX 16-3

Causes of Increased and Decreased Bowel Sounds

CAUSES OF DECREASED BOWEL SOUNDS
Peritonitis
Gangrene
Reflux ileus
Surgical manipulation of bowel
Late bowel obstruction

CAUSES OF INCREASED BOWEL SOUNDS
Early pyloric or intestinal obstruction
Bleeding ulcers or electrolyte disturbances
Bleeding esophageal varices
Diarrhea
Subsiding ileus

STUDY PURPOSE, METHODS, AND FINDINGS

The purpose of this study was to evaluate the reliability and validity of a behavioral numerical pain scale (the Colorado Behavioral Numerical Pain Scale) in the sedated adult patient undergoing gastrointestinal (GI) procedures. Behavioral pain scales are widely used in a variety of settings, including critical care, and accuracy of the scales have been validated. The researchers noted that assessment of pain during GI procedures is often difficult since the patient is often unable to report pain levels while sedated for the procedure.

The scale was developed by experienced endoscopy nurses who provided suggestions and changes of descriptive words for behavioral assessment of pain from a review of relevant literature. Interrater reliability was established by having three nurses simultaneously rate pain using the scale for 30 procedures. Total agreement was achieved among the three raters for 82% of observations. In 17% of the ratings, one of the three persons disagreed on the rating. The scale was also assessed by having 52 nurses from four hospitals and one ambulatory facility evaluate the instrument. Nearly all (98%) of the respondents agreed that the words described what they observed during GI procedures, and 94% believed the tool described pain better than a patient self-report scale. The researchers concluded that the tool was helpful in quantifying pain during GI procedures. Since the patient is sedated, the nurse must assess physical signs and symptoms to quantify pain and discomfort. The Colorado Behavioral Numerical Pain Scale provides a tool for the nurse to assess pain of sedated patients undergoing GI procedures.

STRENGTHS AND LIMITATIONS

A nonnumerical pain scale is needed for this patient population, because it is neither feasible nor practical to wake a patient sedated for a GI procedure for a subjective pain assessment using a numerical or faces scale. The procedures to establish the reliability and validity of the new scale were clearly described and relevant. One weakness of the study is that data are categorical, and more rigorous statistical tests cannot be applied to the data. Another weakness is that although three hospitals and one ambulatory care facility were described in the research design, research nurse observations were conducted only in the hospital settings.

IMPLICATIONS FOR PRACTICE

Federal agencies and accrediting bodies recommend that both organizations and health care professionals provide optimum pain control throughout the hospital stay, and develop a program that provides up-to-date medications and treatment for pain control. Health care professionals must always suspect the presence of pain, and treat pain before procedures. Nurses must be able to assess pain in a variety of patients, including those that are sedated for GI procedures. Although patients are sedated, they may still experience pain during the procedure. The Colorado Behavioral Numerical Pain Scale provides a method for assessing these sedated patients. It is imperative to test optional instruments such as this one for reliability and validity in a variety of patient populations and settings.

Causes of Upper Gastrointestinal Bleeding

- Duodenal ulcer
- Gastric ulcer
- Cushing's ulcer
- Curling's ulcer
- Stress ulcer
- Mallory-Weiss tear
- Gastritis
- Esophagitis
- Esophageal or gastric varices

Dietary Stimulants of Acid Secretion

- Unrefined wheat
- Coffee
- Cola drinks
- Diet colas
- Acid-neutralized coffee
- Clear soft drinks
- Beer
- Tea

Known risk factors for duodenal ulcer disease are listed in Box 16-6. Alcoholic beverages are acid secretion stimulants and in high concentrations damage the gastric mucosal barrier. Intake of alcoholic beverages is associated with duodenal lesions and upper GI bleeding. Aspirin and other nonsteroidal antiinflammatory drugs may cause acute gastric mucosal damage and chronic ulcers and may precipitate upper GI bleeding.

Cigarette smoking has been causally linked to duodenal ulcer disease. Smoking is thought to impair ulcer healing, is associated with recurrences, and increases the patient's risk of complications. It has been proposed that smoking induces bile reflux, stimulates acid secretion, decreases prostaglandin synthesis, and alters gastric blood flow.

Emotional factors also influence gastric function; however, the specific role of personality types and responses to stressful events as mediated by the CNS has not been clearly linked to duodenal ulcer disease and requires further study.

The cause of gastric ulcers is poorly understood. Whether acid and pepsin damage the mucosa or whether acid and pepsin cause the ulceration once mucosal damage occurs is not known. Gastric mucosal ischemia is also believed to be important in pathogenesis of acute mucosal injury (see discussion of stress ulcers). Abnormalities in mucus production or bicarbonate secretion have also been widely studied. Theoretically, patients with gastric ulcers may secrete lower than normal amounts of mucus or bicarbonate, or they may produce an inferior quality of mucus. Gastric ulcers tend to recur frequently, usually at the same site.

Helicobacter pylori bacteria have been associated with the pathogenesis of various gastroduodenal diseases, including duodenal and peptic ulcer formation.

H. pylori infection can be diagnosed by a quantitative serum antibody analysis (Chernecky & Berger, 2004).

Stress Ulcers

A stress ulcer is an acute gastric mucosal erosion that commonly occurs in patients in intensive care units. The lesions are associated with severe trauma, long-term sepsis, severe burns (Curling's ulcer), cranial or CNS disease (Cushing's ulcer), and long-term ingestion of drugs that have known adverse effects on the gastric mucosa. Abnormalities range from small surface hemorrhages to deep ulcerations with massive GI hemorrhage and occasionally perforation. Massive upper GI bleeding usually occurs 3 to 7 days after the initial insult and significantly increases the mortality rate for the critically ill patient.

Factors associated with stress ulcers are reviewed in Box 16-7. Acid hypersecretion is not associated with all causes of stress ulcers, but some amount of acid is necessary for the formation of an ulcer. Cardiogenic shock directly impairs oxygen supply to the stomach and therefore may impair vascular perfusion of the stomach and cause mucosal anoxia. Stress may reduce both the quality and the quantity of mucus in the stomach. Mucus, a natural defense mechanism in the stomach, delays the diffusion of hydrogen ions into the mucosa. Lowered mucosal pH (less than 3.5) and decreased regeneration of mucosal cells also have been implicated in the development of stress ulcers.

Mallory-Weiss Tear

A Mallory-Weiss tear is an arterial hemorrhage from an acute longitudinal tear in the gastroesophageal mucosa and accounts for 10% to 15% of upper GI bleeding episodes. It is associated with long-term nonsteroidal antiinflammatory drug or aspirin ingestion and with excessive alcohol intake. The upper GI bleeding usually occurs after episodes of forceful retching. Bleeding usually resolves spontaneously; however, lacerations of the esophagogastric junction may cause massive GI bleeding, requiring surgical repair.

BOX 16-6

Known Risk Factors For Duodenal Ulcer Disease

- Alcohol
- Drugs
  - Aspirin
  - Nonsteroidal antiinflammatory drugs
  - Corticosteroids (>30 days; >1 g)
- Smoking
- Genetic predisposition
  - Acid hypersecretion
  - Altered mucosa
- Stress

BOX 16-7

Pathogenesis of Stress Ulcers

- Acid hypersecretion
- Gastric anoxia (hypotension)
- Altered mucosal defense mechanisms
- Decreased mucosal pH

Esophageal Varices

In chronic cirrhotic liver failure, liver cell structure and function are impaired, resulting in increased portal venous pressure, which is called portal hypertension (see discussion of liver failure). As a result, part of the venous blood in the splanchnic system may be diverted from the liver to the systemic circulation by the development of connections to neighboring low-pressure veins. This phenomenon is termed *collateral circulation.* The most common sites for the development of these collateral channels are the submucosa of the esophagus and rectum, the anterior abdominal wall, and the parietal peritoneum. Figure 16-6 shows a liver with collateral circulation. The normal portal venous pressure is 2 to 6 mm Hg. As these veins experience increases in pressure, they become distended with blood, the vessels enlarge, and varices develop. Formation of varices requires that this pressure increase to more than 10 mm Hg. The most common sites for the development of these varices are the esophagus and the upper portion of the stomach. These varices tend to have a low tolerance for pressure and thus tend to bleed. Portal venous pressures of at least 12 mm Hg are needed for varices to bleed.

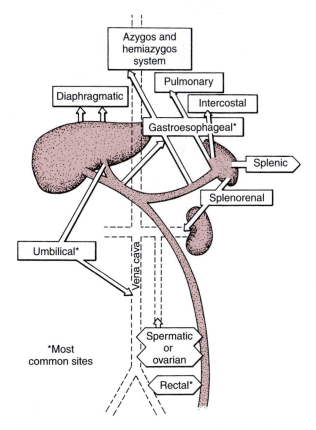

FIGURE 16-6 The liver and collateral circulation.

ASSESSMENT

Clinical Presentation

Patients manifest blood loss from the GI tract in several ways. Hematemesis is bloody vomitus that is either bright red, which indicates fresh blood, or "coffee ground," that is older blood that has been in the stomach long enough for the gastric juices to act on it. Blood may also be passed via the colon. Melena is shiny, black, foul-smelling stool and results from the degradation of blood by stomach acids or intestinal bacteria. Bright red or maroon blood (hematochezia) can also be passed from the rectum. GI blood loss can also be occult, or detected only by testing of the stool with a chemical reagent (guaiac). Stool and nasogastric drainage can test guaiac positive for up to 10 days after a bleeding episode. Hematemesis and melena indicate an episode of acute upper GI bleeding. Hematochezia is usually a sign of lower GI bleeding. When hematochezia is from an upper GI source, it is associated with massive bleeding (greater than 1000 mL). Upper GI bleeding may also be accompanied by mild epigastric pain or abdominal distress, although it is not very common. Pain is thought to arise from the acid's bathing the ulcer crater.

Finally, patients may manifest clinical signs and symptoms of blood loss. The Clinical Alert summarizes the common presenting manifestations of acute upper GI bleeding. Rapid assessment of the patient is undertaken to determine the seriousness of the bleeding, whether it is acute or chronic, and to determine whether the patient is hemodynamically stable or unstable. Patients with acute upper GI bleeding commonly have signs or symptoms of hypovolemic shock. Figure 16-7 describes the pathophysiology of acute upper GI bleeding.

CLINICAL ALERT: CLINICAL SIGNS AND SYMPTOMS OF UPPER GASTROINTESTINAL BLEEDING

- Hematemesis
- Melena
- Hematochezia (massive bleeding)
- Abdominal discomfort
- Signs and symptoms of hypovolemic shock
  - Hypotension
  - Tachycardia
  - Cool, clammy skin
  - Changes in level of consciousness
  - Decreased urine output
  - Decreased gastric motility

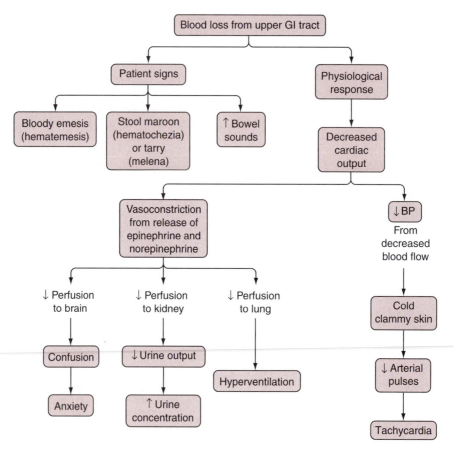

FIGURE 16-7 Pathophysiology flow diagram of acute upper gastrointestinal (GI) bleeding. *BP,* Blood pressure.

Special care should be taken to assess comorbid conditions in the older adult. Such conditions as chronic hypertension or cardiovascular disease could mask signs of shock and make resuscitative attempts difficult.

Nursing Assessment

Assessment of the severity of blood loss is the first priority and includes the frequent monitoring of vital signs and assessments of body systems for signs of shock. Changes in blood pressure and heart rate depend on the amount of blood loss, the suddenness of the blood loss, and the degree of cardiac and vascular compensation. Vital signs should be monitored at least every 15 minutes. As blood loss exceeds 1000 mL, the shock syndrome progresses, causing decreased blood flow to the skin, lungs, liver, and kidneys.

Hypotension is an advanced sign of shock. As a rule, a systolic pressure of less than 100 mm Hg, a postural decrease in blood pressure of greater than 10 mm Hg, or a heart rate of greater than 120 beats per minute reflects a blood loss of at least 1000 mL—25% of the total blood volume.

Hypertension is a common comorbid condition in those at risk of GI bleeding. In the chronically hypertensive patient, normal values for predicting perfusion no longer apply. Emphasis should be placed on other assessment findings, such as level of consciousness and urinary output. As blood pressure decreases, it can be assumed that more blood has been lost.

Rarely, a right atrial or pulmonary artery catheter is inserted to evaluate the patient's hemodynamic response to the blood loss. The electrocardiogram (ECG) may also show ST-segment depression or flattening of the T waves, both of which indicate decreased coronary blood flow.

Abdominal assessment may reveal a soft or distended abdomen. Bowel sounds most often are hyperactive as a result of the sensitivity of the bowel to blood.

In addition to the physical examination, a history is taken to ascertain whether there have been previous episodes of bleeding or surgery for bleeding; a family history of bleeding; or a current illness that may lead to bleeding, such as coagulopathies, cancer, and liver disease. Concurrent diseases also affect the patient's response to the hemorrhage and to the treatment modalities. Patterns of drug or alcohol ingestion and other risk factors need to be assessed and may also help to ascertain the cause.

Medical Assessment

Laboratory studies. The common laboratory studies ordered for a patient with acute upper GI bleeding are listed in Laboratory Alerts. A complete blood count is always ordered. However, the hematocrit (Hct) value does not change substantially during the first few hours after an acute GI bleed. During this time, the severity of the bleeding must not be underestimated. Only when extravascular fluid enters the

---

LABORATORY ALERTS: UPPER GASTROINTESTINAL BLEEDING

Complete Blood Count
Hemoglobin: Normal, then ↓
Hematocrit: Normal, then ↓
White blood cell count: ↑
Platelet count: Initially ↑, then ↓

Serum Electrolyte Panel
Potassium: ↓, then ↑
Sodium: ↑
Calcium: Normal or ↓
Blood urea nitrogen, creatinine: ↑
Ammonia: Possibly ↑
Glucose: Hyperglycemia common
Lactate: ↑

Hematology Profile
Prothrombin time, partial thromboplastin time:
    Usually ↑

Serum Enzyme Levels: ↑

Arterial Blood Gases
Respiratory alkalosis/metabolic acidosis

Gastric Aspirate for pH and Guaiac
Possibly acidotic pH;
Guaiac positive

↑, Increased; ↓, decreased.

---

vascular space to restore volume does the Hct value decrease. This effect is further complicated by fluids and blood that are administered during the resuscitation period. Platelet and white blood cell (WBC) counts may also be increased, reflecting the body's attempt to restore homeostasis. An electrolyte profile is also ordered. Decreases in potassium and sodium levels are common as a result of the accompanying vomiting. Later, serum sodium levels may increase as a result of the loss of vascular volume. Glucose level is often increased related to the stress response. Increases in the BUN and creatinine levels reflect decreased perfusion to the liver and kidneys, respectively. Liver functions tests, clotting profile, and serum ammonia level are ordered to rule out preexisting liver disease. An arterial blood gas analysis is ordered to evaluate the patient's acid-base and oxygenation status. Respiratory alkalosis is common with GI bleeding as a result of the effects of the sympathetic nervous system on the lungs and patient anxiety. As shock progresses, the patient may develop metabolic acidosis as a result of anaerobic metabolism. Hypoxemia may also be present as a result of decreased circulating Hgb levels.

Endoscopy and barium study. The history and physical examination are not definitive diagnostic examinations. Endoscopy is the procedure of choice. Endoscopy allows for direct mucosal inspection with the use of a fiberoptic scope. Flexible scopes allow this test to be performed at the patient's bedside, a preferable approach in an unstable critically ill patient. Endoscopic evaluation of the source of the bleeding is not undertaken until the patient is hemodynamically stable. Barium studies can be performed to help define the presence of peptic ulcers, the sites of bleeding, the presence of tumors, and the presence of inflammatory processes.

NURSING DIAGNOSES

The nursing diagnoses most commonly seen in patients with acute GI bleeding are found in the Nursing Care Plan for the Patient with Acute Gastrointestinal Bleeding.

COLLABORATIVE MANAGEMENT: NURSING AND MEDICAL CONSIDERATIONS

The management of acute GI bleeding initially consists of hemodynamically stabilizing the patient and afterward diagnosing the cause of bleeding and initiating specific and supportive therapies (Box 16-8). The nurse's role during the initial management of acute GI bleeding includes assessing the patient, carrying out prescribed medical therapy, monitoring

Nursing Care Plan for the Patient with Acute Gastrointestinal Bleeding

NURSING DIAGNOSIS: *Fluid volume deficit related to decreased circulating blood volume*

Patient Outcomes	Interventions	Rationales
Circulating body fluid volume will be normal. Hemorrhage will be controlled or resolved. Preload indicators will be WNL. Hct and Hgb levels will be stable. Weight will be stable. I & O will be balanced.	Monitor vital signs for hemodynamic instability, and orthostatic changes. Measure preload indicators: RAP, PAOP. Monitor electrocardiogram, skin, urine output, daily weights, amount and characteristics of GI secretions. Monitor response to blood and fluid replacement. Monitor laboratory values: serial Hct, Hgb, BUN, potassium, sodium.	Early sign of loss of volume and compensatory mechanisms. Preload indicators give information about fluid volume status To monitor volume status and tissue perfusion. This maintains the balance between replacement that is necessary and fluid overload. Hct/Hgb indicate stability of bleeding and outcomes of blood & volume replacement. BUN is the by-product of protein metabolism. Blood being digested in the gut will increase BUN.
	Monitor bowel sounds. Monitor for clinical manifestations of perforation: severe persistent abdominal pain; boardlike abdomen. Gastric lavage as ordered until clear. Administer medications and parenteral fluids. Prepare for endoscopy, assist as necessary, and monitor for complications.	These assess the integrity and function of the gut during an acute episode. Acute events of the gut could lead to perforation, a life-threatening complication of many GI problems. May help to stop or reduce bleeding. To control or stop bleeding and maintain fluid volume status. Especially in patients who are hemodynamically unstable, patients may not tolerate conscious sedation for GI procedures well.

NURSING DIAGNOSIS: *Altered tissue perfusion related to decreased circulating blood volume*

Patient Outcomes	Interventions	Rationales
Signs and symptoms of ↓ perfusion will be absent. ↓ Sensorium, chest pain, renal failure will be absent. Hemodynamics will be stable. Urine output will be > 30 mL/hr.	Monitor for hypoperfusion and hemodynamic instability. Monitor vital signs every 15 min until stable. Measure RAP, PAOP, cardiac output every hour until stable. Monitor for the presence of tachycardia, chest pain, ST-segment elevation, diaphoresis, and cool/clammy extremities.	Prevent end-organ destruction. To assess for hypovolemia and volume status. To assess volume status. GI bleeding can result in low cardiac output and low oxygen-carrying capacity; increased workload of the heart with potentially lowered oxygen delivery can cause myocardial ischemia.

Nursing Care Plan for the Patient with Acute Gastrointestinal Bleeding—cont'd

Patient Outcomes	Interventions	Rationales
Skin will be warm and dry. Bowel sounds will be WNL.	Measure urine output every hour. Monitor level of consciousness. Assess bowel sounds. Monitor for ↑ bilirubin.	Monitor renal tissue perfusion. Monitor tissue perfusion to the brain. Monitor tissue perfusion to the gut itself. Monitor response to blood by-products building in the serum, and liver dysfunction from hypoperfusion in low–cardiac output states.
	Notify the physician of changes and abnormalities.	To promote early intervention and prevent complications.

NURSING DIAGNOSIS: *Anxiety related to hospitalization, hospital regimen*

Patient Outcomes	Interventions	Rationales
Patient and family will demonstrate ↓ anxiety with nursing intervention (e.g., explanations of environment). Patient and family will verbalize understanding of disease, medical and nursing interventions.	Assess the level of anxiety. Explain the critical care unit environment and all procedures. Provide reassurance to the patient and family. Approach the patient and family in a calm, concerned manner. Structure the critical care unit environment to provide rest; limit stimuli as possible. Describe the disease process and all therapeutics instituted. Anticipate treatments and procedures, and provide explanations and reassurance. Provide for patient comfort. Individualize family visitation Involve the patient and family in planning care. Encourage the patient and family to verbalize fears and concerns.	Critical illness produces anxiety, as does the critical care environment. Reassurance and education help to reduce anxiety. Reinforces confidence in the care team. Calming atmosphere is beneficial. Knowledge of current illness and therapies will reduce anxiety. Keep the family informed and less anxious. Comfort may allay anxiety. Maintain a sense of autonomy. Family support and reduce anxiety. Allowing verbalization will reduce anxiety.

NURSING DIAGNOSIS: *Risk for fluid volume excess related to fluid overload from treatment regimen*

Patient Outcomes	Interventions	Rationales
Respiratory pattern will be normal. Lung congestion or pulmonary edema will be absent.	Carefully monitor hemodynamic response to all fluids given. Monitor breath sounds at least every hour during fluid administration.	Monitor for fluid volume excess. Monitor for pulmonary interstitial fluid collection, hypoxia, and signs and symptoms of fluid volume excess.

Continued

Nursing Care Plan for the Patient with Acute Gastrointestinal Bleeding—cont'd

Patient Outcomes	Interventions	Rationales
	Monitor for sudden restlessness or anxiety, dyspnea, tachycardia, coughing, crackles, productive white or pink-tinged frothy sputum, dysrhythmias, abnormal ABG results, blood pressure, ↑ RAP, jugular vein distention.	Symptoms of fluid volume excess.
	Record accurate I & O.	
	Obtain daily weights.	This monitors fluid balance.
	Document and report any abnormalities.	This maintains nurse-physician collaboration.

ABG, Arterial blood gas; *BUN*, blood urea nitrogen; *ECG*, electrocardiogram; *GI*, gastrointestinal; *Hct*, hematocrit; *Hgb*, hemoglobin; *I & O*, intake and output; *PAOP*, pulmonary artery occlusion pressure; *RAP*, right atrial pressure; *WBC*, white blood cell; *WNL*, within normal limits.

the patient's physiological and psychosocial responses to the interventions, monitoring for complications of the disease process or treatment regimen, and providing supportive care. Patient and family support during the acute phase is a nursing priority. Explanations of the diagnostic tests, the medical therapies, and the intensive care environment are extremely important to patients, who are often anxious about their diagnosis and the outcome.

BOX 16-8

Management of Upper Gastrointestinal Bleeding

HEMODYNAMIC STABILIZATION
Colloids
Crystalloids
Blood or blood products

DEFINITIVE AND SUPPORTIVE THERAPIES
Gastric lavage
Pharmacological therapies
  Antacids
  H₂-histamine blockers
  Proton pump inhibitors
  Mucosal barrier enhancers
Endoscopic therapies
  Sclerotherapy
  Heater probe
  Laser
Surgical therapies

Hemodynamic Stabilization

Patients who are hemodynamically unstable need to have immediate venous access (using large-bore intravenous tubes), and administration of fluid must be started. For the restoration of vascular volume, fluids must be infused as rapidly as the patient's cardiovascular status allows and until the patient's vital signs return to baseline. The physician may initially order colloids or crystalloids to achieve this purpose. The nurse's role is to gain venous access and to initiate prompt fluid resuscitation. If massive fluid resuscitation is administered, fluids and blood products should be warmed to prevent hypothermia. Because the blood pressure is the most sensitive measure of adequacy of vascular volume, frequent monitoring of vital signs, at least every 5 to 15 minutes, is a priority. Often, an intraarterial line is inserted for continuous blood pressure monitoring. The goal of fluid therapy is improvement of the circulation of RBCs. Oxygen administration may also be started, which assists in tissue oxygenation.

Patients who continue to bleed or who have an excessively low Hct value (less than 25%) and have clinical symptoms may be resuscitated with blood and blood products. The physician's decision to use blood products is based on laboratory data and clinical examination. Blood is transfused to improve oxygenation (by increasing the number of RBCs) or to improve coagulation (by replacing platelets and plasma). An Hct value may not initially reflect actual blood volume during the first 24 to 72 hours after a hemorrhage and until vascular volume is restored. A reasonable goal for the management of blood transfusions is an Hct value of 30%, but this goal is individually determined for the patient based on clinical assessments. One unit of packed RBCs can be expected to increase the Hgb value by 1 g/dL and the Hct value by 2% to 3%, but this effect is influenced by the patient's intravascular volume status and whether the patient is actively bleeding.

Maintenance of bed rest with the head of the bed elevated is important supportive care geared to prevent further bleeding and to decrease the risk of aspiration. Exertion increases intraabdominal pressure, which predisposes the patient to more bleeding. Keeping the head of the bed elevated also may help prevent reflux of gastric contents into the esophagus. Clearing the nasopharynx of secretions is a nursing priority for the prevention of aspiration, particularly in patients who have an altered level of consciousness and impaired swallowing reflexes. Suction and intubation equipment need to be readily accessible.

In addition to monitoring the effects of fluid resuscitation and blood product administration, the nurse also monitors for complications of the therapy. In patients with preexisting cardiovascular, pulmonary, or renal disease, right atrial or pulmonary artery pressure monitoring may be instituted to prevent fluid administration overload. Frequent assessment of breath sounds by the nurse during fluid administration is an important aspect of care. Careful monitoring for complications of blood transfusion therapy is also important. These complications include hypocalcemia, hyperkalemia, infection, increased ammonia levels, hypothermia, and anaphylactic reactions.

Gastric Lavage

Gastric lavage may be ordered, but this is a controversial therapy in the treatment of upper GI bleeding. Physicians in favor of gastric lavage claim that it helps to indicate the rapidity of the bleeding, helps to ascertain whether there is active bleeding in the GI tract, and serves to cleanse the stomach in preparation for endoscopy. A large-bore nasogastric tube is inserted and is connected to suction. If lavage is ordered, 1000 to 2000 mL of room temperature normal saline is instilled via nasogastric tube and is then gently removed by intermittent suction or gravity, until the secretions are clear. Ice lavage is used in some centers, although this regimen is controversial. After lavage, the nasogastric tube may be left in or removed. Nasogastric tubes left in place may increase hydrochloric acid secretion in the stomach and may cause increased bleeding. Of all upper GI hemorrhages, 80% to 90% are self-limiting and stop with lavage therapy alone or on their own. The nurse must carefully document the nature of the nasogastric secretions or vomitus, such as the color, amount, and pH.

Pharmacological Therapy

Pharmacological agents are used to decrease gastric acid secretion or to reduce acid effects on gastric mucosa. The most common agents used include proton-pump inhibitors, antacids, histamine antagonists (H_2-histamine blockers), and mucosal barrier enhancers. Antacids and antibiotics may also be ordered.

Proton pump inhibitors. Proton pump inhibitors (PPI) are potent and highly specific inhibitors of gastric acid secretion. PPIs (omeprazole or pantoprazole) can be given intravenously followed by continuous infusion for 72 hours in high risk patients, or after endoscopic treatment. PPI can also be given orally in high doses for treatment, followed by maintenance doses (McQuaid, 2004).

Histamine blockers. Histamine blocking agents act to block all factors that stimulate the parietal cells in the stomach to secrete hydrochloric acid. The most common histamine (H_2) blockers are cimetidine, ranitidine, and famotidine. A more recent complication associated with all drugs that increase gastric pH is microbial colonization of the stomach, which may predispose intubated patients to tracheal colonization. This effect may increase the risk for nosocomial pneumonia in these patients.

Mucosal barrier enhancers. Mucosal barrier enhancing agents act on the gastric mucosa to reduce the effects of acid secretion. Prostaglandins are known to improve the mucosal barrier. Sucralfate is a drug used in the treatment of duodenal ulcers and acts to form a protective barrier over the ulcer site. Colloidal bismuth binds to the ulcer base and also stimulates mucus secretion, which prevents further mucosal damage.

Antacids. Antacid agents act as a direct alkaline buffer to control the pH of the gastric mucosa. Administration of antacids is usually ordered every 1 to 2 hours initially. If a nasogastric tube is left in place, antacids may be ordered to maintain the gastric pH at greater than 5. The nurse is responsible for obtaining the gastric pH, for administering the antacid, and for monitoring for side effects of the therapy. The major side effects of antacids include diarrhea, electrolyte disturbances (increased magnesium and sodium ion content), and metabolic alkalosis.

Antibiotics. *H. pylori* infection is often associated with peptic ulcer disease. Triple-agent therapy with a PPI and two antibiotics for 14 days is the recommended treatment for eradication of the *H. pylori* (Wells, et al, 2003).

Endoscopic Therapy

Several endoscopic therapies have been developed for the control of peptic ulcer bleeding. The advantage of these therapies is that they can be applied at the time of diagnosis. Sclerotherapy involves injecting the bleeding ulcer with a necrotizing agent. The most common agents used are morrhuate sodium, ethanolamine, and tetradecyl sulfate. These agents work by traumatizing the endothelium, causing necrosis and eventual sclerosis of the bleeding vessel. Thermal methods of endoscopic therapy include use of the heater probe, laser photocoagulation, and electrocoagulation. All of these therapies act to tamponade the vessel to stop active bleeding. Because they are performed at the patient's bedside, the nurse assists with the procedures and monitors for untoward effects.

Maintenance of airway and breathing during endoscopic procedures is of major concern. Placement of the patient in a left lateral reverse Trendelenburg position can help to prevent respiratory complications. Other common complications of sclerotherapy include fever and oozing from the bleeding site. A more serious complication that can occur when morrhuate sodium is used is the development of acute respiratory distress syndrome (ARDS), which is thought to result from the exposure of lung tissue to fatty substances liberated from the necrotizing agent.

Surgical Therapy

Surgery may be considered in patients who have massive GI bleeding that is immediately life-threatening, in patients who continue to bleed despite medical therapies, and in patients with perforation or unremitting pyloric obstruction. The purpose of emergency surgery in patients with massive upper GI bleeding is the prevention of death from exsanguination. The patient is usually admitted to a critical care unit for initial management and stabilization in preparation for emergency surgery. The most common reason for emergency surgery is massive rebleeding that occurs within 8 hours of admission.

Patients may also become surgical candidates if they continue to bleed despite aggressive medical intervention. Criteria for delayed surgery varies, but it is usually considered in patients who require more than 8 units of blood within a 24-hour period.

Impaired emptying of solids or liquids from the stomach into the small intestine (gastric outlet obstruction) may also necessitate surgical intervention. The major symptoms of obstruction include vomiting and continued ulcer pain that is localized in the epigastrium.

Surgical therapies for peptic ulcer disease include gastric resections (antrectomy, gastrectomy, gastroenterostomy, vagotomy) and combined operations to restore GI continuity (Billroth I, Billroth II) or to prevent GI complications of the surgery (vagotomy and pyloroplasty). An antrectomy may be performed for duodenal ulcers to decrease the acidity of the duodenum by removing the antrum, which secretes gastric acid. A vagotomy decreases acid secretion in the stomach by dividing the vagus nerve along the esophagus. A pyloroplasty may be performed in conjunction with a vagotomy to prevent stomach atony, a common complication of the vagotomy procedure. A Billroth I procedure involves vagotomy, antrectomy, and anastomosis of the stomach to the duodenum. A Billroth II procedure involves vagotomy, resection of the antrum, and anastomosis of the stomach to the jejunum (Figure 16-8). A perforation can be treated by simple closure by use of a patch to cover the gastric mucosal hole (omental patch) or by excision of the ulcer and suturing of the surrounding tissue.

Postoperative nursing care is focused on prevention and monitoring of potential complications. Fluid and electrolyte imbalances are common from loss of fluids during the surgical procedure and drains that are left in place either to decompress the stomach (nasogastric tube) or to drain the surgical site. Additionally, the GI system may not function normally after surgery, with resulting nausea, vomiting, ileus, or diarrhea. Provision of adequate nutrition is essential for proper wound healing. In cases of prolonged ileus after surgery, total parenteral nutrition (TPN) may be considered. Monitoring for proper wound healing is also a nursing responsibility. Signs and symptoms of wound infection (erythema, swelling, tenderness, drainage, fever, increased WBC count) need to be documented and reported. A systemic infection may result from peritonitis in the case of perforation in which stomach or intestinal contents spill into the peritoneum. Postoperative rupture of the anastomosis may also lead to this complication.

Pain is also an important postoperative nursing concern. Abdominal incisions are associated with more postoperative discomfort because of their anatomical location. In addition, postoperative lung infections are more common in patients with abdominal incisions,

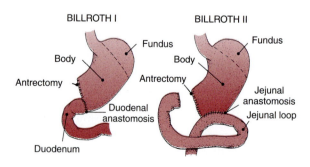

FIGURE 16-8 Billroth I and II procedures.

because incisional pain impairs the ability to cough and breathe deeply.

Specific nursing diagnoses associated with the postoperative care of the patient with upper GI bleeding include the following:

- Risk for infection (wound)
- Risk for infection related to inflammation of the peritoneum
- Risk for altered nutrition (less than body requirements) related to dysfunctional bowel
- Acute pain related to incision
- Impaired gas exchange and ineffective airway clearance related to anesthesia, surgery, decreased activity, pain, and splinting
- Fluid and electrolyte disturbances

Recognition of Potential Complications

Perforation of the gastric mucosa is the major GI complication of peptic ulcer disease. The nurse must be familiar with the signs and symptoms of acute perforation, which are reviewed in the Clinical Alert. The most common signs of this complication are an abrupt onset of abdominal pain, followed rapidly by signs of peritonitis. The goal for the treatment of this patient is preparation for emergent surgery. Fluid and electrolyte resuscitation and treatment of any immediate complications are priorities. These patients almost always have nasogastric tubes placed for gastric decompression. Broad-spectrum antibiotics are also usually prescribed before surgery. Antacids and histamine blockers may or may not be indicated, depending on the cause of the upper GI bleeding. Mortality rates for patients with perforations range from 10% to 40%, depending on the age and condition of the patient at the time of surgery.

TREATMENT OF VARICEAL BLEEDING

Hemorrhaging esophageal or gastric varices are usually a medical emergency because they cause massive upper GI bleeding. The patient typically develops hemodynamic instability and signs and symptoms of shock. Often, the cause of the bleeding is unknown unless the patient has a history of cirrhosis or has previously bled from varices. Initial treatment of patients with esophageal or gastric varices is therefore the same. Top priorities include hemodynamic stabilization and establishment of a patent airway. Gastric lavage may be used to clear the stomach and to document the amount of blood loss. Diagnosis of the cause of the bleeding through endoscopy is the next priority before definitive treatment for the varices can be started.

Somatostatin or ocreotide

Somatostatin or ocreotide (a long-acting somatostatin) are commonly ordered to slow or stop bleeding. Early administration provides for stabilization prior to endoscopy. These drugs decrease splanchnic blood flow and reduce portal pressure, and have minimal adverse effects. Ocreotide is given as an IV bolus of 50 to 100 mcg, followed by an infusion of 25 to 50 mcg/hour. Patients must be monitored for hypoglycemia or hyperglycemia (Wells, et al, 2003).

Vasopressin

Vasopressin (Pitressin) (Box 16-9) is a synthetic antidiuretic hormone. Vasopressin lowers portal pressure

---

CLINICAL ALERT: ACUTE GASTRIC PERFORATION

- Abrupt onset of severe abdominal pain
- Abdominal tenderness
- Boardlike abdomen
- Usually absent bowel sounds
- Leukocytosis
- Presence of free air on x-ray study

BOX 16-9

Vasopressin (Pitressin) Therapy

MECHANISM OF ACTION
Vasoconstrictor: Constricts the splanchnic vascular bed, contracts intestinal smooth muscle, and lowers portal vein pressure.

DOSE
Most commonly given by intravenous (IV) route, although it may be given intraarterially. IV infusion is started at 0.2 units/min. The maximum recommended dose is 0.9 units/min. Vasopressin should be continued for at least 24 hours after bleeding is controlled. Wean slowly.

SIDE EFFECTS
Gastrointestinal: nausea and vomiting, cramping
Cardiovascular: hypertension, cardiac dysrhythmias, exacerbation of heart failure
Neurological: tremors, headache, vertigo, decreased level of consciousness
Integumentary: pallor, localized gangrene

NURSING CONSIDERATIONS
Monitor for angina and dysrhythmias.
Infuse through a central line.
Assess serum sodium.
Assess neurological status.

by vasoconstriction of the splanchnic arteriolar bed. Ultimately, it decreases pressure and flow in liver collateral circulation channels to decrease bleeding. However, vasopressin is not a first-line therapy because of its adverse effects (Wells, et al, 2003).

The critical care nurse's assessments are important during vasopressin administration because this agent has many adverse effects.

Endoscopic Procedures

Sclerotherapy is another option in the treatment of bleeding varices. After the varices are identified, the sclerosing agent is injected into the varix and the surrounding tissue. Usually, several applications of the sclerosing agent several days apart are needed to decompress the bleeding varix.

Endoscopic band ligation is a treatment of varices. Under endoscopy, a rubber band is placed over the varix. This treatment results in thrombosis, sloughing, and fibrosis of the varix. Up to 10 bands can be placed at a time (Savides & Jensen, 2000).

Transjugular Intrahepatic Portosystemic Shunt

Transjugular intrahepatic portosystemic shunting (TIPS) is a nonsurgical treatment for recurrent variceal bleeding after sclerotherapy. Placement of the shunt is performed by use of fluoroscopy. A stainless steel stent is placed between the hepatic and portal veins, to create a portosystemic shunt in the liver and decrease portal pressure (Savides & Jensen, 2000; McQuaid, 2004). Decreasing portal pressure decreases pressure within the varix, thereby decreasing the risk for acute hemorrhage.

TIPS is more effective than sclerotherapy in preventing rebleeding. Its main use is in treatment of patients who do not respond to endoscopic treatment. TIPS has a high rate of reocclusion (50%) within 1 year. Encephalopathy is worsened in about 20% of patients. These risks must be weighed against the risk of bleeding.

Balloon Tamponade

If bleeding continues despite vasopressin therapy, balloon tamponade with a Sengstaken-Blakemore tube may be considered (Figure 16-9). The adult Sengstaken-Blakemore tube has three lumina: one for gastric aspiration, similar to that in a nasogastric tube; one for inflation of the esophageal balloon; and one for inflation of the gastric balloon. A variation of this tube is the Minnesota tube, which has an additional fourth lumen that allows for esophageal aspiration. Inflation of the balloon ports applies pressure to the vessels supplying the varices to decrease blood flow, thereby stopping the bleeding.

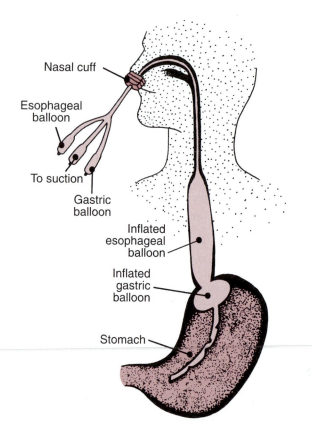

FIGURE 16-9 Sengstaken-Blakemore tube.

The tip of the balloon is inserted into the stomach, and the gastric balloon is inflated and clamped. The tube is then withdrawn until resistance is felt so pressure is exerted at the gastroesophageal junction. Correct positioning and traction are maintained by use of an external traction source or a nasal cuff around the tube at the mouth or nose. External traction can be attached to a helmet or to the foot of the bed. Proper amounts of traction are essential because too little traction lets the balloon fall away from the gastric wall and thereby does not put enough pressure on the bleeding vessels. Too much traction can cause discomfort, gastric ulceration, or vomiting. If bleeding does not stop with inflation of the gastric balloon, the esophageal balloon is inflated and clamped. Normal inflation pressure is 20 to 45 mm Hg. Monitoring of inflation pressures is important for the prevention of tissue damage.

The critical care nurse is responsible for maintaining balloon lumen pressures and patency of the system. The gastric balloon port placement below the gastroesophageal junction must be confirmed by x-ray study. Ideally, the balloons should be deflated every 8 to 12 hours to decompress the esophagus and gastric mucosa. The status of the bleeding varices can also be assessed at this time, and the nurse must be prepared for hematemesis during this procedure. It is crucial that the esophageal balloon be deflated before the gastric balloon is deflated, or else the entire tube will be displaced upward and will occlude the airway.

Spontaneous rupture of the gastric balloon, upward migration of the tube, and occlusion of the airway are other possible complications that need to be assessed. Esophageal rupture may also occur and is characterized by the abrupt onset of severe pain. In the event of either of these two life-threatening emergencies, all three lumina are cut, and the entire tube is removed. For this reason, scissors are generally kept at the patient's beside at all times. Because severe bleeding often results in impaired level of consciousness, the tube inhibits the ability to clear oral secretions. Endotracheal intubation is therefore strongly recommended to protect the airway.

Other complications of the Sengstaken-Blakemore tube include ulcerations of the esophageal or gastric mucosa. Additionally, sores can develop around the mouth and nose as a result of the traction devices. Frequent cleansing and lubrication of these areas can help to prevent skin breakdown. The nasopharynx also requires frequent suctioning because of an increase in secretions and a decreased swallowing reflex. The nasogastric tube should also be irrigated at least every 2 hours to ensure patency and to keep the stomach empty. This measure helps to prevent aspiration and prevents accumulation of blood in the stomach. Ammonia is a by-product of blood breakdown and cannot be detoxified by the patient with liver failure.

Surgical Interventions

Permanent decompression of portal hypertension can be achieved only through surgical procedures that divert blood around the blocked portal system. These are called portacaval shunts. In these operations, a connection is made between the portal vein and the inferior vena cava that diverts blood flow into the vena cava to decrease portal pressure. Several variations of this procedure exist, including the end-to-side shunt and the side-to-side shunt (Figure 16-10). Other surgical techniques for reduction of portal pressure include splenorenal and mesocaval shunting.

Portosystemic shunting reduces portal hypertension and therefore decreases bleeding from esophageal varices. Surgical shunts decrease rebleeding but do not improve survival. The procedure is associated with a higher risk of encephalopathy. The procedure also makes liver transplantation, if needed, more difficult. The nurse needs to be aware that a temporary increase in ascites occurs after all these procedures, and careful assessments and interventions are required in the care of this patient population (see the later discussion of hepatic failure).

PATIENT OUTCOMES

Expected patient care outcomes for each nursing diagnosis for the patient experiencing acute GI bleeding are found in the Nursing Care Plan for the Patient with Acute Gastrointestinal Bleeding.

Acute Pancreatitis

Acute pancreatitis is defined as an acute inflammatory disease of the pancreas. The intensity of the disease ranges from mild, in which the patient develops abdominal pain and elevated blood amylase level, to

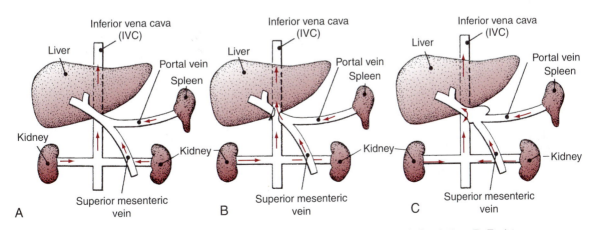

FIGURE 16-10 Types of portacaval shunts. **A,** Normal portal circulation. **B,** End-to-side shunt. **C,** Side-to-side shunt.

extremely severe, which results in multiple organ failure. In 85% to 90% of patients, the disease is self-limiting (mild acute pancreatitis), and patients generally recover rapidly. However, the disease can run a fulminant course and is associated with high mortality rates. Management of this more severe form of the disease requires intensive nursing and medical care.

PATHOPHYSIOLOGY

Acute pancreatitis is an inflammation of the pancreas with the potential for necrosis of pancreatic cells resulting from premature activation of pancreatic enzymes within the pancreas. Normally, pancreatic juices are secreted into the duodenum, where they are activated. These enzymes are essential to normal carbohydrate, fat, and protein metabolism. The way in which the enzymes become prematurely activated has been widely studied, but the exact mechanisms remain unknown. Some theories propose that a toxic agent may alter the way in which the pancreas secretes enzymes. Another theory proposes that duodenal contents that contain activated enzymes enter the pancreatic duct, causing inflammation. Another theory implicates biliary stones that cause obstruction of the biliary ducts and therefore hypertension of the pancreas. Regardless of how the enzymes are activated, enzymatic damage to pancreatic cells (acinar cells) is the outcome of the disease process. Trypsinogen, phospholipase A, and elastase have been proposed as the primary enzymes responsible for the inflammatory process and the resulting systemic complications (Figure 16-11).

Acute pancreatitis has been classified by grading the lesions found in the pancreas. In the mild form, areas of fat necrosis are in and around pancreatic cells along with interstitial edema. This mild form

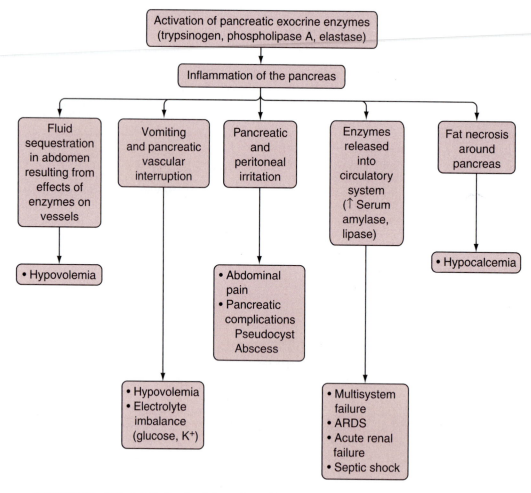

FIGURE 16-11 Pathophysiology flow diagram of acute pancreatitis. *ARDS,* Acute respiratory distress syndrome; *K+,* potassium ion.

may progress to a more severe form, with extensive fat necrosis in and around the pancreas, pancreatic cellular necrosis, and hemorrhage in the pancreas itself. Hemorrhagic pancreatitis is associated with a high mortality rate.

Endocrine and exocrine functions of the pancreas are usually impaired in pancreatitis. Endocrine functions include the secretion of insulin and glucagon. Therefore hyperglycemia, hypoglycemia, and nutritional depletion are commonly seen in all forms of acute pancreatitis.

In most patients, acute pancreatitis resolves spontaneously within 5 to 7 days, with return of normal pancreatic endocrine and exocrine functions. Conversely, severe pancreatitis can affect every organ system in the body. Box 16-10 reviews the major systemic complications of acute fulminating pancreatitis.

It appears that as pancreatic cells are damaged, more digestive enzymes are released, which, in turn, causes more pancreatic damage. Local effects of pancreatitis include inflammation of the pancreas, inflammation of the peritoneum around the pancreas, and fluid accumulation in the peritoneal cavity. Acute pancreatitis can also result in multisystem organ dysfunction syndrome. The release of trypsin is known to cause abnormalities in blood coagulation and clot lysis. Disseminated intravascular coagulation and GI bleeding or infarction can be the result. The release of other enzymes (phospholipases) is thought to cause the many pulmonary complications associated with acute pancreatitis. Respiratory failure and ARDS are the two most common complications. Acute renal failure is thought to be a consequence of alterations in the renin-angiotensin mechanism and of hypotension. Death during the first 2 weeks of acute pancreatitis usually results from pulmonary or renal complications.

Other serious metabolic complications of acute pancreatitis include hypocalcemia and hyperlipidemia, which are thought to be related to the areas of fat necrosis. Hypocalcemia is a major complication and almost always indicates a more serious manifestation of acute pancreatitis. Various hormone imbalances, particularly parathyroid hormone imbalance, are also found.

Occurrence of pancreatic pseudocysts is the most common pancreatic complication and is a part of the necrotizing process. A pseudocyst is a collection of inflammatory debris and pancreatic secretions. The pseudocyst can rupture and hemorrhage or become infected, causing systemic sepsis (see Chapter 10).

Acute pancreatitis has numerous causes, but the most common are alcohol ingestion and gallstone disease. Box 16-11 lists many causes of this disease. Numerous drugs may initiate acute pancreatitis as a result of either ingestion of toxic doses or a drug reaction. Pancreatitis resulting from blunt or penetrating abdominal trauma or occurring after endoscopic exploration of the biliary tree has also been reported.

ASSESSMENT
History and Physical Examination
A diagnosis of acute pancreatitis is based on careful clinical examination and the results of laboratory and radiological tests (see Laboratory Alert). Nurses are responsible for conducting initial and ongoing clinical assessments, for monitoring, recording, and reporting physical and laboratory data, and for coordinating the multidisciplinary plan of care.

In most cases, patients with acute pancreatitis develop severe abdominal pain (Steer, 2000; Friedman, 2004). It is most often midepigastric but may be generalized or localized in the left upper quadrant, often

---

BOX 16-10

Systemic Complications of Acute Pancreatitis

PULMONARY
Hypoxemia
Atelectasis, pneumonia, pleural effusion
Acute respiratory distress syndrome

CARDIOVASCULAR
Hypovolemic shock
Myocardial depression
Cardiac dysrhythmias

HEMATOLOGICAL
Coagulation abnormalities
Disseminated intravascular coagulation

GASTROINTESTINAL
Gastrointestinal bleeding
Pancreatic pseudocyst
Pancreatic abscess

RENAL
Azotemia, oliguria
Acute renal failure

METABOLIC
Hypocalcemia
Hyperlipidemia
Hyperglycemia
Metabolic acidosis

BOX 16-11

Causes of Acute Pancreatitis

- Alcohol
- Biliary disease
    - Gallstones
    - Common bile duct obstruction
- Drugs
    - Thiazide diuretics
    - Furosemide
    - Estrogen
    - Procainamide
    - Tetracycline
    - Sulfonamides
- Hypertriglyceridemia
- Perforation of esophagus, intestine, stomach
- Opiate administration
- Penetrating duodenal ulcer
- Surgery
- Trauma
- Infectious agents
- Tumors, including carcinoma of the
    - Pancreas
    - Lung
- Radiation injury
- Ectopic pregnancy
- Ovarian cyst
- Hypercalcemia
- Heredity
- Idiopathic

LABORATORY ALERT: PANCREATITIS

Serum and urine amylase levels: ↑
Serum lipase level: ↑
White blood cell count: ↑
Hematocrit value: ↑ with dehydration; ↓ with
  hemorrhagic pancreatitis
Calcium level: ↓
Potassium level: ↓
Albumin level: ↓
Glucose level: ↑ with islet cell damage
Bilirubin, AST, LDH levels: ↑
Alkaline phosphatase level ↑ with biliary disease

↑, Increased; ↓, decreased; *AST*, aspartate transaminase; *LDH*, lactate dehydrogenase.

radiating to the back. It usually begins abruptly, commonly after a large meal or alcohol binge. The pain associated with acute pancreatitis is often steady and severe but may increase gradually for several hours. The patient may curl up with both arms over the abdomen to relieve the pain. On physical examination, abdominal tenderness or guarding may be present. Distention of the upper abdomen and tympany may also be present.

Nausea and vomiting are also common symptoms. A hallmark sign of acute pancreatitis is severe abdominal pain that is unrelieved by retching or vomiting. Fever is also a common symptom but is usually less than 39°C (Friedman, 2004). The presence of a temperature higher than 39°C may indicate cholecystitis, peritonitis, or intraabdominal abscess and is associated with more severe forms of the disease.

In severe acute hemorrhagic pancreatitis, the patient exhibits overt signs of dehydration and hypovolemic shock. Patients with more severe pancreatic disease may also have ascites, jaundice, or palpable abdominal masses. A bluish discoloration of the flanks (Grey Turner's sign) or around the umbilical area (Cullen's sign) indicates the presence of hemorrhagic pancreatitis and accumulation of blood in these areas. These signs usually do not appear for 1 to 2 weeks as more of the pancreatic gland is destroyed. Abdominal girth must be measured at least every 4 hours to detect internal bleeding in patients in whom hemorrhagic pancreatitis is suspected (see Clinical Alert).

Diagnostic Tests

The clinical diagnosis of acute pancreatitis requires laboratory and radiological testing because the clinical history, presenting signs and symptoms, and physical findings mimic many other GI and cardiovascular disorders. As an example, the pain associated with acute pancreatitis is like that associated with peptic ulcer disease, gallbladder disease, intestinal obstruction, and acute myocardial infarction. This similarity

CLINICAL ALERT: SIGNS AND SYMPTOMS OF ACUTE PANCREATITIS

- Pain
- Nausea and vomiting
- Fever
- Dehydration
- Abdominal guarding, distention
- Grey Turner's sign
- Cullen's sign

exists because pain receptors in the abdomen are poorly differentiated as they exit the skin surface.

Serum lipase and amylase tests are the most specific indicators of acute pancreatitis because as the pancreatic cells and ducts are destroyed, these enzymes are released. Serum amylase and lipase levels usually increase during the first 24 to 72 hours after the onset of symptoms. In mild pancreatitis, these levels may be close to normal, and if a few days have elapsed since the onset of symptoms, enzyme levels may be completely normal in the presence of acute pancreatitis. Further complicating the diagnosis, an increased serum amylase level is not specific to acute pancreatitis. Other conditions associated with an increased amylase level are listed in Box 16-12. Serum amylase measurement is much more specific if isoenzyme levels (i.e., isoamylase) are increased or urinary amylase level is measured. Serum amylase levels may be falsely decreased in patients with increased blood serum triglyceride levels. Serum lipase level measurement and urine amylase levels are useful in determining a diagnosis (Steer, 2000).

Computed tomography (CT) modalities and magnetic resonance imaging are also used to confirm the diagnosis. These imaging techniques are better than sonography. GI complications of acute pancreatitis, such as pancreatic pseudocyst, abscess or perforation, and obstruction of the biliary tree, are also distinguishable through the use of CT imaging. Endoscopic retrograde cholangiopancreatography (ERCP) combines x-rays with endoscopy and may assist in diagnosis but may also increase the risk for developing pancreatitis (Friedman, 2004). Additionally, x-ray studies of the chest and abdomen are initially obtained in patients presenting with acute abdominal pain to rule out intestinal ileus, perforation, pericardial effusion, and pulmonary disease. Abdominal x-ray studies may also reveal intestinal gas-filled loops, which are signs of paralytic ileus.

Other common laboratory abnormalities associated with acute pancreatitis include an elevated WBC count resulting from the inflammatory process and an elevated serum glucose level, resulting from beta cell damage and pancreatic necrosis. Hypokalemia may be present because of associated vomiting. Hyperkalemia may be a systemic complication in the presence of acute renal failure. Hypocalcemia is common with severe disease and usually indicates pancreatic fat necrosis. Serum albumin and protein levels may be decreased as a result of the movement of fluid into the extracellular space. Increases in serum bilirubin, lactate dehydrogenase (LDH) and aspartate transaminase (AST) levels, and prothrombin time are common in the presence of concurrent liver disease. Triglycerides may increase dramatically and may be a causative factor in the development of the acute inflammatory process. Arterial blood gas analysis may show hypoxemia and retained carbon dioxide levels, which indicate respiratory failure.

Predicting the Severity of Acute Pancreatitis

Patients with acute pancreatitis can develop mild or fulminant disease. As a consequence, research has addressed criteria for predicting the prognosis of patients with acute pancreatitis. The most widely used criteria in this country are those developed by Ranson (1985) (Box 16-13). The number of signs present within the first 48 hours of admission directly relates to the patient's chance of significant morbidity and mortality. In Ranson's (1985) research, patients with fewer than three signs had a 1% mortality rate, those with three to four signs had a 15% mortality rate, those with five to six signs had a 40% mortality rate, and those with seven or more signs had a 100% mortality rate.

High severity of illness scores (APACHE III) and five or more Ranson criteria often predict multiple complications and/or death. Major complications included necrosis, abscess, pseudocyst, hemorrhagic pancreatitis, and ascites.

NURSING DIAGNOSES

Actual or potential nursing diagnoses associated with acute pancreatitis or with systemic complications of the disease process are found in the Nursing Care Plan for the Patient with Acute Pancreatitis.

BOX 16-12

Other Conditions Associated with Increased Serum Amylase Levels

- Salivary gland disease
- Renal insufficiency
- Diabetic ketoacidosis
- Intraabdominal disease (perforations, obstructions, aortic disease, peritonitis, appendicitis)
- Biliary tract disease
- Pregnancy
- Cerebral trauma
- Pneumonia
- Tumors
- Chronic alcoholism
- Burns
- Shock
- Gynecological disorders
- Prostatic disease

Ranson Criteria for Predicting Severity of Acute Pancreatitis*

AT ADMISSION OR ON DIAGNOSIS
Age >55 years (>70)
Leukocyte count >16,000/μL (>18,000)
Serum glucose level >200 mg/dL (>220)
Serum LDH level >350 IU/L (>400)
Serum AST level >250 IU/L

DURING INITIAL 48 HR
Decrease in hematocrit >10%
Increase in blood urea nitrogen level >5 mg/dL (>2)
Serum calcium level <8 mg/dL
Base deficit >4 mEq/L (>5)
Estimated fluid sequestration >6 L (>4)
Partial pressure of arterial oxygen <60 mm Hg

*Criteria values for nonalcoholic acute pancreatitis differing from those in alcohol-related disease are in parentheses.
Modified from Ranson, J. C. (1985). Risk factors in acute pancreatitis. *Hospital Practice, 20*(4), 69-73.
LDH, Lactate dehydrogenase; *AST,* aspartate transaminase.

MEDICAL AND NURSING INTERVENTIONS

Nursing and medical priorities for the management of acute pancreatitis include the following:

- Fluid resuscitation and electrolyte replacement to maintain or replenish vascular volume and electrolyte balance
- Supportive therapies that are aimed at decreasing gastrin release from the stomach and preventing the gastric contents from entering the duodenum (resting the pancreas while maintaining the nutritional status of the patient)
- Analgesics for pain control
- Treatment of systemic complications, the most common being respiratory

Fluid Replacement

In patients with mild or severe acute pancreatitis, some fluid collects in the retroperitoneal space and peritoneal cavity. Initially, most patients develop some degree of dehydration and, in severe cases, hypovolemic shock. Some patients may have sequestered up to 12 L of fluid on presentation of symptoms. Hypovolemia and shock are major causes of death early in the disease process. Fluid replacement becomes a high priority in the treatment of acute pancreatitis.

The intravenous solutions ordered by the physician for fluid resuscitation are usually colloids or lactated Ringer's solution; however, fresh frozen plasma and albumin may also be used. Fluid replacement perfuses the pancreas, an effect that is thought to decrease the severity of the progression of the disease. In addition, the kidneys remain perfused and may prevent the complication of acute renal failure.

Critical assessments for the evaluation of fluid replacement include accurate monitoring of intake and output and daily weights. A decrease in urine output to less than 30 mL per hour is an early and sensitive measure of hypovolemia and hypoperfusion. Vital signs, including blood pressure and heart rate, are also sensitive measures of volume status. Expected patient outcomes must be individualized, but reasonable goals would be maintenance of systolic blood pressure at greater than 100 mm Hg without an orthostatic decrease, a mean arterial pressure of greater than 60 mm Hg, and a heart rate of less than 100 beats per minute. Warm extremities indicate adequate peripheral circulation.

Patients with more severe manifestations of the disease may undergo pulmonary artery pressure monitoring for the evaluation of fluid status and response to treatment. The PAOP is the most sensitive measure of adequacy of volume status and left ventricular filling pressure. A PAOP between 11 and 14 mm Hg is a realistic goal for most patients with this disease.

Patients with severe disease who fail to respond to fluid therapy alone (i.e., hypotension continues) may need medications to support blood pressure (e.g., dopamine, dobutamine). Patients with acute hemorrhagic pancreatitis may also need packed RBCs in addition to fluid therapy to restore intravascular volume.

Electrolyte Replacement

Hypocalcemia (calcium level lower than 8.5 mg/dL) is a common electrolyte imbalance. It is associated with a high mortality rate (see Box 16-13). The exact mechanism for this metabolic complication is not completely understood, but it is thought to be related to decreased binding with proteins in the plasma. Calcium is essential for catalyzing impulses for nerves and muscles, for maintaining the integrity of cell membranes and vessels, for normal clotting of blood, and for strengthening bones and teeth. Calcium is also essential for increasing contractility in the heart. An ECG sign of hypocalcemia is lengthening of the QT interval. Severe hypocalcemia (calcium level less than 6 mg/dL) may cause tetany, seizures, positive Chvostek's and Trousseau's signs, and respiratory distress. Patients with severe hypocalcemia should be placed on seizure precaution status, and respiratory support equipment should be available (e.g., oral airway, suction). The nurse is responsible for monitoring calcium levels, administering replacement, and monitoring the patient's response to any calcium given. Monitoring serum albumin level is also important because true serum calcium levels can be evaluated only in comparison with serum albumin levels. The patient also needs to be monitored for calcium toxicity. Symptoms include lethargy, nausea, shortening of the QT interval, and decreased excitability of nerves and muscles. Hypomagnesemia may also be present in hypocalcemia, and magnesium replacement may be required.

Potassium is another electrolyte that may need to be replaced early in the treatment regimen. Hypokalemia is associated with cardiac dysrhythmias, muscle weakness, hypotension, decreased bowel sounds, ileus, and irritability. Potassium must be diluted and administered via an infusion pump per unit protocol.

Hyperglycemia is, surprisingly, not a common complication of acute pancreatitis because most of the pancreatic gland must be necrosed before the insulin-secreting islet cells are affected. More commonly, hyperglycemia is a result of the normal body stress response to acute illness. Regular insulin, given according to a sliding scale, may be ordered and must be administered cautiously because glucagon levels are only transiently increased in acute pancreatitis.

Resting the Pancreas

Nasogastric suction is used in most patients with acute pancreatitis to suppress pancreatic exocrine secretion by preventing the release of secretin from the duodenum. Normally, secretin, which stimulates pancreatic secretion production, is stimulated when acid is in the duodenum. Nausea, vomiting, and abdominal pain may also be decreased when a nasogastric tube is placed for suctioning early in treatment. A nasogastric tube is also necessary in patients with ileus, severe gastric distention, and decreased level of consciousness to prevent complications resulting from pulmonary aspiration. Oral intake is not usually allowed until the abdominal pain subsides and serum amylase levels have returned to normal. Starting oral intake before these goals are achieved may cause the abdominal pain to return and may induce further inflammation of the pancreas by stimulating the autodigestive disease process. Continuous stimulation of the autodigestive process increases the risk of pancreatic abscess formation. In patients with mild pancreatitis, administration of oral fluids can usually be restarted within 3 to 7 days after onset, with slow advancement of solids as tolerated.

Prolonged NPO (nothing by mouth) status is difficult for patients. Frequent mouth care and maintenance of skin integrity around the nasogastric tube are important nursing actions to prevent injury and to maximize patient comfort. Bed rest is also used to decrease pancreatic secretion stimulation by decreasing the patient's basal metabolic rate.

Nutritional Support

Patients with severe manifestations of the disease may be on prolonged NPO status with nasogastric suction because of paralytic ileus, persistent abdominal pain, pancreatic pseudocyst or abcesses, or other systemic complications. These patients are candidates for TPN. Because patients with acute pancreatitis often have hyperlipidemia as a part of their disease process, lipid supplementation may not be ordered.

Comfort Management

Pain control is a nursing priority in patients with acute pancreatitis not only because the disorder produces extreme patient discomfort but also because pain increases the patient's metabolism and thus increases pancreatic secretions. The pain of pancreatitis is caused by edema and distention of the pancreatic capsule, obstruction of the biliary system, and peritoneal inflammation from pancreatic enzymes. Pain is often severe and unrelenting and is related to the degree of pancreatic inflammation.

A baseline pain assessment is performed early after the patient's admission and includes information about the onset, intensity, duration, and location (local or diffuse) of the pain. Analgesic administration is a nursing priority. Opiate analgesics (e.g., morphine) may cause spasm of the sphincter of Oddi and may exacerbate pain; however, some researchers question whether morphine should be avoided. Meperidine (Demerol) may be ordered in place of morphine if pancreatitis occurs secondary to gallbladder disease (Steer, 2000). Pain medications are administered on a routine schedule, rather than as needed, to prevent uncontrollable abdominal pain. A pain-rating scale, such as a scale of 0 to 10, may also help in determining the amount of analgesia to administer and in evaluating the patient's response to medication. Insertion of a nasogastric tube connected to low intermittent suction may help ease pain. Patient positioning may also relieve some of the discomfort and should be facilitated by the nurse as the patient's hemodynamic status allows.

Pharmacological Intervention

Various pharmacological therapies have been researched in the treatment of acute pancreatitis. Drugs given to rest the pancreas have been studied, specifically anticholinergics, glucagon, somatostatin, cimetidine, and calcitonin, but these have not been shown to be effective. Prevention of stress ulcers, a goal that would be appropriate for this patient population, can be achieved through use of histamine blockers and antacids.

Antibiotics have also been studied in the treatment of inflammation of the pancreas with the idea of preventing pancreatic pseudocysts or abscesses. It is not known whether antibiotics improve survival or merely prevent septic complications (Steer, 2000).

Treatment of Systemic Complications

Multisystemic complications of acute pancreatitis are related to the pancreas's ability to produce many vasoactive substances that affect organs throughout the body. These complications are summarized in Box 16-10.

Peritoneal lavage has been used since the 1960s for the treatment of systemic complications associated with severe acute pancreatitis. The theory behind this therapy is that it removes toxic substances that are released by the damaged pancreas (e.g., trypsinogen, kinins, histamines, and prostaglandins) into the peritoneal fluid. Peritoneal lavage removes these substances before they can be absorbed and exert their systemic effects. It is usually only used when standard therapies are not effective during the first few days of hospitalization. Outcomes of studies show that lavage may be beneficial; however, studies evaluating long-term use need to be done (Steer, 2000).

The procedure for peritoneal lavage involves placement of a peritoneal dialysis catheter. An isotonic solution with dextrose, heparin, and potassium is added. An antibiotic may also be used in the solution. Solution (2 L) is infused over a period of 15 to 20 minutes and then is drained by gravity. This cycle is repeated every 1 to 2 hours for 48 to 72 hours. If peritoneal lavage is effective, the hemodynamic response by the patient is usually immediate.

Close monitoring of respiratory status during peritoneal lavage is essential, because accumulation of fluid in the peritoneum causes restricted movement of the diaphragm. Hyperglycemia may be another effect of this therapy, because dextrose may be absorbed from the fluid into the bloodstream.

Pulmonary complications are common in patients with both mild and severe manifestations of the disease. Arterial hypoxemia, atelectasis, pleural effusions, and pneumonia have been identified in many patients with acute pancreatitis. Arterial oxygen saturation is continuously monitored, and arterial blood gases are assessed as needed. Treatment of hypoxemia includes vigorous pulmonary care, such as deep breathing, coughing, and frequent position changes. Oxygen therapy may also be used to improve overall oxygenation status. Pulmonary emboli have also been documented as a complication of acute pancreatitis. Careful fluid administration is also

necessary for the prevention of fluid overload and pulmonary congestion. Patients with severe disease may develop overt respiratory failure.

Close monitoring and management of other systemic complications of acute pancreatitis, such as coagulation abnormalities and hemorrhage, cardiovascular failure and dysrhythmias, and acute renal failure, are also important. Coagulation defects in acute pancreatitis are associated with a high mortality rate, are similar to disseminated intravascular coagulation, and are treated in the same way. The cardiac depression associated with acute pancreatitis may vary, but hypovolemic shock is a grave presentation. Astute cardiovascular monitoring and volume replacement are required to reverse this serious complication. Impaired renal function has been documented in many patients. Diuretics and vasodilators may be used for the treatment of this complication.

GI complications of acute pancreatitis include pancreatic pseudocyst and abdominal abscess. A pseudocyst should be suspected in any patient who has persistent abdominal pain and nausea and vomiting, a prolonged fever, and an elevated serum amylase level. CT can be helpful in diagnosing the location and size of the pseudocyst. Signs and symptoms of an abdominal abscess include increased WBC count, fever, abdominal pain, and vomiting. CT provides a definitive diagnosis. Early recognition and treatment of a pancreatic pseudocyst are important because this condition is associated with a high mortality rate.

Surgical Therapy

Pancreatic resection for acute necrotizing pancreatitis may be performed to prevent systemic complications of the disease process. In this procedure, dead or infected pancreatic tissue is surgically removed. In some cases, the entire pancreas is removed. Usually, the indication for surgical intervention is clinical deterioration of the patient despite the use of conventional treatments, or the presence of peritonitis.

Surgery may also be indicated for pseudocysts; however, surgery is usually delayed because some pseudocysts resolve spontaneously. Surgical treatment of a pseudocyst can be performed through internal or external drainage or needle aspiration. Acute surgical intervention may be required if the pseudocyst becomes infected or perforated.

Surgery may also be performed when gallstones are thought to be the cause of the acute pancreatitis. A cholecystectomy is usually performed.

PATIENT OUTCOMES

Expected outcomes for the patient with acute pancreatitis are found in the Nursing Care Plan for the Patient with Acute Pancreatitis.

Nursing Care Plan for the Patient with Acute Pancreatitis

NURSING DIAGNOSIS: *Fluid volume deficit related to loss of fluid into peritoneal cavity, dehydration from nausea and vomiting, fever, nasogastric suction, defects in coagulation*

Patient Outcomes	Interventions	Rationales
Heart rate will be < 100. PAOP pressure will be WNL. Urine output will be > 30 mL/hr. Extremities will be warm and dry. Hct and Hgb values will be stable. No bleeding will occur. The patient will be afebrile.	Monitor hemodynamic status closely, VS, pulmonary artery pressures, urine output, I & O, daily weight, and peripheral circulation. Administer fluid replacements, blood or blood products, and monitor patient response to treatment. Monitor for signs and symptoms of hemorrhage, Hct and Hgb values, Cullen's sign, or Turner's sign. Measure abdominal girth every 4 hr. Monitor temperature and treat fever as ordered	Indicates fluid volume status. Appropriate fluid volume to maintain cardiac output and oxygen-carrying capacity. Cullen's and Turner's signs indicate free blood in the retroperitoneal and abdominal cavities. Determine presence of intraabdominal bleeding. High fevers can be associated with pancreatitis.

NURSING DIAGNOSIS: *Pain related to interruption of blood supply to the pancreas, edema and distention of the pancreas, and peritoneal irritation*

Patient Outcomes	Interventions	Rationales
Pain will be within tolerable levels.	Perform a pain assessment, noting onset, duration, intensity, and location. Control pain with the drug of choice: (morphine) or equal analgesic. Schedule pain medication to prevent severe pain episodes. Differentiate pain from cardiac origin. Keep activities at a minimum. Maintain bed rest restriction. Position the patient to optimize comfort. Administer sedation as needed.	Establish baseline assessment. Release of cytokines is due to the acute pain event. Pancreatitis is very painful thus pain management is essential A risk of acute cardiac events exists due to the release of myocardial depressant factor and a low cardiac output state from hypovolemia. Rest the GI tract to rest the pancreas. This promotes comfort. Pain control and comfort measures optimize the patient's outcomes. Anxiety and pain can be experienced from the acute critical illness.

NURSING DIAGNOSIS: *Altered nutrition (less than body requirements) related to nausea and vomiting, depressed appetite, alcoholism, and impaired nutrient metabolism caused by pancreatic injury and altered production of digestive enzymes*

Patient Outcomes	Interventions	Rationales
Positive nitrogen balance will be achieved.	Assess nutritional status through clinical examination and laboratory analysis.	Proper nutrition is one of the key elements of treatment as the digestive enzymes functions are altered.

Continued

Nursing Care Plan for the Patient with Acute Pancreatitis—cont'd

Patient Outcomes	Interventions	Rationales
Serum albumin level will be normal. Weight will be stable.	Calculate caloric needs and compare with actual intake. Provide adequate nutritional intake. Offer nutritional supplements. Administer TPN as ordered. Prevent complications by using aseptic technique for central lines. Monitor glucose and other electrolyte levels.	A high metabolic state results from an acute infectious process. Resting the gut is important treatment in pancreatitis. High risk of line sepsis with central catheters and TPN administration. To assess for complications of TPN.

NURSING DIAGNOSIS: *Impaired gas exchange related to atelectasis, pleural effusions, acute respiratory distress syndrome, fluid overload during fluid administration, pulmonary emboli, and splinting from pain*

Patient Outcomes	Interventions	Rationales
PaO_2 will be >80 mm Hg. $PaCO_2$ will be within normal limits or at baseline. Pulmonary complications will be absent or resolved.	Monitor pulmonary status closely. Auscultate breath sounds every 4 hr. Monitor the respiratory rate. Administer vigorous pulmonary hygiene, coughing and deep breathing, and humidification therapy. Note pulmonary secretions for amount, color, consistency, and presence of an odor. Administer oxygen as prescribed. Monitor ABGs and pulse oximetry values. Administer analgesia to prevent pain caused by splinting. Reposition the patient frequently.	Pulmonary complications can be life-threatening. Tachypnea is an early sign of respiratory compromise. Pulmonary complications are common with fulminate, acute pancreatitis. Pulmonary hygiene reduces these risks. Indicative of pulmonary compromise such as pulmonary edema and pneumonia. Optimize oxygenation. Early indication of improper ventilation. Maintain normal depth of respiration and avoid atelectasis. Turning the patient maximizes ventilation and perfusion and to prevent pooling of secretions.

NURSING DIAGNOSIS: *Electrolyte imbalance related to prolonged nausea and vomiting, gastric suction, autodigestive process, and therapeutic regimen*

Patient Outcomes	Interventions	Rationales
Electrolytes and glucose will be WNL.	Monitor electrolyte balance carefully and administer replacements according to unit protocol. Monitor blood glucose every 6 hr. Assess fluid balance by evaluating electrolyte values.	Electrolyte balance ensures normal cellular environment and functions. Abnormal glucose may occur from disruption of pancreatic functions and TPN. Fluid balance is reflected in electrolyte values.

ABG, Arterial blood gas; *GI,* gastrointestinal; *Hct,* hematocrit; *Hgb,* hemoglobin; *I & O,* intake and output; *PaCO₂,* partial pressure of carbon dioxide in arterial blood; *PaO₂,* partial pressure of oxygen in arterial blood; *PAOP,* pulmonary artery occlusion pressure; *TPN,* total parenteral nutrition; *VS,* vital signs; *WNL,* within normal limits.

Hepatic Failure

PATHOPHYSIOLOGY

Hepatic, or liver, failure results when the liver is unable to perform its many functions. These functions are reviewed in Box 16-2. Liver failure can result from necrosis or a decrease in the blood supply to liver cells. This problem is most often caused by hepatitis or inflammation of the liver. Liver failure can also result from chronic liver disease, in which healthy liver tissue is replaced by fibrotic tissue. This form of liver failure is called *cirrhosis*. Finally, liver cells can be replaced by fatty cells or tissue and is known as *fatty liver disease*.

Hepatitis

Hepatitis is an acute inflammation of liver cells, or hepatocytes. Other cells in the liver may also be inflamed. This inflammation is accompanied by edema, and early in the course of the disease, no disturbance exists in the architecture of the liver. The normal liver architecture is pictured in Figure 16-5 and is characterized by a basic functional unit of the liver called a lobule. The liver lobule is uniquely made in that it has its own blood supply, which allows the liver cells to be exposed continuously to blood. As the inflammation progresses, the normal pattern of the liver is disturbed by the inflammatory process. This interrupts the normal blood supply to liver cells, causing necrosis and breakdown of healthy cells. Blood backs up in the portal system, causing increased pressure, known as portal hypertension. Liver cells have the capacity to regenerate. Over time, liver cells that become damaged are removed by the body's immune system and are replaced with healthy liver cells. Therefore, most patients with hepatitis recover and regain normal liver function.

Hepatitis is most often caused by a viral disease. Several hepatitis viruses have been identified: hepatitis A, B, C, D, E, F, and G. Researchers continue to study other viruses that may be associated with acute hepatitis. Modes of transmission are summarized in Box 16-14.

BOX 16-14

Modes of Transmission For Hepatitis

- Contact with blood
- Contact with blood products
- Contact with semen
- Contact with saliva
- Percutaneously through mucous membranes
- Direct contact with infected fluids or objects

Types of Hepatitis

Hepatitis A. Hepatitis A is the most common type of viral hepatitis. The virus infects the liver and is eliminated by the feces. This virus is primarily spread through oral ingestion of food, water, and shellfish that have been infected by fecal contaminants. This disease is usually mild in presentation; therefore, many persons may have had the disease without being aware of it. The disease is self-limiting.

Hepatitis B. Hepatitis B is usually a more serious form of hepatitis. Persons are considered infectious as long as antigens for the virus are found in the bloodstream. Hepatitis B is spread primarily by blood, blood products, and body fluids or secretions, such as semen. The virus can spread percutaneously (e.g., via contaminated needles), through mucous membranes, through contact with infected fluids, or during childbirth. Health care providers are at risk of contracting this form of hepatitis. Hepatitis B can result in the development of a carrier state, chronic hepatitis, cirrhosis, or liver cancer.

Hepatitis C. Hepatitis C is transmitted through blood or body fluids, and from mother to child during childbirth. This risk of infection is highest in injecting drug users (CDC, 2004). The virus is usually mild in presentation, and 80% of persons do not exhibit symptoms. However, up to 85% of infected persons progress to chronic infection. Hepatitis C is the leading indicator for liver transplants (CDC, 2004).

Hepatitis D. Hepatitis D always occurs in the presence of hepatitis B and relies on the virus to spread. The hepatitis D virus is transmitted in the same way as the hepatitis B virus. Hepatitis D virus can result in the development of chronic liver disease.

Hepatitis E. Hepatitis E refers to an epidemic form of hepatitis that is similar in characteristics to hepatitis A. It is transmitted via the fecal-oral route and does not progress to a chronic phase. The disease is common in developing countries.

Hepatitis F and G. These variations are similar to hepatitis C. Researchers are currently investigating these viruses (Friedman, 2004).

Assessment

Patients with hepatitis are often asymptomatic. In many patients, prodromal symptoms of anorexia, nausea, vomiting, abdominal pain, and fatigue may be present. Symptoms may then progress to a low-grade fever, an enlarged and tender liver, and jaundice (Friedman, 2004; CDC, 2004.)

LABORATORY ALERTS: LIVER FAILURE

Serum or Plasma	Alteration
Albumin	↓
Ammonia	↑
Bile pigments	
Total bilirubin	↑
Direct or conjugated bilirubin	↑
Cholesterol	↑
Coagulation tests	
Prothrombin time	Prolonged
Partial thromboplastin time	Prolonged
Enzymes	
APT	↑
AST	↑
ALT	↑
Urine	
Bilirubin	↑
Urobilinogen	↑

↑, Increased; ↓, decreased; *ALT*, alanine transaminase; *APT*, alkaline phosphatase; *AST*, aspartate transaminase.

Assessment of risk factors often assists in diagnosis of hepatitis. Laboratory tests may show elevated liver function tests. Diagnosis is confirmed by identification of antibodies specific to each type of hepatitis.

Recovery from acute hepatitis usually occurs within 9 weeks for hepatitis A, and 16 weeks for hepatitis B. Hepatitis B, C, D, and G may progress to chronic forms (Friedman, 2004).

CLINICAL ALERT: SIGNS AND SYMPTOMS OF FULMINANT HEPATIC FAILURE

- Hyperexcitability
- Insomnia
- Irritability
- Decreased level of consciousness, coma
- Convulsions
- Sudden onset of high fever
- Nausea and vomiting
- Chills
- Jaundice

NURSING DIAGNOSES

Nursing diagnoses associated with viral hepatitis include the following:
- Activity intolerance related to fatigue, fever, and flulike symptoms
- Altered nutrition (less than body requirements) related to loss of appetite, nausea, vomiting, and loss of liver metabolic functions
- Risk for infection related to loss of liver cell function for phagocytosis of bacteria
- Risk for altered thought processes related to medications that require liver metabolism

MEDICAL AND NURSING INTERVENTIONS

No definitive treatment for acute inflammation of the liver exists. Goals for medical and nursing care include providing rest and assisting the patient in obtaining optimal nutrition.

Rest is important, particularly in the early stages of hepatitis. The patient's severe fatigue often requires frequent periods of rest. Bed rest is generally not required. Most patients can be cared for at home unless the disease becomes prolonged or fulminant failure develops. Medications to help the patient rest or to decrease agitation must be closely monitored because most of these drugs require clearance by the liver, which is impaired during the acute phase.

Maintenance of the nutritional status of the patient is a nursing priority. Loss of appetite, nausea, and vomiting may persist for weeks. Nursing measures such as administration of antiemetics may be helpful. Small, frequent meals and supplements should be offered. Palatable meals should be given as tolerated. Evaluation of nutritional status is ongoing and includes assessments of intake, output, daily weights, serum albumin level, and nitrogen balance. Patients must be instructed not to take any over-the-counter drugs that can cause liver damage. Box 16-15 lists common hepatotoxic drugs. Alcohol should be avoided.

Hepatitis can lead to acute hepatic failure. The clinical manifestations of this disorder are discussed in the section on impaired metabolic processes and impaired bile formation and flow.

Special precautions must be taken to prevent spread of the virus in the care of the patient with hepatitis. These include the following:
- Wearing gloves while handling all items that are contaminated with the patient's body secretions
- Disposable patient care items, such as thermometers, dishes, and eating utensils
- Private room and bathroom for patients who are fecally incontinent
- Gowns when direct patient care is provided

BOX 16-15

Common Hepatotoxic Drugs

- **Analgesics**
  - Acetaminophen (Tylenol)
  - Salicylates (aspirin)
- **Anesthetics**
  - Enflurane (Ethrane)
  - Halothane (Fluothane)
  - Methoxyflurane (Penthrane)
- **Anticonvulsants**
  - Phenytoin (Dilantin)
  - Phenobarbital (Luminal)
- **Antidepressants**
  - Monoamine oxidase inhibitors
  - Amitriptyline (Elavil)
  - Doxepin (Sinequan)
- **Antimicrobial agents**
  - Isoniazid
  - Nitrofurantoin (Macrodantin)
  - Rifampin
  - Sulfonamides (sulfisoxazole acetyl [Gantrisin], silver sulfadiazine [Silvadene])
  - Tetracycline
- **Antipsychotic drugs**
  - Haloperidol (Haldol)
  - Chlorpromazine (Thorazine)
  - Fluphenazine (Prolixin)
  - Prochlorperazine (Compazine)
  - Promethazine (Phenergan)
  - Thioridazine (Mellaril)
- **Cardiovascular drugs**
  - Methyldopa (Aldomet)
  - Quinidine sulfate
- **Hormonal agents**
  - Antithyroid drugs
  - Oral contraceptives
  - Oral hypoglycemics
  - Tolbutamide (Orinase)
  - Chlorpropamide (Diabinese)
- **Sedatives**
  - Chlordiazepoxide (Librium)
  - Diazepam (Valium)
- **Others**
  - Cimetidine (Tagamet)

- Universal precautions for bagging and labeling of linen or any hospital equipment that is contaminated with feces or blood

Teaching the patient and family hand-washing and personal hygiene techniques is important. Counseling may be necessary for patients in whom sexual transmission of the disease is suspected.

Hepatitis B screening is also recommended for all pregnant women and for all patients who test positive for human immunodeficiency virus (HIV).

Prophylaxis is available for hepatitis A and hepatitis B virus in the form of a vaccine. Immune globulin can be administered to persons both before and after exposure to the virus. Preexposure prophylaxis with hepatitis A vaccine is recommended in persons traveling to countries where hepatitis A is prevalent and in high-risk groups. Hepatitis B vaccine is recommended for health care workers and other high-risk groups. Some states have mandated hepatitis B vaccinations for school-age children.

Patients with hepatitis C are often treated to prevent progression of the disease process. The recommended treatment is a combination therapy of pegylated interferon and ribavirin. This drug therapy can rid the virus in 50 to 80% of patients, depending on the genotype of the hepatitis C virus (CDC, 2004; Friedman, 2004). Other therapies are under investigation.

PATIENT OUTCOMES

Resolution of hepatitis can be evaluated based on the following criteria:

- The patient is able to tolerate increasing levels of activity.
- Abdominal pain is absent.
- Liver function test results return to baseline.
- Serological test results indicate the absence of active virus.
- Nutritional status is maintained.
- Infection is absent.
- Thought processes return to baseline.

Cirrhosis

Cirrhosis causes severe alterations in the structure and function of liver cells. It is characterized by inflammation and liver cell necrosis that may be focal or diffuse. Fat deposits may also be present. The enlarged liver cells cause compression of the liver lobule and lead to increased resistance to blood flow and portal hypertension. Necrosis is followed by regeneration of liver tissue, but not in a normal fashion. Fibrous tissue is laid down over time, and this distorts the normal architecture of the liver lobule. These fibrotic changes are usually irreversible, resulting in chronic liver dysfunction.

Four types of cirrhosis exist: (1) alcoholic (Laënnec's), (2) biliary, (3) cardiac, and (4) postnecrotic. Laënnec's cirrhosis, which results from long-term alcohol abuse, is the most common type in the United States. Alcohol is known to be toxic to the liver; however, not all patients with alcoholism develop cirrhosis. Other alcohol-induced injuries of the liver include fatty liver and alcoholic hepatitis. These may occur independently or along with cirrhosis. Acetaldehyde, a toxic metabolite of alcohol ingestion, causes liver cell damage and death. Fibrotic tissue replaces liver cells and ultimately causes the liver to shrink. In end-stage disease, almost all liver cells are replaced by this tissue.

Biliary cirrhosis is caused by a decrease in bile flow, which is most commonly caused by long-term obstruction of bile ducts. It eventually leads to degeneration and fibrosis of the ducts.

Cardiac cirrhosis is most commonly caused by severe long-term right-sided congestive heart failure. Decreased oxygenation of liver cells and cellular death characterize this disease.

Postnecrotic cirrhosis can be a result of exposure to hepatotoxins, chemicals, or infection, or it can be caused by a metabolic disorder. It results in the massive death of liver cells, and it is also associated with the development of liver cancer.

Fatty Liver

Fatty liver is an accumulation of excessive fats in the liver; it is morphologically distinguishable from cirrhosis. Alcohol abuse is the most common cause of this disorder. Other causes include obesity, diabetes, hepatic resection, starvation, and TPN. Damage caused by the fat deposits may result in liver dysfunction, failure, and death.

ASSESSMENT OF HEPATIC FAILURE
Presenting Clinical Signs

Initial clinical signs of hepatic failure are vague and include weakness, fatigue, loss of appetite, weight loss, abdominal discomfort, nausea and vomiting, and change in bowel habits. As destruction in the liver progresses, the systemic effects of the disease become apparent. Impaired liver function results in loss of the normal vascular, secretory, and metabolic functions of the liver (see Box 16-2). The functional sequelae of liver disease can be divided into three categories: (1) portal hypertension, (2) reduced liver metabolic processes, and (3) impaired bile formation and flow. These derangements and their clinical manifestations are summarized in Box 16-16.

Portal hypertension. Portal hypertension causes two main clinical problems for the patient: hyperdynamic circulation and development of esophageal or gastric varices. Liver cell destruction causes shunting of blood and increased cardiac output. Vasodilation is also present, which causes decreased perfusion to all body organs, even though the cardiac output is very high. This phenomenon is known as high-output failure, or hyperdynamic circulation. Clinical signs

---

BOX 16-16

Clinical Signs and Symptoms of Liver Disease

- **Cardiac**
  Hyperdynamic circulation
  Portal hypertension
  Dysrhythmias
  Activity intolerance
  Edema
- **Dermatological**
  Jaundice
  Spider angiomas
  Pruritus
- **Electrolyte**
  Hypokalemia
  Hyponatremia (dilutional)
  Hypernatremia
- **Endocrine**
  Increased aldosterone
  Increased antidiuretic hormone
- **Fluid**
  Ascites
  Water retention
  Decreased volume in vascular space
- **Gastrointestinal**
  Abdominal discomfort
  Decreased appetite
  Diarrhea
  Varices or gastrointestinal bleeding
  Malnutrition
  Nausea and vomiting
- **Hematological**
  Anemia
  Impaired coagulation
  Disseminated intravascular coagulation
- **Immune system**
  Increased susceptibility to infection
- **Neurological**
  Hepatic encephalopathy
- **Pulmonary**
  Dyspnea
  Hyperventilation
  Hypoxemia
  Ineffective breathing patterns
- **Renal**
  Hepatorenal syndrome

---

and symptoms of this disorder are identical to those of heart failure and include jugular vein distention, crackles, and decreased perfusion to all organs. Initially, the patient may have hypertension, flushed skin, and bounding pulses. Blood pressure decreases eventually. Dysrhythmias are also common. Increased portal venous pressure causes the formation of varices that shunt blood to decrease pressure. These varices are problematic because they can bleed, causing massive upper GI bleeding (see the earlier discussion of upper GI bleeding). The most common sites are in the esophageal and gastric areas. Splenomegaly is also associated with portal hypertension.

Impaired metabolic processes. The liver is the most complex organ because of all of its metabolic processes. Liver failure causes the following: altered carbohydrate, fat, and protein metabolism; decreased synthesis of blood clotting factors; decreased removal of activated clotting components; decreased metabolism of vitamins and iron; decreased storage functions; and decreased detoxification functions.

Altered carbohydrate metabolism may result in unstable blood glucose level. The serum glucose level is usually increased to more than 200 mg/dL. This condition is termed *cirrhotic diabetes.* Altered carbohydrate metabolism may also result in malnutrition and a decreased stress response.

Altered fat metabolism may result in a fatty liver. Fat is used by all cells for energy, and altered metabolism may cause fatigue and decreased activity tolerance in many patients. Alterations in skin integrity, which are common in chronic liver disease, are also thought to be related to this metabolic dysfunction. Bile salts are also not adequately produced, and this leads to an inability of fats to be metabolized by the small intestine. Malnutrition can result.

Protein metabolism is also decreased. Albumin synthesis is decreased, and serum albumin level is decreased. Albumin is necessary for colloid oncotic pressure to hold fluid in the intravascular space and for nutrition. Low albumin is also thought to be associated with the development of ascites, a complication of hepatic failure. Globulin is another protein that is essential for the transport of substances in the blood. Fibrinogen is an essential protein that is necessary for normal clotting. A low fibrinogen level, coupled with a decreased synthesis of many blood-clotting factors, predisposes the patient to bleeding. Clinical signs and symptoms range from bruising and nose and gingival bleeding to frank hemorrhage. Disseminated intravascular coagulation may also develop.

Kupffer's cells in the liver play an important role in fighting infections throughout the body. Loss of this function predisposes the patient to severe infections, particularly gram-negative sepsis.

The liver also removes activated clotting factors from the general circulation to prevent widespread clotting in the system. Loss of this function predisposes the patient to emboli, particularly to the lungs.

Decreased metabolism and storage of vitamins A, B_{12}, and D, and of iron, glucose, and fat predispose the patient to many nutritional deficiencies. The liver loses a well-known function of detoxifying drugs, ammonia, and hormones. Loss of ammonia conversion to urea in the liver is responsible for many of the altered thought processes seen in liver failure, because ammonia is allowed to enter the CNS directly. These alterations range from minor sensory perceptual changes, such as tremors, slurred speech, and impaired decision making, to dramatic confusion or profound coma.

Hormonal imbalances are common in liver disease. The most important physiological imbalance is the activation of aldosterone and antidiuretic hormone. Hormones are thought to contribute to some of the fluid and electrolyte disturbances commonly found in liver disease. Sodium and water retention and portal hypertension lead to a third spacing of fluid from the intravascular space into the peritoneal cavity (ascites). The resultant decrease in plasma volume causes activation of compensatory mechanisms in the body to release antidiuretic hormone and aldosterone. This situation causes further water and sodium retention. The renin-angiotensin system is also activated, which causes systemic vasoconstriction. The kidneys are most severely affected, and urine output decreases because of impaired perfusion. Sexual dysfunction is also common in patients with liver disease, and this can lead to self-concept alterations. Dermatological lesions that occur in some patients with liver failure, called "spider angiomas," are thought to be related to an endocrine imbalance. These vascular lesions may be venous or arterial and represent the progression of liver disease.

Impaired bile formation and flow. The liver's inability to metabolize bile is reflected clinically in an increased serum bilirubin level and a staining of tissue by bilirubin, or jaundice. Jaundice is generally present in patients with a serum bilirubin level greater than 3 mg/dL.

NURSING DIAGNOSES

The following nursing diagnoses, actual and potential, can be derived from assessment data in a patient with liver failure. See Nursing Care Plan for the Patient with Hepatic Failure.

MEDICAL AND NURSING INTERVENTIONS

Nursing and medical management of the patient with liver failure is aimed at supportive therapies and early recognition and treatment of complications associated with the disease process (Reynolds, 2000).

Diagnostic Tests

Laboratory findings in patients with liver disease (see Laboratory Alerts) are a direct result of destruction of hepatic cells (liver enzymes) or of the effects of reduced liver metabolic processes.

In addition, parenchymal tests, such as liver biopsy, can be performed to study the liver cell architecture directly. The liver is characteristically small and has a marked decrease in functioning hepatic cell structures. This characteristic allows for a definitive diagnosis of the cause of the hepatic failure. An ultrasound study may detect impaired bile flow.

Supportive Therapy

Hemodynamic instability and decreased perfusion to core organs may be the end result of portal hypertension and hyperdynamic circulation. Invasive monitoring may be used in the very critically ill patient, but it must be weighed in terms of the potential for infection in a patient with an impaired immune response. Administration of vasoactive drugs and fluids may be ordered to support blood pressure and kidney perfusion, which require close monitoring by the nurse. Portal hypertension also predisposes the patient to esophageal and gastric varices, which have the potential to bleed.

Hypoglycemia is common in liver failure. It is caused by depletion of hepatic glycogen stores and loss of ability for gluconeogenesis (Reynolds, 2000). Fingerstick glucose measurements are assessed routinely.

The patient with liver failure is also at risk of bleeding complications because of decreased synthesis of clotting factors. Patients with a prolonged prothrombin time and partial thromboplastin time and a decreased platelet count should be protected from injury through the use of padded side rails and assistance with all activity. Needle sticks should be kept to a minimum. A gentle touch in providing all nursing care also reduces the risk of bleeding. Blood products may be ordered in severe cases. GI bleeding needs to be prevented in these patients because of the associated increase in protein load. Antacids and H_2-blockers may be ordered to prevent gastritis and bleeding from stress ulcers.

Administration of all drugs metabolized by the liver must be restricted. The administration of such drugs could cause acute liver failure in a patient with chronic disease.

Liver Transplantation

Liver transplantation may be warranted in a patient with acute hepatic failure. Patients should be transported to a center that performs transplants for evaluation. Contraindications include HIV infection, malignancy, and significant heart, lung, or kidney dysfunction (Reynolds, 2000).

Experimental Therapies

Trials are ongoing that evaluate extracorporeal liver assist devices to remove toxins. As such devices are perfected, they may provide a bridge to transplantation or may allow time for liver regeneration (Reynolds, 2000).

Treatment of Complications

Ascites. Impaired handling of salt and water by the kidneys and other abnormalities in fluid homeostasis predispose the patient to an accumulation of fluid in the peritoneum, or ascites. Ascites is problematic because as more fluid is retained, it pushes up on the diaphragm, thereby impairing the patient's breathing pattern. Nursing assessment of respiratory status through respiratory rate, breath sounds, and arterial blood gas monitoring is critical. Frequent monitoring of abdominal girth and daily weight alerts the nurse to fluid accumulation. Abdominal girth should be measured at the level of the umbilicus. Positioning the patient in a semi-Fowler's position also allows for free diaphragm movement. Frequent deep-breathing and coughing exercises and changes in position are important to facilitate fuel/optimal breathing. Some patients may require elective intubation until medical management of the ascites is accomplished.

Ascites is medically managed through bed rest, low-sodium diet, fluid restriction, and diuretic therapy. Diuretics must be administered cautiously, however, because if the intravascular volume is depleted too quickly, acute renal failure may be induced. Close monitoring of serum creatinine level, BUN level, and urine output is important for the early detection of renal impairment. Careful monitoring of electrolyte balance, particularly serum potassium and sodium, is also important in diuretic administration.

Paracentesis is another medical therapy for ascites, in which ascitic fluid is withdrawn through percutaneous needle aspiration. Close monitoring of vital signs during this procedure is necessary, especially as fluid is withdrawn. Major complications include sudden loss of intravascular pressure (decreased blood pressure) and tachycardia. One to 2 L of fluid is generally withdrawn at one time to prevent these complications. The amount, color, and character of peritoneal fluid obtained should be documented. Often, a specimen of the fluid is sent to the laboratory for analysis. The patient's abdominal girth should be measured before and after the procedure. Albumin may also be administered to increase colloid osmotic pressure and to decrease loss of fluid into the peritoneal cavity.

Peritoneovenous shunting is a surgical procedure used to relieve ascites that is resistant to other therapies. The LeVeen shunt is inserted by placing the distal end of a tube in the peritoneum and tunneling the other end under the skin into the jugular vein or superior vena cava (Figure 16-12). A valve that opens and closes according to pressure gradients allows ascitic fluid to flow into the superior vena cava. The patient's breathing normally triggers the valve. During inspiration, pressure increases in the peritoneum and decreases vena caval pressure, thereby allowing fluid to flow from the peritoneum into the general circulation. Major complications of this therapy include hemodilution, shunt clotting, wound infection, leakage of ascitic fluid from the incision, and bleeding problems.

A variation of this procedure is use of the Denver shunt, which involves placement of a pump in addition to the peritoneal catheter. Fluid is allowed to flow through the pump from the peritoneum into the general circulation at a uniform rate. The pump also allows the physician or nurse to squeeze the pump percutaneously to increase flow or to clear the catheter of any solid matter.

Portal systemic encephalopathy. Portal systemic encephalopathy, commonly known as hepatic encephalopathy, is a functional derangement of the CNS that causes altered levels of consciousness and cerebral manifestations ranging from confusion to coma. Impaired motor ability is also often present. Asterixis, a flapping tremor of the hand, is an early sign of hepatic encephalopathy that can be assessed by the nurse.

The exact cause of hepatic encephalopathy is unknown, but it is thought to be abnormal ammonia metabolism. Increased serum ammonia levels are thought to interfere with normal cerebral metabolism. In acute liver failure, signs and symptoms of this disorder may appear rapidly, whereas in chronic liver failure, they often occur over time. Many conditions may precipitate the development of hepatic encephalopathy, including fluid and electrolyte and acid-base disturbances, increased protein intake, portosystemic shunts, blood transfusions, GI bleeding, and many drugs, such as diuretics, analgesics, narcotics, and sedatives. Progression of hepatic encephalopathy can be divided into stages (Box 16-17).

Measures for decreasing ammonia production are necessary in the treatment of hepatic encephalopathy. Protein intake is limited to 20 to 40 g per day. Neomycin and lactulose are two drugs that can be administered to reduce bacterial breakdown of protein in the bowel.

Neomycin is a broad-spectrum antibiotic that destroys normal bacteria found in the bowel, thereby decreasing protein breakdown and ammonia production. Neomycin is given orally every 4 to 6 hours.

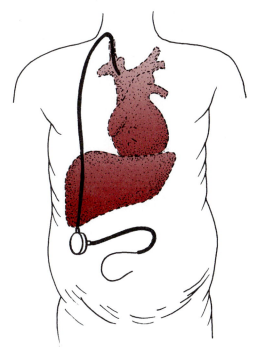

FIGURE 16-12 LeVeen shunt.

BOX 16-17

Stages of Portal Systemic Encephalopathy

STAGE 1
Tremors
Slurred speech
Impaired decision making

STAGE 2
Drowsiness
Loss of sphincter control
Asterixis

STAGE 3
Dramatic confusion
Somnolence

STAGE 4
Profound coma
Unresponsiveness to pain
Gastrointestinal alterations

This drug is toxic to the kidneys and therefore cannot be given to patients with renal failure. Daily renal function studies are monitored when neomycin is administered.

Lactulose creates an acidic environment in the bowel that causes the ammonia to leave the bloodstream and enter the colon. Ammonia is trapped in the bowel. Lactulose also has a laxative effect that allows for elimination of the ammonia. Lactulose is given orally or via a rectal enema.

Restriction of medications that are toxic to the liver is another important treatment. All medications that are metabolized by the liver should be reviewed for their therapeutic effect.

Nursing measures for protecting the patient with an altered mental status from harm are a priority. Many patients with hepatic encephalopathy need to be sedated to prevent them from doing harm to themselves or to others. Oxazepam (Serax), diazepam (Valium), or lorazepam (Ativan) may be used judiciously because these drugs are less dependent on liver function for excretion.

Hepatorenal syndrome. Acute renal failure that occurs with liver failure is called *hepatorenal syndrome*. The pathophysiology of this disorder is not well understood, but it is associated with end-stage cirrhosis and ascites, decreased albumin level, and portal hypertension. Decreased urine output and increased serum creatinine level usually occur acutely. The prognosis for the patient with hepatorenal syndrome is generally poor because therapies to improve renal function usually are ineffective. The goals of general medical therapies are to improve liver function while supporting renal function. Fluid administration and diuretic therapy are used to improve urine output. Administration of drugs that are toxic to the kidney is discontinued. Occasionally, hemodialysis may be used to support renal function if there is a chance for an improvement in liver function. As a result of the poor prognosis, it would be appropriate for the critical care nurse to begin to address end-of-life decisions with the patient and family. This should be done with consideration of the individual nurses' comfort level, as well as organizational policy and family dynamics.

PATIENT OUTCOMES

Patient outcomes for the patient with liver failure are included in the Nursing Care Plan for the Patient with Hepatic Failure.

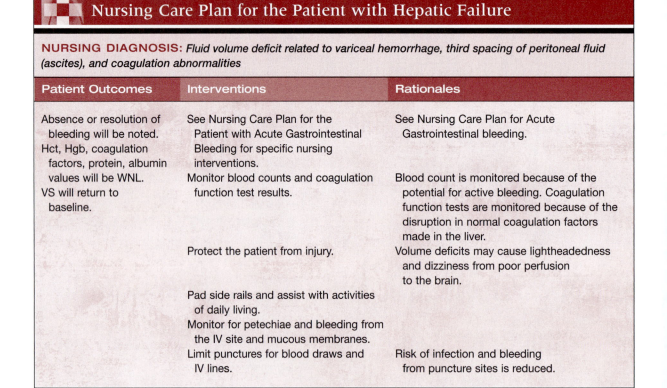

Nursing Care Plan for the Patient with Hepatic Failure

NURSING DIAGNOSIS: *Fluid volume deficit related to variceal hemorrhage, third spacing of peritoneal fluid (ascites), and coagulation abnormalities*

Patient Outcomes	Interventions	Rationales
Absence or resolution of bleeding will be noted. Hct, Hgb, coagulation factors, protein, albumin values will be WNL. VS will return to baseline.	See Nursing Care Plan for the Patient with Acute Gastrointestinal Bleeding for specific nursing interventions.	See Nursing Care Plan for Acute Gastrointestinal bleeding.
	Monitor blood counts and coagulation function test results.	Blood count is monitored because of the potential for active bleeding. Coagulation function tests are monitored because of the disruption in normal coagulation factors made in the liver.
	Protect the patient from injury.	Volume deficits may cause lightheadedness and dizziness from poor perfusion to the brain.
	Pad side rails and assist with activities of daily living. Monitor for petechiae and bleeding from the IV site and mucous membranes. Limit punctures for blood draws and IV lines.	Risk of infection and bleeding from puncture sites is reduced.

Nursing Care Plan for the Patient with Hepatic Failure—cont'd

Patient Outcomes	Interventions	Rationales
	Guaiac specimens to assess for occult blood.	Varices may bleed slightly without being overtly noticeable.
	Administer fluid and blood products as ordered and monitor patient response.	
	Administer vitamin K and other coagulation products.	To promote normal coagulation.

NURSING DIAGNOSIS: *Altered nutrition (less than body requirements) related to altered liver metabolism of food nutrients, insufficient intake, impaired absorption of fat-soluble vitamins, vitamin B_{12} deficiency, and anemia*

Patient Outcomes	Interventions	Rationales
Protein intake will be sufficient for liver regeneration.	Limit protein intake.	Ammonia builds up in body when the liver cannot metabolize protein properly.
No accumulation of nitrogen waste products will be noted.	Monitor serum BUN level.	Determines fluid volume status.
	Administer vitamins synthesized by the liver: A, B, D, and K.	Liver synthesizes these vitamins.
BUN level will be WNL.	Monitor nutritional status through serum albumin level, nitrogen balance, and daily weights.	The liver cannot make albumin and cannot metabolize protein properly. Poor oncotic pressure from low albumin levels increases ascites, noted by increase in weight.
Liver function test results will be WNL.		
Serum albumin level will be WNL.	Consider enteral feeding or TPN if oral intake is insufficient.	Promotes normal nutritional status. Positive nitrogen balance is especially important to patients with liver failure. Positive nitrogen balance will be achieved.

NURSING DIAGNOSIS: *Ineffective breathing pattern and impaired gas exchange related to dyspnea from ascites, increased risk of pulmonary infections from decreased activity of Kupffer's cells*

Patient Outcomes	Interventions	Rationales
Effective lung expansion will occur.	Monitor the patient's respiratory status, including respiratory rate, breath sounds, and depth of respirations.	Early recognition of deteriorating pulmonary status.
Dyspnea will be absent.		
ABGs will be WNL or returned to baseline.	Monitor ABGs for increasing $PaCO_2$ and decreasing PaO_2.	Early recognition of poor ventilatory efforts.
	Encourage the patient to cough and deep breathe.	Mobilizes pulmonary secretions and reduces the risk of pulmonary compromise.
	Perform chest physical therapy (e.g., percussion, vibration, suctioning) as needed.	
	Administer oxygen as ordered according to clinical assessment.	Optimizes oxygenation.

Continued

Nursing Care Plan for the Patient with Hepatic Failure—cont'd

Patient Outcomes	Interventions	Rationales
Effective lung expansion will occur. Dyspnea will be absent. ABGs will be WNL or returned to baseline.—*cont'd*	Administer sedatives and analgesics cautiously so as not to impair respiratory effort. Monitor fluid status and treat ascites. Maintain accurate I & O records. Measure abdominal girth every 4 hr. Monitor daily weights, restrict fluids and sodium, and administer diuretics as ordered. Assist with paracentesis as needed.	Drugs may not be cleared well when liver function is less than optimal. Ascites causes changes in fluid volume status. Assists in monitoring fluid volume status. Assesses ascites. Assesses and manages ascites. Relieves ascites.

NURSING DIAGNOSIS: *Altered thought processes related to impaired handling of ammonia, aggressive diuretic therapy, diet, medications that require liver metabolism, and decreased perfusion states*

Patient Outcomes	Interventions	Rationales
Hepatic encephalopathy will be absent or resolved. BUN level will be stable.	Prevent increased ammonia production via protein restriction. Prevent and treat infection, dehydration, and electrolyte or acid-base disturbances. Use sedatives, narcotic tranquilizers judiciously. Cautiously administer diuretic therapy. Administer lactulose and neomycin and monitor results. Reduce the risk of GI bleeding through antacid and H$_2$-histamine blocker administration. Monitor the patient's response to therapy by checking ammonia levels and through ongoing neurological assessments. Reorient the patient and provide for safety during periods of impaired mentation. Prevent hazards related to immobility.	Ammonia is a by-product of protein metabolism. Reduces complications. The patient is unable to metabolize sedatives and narcotics because of liver disruption. Intravascular dehydration in patients with liver disease is the result of low oncotic pressure with low serum albumin levels. Reduces ammonia levels. Drugs given to treat GI bleeding. The neurological assessment slowly returns to normal as ammonia levels return to normal. High ammonia levels cause disorientation. Maintain a safe environment.

ABG, Arterial blood gas; *BUN,* blood urea nitrogen; *GI,* gastrointestinal; *Hct,* hematocrit; *Hgb,* hemoglobin; *IV,* intravenous; *PaCO$_2$,* partial pressure of arterial carbon dioxide; *PaO$_2$,* partial pressure of oxygen in arterial blood; *TPN,* total parenteral nutrition; *VS,* vital signs; *WNL,* within normal limits.

Trends In Care of The Patient with Gastrointestinal Injury or Illness: Intraabdominal Hypertension and Abdominal Compartment Syndrome

Since the mid-1990s, the phenomenon of intra-abdominal hypertension leading to abdominal compartment syndrome has been recognized as a potentially life-threatening complication of abdominal trauma, massive fluid resuscitation efforts, and some abdominal surgery. Significant increases in morbidity and mortality have been noted in critically ill patients who develop intraabdominal hypertension and abdominal compartment syndrome (Cheatham, White, Sagraves, Johnson, & Black, 2000).

Intraabdominal hypertension is defined as a sustained increase in intraabdominal pressure (Hong et al., 2002). Normal intraabdominal pressure is close to 0. Classification of elevated pressure is as follows: 10 to 20 mm Hg, mildly elevated; 20 to 40 mm Hg, moderately elevated; and greater than 40 mm Hg, severely elevated. Pressure monitoring is accomplished by several methods. Direct methods measure pressure directly in the abdominal cavity itself. Indirect methods include inferior vena cava, intragastric, transgastral, and transvesical techniques. Transvesical (urinary bladder) is the most reliable and easy to perform at the bedside (Wittmann & Iskander, 2000).

Organ dysfunction caused by the consistent increase in pressure is called abdominal compartment syndrome (Hong et al., 2002). Abdominal compartment syndrome occurs more often with acute intraabdominal hypertension and with abdominal trauma with massive resuscitation efforts. Sustained intraabdominal hypertension greater than 35 mm Hg is thought to be one cause of abdominal compartment syndrome (Wittmann & Iskander, 2000). Functional impairments of several organ systems including cardiovascular, respiratory, hepatic, renal, GI, and neurological can occur from abdominal compartment syndrome (Box 16-18). Patients need to be monitored in an intensive care setting where hemodynamic monitoring with pulmonary artery catheters and intraabdominal pressure measurements can be taken.

There is much still not known about intraabdominal hypertension and abdominal compartment syndrome. Some confusion still exists in the terminology surrounding the topics. Therefore, vigilant monitoring of new literature and research studies by those caring for high-risk patients is imperative.

BOX 16-18

Physiological Effects of Abdominal Compartment Syndrome

CARDIOVASCULAR
- Decreased venous return
- Increased systemic vascular resistance and intrathoracic pressure
- Reduction in cardiac output

RESPIRATORY
- Atelectesis
- Pneumonia
- Impaired ventilation
- Respiratory failure

HEPATIC AND RENAL
- Decreased blood flow to liver and kidney
- Functional impairment of both organs

GASTROINTESTINAL
- Impaired lymphatic, venous, and arterial flow
- Poor healing of anastomoses

NEUROLOGICAL
- Simultaneous increased intracranial pressure from both head trauma and intraabdominal hypertension

---

SUMMARY

Acute upper GI bleeding, acute pancreatitis, and liver failure account for potentially life-threatening emergencies that require careful and astute assessments and care by the critical care nurse and medical team. Priorities for care include initial assessments and resuscitation, diagnostic testing for making a definitive diagnosis, and prompt interventions for stabilizing or reversing the pathophysiological process and preventing complications. The nurse's scope of care includes ongoing assessments and monitoring, documentation and reporting of patient responses to diagnostic and treatment regimens, early detection of complications, and supportive care. Patient and family teaching of the intensive care unit routine and all therapies instituted is also a priority. As appropriate, discharge teaching of the underlying pathological process and of the dietary, medication, and activity regimens may also be initiated in the intensive care unit. Successful management of all these patient populations requires a collaborative effort of all disciplines.

Case Study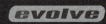

You are working evenings in the intensive care unit and receive report from the emergency department (ED) of a patient to be admitted to the unit. The patient is a 47-year-old man with a week-long history of severe abdominal pain that worsens with food. The pain is associated with nausea and vomiting. The patient is oriented to person and place; however, he is disoriented to day and time and is described as "lethargic." A nasogastric tube and Foley catheter were placed and intravenous access was established in the ED.

Vital signs include the following: heart rate, 110 beats/min; respirations, 30 breaths/min; blood pressure, 104/56 mm Hg, and temperature, 38°C.

Laboratory values include the following: white blood cell count, 19,000/μL; hematocrit, 38%; sodium, 148 mEq/L; potassium, 4.0 mEq/L; chloride, 114 mEq/L; blood urea nitrogen, 25 mg/dL; creatinine, 1.0 mg/dL, glucose, 180 mg/dL; amylase, 500 IU/L; and lipase, 600 IU/L.

QUESTIONS
1. What further data would you like to have from the ED?
2. In addition to management of shock in this patient, what is another priority treatment?
3. What further assessment data would be valuable to the long-term management of this patient?

CRITICAL THINKING QUESTIONS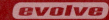

1. You are caring for a patient who is admitted with acute abdominal pain and vomiting. His admission vital signs and laboratory values include the following: blood pressure, 94/72 mm Hg; heart rate, 114 beats per minute; respiratory rate, 32 breaths per minute; potassium level, 3.0 mEq/L; calcium level, 7.0 mg/dL; PaO_2, 58 mm Hg; SaO_2, 88%; serum amylase level, 280 IU/L; and lipase level 32 IU/dL.
   a. What are your priority nursing and medical interventions?
   b. What is the suspected medical diagnosis?
2. A 50-year-old patient is admitted with hematemesis and reports having dark stools for the past 12 hours. Which of the following admission data is the best indicator of the amount of blood lost: blood pressure, 95/60 mm Hg (supine); heart rate, 125 beats per minute; respiratory rate, 28 breaths per minute; Hct value, 27%; or Hgb value, 14 g/dL?

3. A 45-year-old business executive is admitted to your unit. He tells you that he travels a lot for business and has recently returned from a trip to Mexico. During your initial assessment, he tells you that he is not married and he relates stories about some of the women he has met and dated on his many trips. His history includes persistent abdominal pain, nausea with occasional vomiting, fatigue, and decreased appetite. Initial vital signs and laboratory results include the following: heart rate, 70 beats per minute; urine, clear and dark yellow; liver function test results increased (AST level, 20 IU/L; alanine transaminase level, 70 IU/L); albumin level, 3.2 mg/dL; and total bilirubin level, 1.5 mg/dL. What is the most likely diagnosis, and what precautions should you take while caring for this patient?

REFERENCES

Cavanaugh, J., Schmidt, E., & Lord, L. M. (1999). Gastrointestinal problems. In P. Logan (ed.). *Principles of practice for the acute care nurse practitioner.* Stamford, CT: Appleton & Lange.

Centers for Disease Control (CDC). (2004). Hepatitis Fact Sheets. Retrieved from http://www.cdc.gov/hepatitis. Accessed 7/1/2004.

Cheatham, M. L., White, M. W., Sagraves, S. G., Johnson, J. L., & Block, E. F. J. (2000). Abdominal perfusion pressure: A superior parameter in the assessment of intra-abdominal hypertension. *Journal of Trauma Injury, Infection and Critical Care, 49*(4), 621-627.

Chernecky, C. C., & Berger, B. J. (2004). *Laboratory tests and diagnostic procedures.* 4th ed. Philadelphia: W. B. Saunders.

Friedman, L. S. (2004). Liver, biliary tract, & pancreas. (pp. 623-668). In L. M. Tierney, S. J. McPhee, and M. A. Papadakis *2004 Current Medical Diagnosis & Treatment.* New York: McGraw-Hill.

Guyton, A. C. (2001). *Textbook of medical physiology.* 10th ed. Philadelphia: W. B. Saunders.

Hong, J. J., Cohn, S. M., Perez, J. M., Dolich, M. O., Brown, M., & McKenney, M. G. (2002). Prospective study of the incidence and outcome of intra-abdominal hypertension and the abdominal compartment syndrome. *British Journal of Surgery 8,* 591-596.

Jarvis, C. (2004). *Physical examination and health assessment.* 4th ed. Philadelphia: W. B. Saunders.

McQuaid, K. R. (2004). Alimentary tract. (pp. 515-622). In L. M. Tierney, S. J. McPhee, and M. A. Papadakis *2004 Current Medical Diagnosis & Treatment.* New York: McGraw-Hill.

Ranson, J. C. (1985). Risk factors in acute pancreatitis. *Hospital Practice, 20*(4), 69-73.

Reynolds, T. B. (2000). Acute hepatic failure. In A. Grevnik, S. M. Ayres, P. R. Holbrook, & W. C. Shoemaker (eds.). *Textbook of critical care.* 4th ed. Philadelphia: W. B. Saunders.

Savides, T. J., & Jensen, D. M. (2000). Severe gastrointestinal hemorrhage. In A. Grevnik, S. M. Ayres, P. R. Holbrook, & W. C. Shoemaker (eds.). *Textbook of critical care.* 4th ed. Philadelphia: W. B. Saunders.

Steer, M. L. (2000). Acute pancreatitis. In A. Grevnik, S. M. Ayres, P. R. Holbrook, & W. C. Shoemaker (eds.). *Textbook of critical care.* 4th ed. Philadelphia: W. B. Saunders.

Wells, B. G., Dipiro, J. T., Schwinghammer, T. L., & Hamilton, C. W. (2003). *Pharmacotherapy Handbook* (5th ed.). New York: McGraw-Hill.

Wittmann, D. H., & Iskander, G. A. (2000). The compartment syndrome of the abdominal cavity: A state of the art review. *Journal of Intensive Care Medicine, 15*(4), 201-216.

RECOMMENDED READINGS

Walker, J., & Criddle, L. M. (2003). Pathophysiology and management of abdominal compartment syndrome. *American Journal of Critical Care, 12*(4), 367-371.

evolve *Did you remember to check out the bonus material, including free self-assessment exercises, on the Evolve Web site at http://evolve.elsevier.com/Sole/ and on the CD-ROM?*

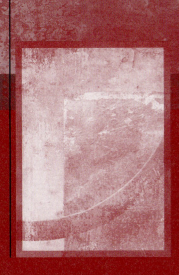

CHAPTER 17

Endocrine Alterations

Zara R. Brenner, BSN, MS, APRN, BC
Sheila A. Myer, MSN, RN

OBJECTIVES

- Analyze disorders resulting from alterations in hormones secreted by the pancreas, adrenal, thyroid, and posterior pituitary glands.
- Describe the feedback mechanisms for regulation of insulin, cortisol, thyroid hormones, and antidiuretic hormone.
- Compare pathophysiology, assessment, nursing diagnoses, interventions and outcomes for hyperglycemic crises, hypoglycemic crisis, adrenal crisis, thyroid storm, myxedema coma, diabetes insipidus, and the syndrome of inappropriate antidiuretic hormone.
- Formulate plans of care for patients with critical alterations in endocrine function.

Introduction

The endocrine glands form a communication network linking all body systems. Hormones from these glands control and regulate metabolic processes governing such activities as energy production, fluid and electrolyte balance, and stress reactions. This system is closely linked to and integrated with the nervous system. In particular, the hypothalamus and pituitary gland play a major role in hormonal regulation. The hypothalamus manufactures and secretes several releasing or inhibiting hormones that are conveyed to the pituitary. The pituitary responds to these hormones by increasing or decreasing hormone secretion, thus regulating circulating hormone levels. This system is designed as a feedback control mechanism. Positive feedback stimulates release of a hormone when serum hormone levels are low. Negative feedback inhibits the release of hormones when serum hormone levels are high. Examples of how these feedback systems work to control circulating levels of cortisol and thyroid hormones are provided in Figures 17-1 and 17-2. This same feedback system also controls the secretion and inhibition of other hormones outside of hypothalamic-pituitary control.

Diseases involving the hypothalamus, the pituitary gland, and the primary endocrine organs (i.e., pancreas, adrenal gland, and thyroid gland) can interfere with normal feedback mechanisms and the secretion of hormones. Crisis states can occur when these diseases are untreated or undertreated, when the patient is stressed, or as the result of a multitude of other factors. This chapter deals with crises that occur as a

evolve *Be sure to check out the bonus material, including free self-assessment exercises, on the Evolve Web site at http://evolve.elsevier.com/Sole/ and on the CD-ROM.*

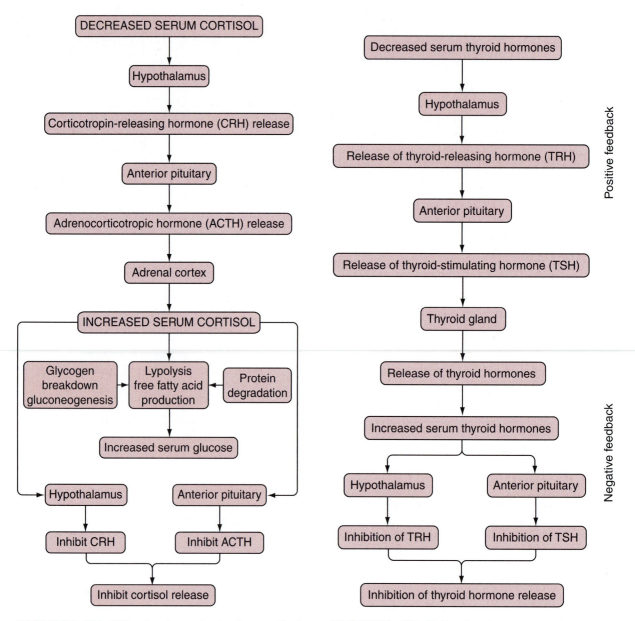

FIGURE 17-1 Feedback systems for cortisol regulation.

FIGURE 17-2 Feedback systems for thyroid hormone regulation.

result of imbalances of hormones from the pancreas, adrenal glands, thyroid gland, and posterior pituitary gland. For a summary of treatment considerations for the older adult, see Geriatric Assessment.

Pancreatic Endocrine Emergencies

REVIEW OF PHYSIOLOGY

Three common critical endocrine disorders associated with the pancreas are diabetic ketoacidosis (DKA), hyperosmolar hyperglycemic nonketotic coma (HHNC), and hypoglycemia, which are acute complications of diabetes mellitus (DM). An understanding of the normal physiology of insulin, as well as of the pathophysiology, critical assessments, and collaborative treatment regimens of the aforementioned disorders, is essential to the management and nursing care of these patients.

In response to increased levels of serum glucose, insulin is released from the pancreas by beta cells in the islets of Langerhans. Insulin is essential to normal carbohydrate, protein, and fat metabolism.

Geriatric Assessment

Pancreas

Elderly patients are more likely to have comorbid conditions, such as cardiac or renal disease, and be taking medications that make them more reactive to electrolyte imbalances. They may also be slower to respond to treatments. Typically, elderly persons are more prone to develop hyperosmolar hyperglycemic nonketotic coma and/or type 2 diabetes mellitus. Elderly patients also are at increased risk of hypoglycemia unawareness.

Adrenal

Utilization and clearance of cortisol decrease with age, and this results in increased serum cortisol levels. Unfortunately, because the feedback systems are intact, a decrease in cortisol secretion takes place, which tends to exacerbate the situation in the elderly (Piano & Huether, 2002).

Thyroid

Recognize that thyroid hormone levels can decrease with age probably as a result of glandular atrophy. Detection of thyroid disease by assessment of signs or symptoms becomes more challenging. Additionally, lower amounts of thyroid replacement are needed, and replacement must be slower to avoid potentially dangerous side effects. Elderly patients are less likely to tolerate urgent treatment with liothyronine sodium.

Older patients may not exhibit the typical signs of thyrotoxicosis. Goiter, hyperactive reflexes, sweating, heat intolerance, tremor, nervousness, and polydipsia are less commonly present. Anorexia, atrial fibrillation, apathy, and weight loss are more common. In the elderly, symptoms of thyroid storm may present as increasing angina or worsening heart failure.

Pituitary

Decreased release of growth hormone and increased sensitivity lead to a decrease in lean body mass and increased blood glucose levels, and they affect the release of thyroid-stimulating hormone, although usually not significantly. An increase in secretion of antidiuretic hormone occurs with advanced age and places the older person at risk of dilutional hyponatremia. Elderly patients are at greater risk of syndrome of inappropriate antidiuretic hormone from any cause than are younger patients. Elderly patients with cognitive impairment have an increased susceptibility to developing diabetes insipidus.

The physiological activity of insulin is summarized in Box 17-1. Insulin is necessary for cellular uptake of glucose by most cells in the body, including muscle, fibroblasts, mammary glands, anterior pituitary, lens of the eye, and aorta. These cells constitute the largest percentage of body mass and expend the most energy. Insulin is not required for glucose to enter liver cells, kidney tubules, neural tissue, retinal cells, erythrocytes, intestinal mucosa, or the beta islet cells.

Other factors affecting control of glucose levels and insulin secretion include glucagon and somatostatin, both secreted by the pancreas, as well as circulating catecholamines, cortisol, and growth hormone. These hormones are released in response to decreased glucose levels and in response to stress. Glucagon, catecholamines, cortisol, and growth hormone promote an increase in serum glucose levels and are often referred to as counterregulatory or stress hormones.

Without insulin, glucose is unable to enter cells, accumulates in the blood (hyperglycemia), and triggers a variety of physiological processes as the cells requiring glucose begin to starve. Levels of circulating insulin that exceed the body's requirement result in decreased serum glucose (hypoglycemia) and changes in the level of consciousness, because glucose is the preferred fuel of the central nervous system.

DM is a metabolic disease of glucose imbalance resulting from alterations in insulin secretion, insulin action, or both. The number of people with DM has been increasing over the years, thus making DKA and HHNC more common in the hospitalized patient. There are several types of DM, the two most common being type 1 and type 2. Type 1 DM (autoimmune-mediated) is primarily caused by pancreatic islet beta-cell destruction resulting in an absolute insulin deficiency and a tendency to ketoacidosis. The most prevalent form is type 2 DM, which involves insulin resistance and an insulin secretory defect, resulting in a relative insulin deficiency. The other types of DM include gestational DM and steroid-induced DM.

There is strong evidence of a genetic factor in the development of type 1 DM. Genetics may also play a role in the development of type 2 DM as well as in those conditions, such as obesity, that are more prevalent in patients with type 2 DM. Certain populations have a higher incidence of DM, thus leading to

BOX 17-1

Physiological Activity of Insulin

CARBOHYDRATE METABOLISM
Increases glucose transport across cell membrane in most cells including muscle and fat

Within liver and muscle, promotes formation of glycogen, the storage form of glucose

Inhibits gluconeogenesis in liver, thus sparing amino acids and glycerol for protein and fatty acid synthesis

FAT METABOLISM
Increases triglyceride synthesis

Increases fatty acid transport into adipose tissue

Inhibits lipolysis of triglycerides stored in adipose tissue

Stimulates fatty acid synthesis from glucose and other substrates

PROTEIN METABOLISM
Increases amino acid transport across cell membrane of muscle and liver

Augments protein synthesis

Inhibits proteolysis

BOX 17-2

Factors Leading to Diabetic Ketoacidosis and Hyperosmolar Hyperglycemic Nonketotic Coma

COMMON FACTORS
Insulin deficiency

HHNC: newly diagnosed type 2 diabetes

DKA: omission of insulin, new onset, noncompliance, inadequate dose

Increased demand from growth in children, exercise

Stress

Infection

Major or acute illness, trauma, surgery, pancreatitis

Preexisting illness such as cardiac, renal

Medications

Thiazide diuretics

Phenytoin

Steroids (especially glucocorticoids)

Beta-blockers

Calcium channel blockers

DKA-SPECIFIC FACTORS
Malfunction of insulin pump or infection at catheter site

Development of insulin resistance: during menstruation or pregnancy

Other endocrine disorders: hyperthyroidism, Cushing's disease, pheochromocytoma

Medications

Psychotropics

Analgesics

Epinephrine

HHNC-SPECIFIC FACTORS
High-calorie parenteral or enteral feedings

Decreased thirst mechanism

Difficult access to fluids (e.g., nursing home resident)

Medications

Cimetidine

Calcium channel blockers

Immunosuppressive agents

Diazoxide

DKA, Diabetic ketoacidosis; *HHNC,* hyperosmolar hyperglycemic nonketotic coma.

an increased awareness of genetic factors and health screening needs for relatives of patients diagnosed with DM. Rates of DM are approximately twice as high in Hispanics and African-Americans than in non-Hispanic whites, and are approximately three times as high in Native American and Alaskan Native adults (Quinn, 2002).

HYPERGLYCEMIC CRISES
Pathogenesis
The basic underlying mechanism for both DKA and HHNC is a reduction in the net effective action of circulating insulin coupled with a concomitant elevation of counterregulatory hormones (ADA, 2003). Together, this hormonal mix leads to increased hepatic and renal glucose production, but it prevents utilization of glucose in the peripheral tissues. DKA and HHNC are endocrine emergencies.

Etiology of diabetic ketoacidosis. Numerous factors can trigger DKA (Box 17-2), the most common being infections and severe stress states (e.g., trauma, surgery, myocardial infarction). Many patients present with DKA as the initial indication of previously undiagnosed type 1 DM. Numerous drugs can trigger an insulin deficiency (Quinn, 2002). The condition may also occur in patients with known DM who fail to administer enough insulin or have increased insulin requirements. Patients using insulin pumps may develop DKA because of a malfunctioning pump system in as little as 12 hours. Lack of knowledge regarding the disease process or insulin administration and lack of compliance with the therapeutic regimen are also possible causes. DKA characteristically develops over a short period, and patients seek medical help early because of the pathophysiological effects.

The incidence of recurrent DKA is higher in female patients and peaks in the early teenage years. The risk of recurrent DKA is higher in those diabetic patients diagnosed at an early age and those of lower socioeconomic background. The cause of recurrent DKA is unclear, but there is support for multiple risk factors including physiological, psychosomatic, and psychosocial elements (Skinner, 2002).

Etiology of hyperosmolar hyperglycemic nonketotic coma.

HHNC is usually precipitated by inadequate insulin secretion or action and is more commonly seen in patients with newly diagnosed type 2 DM. Some patients may have no history of DM. Most patients are elderly, with decreased compensatory mechanisms to maintain homeostasis in hyperosmolar states. A major illness mediated through glucose overproduction resulting from the stress response may contribute to the development of HHNC. High-calorie parenteral and enteral feedings that exceed the patient's ability to metabolize glucose have been known to induce HHNC. Several drugs have also been associated with the development of the disorder. The major etiological factors of HHNC are reviewed in Box 17-2.

Pathophysiology of Diabetic Ketoacidosis

In DKA, high extracellular glucose levels produce an osmotic gradient between the intracellular and extracellular spaces and cause fluid to move out of the cells. This process is called osmotic diuresis. When serum glucose exceeds the renal threshold, glucose is lost through the kidneys (glycosuria). Osmotic diuresis occurs, which leads to urinary losses of water, sodium, potassium, magnesium, calcium, and phosphorus. This cycle of osmotic diuresis causes an increase in serum osmolality, further fluid shifts from the intracellular to the intravascular space, and worsening dehydration.

The typical total body water loss in DKA is 6 L (ADA, 2003). It is also thought that the hyperosmolarity further impairs insulin secretion and promotes insulin resistance. The glomerular filtration rate in the kidney decreases in response to these severe fluid volume deficits. Decreased glucose excretion (causing increased serum glucose) and further hyperosmolarity

result. The altered neurological status frequently seen in these patients is partially the result of cellular dehydration and the hyperosmolar state.

Protein stores are broken down by the liver into amino acids and then into glucose and nitrogen to provide energy. Without insulin, the liberated glucose cannot be used, further increasing serum blood glucose and urine glucose concentrations and worsening osmotic diuresis. As nitrogen accumulates in the periphery, blood urea nitrogen (BUN) rises. Breakdown of protein stores also stimulates the loss of intracellular potassium and increases potassium in the serum (hyperkalemia). This additional circulating potassium may also be lost as a result of osmotic diuresis (hypokalemia). Serum electrolyte levels, particularly potassium, may present a false value in regard to the actual intracellular level. Total body potassium deficits are common and must be considered in the overall management of DKA.

The absence or lack of insulin causes an enhanced decomposition of fat (lipolysis), increased free fatty acid mobilization, and the development of ketosis from impaired metabolism of ketones. Overproduction of fatty acids by the liver leads to increased circulating ketone concentrations and impaired bicarbonate buffering as a result of osmotic diuresis. Ketone bodies likely play an important role in endothelial activation contributing to intracerebral crises (Hoffman, 2002). This process results in metabolic acidosis from increased carbonic acid concentrations. As ketone and hydrogen ions accumulate and acidosis worsens, the respiratory system attempts to compensate for excess carbonic acid by blowing off carbon dioxide, another acid. In addition to carbonic acid, patients with DKA may have an accumulation of lactic acids (lactic acidosis) from the loss of volume because of osmotic diuresis. The resulting dehydration may cause decreased perfusion to core organs, with consequent hypoxemia and worsening of the lactic acidosis.

Excess lactic acid results in what is called an *increased anion gap* (increased body acids). Sodium, potassium, chloride, and bicarbonate are responsible for maintaining a normal anion gap, which is normally less than 18 mEq/L. Ketone accumulation causes an increase in the anion gap greater than 18 (Box 17-3).

Many enzymatic reactions within the body function only within a limited range of pH. As the patient becomes more acidotic and enzymes become more ineffective, body metabolism slows. This situation further decreases ketone metabolism, and acidosis worsens. The stress response also contributes to the metabolic alterations as the liver is stimulated by hormones (glucagon, catecholamines, cortisol, and growth hormones) to break down protein stores, thus increasing serum glucose and nitrogen. Some of

Cl⁻, Chloride; *HCO₃⁻*, bicarbonate; *K⁺*, potassium; *Na⁺*, sodium.

these hormones also decrease cells' ability to use glucose for energy and therefore compound the problem. The central nervous system alterations seen in DKA are thought to be influenced by the acidosis as well as by the dehydration.

In summary, cells without glucose starve and begin to use existing stores of fat and protein to provide energy for body processes (gluconeogenesis). Fats are broken down faster than they can be metabolized, and this results in an accumulation of ketone acids, a by-product of fat metabolism in the liver. Ketone acids accumulate in the bloodstream, where hydrogen ions dissociate from the ketones and cause metabolic acidosis. The more acidotic the patient becomes, the less

able the body is to metabolize these ketones. Acetone is also formed during this process and is responsible for the "fruity breath" found in these patients.

Pathophysiology of Hyperosmotic Hyperglycemic Nonketotic Coma

The pathophysiology of HHNC is similar to that of DKA. However, in HHNC, there are higher levels of hyperglycemia, hyperosmolarity, and severe dehydration; significantly lower levels of free fatty acids, and a lack of ketosis (Figure 17-3). HHNC is referred to by many different acronyms (Box 17-4).

Hyperglycemia results from decreased utilization and/or increased production of glucose. The hyperglycemic state causes an osmotic movement of water from a lesser concentration of solutes to a higher concentration of solutes. This results in expansion of the extracellular fluid volume and intracellular dehydration. The osmotic diuresis and resultant intracellular and extracellular dehydration in HHNC are generally more severe than those found in DKA, because HHNC generally develops insidiously over a period of weeks to months. Alterations in neurological status are common because of cellular dehydration. The typical total body water deficit in HHNC is 9 L (ADA, 2003). By the time these patients seek medical attention, they

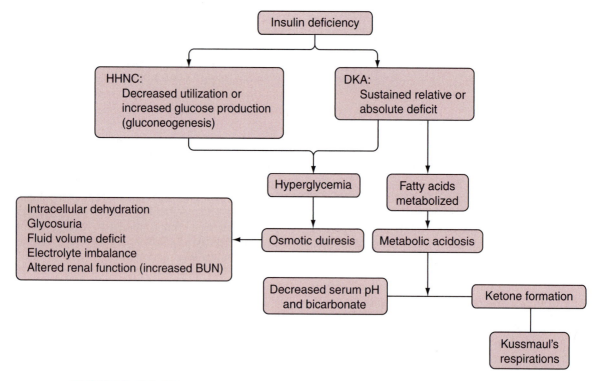

FIGURE 17-3 Pathophysiology of diabetic ketoacidosis (DKA) and hyperosmolar hyperglycemic nonketotic coma (HHNC).

are profoundly dehydrated and hyperosmolar. As a result, the mortality rate of HHNC is higher than that of DKA.

Most commonly, patients who develop HHNC are older. They are also more likely to have other medical problems that affect morbidity and mortality. Issues with mobility and access to health care may also affect the older patient with type 2 DM.

Ketoacidosis is usually not seen in patients with HHNC. It is believed that insulin levels in these patients remain high enough to prevent lipolysis and ketone formation. Glucose counterregulatory hormones that promote lipolysis are lower in patients with HHNC than in those with DKA.

Assessment

Clinical presentation. The presenting symptoms of DKA and HHNC are similar (Table 17-1). Signs of DKA and HHNC are related to the degree of dehydration present and the electrolyte imbalances. The osmotic diuresis occurring from hyperglycemia results in signs of increased thirst (polydipsia), increased urine output (polyuria), and dehydration. Increased hunger (polyphagia) may also be an early sign. Elderly persons have a decreased sense of thirst, so this symptom may not be seen in patients who typically develop HHNC. Signs of intravascular dehydration are also common as these disease processes continue and may include the following:

- Hypotension (orthostatic)
- Tachycardia
- Warm, dry skin
- Dry mucous membranes
- Loss of skin turgor
- Weight loss
- Sunken eyeballs
- Abdominal pain

Hyperglycemia and ketosis both contribute to delayed gastric emptying. Vomiting can occur, which worsens total body dehydration. As a result, urine output decreases. Patients also report symptoms of weakness and anorexia. Abdominal pain and tenderness are common presenting symptoms, particularly in DKA, and are associated with dehydration and underlying pathophysiology, such as pyelonephritis, duodenal ulcer, appendicitis, and metabolic acidosis. Pain associated with DKA most commonly disappears with treatment of dehydration. Weight loss may also occur because of fluid losses and an inability to metabolize glucose. Typically, dehydration is more profound in patients with HHNC.

Altered states of consciousness range from restlessness, confusion, and agitation to somnolence and coma. Visual disturbances are common. Generally, altered levels of consciousness are more pronounced in patients with HHNC. This is related to the severity of hyperglycemia and serum hyperosmolarity. Seizures and focal neurological signs may also be present and often lead to misdiagnosis in patients with HHNC.

In DKA, because of the lack of sufficient insulin, glucose utilization is profoundly impaired and inhibits the peripheral uptake of glucose as well as protein synthesis and lipogenesis. Glucose can still be used in non–insulin-dependent tissues, and free fatty acids are mobilized and transported to the liver for metabolism. The liver becomes overwhelmed and is unable to oxidize the excessive amount of ketones. The excessive production and decreased metabolism of ketone bodies result in ketonuria and loss of bicarbonate, with consequent metabolic acidosis. Nausea is an early sign of DKA and is thought to be a result of retained ketones. Increases in the rate and depth of breathing, called *Kussmaul's respirations*, are common as the patient attempts to compensate for the metabolic acidosis. Later in the disease process, the respiratory status of the patient may be influenced by the neurological status, precipitating impaired breathing patterns and gas exchange. Acetone ("fruity") breath from fat metabolism may be noted. A decreased level of consciousness is also associated with the severe acidotic state (pH less than 7.15). The flushed face associated with DKA is the result of superficial vasodilation.

Laboratory evaluation. Numerous diagnostic studies are used to evaluate for DKA and HHNC, to rule out other diseases, and to detect complications (see Laboratory Alerts: Pancreatic Endocrine Disorders). Additionally, cultures and testing are performed to determine any precipitating factors such as infection or MI.

In DKA, arterial blood gas analysis reflects metabolic acidosis (low pH and low bicarbonate).

TABLE 17-1

Manifestations of Diabetic Ketoacidosis and Hyperosmolar Hyperglycemic Nonketotic Coma

	Diabetic Ketoacidosis	Hyperosmolar Hyperglycemic Nonketotic Coma
Pathophysiology	Insulin deficiency resulting in cellular dehydration and volume depletion, acidosis, and protein catabolism	Insulin deficiency resulting in dehydration and hyperosmolality
Health history	History of type 1 diabetes mellitus (DM) (use of insulin) Signs and symptoms of hyperglycemia prior to admission Can also occur in type 2 DM in severe stress	History of type 2 DM (non–insulin-dependent) Signs and symptoms of hyperglycemia before admission Occurs most frequently in elderly, with preexisting renal and cardiovascular disease
Onset	Develops quickly	Develops insidiously
Clinical presentation	Flushed, dry skin Dry mucous membranes ↓ Skin turgor Tachycardia Hypotension Kussmaul's respirations Acetone breath Altered level of consciousness Visual disturbances Polydipsia Nausea and vomiting Anorexia Abdominal pain	Flushed, dry skin Dry mucous membranes ↓ Skin turgor (may not be present in elderly) Tachycardia Hypotension Shallow respirations Altered level of consciousness (generally more profound and may include absent deep tendon reflexes, paresis, and positive Babinski's sign)
Diagnostics	↑ Plasma glucose (average: 675 mg/dL) and urine glucose levels Arterial pH < 7.30 ↓ Bicarbonate Positive serum and urine ketoacids Azotemia Electrolytes vary with state of hydration; often hyperkalemic Plasma hyperosmolality (Average: 330 mOsm/kg) as a result of hemo-concentration	↑ Plasma glucose (usually >1000 mg/dL) Arterial pH > 7.30 Bicarbonate > 15 mEq/L Absence of significant ketosis Azotemia Electrolytes vary with state of hydration; often hypernatremic Plasma hyperosmolality (Average: 350 mOsm/kg) Hypotonic urine

↑, Increased; ↓, decreased.

The partial pressure of arterial carbon dioxide ($PaCO_2$) may also be low, reflecting the respiratory system's attempt to compensate for the acidosis. As the patient's level of consciousness deteriorates, he or she may develop severe breathing disturbances that cause a precipitous increase in the $PaCO_2$ and a further fall in pH. Severe acidosis is associated with cardiovascular collapse, which can result in death.

In HHNC, the laboratory results are similar to those in DKA, but with four major differences: (1) the serum glucose concentration in HHNC is generally significantly more elevated, (2) plasma osmolality is higher than in DKA and is associated with the degree of dehydration, (3) acidosis is not present or very mild compared with DKA, and (4) ketosis is usually absent or very mild in comparison with DKA.

LABORATORY ALERTS: PANCREATIC ENDOCRINE DISORDERS

Laboratory Test	Critical Value	Significance	Nursing Actions
Serum Glucose	≥ 200 mg/dL (2-hr postprandial or random) >140 mg/dL (fasting)	Combined with symptoms, establishes diagnosis of diabetes mellitus Generally, higher in HHNC	See Nursing Care Plan for the Patient with Hyperglycemic Complications of a Pancreatic Disorder. Administer insulin to correct hyperglycemia. Monitor serum/capillary laboratory values.
	<50 mg/dL	Hypoglycemia	Provide glucose (PO, IM, or IV depending on access or patient's level of consciousness). Monitor serum/capillary laboratory values.
Potassium	>6.5 mEq/L	Potential for heart blocks, bradydysrhythmias, sinus arrest, ventricular fibrillation, or asystole	Cardiac monitoring, IV fluid replacement for rehydration, and monitoring of serum laboratory values.
	<3 mEq/L	Potential for ventricular dysrhythmias	If low, potassium replacement is given either PO or IV.
Sodium	>150 mEq/L	May be a result of stress and dehydration	This usually resolves with IV rehydration and/or replacement. Consider 0.9% NaCl or 0.45% NaCl IV solutions.
BUN	>20 mg/dL	Elevated due to protein breakdown and hemoconcentration	Monitor I & O (especially urine output ≥30 mL/hr) and serum laboratory values.
Bicarbonate	<20 mEq/L	Decreased in DKA due to compensation for acidosis	If not resolved by other measures, consider replacement.
pH	<7.3	Decreased in DKA due to accumulation of acids and dehydration	It should resolve with rehydration, insulin replacement, and return of electrolyte balance.
Osmolality	>330 mOsm/kg H_2O	Elevated in DKA relative to dehydration, higher in HHNC	Rehydration should correct this.

Continued

Serum electrolyte concentrations may be low, normal, or elevated and generally are not reliable indicators of total body stores.

Nursing Diagnoses

The nursing diagnoses that apply to a patient with DKA or HHNC based on assessment data include the following:

- Ineffective breathing pattern related to acidosis (DKA), decreased level of consciousness

- Impaired gas exchange related to decreased level of consciousness
- Deficient fluid volume related to osmotic diuresis and total body loss, ketosis (DKA) and increased lipolysis, vomiting
- Imbalanced electrolytes related to lack of insulin, fluid shifts, acid-base imbalance, vomiting, or nasogastric suction
- Acid-base imbalance: acidosis (DKA only) related to ketosis

LABORATORY ALERTS: PANCREATIC ENDOCRINE DISORDERS—cont'd

Laboratory Test	Critical Value	Significance	Nursing Actions
Phosphorus	<2.5 mg/dL	May result in impaired respiratory and cardiac functions	Potassium phosphate can be used as replacement. Use caution in patients with renal failure. Provide for respiratory support as needed.
Magnesium	<1.3 mEq/L	Depleted by osmotic diuresis May coincide with decreased potassium and calcium; may result in dysrhythmias	Monitor for changes in level of consciousness, increased reflexes, tetany, and take seizure precautions.
Urine Glucose	Positive	Elevated by inadequate utilization, increased serum levels, and increased excretion	Continue to monitor for clearance.
Ketones	Positive	Results from breakdown of fatty acids in DKA	

DKA, Diabetic ketoacidosis; *HHNC*, hyperosmolar hyperglycemic nonketotic coma; *I & O*, intake and output.

- Disturbed thought processes related to hyperglycemia, acidosis (DKA), electrolyte imbalance
- Deficient knowledge: disease process, treatment regimen, sick-day management

Nursing and Medical Interventions

The primary objectives in the treatment of DKA and HHNC include respiratory support, fluid replacement, administration of insulin to correct hyperglycemia, replacement of electrolytes, correction of acidosis in DKA, prevention of complications, and patient teaching and support.

Each year, the American Diabetes Association publishes a supplement to *Diabetes Care* that includes their position statement on the treatment of hyperglycemic crises in patients with DM. The reader is referred to the current issue for the most recent recommendation for treating DKA and HHNC.

Respiratory support. Assessment of the airway, breathing, and circulation is always the first priority in managing life-threatening disorders. Airway and breathing may be supported through the use of oral airways and oxygen therapy. In more severe cases, the patient may be intubated and placed on ventilatory support. Prevention of aspiration is accomplished by elevating the head of the bed. Nasogastric tube suction may be considered in a patient with impaired mentation who is actively vomiting.

Fluid replacement. Dehydration may have progressed to shock by the time of admission. Immediate intravenous (IV) access and rehydration need to be accomplished. In DKA, the typical water deficit approximates 100 mL/kg, and it may be as high as 200 mL/kg in HHNC (ADA, 2003). Monitoring for signs and symptoms of hypovolemic shock is a priority. Vital signs must be recorded at least every hour initially, along with the urine output. Unstable patients require constant monitoring and recording of hemodynamic parameters at least every 15 minutes. Right atrial pressure or pulmonary artery pressure monitoring may also be instituted to evaluate fluid requirements and to monitor the patient's response to treatment. This is particularly true of patients with HHNC, who tend to be elderly and have concurrent cardiovascular and renal disease. Accurate intake, hourly recording of urine output, and daily weights are also essential. Changes in mentation may also indicate a change in fluid status.

Normal saline (0.9% NS) is usually the fluid of choice for initial fluid replacement because it best replaces extracellular fluid volume deficits. Fluid replacement usually starts with an initial bolus of 1 L of 0.9% NS. This is followed by an infusion of 10 to 20 mL/kg during the first hour (ADA, 2003). IV fluids are continued at rapid rates until the patient's blood pressure normalizes. The IV fluid is then changed to hypotonic saline (0.45% NS) at slower rates to replace intracellular fluid deficits. The goal is generally to replace half of the estimated fluid deficit over the first 8 hours. The second half of the fluid deficit should be replaced during the next 16 hours of therapy.

Fluid overload from overaggressive fluid replacement can be prevented by monitoring breath sounds and performing cardiovascular assessments. Signs and symptoms of fluid overload are reviewed in Box 17-5. Rapid fluid administration may also contribute to cerebral edema, a complication associated with DKA. The rapid fall in plasma glucose, combined with rapid fluid administration and concurrent insulin therapy (see next section), may result in movement of water into brain cells, with resulting brain edema.

Insulin therapy. Replacement of insulin is definitive therapy for DKA and HHNC. The goal is to restore normal glucose uptake by cells while preventing complications of excess insulin administration (i.e., hypoglycemia, hypokalemia, and hypophosphatemia). An initial IV bolus of 0.15 units/kg of regular insulin is administered, followed by a continuous infusion of 0.1 units/kg per hour to achieve a steady decrease in serum glucose of 50 to 75 mg/dL per hour.

Serum glucose levels need to be monitored every 1 to 2 hours while the patient is receiving an insulin infusion. One consistent method of monitoring (e.g., fingerstick) must be used. As the serum glucose approaches 250 mg/dL, the primary IV solution is changed to 5% glucose with hypotonic saline (D5 0.45% NS) to replace intracellular fluid volume deficits. The addition of dextrose allows for the continued use of insulin, and prevents hypoglycemia and cerebral edema. While on the insulin infusion, patients are generally allowed nothing by mouth (NPO). Once serum glucose levels are stabilized in a desirable range, the patient is generally managed with subcutaneous insulin based on a sliding scale. Serum glucose levels may then be monitored every 6 to 8 hours.

It is important that serum glucose not be lowered too rapidly, to avoid the potential for cerebral edema, which could result in seizures and coma. Any patient who exhibits an abrupt change in the level of consciousness after initiation of insulin therapy needs to have blood glucose monitoring and protective steps instituted to prevent harm. Seizure precautions should also be started. Treatment of acute cerebral edema usually involves administration of an osmotic diuretic (e.g., 20% mannitol solution).

Electrolyte replacement. Potassium, phosphate, chloride, and magnesium replacement may be required, especially during insulin administration. Osmotic diuresis in DKA and HHNC results in total body potassium depletion ranging from 400 to 600 mEq. Potassium deficit may be greater in HHNC. Potassium therapy is based on serum laboratory results. In the absence of renal disease, potassium monitoring and replacement should begin with fluid therapy. Twenty to 40 mEq of potassium is usually added to each liter of fluid administered. This may be augmented by additional doses of potassium per minibag. The IV site and cardiac function need to be monitored during potassium administration.

Total body phosphorus levels are also depleted by osmotic diuresis. This may result in impaired respiratory and cardiac functions. For this reason, potassium phosphate is often used in treating part of the potassium deficit. Phosphate replacements should not be used in patients with renal failure, because these patients are unable to excrete phosphate and typically suffer from hyperphosphatemia.

Treatment of acidosis. Acidosis is a hallmark feature of DKA. However, multiple studies have shown no benefit and some risk to cerebral function with the administration of sodium bicarbonate. Therefore, sodium bicarbonate is not used to treat acidosis unless the serum pH is 7.0 or less (ADA, 2003). When required, IV bicarbonate is used only to bring the pH up to 7.0, but not to normal levels. Even then, cautious use of sodium bicarbonate is recommended because too rapid correction of acidosis may cause central nervous system acidosis and severe hypoxemia at the cellular level. When administered, the bicarbonate is added to the hypotonic NS and is replaced slowly. Serum arterial blood gas analysis should be done frequently to assess for changes in pH, bicarbonate, an ion gap, $PaCO_2$, and oxygenation status. Once fluid and electrolyte imbalances are corrected and insulin is administered, the kidneys will begin to conserve bicarbonate to restore acid-base homeostasis, and ketone formation will cease.

BOX 17-5

Signs and Symptoms of Fluid Overload

- Tachypnea
- Neck vein distention
- Tachycardia
- Crackles
- Increased pulmonary capillary wedge or right atrial pressures
- Declining level of consciousness in cerebral edema

Patient and family education. Education of patients is key to the prevention of DKA in particular. Medication teaching is a priority. Monitoring of hemoglobin A1C levels, also known as glycosylated or glycated hemoglobin, two to three times a year reflects the patient's long-term control of blood glucose levels. The importance of a regular eating schedule, exercise, rest and sleep, and relaxation needs to be emphasized. Adjustments to the usual diabetic control regimen for illness is known as "sick-day management," and all diabetic patients and families need to learn sick-day management.

Patient Outcomes

Outcomes for a patient with DKA or HHNC include the following:

- Hemodynamic stability
- Fluid balance
- Electrolytes within normal limits
- Serum glucose less than 200 mg/dL, preferably within normal limits
- Serum osmolality within normal limits
- Mental status returned to baseline
- Respiratory parameters returned to baseline
- Nutritional balance
- Verbalization of information needed to comply with discharge regimen
- Verbalization of sick day management for DM
- Arterial blood gases within normal limits or returned to baseline (DKA)

(See Nursing Care Plan for the Patient with Hyperglycemic Complications of a Pancreatic Endocrine Disorder.)

Nursing Care Plan for the Patient with Hyperglycemic Complications of a Pancreatic Endocrine Disorder

NURSING DIAGNOSIS: *Ineffective breathing pattern or impaired gas exchange related to acidosis (DKA), decreased level of consciousness*

Patient Outcomes	Interventions	Rationales

Normal respiratory rate and pattern:
   RR 10-25/min
   Tidal volume >5 ml/kg
Normal PaCO$_2$ on ABG analysis (DKA)
	Assess airway and breathing on admission and every 1-2 hr.
	Provide support as appropriate (e.g., airway, intubation).
	Correlate ABG results with clinical examination.
	Prevent aspiration: head of bed elevated; NG decompression.
		Respiratory changes will stabilize as pH shifts.
		Respiration support is required until breathing pattern is normalized.

NURSING DIAGNOSIS: *Deficient fluid volume related to osmotic diuresis and total body water loss, ketosis and increased lipolysis, vomiting*

Patient Outcomes	Interventions	Rationales

Normal serum glucose
Hemodynamic stability: BP, HR, RAP, PAOP WNL
Normal sinus rhythm
Urine output >30 mL/hr
Balanced I & O
Stable weight
Warm, dry extremities
Presence of normal skin turgor
Moist mucous membranes
	Assess fluid status:
	   Vital signs every 1 hr until stable
	   I & O measurements every 1-2 hr
	   Skin turgor; signs of dehydration
	   Consider insensible fluid losses via skin and lungs
	   Daily weights
	Initiate therapy for dehydration: IV fluid administration; monitor for signs and symptoms of fluid overload; monitor effects.
	Monitor neurological status closely during fluid administration.
		Prevents hypovolemic shock and restores cellular function.

NURSING DIAGNOSIS: *Imbalanced electrolytes related to lack of insulin, fluid shifts, acid/base imbalance, vomiting/NG suction*

Patient Outcomes	Interventions	Rationales

Glucose 70-100 mg/dL
Serum electrolytes WNL:
  Sodium
  Potassium
  Calcium
  Phosphorus
Osmolality WNL
ABGs WNL
	Monitor blood glucose every 1 hr via serum blood glucose or fingersticks, titrate insulin therapy; monitor for signs and symptoms of hypoglycemia.
	Monitor serum electrolytes every 1-2 hr until stable.
	Assess causes of electrolyte loss (e.g., diuresis, vomiting, NG suction).
	Replace electrolytes as needed; individualize according to serum values.
	Monitor for signs and symptoms of hyperkalemia (peaked T wave on ECG).
	Add glucose to maintenance IVs once blood sugar is at 300 mg/dL.
	Take seizure precautions as necessary.
		Sudden shifts in glucose and electrolytes are destabilizing.
		
		Close monitoring achieves gradual return to normal.

NURSING DIAGNOSIS: *Disturbed thought processes related to hyperglycemia, acidosis, electrolyte imbalance*

Patient Outcomes	Interventions	Rationales

Patient alert
Oriented to person, place, and time
Appropriate behavior
	Monitor neurological status every 1 hr until stable, then every 2 hr.
	Monitor for weakness, increasing confusion, lethargy, drowsiness, obtundation.
	Provide orientation cues.
	Take seizure precautions as appropriate.
	Prevent complications related to alterations in consciousness and immobility:
	  Provide mouth and skin care
	  Turn every 1-2 hr
	  Perform passive ROM
	  Provide for elimination
		Neurological status will return to baseline as hypotension and electrolyte balance are restored.
		Monitor for adverse changes signaling cerebral edema.

NURSING DIAGNOSIS: *Deficient knowledge: disease process, treatment regimen, complications of DKA*

Patient Outcomes	Interventions	Rationales

Patient/family able to:
  Describe pathophysiology and causes of DKA and HHNC
  Discuss and follow diet, exercise regimen prescribed
  List signs and symptoms of hypoglycemia, hyperglycemia
	Assess patient/family's ability to learn information and psychomotor and sensory skills.
	Design a teaching program that includes information on pathophysiology and causes of DKA or HHNC; diet and exercise restrictions; signs and symptoms of hyperglycemia and hypoglycemia, including interventions; signs and symptoms of infection.
		DKA and HHNC are prevented with appropriate disease management.

Continued

Nursing Care Plan for the Patient with Hyperglycemic Complications of a Pancreatic Endocrine Disorder—cont'd

Patient Outcomes	Interventions	Rationales
List signs and symptoms of infections that require medical follow-up Demonstrate self-glucose monitoring Demonstrate self-administration of insulin as appropriate Describe sick-day management	Demonstrate methods for blood glucose monitoring; have the patient repeat the demonstration until proficient. If the patient is taking insulin, demonstrate the method of insulin administration; discuss dosage, frequency, action, duration, sites, side effects; discuss situations that require adjustment of insulin dose. Review an insulin pump if used for treatment. Consult with the dietitian. Encourage the use of a diabetic identification bracelet Provide written materials for all content taught; provide means for the patient to get questions answered after discharge. Schedule a follow-up teaching session after discharge.	

ABGs, Arterial blood gases; *BP,* blood pressure; *DKA,* diabetic ketoacidosis; *ECG,* electrocardiogram; *HHNC,* hyperosmolar hyperglycemic nonketotic coma; *HR,* heart rate; *I & O,* intake and output; *IV,* intravenous; *NG,* nasogastric; *PaCO$_2$,* partial pressure of carbon dioxide in arterial blood; *PAOP,* pulmonary artery occlusion pressure; *RAP,* right atrial pressure; *ROM,* range of motion; *RR,* respiratory rate; *WNL,* within normal limits.

HYPOGLYCEMIA

Pathophysiology

A hypoglycemic episode is defined as a decrease in the plasma glucose level to 45 to 60 mg/dL or less, and is sometimes referred to as "insulin shock" or "insulin reaction." Glucose production falls behind glucose utilization, resulting in a change in the level of consciousness. Additionally, there is a rise in counterregulatory hormones (those that work to increase blood glucose levels), including glucagon, epinephrine, cortisol, and growth hormone. Those at highest risk are diabetic patients taking insulin, children and pregnant women with type 1 DM, and older persons with type 1 or type 2 DM (Tkacs, 2002). Hypoglycemia unawareness is a term used to describe those diabetic patients who may not be able to recognize the onset of hypoglycemia. Those at higher risk of hypoglycemia unawareness include the elderly because of their decreased awareness of thirst, and patients with diminished mental function resulting from dementia, concurrent illness, and other factors. Patients taking beta-blockers are also at risk of decreased awareness of the early signs of hypoglycemia.

Cognitive and perceptual changes are common in hypoglycemia, because glucose is the preferred energy source for the brain. Headache, impaired mentation, irritability, inability to concentrate, and dizziness are predominant findings. Prolonged hypoglycemia may lead to irreversible brain damage and coma.

Other systemic clinical manifestations of hypoglycemia are caused by activation of the sympathetic nervous system and the resultant release of epinephrine, which is triggered by a progressive decrease in the glucose supply to the brain. Systemic signs of epinephrine release include cool, clammy skin; pallor; tremors; palpitations; and tachydysrhythmias. The pathophysiologic mechanisms associated with acute hypoglycemia are reviewed in Figure 17-4.

Etiology. Patients receiving insulin therapy need to be closely monitored for hypoglycemia or decreased serum glucose levels, especially when the insulin dose may be greater than the body's requirements or when injection sites are rotated from a hypertrophied area to one with unimpaired absorption. Other causes of hypoglycemia include insufficient caloric consumption because of a missed or delayed meal or snack, insufficient nutrition, and decreased intake because of nausea and vomiting, anorexia, or interrupted tube feedings or total parenteral nutrition. Weight loss and recovery from stress (infections, illness) decrease requirements for exogenous insulin. Strenuous exercise that is not compensated by an increased intake of food or a decrease in insulin dose can also precipitate hypoglycemia. Excessive alcohol consumption produces necrosis of liver cells and fatty infiltration, thereby blocking gluconeogenesis in the liver. The major etiological factors of hypoglycemia are reviewed in Box 17-6.

Careful assessment of a patient with renal and liver dysfunction and use of hypoglycemic medications is necessary. Decreased degradation or excretion of hypoglycemic medications prolongs or potentiates their effects. It is also important to keep in mind other drugs that potentiate the action of antidiabetic medications.

Assessment

Clinical presentation. The most common signs and symptoms of hypoglycemia are summarized in Table 17-2. Symptoms of hypoglycemia can be categorized as (1) mild symptoms from autonomic nervous system stimulation that are characteristic of a rapid decrease in serum glucose and (2) moderate symptoms reflective of an inadequate supply of glucose to neural tissues, associated with a slower, more prolonged decline in glucose. Subjective symptoms of impaired mentation predominate because the brain requires a constant supply of glucose for energy.

With a rapid decrease in serum glucose levels, there is activation of the sympathetic nervous system, mediated by epinephrine release from the adrenal medulla. This compensatory "fight or flight" mechanism may result in symptoms such as tachycardia, diaphoresis, pallor, and dilated pupils. The patient may also report feelings of apprehension, nervousness, headache, tremulousness, and general weakness.

Slower and more prolonged declines in serum glucose result in symptoms related to an inadequate glucose supply to neural tissues (neuroglucopenia).

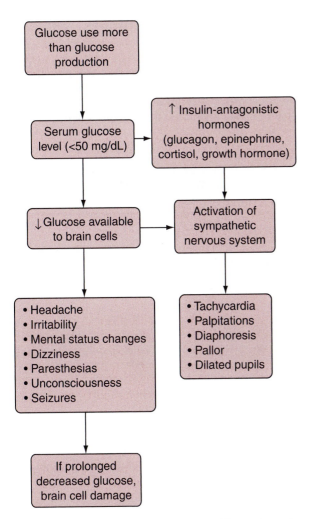

FIGURE 17-4 Pathophysiology of hypoglycemia.

BOX 17-6

Causes of Hypoglycemia

EXCESS INSULIN OR ORAL HYPOGLYCEMICS
Dose of insulin or oral hypoglycemics too high
Islet cell tumors (insulinomas)
Liver disease (impaired metabolism of insulin)
Renal disease (impaired inactivation of insulin)
Autoimmune phenomenon
Drugs that potentiate action of antidiabetic medications (propranolol, oxytetracycline)
Sulfonylureas in elderly patients

UNDERPRODUCTION OF GLUCOSE
Heavy alcohol consumption
Decreased food intake
Drugs: aspirin, disopyramide (Norpace), haloperidol (Haldol)
Decreased production by liver
Hormonal causes

TOO RAPID UTILIZATION OF GLUCOSE
Gastrointestinal surgery
Extrapancreatic tumor
Increased or strenuous exercise

These include restlessness and difficulty in thinking and speaking, and visual disturbances and paresthesias may be present. The patient may also have profound changes in the level of consciousness and/or convulsions. Personality changes and psychiatric manifestations have been reported.

Laboratory evaluation. The confirming laboratory sign of hypoglycemia is a serum or capillary blood glucose level less than 50 mg/dL. The glucose level should be checked on all high-risk patients with the aforementioned clinical signs. In patients with a known history of DM, a thorough history of past experiences of hypoglycemia, including associated signs and symptoms, should be elicited during admission.

Nursing Diagnoses

The nursing diagnoses applicable to a patient with a hypoglycemic episode include the following:
- Imbalanced electrolytes related to excess circulating insulin as compared with glucose
- Disturbed thought processes related to decreased glucose to the brain
- Risk for injury (seizures) related to altered neuronal function associated with hypoglycemia
- Deficient knowledge: prevention, recognition, and treatment of hypoglycemia

Nursing and Medical Interventions

After plasma or capillary glucose levels have been confirmed, carbohydrates must be administered. The patient's neurological status determines the route to be used. Box 17-7 details a protocol for treatment of mild, moderate, and severe hypoglycemia. Common food substances that contain at least 15 g of carbohydrate are listed in Box 17-8. Glucose levels should be reassessed 15 to 20 minutes after treatment. If the blood glucose level remains lower than 70 mg/dL, readminister the same treatment. Ongoing assessment of vital signs and electrocardiogram (ECG) during the acute phase is also a priority. Hypoglycemia is also associated with dysrhythmias in susceptible patients.

In the event of hypoglycemia, insulin should be stopped temporarily. If the patient has an insulin pump, it should be suspended for moderate or severe hypoglycemia. The patient should determine whether to discontinue the pump for mild hypoglycemia.

Neurological assessments are done to detect any changes in cerebral function related to hypoglycemia. It is important to document baseline neurological status, including mental status, cranial nerve function, sensory and motor function, and deep tendon reflexes. There is a potential for seizures related to altered neuronal cellular metabolism during the hypoglycemic phase, so patients should be assessed for seizure activity. Descriptions of the seizure event and associated

---

TABLE 17-2

Signs and Symptoms of Hypoglycemia

Decrease in Blood Sugar	
Rapid	Prolonged
ACTIVATION OF SYMPATHETIC NERVOUS SYSTEM	**INADEQUATE GLUCOSE SUPPLY TO NEURAL TISSUES**
Nervousness	Headache
Apprehension	Restlessness
Tachycardia	Difficulty speaking
Palpitations	Difficulty thinking
Pallor	Visual disturbances
Diaphoresis	Parethesia
Dilated pupils	Difficulty walking
Tremors	Altered consciousness
Fatigue	Coma
General weakness	Convulsions
Headache	Change in personality
Hunger	Psychiatric reactions
	Maniacal behavior
	Catatonia
	Acute paranoia

BOX 17-7

Treatment of Hypoglycemia

MILD HYPOGLYCEMIA
Patient is completely alert. Symptoms may include pallor, diaphoresis, tachycardia, palpitations, hunger, or shakiness. Blood glucose is 60 to 80 mg/dL.
Treatment: 15 g of carbohydrate by mouth

MODERATE HYPOGLYCEMIA
Patient is conscious, cooperative, and able to swallow safely. Symptoms may include difficulty concentrating, confusion, slurred speech, or extreme fatigue. Blood glucose is less than 60 mg/dL.
Treatment: 20 to 30 g of carbohydrate by mouth

SEVERE HYPOGLYCEMIA
Patient is uncooperative or unconscious. Blood glucose is less than 60 mg/dL.
Treatment with intravenous access: ½ ampule of 50% dextrose
Treatment without intravenous access: 1 mg of glucagon subcutaneously

Sources of 15 Grams of Carbohydrates

- 4 oz sweetened carbonated beverage
- 4 oz unsweetened fruit juice
- 1 cup skim milk
- Glucose gels or tablets (follow manufacturer's instructions)

symptoms are important to note. Seizure precautions should be instituted, including padded side rails, oxygen, oral airway, and suction available at the bedside, as well as removal of potentially harmful objects from the environment. Neurological status is the best clinical indicator of effective treatment for hypoglycemia.

Patient and family education about hypoglycemic episodes may also be appropriate in the critical care setting. The patient and family members need to be instructed on the causes, symptoms, treatment, and prevention of hypoglycemia. Principles regarding diet, insulin or oral hypoglycemic agents, and exercise may need to be incorporated into the teaching plan, as appropriate. Instruction on the use of home blood glucose monitoring may also be needed.

Patient Outcomes

Outcomes for a patient with a hypoglycemic episode include the following:
- Plasma or capillary glucose within normal limits
- Absence of signs and symptoms of hypoglycemia
- Mental status returned to baseline
- Absence of seizure activity
- Ability of the patient and family to identify causes of hypoglycemia, state symptoms of hypoglycemia, state type and amount of foods that may be used to treat hypoglycemia, and perform home blood glucose monitoring

Acute Adrenal Insufficiency

ETIOLOGY

Hypofunction of the adrenal gland results from either primary or secondary mechanisms that suppress corticosteroid secretion. Primary mechanisms, resulting in Addison's disease, are those that cause destruction of the adrenal gland itself. At least 90% of the adrenal cortex must be destroyed before clinical signs and symptoms appear. Primary disorders result in deficiencies of both glucocorticoids and mineralocorticoids. Some of the mechanisms that can cause primary adrenal deficiency include autoimmune destruction of the gland (idiopathic), infection, hemorrhagic destruction, and granulomatous infiltration.

Autoimmune destruction of the adrenal gland may have a genetic component. The disease results in hypofunction and eventual atrophy of the gland. Autoantibodies specific to the cells of the adrenal cortex are present in 50% to 70% of patients with this form of Addison's disease (Jones & Huether, 2002). This form of adrenal disease may affect just the adrenal gland or may be part of a constellation of autoimmune problems, such as Hashimoto's thyroiditis or pernicious anemia.

Secondary mechanisms that can produce adrenal insufficiency are those that interfere with adrenocorticotropic hormone (ACTH) secretion or simply suppress normal secretion of corticosteroids. These generally result in deficiencies of only glucocorticoids, because stimulation of the mineralocorticoids is not dependent on ACTH secretion. Mechanisms that can produce secondary adrenal insufficiency include long-term steroid use, pituitary and hypothalamic disorders, infection, and sepsis. A more detailed listing of possible causes of primary and secondary adrenal insufficiency is given in Box 17-9.

Causes of Adrenal Insufficiency

PRIMARY
- Autoimmune disease (idiopathic and polyglandular)
- Granulomatous disease (tuberculosis, sarcoidosis, histoplasmosis, blastomycosis)
- Metastatic cancer
- Hemorrhagic destruction (anticoagulation, trauma, sepsis)
- Sepsis (meningococcal or staphylococcal)
- Acquired immunodeficiency syndrome (AIDS)
- Drugs: ketoconazole, aminoglutethimide, trimethoprim (suppress adrenals); phenytoin, barbiturates, rifampin (increase steroid degradation)
- Developmental or genetic abnormality

SECONDARY
- Long-term steroid use
- Drugs: etomidate, ketoconazole
- Pituitary tumors, hemorrhage, radiation, metastatic cancer
- Systemic inflammatory states (sepsis)
- Infiltrative disorders (sarcoidosis)
- Postpartum hemorrhage (Sheehan's syndrome)
- Trauma or surgery
- Hypothalamic disorders

Patients experiencing acute adrenal insufficiency are most commonly those who are currently receiving, or have recently been withdrawn from, corticosteroid therapy. Corticosteroids are used in the treatment of various inflammatory, allergic, and immunoreactive disorders (Box 17-10). Long-term steroid use suppresses the normal corticotropin-releasing hormone (CRH)-ACTH-adrenal feedback systems (see Figure 17-1) and can result in adrenal suppression. There is insufficient evidence to predict accurately the amount of adrenal suppression in patients receiving exogenous glucocorticoid therapy. Longer-acting agents such as dexamethasone are more likely to produce suppression than are shorter-acting steroids such as hydrocortisone. It may take several months for normal secretion of corticosteroids to return in patients in whom corticosteroid administration has been tapered off in the previous 9 months. Once corticosteroid use has been tapered off, it may take several months for these patients to resume normal secretion of corticosteroids. Thus, it is important to be familiar with disorders that may be treated with corticosteroids, because the resulting adrenal suppression may prevent a normal stress response in these patients and may put them at risk of an adrenal crisis.

Infection is one of the most common causes of adrenal insufficiency in the critical care setting. Patients with human immunodeficiency virus (HIV) infection are at risk of developing adrenal insufficiency. In fact, approximately 33% of patients with HIV infections who are admitted to the intensive care unit have adrenal insufficiency (Zaloga & Marik, 2001). The adrenal glands may also be the site of cytomegalovirus infection in as many as 50% of patients with HIV. Although adrenal involvement is common, it is rare for HIV-infected patients to have more than 90% destruction of the adrenal gland.

Addison's disease, or primary adrenal insufficiency, is a less common cause of adrenal insufficiency or adrenal crisis than either corticosteroid therapy or HIV infection. Damage to the adrenal gland in approximately 50% to 70% of patients with Addison's disease is the result of idiopathic autoimmune destruction (Jones & Huether, 2002). Tuberculosis is now a rare cause of adrenal insufficiency in the United States. The autoimmune form of the disease is frequently associated with other autoimmune diseases such as Hashimoto's thyroiditis, pernicious anemia, idiopathic hypoparathyroidism, and type 1 DM. Young women with spontaneous premature ovarian failure are at increased risk of developing the autoimmune form of adrenal insufficiency (Bakalov, Vanderhoof, & Bondy, 2002).

Hemorrhagic destruction of the adrenal gland has been reported with anticoagulation therapy, after surgical procedures, and during infection. Anticoagulation therapy with heparin can cause selective hypoaldosteronism and, more rarely, cases of hemorrhage resulting in both mineralocorticoid and glucocorticoid deficiencies. A common complication of meningococcal meningitis is massive adrenal hemorrhage, which can result in lethal adrenal insufficiency.

Adrenal crisis can be precipitated in any patient with chronic adrenal insufficiency by providing inadequate hormone replacement during times of acute stress such as infection, trauma, or surgery or after sudden withdrawal of steroids in a patient receiving long-term therapy. It is also recognized that many seriously ill patients are often found to have occult or unrecognized adrenal insufficiency, especially patients with sepsis, septic shock, or severe trauma (Rivers et al., 2001). During periods of stress, the adrenal

---

BOX 17-10

Therapeutic Uses of Corticosteroids

- Replacement therapy in patients with primary or secondary adrenal cortical insufficiency
- Symptomatic treatment of inflammatory, allergic, or immunological disorders, including the following:
  Rheumatic: rheumatoid arthritis, osteoarthritis, acute gouty arthritis, ankylosing spondylitis, systemic lupus erythematosus
  Allergic: allergic rhinitis, bronchial asthma, dermatitis, serum sickness, drug hypersensitivity, anaphylactic shock
  Ophthalmic: conjunctivitis, keratitis, iritis, uveitis, acute optic neuritis, chorioretinitis, allergic corneal marginal ulcers
  Gastrointestinal: ulcerative colitis, regional enteritis, chronic active hepatitis
  Hematological/neoplastic: thrombocytopenic purpura, hemolytic anemia, leukemia, Hodgkin's disease, multiple myeloma
  Other: nephrotic syndrome, gout, hypercalcemia, multiple sclerosis, tuberculosis, meningitis
- Supportive use in acute disorders, including the following:
  Septic shock
  Neurological emergencies (to treat cerebral edema): head trauma, cerebral hypoxia, tumors, hemorrhage, infection
  Pulmonary disorders: asthma, chronic bronchitis, acute respiratory distress syndrome

cortex is able to increase the production of cortisol up to 10 times the normal rate, if necessary. Patients with inadequate adrenal cortex function are unable to increase production and thus develop an acute, life-threatening crisis.

REVIEW OF PHYSIOLOGY

Persons who have suppression or an absolute lack of secretion of corticosteroids are candidates for an adrenal crisis, which represents a life-threatening endocrine emergency. The manifestations of adrenal crisis result from insufficient secretion by the adrenal cortex of glucocorticoids (primarily cortisol) and/or mineralocorticoids (primarily aldosterone). The deficiency of glucocorticoids is especially significant, because their influence on the defense mechanisms of the body and its response to stress makes them essential for life. An insufficiency of adrenal androgens may also exist, but the manifestations are not clinically significant.

Cortisol, which is the strongest of the glucocorticoids synthesized by the adrenal cortex, is normally released in response to stimulation by ACTH from the anterior pituitary gland (see Figure 17-1). ACTH is stimulated by CRH from the hypothalamus, which is influenced by circulating cortisol levels, circadian rhythms, and stress. Circadian rhythms affect ACTH, and thus cortisol levels, diurnally, creating peak levels of cortisol in the morning and the lowest levels around midnight. This normal rhythm can be overridden by stress. During stress, plasma cortisol may increase as much as 10 times its normal level. Increased release of cortisol increases blood glucose concentration by promoting glycogen breakdown and gluconeogenesis in the liver, increases lipolysis and free fatty acid production, increases protein degradation, and inhibits the inflammatory and immune responses. Additional effects are summarized in Box 17-11.

Mineralocorticoids regulate the body's electrolyte and water balance, and aldosterone is the most important of the mineralocorticoids synthesized by the adrenal cortex. Secretion of aldosterone is regulated primarily by the renin-angiotensin system. Renin is an enzyme stored in the cells of the juxtaglomerular apparatus in the kidneys. Its release occurs in response to decreased plasma sodium, increased plasma potassium, decreased extracellular fluid volume, and decreased blood pressure. Once released, renin cleaves angiotensinogen in the plasma to form angiotensin I. Angiotensin I is then converted to angiotensin II in the lungs under the influence of angiotensin-converting enzyme. Angiotensin II stimulates the secretion of aldosterone by the adrenal cortex and is also a potent vasoconstrictor. Aldosterone acts in the kidneys on the ascending loop of Henle, the distal convoluted tubule, and the collecting ducts to increase sodium ion reabsorption and to increase potassium and hydrogen ion excretion. Because reabsorption of sodium creates an osmotic gradient across the renal tubular membrane, antidiuretic

---

BOX 17-11

Physiological Effects of Glucocorticoids (Cortisol)

- Protein metabolism: promotes gluconeogenesis, stimulates protein breakdown, and inhibits protein synthesis
- Fat metabolism: ↑ lipolysis and free fatty acid production, promotes fat deposits in face and cervical area
- Opposes action of insulin: ↓ glucose transport and utilization in cells
- Inhibits inflammatory response
  Suppresses mediator release (kinins, histamine, interleukins, prostaglandins, leukotrienes, serotonin)
  Stabilizes cell membrane and inhibits capillary dilation
  ↓ Formation of edema
  Inhibits leukocyte migration and phagocytic activity
- Immunosuppression
  ↓ Proliferation of T lymphocytes and killer cell activity
  ↓ Complement production and immunoglobulins
- ↑ Circulating erythrocytes
- Gastrointestinal effects: ↑appetite; increases rate of acid and pepsin secretion in stomach
- ↑ Uric acid excretion
- ↓ Serum calcium
- Sensitizes arterioles to effects of catecholamines; maintains blood pressure
- ↑ Renal glomerular filtration rate and excretion of water

↑, Increases; ↓, decreases.

hormone (ADH) is activated, causing water to be reabsorbed with sodium. The physiology of aldosterone release is summarized in Figure 17-5.

PATHOPHYSIOLOGY

Acute adrenal insufficiency is produced by an absolute or relative lack of cortisol (glucocorticoid) and aldosterone (mineralocorticoid) (Figure 17-6). A deficiency of cortisol results in decreased production of glucose, decreased metabolism of protein and fat, decreased appetite, decreased intestinal motility and digestion, decreased vascular tone, and diminished effect of catecholamines. If a patient with deficient cortisol is stressed, this deficiency can produce profound shock because of significant decreases in vascular tone and the diminished effects of catecholamines (Zaloga & Marik, 2001).

Deficiency of aldosterone results in decreased retention of sodium and water, decreased circulating

volume, and increased potassium and hydrogen ion reabsorption. These effects are seen in patients with underlying primary adrenal insufficiency but not secondary adrenal insufficiency (decreased ACTH), because aldosterone secretion is not dependent on ACTH. A summary of pathophysiological effects of adrenal insufficiency can be found in Figure 17-6.

ASSESSMENT
Clinical Presentation

Acute adrenal crisis requires astute and rapid data collection. Box 17-12 gives a risk factor analysis for adrenal crisis. Features of adrenal crisis are nonspecific and may be attributed to other medical disorders. Signs and symptoms vary (see Figure 17-6). Because this condition is a medical emergency, the diagnosis should be considered in any patient acutely ill with fever, vomiting, hypotension, shock, decreased sodium, increased potassium, or hypoglycemia (see Laboratory Alerts: Adrenal Disorders). Specific system disturbances are widespread.

Cardiovascular system. Cardiovascular signs and symptoms in acute adrenal crisis are related to hypovolemia (decreased water reabsorption), decreased vascular tone (decreased effectiveness of catecholamines), and hyperkalemia. The most common presentation of adrenal insufficiency in the intensive care unit is hypotension refractory to fluids and requiring vasopressors. The patient may also have symptoms of decreased cardiac output: weak, rapid pulse; dysrhythmias; and cold, pale skin. The chest x-ray study may show decreased heart size. Changes in the ECG may result if hyperkalemia is significant. These changes include narrow and taller T waves with a shortened QT interval with mild hyperkalemia and, with severe hyperkalemia (levels of 6.0 mEq/L or higher), depressed ST segment, prolonged PR interval, and widened QRS complex may be seen. Hypovolemia and vascular dilation may be severe enough in crisis to cause hemodynamic collapse and shock.

Neurological system. Neurological manifestations in acute adrenal crisis are related to decreases in glucose levels, protein metabolism, volume and perfusion, and sodium concentrations. Patients may complain of headache, fatigue that worsens as the day progresses, and severe weakness. They may also suffer from mental confusion, listlessness, lethargy, apathy, psychoses, and emotional lability.

Gastrointestinal system. The gastrointestinal (GI) signs and symptoms in acute adrenal crisis are related to decreased digestive enzymes and to decreased intestinal motility and digestion. Anorexia, nausea,

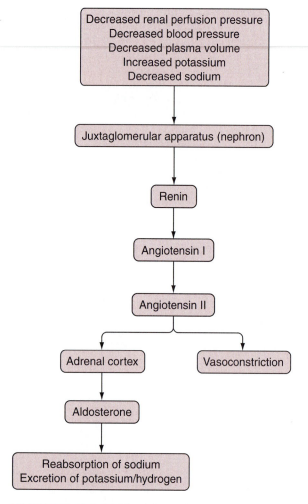

FIGURE 17-5 Physiology of aldosterone release.

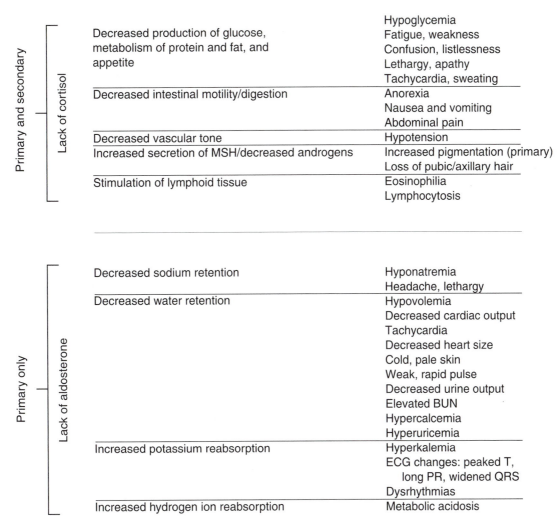

FIGURE 17-6 Pathophysiological effects of adrenal insufficiency. *BUN,* Blood urea nitrogen; *ECG,* electrocardiogram; *MSH,* melanocyte-stimulating hormone.

BOX 17-12

Risk Factor Analysis for Adrenal Crisis

When collecting the patient database, look carefully at patients who are at risk, have predisposing factors, or have physical findings associated with chronic adrenal insufficiency. Some of the historical data to look for include the following:

- *Drug history:* steroids in the past year, phenytoin, barbiturates, rifampin
- *Illness history:* infection, cancer, autoimmune disease, diseases treated with steroids, radiation to head or abdomen, human immunodeficiency virus–positive status
- *Family history:* autoimmune disease, Addison's disease
- *Nutrition:* weight loss, decreased appetite
- *Miscellaneous:* fatigue, dizziness, weakness, darkening of skin, low blood glucose that does not respond to therapy, salt craving (dramatic craving such as drinking pickle juice or eating salt from the shaker)

LABORATORY ALERTS: ADRENAL DISORDERS

Laboratory Test	Critical Value	Significance	Nursing Actions
Serum Glucose	<50 mg/dL	Hypoglycemia	Provide a form of glucose (PO, IM, or IV depending on access or patient's level of consciousness). Monitor serum/capillary laboratory values.
Cortisol	<10 mcg/dL	In severely ill patient or stressed patient indicates insufficiency	Replace hormones (specifically, glucocorticoids). Monitor serum cortisol levels.
Potassium	>6.5 mEq/L	Potential for heart blocks, brady-dysrhythmias, sinus arrest, ventricular fibrillation, or asystole	Use close cardiac monitoring, IV fluid replacement for rehydration, and monitoring of serum laboratory values. If low, potassium replacement is given either PO or IV depending on circumstances.
	<3.0 mEq/L	Potential for ventricular dysrhythmias	
Sodium	>150 mEq/L	May be a result of stress and dehydration	This usually resolves with IV rehydration and/or replacement. Adjust sodium replacement in IV therapy.
	<130 mEq/L	Resulting from hydration therapy	
BUN	>20 mg/dL	↑ From protein breakdown and hemoconcentration	Monitor I & O (especially urine output ≥30 mL/hr) and serum laboratory values.
pH	<7.3	↓ From accumulation of acids and dehydration	This should resolve with rehydration and return of electrolyte balance. If it is not resolved by other measures, consider bicarbonate replacement.

↑, Increased; ↓, decreased; *BUN*, blood urea nitrogen, *I & O*, intake and output; *IM*, intramuscular; *IV*, intravenous; *PO*, orally.

vomiting, diarrhea and vague abdominal pain are present in the majority of patients (Jones & Huether, 2002).

Genitourinary system. Decreased circulation to the kidneys from diminished circulating volume and hypotension causes decreases in the glomerular filtration rate and in renal perfusion. Urine output may decline as a result.

Box 17-13 lists the signs associated with progressive onset of chronic adrenal insufficiency.

Laboratory Evaluation

Typical laboratory findings in a patient with acute adrenal crisis include hypoglycemia, hyponatremia, hyperkalemia, eosinophilia, increased BUN, and metabolic acidosis. Hypercalcemia or hyperuricemia are possible as a result of volume depletion (see Laboratory Alerts: Adrenal Disorders).

Diagnosis of adrenal insufficiency is made by evaluating plasma cortisol levels. A decreased plasma cortisol level is indicative of adrenal insufficiency but does not differentiate between primary and secondary adrenal insufficiency. A "normal" plasma cortisol level in a stressed patient is considered abnormally low and may indicate adrenal insufficiency; it should be higher during stress. ACTH levels vary, depending on whether the adrenal insufficiency is primary (increased) or secondary (decreased) and can assist in diagnosis. In acute adrenal crisis, there is no time to wait for the laboratory results to confirm the

BOX 17-13

Progressive Signs of Chronic Adrenal Insufficiency

- Weakness
- Fatigue
- Weight loss
- Anorexia
- Hyperpigmentation, especially in the mucous membranes, in scars, and over joints, related to the increased secretion of melanocyte-stimulating hormone that occurs with increases in adrenocorticotropic hormone secretion
- Loss of pubic and axillary hair related to decreased levels of adrenal androgens

diagnosis before beginning treatment. If possible, a cosyntropin (a synthetic ACTH; Cortrosyn) stimulation test is done to determine adrenal insufficiency. The technique for performing this test is outlined in Box 17-14. Dexamethasone is given to the patient during the test to provide the necessary glucocorticoid support while the test is being run.

Box 17-14 also outlines a newer rapid, low-dose ACTH stimulation test. The lower-dose test better detects subtle cases of adrenal insufficiency. The test is done by administering 1 mcg of cosyntropin. Serum cortisol levels are evaluated before administration and 30 and 60 minutes after the drug is given (Marik & Zaloga, 2003; Offner, Moore, & Ciesla, 2002).

NURSING DIAGNOSES

The nursing diagnoses that may apply to a patient with acute adrenal crisis based on the assessment data include the following:

- Deficient fluid volume related to deficiency of aldosterone hormone (mineralocorticoid) and decreased sodium and water retention
- Ineffective tissue perfusion related to cortisol deficiency, resulting in decreased vascular tone and decreased effectiveness of catecholamines
- Disturbed thought processes related to decreased glucose levels, decreased protein metabolism, decreased perfusion, and decreased sodium
- Imbalanced nutrition (less than body requirements) related to cortisol deficiency and resultant decreased metabolism of protein and fats, decreased appetite, and decreased intestinal motility and digestion
- Deficient knowledge: proper long-term corticosteroid management
- Activity intolerance related to use of endogenous protein for energy needs and loss of skeletal muscle mass, as evidenced by early fatigue, weakness, and exertional dyspnea

NURSING AND MEDICAL INTERVENTIONS

Adrenal crisis requires immediate recognition and intervention if the patient is to survive. Primary objectives in the treatment of adrenal crisis include identifying and treating the precipitating cause, replacing fluid and electrolytes, replacing hormones, and educating the patient and family.

Fluid and Electrolyte Replacement

Fluid losses should be replaced with 5% dextrose and NS until signs and symptoms of hypovolemia stabilize. This not only reverses the volume deficit but also provides glucose to minimize the hypoglycemia. The patient may need as much as 5 L of fluid in the first 12 to 24 hours to maintain an adequate blood pressure and urine output and to replace the fluid deficit.

Hyperkalemia frequently responds to volume expansion and glucocorticoid replacement and may require no further treatment. In fact, the patient may become hypokalemic during therapy and may require potassium replacement. The acidosis also usually

BOX 17-14

Cosyntropin Stimulation Tests

Traditional Method

Obtain baseline serum cortisol level
Administer 250 mcg cosyntropin IV (synthetic ACTH)
Obtain serum cortisol level 30 and 60 min after cosyntropin
To cover adrenal insufficiency, may give dexamethasone (Decadron) 2-8 mg IV (does not affect serum cortisol)
Normal response: Two- to threefold increase in cortisol over baseline, or cortisol level >20 mcg/dL

Rapid Test

Obtain baseline serum cortisol level
Administer 1-2 mcg cosyntropin IV
Obtain serum cortisol level 30 and 60 min after cosyntropin
Normal response: Circulating cortisol level >25-30 mcg/dL

Doses are approximate and may vary based on the individual situation.

corrects itself with volume expansion and glucocorticoid replacement. However, if the pH is less than 7.1 or bicarbonate is less than 10 mEq/L, the patient may require sodium bicarbonate.

Hormonal Replacement

If adrenal insufficiency has not been previously diagnosed and the patient's condition is unstable, dexamethasone phosphate (Decadron), 4 mg by IV bolus, then 4 mg every 8 hours, can be given until the cosyntropin test has been done. This drug does not significantly cross-react with cortisol in the assay for cortisol and therefore can be administered to patients pending adrenal testing results.

Initially, glucocorticoid replacement is the most important type of hormonal replacement. Hydrocortisone sodium succinate (Solu-Cortef) is the drug of choice, because it has both glucocorticoid and mineralocorticoid activities in high doses. After a bolus dose, an infusion is administered for at least 24 hours or until the patient has stabilized. Cortisone acetate may be given intramuscularly if the IV route is not available.

TABLE 17-3

DRUGS USED TO TREAT ADRENAL CRISIS

Drug	Action/Uses	Dosage/Route	Side Effects	Nursing Implications
Hydrocortisone sodium succinate (Solu-Cortef)	Same as cortisol Antiinflammatory and immunosuppressive effects Salt-retaining (mineralocorticoid) effects in high doses	Individualized: adrenal crisis: 100-300 mg IV bolus; 100 mg every 6 hr in continous infusion	Vertigo, headache, insomnia, menstrual abnormalities, fluid and electrolyte imbalance, hypertension, HF, peptic ulcers, nausea and vomiting, immunosuppression, impaired wound healing, increased serum glucose, cushingoid state	Institute prophylactic measures against GI bleeding. Be aware of multiple drug-drug interactions, especially with IV route: oral contraceptives, phenytoin, digoxin, phenobarbital, theophylline, insulin, anticoagulants, salicylates. Avoid abrupt discontinuation. Monitor serum glucose and electrolytes. Watch for signs of fluid overload. Watch for signs of infection (may mask). Maintain adequate nutrition to avoid catabolic effects. Provide meticulous mouth care.
Cortisone acetate (Cortone)	Same as hydrocortisone	Individualized: crisis: 50 mg IM every 12 hr	Same as hydrocortisone	These are the same as for hydrocotisone.
Dexamethasone (Decadron)	Has only glucocorticoid effects	Give only during cosyntropin test; 4 mg IV push every 8 hr until test done	Same as hydrocortisone	These are the same as for hydrocortisone
Fludrocortisone acetate (Florinef)	Increases sodium reabsorption in renal tubules and increases potassium, water, and hydrogen loss	0.05-0.2 mg/day PO	Increased blood volume, edema, hypertension, HF, headaches, weakness of extremities	Assess for signs of fluid overload, HF. Monitor serum sodium and potassium. Use only in conjunction with glucocorticoids. Restrict sodium intake if the patient has edema or fluid overload. This is not used to treat acute crisis, but added as glucocorticoid is decreased toward maintenance level

GI, Gastrointestinal; *HF*, heart failure; *IM*, intramuscular; *IV*, intravenous.

Once the patient improves, the dose of hydrocortisone is decreased 20% to 40% daily until a maintenance dose is achieved. The patient can be switched to oral replacement once oral intake is resumed. At lower doses (less than 300 mg hydrocortisone/day), a patient with primary adrenal insufficiency may also require mineralocorticoid replacement. Fludrocortisone, 0.1 to 0.2 mg daily, is then added. A nutritional consideration if the patient is experiencing excessive sweating or diarrhea would be to increase sodium intake to 15 mEq of sodium/day. Table 17-3 describes the drugs used in the treatment of acute adrenal crisis. Box 17-15 contains a summary of the treatment of adrenal crisis.

Patient and Family Education

In a patient with known adrenal insufficiency and/or on corticosteroid therapy, adrenal crisis is preventable. Education of patients, family, and significant others is the key to prevention. See Nursing Care Plan for the Patient in Acute Adrenal Crisis discharge goals and interventions.

PATIENT OUTCOMES

Patient care outcomes for a patient with adrenal crisis include the following:
- Return of fluid and electrolyte balance
- Adequate central and peripheral perfusion
- Hemodynamic stability
- Return of mentation to baseline
- Adequate nutritional balance and stable weight
- Ability of the patient and family to state activities necessary to prevent adrenal crisis
- Increased physical activity

(See Nursing Care Plan for the Patient in Acute Adrenal Crisis; see also Research Analysis.)

Thyroid Crises

REVIEW OF PHYSIOLOGY

Like adrenal insufficiency, thyroid disorders that have been previously diagnosed and adequately treated do not generally result in crisis states. However, if patients with thyroid disorders, especially undiagnosed thyroid disorders, are stressed either physiologically or psychologically, the results can be life-threatening.

Deficient or excessive thyroid hormones can produce dysfunction in all body systems. The thyroid hormones thyroxine (T_4) and triiodothyronine (T_3) are secreted by the thyroid gland under the influence of the anterior pituitary gland via secretion of thyroid-stimulating hormone (TSH) from the hypothalamus. Regulation of these hormones occurs via the positive and negative feedback mechanisms discussed earlier (see Figure 17-2).

T_4 accounts for more than 95% of circulating thyroid hormone, but half of all thyroid activity comes from T_3. T_3 is five times more potent, acts more quickly, and enters cells more easily than T_4. T_3 is derived from conversion of T_4 in nonthyroid tissue. Certain conditions and drugs can block the conversion of T_4 to T_3, creating a potential thyroid imbalance. Possible causes for blocked conversion are listed in Box 17-16.

To understand the pathogenesis, clinical manifestations, and management of thyroid disease, particularly thyroid crises, it is necessary to understand the effects of thyroid hormones on the body. Box 17-17 lists some of the physiological effects of thyroid hormones.

BOX 17-15

Treatment of Adrenal Crisis

- Identify and treat precipitating event
- Replace fluid and electrolytes
  Give 5% dextrose in normal saline until hypotension improves
  Acidemia usually corrects with volume expansion; if pH <7.1, bicarbonate <10 mEq/L, give sodium bicarbonate
  Hyperkalemia responds to volume expansion and glucocorticoids
- Hormonal replacement
  Hydrocortisone (Solu-Cortef) 100 mg IV immediately; then 100 mg every 8 hr
  Cortisone acetate 50 mg IM every 12 hr (in case IV route faulty)
  Continue IV replacement at least 24 hr after recovery from acute phase
  After stabilized, decrease hydrocortisone dose 20% to 40% daily until maintenance dose reached (25.0-37.5 mg/day)
  When dose <100-150 mg/day, add fludrocortisone acetate (oral mineralocorticoid)
- Patient education
  Identification bracelet
  Awareness of signs and symptoms of insufficiency
  Doubling dose with minor stress

Doses are approximate and may vary based on the individual situation.

Nursing Care Plan for the Patient in Acute Adrenal Crisis

NURSING DIAGNOSIS: *Deficient fluid volume related to deficiency of aldosterone hormone (mineralocorticoid), decreased sodium, and water retention*

Patient Outcomes	Interventions	Rationales
Fluid balance restored Electrolyte balance restored: 　Na, 135-145 mEq/L 　K, 3.5-5.0 mEq/L Urine output >30 mL/hr BP WNL/returned to baseline Warm, pink skin HR 60-100 beats/min	Administer IV fluids and electrolytes as ordered; (D$_5$NS until signs and symptoms of hypovolemia stabilized; initial fluids will be administered rapidly; monitor for signs of overload). Monitor vital signs, orthostatic changes, hemodynamics (preload indicators with hemodynamic catheter in place; RAP/PAOP), central and peripheral perfusion (MAP/CO). Monitor fluid balance (I & O) and daily weight. Monitor heart rate and rhythm at least every 1 hr (every 15 min in unstable patients). Monitor Glucose, K, and N every 2 hr until stable. Monitor renal function: BUN, creatinine, urine output, specific gravity, urine Na and K. Administer scheduled doses of IV glucocorticoids and assess response. Avoid abrupt changes in position (to upright) until fluid balance is restored. Explain diagnostic tests to the patient/family. Prevent adrenal crisis by ensuring patients at risk receive exogenous cortisol in stress states.	Combats shock and restores circulation Detect inadequate fluid volume status. Assess patient progress.

NURSING DIAGNOSIS: *Altered tissue perfusion (decreased) related to cortisol deficiency resulting in decreased vascular tone, decreased effectiveness of catecholamines*

Patient Outcomes	Interventions	Rationales
Adequate central and peripheral perfusion and hemodynamic stability as evidenced by the following: Palpable peripheral pulses (2+) Warm/dry skin Adequate urine output (30 mL/hr) Usual mentation Systolic BP >90 mm Hg MAP >60 mm Hg CI >2.5 L/min/m^2 RAP 0-8 mm Hg SVR 900-1400 dynes/sec/cm^{-5} Absence of respiratory distress	Monitor changes in mental status (anxiety, confusion, lethargy, coma), personality changes. Inspect skin for pallor, mottling, cyanosis; note color and temperature. Provide skin care, change position every 2 hr, keep skin clean, dry. Monitor the respiratory rate. Monitor for changes in blood pressure. Assess GI function: decreased bowel sounds, nausea and vomiting, abdominal distention; anorexia; insert NG tube as needed. Monitor laboratory data: serum and urine electrolytes, BUN, creatinine. Note hourly changes in urine output; record specific gravity.	Determine perfusion to brain. Detect changes in tissue perfusion. Promote blood flow. Detect problems early.

Nursing Care Plan for the Patient in Acute Adrenal Crisis—cont'd

NURSING DIAGNOSIS: *Altered thought processes related to decreased glucose levels, decreased protein metabolism, decreased perfusion, decreased sodium*

Patient Outcomes	Interventions	Rationales
Mentation returned to baseline Alert/oriented	Assess the patient's level of consciousness, ability to speak, response to stimuli/commands. Observe behavioral responses: disorientation, confusion, irritability. Provide a quiet environment; speak in a calm, quiet voice. Provide consistent caregivers whenever possible. Encourage family/significant others to stay with patient. Provide frequent reality orientation. Provide for environmental safety, soft restraints; minimize stressful situations, promote rest. Monitor electrolytes, BUN, liver function tests.	Decrease stress and O_2 Provide safe and effective care environment.

NURSING DIAGNOSIS: *Imbalanced nutrition (less than body requirements) related to deficiency of cortisol and resultant decreased metabolism of protein and fat, decreased appetite, decreased intestinal motility and digestion*

Patient Outcomes	Interventions	Rationales
Normal protein and fat metabolism is restored Adequate nutrition is re-established as evidenced by positive nitrogen balance; weight WNL	Note admission weight/height, daily weight. Document oral intake, food history, calorie counts. Promote optimal environment during attempts at oral intake; provide assistance with eating as necessary. Assess the presence/character of bowel sounds; assess GI losses (i.e., vomiting, diarrhea). Provide small, frequent meals. Ensure the parenteral/enteral nutrition solutions are delivered as prescribed; assess tolerance. Refer to nutritional team/registered dietitian. Provide antacids/histamine antagonists as ordered. Assess metabolic response to nutritional support; monitor laboratory studies.	Establish baseline. Provide record. Enhance appetite, facilitate digestion.

NURSING DIAGNOSIS: *Deficient knowledge: proper long-term corticosteroid management*

Patient Outcomes	Interventions	Rationales
Patient/family able to state activities necessary to prevent adrenal crisis: Pathophysiology and therapy for chronic adrenal insufficieny. Rationale for and long-term effects of corticosteroid therapy.	Provide medication instructions: action, name, dose, schedule, importance of adherence, lifelong need for drug. Instruct patient/family on administration of corticosteroids in stress states: Define stress; identification and reduction; minor vs. severe. Instruct patient to call physician for temporary increase in glucocorticoid dose; double dose for minor stress.	Gain patient involvement. Promote compliance.

Continued

Nursing Care Plan for the Patient in Acute Adrenal Crisis—cont'd

Patient Outcomes	Interventions	Rationales
Signs and symptoms of acute adrenal insuffiency. Doubling of corticosteroids during minor stress. Notification of physician during major stress situations.	If the patient is vomiting, instruct patient to call physician (for parenteral administration); instruct in parenteral hydrocortisone at home. Instruct patient to inform all health care providers of corticosteroid use; carry ID card. Instruct the patient/family on importance of gradual corticosteroid tapering and to seek medical attention in event of stress state (Note: Patients who have been on long-term corticosteroid therapy should receive glucocorticoids during periods of stress for at least 1 yr after the drugs are discontinued).	Prevent further fluid loss. To manage disease process.

NURSING DIAGNOSIS: *Activity intolerance related to use of endogenous protein for energy needs and loss of skeletal muscle mass as evidenced by early fatigue and weakness, exertional dyspnea*

Patient Outcomes	Interventions	Rationales
Demonstrates increased physical activity as evidenced by: BP, HR, RR WNL Verbalizes decreased fatigue	Provide passive/active ROM exercises. Assist with ambulation, activities of daily living. Monitor patient response to increased activity: monitor BP, heart rhythm, respirations; note tachycardia, dysrhythmias, dyspnea, diaphoresis, pallor. Check vital signs before and immediately after each activity. Assess for other causes of fatigue (i.e., treatments, medications). Restrict activity; space with rest periods. Provide for nutrition (see above). Encourage verbalization of feelings regarding limitations.	Promote safety. Psychological support.

BP, Blood pressure; *BUN,* blood urea nitrogen; *CI,* cardiac index, *CO,* cardiac output; *D₅NS,* 5% dextrose in normal saline; *GI,* gastrointestinal; *HR,* heart rate; *ID,* identification; *I & O,* intake and output; *IV,* intravenous; *K,* potassium; *MAP,* mean arterial pressure; *Na,* sodium; *NG,* nasogastric; *PAOP,* pulmonary artery occlusion pressure; *RAP,* right atrial pressure; *ROM,* range of motion; *RR,* respiratory rate; *SVR,* systemic vascular resistance; *WNL,* within normal limits.

ETIOLOGY

Hyperthyroidism is a common and usually benign illness. The most common types of hyperthyroidism are toxic diffuse goiter and toxic multinodular goiter.

The most frequent form of hyperthyroidism is toxic diffuse goiter, also known as Graves' disease. It occurs most frequently in young (third or fourth decade), previously healthy women. A family history of hyperthyroidism is often present. Graves' disease is an autoimmune disease, and affected patients have abnormal thyroid-stimulating immunoglobulins. These immunoglobulins mimic TSH, producing thyroid inflammation, diffuse enlargement, and hyperplasia of the gland (Fisher, 2002).

Toxic multinodular goiter is the second most common cause of hyperthyroidism. It also occurs more commonly in women, but these patients are generally older (fourth to seventh decades). Crises in patients with toxic multinodular goiter are more commonly associated with heart failure or severe muscle weakness. These and other possible causes of hyperthyroidism are listed in Box 17-18.

Hyperthyroidism is seen as secondary to exposure to radiation (Grossman, Nussbaum, & Nussbaum, 2002)

RESEARCH ANALYSIS

ARTICLE REFERENCE
Marik, P. E., & Zaloga, G. P. (2003). Adrenal insufficiency during septic shock. *Critical Care Med, 31*(1), 141-145.

PURPOSES AND METHODS
The purpose of the study was to compare the ability of a random serum cortisol concentration with the commonly used low-dose (LD) and high-dose (HD) corticotropin stimulation tests to diagnose adrenal insufficiency in patients with septic shock. Researchers used a cortisol concentration of less than 25 mcg/dL as the baseline reference measurement.

Fifty-nine adult patients who met the criteria for septic shock were studied. Of the group, 29 were men and 30 were women; the mean age was 57 years. Excluded from the study were patients with human immunodeficiency virus infection, a history of adrenal insufficiency, or a history of receiving corticosteroids during the previous year. Patients had not received any drugs known to suppress adrenal function. All patients were given norepinephrine as a vasopressor. Within 48 hours of admission to the medical intensive care unit, all patients had a baseline serum cortisol level drawn, followed by LD (1 mcg), then HD (249 mcg) corticotropin stimulation testing. Specifically, a patient received 1 mcg of corticotropin. At 30 and 60 minutes, serum cortisol concentrations were drawn. Sixty minutes after the 1-mcg dose, a 249-mcg dose of cortisol was given. Serum cortisol concentrations were drawn 30 and 60 minutes later. All patients were then given 100 mg hydrocortisone intravenously every 8 hours. Patients able to have their vasopressor (norepinephrine) discontinued within 24 hours of the first dose of hydrocortisone were defined as being steroid responsive.

STUDY FINDINGS
Of the 59 patients in the study, 28 (47%) died. Sixty-one percent of patients had adrenal insufficiency as defined as baseline cortisol concentration of less than 25 mcg/dL. When the standard threshold of less than 18 mcg/dL was used, only 22% of patients in the LD test group and 8% of patients in the HD test group met the criteria for adrenal insufficiency. When a baseline cortisol concentration of less than 25 mcg/dL was used, 62% of the LD group and 24% of the HD group were identified with adrenal insufficiency. A stress cortisol concentration of 23.7 mcg/dL was found to have the best discriminating power for identifying hemodynamic response to steroid therapy.

STUDY STRENGTHS
This study is a good example of taking a new look at accepted practices. It examines commonly used tests and reference standards to identify adrenal insufficiency. The literature was reviewed to explain the rationale for currently used tests. The study appears to use statistical methods and interpretations accurately and rigorously.

STUDY LIMITATIONS
As the authors correctly identify, there is no exact way to measure success of steroid treatment for acute adrenal insufficiency. Hemodynamic response was used in this study, an end point commonly used by other researchers examining treatment strategies for septic shock.

IMPLICATIONS FOR PRACTICE
The implications of this study for nursing practice include the understanding that the determination of patients with adrenal insufficiency very much depends on the choice of diagnostic test and criteria. Nurses frequently administer the LD and HD corticotropin stimulation tests. This study may change practice and may cause patients who are critically ill with sepsis to be identified earlier as having adrenal insufficiency. A random baseline cortisol concentration may become a useful diagnostic tool in the critical care unit.

BOX 17-16

Causes of Blockage of Conversion from Thyroxine to Triiodothyronine

- Severe illness: chronic renal failure, cancer, chronic liver disease
- Trauma
- Malnutrition, fasting
- Drugs: glucocorticoids, propranolol (Inderal), propylthiouracil, amiodarone
- Radiopaque dyes
- Acidosis

---

or to interferon-alpha therapy for viral hepatitis (Wong, Fu, George, & Cheung, 2002). With the increasing use of amiodarone (a heavily iodinated compound) for control of tachyarrhythmias, the incidence of hyperthyroidism as an adverse effect of amiodarone is increasing (Leung, Quinn, & Belchetz, 2002).

Thyroid storm usually occurs in untreated or inadequately treated patients with hyperthyroidism; it is rare in patients who have had previously normal

---

BOX 17-17

Physiological Effect of Thyroid Hormones

MAJOR EFFECTS
↑ Metabolic activities of all tissues
↑ Rate of nutrient use for energy production
↑ Rate of growth
↑ Activities of other endocrine glands

OTHER EFFECTS
Regulate protein synthesis and catabolism
Regulate body heat production and dissipation
↑ Gluconeogenesis and utilization of glucose
Maintain appetite and gastrointestinal motility
Maintain calcium metabolism
Stimulate cholesterol synthesis
Maintain cardiac rate, contractility, and output
Affect respiratory rate, oxygen utilization, and carbon dioxide formation
Affect red blood cell production
Affect central nervous system development and cerebration
Are necessary for muscle tone and vigor and normal skin constituents

↑, Increase; ↓, decrease.

BOX 17-18

Causes of Hyperthyroidism

MOST COMMON
Toxic diffuse goiter (Graves' disease)
Toxic multinodular goiter
Toxic uninodular goiter

OTHER CAUSES
Factitious hyperthyroidism
Triiodothyronine
Exogenous iodine in patient with preexisting thyroid disease: exposure to iodine load from radiographic contrast dyes, medications (amiodarone, organidine)
Thyroiditis (transient)
Postpartum thyroiditis

RARE CAUSES
Toxic thyroid adenoma
Metastatic thyroid cancer
Malignancies with circulating thyroid stimulators
Pituitary tumors producing thyroid-stimulating hormone
Acromegaly

ASSOCIATED WITH OTHER DISORDERS*
Pernicious anemia, idiopathic Addison's disease, myasthenia gravis, sarcoidosis, Albright's syndrome

---

*The presence of these disorders in a patient in crisis increases the likelihood that the patient has hyperthyroidism.

---

thyroid glands. Most of these patients have had Graves' disease for at least several months. The crisis is often precipitated by stress related to an underlying illness, general anesthesia, surgery, or infection. Mortality is more often the result of the underlying illness rather than the thyrotoxic state.

THYROTOXIC CRISIS (THYROID STORM)

Pathophysiology

Thyroid storm is a rare emergency that can result in death within 48 hours without treatment. Thyroid hormones are highly bound to globulin, T_4-binding prealbumin, and albumin. Only the unbound (or free) fraction of the circulating hormone is biologically active. The specific mechanism that produces thyroid storm is unknown. It is believed that the rapidity with which hormone levels rise may be more important than the absolute levels. Theories regarding the

TABLE 17-4	
Clinical Manifestations of Thyroid Storm and Myxedema Coma	
Thyroid Storm	**Myxedema Coma**
↑ Metabolic rate	↓ Metabolic rate
↑ Temperature, heat intolerance, diaphoresis	↓ Temperature, cold intolerance
Tachycardia	Distant heart sounds
Widened pulse pressure	Bradycardia
Palpitations	Pericardial effusion
Dysrhythmias	Lethargy, somnolence
Agitation, delirium, psychoses	Dyspnea on exertion
	↓ Respiratory rate
Fine tremor	Mucinous edema
Exaggerated reflexes	↓ Bowel movements
Dyspnea	Slow speech, coarse voice
↑ Respiratory rate	

↑, Increased; ↓, decreased.

onset of thyroid storm include (1) a change in the binding of thyroid hormone to circulating proteins, (2) a change in thyroid hormone receptors in the target tissues, and (3) exaggerated response to sympathetic activity (Ringel, 2001).

Certain enzymes may be the key to the dramatic increase in metabolic rate that occurs in thyroid storm. Thyroid hormones normally increase the synthesis of enzymes that stimulate cellular mitochondria and energy production. When excess thyroid hormones are present, as in thyroid storm, the increased activity of these enzymes produces excessive thermal energy and fever.

Thyroid hormones play a major role in regulating body metabolism; as a result, they affect most body systems. Thus, hyperthyroidism can produce a hyperdynamic, hypermetabolic state that results in disruption of many major body functions. Common findings in patients with thyroid storm are listed in Table 17-4 and are discussed later.

Assessment

Clinical presentation. The excess thyroid hormone activity of hyperthyroidism affects the body in many ways over time. Box 17-19 gives signs associated with chronic hyperthyroidism.

Thyroid storm has an abrupt onset and is best characterized as a state of unregulated hypermetabolism. The signs and symptoms of thyroid storm are variable and nonspecific (see Clinical Alerts: Thyroid Disorders). The most prominent clinical features of thyroid storm are severe fever, marked tachycardia, tremors, delirium, stupor, and coma. Untreated patients succumb in

BOX 17-19	
Progressive Signs of Hyperthyrodism	

- *Cardiovascular:* Increased heart rate and palpitations. Hyperthyroidism may present as sinus tachycardia in a sleeping patient or as atrial fibrillation with a rapid ventricular response.
- *Neurological:* Increased irritability, hyperactivity, decreased attention span, and nervousness. In an elderly patient, these signs may be masked, and depression or apathy may be present.
- *Temperature intolerance:* Increased cold tolerance, heat intolerance, fever, excessive sweating, and warm, moist skin. Older patients may naturally lose their ability to shiver and may be less comfortable in the cold.
- *Respiratory:* Increased respiratory rate, weakened thoracic muscles, and decreased vital capacity are evident.
- *Gastrointestinal:* Increased appetite, decreased absorption (especially of vitamins), weight loss, and increased stools. Diarrhea is not common. Elderly patients may be constipated.
- *Musculoskeletal:* Fine tremors of tongue or eyelids, peripheral tremors with activity, and muscle wasting are noted.
- *Integumentary:* Thin, fine, and fragile hair, soft friable nails, and petechiae. Young women generally have the more classic findings. Young men may notice an increase in acne and sweating. An elderly patient with dry, atrophic skin may not have significant skin changes.
- *Hematopoietic:* Pernicious anemia and jaundice. Splenomegaly occurs in about 50% of patients. About 10% of patients have a decrease in neutrophils.
- *Ophthalmic:* Pathological features result from edema and inflammation. Physical findings may include upper lid retraction, lid lag, extraocular muscle palsies, and sight loss. Exophthalmos is found almost exclusively in Graves' disease.

CLINICAL ALERTS: THYROID DISORDERS

Clinical Concerns	Significance	Nursing Actions
Thyroid Storm Alterations in level of consciousness	Symptoms can be confused with other disorders (e.g., paranoia, psychosis, depression), especially in the elderly	Assess and maintain patient safety. Attempt to control environmental influences.
↑ Cardiac workload due to hypermetabolic state; ↓ cardiac output	Can lead to heart failure and collapse	Perform cardiac monitoring for dysrhythmias (e.g., atrial fibrillation or flutter) and tachycardia, and blood pressure monitoring for widening pulse pressure. Auscultate for the development of S_3.
↑ Oxygen demand due to hypermetabolic state; ineffective breathing pattern	↑ Respiratory rate and drive can lead to ↑ fatigue and hypoventilation	Provide supplemental oxygen as needed. Monitor respiratory rate and effort. Monitor oxygen saturation via pulse oximeter.
Loss of ability to regulate temperature	Inability to respond to fever exacerbates hypermetabolic demands	Monitor temperature and treat with acetaminophen and/or a cooling blanket as needed.
Myxedema Coma Alterations in level of consciousness	Ranges from difficulty concentrating to coma Seizures can occur	Assess and maintain patient safety.
↓ Cardiac function	Hypotension and potential to develop pericardial effusion	Perform cardiac monitoring (look for ↓ voltage, indicating effusion). Auscultate for diminished heart sounds. Monitor blood pressure for signs of hypotension.
Muscle weakness, hypoventilation, pleural effusion; ineffective breathing	Potential for respiratory acidosis and hypoxemia	Auscultate the lungs frequently. Monitor respiratory effort (rate and depth) and pattern. Maintain I & O (probable need for fluid restriction). Monitor ABGs/pulse oximetry and CBC (for anemia). Position for optimum respiratory effort.
Loss of ability to regulate temperature	Inability to respond to cold	Monitor temperature. Control room temperature, provide rewarming measures.

↑, Increased; ↓, decreased; *ABGs,* arterial blood gases; *CBC,* complete blood count; *I & O,* intake and output.

1 to 2 days to extreme hyperpyrexia and cardiovascular collapse.

Cardiovascular disturbances. Thyroid hormones play a role in maintaining cardiac rate, force of contraction, and cardiac output. The increase in metabolism and the stimulation of catecholamines produced by thyroid hormones cause a hyperdynamic heart. Contractility, heart rate, and cardiac output increase as peripheral vascular resistance decreases. These effects are magnified by the body's increased demand for oxygen and nutrients. In thyroid storm, the increased demands on the heart may be severe enough to produce high-output heart failure and cardiovascular collapse if the crisis is not recognized and treated.

Patients experience palpitations, tachycardia (out of proportion to the fever), and a widened pulse pressure. A prominent third heart sound may be heard as well as a systolic murmur over the pulmonic and/or aortic areas. Occasionally, a pericardial rub may be heard. The most common dysrhythmias are frequent premature atrial contractions, atrial fibrillation, and atrial flutter. In an elderly patient with underlying heart disease, worsening of angina or severe heart failure may herald thyroid storm.

Neurological disturbances. The thyroid hormones normally maintain central nervous system cerebration. The hypermetabolism and resultant increased cerebration produced by excess thyroid hormones cause hyperactivity of the nervous system both psychologically and physiologically. Thyroid storm may be heralded by the onset of wide mood swings, fear or paranoia, delirium, overt psychosis, convulsions, stupor, or coma.

Pulmonary disturbances. Thyroid hormones affect respiratory rate and depth, oxygen utilization, and CO_2 formation. Tissues need more oxygen as a result of hypermetabolism. This increased need for oxygen stimulates the respiratory drive and increases respirations. However, increased protein catabolism reduces protein in respiratory muscles (diaphragm and intercostals). As a result, even with increased respirations, muscle weakness may prevent the patient from meeting the oxygen demand and may cause hypoventilation, CO_2 retention, and respiratory failure.

Temperature regulation is lost. The patient's body temperature may be as high as 106°F (41.1°C). The increase in heat production and metabolic end products also causes the blood vessels of the skin to dilate. This enhances oxygen and nutrient delivery to the peripheral tissues and accounts for the patient's warm, moist skin.

Gastrointestinal disturbances. Excess thyroid hormones increase metabolism and accelerate protein and fat degradation. Thyroid hormones also increase GI motility, which may result in abdominal pain, nausea, jaundice, vomiting, and/or diarrhea. The latter two problems contribute to volume depletion during thyroid crises.

Muscle weakness and fatigue result from increased protein catabolism. Skeletal muscle changes are manifested as tremors. Thoracic muscles are weak, causing dyspnea and affecting proximal muscles. In thyroid crises, patients are prescribed bed rest to reduce metabolic demand.

The patient's ability to survive thyroid storm is determined by the severity of the hyperthyroid state and the patient's general health. The severity of the hyperthyroid state is not necessarily indicated by the serum levels of thyroid hormones but rather by tissue and organ responsiveness to the hormones.

Laboratory evaluation. There are no laboratory tests that separate thyroid storm from uncomplicated hyperthyroidism. TSH, T_3, and T_4 levels should be measured, as well as resin T_3 uptake. Resin T_3 uptake is an indirect measure of free T_4 levels (free T_4 is the portion that is biologically active) and is elevated in hyperthyroid states. Although an elevation of thyroid hormones is to be expected, these levels are generally no higher than those normally found in uncomplicated hyperthyroidism. In any event, the patient must be treated before these results are available. (See Laboratory Alerts: Thyroid Disorders for possible laboratory abnormalities that may occur in thyroid storm.)

Nursing Diagnoses

The nursing diagnoses that may apply to a patient with thyroid storm are based on assessment data and include the following:
- Decreased cardiac output related to increased metabolic demands on the heart, extreme tachycardia, dysrhythmias, heart failure
- Disturbed thought processes related to hypermetabolism and increased cerebration, agitation, delirium, psychosis
- Hyperthermia related to loss of temperature regulation, increased metabolism, increased heat production
- Ineffective breathing pattern related to muscle weakness and decreased vital capacity resulting in hypoventilation and CO_2 retention, increased oxygen need from hypermetabolism
- Imbalanced nutrition: less than body requirements related to increased requirement, increased peristalsis, decreased absorption

LABORATORY ALERTS: THYROID DISORDERS

Laboratory Test	Critical Value	Significance	Nursing Actions
Thyroid Storm T_3, free (triiodothyronine) T_3, resin uptake T_4 (thyroxine) TSH	>0.52 ng/dL > 35% of total > 12 mcg/dL <0.01 mU/L	Hyperthyroidism	See Nursing Care Plan for the Patient with Thyroid Storm Beta-blockers are given to offset effects of elevated thyroid hormones. Correct the underlying cause.
Glucose	≥ 200 mg/dL (2 hr postprandial or random) >140 mg/dL (fasting)	↑ Insulin degradation	Monitor serum/capillary laboratory values; IV replacement of fluids and electrolytes should resolve the problem.
Sodium	> 150 mEq/L	May be a result of stress, dehydration, and/or hypermetabolic state	This usually resolves with IV rehydration (once the underlying cause is corrected).
BUN	>20 mg/dL	↑ Due to protein breakdown and hemoconcentration	Monitor I & O (especially urine output ≥ 30 mL/hr) and serum laboratory values.
CBC	↓ RBCs ↑ WBCs	Normocytic, normochromic anemia	Correct underlying cause.
Calcium	>10.2 mg/dL	Excess bone resorption	Correct underlying cause.
Myxedema Coma T_3, Free (triiodothyronine) T_3, resin uptake T_4 (thyroxine) TSH	<0.2 mg/dL <25% of total <5 mcg/dL >25 mU/mL	Hypothyroidism	
Sodium	<130 mEq/L	Dilutional from increased total body water	Usually responds to thyroid replacement and fluid restriction.
Glucose	<50 mg/dL	Hypoglycemia due to hypermetabolic state	Provide a form of glucose (PO, IM, or IV). Monitor serum/capillary laboratory values.
CBC	↓ RBCs	Anemia due to vitamin B_{12} deficiency, inadequate folate or iron absorption	Correct underlying cause; may require therapy with vitamin B_{12}, folate, or iron.
Platelets	<150,000 cells/µL	Risk for bleeding	Take bleeding precautions.
pH	<7.35	Respiratory acidosis from hypoventilation	Optimize ventilatory effort and rate.

↑, Increased; ↓, decreased; *BUN,* blood urea nitrogen; *CBC,* complete blood count; *IM,* intramuscular; *I & O,* intake and output; *IV,* intravenous; *PO,* orally; *RBCs,* red blood cells; *TSH,* thyroid-stimulating hormone; *WBCs,* white blood cells.

- Activity intolerance related to muscle weakness, tremors, anemia, fatigue, and extreme energy expenditure
- Deficient knowledge: disease process, therapeutic regimen, prevention of complications

Nursing and Medical Interventions

Thyroid storm requires immediate intervention if the patient is to survive. The primary objectives in the treatment of thyroid storm are inhibiting thyroid hormone biosynthesis, blocking thyroid hormone release, antagonizing peripheral effects of thyroid hormone, providing supportive care, identifying and treating the precipitating cause, and providing patient and family education. Box 17-20 details the treatment of thyroid storm.

Inhibition of thyroid hormone biosynthesis. Two drugs may be used to inhibit thyroid hormone biosynthesis: propylthiouracil and methimazole (Tapazole). Neither of these drugs is available in IV form. Propylthiouracil is the drug of choice because in large doses it inhibits conversion of T_4 to T_3 in peripheral tissues, and results in a more rapid reduction of circulating thyroid hormone levels.

Both propylthiouracil and methimazole lack immediate effects. They do not block the release of thyroid hormones already stored in the thyroid gland and may take weeks or even months to lower thyroid hormone levels to normal.

Block release of thyroid hormone. Iodide agents inhibit the release of thyroid hormones from the thyroid gland, and at high doses, they may also inhibit thyroid hormone production. Serum T_4 levels fall approximately 30% to 50% with any of these drugs, with stabilization in 3 to 6 days.

Sodium iodide is administered by slow IV drip. Alternatively, saturated solution of potassium iodide or Lugol's solution may be given orally. All these drugs must be given 1 to 2 hours after antithyroid drugs (propylthiouracil or methimazole) to prevent the iodide from being used to synthesize more T_4. Ipodate (Oragrafin) and iopanoic acid (Telepaque) are radiographic contrast media that may also be used to block thyroid hormone release. Lithium carbonate also inhibits the release of thyroid hormones but is more toxic, so it is used only in patients with an iodide allergy. Lithium carbonate is given orally or by nasogastric tube at doses of 300 mg every 6 hours and adjusted to maintain therapeutic serum levels.

Antagonism of peripheral effects of thyroid hormones. Because it may take days or longer for the foregoing treatments to have full effect, immediate action is necessary to minimize the dramatic

---

BOX 17-20

Treatment of Thyroid Storm

IDENTIFY AND TREAT PRECIPITATING CAUSE

Inhibit hormone biosynthesis
Propylthiouracil: PO loading dose of 200-250 mg, then every 6 hr until thyrotoxicosis controlled, or
Methimazole (Tapazole): 60-100 mg PO loading dose; 20 mg PO every 4 hr

BLOCK THYROID HORMONE RELEASE

Give 1-2 hr after propylthiouracil or methimazole loading dose
Sodium iodide: 0.5 g IV infusion over 24 hr, or
Saturated solution of potassium iodide: 15 drops every 8 hr, or
Lugol's solution: 30 drops daily PO in 3-4 doses, or

Secondary options
Iopanoic acid: 1 g every 8 hours times 24 hours, 0.5 g PO twice daily

ANTAGONIZE PERIPHERAL EFFECTS OF THYROID HORMONE

Propranolol (Inderal): 1-2 mg IV boluses every 10-15 min up to 15-20 mg IV or 160-480 mg daily PO; individualized to response
If beta-blocker contraindicated, give reserpine or guanethidine

SUPPORTIVE THERAPY

Hydrocortisone: 200-300 mg IV drip over 24 hr, or dexamethasone: 0.5 mg PO every 6 hr
Digoxin for heart failure or tachydysrhythmias
Correct fluid and electrolyte imbalance
Treat hyperthermia (avoid aspirin)
High-calorie, high-protein diet

PATIENT AND FAMILY EDUCATION

Doses are approximate and may vary based on the individual situation.

TABLE 17-5

DRUGS USED TO TREAT THYROID STORM

Drug	Action/Uses	Dosage/Route	Side Effects	Nursing Implications
Propylthiouracil (PTU)	Inhibits synthesis of thyroid hormones; inhibits peripheral conversion of T_4 to T_3	200 mg PO every 6 hr until thyrotoxicosis is controlled	Granulocytopenia, thrombocytopenia, bleeding, paresthesias, vertigo, drowsiness, nausea and vomiting, rash, edema	Monitor for bleeding tendencies and decreased platelet count. Provide small, frequent meals if the patient has problems. Monitor for neurological changes and provide safety measures. Provide frequent skin care.
Methimazole (Tapazole)	Inhibits synthesis of thyroid hormones	15-60 mg/day PO loading dose; 5-15 mg/day	Same as above	Same as above.
Sodium Iodide	Inhibits synthesis of thyroid hormones and their release into circulation	0.5 g IV infusion over 24 hrs	Same as above	Monitor for allergic reactions; give 1-2 hrs after antithyroid drugs.
Lugol's solution, saturated solution of potassium iodide (SSKI)	Inhibit synthesis of thyroid hormones and their release into the circulation	Lugol's: 30 drops PO daily in 3-4 doses SSKI: 5 drops every 8 hr	Rash, metallic taste, burning mouth, sore teeth/gums, inflammation of salivary glands, headaches, gastritis, diarrhea, allergic reactions	Monitor for allergic reactions; acute toxicity (vomiting, abdominal pain, diarrhea, circulatory collapse). Provide frequent mouth care; dilute with fruit juice or water to improve taste Provide small, frequent meals if GI problems are present. Give 1-2 hr after antithyroid drugs
Ipodate, iopanoic acid	Inhibit peripheral conversion of T_4 to T_3; block release into circulation; may inhibit binding of hormone to cell receptors	Ipodate: 0.5-3 g PO daily Iopanoic acid: 0.5 g bid	Flushing, warmth, tingling sensations, vertigo, nausea, metallic taste, allergic reaction, apprehension, restlessness, hypotension	Monitor for allergic reactions; acute toxicity (vomiting, abdominal pain, diarrhea, shock). Provide frequent mouth care. Provide small, frequent meals Give 1-2 hr after antithyroid drugs.
Propranolol (Inderal)	Blocks beta-adrenergic receptors in heart and juxtaglomerular apparatus; ↓ sympathetic influence, partially inhibits peripheral conversion of T_4 to T_3 Rapidly acting agents such as esmolol may be used based on symptoms.	IV: 1-2 mg bolus every 10-15 min up to 15-20 mg PO: 60-120 mg every 6 hr	Bradycardia, heart failure, dysrhythmias, hypotension, dizziness, vertigo, tinnitus, bronchospasm, dyspnea, rhinitis GI upset: pain, nausea, vomiting, anorexia	Contraindicated in patients with chronic lung disease, hypotension, pulmonary edema, or heart block. Use caution in patients on insulin, oral hypoglycemic agents, and monoamine oxidase inhibitors, and in pregnant women. Cardiac monitoring and frequent blood pressure monitoring when giving IV. Give with food if administering orally. Report side effects.
Digoxin	For control of atrial fibrillation and to control/convert atrial tachydysrhythmias	0.25 mg IV, frequency based on symptoms	Bradycardia, atrioventricular block, GI distress	Monitor serum renal findings, and therapeutic level.

↑, Increased; ↓, decreased; *GI*, gastrointestinal; *IM*, intramuscularly; *IV*, intravenously; *PO*, orally, T_3, triiodothyronine; T_4, thyroxine.

effects of thyroid storm on the major organ systems. The mortality rate of thyroid storm has been significantly reduced with the introduction of beta-blockers to block the peripheral effects of thyroid hormones. The drug used most frequently is oral propranolol (Inderal). Other beta-blockers such as esmolol hydrochloride (Brevibloc) or atenolol (Tenormin) may also be used. Results should be seen within minutes using the IV route and within 1 hour after the oral route. IV effects should last 3 to 4 hours.

High-dose glucocorticoids are administered to block the conversion of T_4 to T_3 and therefore thyroid hormone effects on peripheral tissues. Drugs used to treat thyroid storm are summarized in Table 17-5.

Supportive Care

Symptoms are aggressively treated. Cardiac complications are treated with digitalis and other pharmacotherapy. Acetaminophen is used as an antipyretic. Cooling blankets may be used. Oxygen is administered to support the respiratory effort. The large fluid losses are replaced. Hemodynamic monitoring may be required. Nutritional support is provided.

Precipitating factors are identified and treated and/or removed.

Patient and family education. Education of patients, families, and significant others is crucial in identifying and preventing episodes of thyroid storm. Teaching varies, depending on the long-term therapy chosen for each patient (e.g., drugs versus radioactive iodine or surgery).

Patient Outcomes

Outcomes for a patient with thyroid storm include the following:

- Stable hemodynamics within normal limits
- Return to baseline mentation and personality
- Temperature within normal range
- Effective breathing pattern
- Nutritional needs met and weight maintained
- Return to baseline activity level
- Verbalization by the patient and significant others of an understanding of the patient's illness, anticipated treatment, and potential complications

(See Nursing Care Plan for the Patient with Thyroid Storm.)

Nursing Care Plan for the Patient with Thyroid Storm

NURSING DIAGNOSIS: *Decreased cardiac output related to increased metabolic demands on heart, extreme tachycardia, dysrhythmias, heart failure*

Patient Outcomes	Interventions	Rationales
Stable hemodynamic parameters and metabolic rate as evidenced by: CO 4-8 L/min; CI 2.8-4.2 L/min/m² PAP, PAOP, and RAP within normal range Return to baseline BP for patient; HR 60-100 beats/min Control of dysrhythmias Urine output >30 mL/hr	Control temperature (see nursing diagnosis of hyperthermia). Assess/monitor for signs and symptoms of cardiac compromise: BP, pulse pressure Apical pulse, resting heart rate, heart sounds Pulmonary artery occlusion pressure, RAP CO, CI, SVR RR, breath sounds, secretions Dysrhythmias Complaints of chest pain, palpitations, shortness of breath, signs of ischemia Hourly urine output Administer antithyroid medications. Provide adequate hydration, monitor hemodynamic response to fluid therapy. Monitor electrolyte status, potassium and calcium Administer digoxin as ordered and monitor response Minimize the demand on the heart by controlling activity	Excess thyroid hormones and treatment can result in hemodynamic instability. Close monitoring allows rapid supportive treatment.

Continued

Nursing Care Plan for the Patient with Thyroid Storm—cont'd

NURSING DIAGNOSIS: *Disturbed thought processes related to hypermetabolism and increased cerebration, agitation, delirium, psychosis*

Patient Outcomes	Interventions	Rationales

Return to baseline mentation and behavior
Return to normal personality (*per family/significant others*)
	Provide a safe environment.
	Take seizure precautions.
	Assess for degree of physiological/psychological dysfunction:
	  Orientation
	  Irritability, nervousness, agitation
	  Memory, attention span
	  Mood swings, fear, paranoia
	  Convulsions, stupor, coma
	  Tremors: tongue, eyelids, peripheral
	  Muscle weakness
	Minimize effects of environment on mental status:
	  Reorient patient frequently.
	  Maintain quiet environment, minimizing extraneous stimuli.
	  Provide simple, brief explanations of activities, procedures, or equipment.
	  Provide meaningful, relaxing stimuli to patient.
		Support the patient until the adverse effects of excess thyroid hormones on mental status function are reversed.

NURSING DIAGNOSIS: *Hyperthermia related to loss of temperature regulation, increased metabolism, increased heat production*

Patient Outcomes	Interventions	Rationales
Temperature return to normal value: 98.6°F (37°C)	Monitor the patient's temperature every 1 hr; continuously with a probe if possible. Assess fluid status: hourly I & O, daily weights, diaphoresis, skin turgor, mucous membranes. Use cooling measures and administer acetaminophen. Administer and monitor effects of drugs used to combat thyroid hormone effects. Administer antibiotics if infection is a precipitator.	Decreasing temperature decreases cardiac workload.

NURSING DIAGNOSIS: *Ineffective breathing pattern related to muscle weakness and decreased VC resulting in hypoventilation and CO_2 retention, increased oxygen need from hypermetabolism*

Patient Outcomes	Interventions	Rationales
Effective breathing pattern as evidenced by: Normal respiratory rate, depth, and pattern ABGs WNL or return to patient baseline ABG	Assess respiratory status every 4 hr; every 1-2 hr in a patient with an altered level of consciousness. Obtain ABGs as ordered and as needed. Obtain pulmonary function parameters: V_T, VC Assess subjective complaints of shortness of breath, dyspnea on exertion.	Respiratory support needs vary with thyroid hormone levels.

Nursing Care Plan for the Patient with Thyroid Storm—cont'd

Patient Outcomes	Interventions	Rationales

PaO$_2$ >60 mm Hg
Normal VC, V$_T$
Resolution of muscle weakness
Patient reports breathing easier
	Provide supportive measures to facilitate respiratory effort:
	  Airway, supplementary oxygen, suctioning, intubation, ventilation.
	  Position patient for ease of respiratory effort;
	  Quiet, restful environment
	  Frequent rest periods.
	  Minimize activity to decrease oxygen need.	

NURSING DIAGNOSIS: *Imbalanced nutrition of less than body requirements related to increased requirements, increased peristalsis, decreased absorption*

Patient Outcomes	Interventions	Rationales

Body weight will stabilize at patient's normal level
Nutritional needs met:
  Serum albumin 3.5-5.5 g/dL
  Serum glucose 70-110 mg/dL
	Assess effects of thyroid hormone on GI system:
	  Bowel sounds; abdominal pain
	  Nausea and vomiting
	  Number/frequency of bowel movements
	  Weight
	  Serum albumin level
	  Fatigue, weakness
	  Liver function tests, BUN
	Provide adequate glucose to support energy needs:
	  Provide adequate dextrose in IV fluids.
	  Administer hydrocortisone as ordered.
	  Monitor for signs and symptoms of hypoglycemia and hyperglycemia.
	  Monitor serum glucose levels.
	Provide adequate nutrition
	High-calorie, high-protein intake.
	Vitamin and mineral supplements.
	Frequent, small feedings as tolerated.
	Skin care to protect fragile skin.
	Minimize activity to decrease energy needs.
		Nutritional support enhances the body's ability to deal with metabolic demands.

NURSING DIAGNOSIS: *Activity intolerance related to muscle weakness, muscle wasting, tremors, fatigue, anemia, and extreme energy expenditure*

Patient Outcomes	Interventions	Rationales

Patient will return to baseline activity level	During acute crisis, minimize physical activity:
	  Provide all daily care for patient.
	  Maintain on bed rest.
	  Allow for adequate rest/sleep periods.
	Provide patient with calming diversional activities
	Provide adequate nutrition
	Increase activity gradually after acute crisis abates; monitor physical response to activity
	Administer oxygen during activity.
		The metabolic rate is so high that added physical activity will not be tolerated.

Continued

Nursing Care Plan for the Patient with Thyroid Storm—cont'd

NURSING DIAGNOSIS: *Deficient knowledge related to disease process, therapeutic regimen, prevention of complications*

Patient Outcomes	Interventions	Rationales
Patient/family member/ significant other will verbalize an understanding of the patient's illness, anticipated treatment, and potential complications	Assess the patient/family's current level of knowledge and readiness to learn Design a teaching program that includes the following information as appropriate: Pathophysiology of hyperthyroidism Signs and symptoms associated with crisis Situations that require notification of physician Rationale for and appropriate administration of drugs, side effects Provide written materials for all content taught; provide means for the patient to get questions answered after discharge. Schedule a follow-up teaching session after discharge.	Hyperthyroidism is a chronic illness that requires lifelong management.

ABGs, Arterial blood gases; *BP,* blood pressure; *BUN,* blood urea nitrogen; *CI,* cardiac index; *CO,* cardiac output; *CO₂,* carbon dioxide; *CVP,* central venous pressure; *GI,* gastrointestinal; *HR,* heart rate; *I & O,* intake and output; *IV,* intravenous; *PaCO₂,* partial pressure of carbon dioxide in arterial blood; *PaO₂,* partial measure of oxygen in arterial blood; *PAP,* pulmonary artery pressure; *PAOP,* pulmonary artery occlusion pressure; *RAP,* right atrial pressure; *RR,* respiratory rate; *SVR,* systemic vascular resistance; *VC,* vital capacity; *V_T,* tidal volume; *WNL,* within normal limits.

MYXEDEMA COMA

Pathophysiology

Myxedema coma in the absence of an associated stress or illness is uncommon, with infection being the most frequent stressor. The addition of stress to an already hypothyroid patient accelerates the metabolism and clearance of whatever thyroid hormone is present in the body. Thus, the patient experiences increased hormone utilization but decreased hormone production, which precipitates a crisis state.

As in hyperthyroidism, low levels of thyroid hormones also disrupt the normal physiology of most body systems. Hypothyroidism produces a hypodynamic, hypometabolic state. Myxedema coma is a magnification of these disruptions initiated by some type of stressor. This condition takes many months to develop and should be suspected in patients with a known thyroid history, with a surgical scar on the lower neck, or in those who are unusually sensitive to medications or narcotics. Common findings in patients with myxedema coma are discussed later and are contrasted with those of thyroid storm in Table 17-4.

Etiology

The underlying causes of myxedema coma are those that produce hypothyroidism. Most cases occur either in patients with long-standing autoimmune disease of the thyroid (Hashimoto's thyroiditis) or in patients who have received surgical or radioactive iodine treatment for Graves' disease and have received inadequate hormone replacement. The disorder is rarely associated with hypothyroidism produced by pituitary or hypothalamic disorders. These and other less common causes of hypothyroidism are listed in Box 17-21.

Myxedema coma is the end stage of improperly treated, neglected, or undiagnosed hypothyroidism. It is a life-threatening emergency with a mortality rate as high as 50% despite appropriate therapy. Much of this mortality can be attributed to underlying illnesses. Most patients who develop myxedema coma are elderly women. It is rarely seen in young persons. It occurs more frequently in winter as a result of the increased stress of exposure to cold in a person unable to maintain body heat. Known precipitating factors include hypothermia, infection, cerebral vascular accidents, trauma, and critical illness. Medications that may precipitate myxedema coma include those that affect the central nervous system such as analgesics, anesthesia, barbiturates, narcotics, sedatives, tranquilizers and lithium. The most recent addition to the list of medications that may cause myxedema coma is amiodarone (Ringel, 2001).

BOX 17-21

Causes of Hypothyroidism

PRIMARY THYROID DISEASE
Autoimmune (Hashimoto's thyroiditis)
Radioactive iodine treatment of Graves' disease
Thyroidectomy
Congenital enzymatic defect in thyroid hormone biosynthesis
Inhibition of thyroid hormone synthesis or release
Antithyroid drugs
Iodides
Lithium carbonate
Oral hypoglycemic agents
Idiopathic thyroid atrophy

SECONDARY (PITUITARY) OR TERTIARY (HYPOTHALAMUS) DISEASE
Tumors
Infiltrative disease (sarcoidosis)
Hypophysectomy
Pituitary irradiation
Head injury
Cerebrovascular accidents
Pituitary infarction

Assessment

Clinical presentation. Many patients may have had vague signs and symptoms of hypothyroidism for several years. Box 17-22 gives progressive signs of hypothyroidism. Many of the manifestations are attributable to the development of mucinous edema. This interstitial edema is the result of water retention and decreased protein. Fluid collects in soft tissue such as the face and in joints and muscles, and it can also produce pericardial effusion. The clinical picture of myxedema coma varies with the rate of onset and severity. Diagnosis is based on the clinical signs and symptoms, a high index of suspicion, and a careful history and physical examination.

Neurological disturbances. The low metabolic rate and resulting decreased mentation produce both psychological and physiological changes. The patient in hypothyroid crisis may present with somnolence, delirium, or coma. Grand mal seizures can occur. Personality changes such as paranoia and delusions may be evident.

Patients with hypothyroidism are unable to maintain body heat because of the decreased metabolic rate and production of thermal energy. Because of this, patients may present in crisis after being stressed by exposure to cold. Hypothermia is present in 80% of patients in myxedema coma, with temperatures as low as 80°F (26.7°C). Patients with temperatures less than 88.6°F (32°C) have a grave prognosis. If a patient with myxedema coma has a temperature

BOX 17-22

Progressive Signs of Hypothyrodism

- *Earliest signs:* Fatigue, weakness, muscle cramps, intolerance to cold, and weight gain.
- *Cardiovascular:* Bradycardia and hypotension.
- *Neurological:* Difficulty concentrating, slowed mentation, depression, lethargy, slow and deliberate speech, coarse and raspy voice, hearing loss, and vertigo.
- *Respiratory:* Dyspnea on exertion.
- *Gastrointestinal:* Decreased appetite, decreased peristalsis, anorexia, decreased bowel sounds, constipation, and paralytic ileus. However, the decreased metabolic rate also leads to weight gain.
- *Musculoskeletal:* Fluid in joints and muscles results in stiffness and muscle cramps.
- *Integumentary:* Dry, flaky, cool, coarse skin; dry, coarse hair; and brittle nails. The face is puffy and pallid, the tongue may be enlarged. The dorsa of the hands and feet are edematous. There may be a yellow tint to the skin from depressed hepatic conversion of carotene to vitamin A. Ecchymoses may develop from increased capillary fragility and decreased platelets.
- *Hematological:* Normochromic normocytic anemia and leukocytosis may occur.
- *Ophthalmic:* Generalized mucinous edema in the eyelids and periorbital tissue.
- *Metabolic:* Elevated creatine phosphokinase, aspartate aminotransferase, lactate dehydrogenase, cholesterol, and triglycerides. Elevated cholesterol and triglycerides predispose persons with hypothyroidism to the development of atherosclerosis.

greater than 98.6°F (37°C), underlying infection should be suspected.

Cardiovascular disturbances. Cardiac function is depressed, resulting in decreases in heart rate, contractility, stroke volume, and cardiac output, as well as hypotension. The patient may develop a pericardial effusion, making heart tones distant. The ECG has decreased voltage as a result of the pericardial effusion.

Pulmonary disturbances. Respirations are depressed, producing hypoventilation and CO_2 retention. CO_2 narcosis may contribute to decreased mentation. As part of the picture of generalized mucinous edema and fluid retention, these patients may also develop pleural effusions or upper airway edema, further restricting their breathing.

Gastrointestinal disturbances. Chronic low thyroid hormone levels lead to decreased cardiac output, which causes fluid retention and ascites.

Skeletal muscle disturbances. Slowed motor conduction produces decreased tendon reflexes and sluggish, awkward movements.

Laboratory evaluation. Serum T_4 and T_3 levels and resin T_3 uptake are low in patients with myxedema coma. In primary hypothyroidism, TSH levels are high. If hypothyroidism is the result of disease of the pituitary gland or hypothalamus (secondary and tertiary hypothyroidism), TSH levels are inappropriately normal or low. However, as in patients with thyroid storm, if myxedema coma is suspected, treatment should not be delayed while awaiting these results to confirm the diagnosis.

Serum sodium levels may be low as a result of impaired water excretion and resultant water retention. Impaired water excretion is the result of the inappropriate ADH secretion and cortisol deficiency that frequently accompany hypothyroidism. The patient should be monitored for signs and symptoms related to hyponatremia such as weakness, muscle twitching, seizures, and coma.

Hypoglycemia is common and may also be related to pituitary or hypophyseal disorders and/or adrenal insufficiency. Adrenal insufficiency may also result in serum cortisol levels that are inappropriately low for stress. Laboratory manifestations of myxedema coma are summarized in Laboratory Alerts: Thyroid Disorders.

Nursing Diagnoses

The nursing diagnoses that may apply to a patient in myxedema coma are based on assessment data and include the following:

- Disturbed thought processes related to slowed metabolism and cerebration, hyponatremia
- Hypothermia related to inability of body to retain heat
- Excess fluid volume related to impaired water excretion
- Decreased cardiac output related to decreased contractility, decreased heart rate, decreased stroke volume, pericardial effusion, dysrhythmias
- Ineffective breathing pattern related to hypoventilation, muscle weakness, decreased respiratory rate, ascites, pleural effusions
- Risk for injury related to edema, decreased platelets
- Activity intolerance related to muscle weakness
- Imbalanced nutrition: less than body requirements related to decreased appetite, decreased carbohydrate metabolism, hypoglycemia
- Deficient knowledge: disease process, therapeutic regimen, prevention of complications

Nursing and Medical Interventions

Myxedema coma requires immediate intervention if the patient is to survive. The primary objectives in the treatment of myxedema coma are identifying and treating the precipitating cause, providing thyroid replacement, restoring fluid and electrolyte balance, providing supportive care, and providing patient and family education. Box 17-23 details the treatment of myxedema coma.

Thyroid replacement. The best method of thyroid replacement is controversial. Either liothyronine sodium (Cytomel; T_3) or levothyroxine sodium (Synthroid; T_4) can be used. T_3 is more potent than T_4, and most of T_3 comes from peripheral conversion of T_4 to T_3. Thus, liothyronine requires lower doses, and levothyroxine ultimately provides the patient with both T_4 and T_3 replacement.

Levothyroxine sodium is the more commonly used drug. It has a smoother effect and a longer activity, and a portion of it is converted to T_3 in peripheral tissues. The preferred route is IV, because absorption of oral or intramuscular levothyroxine is variable. The initial dose may be decreased if the patient has underlying factors such as angina, dysrhythmias, or other heart disease.

Liothyronine sodium has heightened metabolic effects, a more rapid onset (6 hours), and a shorter half-life (1 day) than levothyroxine. Because of liothyronine's potency, its administration may be complicated by angina, myocardial infarction, and cardiac irritability. Thus, it is generally avoided in older populations.

BOX 17-23

Treatment of Myxedema Coma

- Identification and treatment of underlying disorder
- Thyroid replacement: levothyroxine sodium 300-500 mcg IV loading dose; 50 mcg/day IV
- Restoration of fluid and electrolyte balance
- Cautious administration of vasopressors
- Hyponatremia: <115 mEq/L, hypertonic saline; <120 mEq/L, fluid restriction
- Hypoglycemia: IV glucose
- Adrenal hormone replacement: hydrocortisone 100 mg IV bolus; 100 mg every 8 hr; taper dose as patient recovers
- Supportive care
- Passive warming with blankets (do not actively warm)
- Ventilatory assistance
- Avoidance of narcotics and sedative drugs
- Chest x-ray or ultrasound study of the chest possibly needed to assess pleural effusion
- Echocardiogram possibly needed to assess cardiac function and/or pericardial effusion
- Patient and family education

Doses are approximate and may vary based on the individual situation.

The effects of levothyroxine are not as rapid as those of liothyronine, but its cardiac toxicity is lower. Serum levels of T_4 reach normal in 1 to 2 days. Levels of TSH begin to fall within 24 hours and return to normal in 7 to 10 days. Drugs used to treat myxedema coma are summarized in Table 17-6.

Fluid and electrolyte restoration. If the patient is hypotensive or in shock, thyroid replacement usually corrects this, but cautious volume expansion with saline also helps. Vasopressors should be used with extreme caution, because patients in myxedema coma are unable to respond to vasopressors until they have adequate levels of thyroid hormones available. Simultaneous administration of vasopressors and thyroid hormones is associated with myocardial irritability.

Hyponatremia usually responds to thyroid replacement and water restriction; the patient can be rid of free water once thyroid hormones are replaced. If hyponatremia is severe (less than 110 mEq/L) or the patient is having seizures, hypertonic saline with or without furosemide (Lasix) may be administered, but only until symptoms disappear or the sodium level is 120 mEq/L.

Glucose should be added to IV fluids to provide support to a patient with hypoglycemia and/or concomitant adrenal insufficiency. Hydrocortisone, 100 mg, is given initially, followed by 50 to 100 mg every 6 hours in the first 24 hours. Subsequently, the dose is 50 to 100 mg every 8 hours for 7 to 10 days. The adrenal abnormality may last several weeks after thyroid replacement is begun, so this support should be continued during that time.

Supportive Care

Symptoms are aggressively treated. Hypothermia is treated by keeping the room warm and using warmed blankets. Electric heating blankets are not used because active heat in the presence of vasodilation may lead to vascular collapse. Mechanical ventilation is frequently required. Cardiac function is assessed and treated.

TABLE 17-6

DRUGS USED TO TREAT MYXEDEMA COMA

Drug	Action/Uses	Dosage/Route	Side Effects	Nursing Implications
Levothyroxine sodium (Synthroid)	Same as thyroid hormone	300-500 mcg IV loading dose then 50-200 mcg/day	Symptoms of hyperthyroidism, allergic skin reactions	Monitor for signs and symptoms of hyperthyroidism. Monitor cardiac response closely
Liothyronine sodium (Cytomel)	Same as thyroid hormone	25 mcg IV every 8 hr for 24-48 hr; then 12.5 mcg every 8 hr	Same as levothyroxine plus angina, myocardial infarction, cardiac irritability	Same as levothyroxine
Hydrocortisone	If patient has central hypothyroidism, provides stress dose corticosteroid	100 mg IV every 8 hr	Hyperglycemia, sodium retention, hypertension are immediate effects	Taper dose as patient recovers.

IV, Intravenous.

Patient and family education. The education of patients, family, and significant others is critical in identifying and preventing episodes of myxedema coma.

Patient Outcomes

Outcomes for a patient with myxedema coma include the following:

- Return to baseline mentation and personality
- Maintenance of temperature within normal range
- Normal fluid volume balance and absence of edema
- Stable hemodynamics within normal limits
- Effective breathing pattern
- Intact skin without edema or bleeding
- Return to baseline activity level
- Adequate nutrition and stable body weight
- Verbalization by the patient and/or significant other of an understanding of disease, therapeutic regimen, and prevention of complications

Antidiuretic Hormone Disorders

REVIEW OF PHYSIOLOGY

The primary function of ADH is regulation of water balance and serum osmolality. ADH (also known as arginine vasopressin) is produced in the supraoptic nuclei and paraventricular nuclei of the hypothalamus. These nuclei are positioned near the thirst center and osmoreceptors in the hypothalamus (Figure 17-7).

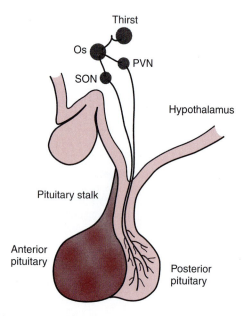

FIGURE 17-7 Hypothalamic–posterior pituitary system. *Os,* Osmoreceptors; *PVN,* paraventricular nucleus; *SON,* supraoptic nucleus.

Once produced, ADH is stored in neurons in the posterior pituitary. If the supraoptic and paraventricular nuclei are stimulated (via mechanisms described later), their discharge stimulates the nerve endings in the posterior pituitary to release ADH. This stimulation occurs in response to both osmotic and nonosmotic forces: osmoreceptors in the hypothalamus respond to changes in extracellular osmolality, and stretch receptors in the left atrium and baroreceptors in the carotid sinus and aortic arch respond to changes in circulating volume and blood pressure, respectively.

Once released, ADH acts on the renal distal and collecting tubules to cause water reabsorption. In high concentrations, ADH also acts on smooth muscles of the arterioles to produce vasoconstriction. Normally, ADH is released in response to increased serum osmolality (primary stimulus), elevated serum sodium, decreased blood volume (10% drop), decreased blood pressure (5% to 10% drop), stress, trauma, hypoxia, pain, and anxiety. Certain drugs, such as narcotics, barbiturates, anesthetics, and chemotherapeutic agents, are also known to stimulate ADH release. The physiology of ADH release is summarized in Figure 17-8. Two common disturbances of ADH are diabetes insipidus (DI) and the syndrome of inappropriate ADH (SIADH).

DIABETES INSIPIDUS
Etiology

Various disorders can produce neurogenic DI (Box 17-24), but the primary cause is traumatic injury to the posterior pituitary or hypothalamus as a result of head injury or surgery. Transient DI may occur after pituitary surgery or trauma resulting from manipulation of the pituitary stalk or cerebral edema. Permanent DI occurs when more than 80% to 85% of the supraoptic or paraventricular nuclei or the proximal end of the pituitary stalk is destroyed.

Nephrogenic DI may occur in genetically predisposed persons or may be acquired from chronic renal disease, drugs, or other conditions that produce permanent kidney damage or inhibit the generation of cyclic adenosine monophosphate in the tubules.

Pathophysiology

DI results from an ADH deficiency (neurogenic or central DI), ADH insensitivity (nephrogenic DI), or excessive water intake (secondary DI). Regardless of the cause, the result is impaired renal conservation of water and polyuria (greater than 3 L in 24 hours). As long as the thirst center remains intact and the person is able to respond to this thirst, fluid volume can be maintained. If the patient is unable to respond, severe dehydration can result if fluid losses are not replaced. This defect may be permanent or transient.

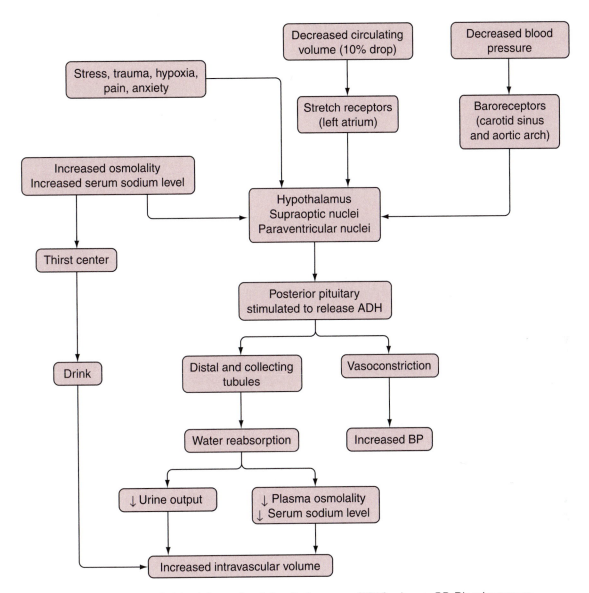

FIGURE 17-8 Physiology of antidiuretic hormone (ADH) release. *BP,* Blood pressure.

Neurogenic DI is the type most frequently encountered in clinical practice.

In neurogenic DI, absent or diminished release of circulating levels of ADH from the posterior pituitary produces free water loss and causes serum osmolality and serum sodium to rise. The posterior pituitary is unable to respond by increasing ADH levels; thus, the kidneys are not stimulated to reabsorb water, and excessive water loss results. Neurogenic DI occurs as the result of disruption of the neural pathways or structures involved in ADH production, synthesis, or release.

In nephrogenic DI, the kidney collecting ducts and distal tubules are unresponsive to ADH; thus, adequate levels of ADH may be synthesized and released, but the kidneys are unable to conserve water in response. In patients with secondary DI, compulsive volume consumption causes polyuria.

Assessment

Clinical presentation. Neurogenic DI usually occurs suddenly with an abrupt onset of polyuria, as much as 5 to 40 L in 24 hours. The urine is pale and dilute. The thirst mechanism is activated in conscious

Causes of Diabetes Insipidus

ANTIDIURETIC HORMONE DEFICIENCY (NEUROGENIC DIABETES INSIPIDUS)

Idiopathic: familial or congenital
Intracranial surgery: especially in region of pituitary
Tumors: craniopharyngioma, pituitary tumors, metastases to hypothalamus
Infections: meningitis, encephalitis, syphilis, mycoses, toxoplasmosis
Granulomatous disease: tuberculosis, sarcoidosis, histiocytosis
Severe head trauma or any disorder that causes increased intracranial pressure

ANTIDIURETIC HORMONE INSENSITIVITY (NEPHROGENIC DIABETES INSIPIDUS)

Hereditary: idiopathic
Renal disease: pyelonephritis, amyloidosis, polycystic kidney disease, obstructive uropathy, transplantation
Multisystem disorders affecting kidneys: multiple myeloma, sickle cell disease, cystic fibrosis
Metabolic disturbances: chronic hypokalemia or hypercalcemia
Drugs: ethanol, phenytoin, lithium carbonate, demeclocycline, amphotericin, methoxyflurane

SECONDARY DIABETES INSIPIDUS

Idiopathic
Psychogenic polydipsia
Hypothalamic disease: sarcoidosis
Excessive intravenous fluid administration
Drug-induced disease: anticholinergic, tricyclic antidepressant

greater than 295 mOsm/kg H_2O, and serum sodium is greater than 145 mEq/L. The presence of hypokalemia or hypercalcemia suggests nephrogenic DI. Other values such as BUN and creatinine may be elevated as a result of hemoconcentration. Plasma ADH may be measured to evaluate the cause of the DI. The level is decreased in neurogenic DI and increased in nephrogenic DI.

If the cause of polyuria is unclear, additional diagnostic testing may be needed. A water deprivation test is typically done to determine whether the patient responds to hyperosmolality with the release of ADH. Water intake is restricted, and urine volume and serum osmolality are measured for 6 to 8 hours. If the urine remains dilute (urine osmolality less than 100 mOsm/kg H_2O, specific gravity less than 1.005) and polyuria continues in spite of increasing serum osmolality (greater than 300 mOsm/kg H_2O), the patient has DI. To differentiate neurogenic DI from nephrogenic DI, vasopressin 10 milliunits/kg or 1 mcg desmopressin is given intranasally. Urine is collected at 30-, 60-, 90-, and 120-minute intervals, and osmolality is measured. If urine volume decreases and the urine osmolality rises more than 50%, the patient has neurogenic DI. A patient with nephrogenic DI will not respond. Careful monitoring of the patient is mandatory during this testing to avoid dehydration and hypotension (see Laboratory Alerts: Pituitary Disorders).

Nursing Diagnoses

The nursing diagnoses that may apply to a patient with DI include the following:

- Deficient fluid volume related to deficient ADH, renal cells insensitive to ADH, polyuria, and inability to respond to thirst
- Disturbed thought processes related to decreased cerebral perfusion, cerebral dehydration, and hypernatremia

Nursing and Medical Interventions

The primary goals of treatment are to identify and correct the underlying cause and restore normal fluid volume and osmolality and electrolyte balance. Identifying the underlying cause is a necessary part of determining appropriate treatment, particularly drug therapy.

Volume replacement. If the patient is alert and able to respond to thirst, he or she will generally drink enough water to avoid symptomatic hypovolemia. However, patients in critical care units who develop DI and elderly patients with cognitive impairments are frequently unable to respond to or recognize thirst, so fluid replacement is essential.

patients and polydipsia occurs. If the patient is unable to replace the water lost by responding to thirst, signs of hypovolemia will develop: hypotension, decreased skin turgor, dry mucous membranes, tachycardia, weight loss, and low central venous and pulmonary artery occlusion pressures. Neurological signs and symptoms may be produced by hypovolemia and hypernatremia. A detailed listing of signs and symptoms of DI is found in Table 17-7.

Laboratory evaluation. One of the classic signs of DI is the finding of an inappropriately low urine osmolality in the face of a high serum osmolality. Corresponding with the low urine osmolality is a decreased urine specific gravity. Serum osmolality is

TABLE 17-7

Comparison of Signs and Symptoms of Abnormal Antidiuretic Hormone Secretion

System	Diabetes Insipidus	Syndrome of Inappropriate Antidiuretic Hormone
Cardiovascular	Weight loss Hypotension Tachycardia ↓ Skin turgor Dry mucous membranes RAP <2 mm Hg PAOP <8 mm Hg	Weight gain Hypertension RAP >10 mm Hg PAOP >12 mm Hg
Neurological	Confusion Restlessness Lethargy Irritability Seizures Coma	Confusion Restlessness Lethargy Weakness Difficulty concentrating Headache Seizures Coma
Renal	Pale, dilute urine Polyuria	Concentrated urine ↓ Output
Gastrointestinal	Constipation	Nausea and vomiting Anorexia Muscle cramps ↓ Bowel sounds
Pulmonary	Thick, tenacious secretions	Tachypnea Dyspnea Adventitious sounds Frothy, pink sputum
Laboratory values	Serum sodium >145 mEq/L Serum osmolality >295 mOsm/kg H_2O Urine osmolality ↓	Serum sodium <135 mEq/L Serum osmolality <275 mOsm/kg H_2O Urine osmolality ↑

↑, Increased; ↓, decreased; *PAOP,* pulmonary artery occlusion pressure; *RAP,* right atrial pressure.

If the patient already has symptoms of hypovolemia, the volume already lost must be replaced. In addition, fluid is replaced every hour to keep up with current urine losses. Correction of hypernatremia and replacement of free water are achieved using hypotonic dextrose in water solutions. However, if the patient has circulatory failure, isotonic saline may be administered until hemodynamic stability and vascular volume have been restored.

Monitoring for signs and symptoms of hypovolemia is a priority. Vital signs must be recorded at least every hour, along with urine output. Hemodynamic monitoring may be instituted to evaluate fluid requirements and to monitor the patient's response to treatment. This is particularly important in elderly patients who are likely to have concurrent cardiovascular and renal disease. Accurate intake and output and daily weights are essential. Measurement of urine specific gravity assists in evaluating the patient's response to treatment. Once drug therapy has been instituted, the urine should become more concentrated and the specific gravity should increase.

Frequent monitoring of the patient's neurological status is also critical because changes may indicate a change in fluid and/or electrolyte status (e.g., sodium). Fluid overload from overaggressive fluid replacement, particularly once drug therapy has been instituted, must be assessed.

Hormone replacement. Neurogenic DI is controlled primarily with exogenous ADH preparations (Holcomb, 2002). These drugs replace ADH and enable

LABORATORY ALERTS: PITUITARY DISORDERS

Laboratory Test	Critical Value	Significance	Nursing Actions
Diabetes Insipidus **Serum** Sodium	>145 mEq/L	Absent or diminished release of ADH or lack of response by the kidneys leads to free water loss	IV fluid replacement should correct In secondary DI, fluid restriction
Osmolality ADH	>295 mOsm/kg H_2O	Low (neurogenic) High (nephrogenic) Normal (secondary)	
Urine Osmolality Specific gravity	<100 mOsm/kg H_2O <1.005		
Syndrome of Inappropriate Antidiuretic Hormone **Serum** Sodium	<135 mEq/L	Oversecretion of ADH and failure of negative feedback system leading to free water retention	Mild: Fluid restriction, I & O, liberal dietary salt/protein Monitor serum sodium, osmolality and weight Severe: Hypertonic saline IV, fluid restriction, I & O, daily weight; treat underlying cause
Osmolality ADH	<275 mOsm/kg H_2O High		
Urine Sodium	>20 mEq/L	Used as differential for other causes of hypo-osmolality (e.g., HF)	

ADH, Antidiuretic hormone; *HF,* heart failure; *DI,* diabetes insipidus; *I & O,* intake and output; *IV,* intravenous.

the kidneys to conserve water. They can be administered by the IV route or intramuscularly, intranasally, or subcutaneously. Injectable forms are generally more potent than intranasal, and absorption is more reliable through the IV route.

The drug most commonly used for management is desmopressin (DDAVP), a synthetic analogue of vasopressin. Unlike aqueous vasopressin and lysine vasopressin, desmopressin is devoid of any vasoconstrictor effects and has a longer antidiuretic action (12 to 24 hours). It also has infrequent and mild side effects: headache, nausea, and mild abdominal cramps. Table 17-8 gives specific dosages of this and other drugs used to treat DI.

Aqueous vasopressin is used primarily for diagnostic purposes or in patients whose DI is expected to be temporary (such as those with head injuries). Its shorter duration of action (3 to 6 hours) enables detection of the return of ADH function. Lysine vasopressin is generally used in patients who are refractory to desmopressin or who demonstrate significant side effects.

Aqueous vasopressin and lysine vasopressin can cause vasoconstrictive side effects in high doses, but patients with preexisting vascular disease (particularly coronary artery disease) may experience these side effects even with small doses. Tachycardia, hypertension, dysrhythmias, angina, and myocardial infarction may occur. Careful hemodynamic and cardiac monitoring of these patients is required. When these drugs are used, a nitroglycerin infusion may be started to counteract the potential cardiac effects.

TABLE 17-8
DRUGS USED TO TREAT DIABETES INSIPIDUS

Drug	Dosage/Route	Side Effects	Nursing Implications
Aqueous vasopressin	IM/subcu: 5-10 units every 6-12 hr IV: 0.2-0.4 units/min, up to 0.9 units/min	Water intoxication, circumoral pallor, sweating, tremor, head pounding, abdominal cramps, flatus, vertigo, nausea and vomiting Large doses or patients with cardiac history: hypertension, dysrhythmias, angina, myocardial infarction	Monitor for signs of water intoxication: lethargy, behavioral changes, disorientation, neuromuscular excitability. Monitor I & O, daily weight, and specific gravity. Monitor BP, HR, and ECG rhythm.
Lysine vasopressin	Intranasal: 5-10 units several times a day	Same as above	Same as above
Desmopressin (DDAVP)	Subcu/IM/IV: 1-4 mcg/day Intranasal: 10-40 mcg/day	Infrequent and mild: headache, nausea, abdominal cramps	Monitor for signs of water intoxication. Monitor I & O and daily weight
Chlorpropamide (Diabinese)	125-500 mg/day	Hypoglycemia, headache, weakness, dizziness, drowsiness	Monitor blood glucose. Monitor I & O and daily weight. Monitor for signs of water intoxication.
Carbamazepine (Tegretol)	400-600 mg/day	Water intoxication, thrombocytopenia, leukocytosis, anemia, HF, hypertension, syncope, edema	Monitor I & O and daily weight. Monitor CBC and platelet count. Monitor for signs of water intoxication.
Clofibrate (Atromid-S)	2 g/day	Most common: nausea Less common: rash, myalgias, arthralgias, muscle weakness	Monitor renal/hepatic function (contraindicated in hepatic or renal disease). If GI symptoms, are present, the patient should take the drug with meals.

BP, Blood pressure; *CBC*, complete blood count; *ECG*, electrocardiogram; *GI*, gastrointestinal; *HF*, heart failure; *HR*, heart rate; *IM*, intramuscular; *I & O*, intake and output; *IV*, intravenous; *subcu*, subcutaneous.

Overmedication with an ADH preparation can also produce water overload. The patient should be monitored for signs of dyspnea, hypertension, weight gain, hyponatremia, headache, or drowsiness.

Nephrogenic diabetes insipidus. Treatment of nephrogenic DI relies primarily on solute restriction and the administration of thiazide diuretics. Sodium depletion causes a fall in the glomerular filtration rate, enhanced reabsorption of fluid, and a reduced capacity to dilute the urine.

Patient and family education. Patients who have a permanent ADH deficit require education regarding the following:
- Pathogenesis of DI
- Dose, side effects, and rationale for prescribed medications
- Parameters for notifying the physician
- Importance of adherence to medication regimen
- Importance of recording daily weight measurements to identify weight gain
- Importance of wearing a Medic-Alert identification bracelet
- Importance of drinking according to thirst and avoiding excess drinking

Patient Outcomes
Outcomes for a patient with DI include the following:
- Serum osmolality 275 to 295 mOsm/kg H_2O
- Stable weight and balanced intake and output
- Serum sodium 135 to 145 mEq/L
- Return to baseline mentation

SYNDROME OF INAPPROPRIATE ANTIDIURETIC HORMONE
Etiology
The most common cause of SIADH is ectopic production of ADH by malignant disease, especially small cell carcinoma of the lung (Miller, 2001). The malignant

cells themselves actually synthesize, store, and release ADH and thus place control of ADH outside the normal pituitary-hypothalamus feedback loops. Other types of malignancies known to produce SIADH include pancreatic and duodenal carcinoma, Hodgkin's lymphoma, sarcoma, and squamous cell carcinoma of the tongue.

Nonmalignant pulmonary conditions such as tuberculosis, pneumonia, lung abscess, and chronic obstructive pulmonary disease can also produce SIADH. As with malignant cells, it is believed that benign pulmonary tissue is capable of synthesizing and releasing ADH in certain disease states.

Central nervous system disorders such as head injuries, infections, hemorrhages, surgery, and cerebrovascular accidents can produce SIADH. The problem is caused by stimulation of the hypothalamic and/or pituitary systems.

Many medications are associated with SIADH (Kokko, Hall, & Afrin, 2002; Patel & Kasiar, 2002). The mechanisms involved include increasing or potentiating the action of ADH, acting on the renal distal tubule to decrease free water excretion, or causing central release of ADH.

Pathophysiology

SIADH occurs when the body secretes excessive ADH unrelated to plasma osmolality; that is, a failure in the negative feedback mechanism that regulates the release and inhibition of ADH. The results are an inability to secrete a dilute urine, fluid retention, and dilutional hyponatremia. SIADH may result from a clinical disorder or may be pharmacologically induced (Box 17-25).

Assessment and Clinical Presentation

ADH stimulation produces a clinical picture of water intoxication. The clinical manifestations are primarily the result of water retention, hyponatremia, and hypo-osmolality of the serum. The severity of the signs and symptoms is related to the rate of onset and the severity of the hyponatremia.

Central nervous system. Manifestations such as weakness, lethargy, mental confusion, difficulty concentrating, restlessness, headache, seizures, and coma may occur in response to hyponatremia and hypo-osmolality. Hypo-osmolality disrupts the intracellular-extracellular osmotic gradient and causes a shift of water into brain cells, cerebral edema, and increased intracranial pressure. If the serum sodium falls to less than 120 mEq/L in 48 hours or less, there are usually serious neurological symptoms and a mortality rate as high as 50%. If hyponatremia develops more slowly, the body is able to protect against cerebral

---

BOX 17-25

Causes of Syndrome of Inappropriate Antidiuretic Hormone

ECTOPIC ANTIDIURETIC HORMONE PRODUCTION
Small cell carcinoma of lung
Cancer of prostate, pancreas, or duodenum
Hodgkin's disease
Sarcoma, squamous cell carcinoma of the tongue, thymoma
Nonmalignant pulmonary disease: viral pneumonia, tuberculosis, chronic obstructive pulmonary disease, lung abscess

CENTRAL NERVOUS SYSTEM DISORDERS
Head trauma
Infections: meningitis, encephalitis, brain abscess
Intracranial surgery, cerebral aneurysm, brain tumor, cerebral atrophy, cerebrovascular accident
Guillain-Barré syndrome, lupus erythematosus

DRUGS
Amiodarone
Analgesics and narcotics: morphine, fentanyl, acetaminophen
Antineoplastics: vincristine, cyclophosphamide, vinblastine, cisplatin
Barbiturates
Carbamazepine (Tegretol)
Chlorpropamide (Diabinese)
General anesthetics
Mizoribine
Nicotine
Pentamidine
Serotonergic agents: 3-4,-methylenedioxymethamphetamine (MDMA; Ecstasy), selective serotonin reuptake inhibitors
Thiazide diuretics
Tricyclic antidepressants

POSITIVE-PRESSURE VENTILATION

edema, and the patient may remain asymptomatic even with a very low sodium level.

Gastrointestinal system. Congestion of the GI tract and decreased motility because of electrolyte imbalance (hyponatremia) can produce nausea and vomiting, anorexia, muscle cramps, and decreased bowel sounds.

Cardiovascular system. In the cardiovascular system, water retention produces weight gain, increased blood pressure, and elevated central venous and pulmonary artery occlusion pressures.

Pulmonary system. Fluid overload in the pulmonary system can produce increased respirations, dyspnea, adventitious lung sounds, and frothy, pink sputum.

Laboratory Evaluation

The hallmark of SIADH is hyponatremia and hypo-osmolality in the presence of an inappropriately concentrated urine (a low serum osmolarity should trigger inhibition of ADH, resulting in the loss of water through the kidneys and a dilute urine). Hyponatremia (less than 135 mEq/L) and hypo-osmolality (less than 275 mOsm/kg) result from water retention.

High urinary sodium levels (greater than 20 mEq/L) help to differentiate SIADH from other causes of hypo-osmolality, hyponatremia, and volume overload (such as heart failure). In SIADH, renal perfusion (a major stimulus for sodium reabsorption) is usually adequate, so sodium is not conserved. In a disorder such as heart failure, renal perfusion is low because of decreased cardiac output, triggering reabsorption of sodium.

Hemodilution may also decrease other laboratory values such as BUN, creatinine, and albumin. SIADH should be suspected in a patient with evidence of hemodilution and urine that is hypertonic relative to plasma.

If the cause of hyponatremia and hypo-osmolality is unclear, a water load test may be performed to establish the diagnosis of SIADH. In this test, an oral water load is administered over 15 to 20 minutes. Water volume and urine osmolality are then measured. Normally, 80% of the water load is excreted in 5 hours, and the urine becomes more dilute. If the patient has SIADH, less than 40% of the water is excreted in 5 hours, and the urine osmolality does not drop significantly. The serum sodium should be corrected to at least 125 mEq/L before performing this test.

Nursing Diagnoses

The nursing diagnoses that may apply to a patient with SIADH include the following:

- Excess fluid volume related to excess water retention from excess ADH
- Disturbed thought processes related to brain swelling and fluid shift into cerebral cells

Nursing and Medical Interventions

The primary goals of therapy are to treat the underlying cause, to eliminate excess water, and to increase serum osmolality. In many instances, treatment of the underlying disorder (e.g., discontinuation of a responsible drug) is all that is needed to return the patient's condition to normal.

Fluid balance. In mild to moderate cases (serum sodium 125 to 135 mEq/L), fluid intake is restricted to 800 to 1000 mL/day, with liberal dietary salt and protein intake. The patient's response is evaluated by monitoring serum sodium, serum osmolality, and weight loss for a gradual return to baseline.

In severe, symptomatic cases (coma, seizures, sodium less than 110 mEq/L), hypertonic 3% or 5% saline (200 to 500 mL) may be given over a period of 3-4 hours, followed by infusion at 75 to 100 mL per hour until sodium goal has been reached. Fluid intake is restricted to 500 mL/day. However, hypertonic saline administration may not be successful because the additional sodium may be excreted rapidly. Hypertonic saline administration should be no faster than 1 to 2 mL/kg per hour to raise the serum sodium no faster than 0.5 to 2 mEq/L per hour. Serum sodium should be checked at 1- to 2-hour intervals to guide initial therapy. Sodium should be corrected to a serum level of 120 mEq/L (lower if the symptoms resolve) with hypertonic solutions. Administering hypertonic saline too rapidly and/or correcting serum sodium too rapidly can result in central pontine myelinolysis, a severe neurological syndrome that can result in permanent brain damage or death. The risk of heart failure is also significant. A diuretic such as furosemide may be given during hypertonic saline administration to promote diuresis and free water clearance. Treatments for chronic or resistant SIADH are listed in Box 17-26.

Nursing. Prevention of SIADH may not be possible, but early detection and treatment may prevent more serious sequelae from occurring. Thus, being aware of the populations at risk and monitoring at-risk populations for clinical signs are key roles for the critical care nurse.

Close monitoring of fluid and electrolyte balance is required. Daily weight, intake and output, and urine

BOX 17-26

Treatments for Chronic or Resistant Syndrome of Inappropriate Antidiuretic Hormone

- Water restriction of 800-1000 mL/day.
- Butorphanol (Stadol) to inhibit ADH secretion for central nervous system causes.
- Demeclocycline is an antibiotic that also decreases renal tubule responsiveness to ADH. Doses of 600 to 1200 mg are given in divided doses bid. Its onset is delayed for several days, and it may not be completely effective for 2 weeks, evidenced by a decrease in urine osmolality to therapeutic range. The major side effects are azotemia (nephrotoxicity) and risk of infection.
- Administration of loop diuretics in conjunction with increased salt and potassium intake is the safest method for treating chronic hyponatremia. The diuretic prevents urine concentration, and the increased salt and potassium intake increases water output by increasing delivery of solutes to the kidney.

ADH, Antidiuretic hormone.
Doses are approximate and may vary based on the individual situation.

specific gravity should be measured. Fluid overload may occur from hypervolemia or too rapid administration of hypertonic saline. Cardiovascular symptoms such as tachycardia, increased blood pressure, increased hemodynamic pressures, full bounding pulses, and distended neck veins are all indicators of fluid overload. Respiratory function should be monitored for signs of tachypnea, labored respirations, shortness of breath, or fine crackles. Careful monitoring of potassium and magnesium levels is necessary to replace diuresis-induced losses.

Adherence to fluid restrictions is critical but difficult for patients. The nurse should ensure that the patient and the family understand the importance of the restriction and that they are included in planning types and timing of fluids. Patients should be encouraged to choose fluids high in sodium content such as milk, tomato juice, and beef and chicken broth. Measures that can relieve some of the discomfort caused by fluid restriction include frequent mouth care, oral rinses without swallowing, using chilled beverages, and sucking on hard candy.

Assessment of the patient's neurological status is also critical to monitor the effects of treatment and to watch for complications. The patient should be assessed for subtle changes that may indicate water intoxication, such as fatigue, weakness, headache, or changes in level of consciousness. Strict adherence to administration rates of hypertonic (3% to 5%) saline solutions and measurement of serial

Case Study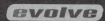

J. O., a 72-year-old woman, comes to the emergency room with complaints of heart "palpitations," weakness, shortness of breath, abdominal pain, and a history of fever, nausea, vomiting, and constipation for the last week. She denies cigarette use. On questioning, she states she has lost about 15 lb, unintentionally, in the last month. She shares that her husband passed away approximately a month ago after more than 50 years of marriage. She also reports that her ankles have been swollen recently. On examination, her blood pressure is 130/72 mm Hg, her heart rate is 130 beats/min and irregular, and her respiratory rate is 32 breaths/min. Her temperature is 104.6°F. Her electrocardiogram shows atrial fibrillation, which is a change from her last electrocardiogram. An arterial blood gas determination reveals the following: pH, 7.32; PaO_2, 70 mm Hg; $PaCO_2$, 55 mm Hg, bicarbonate, 25 mEq/L on room air. Chest x-ray study reveals the beginning stages of heart failure. Other abnormal laboratory

results reveal the following: blood glucose, 223 mg/dL; potassium, 3.0 mEq/L; calcium, 11 mg/dL; blood urea nitrogen, 22 mg/dL; and white blood cell count, 17,000/μL. Previous medications include propranolol (Inderal) and hydroclorothiazide since the age of 56 years.

CRITICAL THINKING QUESTIONS

1. What do you suspect this patient is experiencing? Why?
2. What other physical findings would you expect?
3. What other laboratory studies would you want? What would you expect these results to show?
4. Would you wait for these laboratory results to treat the patient? Why?
5. What would your initial actions be?
6. What are this patient's learning needs?
7. What discharge needs does this patient have?

serum sodium levels are essential to prevent neurological sequelae. Seizure precautions should be instituted if the patient's sodium level falls to less than 120 mEq/L.

Patient and family education. In some patients, SIADH may require long-term treatment and/or ongoing monitoring. These patients and their families require instruction regarding the following:
- Early signs and symptoms to report to the health care provider: weight gain, lethargy, weakness, nausea, mental status changes
- The significance of adherence to fluid restriction
- Dose, side effects, and rationale for prescribed medications
- Importance of daily weights

Patient Outcomes
Outcomes for a patient with SIADH include the following:
- Serum osmolality, 275 to 295 mOsm/kg H$_2$O
- Serum sodium, 135 to 145 mEq/L

- Hemodynamic measurements that are within normal limits
- Return of vital signs to patient baseline
- Return of mental status to patient baseline
- Ability of the patient and family to verbalize an understanding of SIADH, therapeutic regimen, and prevention of complications

SUMMARY
Various endocrine disorders are seen in critical care. Patients may be admitted to the critical care unit for treatment of an endocrine disorder (e.g., DKA) or a disorder secondary to another problem (e.g., SIADH after a head injury). Preexisting disorders (e.g., hypothyroidism) may become secondary during treatment of a critical illness. The stress of critical illness can affect the endocrine system. The critical care nurse must be knowledgeable about the endocrine system, its feedback mechanisms, and its role in maintaining homeostasis. Nursing assessments and interventions can assist in prevention, detection, and early treatment of endocrine imbalance.

CRITICAL THINKING QUESTIONS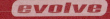

1. Insulin therapy is a critical intervention in the treatment of DKA. What crucial parameters must be monitored to ensure optimal patient outcomes?
2. What is the critical assessment parameter to differentiate DKA from HHNC?
3. Which organ system is most affected by a slower, more prolonged fall in serum glucose, and what nursing interventions are most critical to prevent harm to this patient?
4. Features of adrenal crisis are nonspecific and may be attributed to other medical disorders. What clinical indicators should make you consider this diagnosis? What would you look for in the patient's history?

5. Which medication or combination of medications should be used with caution in critically ill patients because of the risk of SIADH?
6. An order has been placed for your patient in thyroid crisis. The order reads: propylthiouracil 250 mg orally loading, followed by 250 mg orally every 6 hours, and saturated solution of potassium iodide five drops every 6 hours. How should you time the medication administration, and why?
7. What are the major cardiac manifestations of myxedema coma, and what medical and nursing interventions are most important to prevent more-serious sequelae?

REFERENCES
American Diabetes Association (ADA). (2003). Hyperglycemic crises in patients with diabetes mellitus. *Diabetes Care, 20*[Suppl 1], S109-S117.

Bakalov, V. V., Vanderhoof, V. H., & Bondy, C. A. (2002). Adrenal antibodies detect asymptomatic auto-immune adrenal insufficiency in young women with spontaneous premature ovarian failure. *Human Reproduction, 17*(8), 2096-2100.

Fisher, J. N. (2002). Management of thyrotoxicosis. *Southern Medical Journal, 95*(5), 493-505.

Grossman, C. M, Nussbaum, R. H., & Nussbaum, F. D. (2002). Thyrotoxicosis among Hanford, Washington,

Downwinders: A community-based health survey. *Archives of Environmental Health, 57*(1), 9-15.

Hoffman, W. H. (2002). Acetoacetate increases expression of intracellular adhesion molecule-1 (CAM-1) in human brain microvascular endotheial cells. *Neuroscience Letters, 334*(2), 71-74.

Holcomb, S. S. (2002). Diabetes insipidus. *Dimensions of Critical Care Nursing, 21*(3). 94-97.

Jones, R. E., & Huether, S. E. (2002). Alterations in hormonal regulation. In K. L. McCance & S. E. Huether (eds.). *Pathophysiology: The biologic basis for disease in adults and children* [pp. 624-669]. 4th ed. St. Louis: Mosby.

Kokko, H., Hall, P. D., & Afrin, L. B. (2002). Fentanyl-associated syndrome of inappropriate antidiuretic hormone secretion. *Pharmacotherapy, 22*(9), 1188-1192.

Leung, P. M., Quinn, N. D., & Belchetz, P. E. (2002). Amiodarone-induced thyrotoxicosis is not a benign condition. *International Journal of Clinical Practice, 56*(1), 44-46.

Marik, P. E., & Zaloga, G. P. (2003). Adrenal insufficiency during septic shock. *Critical Care Medicine, 31*(1), 141-145.

Miller, M. (2001). Syndromes of excess antidiuretic hormone release. *Critical Care Clinics, 17*(1), 11-23.

Offner, P. J., Moore, E. E., & Ciesla, D. (2002). The adrenal response after severe trauma. *American Journal of Surgery, 184*, 649-654.

Patel, G. P., & Kasiar, J. B. (2002). Syndrome of inappropriate antidiuretic hormone-induced hyponatremia associated with amiodarone. *Pharmacotherapy, 22*(5), 649-651.

Piano, M. R., & Huether, S. E. (2002). Mechanisms of hormonal regulation. In K. L. McCance & S. E. Huether (eds.). *Pathophysiology: The biologic basis for disease in adults and children* [pp. 597-623]. 4th ed. St. Louis: Mosby.

Quinn, L. (2002). Pharmacologic treatment of the critically ill patient with diabetes. *Critical Care Nursing Clinics of North America, 14*(1), 81-98.

Ringel, M. D. (2001). Management of hypothyroidism and hyperthyroidism in the intensive care unit. *Critical Care Clinics, 17*(1), 59-74.

Rivers, E. P., et al. (2001). Adrenal insufficiency in high-risk surgical ICU patients. *Chest, 119*(3), 889-896.

Skinner, T. C. (2002) Recurrent diabetic ketoacidosis: Causes, prevention and management. *Hormone Research, 57*[Suppl 1], 78-80.

Tkacs, N. C. (2002). Hypoglycemia unawareness: Your patients with diabetes won't always know when their blood sugar is low. *American Journal of Nursing, 102*(2), 34-41.

Wong, V. F., Fu, A., George, J., & Cheung, N. W. (2002). Thyrotoxicosis induced by alpha-interferon therapy in chronic viral hepatitis. *Clinical Endocrinology, 56*(6), 793-798.

Zaloga, G. P., & Marik, P. (2001). Hypothalamic-pituitary-adrenal insufficiency. *Critical Care Clinics, 17*(1), 25-41.

RECOMMENDED READINGS

Gillespie, G. L, & Campbell, M. (2002). Diabetic ketoacidosis. *American Journal of Nursing, 102*[9 Suppl], 13-17.

Holcomb, S. S. (2002) Thyroid diseases: A primer for the critical care nurse. *Dimensions of Critical Care Nursing, 21*(4), 127-133.

McConnell, E. A. (2002). Myths and facts...about Addison's disease. *Nursing, 32*(8), 79.

evolve *Did you remember to check out the bonus material, including free self-assessment exercises, on the Evolve web site at http://evolve.elsevier.com/Sole/ and on the CD-ROM?*

CHAPTER **18**

Surgical and Trauma Management

Pamela J. Bolton, MS, RN, CCRN, CNS
Deborah G. Klein, MSN, RN, CCRN, CS

OBJECTIVES

- Describe a systems approach to trauma care.
- Identify mechanisms of traumatic injury commonly seen in the critical care setting.
- Discuss prehospital, emergency, and resuscitation care of the trauma patient.
- Describe assessment and management of common traumatic injuries.
- Explain the priorities of care for the postoperative surgical patient.
- Discuss nursing interventions for care of the trauma patient, including prevention of complications.

Introduction

The incidence of trauma in the United States is a major health care and economic issue. Trauma continues to be the fourth leading cause of death for all ages. Only heart disease, cancer, and strokes result in a higher death rate. Trauma is the leading cause of death for persons less than 44 years of age (Beachley, 2002). Motor vehicle crashes are the most common cause of death for ages 1 to 34 years (Beachley, 2002). Nearly half of all traumatic incidents involve the use of alcohol, drugs, or other substance abuse (Centers for Disease Control and Prevention, 2002).

There are significant economic factors to consider as the direct and indirect costs of trauma-related expenses exceed $400 billion annually (American College of Surgeons, 1997). Nearly 9 million Americans sustain injuries that result in a disability (American College of Surgeons, 1997). Trauma is responsible for the loss of significant productive work years as it is predominantly a disease of the young and carries the potential for permanent disability. Unlike cardiovascular disease, cancer, and strokes, trauma is thought to be preventable. Advocates of organized trauma systems identify prevention as an essential component of a structured approach to trauma.

Systems Approach to Trauma Care

TRAUMA SYSTEM

A model trauma system is defined as an organized approach to trauma care that includes components of prevention, access, acute hospital care, rehabilitation, and research activities (American College of Surgeons, 1997). Regional and state trauma systems provide comprehensive processes to deliver optimal care using priorities, trauma teams, appropriate resources, and an organized plan. This type of a process is required for the delivery of quality care to

evolve *Be sure to check out the bonus material, including free self-assessment exercises, on the Evolve Web site at http://evolve.elsevier.com/Sole/ and on the CD-ROM.*

trauma patients when one considers the trimodal distribution of death that trauma victims confront.

The trimodal distribution of death caused by injury was first described in 1982 (American College of Surgeons, 1997). Death caused by injury occurs in one of three time periods. The first peak of death occurs within seconds to minutes from the time of injury. Death is caused by severe injuries, such as lacerations of the brain, brainstem, high spinal cord, heart, aorta, and large blood vessels. The second peak occurs within minutes to several hours after injury. Death is the result of subdural and epidural hematomas, hemopneumothorax, ruptured spleen, liver lacerations, pelvic fractures, and/or other multiple injuries associated with significant blood loss. This first hour of care focuses on rapid assessment, resuscitation, and treatment of life-threatening injuries. The third peak occurs several days to weeks after the initial injury and is most often the result of sepsis and multiple organ failure. Patient outcomes at this stage are affected by the care provided previously. This trimodal distribution of death supports the concept of an organized trauma system to prioritize and allocate proper resources and personnel, as well as to determine the most appropriate facility to manage the trauma patient.

Levels of Trauma Care

Formal categorization of trauma care facilities is essential for the development, implementation, and improvement of systems to provide optimal care of the injured patient. The goal of every system is to match the needs of injured patients to the capabilities of the trauma facility. The American College of Surgeons Committee on Trauma devised a system to identify a trauma center's expected level of care based on categorization as level I, II, III, or IV (American College of Surgeons, 1998). Level I facilities are the most sophisticated and care for the patient in every aspect from prevention and acute care to rehabilitation. Level II and III centers are similar in that prompt assessment, resuscitation, emergency operations, and stabilization may be provided to the trauma patient. Differences exist between a level II and a level III facility in the type of care provided. A level II center may care for complex patients yet may transport patients to a level I facility if advanced and extended surgical care is required. Level III facilities are often in communities where no level I or II facilities exist. Level IV facilities provide advanced trauma life support and prepare for immediate transport. The level I through IV designations are important in determining the facilities needed in each state (American College of Surgeons, 1998). All states with an identified trauma system are divided into regions. Each region has an identified lead trauma hospital. The lead

hospital is usually the level I trauma center (American College of Surgeons, 1998).

Trauma Team Concept

The term *trauma team,* similar to a code team, refers to health care professionals who respond immediately to and participate in the initial resuscitation and stabilization of the trauma victim. Box 18-1 lists the composition of a typical trauma team. Essential to the team approach is that each team member is preassigned and understands the specific responsibilities inherent in a particular team role. The trauma surgeon is ultimately responsible for the activities of the trauma team and acts as the team leader in establishing resuscitation, stabilization, and intervention priorities. Other team members, such as emergency room physicians, consulting physicians (e.g., orthopedic surgeons, neurosurgeons, otolaryngologists, thoracic surgeons, ophthalmologists, plastic surgeons), nurses, social workers, respiratory therapists, and interventional radiologists have specific responsibilities and may receive additional direction from the trauma surgeon. Each member of the trauma team is vital to meeting the needs of a multitraumatized patient.

Trauma Triage

Triage of an injured patient to the appropriate care facility with the necessary personnel is an essential component and is the hallmark of a successful trauma system. Triage means sorting the patients to determine which patients need specialized care for actual or potential injuries. Determining the type of patient

---

BOX 18-1

Multidisciplinary Trauma Team

- Trauma surgeon (team leader)
- Emergency physician
- Anesthesiologist
- Trauma nurse team leader (coordinates and directs nursing care)
- Trauma resuscitation nurse (hangs fluids, blood, and medications; assists physicians)
- Trauma scribe (records all interventions on the trauma flowsheet)
- Laboratory phlebotomist
- Radiological technologist
- Respiratory therapist
- Social worker/pastoral services
- Hospital security officer
- Physician specialists (neurosurgeon, orthopedic surgeon, urological surgeon)

who requires transport to a trauma center rather than a basic emergency care facility occurs according to established protocols, policies, and procedures. Triage decisions are often made by prehospital personnel based on knowledge of the mechanisms of injury and rapid assessment of the patient's clinical status. Medical direction of this process occurs through voice communication and medical review of triage decisions.

Trauma injury resulting from an external force may be accidental, self-inflicted, or the result of an act of violence. Trauma may be classified as major or minor depending on the severity of injury. Minor trauma refers to a single-system injury that does not pose a threat to life or limb and can be appropriately treated in a basic emergency facility. Major trauma refers to serious multiple system injuries that require immediate intervention to prevent disability, loss of limb, or death. The development of and adherence to established triage criteria are essential for maintaining an effective system of optimal care for the trauma patient. Triage decisions may be based on abnormal findings in the patient's physiological functions, the severity of the mechanism of injury, the anatomical area of injury, or evidence of risk factors such as age and preexisting disease. Identified triage criteria, such as a systolic blood pressure of less than 90 mm Hg in an adult trauma patient, are considered absolute and should always result in transport to a trauma care facility. Other criteria, such as passenger space intrusion and a 30-inch deformity of an automobile, may be guidelines to consider triage to a trauma center. Prehospital personnel may elect to transport the patient to a trauma center in the absence of accepted triage criteria. This is most often based on visualization of the trauma incident and the patient's actual clinical condition.

Mechanisms of Injury

Injury and death result from both unintentional (vehicle collisions and sports activities) and deliberate (violent aggression and suicide) events. Questions regarding mechanisms of injury are directed to the patient (if applicable), prehospital care providers, enforcement personnel, or bystanders in an attempt to reenact the scene of the trauma. Obtaining information on the mechanism of injury is vital to the initial assessment and may raise suspicions about the patient's injury pattern. For example, injuries such as anterior flail chest, blunt cardiac injury, pneumothorax, or femur fracture should be considered in a patient involved in a frontal impact automobile collision.

Injuries, such as those previously described, occur when an uncontrolled source of energy comes into contact with the body. Energy may be kinetic (mechanical), thermal, chemical, electrical, or from radiation. Incidents involving kinetic energy (crashes, falls, and gunshot wounds) account for the majority of injury-related deaths and nonfatal injuries. Kinetic energy is defined as mass times velocity squared, divided by 2. Therefore, the greater the mass and velocity (speed), the more significant is the displacement of kinetic energy to the body structures, resulting in severe injury. The effects of the energy released and the resultant injury depend on the force of impact, the duration of impact, the body part involved, the injuring agent, and the presence of associated risk factors. The personal and environmental risk factors include patient age, sex, race, income, alcohol or substance abuse, geography, and temporal variation. Temporal variation describes the pattern and timing of trauma. For example, injury deaths occur most frequently on weekends, unintentional injuries occur during recreational activities, and suicides occur more frequently on Mondays (Weigelt & Klein, 2002). Injury may also occur when patients are deficient in oxygen, with resulting drowning or suffocation, or in the presence of a lack of heat leading to frostbite.

It is also important to determine whether the mechanism of traumatic injury was blunt or penetrating. The incidence of blunt trauma is usually greater in rural and suburban areas, whereas penetrating trauma occurs more frequently in inner-city urban neighborhoods.

BLUNT TRAUMA

Blunt trauma most often results from motor vehicle accidents, but it may also occur from assaults with blunt objects, falls from heights, and sports-related activities. The severity of injury depends on the amount of kinetic energy dissipated to the body and its underlying structures. Blunt trauma may be caused by accelerating, decelerating, shearing, crushing, and compressing forces. Vehicular trauma often results from a mechanism of acceleration-deceleration forces. The vehicle and the body accelerate and travel at an identified speed. In normal circumstances, the vehicle and body slow to a motionless state in a timely manner. However, when the vehicle stops abruptly, as in a collision, the body continues to travel forward until it comes into contact with a stationary object such as the dashboard, windshield, or steering column. Bodily injury occurs in the presence of rapid deceleration, when the movement ceases and contents within the body continue to travel within an enclosed space or compartment. An example of this occurs when the patient's head strikes the windshield after impalement of the automobile into a cement barrier. The brain tissue strikes the cranium and is thrown back against the opposite side of the cranial vault, with a resulting coup-contrecoup injury. In addition to the shearing forces of the cerebral tissue over the skull, vessels may undergo stretching exceeding the vessel elasticity that results in tears, dissection, or rupture.

Body tissues and structures respond to kinetic energy in different ways. Low-density porous tissues and structures, such as the lungs, tolerate energy transference and often experience little damage because of their elasticity. Conversely, organs such as the heart, spleen, and liver, are less resilient because of the high-density tissue and the decreased ability to release energy without resultant tissue damage. These types of organs often present with fragmentation or rupture. The severity of injury resulting from a blunt force is contingent on the duration of energy exposure, the body part involved, and the underlying structures.

Blunt trauma requires expert clinical judgment to assess and diagnose actual and potential injury. An awareness of the mechanism of injury is vital in the care of the patient who has undergone blunt trauma because minimal external signs on the body are often visible to alert the practitioner to a serious problem.

PENETRATING TRAUMA

Penetrating trauma results from the impalement of foreign objects (knives or bullets) into the body. Penetrating injuries may be more easily diagnosed and treated because of the obvious signs of injury.

Stab wounds are low-velocity injuries because the velocity is equal only to the speed with which the object is thrust into the body. The direct path of injury occurs when the impaled object comes into contact with underlying vessels and tissues. Important considerations in stabbings are the length and width of the impaling object and the presence of vital organs in the area of the stab wound. Gender differences are seen and may provide information on the trajectory of the injury. Women tend to stab with a downward thrust, whereas an upward force is used by male assailants.

Ballistic trauma may consist of either low- or high-velocity injuries. Low-velocity weapons deliver bullets at approximately 1000 feet per second and include weapons such as the 0.22-caliber pistol. Missile speeds of approximately 3000 feet per second are considered high-velocity injuries and may be caused by 0.45-caliber semiautomatic weapons (Weigelt & Klein, 2002). High-velocity injuries result in greater dissipation of the kinetic energy and more significant bodily injury. A high-velocity missile creates a cavity as tissues and vessels are stretched and compressed, known as a cavitation. Depending on the range, the distance from the weapon to the point of impact, and the velocity of the missile, the cavitation may be as great as 30 times the diameter of the bullet. These wounds are often more extensive and require tissue debridement. A second issue to consider in high velocity tissue destruction is the degree of bullet yaw or tumbling. The greater the yaw is, the more significant is the kinetic energy lost to the tissue, and more significant tissue damage will result.

Missiles or bullets that come into contact with internal structures that produce a change in pathway release more energy and result in more damage than missiles passing through the body in a direct path. Bullet design is important in determining the injuring capability of a gunshot wound. Solid-point bullets remain intact limiting tissue damage, whereas hollow-point bullets tend to break apart or fragment, resulting in more severe tissue injury.

Missile injuries must be monitored closely for subsequent complications. As a bullet enters the body and travels to its point of impact, it may pass through clothing, glass, wood, or other objects. These foreign objects are often carried into the body and cause additional injury and/or infection.

Prehospital Care and Transport

Reduced morbidity and mortality can be achieved with rapid assessment in the field by prehospital personnel and immediate transport of the trauma victim to an appropriate care facility. Once prehospital personnel arrive at the scene of a traumatic incident, they direct the situation and prepare the patient for transport. The time from injury to definitive care is a determinant of survival in many critically injured patients, particularly those with major internal hemorrhage (American College of Surgeons, 1998). Treatment of life-threatening problems are provided at the scene, with careful attention given to the airway with cervical spine immobilization, breathing, and circulation (ABCs). Interventions to be considered include establishing an airway, immobilizing the complete spine, providing ventilation, controlling hemorrhage, and stabilizing fractures (American College of Surgeons, 1998). The current process of spinal immobilization is being challenged and reexamined. These issues include the necessity of spinal immobilization in all trauma patients, the appropriateness of prehospital care providers to assess for spine abnormalities, and the concern with the number of false-positive results that occur with prolonged spine immobilization (Cornwell et al., 2001; Hauswald, 2002; March, 2002). Although these debates continue, current guidelines support complete spinal immobilization in trauma patients with protocols to direct the use of diagnostic studies for spinal clearance (Anderson et al., 1999; Anonymous, 2002; Eastern Association for the Surgery of Trauma, 2000). Additional lifesaving prehospital interventions that may be initiated, depending on protocols, include occlusive dressings on open chest wounds, needle thoracotomy to relieve tension pneumothorax, endotracheal intubation, or cricothyrotomy.

Traditional prehospital management includes large-bore venous access and administration of crystalloid solution to restore blood volume and to maintain systemic arterial blood pressure. However, research has illustrated increased mortality rates if intravenous fluids are provided before hemorrhage is controlled, especially in victims of penetrating trauma (Fowler & Pepe, 2002). Therefore, transport is not delayed to initiate intravenous access.

Ground or air transport is appropriate for the trauma patient from the scene of the injury to the trauma center. Considerations in the choice of transport include travel time, terrain, availability of air and ground units, capabilities of transport personnel, and weather conditions. Once the decision is made to transport a patient to a trauma center, the trauma team is notified. In most trauma centers, the initial resuscitation and stabilization of the trauma patient occur in a designated resuscitation area, usually within the emergency department. Optimally, the trauma team responds before the patient's arrival and begins preparations based on the report of the patient's injuries and clinical status. Trauma patients in unstable condition may be admitted directly to the operating room for resuscitation and immediate surgical intervention.

Emergency Care Phase

PREPARATION FOR PATIENT ADMISSION

Data obtained during the prehospital phase provide essential information to ensure a coordinated, lifesaving approach to the care of the trauma patient. Most traumatic events are considered "scoop and run" situations with short transport times, but other patients may come to the hospital by private car. For these reasons, the resuscitation area must always be in a state of readiness for the next trauma patient. Equipment needed for management of the airway with cervical spine immobilization, breathing, circulatory support, and hemorrhage control must be immediately available and easily accessible. Delays in implementing definitive critical interventions adversely affect patient outcomes. The latest standards require that surgeons be present when the trauma patient arrives, during

the operation, and during critical care interventions. This continuum of early surgical involvement has resulted in improved outcomes (American College of Surgeons, 1998, Orlinsky, Shoemaker, Reis, & Kerstein, 2001).

INITIAL PATIENT ASSESSMENT

Patient survival after a serious traumatic event depends on prompt, rapid, and systematic assessment in conjunction with immediate resuscitative interventions. Priorities of care are based on the patient's clinical presentation, physical assessment, history of the traumatic event, and preexisting disease. Patients' preexisting illnesses can predict outcome (Ferrera, Bartfield, & D'Andrea, 2000; Grossman, 2002). Evaluation of airway patency, ventilation, and venous access with circulatory support are of prime importance and take precedence over other diagnostic or definitive interventions. Adherence to established protocols for patient assessment and intervention is essential to ensure that management priorities are addressed in an appropriate manner.

PRIMARY SURVEY

The primary survey is the most crucial assessment tool in trauma care. This rapid, 1- to 2-minute evaluation is designed to identify life-threatening injuries accurately, establish priorities, and provide simultaneous therapeutic interventions. The primary survey is a systematic survey of the patient's airway with cervical spine immobilization, breathing and ventilation, circulation with hemorrhage control, and disability or neurological status (ABCDs) (American College of Surgeons, 1998; Emergency Nurses Association, 2000). Table 18-1 details the critical assessment parameters included in the primary survey. All major life-threatening conditions must be treated before one proceeds with the secondary survey.

Resuscitation Phase

SECONDARY SURVEY

The secondary survey is initiated after the primary survey has been accomplished and all the actual or potential life-threatening injuries have been identified and addressed. Temperature, heart rate, respiratory effort, and auscultated blood pressure are obtained as a baseline for analysis of trends during the resuscitation phase.

The secondary survey is a methodical head-to-toe evaluation of the patient using the assessment techniques of inspection, palpation, percussion, and auscultation to identify all injuries. A mnemonic *(E through I)* may be used to remember the features

TABLE 18-1

Primary Survey

Assessment		Observations Indicating Impaired ABCs
A = Airway	Open and patent Maintain cervical spine immobilization	Shallow, noisy breathing Stridor Cyanosis Nasal flaring Accessory muscle use Inability to speak Drooling Anxiety Decreased level of consciousness Trauma to face, mouth, neck Debris or foreign matter in mouth or pharynx
B = Breathing	Presence and effectiveness Presence of external haemorrhage	Asymmetrical rise and fall of chest Absent, decreased, or unequal breath sounds Open sucking chest wounds Blunt chest injury Dyspnea Cyanosis Respiratory rate <8 to 10/min or >40/min Accessory muscle use Anxiety Tracheal shift Distended neck veins Paradoxical chest wall motion
C = Circulation	Presence of major pulses	Weak, thready pulse >120 beats/min Pallor Blood pressure <90 mm Hg Capillary refill >2 sec Obvious external hemorrhage Decreased level of consciousness Distended neck veins
D = Disability	Gross neurological status Pupil size, equality, and reactivity to light	Glasgow Coma Scale score ≤11 Agitation

of the secondary assessment (Emergency Nurses Association, 2000). *Exposing* the patient and providing environmental control with warmed blankets, intravenous solutions, or overhead radiant warmers to prevent hypothermia are the first or E aspects of the secondary survey. There are three aspects of F. These include *full set of vital signs, five interventions* (cardiac monitor, pulse oximetry, urinary catheter, gastric tube if not contraindicated, laboratory studies), and *facilitating family presence*. G refers to *giving comfort measures* to reassure the patient and to facilitate pain control. *History* and *head-to-toe assessment* are the H considerations. Finally, patients are log rolled to each side and the *posterior side is inspected* (I) for hidden injuries (Table 18-2). Information about actual

and potential injuries is noted and is used to establish diagnostic and treatment priorities. Radiological studies are completed according to a standardized trauma protocol or based on assessment of suspected injuries. The sequence of diagnostic procedures is influenced by the level of consciousness, the stability of the patient's condition, the mechanism of injury, and identified injuries. As data are obtained, the team leader determines the need for consultation with specialty physicians such as neurosurgeons, orthopedists, urologists, or others. Supportive interventions such as splinting of extremities, wound care, and administration of tetanus prophylaxis and antibiotics are done at this time. Finally, the secondary survey provides data that enable the team leader to

TABLE 18-2

Secondary Assessment

Mnemonic*	Actions	Inspection	Palpation	Ausculation
E = Expose Patient/ Environmental Control	Remove patient's clothing Rewarm with blankets, warming lights, fluid-filled or air convection warming blankets	Inspect for soft tissue injury Inspect for deformities Inspect for edema	Palpate bony deformities Palpate for crepitus	
F = Full Set of Vital Signs/Five Interventions/ Facilitate Family Presence	Obtain full set of vital signs (blood pressure, heart rate, respiratory rate, temperature) Insert nasogastric tube, Foley catheter Obtain oxygen saturation via pulse oximetry Connect to cardiac monitor Obtain blood and urine for laboratory studies Identify family, provide updates, and facilitate visitation with patient	Inspect perineal area during insertion of Foley catheter Inspect digits to ensure adequate vascular flow to obtain accurate oxygen saturation	Palpate for radial pulse Palpate for vein to access for blood studies	Auscultate for blood pressure Auscultate placement of nasogastric tube
G = Give Comfort Measures	Provide emotional reassurance Administer narcotics as ordered by trauma surgeon	Inspect patient for relief of pain	Provide touch to facilitate patient comfort and reassurance	
H = History/ Head-to-Toe Assessment	Perform head-to-toe assessment	HEAD/FACE: Inspect for wounds, ecchymosis, deformities, drainage, pupillary reaction NECK: Inspect for wounds, ecchymosis, deformities, distended neck veins CHEST: Inspect for breathing rate and depth, wounds, deformities, ecchymosis, use of accessory muscles, paradoxical movement	HEAD/FACE: Palpate for tenderness, crepitus, deformities NECK: Palpate for tenderness, crepitus, deformity, tracheal position CHEST: Palpate for tenderness, crepitus, subcutaneous emphysema, deformities	CHEST: Auscultate breath and heart sounds ABDOMEN: Auscultate bowel sounds in all four quadrants

Continued

TABLE 18-2

Secondary Assessment—cont'd

Mnemonic*	Actions	Inspection	Palpation	Auscultation
		ABDOMEN: Inspect for wounds, distention, ecchymosis, scars PELVIS/PERINEUM: Inspect for wounds, deformities, ecchymosis, priapism, blood at the urinary meatus or in the perineal area EXTREMITIES: Inspect for ecchymosis, movement, wounds, deformities	ABDOMEN: Palpate all four quadrants for tenderness, rigidity, guarding, masses, femoral pulses PELVIS/PERINEUM: Palpate the pelvis and anal sphincter tone EXTREMITIES: Palpate for pulses, skin temperature, sensation, tenderness, deformities, crepitus	
I = Inspect Posterior Surfaces	Maintain cervical spine stabilization Log roll using three hospital personnel	Inspect posterior surfaces for wounds, deformities, and ecchymosis	Palpate posterior surfaces for deformities and pain Assist the physician with the rectal examination, if not previously completed	

*Mnemonic from Emergency Nurses Association. (2000). *Trauma nursing core course: Provider manual.* 5th ed. Des Plaines, IL: Emergency Nurses Association.

establish priorities for definitive care and ongoing management of the trauma patient.

MAINTAIN AIRWAY PATENCY

Maintaining a patent airway and adequate ventilation is an essential element of trauma management. Every trauma patient has the potential for airway obstruction, whether it occurs at the time of injury or develops during resuscitation. The tongue, because of posterior displacement, is the most common cause of airway obstruction. Other causes of obstruction are foreign debris (blood or vomitus) or secretions resulting from maxillofacial fractures. Direct injuries to the throat or neck can structurally impair the airway in patients with a depressed sensorium or absent gag reflex.

Opening the airway is easily accomplished by the simple manual technique of a jaw thrust or chin lift. These maneuvers do not hyperextend the neck or compromise the integrity of the cervical spine. These are temporary interventions that serve to move the mandible anteriorly and create a patent airway. The airway must be cleared of any foreign material such as blood, vomitus, bone fragments, or teeth by a finger sweep or gentle suction with a tonsillar tip catheter.

Nasopharyngeal and oropharyngeal airways are the simplest artificial airway adjuncts used in patients with spontaneous respirations and adequate ventilatory effort. Both devices help to maintain a patent airway by preventing posterior displacement of the tongue. Responsive patients are best served with the nasopharyngeal airway. The oropharyneal airway is not used in the conscious patient because it may induce gagging, vomiting, and aspiration.

Endotracheal intubation is the definitive nonsurgical airway management technique and allows for complete control of the airway. Both the oral and nasal routes may be used for intubation. Nasotracheal intubation is indicated for the spontaneously breathing patient and is contraindicated for patients with facial, frontal sinus, basilar skull, or cribriform plate fractures (American College of Surgeons, 1997). It is used when the urgency of the resuscitation procedure does not allow time to obtain preliminary cervical spine x-ray studies. Disadvantages of nasal intubation are epistaxis, injury to the nasal turbinates, and introduction of infection. In the presence of documented or suspected cervical spine injury, oral tracheal intubation must be performed carefully to prevent manipulation of the neck. Manual immobilization of the neck must be provided by an assistant. Disadvantages of oral tracheal intubation include possible manipulation of the cervical spine, incorrect tube placement in the esophagus or right mainstem bronchus, vocal cord trauma, and injury to the intraoral structures.

Before intubation, patients are preoxygenated with 100% oxygen via a bag-valve mask. Experienced practitioners may choose to use rapid sequence intubation in which there is sequential administration of a sedative or anesthetic and a neuromuscular blocking agent to facilitate the procedure. Correct position of the tube is verified by auscultation of bilateral breath sounds, chest x-ray study, and use of an end-tidal carbon dioxide detector. If carbon dioxide is detected in exhaled air, the tube is in the airway. Mechanical ventilation with 100% oxygen is initiated immediately after intubation.

Inability to intubate the trauma patient is an indication for surgical intervention (cricothyrotomy) to control the airway. Conditions that may require cricothyrotomy are maxillofacial trauma, laryngeal fractures, facial or upper airway burns, and severe oropharyngeal hemorrhage. The adult cricothyroid membrane is located inferior to the thyroid cartilage and superior to the cricoid cartilage (Figure 18-1). The anatomical position of the avascular cricoid membrane makes this a relatively bloodless, safe, and rapid procedure. Access to the trachea through the cricothyroid membrane can be accomplished by either needle cricothyrotomy or surgical cricothyrotomy.

The choice of airway management technique is based on familiarity with the procedures, the clinical condition of the patient, and the degree of hemodynamic stability. The nurse has an important responsibility in assessing and maintaining a patent airway. A patent airway is the cornerstone of successful trauma resuscitation.

INEFFECTIVE BREATHING PATTERNS

Interventions to restore normal breathing patterns are directed toward the specific injury or underlying

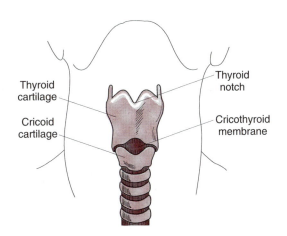

FIGURE 18-1 Location of the cricothyroid membrane.

cause of respiratory distress, with the goal of improving ventilation and gas exchange. Basic nursing interventions include application of supplemental oxygen with ventilatory assistance (if applicable), preparation for intubation, and evaluation of specific interventions. Ineffective breathing patterns are the result of certain traumatic injuries. These injuries and specific interventions are listed in Table 18-3.

The nurse monitors the patient frequently to assess respiratory rate and effort, heart rate rhythm, breath sounds, skin color, temperature, tracheal position, and neck vein distention. When spontaneous breathing is present but ineffective, a life-threatening condition must be considered if any of the following are present: altered mental status (agitation), cyanosis (nail beds and mucous membranes), asymmetrical expansion of the chest wall, use of accessory and/or abdominal muscles, sucking chest wounds, paradoxical movement of the chest wall during the inspiration and expiration, tracheal shift from midline position, distended jugular veins, or diminished/absent breath sounds. Arterial blood gases and diagnostic studies, including chest x-ray and chest computed tomography (CT) imaging, may be completed to assist in determining the effectiveness of specific interventions.

IMPAIRED GAS EXCHANGE

Impaired gas exchange follows airway obstruction as the most crucial problem of the trauma patient. Causes of impaired gas exchange include a decrease in inspired air, retained secretions, lung collapse or compression, atelectasis, or accumulation of blood in the thoracic cavity. Any patient presenting with multiple systemic injuries, hemorrhagic shock, chest trauma, and/or central nervous system trauma must be assessed for the potential for impaired gas exchange. These conditions have the potential to affect the patient's volume status and oxygen-carrying capacity, to

---

TABLE 18-3

Specific Interventions for Ineffective Breathing Patterns

Etiology	Interventions
Tension pneumothorax	Prepare for decompression by needle thoracostomy with a 14-gauge needle in second intercostal space in midclavicular line on affected side. Prepare for chest tube insertion.
Pneumothorax	Prepare for chest tube insertion on affected side.
Open sucking wound	Seal the wound with an occlusive dressing and tape on three sides. Prepare for chest tube insertion.
Massive hemothorax	Establish two 14-gauge to 16-gauge IV lines for crystalloid infusion. Obtain blood for type and crossmatch. Prepare for chest tube insertion. Prepare the autotransfusion device. Administer blood or blood products as ordered. Anticipate and prepare for emergency open thoracotomy.
Pulmonary contusion	Prepare for early intubation and mechanical ventilation. Administer IV crystalloids at a rate guided by the absence of signs of shock.
Flail chest	Prepare for early intubation and mechanical ventilation. Administer IV crystalloids at a rate guided by the absence of signs of shock. Administer analgesics as ordered.
Spinal cord injury	Avoid hyperextension or rotation of the patient's neck. Maintain complete spinal immobilization. Prepare for application of cervical traction tongs or a halo device. Monitor motor and sensory function. Monitor for signs of neurogenic shock.
Decreased level of consciousness	Position the patient's head midline with the head of the bed elevated. Anticipate a computed tomography scan. Administer osmotic diuretics. Prepare for intubation and mechanical ventilation.

interfere with the mechanics of ventilation, or to interrupt the autonomic control of respirations. Immediate intervention is required to prevent these potential adverse effects.

Interventions are directed toward maintaining a patent airway and optimizing gas exchange. In addition to providing the trauma patient with high-flow supplemental oxygen, the nurse monitors the patient's respiratory rate, use of accessory muscles, depth of breathing, oxygen saturation, and need for secretion removal. The nurse must be prepared to assist with intubation and subsequent mechanical ventilation, needle thoracostomy, chest tube insertion, and restoration of circulating blood volume. These interventions will serve to restore the patient to a state of adequate oxygenation and gas exchange.

DECREASED CARDIAC OUTPUT AND HYPOVOLEMIA

The most common cause of impaired cardiac output in the trauma patient is hypovolemic shock resulting from acute blood loss. The causes may be external (hemorrhage) or internal (hemothorax, hemoperitoneum, long bone or massive pelvic fractures). In the presence of significant intraabdominal, pelvic, or lower extremity bleeding, the pneumatic antishock garment (PASG) may be applied as an external pressure device used to control hemorrhage in addition to fluid resuscitation. It also provides splinting and stabilization of pelvic and leg fractures. When inflated, the PASG compresses the legs and abdomen, results in increased venous return and systemic vascular resistance, and thus prevents further blood loss into the abdomen and legs. It may also provide translocation of a small amount (130 to 150 mL) of blood into the central circulation, thereby elevating the systemic arterial blood pressure. This increase in blood pressure may be seen as beneficial. However, blood pressure elevation in the presence of hemorrhage without definitive control may be fatal (Fowler & Pepe, 2002). The use of PASGs remains controversial and is not considered a first-line management strategy. Two additional causes of diminished cardiac output are impairment of venous blood return to the heart secondary to tension pneumothorax and decreased filling and ventricular ejection fraction resulting from pericardial tamponade. Table 18-4 demonstrates the stages of predictability in hemorrhagic shock, as it relates to the patient's presentation to guide in early recognition and management (American College of Surgeons, 1997).

Priority interventions involve ensuring that the patient has a patent airway, maintaining adequate ventilation, and providing adequate gas exchange. Subsequent interventions are directed toward controlling the hemorrhage and replacing circulating blood volume to restore adequate tissue perfusion. Blood loss caused by obvious external hemorrhage is controlled with direct pressure, elevation of an extremity, or compression of pressure points. Tourniquets are avoided to prevent compromise of circulation to the extremity and possible loss of the limb. Internal hemorrhage must be controlled with identification and correction of the underlying problem.

TABLE 18-4

Estimated Fluid and Blood Requirements* (Based on Patient's Initial Presentation)

	Class I	Class II	Class III	Class IV
Blood loss (mL)	Up to 750	750-1500	1500-2000	2000 or more
Blood loss (% blood volume)	Up to 15	15-30	30-40	40 or more
Pulse rate (beats/min)	<100	>100	>120	140 or higher
Blood pressure	Normal	Normal	↓	↓
Pulse pressure	Normal or ↑	↓	↓	↓
Respiratory rate (breaths/min)	14-20	20-30	30-40	>35
Urine output (mL/hr)	30 or more	20-30	5-15	Negligible
Central nervous system: mental status	Slightly anxious	Mildly anxious	Anxious and confused	Confused and lethargic
Fluid replacement (3:1 rule)	Crystalloid	Crystalloid	Crystalloid + blood	Crystalloid + blood

*For a 70-kg male patient.
↑, Increased; ↓, decreased.
Modified from the American College of Surgeons, Committee on Trauma. (1997). *Advanced trauma life support for doctors: Instructor course manual.* Chicago: American College of Surgeons.

Venous access and infusion of volume are the keys to optimal fluid resuscitation in the patient with hemorrhagic shock. At least two large-bore (14-gauge to 16-gauge) peripheral intravenous lines are necessary. The forearm or antecubital veins are preferred sites for peripheral lines. A central venous line or a venous cutdown may be necessary because of vasoconstriction and venous collapse. A central line (single- or multiple-lumen line) is more beneficial as a resuscitation monitoring tool. A pulmonary artery catheter may be inserted in the critical care unit to evaluate the response to fluid resuscitation. As a general rule, venous access is achieved rapidly with the largest-bore catheter possible to initiate early resuscitation.

Isotonic electrolyte solutions are used for initial fluid resuscitation. Ringer's lactate solution is the fluid of choice, followed by normal saline. An initial fluid bolus of 2 L for an adult is given as rapidly as possible. Alterations in the amount of the bolus may be necessary for certain trauma populations, such as the patient with cardiac disease. Large-bore intravenous catheters, short intravenous tubing, and a rapid infuser device are often used to facilitate rapid infusion of warm, intravenous fluids. The American College of Surgeons (1997) recommends replacing each milliliter of blood loss with 3 mL of crystalloid (3:1 rule). The patient's response to the initial fluid administration is monitored using urine output (50 mL per hour in the adult), level of consciousness, heart rate, blood pressure, and capillary refill.

Three response patterns are used to determine further therapeutic and diagnostic decisions. These response patterns to initial fluid administration are rapid, transient, or no response (Table 18-5) (American College of Surgeons, 1997). *Rapid responders* react quickly to the initial bolus and remain hemodynamically stable when the initial fluid bolus has been completed. Fluids are then slowed to maintenance rates. *Transient responders* improve in response to the initial fluid bolus. However, these patients begin to show deterioration in perfusion when fluids are slowed to maintenance rates. This finding indicates ongoing blood loss or inadequate resuscitation. Continued fluid administration and blood transfusion are indicated. If the patient continues to respond in a transient manner, the patient is probably bleeding and requires rapid surgical intervention. *Minimal* or *no responders* fail to respond to crystalloid and blood administration in the emergency department, and surgical intervention is needed immediately to control hemorrhage.

The decision to administer blood is based on the patient's response to initial fluid therapy (American College of Surgeons, 1997). If the patient is unresponsive to intravenous fluid therapy, type-specific blood may be administered. In the event of life-threatening blood loss, the physician may request unmatched, type-specific or type O (universal donor) blood. Crossmatched, type-specific blood should be instituted as soon as it is available. Autotransfusion of shed blood, or autologous blood, is an alternative method of blood replacement that may be used in the patient with hemorrhage caused by hemothorax or other intrathoracic injuries. This inexpensive, safe, and rapid technique involves accumulation of the patient's own blood into an autotransfusion device. The blood is

---

TABLE 18-5

Responses to Initial Fluid Resuscitation*

	Rapid Response	Transient Response	No Response
Vital signs	Return to normal	Transient improvement; recurrence of ↓BP and ↑HR	Remain abnormal
Estimated blood loss	Minimal (10%-20%)	Moderate and ongoing (20%-40%)	Severe (> 40%)
Need for more crystalloid	Low	High	High
Need for blood	Low	Moderate to high	Immediate
Blood preparation	Type and crossmatch	Type-specific	Emergency blood release
Need for operative intervention	Possibly	Likely	Highly likely
Early presence of a surgeon	Yes	Yes	Yes

*2000 mL Ringer's lactate solution in adults, 20 mL/kg Ringer's lactate bolus in children.
↑, Increased; ↓, decreased; *BP,* blood pressure; *HR,* heart rate.
Modified from the American College of Surgeons, Committee on Trauma. (1997). *Advanced trauma life support for doctors: Instructor course manual.* Chicago: American College of Surgeons.

then anticoagulated and filtered and is immediately available for reinfusion. Autotransfusion is an excellent way to provide fresh, warm blood that carries no risk of compatibility problems and eliminates the risk of transmittable infectious diseases.

Determining the cause of bleeding is imperative. Diagnostic testing including chest and pelvis x-ray studies, abdominal ultrasound, and x-ray studies of suspected extremity fractures are commonly completed early in the resuscitative phase to determine injuries and potential sources of bleeding. An abdominal CT scan may be completed to assist in identifying a specific source of intraperitoneal bleeding. However, an abdominal CT scan is not the diagnostic test of choice in the presence of hemodynamic instability. In this case, a quick invasive procedure identified as diagnostic peritoneal lavage may be performed by the surgeon. This procedure involves the insertion of a lavage catheter into the peritoneum with subsequent gentle syringe aspiration. If frank blood is obtained, the patient is prepared for emergency laparotomy. If less than 10 mL of blood is aspirated, 1 L of warmed Ringer's lactate or 0.9% normal saline is infused into the peritoneal cavity. The abdomen is gently agitated to distribute the fluid throughout the peritoneal cavity and is then drained via gravity. A sample of the fluid is then sent for evaluation of red blood cells, white blood cells, amylase, bile, bacteria, fecal material, or food particles to determine the need for immediate operative intervention.

Hypothermia is a universal problem that may occur year round and especially in the presence of cooler atmospheric temperatures, in the presence of a patient's submersion in water, and with rapid infusion of room temperature fluids. It is desirable to warm any fluid to prevent the hazardous effects of cold fluid on the myocardium and coagulation system. Crystalloids may be warmed in a microwave, small warming ovens, or through a fluid-warming rapid infusion device. The ability instantaneously to infuse and simultaneously to warm intravenous fluids makes the rapid infusion devices preferable to other methods.

Patients may present with ongoing signs and symptoms of shock (decreased hemoglobin or hematocrit, deteriorating arterial oxygen tension [PaO_2] and pH, rising base deficits, diminished urine output [less than 0.5 mL/kg per hour in the adult], and increasing arterial lactate levels) despite resuscitation measures. These signs and symptoms are indicative that a more aggressive approach to resuscitation is required. Initial hemoglobin and hematocrit values may require up to 4 hours to reequilibrate and therefore may be unreliable in gauging the degree of shock. Ongoing metabolic acidosis indicates inadequate

tissue perfusion and anaerobic metabolism. Anaerobic metabolism is a very inefficient process for adenosine triphosphate production and subsequent cellular metabolism. It is imperative that this cycle be interrupted to prevent cellular dysfunction, swelling, rupture, and death.

MASSIVE FLUID RESUSCITATION

Massive fluid resuscitation is defined as the administration of greater than 10 units of packed red blood cells given over 24 hours or the replacement of a patient's total blood volume in less than 24 hours, and it is associated with poor patient outcomes (Drummond & Petrovitch, 2001). The purpose of massive fluid resuscitation after traumatic injury is to rapidly restore oxygen transport to the body tissues, stop the progression of shock, and prevent complications. Potential complications of massive fluid resuscitation include acid-base changes, electrolyte imbalances, hypothermia, dilutional coagulopathy, volume overload, systemic inflammatory response syndrome (SIRS), acute respiratory distress syndrome (ARDS), and multiple organ dysfunction syndrome (MODS).

Metabolic acidosis is the result of hypovolemia and hypoxemia, which lead to a change in cellular metabolism. In this setting, oxygen debt occurs, causing a shift from aerobic to anaerobic metabolism resulting in excessive production of lactic acid. Reversal of this process must occur to prevent cellular destruction and death. Electrolyte imbalances that may develop during massive fluid resuscitation include hypocalcemia, hypomagnesemia, and hyperkalemia. These imbalances may lead to changes in myocardial function, laryngeal spasm, and neuromuscular and central nervous system hyperirritability (Tierney, McPhee, & Papadakis, 2002).

As changes in cellular metabolism occur and patients are aggressively fluid resuscitated, vessels become more permeable to fluid and molecules. This change leads to the movement of fluid from the intravascular space into the interstitial spaces (third spacing). Patients become intravascularly hypovolemic and require a larger volume of fluid replacement. Another contributing factor to the development of hypovolemia is dilutional coagulopathy. Massive transfusions of fluid and blood produce dilutional thrombocytopenia and a reduction in fibrinogen, factor V, factor VIII, and other clotting components. High levels of citrate in banked blood may induce transient hypocalcemia. Decreased calcium may lead to an ineffective coagulation system because it is a necessary cofactor in the coagulation cascade. Further inhibition of the clotting cascade is observed when platelet dysfunction develops secondary to hypothermia or metabolic acidosis. Management focuses on improving perfusion to the body tissues, increasing the patient's body temperature, and administering clotting factors (fresh frozen plasma, cryoprecipitate, and platelets). Monitoring of hemoglobin, hematocrit, fibrinogen, platelet count, prothrombin time, and partial thromboplastin time is essential. These changes in the coagulation cascade incite the inflammatory process with release of a multitude of inflammatory mediators. These inflammatory mediators are initially helpful, but over time they become devastating to the healing process. The end result is the early (within hours of injury) or late (within days to weeks after injury) development of SIRS, ARDS, and MODS (Mattox, Brundage, & Hirshberg, 1999).

Hypothermia, defined as a core body temperature less than 35°C, is caused by a combination of accelerated heat loss and decreased heat production. A person is more susceptible to hypothermia after severe injury, geriatric trauma, excessive blood loss, alcohol or sedative use, and massive transfusions (Biem, Koehncke, & Dosman, 2003). Body temperature continues to fall after clothing removal, exposure to wet, bloody linens, and surgical exposure of body cavities during the patient's initial assessment. Prolonged exposure to hypothermia is associated with the development of myocardial dysfunction, coagulopathies, reduced perfusion, and dysrhythmias (bradycardia and atrial or ventricular fibrillation), as well as impaired citrate, lactate, and drug metabolism. Implementation of rewarming strategies is imperative to prevent the triad of hypothermia, coagulopathy, and acidosis. Suggested techniques for rewarming are listed in Table 18-6.

Assessment and Management of Specific Organ Injuries

CHEST INJURIES

Tension Pneumothorax

Tension pneumothorax is a rapidly fatal emergency that is easily resolved with early recognition and intervention. It occurs when an injury to the chest allows air to enter the pleural cavity without a route for escape. With each inspiration, additional air accumulates in the pleural space, thus increasing intrathoracic pressure that leads to lung collapse. The increased pressure then causes compression of the heart and great vessels toward the unaffected side, as evidenced by mediastinal shift and distended neck veins. The resulting decreased cardiac output and alterations in gas exchange are manifested by severe respiratory distress, chest pain, hypotension, tachycardia, absence of breath sounds on the affected side, and tracheal deviation. Cyanosis is a late manifestation of this

TABLE 18-6	
Rewarming Strategies	
Type	**Interventions**
Passive external	Removal of wet clothing
	Warm room
	Decrease airflow over patient
	Blanklets
	Head coverings
Active external	Radiant lights
	Fluid-filled warming blankets
	Convection air blankets
Active internal	Warmed gases to respiratory tract
	Warmed intravenous fluids, including blood
	Body cavity irrigation (peritoneal, mediastinal, pleural, gastric)
	Continuous arteriovenous rewarming
	Cardiopulmonary bypass

life-threatening clinical situation. Diagnosis of tension pneumothorax is based on the patient's clinical presentation. Treatment is never delayed to confirm presence with a chest x-ray study. After recognition of tension pneumothorax, immediate decompression of the intrathoracic pressure is accomplished by needle thoracostomy. A 14-gauge needle is inserted in the second intercostal space in the midclavicular line on the injured side. This procedure converts a tension pneumothorax to a simple pneumothorax. Subsequent definitive treatment will be required with placement of a chest tube.

Hemothorax

Hemothorax is a collection of blood in the pleural space resulting from injuries to the heart, great vessels, or the pulmonary parenchyma. Bleeding can be moderate (from intercostal vessels) or massive (from the aorta or from subclavian or pulmonary vessels). Decreased breath sounds, dullness to percussion on the affected side, hypotension, and respiratory distress may be seen. Placement of a chest tube facilitates removal of blood from the pleural space with resolution of ventilation and gas exchange abnormalities.

Open Pneumothorax

Open pneumothorax results from penetrating trauma that allows air to pass in and out of the pleural space. The normal pressure gradient between the atmosphere and intrathoracic space no longer exists. Patients present with hypoxia and hemodynamic instability. Management of the open wound is accomplished with a three-sided occlusive dressing. The fourth side is left open to allow for exhalation of air within the pleural cavity. If the dressing becomes completely occlusive on all sides, tension pneumothorax may occur. A chest tube is inserted on the affected side, and a chest x-ray study is obtained to determine proper placement and to determine if there is resolution of the pneumothorax.

Cardiac Tamponade

Cardiac tamponade is a life-threatening condition caused by rapid accumulation of fluid (usually blood) in the pericardial sac. As the intrapericardial pressure increases, cardiac output is impaired because of decreased venous return. The development of pulsus paradoxus may occur with a decrease in systolic blood pressure during spontaneous inspiration. Blood, if unable to flow into the right side of the heart, causes increased right atrial pressure and distended neck veins. Classic signs of this injury are hypotension, muffled or distant heart sounds, and elevated venous pressure (Beck's triad). Beck's triad may not be present until the patient is hypotensive and hypovolemic.

Cardiac tamponade is generally caused by penetrating trauma to the chest. However, it should also be suspected in any patient with blunt trauma to the chest and multisystemic injuries who presents in shock without a response to aggressive fluid resuscitation. Pericardial tamponade is often difficult to diagnose in the presence of other injuries that may also contribute to the source of decreased cardiac output. Cardiac tamponade is diagnosed using the focused abdominal sonography for trauma (FAST) or pericardiocentesis. The pericardiocentesis may also provide therapeutic intervention by decompressing the pericardium. Needle aspiration of the pericardial sac is done with a 16- to 18-gauge over-the-needle catheter attached to a 35-mL syringe with a three-way stopcock. Aspirated pericardial blood usually will not clot unless the heart itself has been penetrated. Arterial blood pressure may dramatically improve with removal of as little as 15 to 20 mL of blood. Nurses should anticipate and obtain equipment for an emergency thoracotomy in the event of cardiac arrest. After the pericardocentesis, immediate operative intervention is required for definitive repair. Trauma surgeons are currently debating the effectiveness of pericardiocentesis. Some believe that pericardiocentesis should be abandoned and the surgeon should proceed with immediate operative repair.

Pulmonary Contusion

Pulmonary contusion occurs as a result of blunt or penetrating trauma to the chest. It is one of the most common causes of death after chest trauma, and it predisposes the patient to pneumonia or ARDS.

It can be difficult to detect because the initial chest x-ray study may be normal. The appearance of infiltrates on chest x-ray films and hypoxemia may not be present until hours or days after injury. Rib fractures and flail chest are often associated with a pulmonary contusion. The clinical presentation of this condition includes chest wall abrasions, ecchymosis, bloody secretions, and a PaO_2 less than 60 mm Hg on room air. The bruised lung tissue becomes edematous, resulting in hypoxia and respiratory distress. Ventilatory support is needed to promote healing of the lung with careful administration of fluid to avoid further lung edema. Adequate pain relief, with intravenous narcotics or epidural infusion, is essential to optimize lung expansion and respiratory effort and to prevent the complications.

Rib Fractures

Rib fractures are the most common injury after chest trauma. Rib fractures may lead to significant respiratory dysfunction and indicate a serious underlying injury. The diagnosis of rib fractures is frequently made following a chest x-ray study. However, there are situations in which rib fractures are not visualized on chest x-ray films, and the diagnosis is made through clinical assessment. A high-impact force is needed to fracture the short, thick first and second ribs. Patients with fractures of these ribs require careful assessment for hemodynamic instability, which may indicate in the presence of major vessel injury, such as aortic disruption or injury to the subclavian artery. Injury to the liver, spleen, or kidney may accompany fractures of ribs 10 through 12.

The management of rib fractures is dependent on the number of ribs fractured, the degree of underlying injury, and the age of the patient. A young, healthy patient with a single rib fracture may be treated in an outpatient setting. It is important to educate the patient on proper pain control, pillow splinting, and ambulation and on not to restrict the chest movement with restraining devices, such as a corset or elastic (Ace) bandages. An elderly patient with multiple rib fractures usually requires hospital admission, cardiac monitoring, and/or respiratory support. Treatment focuses on adequate ventilation and gas exchange, ambulation, secretion removal, and pain relief. Systemic narcotics (fentanyl [Sublimaze], morphine), nonsteroidal antiinflammatory agents (ibuprofen, ketorolac [Toradol]), epidural catheters, and intercostal nerve blocks are options for reducing pain and for promoting positive patient outcomes.

Flail Chest

A flail chest is produced when three or more adjacent ribs fracture in more than one location. Blunt forces are the most common cause of injury. For example, the chest wall strikes the steering wheel or dashboard. The flail segment "floats" freely and results in paradoxical chest movement. The flail segment contracts inward with inhalation and expands outward with exhalation. The uncoordinated chest movement, underlying chest injury, and associated pain contribute to impaired ventilation and subsequent hypoxemia. Treatment includes nonoperative management with intubation and mechanical ventilation, frequent pulmonary care, and aggressive pain management including the use of an epidural catheter.

Aortic Disruption

Aortic disruption is produced by blunt trauma to the chest. Rapid deceleration forces produced by a head-on motor vehicle crash, ejection, or falls can dissect the aorta in four common sites. These sites are just distal to the left subclavian artery at the level of the ligamentum arteriosum, the ascending aorta, the lower thoracic aorta above the diaphragm, and avulsion of the innominate artery at the aortic arch (Sherwood & Hartsock, 2002). Often the outer two layers of the aorta are torn, leaving the innermost layer intact. Although this is considered a lethal injury, early diagnosis can prevent tearing of the innermost layer, exsanguination, and death. Signs of aortic disruption include weak femoral pulses, dysphagia, dyspnea, hoarseness, and pain. A chest x-ray study may demonstrate a widened mediastinum (greater than or equal to 8 mm), tracheal deviation to the right, depressed left mainstem bronchus, first and second rib fractures, and left hemothorax. Diagnosis is confirmed by an aortogram. The rupture will require definitive surgical resection and repair.

SPINAL CORD INJURY

Mechanisms of injuries that may result in spinal cord injury (SCI) include hyperflexion, hyperextension, axial loading, rotation, and penetrating trauma. The initial treatment of a patient suspected of having an SCI includes the ABCs of resuscitation, spinal immobilization, prevention of further injury, and appropriate triage to a facility with capabilities to care for patients with SCIs. Immobilization initiated in the field by prehospital personnel is maintained during the initial assessment and resuscitation efforts. Conscious patients are reassured, with an emphasis on complete cooperation with spinal immobilization.

A complete sensory and motor neurological examination is performed after the ABC components of the primary survey. Portable lateral x-ray studies of the cervical spine are obtained, and the patient is prepared for a possible spinal CT scan to rule out occult injury. Dislocations of the spine are reduced as soon as possible by means of postural reduction including

cervical traction tongs, halo traction devices, or surgical fusion. The administration of intravenous methylprednisolone initiated within 8 hours of injury has been shown to improve outcomes after SCI. The use of glucocorticoids reduces the acute inflammatory response and thereby reduces secondary SCI (King, Gupta, & Narayan, 2000).

Ongoing assessment includes evaluation of airway and ventilatory function, heart rate and rhythm, blood pressure, and urine output. With the loss of sympathetic output after a cervical spine injury, most patients will develop neurogenic shock with hypotension and bradycardia. Blood pressure may respond initially to fluid resuscitation, but patients often require vasopressor support to compensate for the loss of sympathetic innervation and resultant vasodilation. Atropine may be used to treat symptomatic bradycardia. In addition, the patient must be closely monitored for further deterioration in spinal cord function resulting from secondary injury or ascending cord edema. Potential complications associated with SCI include impaired gastrointestinal functioning, autonomic dysreflexia, deep vein thrombosis (DVT), orthostatic hypotension, loss of bowel and bladder function, immobility, spasticity, and contractures. It is important to ensure that interventions are taken to prevent these potential complications. All patients have a Foley catheter inserted, started on daily bowel stimulants, given DVT prophylaxis, have a consultation for a physical or occupational therapy evaluation (if indicated), and have precautions taken to prevent the development of autonomic dysreflexia. Early consultation with physical medicine and rehabilitative specialists is vital in obtaining positive patient outcomes. The patient with an SCI presents complex issues for the trauma team and the patient's support systems. Proactive, aggressive, and comprehensive care is necessary to help the patient to achieve optimal functional outcomes (see Chapter 12).

HEAD INJURY

Injuries to the head are caused by blunt or penetrating trauma. Lacerations to the scalp may result in significant bleeding. These wounds are cleaned, debrided, and sutured. Fractures of the skull may be linear, basilar, closed depressed, open depressed, or comminuted. Underlying brain injury may also occur. Interventions are necessary when the fracture crosses arterial grooves or vascular sinuses, owing to the increased risk of epidural bleeding.

Basilar skull fractures are located at the base of the cranium and potentially involve the five bones that form the skull base. Diagnosis is based on the presence of cerebrospinal fluid in the nose (rhinorrhea) and/or ears (otorrhea), ecchymosis over the mastoid area (Battle's sign), or hemotympanum (blood in the middle ear). Raccoon eyes or periorbital ecchymoses are present after a cribriform plate fracture. Two potential complications that may develop following a basilar skull fracture are infection and cranial nerve injury. Infection occurs as a result of straightforward access to the cranium by organisms through the cerebrospinal fluid drainage pathway. Cranial nerve injury may result from the close proximity of these nerves to the fracture sites. Therefore, it is important to monitor the patient closely for an intracerebral infection or a cranial nerve injury.

Primary head injury occurs in the presence of acceleration, deceleration, or rotational forces. Injury may be focal or diffuse. Secondary head injury refers to the systemic (hypotension, hypoxia, anemia, hypocapnia, hyperthermia) or intracranial (edema, intracranial hypertension, seizures, vasospasm) changes that result in alteration in the nervous system tissue (Emergency Nurses Association, 2003; Littlejohns, Bader, & March, 2003). The effects of these secondary injuries are certain chemical alterations in the cerebral tissue. These result from interference in cerebral blood flow and oxygen supply to the brain cells. Patients with secondary injury often have poor outcomes, including death. Therefore, interventions are directed toward restoring circulating blood volume and maintaining adequate cerebral perfusion, oxygenation, and gas exchange to minimize the effects of secondary brain insults (Zink, 2001; Emergency Nurses Association, 2003).

The prehospital phase is considered the most critical interval in determining the ultimate outcome after severe head injury (Bulger et al., 2002). Rapid interventions to prevent secondary brain injury are critical to the outcome of these patients. Supplemental oxygen is essential, and tracheal intubation with mechanical ventilation is often required to prevent hypoxia. Aggressive volume resuscitation is necessary to return the patient in hemorrhagic shock rapidly to a normotensive state and to maintain cerebral perfusion. Care must be exercised, however, to avoid overhydration and subsequent intracranial hypertension. The most common fluid for prehospital resuscitation is isotonic crystalloid solution. However, resuscitation using small-volume hypertonic saline has demonstrated positive results (Brain Trauma Foundation, 2000). Hypertonic saline solutions restore blood pressure and cardiac output and may decrease intracranial pressure (ICP) with less volume and lower capillary hydrostatic pressure than with lactated Ringer's solution (Klein, 1999).

ICP monitoring is indicated in any severely head-injured patient (Glasgow Coma Scale [GCS] less than or equal to 8) with an abnormal CT scan.

ICP monitoring is warranted in patients with severe head injuries with a normal CT scan if two or more of the following are present on admission: age older than 40 years, unilateral or bilateral motor posturing, and systolic blood pressure less than 90 mm Hg (Brain Trauma Foundation, 2000; Bulger et al., 2002). The goal is an ICP of less than 20 mm Hg to prevent cerebral ischemia and subsequent secondary brain injury. Preservation of the patient's cerebral perfusion pressure (Cerebral perfusion pressure = Mean arterial pressure – Mean ICP) at 70 mm Hg or greater has been shown to decrease neurological disability. However, there is a concern that the increased fluid resuscitation required to maintain the cerebral perfusion pressure at 70 mm Hg or higher may be a contributing factor in the development of ARDS (Bulger et al., 2002). Management strategies for the patient with intracranial hypertension include the administration of osmotic (mannitol) and loop (furosemide) diuretics to maintain a serum osmolality of less than 320 mOsm, cerebral spinal fluid drainage with an intraventricular catheter, sedation, and adequate oxygenation (Brain Trauma Foundation, 2000). Hyperventilation to reduce the $PaCO_2$ level to 35 mm Hg or less may be used during brief periods in the presence of acute neurological deterioration or when intracranial hypertension is refractory to sedation, paralysis, cerebrospinal fluid drainage, or osmotic diuretics (Brain Trauma Foundation, 2000). Hyperventilation results in vasoconstriction of cerebral vessels and allows more space for brain tissue swelling. However, the Brain Trauma Foundation guidelines (2000) suggest that the use of prophylactic hyperventilation during the first 24 hours after injury be avoided because this therapy may compromise cerebral perfusion further in a time when cerebral blood flow is already reduced. Pharmacologically induced coma, with pentobarbital, may be used as a final intervention in situations of severe intracranial hypertension. Future research will continue to evaluate the effectiveness of hypothermia induction to treat severe traumatic brain injury. Currently, there are varying degrees of success, and thus the efficacy and safety of this therapy remain under investigation (Inamasu & Ichikizaki, 2002; Zink, 2001).

Monitoring of jugular venous oxygen saturation (SjO_2) provides valuable information regarding the balance between cerebral oxygen delivery and consumption. A fiberoptic catheter placed in the jugular bulb (a dilation of the internal jugular vein near the base of the skull) provides continuous measurements of SjO_2. The optimal SjO_2 value is between 55% and 75%, reflecting oxygen saturation of the venous blood as it leaves the brain. It is thought that changes in SjO_2 will be seen before changes in ICP. This early sign of adverse changes may assist in implementing interventions to prevent the deleterious effects of increased ICP. Additionally, monitoring of the partial pressure of brain tissue oxygen (PbtO$_2$) has been shown to assist in the identification of hypoxic events and has resulted in timely targeted interventions and improved patient outcomes (Littlejohns, Bader, & March, 2003). These monitoring devices measure brain temperature and oxygen values. Brain temperature is measured in an effort to control a febrile state more closely and to prevent deleterious outcomes. Monitoring of PbtO$_2$ provides valuable information to the medical team regarding the necessity to intervene in an effort to maintain adequate oxygen, blood flow, and carbon dioxide levels to the brain. Maintaining PbtO$_2$ at a level of greater than 20 mm Hg has been shown to have improved patient outcomes. Partial pressure of brain tissue oxygen levels of less than 15 mm Hg during the resuscitation phase of traumatic brain injury represent a poor predictive outcome (Littlejohns, Bader, & March, 2003). Early identification of impaired brain tissue oxygenation provides an additional dimension when monitoring, intervening, and evaluating a patient with severe traumatic brain injury.

Nursing care for the patient with a traumatic head injury is directed at maintaining a patent airway, providing adequate ventilation and gas exchange, clearance of pulmonary secretions, proper head alignment to maximize venous drainage, and close monitoring of neurological functioning. Pulmonary complications are common in the neurologically impaired patient. Aggressive pulmonary hygiene is vital. Careful consideration must be given to the position of the patient's head, neck, and body during the acute critical phase of care. Although multiple methods of patient positioning have been suggested, current recommendations include head elevation to 30 degrees, avoidance of aggressive hip flexion, and maintenance of neck alignment to optimize cerebral venous drainage (Emergency Nurses Association, 2003). All nursing care is assessed for the patient's tolerance and its effect on intracranial hemodynamics (ICP and cerebral perfusion pressure) (see Chapter 12).

MUSCULOSKELETAL INJURIES

Musculoskeletal trauma is a significant problem that results in 33 million injuries annually (Walsh, 2002). It may involve only a single system or may occur in combination with injuries to other systems. The injuries may be blunt or penetrating and may involve bone, soft tissue, muscle, nerves, and/or blood vessels. Injuries may be classified as fractures, fracture-dislocations, amputations, and tissue trauma (crushing injuries of the soft tissue, nerves, vessels, or tendons).

TABLE 18-7	
Types of Fractures	
Type of Fracture	**Description**
Open	Skin integrity over or near fracture site is disrupted
Closed	Skin integrity over or near fracture site is intact
Complete	Total interruption in bony continuity
Incomplete	Incomplete interruption in bony continuity
Comminuted	Splintering of bone into fragments
Greenstick	Bone buckles or bends; fracture does not go through the entire bone
Impacted	Distal and proximal fracture sites are wedged into each other
Displaced	Proximal and distal fracture sites are out of alignment

Fractures involve a disruption of bony continuity. Table 18-7 describes types of fractures. Open and closed fractures are further classified into grades based on the degree of bony, soft, and vascular tissue and nerve damage. Extremity assessment is often described by the five Ps: *pain, pallor, pulses, paresthesia,* and *paralysis.* This process of assessment describes the neurovascular status of the injured extremity. When possible, the injured extremity is compared with the opposite uninjured extremity.

Treatment

Fractures are treated with reduction. Closed reduction is appropriate for closed fractures because good alignment can be achieved with casts or splints. Open reduction is necessary for open fractures. Fracture wounds are debrided, and the fracture is reduced within 18 hours of injury to prevent infection and nonunion. In the event that the patient's hemodynamic status precludes immediate repair of the fracture, skeletal traction to realign the extremity may be instituted to provide continuous reduction using weights and counterweights. Once reduction occurs, bleeding and pain are lessened.

Pelvic fractures are considered to be stable or unstable. Unstable fractures can be life-threatening and are often accompanied by severe hemorrhage or exsanguination, damage to the genitourinary system, or sepsis (American College of Surgeons, 1997). A fracture of the pelvis may produce significant venous bleeding caused by a disruption of pelvic veins potentially resulting in hypovolemic shock. Temporary control of the bleeding may be obtained with use of the PASG. However, definitive treatment must be accomplished though interventional radiology techniques or operative repair. The radiological techniques assist in resolution of vessel bleeding through embolization and coil occlusion. Operative repair may be required for internal or external fixation of complex pelvic fractures.

Traumatic soft tissue injuries are categorized as contusions, abrasions, lacerations, puncture wounds, hematomas, amputations, and avulsion injuries (Casper & Joshi, 2002). Mechanism of injury, time from injury to definitive care, and periods of hypotension or hypoxia are considered when evaluating the patient with traumatic soft tissue injuries. Patients with severe soft tissue injuries may quickly develop signs and symptoms of hypotension, oxygen deprivation, and metabolic acidosis. Thus, it is important to first assess and determine the extent of soft tissue injury. Amputation produces a well-defined wound edge with localized injury to soft tissue, nerves, and vessels. These wounds usually require debridement and surgical closure. Avulsion injuries result in stretching and tearing of the soft tissue and may tear nerves and vessels at different levels other than the actual site of bone and tissue trauma. A crush injury may produce local soft tissue trauma or extensive damage distant from the site of injury. Crush injuries of the pelvis and/or both lower extremities or a prolonged entrapment may be life-threatening. Prolonged compression produces ischemia and anoxia of the affected muscle tissue. Third spacing of fluid, localized edema, and increased compartment pressures cause secondary ischemia. Without aggressive intervention, these injuries can result in irreversible complications.

All wounds are considered contaminated with microorganisms at the time of injury. An increased risk of infection is observed the greater the time from injury to treatment. Irrigation, debridement, and appropriate wound care may reduce the risk of infection. Tetanus toxoid administration and antibiotic therapy must always be considered.

After musculoskeletal injury, the patient is monitored for signs of hemorrhage and development of neurovascular compromise. Pelvic fractures can result in 750 to 6000 mL of blood loss. Femur fractures can result in the loss of 500 to 3000 mL of blood. Volume replacement, fracture stabilization, and pressure dressings may reduce the risk of hemorrhagic shock. Patients with musculoskeletal injury are at risk of developing neurological and/or vascular compromise. Patients at high risk include those with soft tissue injuries, arterial injury, dislocations, use of PASG, open or closed fractures, or compression or crush injuries. Patients are monitored continuously for changes in motor or sensory status. Proper alignment, immobilization, and elevation help to prevent neurovascular damage.

Complications

Rhabdomolysis. Complications of musculoskeletal injury include the systemic effects that may occur after a crush injury, including rhabdomyolysis, compartment syndrome, and fat embolism syndrome. Rhabdomyolysis is a complication of crush injuries, resulting from marked vasoconstriction and hypotension followed by acute renal failure (ARF) (Beetham, 2000). It results from muscle destruction from the primary and secondary injury. Myoglobin and potassium are released from the damaged muscles. Excessive release of potassium predispose the patient to the life-threatening effects of hyperkalemia. Myoglobinuria (myoglobin excreted through the urine), when combined with hypovolemia, produces ARF and acute tubular necrosis in the absence of aggressive, rapid intervention. Additional sequelae include hyperuricemia, hypocalcemia, intravascular coagulation, and metabolic acidosis (Beetham, 2000). Institution of aggressive saline replacement, urine alkalinization, and osmotic diuresis are necessary to support the circulation, decrease cast formation, and reduce muscle damage. These interventions will lessen the risk of developing ARF. This regimen continues to be extensively used in today's clinical environment in the absence of controlled research trials.

Compartment syndrome. Compartment syndrome places the patient at risk of losing a limb. It occurs more frequently in the muscles of the lower leg or forearm, but it may involve any fascial compartment. The closed muscle compartment contains neurovascular bundles that are tightly covered by fascia. An increase in pressure within the compartment, from internal or external sources, produces the syndrome. Internal sources include hemorrhage, edema, open or closed fractures, or crush injuries that increase muscle compartment content. Skeletal traction, casts, air splints, and PASGs are external sources that decrease the size of the compartment. If the pressure is not relieved, compression of nerves, blood vessels, and muscle occurs, with resulting ischemia, necrosis, and scarring of muscle and nerve tissue.

Patients with compartment syndrome complain of throbbing pain disproportionate to the injury. Narcotic administration does not relieve the pain. The pain is localized to the involved compartment and increases with passive muscle stretching. The area affected is firm to the touch. Paresthesia distal to the compartment, pulselessness, and paralysis are late signs and must be reported immediately to prevent loss of the extremity. The affected limb is elevated to heart level to promote venous outflow and to prevent further swelling. Compartmental pressure monitoring may be performed to diagnosis this syndrome definitively. Treatment of compartment syndrome is immediate surgical fasciotomy in which the fascial compartment is opened to relieve the pressure.

Fat embolism. Development of fat embolism syndrome is a risk factor that accompanies traumatic injury of the long bones, pelvis, and multiple skeletal fractures. The syndrome develops between 24 and 48 hours after injury. Two theories exist to describe the origin of fat emboli syndrome. The mobilization theory focuses on recruitment of fat globules at the time of injury. As a bone is stressed or injured, bone marrow fat globules from the fracture site are released into torn vessels and the systemic circulation. A second theory is based on the production and release of free fatty acids in abnormal amounts after skeletal injury. This alteration in fatty acid metabolism is implicated in the destruction of pulmonary endothelial tissue and the development of pulmonary edema. The physiological changes that occur are the same regardless of the etiological process.

Hallmark clinical signs that accompany fat embolism syndrome begin with development of a low-grade fever followed by a new-onset tachycardia, dyspnea, increased respiratory rate and effort, abnormal arterial blood gas studies, thrombocytopenia and petechiae (Box 18-2). If pulmonary distress continues, the patient will begin to demonstrate symptoms of cerebral hypoxia, such as changes in level of consciousness or coma. Electrocardiogram (ECG) findings include development of a right bundle-branch block, S waves of prominent size in lead I, Q waves in lead III, T-wave inversion, depressed ST segments,

and dysrhythmias. Development of lipuria (fat in the urine) indicates a severe case of fat embolism syndrome.

Prevention of fat embolism is the best treatment. Stabilization of extremity fractures to minimize both bone movement and the release of fatty products from the bone marrow must be accomplished as early as possible. Either internal or external fixation devices may be used, depending on the location and extent of the fractures. Treatment of fat embolism syndrome is directed toward the preservation of pulmonary function and maintenance of cardiovascular stability. Administration of supplemental oxygen, intubation with mechanical ventilation, and use of positive end-expiratory pressure (PEEP) may be required to restore or maintain pulmonary perfusion and ventilation. Monitoring the patient's cardiovascular stability must be continued throughout the critical care phase, with particular attention paid to ECG and hemodynamic changes.

ABDOMINAL INJURIES

Abdominal injuries are often difficult to diagnose. A normal initial examination does not necessarily rule out intraabdominal injury. The classic sign of abdominal injury is pain. However, it cannot be used as an assessment tool if the patient has an altered sensorium, drug intoxication, or SCI with impaired sensation.

The liver is the most commonly injured organ after blunt or penetrating trauma. Hemorrhage is the primary cause of death after liver injury. The patient may present with a history of right lower thoracic trauma, fractured lower right ribs, right upper quadrant ecchymosis, right upper quadrant tenderness, and hypotension. The diagnosis is confirmed with the use of the FAST, abdominal CT, and/or diagnostic peritoneal lavage. The degree of liver injury is graded on a scale of I to VI, with I representing a nonexpanding subcapsular hematoma and VI signifying hepatic avulsion. Grade I through IV injures may be treated with close monitoring (serial abdominal assessment and serial hemoglobin and hematocrit) and bed rest for 5 days. Surgical management is indicated for grades IV through VI in which there is expansion of the hemorrhage, large laceration, or complete avulsion of the liver from its vascular supply.

Splenic injury occurs most often as a result of blunt trauma to the abdomen. However, penetrating trauma to the left upper quadrant of the abdomen or fracture of the anterior left lower ribs also contributes to splenic injuries. The patient may present with left upper quadrant tenderness, peritoneal irritation, referred pain to the left shoulder (Kehr's sign), hypotension, or signs of hemorrhagic shock.

BOX 18-2

Clinical Manifestations of Fat Embolism Syndrome

- Tachycardia (>100 beats/min)
- Hypotension
- Abrupt change in behavior or mentation
- Dyspnea
- Tachypnea
- Hypoxemia
- Radiological evidence of pulmonary infiltrates
- Productive cough

An encapsulated hemorrhage of the spleen produces no immediate signs of bleeding. The diagnosis is confirmed using the same tests as for liver injuries. The degree of splenic injury is graded on a scale from I to V. Grade I is a subcapsular, nonexpanding hematoma or a laceration involving less than 1 cm of spleen parenchyma. The completely shattered spleen with devascularization is considered a grade V spleen injury. Management of splenic injury is similar to that of liver injuries. Close monitoring of the patient is vital. This includes assessment of the patient's hemodynamic status, the presence of guarding, rebound tenderness, rigidity, or distention of the abdomen, and/or alteration in the patient's hemoglobin and hematocrit. Bed rest for 5 days may be appropriate for grade I to III splenic injuries. Operative intervention is often necessary for grade IV and V injuries. Every effort is made to preserve splenic tissue because of its role in immune function. Overwhelming postsplenectomy infection has been seen after removal of the spleen. Patients undergoing splenectomy are susceptible to pneumococcal infections. The administration of the pneumococcal vaccine within the first few days postoperatively is recommended. Spleen injury may continue to bleed slowly, and the spleen may ultimately rupture days to weeks after the initial injury. This is a life-threatening situation necessitating immediate surgical intervention.

Injury to the kidneys occurs most frequently after blunt trauma to the abdomen and usually affects a single kidney. Renal trauma can be classified as minor, major, or critical (life-threatening). The patient may present with costovertebral tenderness, microscopic or gross hematuria, bruising or ecchymosis over the eleventh and twelfth rib, hemorrhage, and/or shock. Diagnostic studies include CT scan, angiography, intravenous pyelogram, and cystoscopy. For minor injuries, management focuses on bed rest, hydration, and monitoring of renal function, including hematuria, urine output, urinalysis, serum blood urea nitrogen (BUN), electrolytes, and complete blood count. Management of major and critical renal injuries focuses on surgical intervention including control of bleeding, repair of the injury, renorrhaphy, or nephrectomy. Postsurgical complications include refractory hypertension, hemorrhage, fistula formation, and infection.

Critical Care Phase

POSTOPERATIVE MANAGEMENT

Postoperative management of a critically ill patient involves the systematic assessment and monitoring of respiratory and cardiovascular function, neuromuscular abilities, mental status, temperature, pain, drainage and bleeding, urine output, and resuscitation efforts (Silverstein, Apfelbaum, Barlow, et al., 2002). Initial attention in the care of the postoperative surgical patient is directed toward airway and breathing. It is important to ascertain from the physician the plan for airway management. Patients usually present to the critical care unit intubated for postoperative recovery monitoring. Patients not requiring extended mechanical ventilation may be extubated within minutes to hours of admission, depending on the patient's ability to protect the airway after the reversal of anesthesia and neuromuscular blocking agents. Other critically ill patients are maintained on mechanical ventilation until hemodynamic stability is attained and their injuries are definitely repaired and/or there is resolution of the patient's pulmonary pathological process. This will require ongoing monitoring of the patient's oxygenation and ventilation status with potential modifications in the ventilatory modes, adjuncts, and fraction of inspired oxygen (FiO_2).

After stability of the patient's airway, attention is focused on hemodynamic assessment. This includes the observation of heart rate, cardiac rhythm, blood pressure, respiratory rate, pulse oximetry, temperature, drainage monitoring (e.g., chest tubes, drains, urinary output), intravenous fluids, and vasoactive medications. The postoperative standard for monitoring these values is as follows: every 5 minutes for three measurements, every 15 minutes for three measurements, every 30 minutes for 1 hour, with hourly vital sign measurements thereafter. More frequent monitoring may be indicated if the patient becomes hemodynamically unstable. Additional hemodynamic values may be obtained if the patient has a pulmonary artery catheter or an ICP monitor. Temperature is measured on admission and is monitored at regular intervals. In the event of hypothermia, passive and active rewarming strategies are used to rewarm the patient to a normothermic state. Refer to Table 18-6 for rewarming strategies. Shivering is avoided because it leads to elevations in the patient's metabolic rate and results in increased oxygen demands. In a compromised patient, this leads to further hemodynamic instability. The patient is monitored for decreased blood pressure during the rewarming process. This decline in blood pressure is related to vasoconstriction during hypothermia and the vasodilation during the rewarming process.

Physical assessment is the next priority of care for the postoperative surgical patient. It is important to perform a full-body assessment including the evaluation of all body systems (neurological, cardiovascular, pulmonary, gastrointestinal, renal, hematological, immune, musculoskeletal, and integumentary) and invasive line access. Continual collection of assessment data is required to guide therapies aimed at correcting identified problems or injuries and preventing or minimizing postinjury complications. Elderly patients are at increased risk of complications after traumatic injury because of age-related changes (see Geriatric Assessment). In all patients, it is especially important to assess the patient's mental status to ensure that a neurological event did not occur intraoperatively. Report from the anesthesiologist should include whether or not the anesthesia was reversed

pharmacologically and the most recent times for administration of analgesic, amnesic, or sedative medications. This will provide information on the estimated time of patient wakefulness. Once awake, the patient is assessed for alertness and for orientation to person, place, and time, as well as for the ability to follow commands. In the event that the patient does not awaken, measures must be taken to determine the cause of the comatose state. The medical team must determine whether the anesthetic agents, sedation, or analgesic medications are contributing factors. If it

Geriatric Assessment

- Falls, resulting in hip, arm, hand, leg, feet, pelvic, ribs, and vertebral fractures, are the most frequent cause of injury for the elderly population.
- The elderly patient has three major factors influencing care needs after traumatic injury: known preexisting disease, diminished physiological capacity, and occult disease. The effects of trauma may be exacerbated by decreased physiological reserve and host resistance that occur with aging. (Yoshikawa & Norman, 2000). Thus, these patients may present with hemodynamic instability, diminished organ function, and delayed healing.
- The cardiopulmonary effects of aging affect the patient's ability to respond to the pathophysiologic effects of trauma. These include decreased sensitivity to catecholamines; stiffened left ventricle; rigid cardiac valves; decreased arterial wall elasticity; increased incidence of atrial fibrillation, premature atrial or ventricular contractions and heart blocks; decreased vital capacity; decline in respiratory muscle strength; and increased work of breathing. These patients often present with decreased cardiac output, have a risk of volume overload with fluid resuscitation, and have a lack of compensatory response to altered hemodynamics.
- It is vital to obtain a list of current medications because there may be increased risk of complications. The following drugs may contribute to patient complications:

Medications	Complication
Aspirin (ASA), warfarin (Coumadin), and antiplatelet medications	Increase risk of bleeding
Nonsteroidal antiinflammatory drugs [NSAIDS]	Gastrointestinal bleeding
Steroids	Delay in healing
Beta-blockers and calcium channel blockers	Inadequate hemodynamic response
Herbal therapies	Multiple severe drug interactions

- Decreased brain mass, increased neuronal death, decline in sensory nerve function, decreased cerebral perfusion, and autoregulation contribute to the changes seen in neurological assessment of the elderly patient. Patients may present with changes in level of consciousness (agitation or coma), more pronounced neurological impairments after intracranial bleeding because of a larger compartment available for blood to accumulate, and an inability to report acute changes in painful stimuli.
- Other physiological changes that must be considered in the assessment and treatment of an elderly patient's response to trauma include decreased renal blood flow and glomerular filtration rate, increased susceptibility to infection, decreased hematopoiesis, increased insulin resistance, decreased insulin release, diminished bowel motility, delayed wound healing, increased osteoporosis, decreased inflammatory response, and loss of subcutaneous fat (more prone to pressure). These physiological changes will alter the elderly patient's ability to respond to the trauma. Thus, these patients must be monitored closely for the development of decreased urinary output, diminished hemoglobin or hematocrit, increased blood glucose levels, development of ileus, signs and symptoms of infection, increased number of bony fractures, and alteration in skin integrity.
- Elderly patients often have limitations in mobility and joint flexibility, muscle atrophy, osteoarthritis, and preexisting deformities, which complicate their ability to participate in physical and/or occupational therapy and delay the return to pretraumatic functional status.

is determined that medications are not the contributing cause of the neurological impairment, the patient may require additional diagnostic tests, such as a CT scan of the head. Any alterations in the patient's clinical assessment must be analyzed to determine whether intervention is necessary. This may require interdisciplinary collaboration with surgeons, advanced practice nurses, respiratory therapy, and consulting physicians.

Patients must be assessed to determine their level of pain. Multiple pain scales are available to assess the degree of pain. Individual institutions will determine the most appropriate pain scale for use with their patient population. All postoperative orders must include analgesic medication to be administered orally or intravenously as needed or as a continuous infusion. If clinicians are unable to assess the patient's pain postoperatively because of the patient's lack of wakefulness or secondary to a neurological event, the pain level is evaluated using other physiological values (e.g., alterations in heart rate and blood pressure, anxiety, facial grimacing, decreasing oxygen levels, ventilator asynchrony). After administration of analgesia, the patient's pain level must be reassessed. The inability to control a patient's pain will result in worsening anxiety and an inability to wean the patient from ventilatory support and may contribute to the development of chronic pain syndrome.

Resuscitative efforts are evaluated postoperatively to determine the effectiveness of fluid management. The establishment of baseline hemodynamic status, laboratory values (complete blood count, complete metabolic panel, coagulation studies, lactate, arterial blood gas with base deficit or excess), and intake and output will assist the practitioner in determining the patient's fluid volume status and the degree of successful resuscitation. Hemoglobin, hematocrit, and coagulation studies provide valuable information on whether the patient is bleeding or has a high probability of bleeding because of unavailable or ineffective clotting factors. Determining whether the patient is adequately resuscitated may be assessed using the lactate level and base deficit values. Inadequate resuscitation resulting in anaerobic metabolism is indicated by a higher lactate level and/or a more negative base deficit value. The presence of abnormal values indicates the need for more aggressive resuscitation.

Ongoing patient care priorities evolve from the patient's diagnosis and/or surgical procedure. Careful attention must be given to anticipating potential and intervening on actual patient problems. A comprehensive reassessment every 4 hours will guide the nurse in identifying changes in the patient's status, preparing for additional diagnostic procedures, and intervening appropriately. It is vital to evaluate continually for alterations in the patient's oxygenation, ventilation, acid-base balance, perfusion, and infection, metabolic, and hemodynamic status. In the event that the patient is unable to be extubated within 24 hours, consideration must be given to initiating nutrition. For additional information, refer to Chapter 5. Ensuring that the patient has pharmacological prophylaxis for DVT and gastrointestinal ulceration, as well as an aggressive protocol for mobilization, may prevent untoward complications. Additionally, research has illustrated improvements in critical care mortality rates of bloodstream infections, number of patients with ARF who require dialysis, need for red cell transfusions, and incidence of critical illness polyneuropathy when an intensive insulin therapy protocol was used on mechanically ventilated patients to maintain glucose levels between 80 and 110 mg/dL (Van Den Berghe et al., 2001). Addressing these care priorities will assist in preventing adverse complications and improving patient outcomes.

Damage-Control Surgery

Since the early 1990s, patients undergoing extensive surgical repair have developed severe complications that contributed to their ultimate demise. These complications, now recognized as the leading cause of death in multitraumatized patients, include the triad of hypothermia, acidosis, and coagulopathy. These complications and resultant mortality have changed the current surgical focus to a new approach known as damage-control surgery or a staged laparotomy. This strategy sacrifices the completeness of immediate repair. The first stage includes the operative repair of life-threatening injuries only. Patients are then returned to the critical care unit (second stage) for aggressive rewarming, ongoing resuscitation, and attainment of hemodynamic stability (Kouraklis, 2002). The third stage occurs usually within 24 to 48 hours after the initial operation. This involves the return to the operating room for definitive repair of the intraabdominal injuries. This three-stage approach allows for stabilization of hemodynamics, correction of coagulopathy, rewarming, and optimization of pulmonary function (Kouraklis, 2002; Mikhail, 1999). The damage-control concept has been shown to improve the outcomes of critically ill patients with severe intraabdominal injuries.

The patient with multisystemic injuries is at risk of developing a myriad of complications because of the body's compromised condition, prolonged immobility, and the long-term rehabilitation associated with trauma care. The most common secondary complications encountered during this critical phase of care are related to respiratory impairment, infection, acute renal failure, high nutritional demands, and MODS.

RESPIRATORY IMPAIRMENT
Acute Respiratory Distress Syndrome

ARDS is a syndrome of lung injury characterized by dyspnea, severe hypoxemia, decreased lung compliance, and diffuse bilateral pulmonary infiltrates (Udobi, Childs, & Touijer, 2003) (see Chapter 13). This cluster of symptoms may occur physiologically 2 to 48 hours after a traumatic injury. However, recognizable clinical symptoms may not occur for 5 or more days after injury. The etiology of ARDS can be divided into direct and indirect causes. Direct causes of ARDS in trauma patients include aspiration of gastric contents, pulmonary contusion, pneumonia, inhalation injury, multiple fractures, and/or fat or air embolism. Indirect causes involve the release of mediators from systemic injuries, including sepsis, cardiogenic or hemorrhagic shock, multiple trauma, disseminating intravascular coagulation, massive blood resuscitation, and burns (Sherwood & Hartsock, 2002). The critical care nurse must identify those patients at risk of developing ARDS, because early initiation of therapy is crucial for successful recovery.

Clinical manifestations. The symptoms associated with the development of ARDS usually occur in the critical care phase. They may include hypoxemia (PaO_2 lower than 50 mm Hg with FiO_2 greater than 0.6 or a PaO_2/FiO_2 ratio of less than 200 mm Hg with mechanical ventilation), rising carbon dioxide levels, increased respiratory distress (tachypnea, dyspnea), pulmonary hypertension (systolic pulmonary artery pressure greater than 30 mm Hg), decreased static lung compliance, and new diffuse bilateral chest infiltrates (Sherwood & Hartsock, 2002).

Treatment. Treatment of ARDS is directed toward correcting the underlying cause, maximizing oxygen delivery to the tissues, decreasing pulmonary congestion, preventing further lung damage and organ dysfunction, and supporting the patient's cardiovascular system. Chest injuries or fluid overhydration must be corrected. Mechanical ventilation, if not instituted during the resuscitative phase, is required in a majority of patients with ARDS. PEEP is indicated to increase the patient's PaO_2 levels while using a lower inspired concentration of oxygen. Other approaches to improving ventilation and oxygenation include pressure-control ventilation, inverse-ratio ventilation, high-frequency ventilation, permissive hypercapnia, protective lung strategies (6 mL/kg tidal volumes), and prone positioning (Bower, Ware, Berthiaume, & Matthay, 2001; Udobi, Childs, & Touijer, 2003).

Cardiovascular compromise can result from the use of positive-pressure ventilation. It is imperative that cardiac output be maintained to prevent further deterioration of the patient's condition. Manipulation of preload, contractility, and afterload through administration of pharmacological agents may be necessary. Fluid therapy in the trauma patient with ARDS requires careful monitoring. A balanced electrolyte solution is the most common type of fluid used to correct the hypovolemia associated with trauma patients. The amount of infused fluid must be sufficient to maintain the patient's cardiac output and intravascular volume without increasing intrapulmonary edema. Monitoring of the patient's pulmonary artery pressure, pulmonary artery occlusion pressure, and daily weight helps to monitor trends in response and to guide fluid therapy. Transfusion of red blood cells may be required not only to provide cardiovascular support, but also to augment oxygen delivery and minimize cellular oxygen debt.

Deep Vein Thrombosis

DVT is a significant complication of traumatic injury. The risk of DVT in young patients with multiple trauma has been estimated to be 20%. Patients with acute head injury or SCIs have at least a 40% chance of developing DVT and a 1% to 4% risk of a fatal pulmonary embolism (PE). A reduction in DVT will result in a decrease in PEs, because DVT is a marker for PE. Advanced age, type and severity of injury, obesity, malignancy, pregnancy, heart failure, SCI, sepsis or shock states, recent surgery, complex lower extremity fractures, pelvic fractures, direct vascular injury necessitating operative repair, history of thromboembolic disease, prolonged immobilization, respiratory failure, number of blood transfusions, and central venous catheterization are associated with an increased incidence of DVT in trauma patients (Rocha & Tapson, 2003; Walsh, 2002).

DVT usually occurs in the lower extremities. Thrombus formation is enhanced in the presence of vessel damage, venous stasis, and hypercoagulability (Virchow's triad). The thrombus may be dislodged by increased venous pressure, direct trauma, or sudden muscle action. The dislodged clot becomes an embolus and travels through the body's vasculature until it lodges in either the pulmonary artery or its smaller branches. Once the embolus becomes lodged, blood flow is obstructed distally, and tissues distal to the obstruction become hypoxic. Pulmonary vessels constrict in response to the hypoxia and the result is a ventilation-perfusion mismatch (ventilation greater than perfusion), causing hypoxemia.

Clinical manifestations. Clinical manifestations of DVT are outlined in Box 18-3. Although clinical assessment is helpful, early aggressive diagnostic screening is important to prevent complications

BOX 18-3

Clinical Manifestations of Deep Vein Thrombosis

- Pain and tenderness
- Swelling
- Fever
- Homans' sign (discomfort in calf on forced dorsiflexion of foot)
- Venous distention
- Palpable cord
- Discoloration

BOX 18-4

Clinical Manifestations of Pulmonary Embolism

- Dyspnea: sudden onset
- Chest pain: sudden onset
- Rapid, shallow respiratory rate
- Shortness of breath
- Auscultation of bronchial breath sounds
- Pale, dusky, cyanotic skin coloring
- Increased anxiety
- Decreased level of consciousness
- Other signs of hypovolemic shock
  Decreased systolic blood pressure
  Narrowing pulse pressure
  Tachycardia

of DVTs. DVT prophylaxis in high-risk patients is both safe and effective in reducing the incidence of DVT (Rocha & Tapson, 2003).

Diagnosis and treatment. Patients at high risk of DVT can be screened noninvasively with venous Doppler flow studies, duplex scanning (compression ultrasound), or impedance plethysmography (two-dimensional ultrasound). In addition, DVT prophylaxis is recommended for the high-risk trauma patient. This includes early ambulation, sequential compression devices, low-dose subcutaneous anticoagulant, and/or the placement of a filter in the inferior vena cava to prevent migration of the emboli to the pulmonary vasculature. Special attention is required for patients with the potential for bleeding. These trauma patients may have to forgo initial treatment with anticoagulation until the risk of bleeding is minimized.

Pulmonary Embolism

PE is often a fatal complication of DVT. Therefore, high-risk patients are continuously monitored for signs and symptoms associated with PE. These include new-onset dyspnea, changes in respiratory rate and effort, hemoptysis, pleuritic pain, fever, and changes in cerebral and tissue perfusion (Box 18-4).

Clinical manifestations. The supporting laboratory data demonstrate changes in the patient's arterial blood gas values. Hypoxemia, hypocapnia, decreased oxygen saturation, and an alkalotic pH are associated with the development of PE. ECG changes include development of tachycardia, peaked T waves, a widened QRS complex, ST- and T-wave changes, and right axis deviation. Chest x-ray studies may be normal initially with evidence of atelectasis or infiltrates. A ventilation-perfusion lung scan may be either normal or may indicate a perfusion defect. The gold standard diagnostic test is a pulmonary angiogram to define the area of obstruction.

Treatment. Therapy for PE is directed toward improving gas exchange and pulmonary tissue perfusion. Positioning the patient in a high-Fowler's position facilitates breathing and increases diaphragmatic excursion. Administration of supplemental oxygen corrects the impaired gas exchange and enhances tissue perfusion. Analgesics may be required in an attempt to relieve the patient of chest pain. Patients with severe PE may require additional interventions of intubation, mechanical ventilation, vasopressor support, inotropic agents, volume resuscitation, and institution of PEEP. Dissolution of the embolus using anticoagulant or thrombolytic therapy is desirable.

INFECTION

Trauma patients are at high-risk of developing infection because of the presence of open wounds, open fractures, and massive tissue injury that provide a site for the introduction of microorganisms. Nosocomial infections are a major source of sepsis in the trauma patient. The development of infection requires both a susceptible host and the presence of microorganisms. Infection in the trauma patient can be viewed as a failure of the host's immune defenses resulting from either impaired immune function or an overwhelming presence of microorganisms. The magnitude of the immune response after trauma is directly related to the extent of injury (Deitch, Livingston, & Hauser, 1999). However, the immune response can also be affected by age, nutritional status, and preexisting conditions including diabetes mellitus, heart failure, liver disease, and heart disease. Therefore, management of infection in the trauma patient focuses on both eradicating the invading microorganism and increasing the patient's resistance to infection. These strategies include identification of the microorganism through blood, sputum, and urine cultures, appropriate fluid resuscitation to improve oxygen delivery to the body tissues, early stabilization of fractures, removal of necrotic tissue, appropriate antibiotic therapy, and aggressive early nutrition.

Pulmonary Infection

Pulmonary infection, the most common infectious complication after injury, occurs in 20% to 40% of all critically ill trauma patients. (Deitch, Livingston, & Hauser, 1999). The most common cause of pneumonia in the trauma patient is aspiration at the time of injury. Other risk factors that increase the development of pneumonia after injury include direct injury to the lungs, prolonged immobility, and the use of antacids or H_2-blockers to prevent stress bleeding. Management includes antibiotic therapy, aggressive pulmonary care, and meticulous mouth care. Strategies are taken to prevent pneumonia, because it is a serious condition that results in increased mechanical ventilation time, length of stay in the critical care unit and hospital, and mortality rate.

Catheter Sepsis

The widespread use of intravascular catheters in trauma patients has resulted in their being the most frequent site of bacterial infection. Catheter sepsis is iatrogenic in origin. Therefore, it is considered a preventable condition. Catheter sepsis may originate from any type of catheter. However, it is most commonly associated with central venous catheters, as well as lines inserted in the femoral vein (O'Grady et al., 2002). Mechanisms of infection include contamination at the time of placement, entrance of skin flora along the catheter from the skin entry site, and breaks in technique that allow bacteria to enter the catheter at the hub. In addition, the longer the indwelling time is, the greater is the risk of catheter-related sepsis.

The best method to reduce the incidence of catheter sepsis is to ensure that the appropriate patients receive the appropriate catheter for the shortest time possible. Groin vascular access should be avoided whenever possible. The insertion site should be dressed to avoid excess moisture and maceration. Frequent assessment of the site for redness, swelling, or drainage is essential to recognize a potential infection.

Sinusitis

Sinusitis in trauma patients occurs as the result of devices and procedures in the nasopharynx. These include nasotracheal and nasogastric tubes, intranasal packing to control bleeding, and pooling of blood and clots in the sinuses secondary to facial injury. These devices and conditions impede normal drainage of the sinuses and result in bacterial overgrowth. Purulent nasal discharge around an indwelling nasotracheal or nasogastric tube is highly suggestive of sinusitis. Management of sinusitis focuses on prevention and treatment. A nasotracheal tube is converted to an orotracheal tube as soon as possible. When long-term tube feeding is anticipated, nasogastric or naso-duodenal tubes should be converted to an abdominal feeding site through a percutaneous endoscopic gastrojejunostomy (PEG/jejunostomy) tube. Antibiotic therapy is instituted, and aspiration and/or irrigation of the affected sinus may be indicated.

ACUTE RENAL FAILURE

Renal function may be impaired in the trauma patient as a result of either the systemic effects of trauma or actual injury to the renal system. ARF occurs as a result of sustained circulating volume loss (prerenal failure), direct injury to the kidney (intrarenal failure), or obstruction in the drainage system (postrenal failure). The trauma patient is at risk of developing ARF from any of these causes.

Trauma and surgical patients develop a reduction in renal blood flow with the advent of shock or a low cardiac output state. This decreased blood flow reduces the normal glomerular filtration rate and urine production, thereby leading to prerenal failure. Prerenal failure is best managed with intravenous fluids to improve cardiac output and to improve renal perfusion. Intrarenal failure is caused by damage of the renal tissue. This may occur in the presence of untreated prerenal failure, from nephrotoxicity resulting from the administration of nephrotoxic antibiotics, or the with development of rhabdomyolysis. Obstructive processes are common causes of postrenal failure. Situations such as increased pressure, obstruction from displaced postrenal structures, and administration of certain medications (ganglionic blocking agents or antihistamines) may interrupt the autonomic nervous supply to the postrenal structures and may lead to renal obstruction.

Clinical Manifestations

Assessment data must be continually monitored to analyze the trends of renal function. A decrease in urine output is a hallmark sign of ARF. Urinalysis provides information regarding specific gravity and the presence of substances such as protein, myoglobin, nitrite, leukocyte esterases, and white or red blood cells. The presence of nitrite, leukocyte esterases, and white blood cells indicates a urinary tract infection. Serum creatinine and BUN levels are indicators of renal function. Elevated levels of creatinine and BUN are indicative of decreased renal function. Creatinine clearance is a direct reflection of glomerular filtration and is therefore the standard for monitoring renal function.

Treatment

Treatment for trauma patients with ARF depends on the cause and severity of the failure. Goals of management focus on compensating for the deterioration in renal function. Fluid, electrolyte, and pH balance may be exacerbated by postresuscitation fluid overload, thus making management particularly difficult. Trauma patients have high protein requirements as a result of stress and wound healing. Protein produces urea as a metabolic end product. When levels are elevated, urea can contribute to azotemia. Continuous renal replacement therapy for hemodynamically unstable patients or hemodialysis for the stable trauma patient may be used to manage azotemia. These therapies are initiated early, to optimize the patient's renal function (see Chapter 14).

ALTERED NUTRITION

Nutritional demands of the trauma patient are significantly increased by alterations in metabolism. The critically injured patient develops high energy demands and metabolic alterations leading to a nutritional imbalance. The body's metabolism is increased by activation of the sympathetic response. Other conditions such as hypoxia, pain, decreased fluid volume, anxiety, tissue injury, and decreased resistance to infection further stimulate the sympathetic response, and a hypermetabolic stress state is induced. Available glucose is used rapidly as the provider substrate for energy, followed by initiation of glycogenolysis, and the metabolism of glycogen stores. As high energy demands continue, formation of glucose from stored protein and fats (gluconeogenesis) occurs. This period of metabolic response to injury has been termed the *ebb* or *shock phase* and encompasses a period during the first 24 to 48 hours after injury. During the ebb phase, there may actually be an overall weight gain as a result of fluid retention.

The second, or flow phase, begins at the end of the ebb phase and lasts until recovery. This is a catabolic process. The patient's metabolic rate increases and usually peaks 5 to 10 days after injury. The average increase in metabolic rate ranges from 12% to 20%. During the flow phase, protein catabolism is continuous, and fat often acts as the main energy substrate. Nutritional imbalances easily result from the body's increased caloric and protein needs and the patient's inability to ingest nutritional supplements. Patients may demonstrate decreased body mass, increased metabolic needs, increased oxygen consumption, increased carbon dioxide production,

delayed wound healing, and a weakened immune system (Mechanick & Brett, 2002).

Nutritional Assessment

Baseline nutritional assessments are done early in the critical care phase (see Chapter 5). Assessment data should include a history of the patient's eating habits, weight loss or gain, caloric and protein intake, weight-to-height ratios, anthropometric measures of the triceps skinfold or midarm circumference, and biochemical measures such as creatinine-height index, serum proteins, nitrogen balance, total lymphocyte count, and metabolic rate (Dabrowski & Rombeau, 2000; Mechanick & Brett, 2002).

Nutritional Replacement

Nutritional replacement for the trauma patient should be instituted within 24 to 48 hours of injury. Patients who receive less than required nutritional support for a prolonged period are susceptible to the development of infection, including bacteremia and pneumonia. The route of administration (oral, enteral, or parenteral) and the rate and concentration of nutritional replacement used depend on the severity and type of injury and the expected recovery period. These decisions are best accomplished using a team approach.

Enteral route. The enteral route includes the use of an oronasal gastric feeding tube or, for long-term use, a jejunostomy tube or a PEG tube. If the oronasal gastric feeding route is used, care must be taken to place the tube correctly. This can be accomplished by visualizing the feeding tube on an x-ray film. A weighted Silastic tube in a small French size is ideal because it prevents unnecessary pressure on the nostrils and esophagus. Patients who are receiving nutritional support through the enteral route are monitored for tolerance to the supplements. Intolerance to nutritional formulas is demonstrated by patient complaints of nausea or vomiting, abdominal distention, diarrhea, or abdominal pain. If the patient is unable to communicate, tolerance of the tube feeding is evaluated by assessing for abdominal distention and monitoring of tube feeding residuals every 4 hours as needed. The head of the bed is elevated to 45 degrees to facilitate infusion of the solution and to prevent aspiration. Feedings may be administered by either bolus or continuous infusion. Osmolality of the feeding formula may range from 300 mOsm (isotonic) to 850 mOsm (hypertonic). The starting formula osmolality is usually isotonic.

Parenteral route. Parenteral nutritional support is administered by either partial or total methods.

Partial parenteral nutritional support is infused through the peripheral veins. It is a short-term administration method and must be used in conjunction with administration of lipids. Total parenteral nutritional (TPN) support is instituted in patients who are unable to resume gastrointestinal nutritional intake for a minimum of 5 days because of gastrointestinal trauma, paralytic ileus, bowel obstruction, and/or small bowel fistulas. Lipid administration occurs in conjunction with TPN nutritional support. Electrolyte levels and liver function tests are monitored frequently. Total parenteral nutrition can cause alterations in liver function. Urine urea nitrogen levels and serum prealbumin levels are monitored weekly. Serial serum glucose monitoring every 6 hours may be required to avoid unexpected elevations resulting from the glucose content in the TPN.

Decisions about nutritional support for the trauma patient are made on an individual basis. The goal is to provide the patient with balanced nutritional support. Excess replacement can produce physiological stress on the body by increasing oxygen consumption and carbon dioxide production. Additionally, fatty infiltrates may develop in the liver, thus producing other complications. Inadequate replacement often results in body protein loss, delayed wound healing, and decreased resistance to infectious processes.

MULTIPLE ORGAN DYSFUNCTION SYNDROME

Traumatic injury results in inflammatory, immune, and hormonal responses to the injury. The inflammatory process is necessary for healing. However, excessive inflammation with the release of mediators and activation of lymphocytes results in vasodilation, increased vascular permeability, coagulopathy, and decreased organ perfusion. Decreased organ perfusion occurring within hours of injury results in SIRS and sepsis. Decreased organ perfusion occurring days to weeks after injury may result in MODS (Mattox, Brundage, & Hirshberg, 1999).

MODS is defined as the presence of altered organ function in an acutely ill patient (Casper & Joshi, 2002). Organ systems affected by MODS include the pulmonary, cardiac, gastrointestinal, renal, and neurological systems. The severity of MODS varies from mild transient dysfunction to overwhelming, irreversible failure. Risk factors associated with multiple organ failure in the trauma patient include the presence of SIRS, sepsis, extensive tissue damage and/or necrotic tissue, multiple trauma, hypotensive episodes, inadequate fluid resuscitation, hemorrhagic shock, and multiple transfusions.

A significant problem in treating MODS is an incomplete understanding of its pathophysiology. Bacterial infection is the most common event leading to MODS. Multiple organ failure may occur after a single initial, severe insult (one-hit model) or after a series of insults (two-hit or second-hit model). The first hit (massive tissue injury, hypovolemic shock) activates the inflammatory response with the development of SIRS and, if the initial insult is severe and prolonged, early MODS. The second hit (hypotension, hypoxia, infection) occurs days to weeks after injury and results in an overwhelming inflammatory response producing MODS (Kerton & Civetta, 1999).

Management focuses on prevention, early identification of those patients at risk of developing MODS, elimination of the source of infection, maintenance of tissue oxygenation, and nutritional support. Research continues to evaluate drotrecogin alfa (Xigris) and its effects on outcomes in patients with severe sepsis. It is speculated that the antiinflammatory, antithrombotic, and profibrinolytic properties of the drug are responsible for the reduction in patient mortality (Bernard, 2003).

RESEARCH ANALYSIS

ARTICLE REFERENCE
Epstein, C. D., Peerless, J., & Malangoni, M. (2002). Oxygen transport and organ dysfunction in the older trauma patient. *Heart and Lung, 31*(5), 315-326.

STUDY OVERVIEW
This study was conducted to determine baseline values of cardiac index and oxygen transport variables in the older patient with multiple trauma within 24 hours of admission. The goal of the study was to examine the clinical management of older trauma patients to determine their response to injuries and the pattern of oxygen transport in patients who survived and those who succumbed to their traumatic event. Specific interventions to achieve supranormal levels of oxygen transport were not performed.

Continued

The researchers conducted a descriptive, correlational study of 38 multitraumatized patients who were admitted to a level I trauma center. Subjects were 18 years or older with multiple anatomical regions of injury, blunt mechanism of injury, and pulmonary artery monitoring. Furthermore, patients were distributed by age in the following manner: (1) 18 to 30 years, (2) 31 to 49 years, (3) 50 to 64 years, (4) 65 to 74 years, and (5) older than 74 years.

Data were collected over a 24-month period. The average subject age was 59 years, with 74% of the sample older than 50 years of age. The Injury Severity Score was calculated on all patients and indicated that the more severe the injury was, the higher the score was. Older patients had higher scores than their younger counterparts (13 to 30 years, 20; 31 to 49 years, 15; 50 to 64 years, 40; 65 to 74 years, 26; and older than 74 years, 38). Cardiac index, oxygen delivery (DO_2), and oxygen consumption (VO_2) for patients 50 years and older were significantly lower. Younger patients were able progressively to increase their cardiac index, whereas the older population began low and remained at that level. Similarly, DO_2 values were higher in the younger population when compared with patients who were older than 50 years of age. Patients in each age group were hypermetabolic, as indicated by VO_2 levels. However, older patients exhibited a much lower hypermetabolic response. Older patients had lower values of oxygen transport than did their younger counterparts, yet 20 of 28 older patients survived their serious injuries. The overall mortality rate was 21% (8 of 38 patients). All nonsurvivors were 50 years of age or older. The causes of death were as follows: massive pulmonary embolism (n = 1), cardiogenic shock (n = 1), adult respiratory distress syndrome (n = 1), and multiple organ dysfunction syndrome (n = 5). These data were consistent with the calculation of the Multiple Organ Failure Score. The mean score of survivors was 5.5, compared with 17.7 for nonsurvivors. The results of this study highlight the vulnerability of older trauma patients to poor outcomes. Therefore, additional research is needed to determine the cardiovascular response to resuscitation and the most effective method of management in the elderly patient population.

CRITIQUE

This study highlights the physiological response to trauma in the older patient population and provides a direction for future research needs to determine the best care approach for these patients. Study methods were identified clearly and allow for replication. However, no specific intervention was tested. Sample size was small (n = 38), and factors such as levels of injury, time to definitive treatment, and levels of inotropic agents were not controlled. The researchers identified additional limitations to the study. These include nonprobability sampling and lack of inclusion of patients with injuries of more than 24 hours' duration. Additionally, the characteristics of the patients may have been skewed because most of the patients were older, from outlying facilities, and had a greater degree of underlying medical history, more severe injuries, and greater involvement in transportation-related injuries.

NURSING IMPLICATIONS FOR PRACTICE

Providing adequate oxygenation and ensuring tissue perfusion remain the primary priorities for the critical care nurse. Current trends in critical care are to prevent untoward patient events through the prevention, detection, and intervention of inadequate tissue perfusion. Monitoring of oxygen transport variables such as cardiac output, cardiac index, DO_2, and VO_2 provides the practitioner with opportunities to intervene and correct abnormal perfusion indicators to prevent the sequelae of organ failure with resultant multiple organ dysfunction syndrome. This research has demonstrated the need for aggressive monitoring to detect inadequate global perfusion abnormalities in the older population. These subjects illustrated a decreased ability to compensate for their injuries and inadequate perfusion as compared with their younger counterparts. Nurses must recognize cardiac dysfunction, inadequate DO_2 and delivery of substrate to the tissues, and ineffective utilization of those substrates. This research has highlighted the need for further research to address the most effective method to treat the older population in the event of inadequate tissue perfusion.

CONTINUING CARE

Trauma patients require specialized nursing care during their critical care hospitalization. Nurses play a pivotal role in the care of the multitraumatized patient in the acute care setting. Prevention of complications that prolong hospitalization and delay rehabilitation is imperative. The initiation of the rehabilitative process begins the moment the patient is admitted to the trauma center. Early involvement of the physical, medicine, and rehabilitation personnel is vital to positive functional patient outcomes.

Patients should minimally be evaluated weekly to identify rehabilitation needs, and the plan of care should be modified to optimize the patient's rehabilitative goals.

Positive rehabilitation outcomes can be achieved with early mobilization, nutritional support, education, and psychological support. This process is best accomplished by a multidisciplinary approach involving the physician, nursing staff, social service, physical therapists, occupational therapists, and family members.

 ## Case Study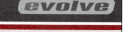

B. G., a 24-year-old male and minor league baseball player, was a restrained driver involved in a high-speed motor vehicle crash on April 20. B. G. was hit on the driver's side by the other automobile and subsequently collided with a tree. Glasgow Coma Score (GCS) at the scene was 3T (Eye [E]: 1, Motor [M]: 1, Verbal [V]: 1, Tubed [T], unresponsive). Extrication time was prolonged at 30 minutes. The patient's initial vital signs were as follows: blood pressure (BP), 112/54 mm Hg; heart rate (HR), 136 beats/min; and respiratory rate, 30 breaths/min. At the scene, intravenous (IV) access was established, and he was intubated. The patient was transported via helicopter to a level I trauma center. During transport, he developed a transient decline of his vital signs with a decrease in HR to 112 beats/min, BP to 98/50 mm Hg, and RR of 20 to 26 breaths/min via a resuscitative bag. He responded to an increase in fluid rate and received 1 L of IV lactated Ringer's solution during transport. His vital signs on arrival in the emergency department were as follows: HR, 101 beats/min; BP, 120/58 mm Hg; and pulse oximetry oxygen saturation, 100%. Lungs were clear to auscultation bilaterally, and bilateral pulses were present in all four extremities. GCS remained at 3T. Pupils were unequal, with the left pupil approximately 5 mm in size and the right approximately 3 mm in size. Both pupils were sluggishly reactive to light. On secondary survey, a 6-cm laceration was present in the right frontal temporal area of his head with significant active bleeding. His upper teeth were broken, and he had a possible maxillary fracture. Examination of the neck was unremarkable. His trachea was midline. There were no obvious deformities of the cervical spine. A left chest contusion was present, and a right clavicular deformity was visualized. His abdomen was soft and nondistended, with audible bowel sounds. His pelvis was stable to palpation. A rectal examination revealed decreased tone,

and stool was guaiac negative. Contusion and ecchymoses were seen on his left upper arm, left upper thigh, and the anterior aspect of his right lower extremity. No gross deformities were visualized.

A focused abdominal sonography for trauma (FAST) examination was completed in the emergency department and showed no signs of intraabdominal free fluid. Initial arterial blood gases (ABGs) showed the following: pH, 7.42; $PaCO_2$, 29 mm Hg; PaO_2, 200 mm Hg; HCO_3^-, 22; base deficit, −1. Chest x-ray study showed a right clavicular fracture and left eleventh rib fracture without evidence of pneumothorax or effusion. Cervical spine films from C1 to T1 showed no fracture or subluxation. Pelvic x-ray film showed left superior and bilateral inferior pubic rami fractures and a left sacral fracture. A questionable fracture in the trochanter area of the left femur was visualized. Hemostasis of the right frontal temporal laceration was obtained with manual pressure and subsequent surgical repair.

A Foley catheter was placed, with some gross hematuria, which immediately cleared. Mannitol, 25 g IV, was given for unequal pupillary size. A 12-lead electrocardiogram (ECG) was performed and showed sinus tachycardia. B. G. also received a tetanus toxoid injection and cefazolin (Kefzol), 1 g IV. He was transferred to the radiology department for a head and abdominal computed tomography (CT) scan and then to the surgical intensive care unit (SICU). The head CT scan revealed right caudate and right frontal contusions with a significant subarachnoid hemorrhage and intraventricular hemorrhage. A facial CT scan confirmed bilateral maxillary fractures. Abdominal CT scan confirmed a pelvic fracture with a small pelvic hematoma and a left renal contusion.

On B. G.'s arrival in the SICU, physicians from the neurosurgery, orthopedics, and physical medicine and rehabilitation departments were consulted.

Continued

Case Study—cont'd

Decorticate posturing was noted during the neurological assessment, and a fiberoptic intracranial pressure (ICP) monitor was inserted with an opening pressure of 7 mm Hg. The orthopedic surgeons decided to manage his pelvic fractures medically with non–weight bearing bilaterally for 6 weeks. Fluid resuscitation continued through his first 24 hours of admission, and his ICP ranged from 3 to 18 mm Hg. Over the next 3 days, his neurological function slowly improved to a GCS of 3T to 7T (E: 2, M: 4, V: 1T, intubated). The patient's ICP remained less than 20 mm Hg. Flexion withdrawal to pain was noted. A magnetic resonance imaging scan of the head was done on April 24 and showed multiple areas of hemorrhagic and nonhemorrhagic contusions with no signs of significant brainstem injury. On day 5, heparin, 5000 units subcutaneously, was ordered for DVT prophylaxis. His prognosis for recovery was guarded, although significant recovery could occur after several months of rehabilitation.

B. G. remained ventilator dependent. Twenty days after admission, a tracheotomy and a percutaneous endoscopic gastrostomy (PEG) were placed. Internal maxillary fixation was performed in the operating room with a mechanical fixator. His GCS improved from 7T to 9T (E: 3, M: 5, V: 1T, tracheostomy). He developed a fever, and pneumonia was diagnosed. He remained hemodynamically stable, and his ICP monitor was discontinued. A venous duplex examination was negative for DVT. On day 9 of his hospitalization, he developed a sudden rise in his temperature to 39.4°C, and he had a heart rate of 180 beats/min and a respiratory rate of 32 breaths/min. Cultures of the patient's blood, sputum, and urine were obtained, and the patient was started on a broad-spectrum antibiotic. ABGs revealed the following: pH, 7.37; $PaCO_2$, 33 mm Hg; PaO_2, 63 mm Hg; HCO_3^- 25, base excess, +1; and SaO_2 91%. Appropriate changes were made to his ventilator to improve oxygenation. His HR increased quickly to 220 beats/min and was identified on a 12-lead ECG as supraventricular tachycardia. Adenosine, 6 mg IV, was given, followed immediately by a 10 mL saline bolus to slow his HR. An esmolol infusion was started, and acetaminophen (Tylenol) was given per rectum. A ventilation/perfusion scan showed an intermediate probability of a pulmonary embolism (PE), and a pulmonary angiogram was negative for a PE. On April 30, an inferior vena cava (IVC) filter was placed prophylactically to prevent a PE.

Over the next several days, his neurological status slowly improved (GCS 10T: E: 4, M: 5, V: 1T), and he was weaned from mechanical ventilation. The esmolol infusion was stopped. However, he remained febrile. A search for an infection as a source of his fever continued, and the infectious disease experts were consulted. A repeat chest CT scan revealed a left lower lobe infiltrate and a small pleural effusion. Sinusitis was diagnosed after the development of brown purulent drainage from his bilateral nares. The patient's sinuses were drained by the ear, nose, and throat physicians. Antibiotics were changed, and his fevers diminished. On May 7, he was transferred to the stepdown unit. On May 9, B. G. was afebrile for the first time for more than 24 hours, and on May 14, he was transferred to the physical medicine and rehabilitation service. His GCS was 11T (E: 4, M: 6, V 1T). At this time, he was able to follow some commands with his right arm. He did not attempt to speak or mouth words. He required maximum assistance for all self-care skills and wheelchair skills. He was non–weight bearing on the left leg because of his pelvic fracture. He had decreased attention and poor object recognition. Tube feedings were provided through his PEG tube. Airway management with humidified oxygen was maintained through the tracheotomy tube. A modified barium swallow showed a normal swallow mechanism with some difficulty in the oral phase because of the mechanical fixator. A blenderized diet was begun, with tube feeding infusion for only 18 hours each day. On May 30, the rubber bands were removed from his jaw wiring, and opening and closing exercises were initiated with his mandible. On June 5, his tracheotomy tube was removed. Standing and walking exercises were begun. On June 20, the PEG tube was removed. On July 5, B. G. went home with his wife on a weekend pass, with no problems reported. B. G. was discharged home on July 11 and required minimal assistance for self-care skills and walking. He did require a wide-based quad cane. He continued to receive outpatient physical therapy, occupational therapy, and speech therapy and was followed-up by the traumatic brain injury clinic.

QUESTIONS

1. Describe the priorities for care based on the patient's primary and secondary survey.
2. List the injuries B. G. had and describe the potential complications.
3. What interventions contributed to B. G.'s positive outcome?

SUMMARY

Trauma is a leading cause of death in people between the ages of 1 and 44 years. It is considered to be preventable, unlike cardiovascular disease, cancer, and cerebrovascular accidents. Patient survival after traumatic injury depends on prompt, rapid, systematic assessment in conjunction with immediate resuscitative interventions. Evaluation of airway patency, ventilation, and venous access with circulatory support takes precedence over other diagnostic interventions. The goal is to restore oxygen to the body tissues, to stop the progression of shock, and to prevent long-term complications.

CRITICAL THINKING QUESTIONS
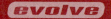

1. A patient presents to the critical care unit with a gunshot wound to the left lower anterior chest from a 0.45-caliber semiautomatic weapon. What additional prehospital information would be helpful? Considering the mechanism of injury and location of the entrance wound, describe the potential patterns of injury. What are the immediate management priorities?

2. After operative repair, this patient is admitted to the critical care unit. Describe the assessment and intervention priorities during the first postoperative hour.

3. Massive fluid resuscitation may be necessary after traumatic injury. What are the complications of massive fluid resuscitation?

4. What are the management priorities for a patient with a traumatic brain injury?

REFERENCES

American College of Surgeons, Committee on Trauma. (1997). *Advanced trauma life support for doctors: Instructor's course manual.* 6th ed. Chicago: American College of Surgeons.

American College of Surgeons, Committee on Trauma. (1998). *Resources for optimal care of the injured patient 1999.* Chicago: American College of Surgeons.

Anderson, R. E., Drayer, B. P., Braffman, B., et al. (1999). ACR appropriateness criteria for spine trauma. Retrieved from http://guidelines.gov. Accessed 7/8/2004. Also in *Radiology, 215*[Suppl], 589-595.

Anonymous. (2002). Cervical spine immobilization before admission to the hospital. *Neurosurgery, 50*[3 Suppl], S7-S17.

Beachley, M. (2002). Evolution of the trauma cycle. In K. A. McQuillan, K. T. Von Rueden, R. L. Hartsock, M. B. Flynn, & E. Whalen (eds.). *Trauma nursing from resuscitation through rehabilitation* [pp. 2-18]. Philadelphia: W. B. Saunders.

Beetham, R. (2000). Biochemical investigation of suspected rhabdomyolysis. *Annals of Clinical Biochemistry, 37,* 581-587.

Bernard, G. R. (2003). Drotrecogin alfa (activated) (recombinant human activated protein C) for the treatment of severe sepsis. *Critical Care Medicine, 31*(1), S85-S93.

Biem, J, Koehncke, N, & Dosman, J. (2003). Out of the cold: Management of hypothermia and frostbite. *Canadian Medical Association Journal, 168*(3), 305-311.

Bower, R. G, Ware, L. B, Berthiaume, Y., & Matthay, M. A. (2001). Treatment of ARDS. *Chest, 120*(4), 1347-1367.

Brain Trauma Foundation. (2000). Guidelines for prehospital management of traumatic brain injury. Retrieved from http://guidelines.gov. Accessed 7/8/2004.

Bulger, E. M., Nathens, A. V., Rivara, F. P., Moore, M., MacKenzie, E. J., Jurkovich, G. J. (2002). Management of severe head injury: Institutional variations in care and effect on outcome. *Critical Care Medicine, 30*(8), 1870-1876.

Casper, P. B., & Joshi, M. (2002). Infection and infection control. In K. A. McQuillan, K. T. Von Rueden, R. L. Hartsock, M. B. Flynn, & E. Whalen (eds.). *Trauma nursing from resuscitation through rehabilitation* [pp. 222-239]. Philadelphia: W. B. Saunders.

Centers for Disease Control and Prevention. (2002). Centers for Disease Control: Injury fact book 2001-2001. Retrieved from http://www.cdc.gov. Accessed 7/8/2004.

Cornwell, E. E., Chang, D. C., Donar, J. P., et al. (2001). Thoracolumbar immobilization for trauma patients with torso gunshot wounds. Is it necessary? *Archives of Surgery, 136,* 324-326.

Deitch, E. A., Livingston, D. H., & Hauser, C. J. (1999). Septic complications in the trauma patient. *New Horizons, 7*(1), 158-172.

Dabrowski, G. P., & Rombeau, J. L. (2000). Practical nutritional management in the trauma intensive care unit. *Surgical Clinics of North America, 80*(3), 921-932.

Drummond, J. C., & Petrovitch, C. T. (2001). The massively bleeding patient. *Anesthesiology Clinics of North America, 19*(4), 633-649.

Eastern Association for the Surgery of Trauma. (2000). Determination of cervical spine stability in trauma patients. Retrieved from http://guidelines.gov. Accessed 7/8/2004.

Emergency Nurses Association. (2000). *Trauma nursing core course: Provider manual.* 5th ed. Des Plaines, IL: Emergency Nurses Association.

Emergency Nurses Association. (2003). *Course in advanced trauma nursing. II: A conceptual approach to injury and illness.* 2nd ed. Dubuque, IA: Kendall/Hunt.

Ferrera, P. C., Bartfield, J. M., & D'Andrea, C. C. (2000). Outcomes of admitted geriatric trauma victims. *American Journal of Emergency Medicine, 18*(5), 575-580.

Fowler, R., & Pepe, P. E. (2002). Prehospital care of the patient with major trauma. *Emergency Medicine Clinics of North America, 20*(4), 953-974.

Grossman, M. D. (2002). When is an elder old? Effect of preexisting conditions on mortality in geriatric trauma. *Journal of Trauma, 52*(2), 242-246.

Hauswald, M. (2002). Spine immobilization in trauma patients: Is it really necessary? *Current Opinion in Critical Care, 8*(6), 566-570.

Inamasu, J., & Ichikizaki, K. (2002). Mild hypothermia in neurologic emergency: An update. *Annals of Emergency Medicine, 40*(2), 220-230.

Kerton, O. C., & Civetta, J. M. (1999). Ischemic reperfusion in the critically ill: A progenitor of multiple organ failure. *New Horizons, 7*(1), 87-95.

King, B. S., Gupta, R., & Narayan, R. K. (2000). Early issues in the intensive care unit: The second golden hour. *Surgical Clinics of North America, 80*(3), 855-870.

Klein, D. G. (1999). Management strategies for improving outcome following severe head injury. *Critical Care Nursing Clinics of North America, 11*(2), 209-225.

Kouraklis, G. (2002). Damage control surgery: An alternative approach for the management of critically injured patients. *Surgery Today, 32*(3), 195-202.

Littlejohns, L. R., Bader, M. K., & March, K. (2003). Brain tissue oxygen monitoring in severe brain injury. I. Research and usefulness in critical care. *Critical Care Nurse, 23*(4), 17-25.

March, J. A. (2002). Changes in physical examination caused by use of spinal immobilization. *Prehospital Emergency Care, 6*(4), 421-424.

Mattox, K. L., Brundage, S. I., & Hirshberg, A. (1999). Initial resuscitation. *New Horizons, 7*(1), 4-9.

Mechanick, J. I., & Brett, E. M. (2002). Nutrition support of the chronically ill patient. *Critical Care Clinics, 18*(3), 597-618.

Mikhail, J. (1999). The trauma triad of death: Hypothermia, acidosis, and coagulopathy. *AACN Clinical Issues, 10*(1), 85-94.

O'Grady, N. P., Alexander, M., Dellinger, E. P., et al. (2002). Guidelines for the prevention of intravascular catheter-related infections. *Morbidity and Mortality Weekly Report, 52*(10), 1-29.

Orlinsky, M., Shoemaker, W., Reis, E. D., Kerstein, M. D. (2001). Current controversies in shock and resuscitation. *Surgical Clinics of North America, 81*(6), 1217-1262.

Rocha, A. T., & Tapson, V. F. (2003). Venous thromboembolism in intensive care patients. *Clinics in Chest Medicine, 24*(1), 103-133.

Sherwood, S. F., & Hartsock, R. L. (2002). Thoracic injuries. In K. A. McQuillan, K. T. Von Rueden, R. L. Hartsock, M. B. Flynn, & E. Whalen (eds.). *Trauma nursing from resuscitation through rehabilitation* [pp. 543-590]. Philadelphia: W. B. Saunders.

Silverstein, J. H., Apfelbaum, J. L., Barlow, J. C., et al. (2002). Practice guidelines for postanesthetic care. *Anesthesiology, 96*, 742-752.

Tierney, L. M., McPhee, S. J., & Papadakis, M. A. (2002). *Current medial diagnosis and treatment: Adult ambulatory and inpatient management.* New York: Lange Medical Books/McGraw-Hill.

Udobi, K. E, Childs, E., & Touijer, K. (2003). Acute respiratory distress syndrome. *American Family Physician, 67*(2), 315-322.

Van Den Berghe, G., Wouers, P., Weekers, F., et al. (2001). Intensive insulin therapy in critically ill patients. *New England Journal of Medicine, 345*(19), 1359-1367.

Walsh, C. R. (2002). Musculoskeletal injuries. In K. A. McQuillan, K. T. Von Rueden,, R. L. Hartsock, M. B. Flynn, & E. Whalen (eds.). *Trauma nursing from resuscitation through rehabilitation* [pp. 646-689]. Philadelphia: W. B. Saunders.

Weigelt, J. A., & Klein, J. D. (2002). Mechanisms of injury. In K. A. McQuillan, K. T. Von Rueden,, R. L. Hartsock, M. B. Flynn, & E. Whalen (eds.). *Trauma nursing from resuscitation through rehabilitation* [pp. 149-172]. Philadelphia: W. B. Saunders.

Yoshikawa, T. T., & Norman, D. C. (2000). *Acute emergencies and critical care of the geriatric patient.* New York: Marcel Dekker.

Zink, B. J. (2001). Traumatic brain injury outcome: Concepts for emergency care. *Annals of Emergency Medicine, 37*(3), 318-322.

RECOMMENDED READINGS

Krajewski, B. (2002). Emergency nurse's response to terrorism. *International Journal of Trauma Nursing, 8*(2), 62-64.

Matthews, B. G. (2002). Should families be allowed in trauma resuscitations? *International Journal of Trauma Nursing, 8*(3), 84-85.

evolve *Did you remember to check out the bonus material, including free self-assessment exercises, on the Evolve Web site at http://evolve.elsevier.com/Sole/ and on the CD-ROM?*

CHAPTER **19**

Burns

Karla S. Ahrns, BSN, RN, CCRP

OBJECTIVES

- Review the anatomy and physiology of the integumentary system.
- Describe the pathophysiology of burns.
- Compare the types of burn injuries.
- Discuss the primary and secondary survey assessments during resuscitation and the acute phases of burn management.
- Formulate a plan of care for the patient with a burn injury.
- Relate the nursing diagnoses, outcomes, and interventions for the burned patient.

Introduction

There is no greater challenge in critical care nursing than caring for a severely burned patient. It is estimated that burns result in 4500 deaths, 61,000 acute hospital admissions, and 700,000 total injuries annually in the United States (Brigham & Quinn, 2003). Initial management of the seriously injured burn patient can dramatically affect the patient's long-term outcome. Therefore, many burn patients are treated in hospitals with special capabilities for managing extensive burn injuries. However, even with the expanded network of burn center facilities, most patients are first seen in the community hospital. Consequently, it is crucial that emergency department (ED) and critical care nurses have the skills necessary to provide initial resuscitative care to

burn-injured patients. Care of the burned patient requires a multidisciplinary team approach to maximize favorable patient outcomes.

Burn injuries have significant economic and social consequences, as well as marked morbidity and mortality. Historically, burn injuries have been one of the most lethal forms of trauma. However, application of research-based advances in fluid resuscitation, early excision and closure of the wound, respiratory and metabolic support, microbial surveillance, and infection control have dramatically improved survival and recovery from burn injury (Barret & Herndon, 2003a; Redlick et al., 2002; Wraa, 2003). Even with these improvements, morbidity and mortality remain significant in patients with burns greater than 50% of total body surface area (TBSA) (ABA, 2002).

evolve Be sure to check out the bonus material, including free self-assessment exercises, on the Evolve Web site at http://evolve.elsevier.com/Sole/ and on the CD-ROM.

Elderly and young patients with a smaller percentage of burned areas involved are also at considerable risk of mortality (ABA, 2002; Brandt, Ahrns, & Wahl, 2003). Knowledge of the physiological changes and the potential complications associated with burn injury prepares the critical care nurse to care for these complex patients and to optimize their outcome.

Review of Anatomy and Physiology of the Skin

The skin, also called the integumentary system, is the largest organ of the body. It is a vital organ because of its many functions, including protective barrier status against infection and injury, regulation of fluid loss, thermoregulatory (or body heat) control, synthesis of vitamin D, sensory contact with the environment, determination of identity, and presentable cosmetic appearance. The skin is composed of two layers, the *epidermis* and the *dermis*, with an underlying *subcutaneous* fat tissue layer that binds the dermis to organs and tissues of the body (Figure 19-1). The epidermis

is the outermost and thinnest skin layer. The dermis is considerably thicker and contains collagen and elastic fibers, blood and lymph vessels, sweat glands, hair follicles, sebaceous glands, and sensory fibers for the detection of pain, pressure, touch, and temperature. The underlying subcutaneous tissue is a layer of connective tissue and fat deposits. When an extensive amount of skin is damaged from burn injury, alterations of these multiple physiological and psychological characteristics place the patient at risk for complications and/or poor outcome.

Mechanisms of Injury

There are three types of burn injuries: thermal, chemical, and electrical. These types of injuries can also occur in conjunction with inhalation injury. Inhalation injury is observed in 20% to 50% of patients admitted to burn centers and significantly increases the risk of death (ABA, 2001). Approximately 90% of burn injuries are thermally induced. Chemical and electrical burns account for the remaining 10% of the injuries (ABA, 2001). Although the primary principles

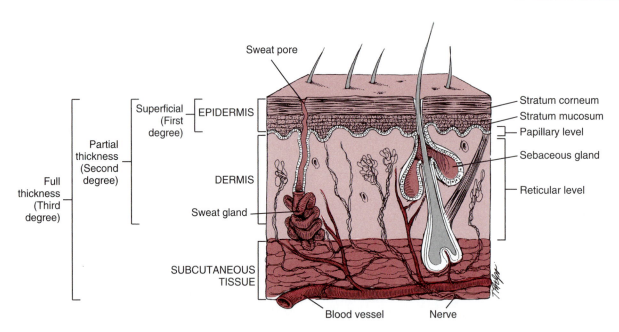

FIGURE 19-1 Anatomy of the skin. The depth of the injury determines whether a burn will heal or require skin grafting. First- and second-degree burns heal because they are superficial and partial-thickness burns; thus, the elements necessary to generate new skin remain. Often, deep partial-thickness injuries are grafted for improved functional and cosmetic reasons. Full-thickness injury destroys all dermal appendages and requires skin grafting for achievement of wound closure. (Modified from Flynn, M. B. [2002]. Wound healing. In K. A. McQuillan, K. T. Von Rueden, R. L. Hartsock, M. B. Flynn, & E. Wahlen [eds.]. *Trauma nursing: From resuscitation through rehabilitation*. 3rd ed. Philadelphia: W. B. Saunders.)

of care are the same for all burn injuries regardless of cause, chemical and electrical burns require special initial management and ongoing assessment, as discussed later in this chapter.

THERMAL INJURIES

Thermal injury is caused when the skin comes in contact with a source of sufficient temperature to cause cell injury by coagulation. This can occur from flame (e.g., house fires, ignition of clothing, explosion of gases), scalding liquids (e.g., water, cooking oil, grease), steam (e.g., car radiators, cooking pots, industrial equipment), or direct contact with a heat source (e.g., space heater, metal). The severity of injury is related to heat intensity and duration of contact. For example, a heat source of less than 40° C (111.2° F) does not cause a burn regardless of the length of exposure. However, the extent of damage increases with temperatures greater than this level, in direct proportion to the duration of exposure. Exposure to temperatures of 60° C (140° F) causes full-thickness tissue destruction (third-degree burns) in as little as 3 to 5 seconds. This poses an interesting injury prevention issue, because 140° F is a common setting for home water heaters despite recommendations of maintaining temperature settings of less than 120° F (49° C). Children and the elderly are at greater risk of thermal injury at lower temperatures because of their thinner skin and their decreased agility in moving to avoid harm.

CHEMICAL INJURIES

Chemical burns can be caused by contact, inhalation of fumes, ingestion, or injection. Although chemical injuries account for only a small percentage of admissions to burn centers, they can be severe, and they have both local and systemic effects. The severity of injury is related to type, volume, duration of contact, and concentration of the agent. Tissue damage from chemical burns continues until the chemical is completely removed or neutralized. Chemical agents are part of our lifestyle. Thus, the potential for injury from exposure is great. Occupational Safety and Health Administration law requires that employees receive educational training regarding hazardous materials in the workplace and that Material Safety Data Sheets (MSDSs) are posted in work areas. MSDSs list specific information on all chemicals in the workplace including composition, side effects, and potential for systemic toxicity. The Joint Commission on the Accreditation of Healthcare Organizations also monitors compliance with this mandatory regulation in the hospital environment.

Three categories of chemical agents exist: alkalies, acids, and organic compounds. Alkalies are commonly found in cleaning products used in the home and industry, such as oven cleaners, wet cement, and fertilizers. This category of chemical agents can produce far more damage than acids because alkalies loosen tissue by protein denaturation and liquefaction necrosis, thereby allowing the chemical to diffuse more deeply into the tissue. Furthermore, alkalies bind to tissue proteins and make it more difficult to stop the burning process.

Acids are found in many household and industrial products, such as bathroom cleansers, rust removers, and acidifiers for home swimming pools. Depth of burn injury from acids (except hydrofluoric acid) tends to be more limited because acids cause coagulation necrosis of tissue and precipitation of protein. Hydrofluoric acid is a weak acid. However, the fluoride ion is very toxic because it causes hypocalcemia by rapidly binding to free calcium in the blood.

Organic compounds, such as phenols and petroleum products (e.g., gasoline, chemical disinfectants), can produce cutaneous burns as well as be absorbed and have systemic effects. Phenols cause severe coagulation necrosis of dermal proteins and can produce a layer of thick, nonviable tissue called *eschar* (ABA, 2001). Petroleum products such as gasoline promote cell membrane injury and dissolution of lipids with resulting skin necrosis. Systemic effects such as central nervous system depression, hypothermia, hypotension, pulmonary edema, and intravascular hemolysis may be severe or even fatal. Chemical pneumonitis and bronchitis may occur from inhalation of fumes. Other complications observed with gasoline burns include hepatic and renal failure and sudden death (ABA, 2001).

ELECTRICAL INJURIES

Electrical injury is caused by contact with such varied sources as household current, car batteries, electrosurgical devices, high-tension electric lines, and lightning. Injuries are arbitrarily classified as high-voltage (more than 1000 volts) or low-voltage (less than 1000 volts) injuries (ABA, 2001; Koumbourlis, 2002). Tissue damage is the result of conversion of energy into heat. Many factors can affect the degree of injury: type and pathway of current, duration of contact, environmental conditions, and the resistance offered by body tissues. Electricity follows the path of least resistance, with nerve tissue offering the least resistance and bone tissue the greatest resistance. Therefore, nerves, blood vessels, and muscles are at high risk of damage or degeneration (Wraa, 2003). Current density and thus the greatest heat dissipation are at the point of entry or exit, which is typically on the extremities. Although alternating (AC) and direct current (DC) are both dangerous, AC has a greater probability of producing cardiopulmonary arrest by fibrillation and has a tetanic muscle contraction effect that may "lock" the patient to the source of electricity and cause respiratory muscle paralysis. Electrical injury wounds are extremely variable in presentation. There may be a small burn at the point of contact, or there may be a craterlike "blowout" wound. Even though the wound may appear minimal or superficial on initial presentation, it may manifest as an extensive, deep wound with neurological impairment several days or weeks later. This occurs as high-voltage current ceases, and the superficial tissues begin to cool more rapidly than the deeper tissues and bony structures (Koumbourlis, 2002). Consequently, deep tissue necrosis occurs beneath viable more superficial tissue.

Lightning injury is caused by a direct strike or a side flash that causes a flow of current between the person and a close object that is struck by lightning (ABA, 2001). Cutaneous injury is often superficial because the current travels on the surface of the body rather than through it. Lightning injuries frequently result in cardiopulmonary arrest. Approximately 70% of survivors suffer transient but severe central nervous system deficits (ABA, 2001).

INHALATION INJURY

Lung injury secondary to the inhalation of smoke and products of incomplete combustion is associated with increased mortality (ABA, 2001). Inhalation injury is classified as (1) injury from carbon monoxide (CO), (2) injury above the glottis, and (3) injury below the glottis (ABA, 2001). Table 19-1 summarizes characteristics of each type of injury. Inhalation injury may be the reason for admission to a critical care unit, even when there are no cutaneous surface burns.

Carbon Monoxide Poisoning

CO poisoning is the most frequent cause of death at the burn scene (ABA, 2001). CO is released when organic compounds, such as wood or coal, are burned. CO has an affinity for hemoglobin 200 times greater than that of oxygen (ABA, 2001). Therefore, when CO is inhaled, it binds to hemoglobin (*carboxyhemoglobin* [COHgb]) and prevents the red blood cell from transporting oxygen to body tissues, thus leading to hypoxia. CO poisoning can be difficult to detect, because it may not present with significant clinical findings. Therefore, it is important to measure COHgb levels, which are reported as a percentage of hemoglobin molecules bound with CO. Death generally ensues with COHgb levels greater than 60%. Loss of consciousness occurs at COHgb levels of 40% to 60%. Central nervous system dysfunction of varying

TABLE 19-1	
Types of Smoke Inhalation Injury	
Type of Injury	**Pathology**
Carbon monoxide poisoning	Carbon monoxide binds to hemoglobin molecules more rapidly than does oxygen molecules; tissue hypoxia results
Inhalation injury above the glottis	Most often a thermal injury; heat absorption and damage occur mostly in the pharynx and larynx; may cause obstruction after resuscitation is initiated
Inhalation injury below the glottis	Usually a chemical injury that produces impaired ciliary activity, erythema, hypersecretion, edema, ulceration of mucosa, increased blood flow, and spasm of bronchi and/or bronchioles

Modified from American Burn Association. (2001). *Advanced burn life support course: Instructor's manual*. Chicago: American Burn Association.

degrees (e.g., restlessness, confusion) occurs at levels of 15% to 40%. Levels lower than 10% to 15% can be found in mild CO poisoning, but they are also commonly associated with heavy smokers (see Laboratory Alerts: Carboxyhemoglobin).

Injury Above the Glottis

Inhalation injuries above the glottis, also referred to as upper airway injuries, are caused by breathing in heat or noxious chemicals produced during the burning process. The nose, mouth, and throat dissipate the heat and prevent damage to lower airways. However, the resulting upper airway thermal injury causes edema, thereby placing the patient at high risk of airway obstruction. Airway obstruction clinically presents as hoarseness, dry cough, labored or rapid breathing, difficulty swallowing, or stridor.

Injury Below the Glottis

Injuries below the glottis are almost always caused by breathing noxious chemical by-products of burning materials and smoke, and these injuries can cause extensive damage to alveoli and impair pulmonary functioning (see Table 19-1). A hallmark sign is *carbonaceous sputum* (soot or carbon particles in

LABORATORY ALERTS: CARBOXYHEMOGLOBIN

Carboxyhemoglobin Level*	Clinical Presentation
<10% to 15%	Commonly associated with heavy smokers; may indicate mild carbon monoxide poisoning: headache, flushing, impaired visual acuity
15% to 40%	Central nervous system dysfunction: restlessness, confusion, impaired dexterity, dizziness, nausea/vomiting
40% to 60%	Loss of consciousness, tachycardia, tachypnea
>60%	Coma; death generally ensues

*Percentage of hemoglobin molecules bound with carbon monoxide.

secretions). Tracheal and bronchial/bronchiolar constriction and spasms with resulting wheezing can occur within minutes to several hours after injury (ABA, 2001). Acute respiratory failure and acute respiratory distress syndrome may develop within the first few days. Respiratory tract mucosal sloughing may occur within 4 to 5 days. Admission chest x-rays are typically normal. However, later x-rays may display reduced lung expansion, collapse of alveoli (atelectasis), and diffuse lung edema or infiltrates. Fiberoptic bronchoscopy or ventilation/perfusion lung scanning (with xenon or technetium) may be indicated to provide a definitive diagnosis of injury below the glottis (ABA Evidence-Based Guidelines Group, 2001).

Burn Classification and Severity

Burn injury severity is determined by the type of burn injury, burn wound characteristics (depth, extent, body part burned), concomitant injuries, patient age, and preexisting health status. Properly classifying and assessing the severity of injury allow appropriate triage and transfer of patients to a burn center (Clinical Alert: Guidelines for Burn Center Referral). The extent and depth of burn injury are affected by duration of contact with the injuring agent, the temperature of the agent, the amount of tissue exposed, and the ability of the agent and tissue to dissipate the thermal energy.

DEPTH OF INJURY

Burn depth predicts wound care treatment requirements, determines the need for skin grafting, and affects scarring, cosmetic, and functional outcomes. Burn injuries are commonly classified as first-, second-, or third-degree burns. However, using the terms *superficial, partial-thickness,* or *full-thickness* burns more closely correlates with burn injury pathophysiology and the level of affected skin layer involvement (see Figure 19-1). Accurate depth assessment may be difficult to determine initially, because progressive edema formation and compromised wound blood flow during the first 48 to 72 hours after injury may increase the definitive burn depth. Physiological changes associated with burn injury are discussed later in the chapter.

Superficial burns involve only the first layer of skin or the epidermis (hence termed first-degree injury), and typically heal in 3 to 5 days without treatment. Because superficial burn injuries (e.g., sunburns) only cause erythema and do not involve the dermis, they are not included in the calculation of size of burn (extent of injury) used for fluid resuscitation requirements. *Partial-thickness* burns involve injury of the

CLINICAL ALERT: GUIDELINES FOR BURN CENTER REFERRAL

- Partial-thickness burns >10% total body surface area
- Full-thickness burns
- Burns involving the face, hands, feet, genitalia, perineum, or major joints
- Chemical and electrical (including lightning) burns
- Presence of inhalation injury
- Preexisting medical conditions
- Associated trauma
- Hospitals without qualified personnel or equipment to care for burn-injured children

TABLE 19-2

Depth of Burn Injury

Degree of Injury	Morphology	Healing Time	Wound Characteristics
Superficial (First degree)	Destruction of epidermis only	3 to 5 days	Red, dry, painful; blisters rarely present
Superficial partial-thickness (Second degree)	Destruction of epidermis and some dermis	10 to 21 days	Moist, pink or mottled red; very painful; blisters; blanches with pressure
Deep partial-thickness (Second degree)	Destruction of epidermis and most of dermis; some skin appendages remain	3 to 6 weeks	Pale, mottled, pearly red/white; moist or somewhat dry; typically less painful; blanching decreased and prolonged; difficult to distinguish from full-thickness injury
Full-thickness (Third degree)	Destruction of epidermis, dermis, and underlying subcutaneous tissue	Does not heal; requires skin grafting	Thick, leathery eschar; dry; white, cherry-red or brown-black; painless; does not blanch with pressure; thrombosed blood vessels

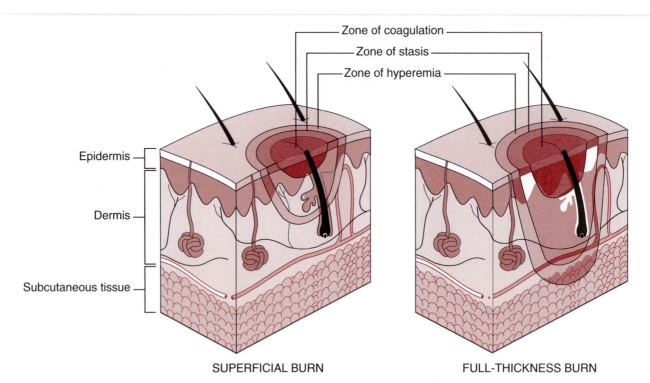

FIGURE 19-2 Zones of thermal injury. The zone of coagulation is the site of irreversible skin death. The zone of hyperemia is the site of minimal cell involvement and early spontaneous recovery. In the zone of stasis, secondary insults such as inadequate resuscitation or infection result in conversion of this potentially salvageable area to full-thickness skin destruction with irreversible cell death. (Modified from Cornwell, P. & Gregory, C. Management of clients with burn injury. In J. M. Black and J. H. Hawks. [eds.] [2005]. *Medical-surgical nursing: Clinical management for positive outcomes.* 7th ed. Philadelphia: W. B. Saunders.)

second skin layer or dermal layer (hence a second-degree injury), and are further subdivided into superficial and deep classifications. *Superficial partial-thickness* injuries that involve the epidermis and a limited portion of the dermis heal by growth of undamaged basal cells within 10 to 21 days. *Deep partial-thickness* injuries involve destruction of the epidermis and most of the dermis. Although such wounds may heal spontaneously within 3 to 6 weeks, they are typically excised and grafted to achieve better functional and cosmetic results and to decrease the length of healing time and hospitalization. Destruction of all layers of the skin down to or past the subcutaneous fat, fascia, muscles, or bone is defined as a *full-thickness* injury (third-degree injury). A thick, leathery, nonelastic, coagulated layer of necrotic tissue called *eschar* is created. The nerves are destroyed, resulting in a painless wound. These injuries always require skin grafting for permanent wound closure. Table 19-2 describes the characteristics of superficial, partial-thickness, and full-thickness burn injuries.

Initially, differentiating partial-thickness from full-thickness injuries may be difficult, particularly in the elderly or in children because burn wounds can mature or progress within the first few days. The three zones of thermal injury explain this phenomenon by illustrating the relationship of depth and extent of injury with injured tissue viability (Figure 19-2). The outermost area of minimal injury is termed the *zone of hyperemia* and is similar to a superficial burn. The greatest area of tissue necrosis is at the core of the wound or the *zone of coagulation*. Peripheral to this area is a *zone of stasis*, where vascular damage (and therefore reduced blood flow) with potentially reversible tissue injury has occurred. Without optimal conditions, including proper wound care and adequate resuscitation, this labile area may progress to tissue necrosis or death.

EXTENT OF INJURY

The extent of injury or size of a burn is expressed as the percentage of TBSA (%TBSA). The quickest method to initially calculate %TBSA is the rule of nines. This technique divides the TBSA into areas representing 9% or multiples of 9% (Figure 19-3). By summing all areas of partial- and full-thickness burns (superficial burns are *not* included), the %TBSA burned can be quickly estimated. For evaluations of injury extent in irregular or scattered small burns, the size of the patient's palm (including fingers) may be used for measurement and represents 1% TBSA (ABA, 2001). The rule of nines varies between adult and pediatric patients because of the difference in head surface area proportion in children compared with that in adults. Another surface area assessment method

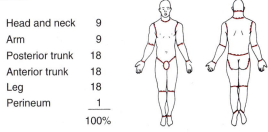

ADULT:

Head and neck	9
Arm	9
Posterior trunk	18
Anterior trunk	18
Leg	18
Perineum	1
	100%

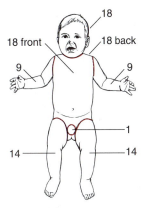

CHILD:

18
18 front
18 back
9   9
1
14 — 14

EXAMPLE: An adult with superficial burns to the face and partial-thickness circumferential burns to the lower half of the right arm, entire left arm, and chest (upper anterior trunk).
4.5% (lower right arm) + 9% (entire left arm) + 9% (upper anterior trunk) = 22.5% TBSA (the superficial burns to the face are not included in the calculation)

FIGURE 19-3 The rule of nines is a commonly used assessment tool that permits rapid estimation of the size and the extent of burn injury. Small children and infants have a proportionately larger head size compared with adults; therefore, an adjusted rule of nines is required.

called the Lund and Browder chart (Figure 19-4) provides a more accurate determination of the extent of burn injury by correlating body surface area with age-related proportions. This is the method used most frequently in a burn center. Accurate calculation of extent of injury is important for assessing burn severity and for estimating fluid resuscitation requirements.

Physiological Responses to Burn Injury

The body responds to major burn injuries with significant hemodynamic, metabolic, and immunological effects that occur locally and systemically as a result of cellular damage from heat (Figures 19-5 and 19-6).

Text continued on page 686

Burn Estimate and Diagram

Age vs. Area

Area	Birth 1 yr	1–4 yr	5–9 yr	10–14 yr	15 yr	Adult	2°	3°	Total	Donor Areas
Head	19	17	13	11	9	7				
Neck	2	2	2	2	2	2				
Ant. Trunk	13	13	13	13	13	13				
Post. Trunk	13	13	13	13	13	13				
R. Buttock	2 ½	2 ½	2 ½	2 ½	2 ½	2 ½				
L. Buttock	2 ½	2 ½	2 ½	2 ½	2 ½	2 ½				
Genitalia	1	1	1	1	1	1				
R. U. Arm	4	4	4	4	4	4				
L. U. Arm	4	4	4	4	4	4				
R. L. Arm	3	3	3	3	3	3				
L. L. Arm	3	3	3	3	3	3				
R. Hand	2 ½	2 ½	2 ½	2 ½	2 ½	2 ½				
L. Hand	2 ½	2 ½	2 ½	2 ½	2 ½	2 ½				
R. Thigh	5 ½	6 ½	8	8 ½	9	9 ½				
L. Thigh	5 ½	6 ½	8	8 ½	9	9 ½				
R. Leg	5	5	5 ½	6	6 ½	7				
L. Leg	5	5	5 ½	6	6 ½	7				
R. Foot	3 ½	3 ½	3 ½	3 ½	3 ½	3 ½				
L. Foot	3 ½	3 ½	3 ½	3 ½	3 ½	3 ½				
						Total				

Burn Diagram

Age _____

Sex _____

Weight _____

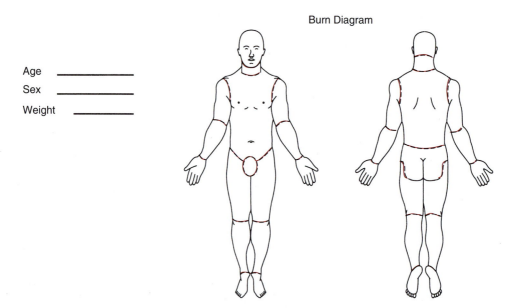

FIGURE 19-4 Burn estimate and diagram. The form was developed and is used by the United States Army Institute of Surgical Research. Based on the Lund and Browder chart with Berkow's formula, it allows for more accurate assessment of the extent of burn injury based on age and depth of injury. *Ant.,* Anterior; *Post.,* posterior; *L.,* left; *R.,* right; *R.U.,* right upper; *R.L.,* right lower; *L.U.,* left upper; *L.L.,* left lower.

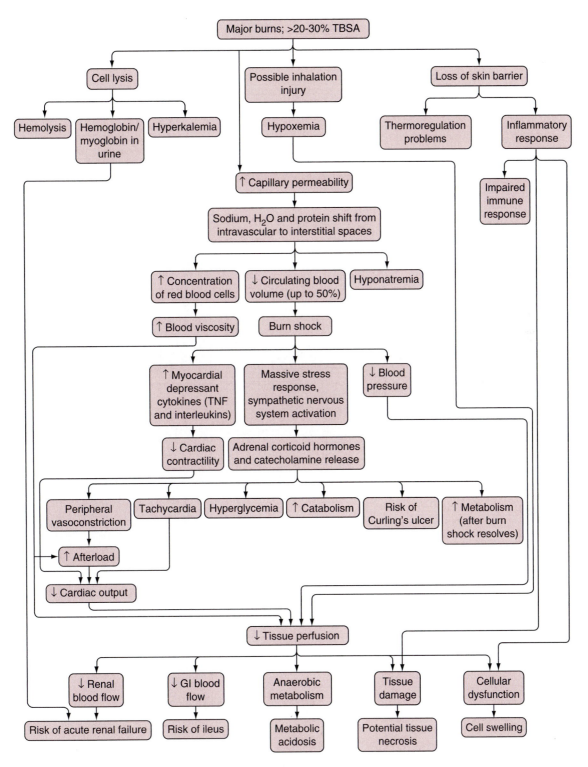

FIGURE 19-5 Overview of physiological changes that occur after acute burn injury. *TBSA,* Total body surface area; *TNF,* tumor necrosis factor. (Modified from Byers, J. F., & LaBorde, P. J. [2004]. Management of patients with burn injury. In S. C. Smeltzer & B. G. Bare [eds.]. *Brunner & Suddarth's textbook of medical-surgical nursing.* 10th ed. Philadelphia: Lippincott, Williams & Wilkins.)

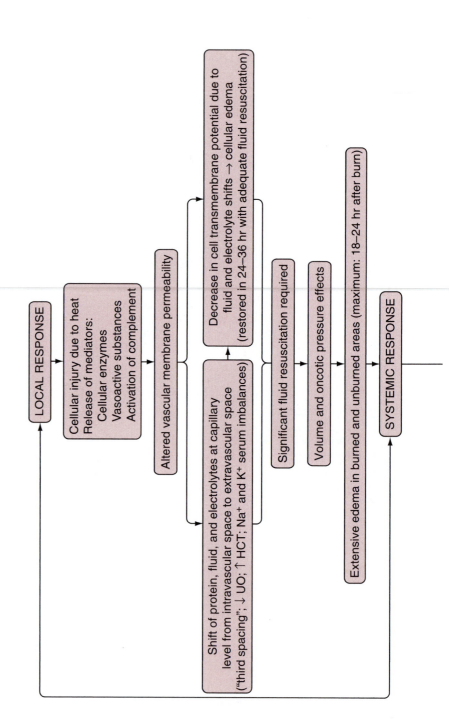

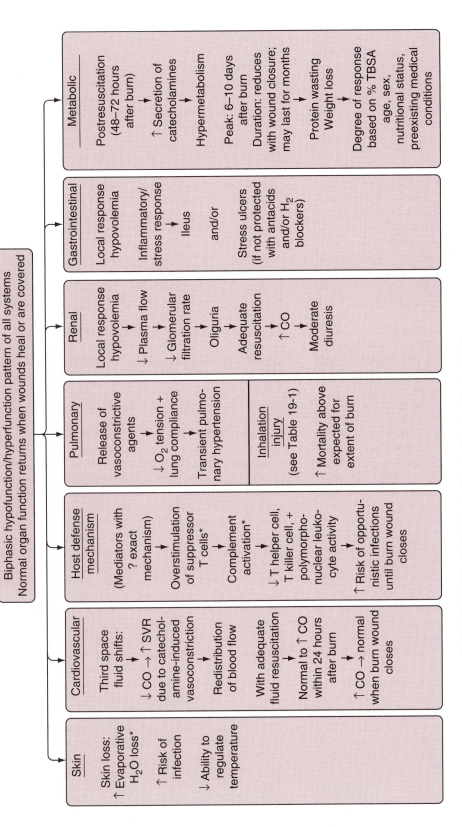

FIGURE 19-6 Pathophysiology of extensive burn injury.

*A response associated with burn injury greater than 20% to 25% total body surface area (%TBSA).

CO, Cardiac output; HCT, hematocrit; SVR, systemic vascular resistance; UO, urinary output.

The magnitude and duration of the systemic response and the degree of physiological change are proportional to the extent of body surface area (%TBSA) injured. Direct thermal damage to blood vessels causes intravascular coagulation, with arterial and venous blood flow ceasing in the wound injury area. The damaged and ischemic cells release *mediators*. These are endogenously produced substances that the body secretes to initiate a protective inflammatory response. Mediators such as histamine, prostaglandins, bradykinins, catecholamines, and cytokines are stimulated and released, causing myriad vasoactive, cellular, and cardiovascular effects. Gaps between endothelial cells in vessel wall membranes develop, making vessel walls porous or "leaky." This *increased capillary membrane permeability* allows a significant shift of protein molecules, fluid, and electrolytes from the *intravascular space* (inside the blood vessels) into the *interstitium* (the space between cells and the vascular system) in a process also referred to as *third spacing* (Figure 19-7). There is rapid and dramatic edema formation. Cellular swelling (and thus, increased tissue edema) may also occur as a result of a decrease in cell transmembrane potential and a shift of extracellular sodium and water into the cell (Cope & Moore, 1947). The leaking of proteins into the interstitium dramatically lowers intravascular *oncotic pressure*, which draws even more intravascular fluid into the interstitium and contributes to development of edema and *burn shock* (shock from intravascular volume loss, created by the sudden fluid and solute shifts immediately after burn injury). In burns greater than 20% TBSA, the increased capillary permeability and edema formation process not only occur locally at the site of burn injury, but also systemically in distant unburned tissues and organs (ABA, 2001; Sheridan, 2002; Wraa, 2003). Edema may be further exacerbated as lymph drainage flow is obstructed from either direct damage of lymphatic vessels or from blockage by serum proteins that have leaked into the interstitium. Edema is a natural inflammatory response to injury that aids transport of white blood cells to the site of injury for bacterial digestion; however, the extent and rate of edema formation associated with major burn injury far exceed the intended beneficial inflammatory effect (Ahrns, 2004). A hallmark study by Demling, Mazess, Witt, and Wolberg (1978) found that edema continues to expand until it reaches a maximum at approximately 24 hours after burn injury. Edema resolution and reabsorption then typically begin 1 to 2 days after a burn injury.

Intravascular fluid volume lost into the interstitium causes a unique phenomenon called *burn shock*. Burn shock can be described as a combination of *distributive* and *hypovolemic shock*. There is a distributive component because third spacing greatly expands the area in which total body fluid is contained, to include the intravascular space, plus intracellular and interstitial spaces. The hypovolemic component is caused by massive loss of intravascular fluid from increased vessel membrane permeability and evaporative losses through the open wound beds. Burn shock ensues when plasma or intravascular volume becomes insufficient to maintain circulatory support and adequate preload, causing cardiac output to decrease and impairing tissue perfusion. Fluid resuscitation is a crucial part of burn management because it directly replaces plasma fluid losses, fills the newly increased body fluid reservoir, and restores preload deficits.

In summary, significant burn injuries trigger local and systemic responses involving a multitude of complex mechanisms and cascades of physiological events that stress all body systems. The magnitude of physiological response is unique to burn injury and is characterized by dramatic shifts in intravascular fluid, mediator activation, hyperexaggerated inflammatory cascade reaction, and impressive edema formation. The specific organ system responses are summarized in the following sections and in Figure 19-6.

CARDIOVASCULAR RESPONSE

Loss of intravascular volume after major burn injury produces a decrease in cardiac output and oxygen delivery to the body tissues. The sympathetic nervous system is activated as a compensatory mechanism, with the release of catecholamines causing tachycardia and vasoconstriction to maintain arterial blood pressure. Tissue perfusion and organ perfusion are altered as a redistribution of blood flow occurs early in the postburn period to perfuse essential organs such as the heart and brain. Early postburn myocardial depression is observed and exerts a negative inotropic effect on myocardial tissues. The magnitude of myocardial depression exceeds that which would be explained by intravascular fluid volume loss. Inflammatory cytokine mediators such as tumor necrosis factor and interleukins secreted locally within the myocardium have been implicated as the major contributors to this progressive cardiac contractile dysfunction (Maass, White, & Horton, 2002). Cardiac instability in burn patients can be caused by underresuscitation (hypovolemia), overresuscitation (hypervolemia), or increased afterload. With adequate fluid resuscitation, cardiac output normalizes approximately 24 hours after burn injury and becomes supranormal thereafter until the burns are closed (Ahrns & Harkins, 1999; Mikhail, 1999).

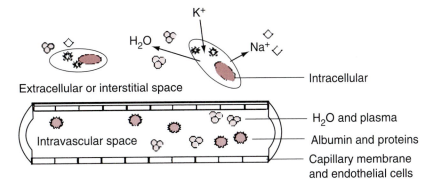

NORMAL PHYSIOLOGY BEFORE BURN INJURY
Intact capillary wall membranes keep large protein molecules within the blood vessels or intravascular space. This maintains normal protein oncotic pressure and retains intravascular fluid volume.

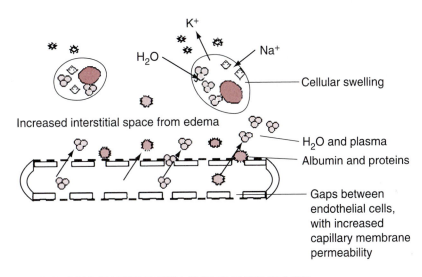

PHYSIOLOGIC CHANGES FOLLOWING BURN INJURY
Gaps develop between endothelial cells causing increased capillary membrane permeability. Intravascular proteins and fluids flow into the interstitium in a process called third-spacing and produces tissue edema. Loss of intravascular proteins decreases intravascular oncotic pressure, pulls additional fluid into the interstitium, and reduces intravascular fluid volume. Decreased cell transmembrane potential shifts sodium into the cells, drawing in water and producing cellular swelling and further tissue edema.

FIGURE 19-7 Burn edema and shock development. H_2O, Water; K^+, potassium; Na^+, sodium.

HOST DEFENSE MECHANISMS

With the loss of skin from burn injury, the primary barrier to microorganisms is destroyed. Tissue damage invokes simultaneous activation of all inflammatory response cascades including the complement, fibrinolytic, clotting, and kinin systems. The exact mechanism by which postburn immune defects occur remains ambiguous, because inflammatory mediators and cytokines exert numerous, varied, and interrelated effects. However, the end results are overstimulation of suppressor T-cells and depression of other components, such as helper T-cell, killer T-cell, and polymorphonuclear leukocyte activity. This immuno-suppression interferes with the ability of the patient's host defense mechanisms to fight invading microorganisms and thus places the patient at high risk of developing infection and sepsis.

PULMONARY RESPONSE

Release of vasoconstrictive mediator substances causes an initial transient pulmonary hypertension that may be associated with a modest decrease in oxygen tension and lung compliance (Pruitt, Goodwin, & Cioffi, 1995). The impact of inhalation injury on the pulmonary system is described in Table 19-1.

RENAL RESPONSE

The renal circulation is sensitive to decreasing cardiac output. Hypoperfusion and decreased glomerular filtration rate signal the nephrons to initiate the renin-angiotensin-aldosterone cascade. Sodium and water are retained to preserve intravascular fluid in an attempt to increase cardiac preload. Oliguria occurs, and urine becomes more concentrated. If fluid resuscitation is inadequate, acute renal failure can develop. With resuscitation, approximately 48 hours after injury, diuresis occurs secondary to an increase in cardiac output.

GASTROINTESTINAL RESPONSE

As a consequence of the inflammatory response and hypovolemia after major burn injury, the gastrointestinal (GI) circulation undergoes compensatory vasoconstriction and redistribution of blood flow to preserve core perfusion to the brain and heart. The resulting ischemia of the stomach and duodenal mucosa places burn patients at high risk of developing a duodenal ulcer, called a stress ulcer or *Curling's ulcer*. GI motility or peristalsis is also decreased, creating a *paralytic ileus*. The ileus clinically presents as decreased bowel sounds, gastric distention, nausea, or vomiting.

METABOLIC RESPONSE

There are two phases of dysfunction after a major burn injury. First, a decreased response in organ function occurs, followed by a second phase of hypermetabolic and hyperfunctional response of all systems. Hypermetabolism begins as resuscitation is completed and is one of the most significant and persistent alterations observed after burn injury. The postburn hypermetabolic response is greater than that seen in any other forms of trauma (Wraa, 2003). Patients with severe burns have metabolic rates that are 100% to 200% above their basal (baseline) rates, with some degree of elevation continuing for up to 9 to 12 months after injury (Hart et al., 2000; Sheridan, 2001). The rapid

metabolic rate is caused by the secretion of inflammatory response mediators or catabolic hormones, such as catecholamines, cortisol, and glucagon, in an effort to support tissue remodeling and repair (Barret & Herndon, 2003b). The hypermetabolic state produces a catabolic effect on the body, with skeletal muscle breakdown, decreased protein synthesis, increased glucose utilization, and rapid depletion of glycogen stores (Wraa, 2003). The amount of protein wasting and weight loss that occurs is affected by several factors including %TBSA burned, age, sex, preburn nutritional status, other health problems, and nutrient intake. Wound closure reduces metabolic expenditure (Barret & Herndon, 2003b; Hart et al., 2000).

Phases of Burn Care Assessment and Collaborative Interventions

Assessment and management of the burn-injured patient can be categorized into three phases of care: (1) resuscitative, (2) acute, and (3) rehabilitative. The *resuscitative phase* or emergency phase begins at the time of injury and continues for approximately 48 hours until the massive fluid and protein shifts have stabilized. The primary focus of assessment and intervention is on maintenance of the ABCs (airway, breathing, and circulation) and prevention of burn shock. The resuscitative phase spans care in the prehospital setting, in the ED, and transfer to a burn center. With the onset of diuresis approximately 48 to 72 hours after injury, the *acute phase* begins and continues until wound closure occurs. This phase typically occurs in a burn center and may last for weeks or months. Nursing care focuses on the promotion of wound healing, the prevention of infections and complications, and the provision of psychosocial support. Although the critical care nurse is rarely involved in the *rehabilitative phase*, the care given in the first two phases is instrumental in achieving optimal final rehabilitative outcomes. The primary goal in this final phase is to restore the patient's ability to function in society and to return to an established family role and vocation. Critical care activities usually occur in the resuscitative and acute phases. In both these phases, patient assessment and management are prioritized and guided by following the primary and secondary surveys as described in the Advanced Burn Life Support Course (ABA, 2001). Pain control, wound management, infection control, special considerations for unique burn injuries, and psychosocial concerns are important issues throughout all the phases of burn care.

RESUSCITATIVE PHASE: PREHOSPITAL

Primary Survey

Prehospital personnel (e.g., flight nurses, emergency medical technicians) are the first health care providers to arrive at the scene of injury. Care rendered in the first few hours after a significant burn injury greatly affects the patient's likelihood of survival. The priorities of prehospital care and management are to extricate the patient safely, to stop the burning process, to identify life-threatening injuries, and to minimize time on the scene by rapidly transporting the patient to an

---

RESEARCH ANALYSIS

ARTICLE REFERENCE

Carrougher, G. J., Ptacek, J. T., Sharar, S. R., et al. (2003). Comparison of patient satisfaction and self-reports of pain in adult burn-injured patients. *Journal of Burn Care and Rehabilitation, 24*(1):1-8.

PURPOSES AND METHODS

The Joint Commission on Accreditation of Healthcare Organizations has mandated that pain assessment and treatment be patient care priorities in all hospitals. One method of complying with this mandate is to develop a pain management plan with every patient and to evaluate and alter pain treatment to achieve the stated goals. There has been considerable research published on assessing pain level intensity with pain scales (visual analogue scales, numerical rating scales, graphic rating scales) and developing caregiver-driven pain management goals. However, there is limited burn-related literature on using these scales to develop patient-derived pain relief goals and to analyze patient satisfaction with pain management. The purpose of this nonexperimental correlational study was to analyze the relationship of procedural and background pain scores to patient-identified pain management goals (the level of pain patients report they would be satisfied experiencing) and patient satisfaction scores. The authors hypothesized that patient satisfaction with pain management plans would be highest in those who experienced the least amount of pain and/or in patients whose pain intensity scores most closely matched their pain treatment goals.

The investigators used a prospective convenience sample of adult (≥18 years old) burn patients admitted to a university-based verified burn center. Inclusion consisted of those patients anticipated to require analgesic premedication with opioids for wound care. Excluded were those patients treated for alcohol withdrawal and those already participating in pain study evaluating hypnosis. Approval was obtained from the researching institution's human subject review board. Patients underwent standard burn care for the unit. Analgesic and anxiolytic medications were selected and administered according to existing burn unit guidelines. Subjects were assessed twice weekly until discharge for worst and average procedural (wound care) pain, average background pain for the previous 24 hours, personal pain treatment goals, and overall satisfaction with their pain management. A 0- to 10-cm/point graphic rating scale (GRS) was used for all ratings. Opioid administration and anxiolytic administration were retrospectively abstracted from patient medication administration records. Opioid equivalents or "morphine equivalents" were calculated.

STUDY FINDINGS

Eighty-four patients participated in the study over a 29-month period. Sixty-seven (80%) of the subjects were men. The mean patient age was 36.9 years, with a mean total body surface area burn of 13.3% and an average hospital length of stay of 18 days. Most burn injuries in the study participants were caused by scald (43%) and by flame or flash (37%); 351 pain assessments were collected, ranging from 1 to 9 assessments per subject. Only the first 4 assessments of each patient (274 out of 351 total assessments) were used in the final analyses, because of a decrease in subject reports after the first 4 assessments. The majority (58% to 70%, depending on the day queried) of subjects reported that they did not expect to be completely pain free and stated that they would be satisfied experiencing some degree (GRS pain level score of 1 to 6) of procedural and background pain. Procedural and background pain levels reported by patients were found to be significantly and consistently higher than the patient's

Continued

RESEARCH ANALYSIS—cont'd

stated treatment goals. Additionally, both types of pain did not significantly decrease over time. Although 91% of subjects received analgesic medications consistent with the burn unit's pain treatment guidelines, opioid equivalent dosing or the amount of opioids administered did not correlate or change with reported procedural and background pain ratings or treatment goals. Anxiolytics were used during wound care in only 13% to 15% of subjects. Patient satisfaction did not correlate with how closely a patient's pain treatment goal matched the reported pain intensity scores. Rather, a negative correlation was shown between pain scores and satisfaction (i.e., those with the highest pain levels reported the lowest satisfaction with pain management).

STUDY STRENGTHS

This is a fine example of a collaborative multidisciplinary burn team project led by a nurse investigator. This is the first analysis documented in the burn literature of quantifying and evaluating patient self-reported pain management goals. Using a standardized, validated GRS pain scale for data collection produced a study with high instrument reliability that may be easily replicated by other researchers.

STUDY LIMITATIONS

The study was limited by its convenience sampling method. Because the total number of burn patients admitted during the study period was not described, it is not possible to determine the percentage of the total population the subject sample comprised, nor whether the sample and its size accurately represented the composition of the total burn patient population (i.e., gender, age, injury severity). Details were not provided regarding consistent utilization of specific personnel trained to administer study instruments for the pain assessment collection; therefore, interrater reliability could not be confirmed. Anxiolytics have been previously described to reduce pain score ratings during burn wound care. Therefore, it is not clear how the infrequent use of anxiolytics reported in this study may have affected pain and satisfaction scores.

IMPLICATIONS FOR PRACTICE

Effective pain management in the burn-injured patient continues to be a challenge to the burn management team. Even though burn patients express willingness to experience some degree of pain during their hospital stay, overall pain management satisfaction is highest when they have the least amount of pain. Therefore, nurses must continually assess for the presence of pain and must implement appropriate relief interventions to strive maximally to reduce pain intensity. Acknowledging the multiple forms of burn pain by assessing both worst and average procedural and background pain will assist the nurse to provide more comprehensive pain monitoring and management. Reviewing the overall trend in patient reports of background and procedural pain and the dosing of analgesics and anxiolytics administered will provide the nurse with vital information on whether the patient's pain is effectively being decreased. Analgesic dosing should be reassessed frequently and adjusted to reflect the level of pain a patient reports. Because patient satisfaction was most strongly affected by the level of pain experienced during hospitalization, further studies are needed to determine how patient satisfaction scoring tools should be used to direct changes in analgesic therapy and pain management.

appropriate care facility. As with any other type of trauma, the primary survey is used to provide a fast systematic assessment that prioritizes evaluation of the patient's airway, breathing, and circulatory status (Figure 19-8).

Stopping the burning process. The first priority of patient care is stopping the burning process by removing the patient from the source of burning while preventing further injury to the patient or staff (ABA, 2001). It is crucial that this step be performed safely, but quickly, because interventions aimed to stop the burning should not greatly delay continuing to the next assessment phases of the primary survey.

Flame burns are extinguished by rolling the patient on the ground, smothering the flames with a blanket or other cover, or dousing the flames with water. Ice is never applied to the wounds, because further tissue damage may occur as a result of vasoconstriction and hypothermia. Jewelry is immediately removed, because metal retains heat and can cause continued burning. Scald, tar, and asphalt burns are

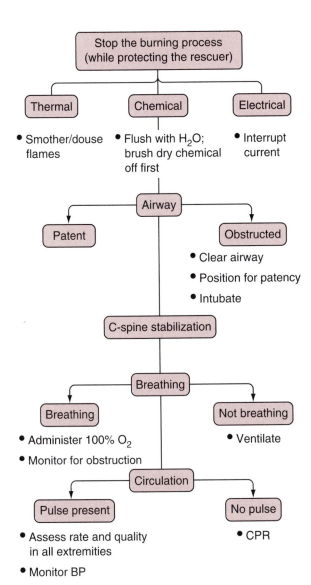

FIGURE 19-8 Major burn injury: primary survey. *BP*, Blood pressure; *CPR*, cardiopulmonary resuscitation.

treated by immediate removal of the saturated clothing and/or immediate cooling with water if available. No attempt is made to remove adherent tar at the scene. Adherent clothing (clothing that is burned into and stuck to the skin) is not removed because increased tissue damage and bleeding may occur; however, water is applied to cool the clothing material. Immediate treatment of electrical injuries involves prompt removal of the patient from the electrical source while protecting the rescuer. The burning process of chemical injuries continues as long as the chemical is in contact with the skin. All the patient's clothing (including gloves, shoes, and underwear) is

immediately removed, and water lavage is instituted before and during transport. Powdered chemicals are first brushed from the clothing and skin before lavage is performed. Clean water is the lavage solution of choice. If the chemical is in or near the eyes, remove contact lenses if applicable, and then irrigate the eyes with saline or clean water. Cross-contamination of the opposite eye is avoided during lavage by irrigating in the direction from inner to outer canthus. Do not attempt to use neutralizing agents on chemical burns. When neutralizing agents come in contact with chemicals, increased heat production occurs and can further increase the depth of injury. Health care providers must prevent exposure to themselves during initial treatment and lavage of chemical injuries by wearing protective barrier garments such as plastic gowns, gloves, goggles, and a face shield.

Airway (with cervical spine precautions). A history of the injury event occurring in a closed space should alert the clinician to the high potential for inhalation injury. Any suspicion of inhalation injury requires immediate intervention for airway control while maintaining cervical spine immobilization precautions (as indicated by the injury event). Refer to Clinical Alert: Clinical Indicators of Inhalation Injury for clinical findings indicative of respiratory injury. Respiratory stridor indicates airway obstruction and mandates immediate endotracheal intubation at the scene. Patients with severe facial burns are prophylactically intubated because delayed or later endotracheal intubation will be difficult or impossible as edema develops.

Breathing. The half-life of CO is reduced to 45 minutes in the presence of an oxygen concentration of

CLINICAL ALERT: CLINICAL INDICATORS OF INHALATION INJURY

- Facial burns
- Presence of soot around the mouth and nose and in sputum (carbonaceous sputum)
- Signs of hypoxemia (tachycardia, dysrhythmias, anxiety, lethargy)
- Signs of respiratory difficulty (change in respiratory rate, use of accessory muscles for breathing, intercostal or sternal retractions, stridor, hoarseness)
- Abnormal breath sounds
- Abnormal blood gas values
- Singed nasal hairs
- Elevated carboxyhemoglobin levels

100% (versus a half-life of 2.5 hours on room air). Therefore, all patients with suspected smoke inhalation are treated at the scene with 100% humidified oxygen delivered by nonrebreathing face mask or endotracheal tube. Patients are monitored for clinical signs of decreasing oxygenation such as changes in respiratory rate or neurological status. Pulse oximetry may not be accurate in acute inhalation injuries, because the pulse oximeter cannot distinguish between the presence of CO and that of oxygen attached to the hemoglobin, thus leading to falsely high oxygen saturation readings.

Circulation. All restrictive clothing and jewelry are removed to prevent constriction and ischemia to distal extremities secondary to edema formation during fluid resuscitation. Intravenous (IV) therapy is initiated with insertion of two large-bore (14- or 16-gauge) IV lines, preferably through nonburned tissue, and infusion of lactated Ringer's (LR) solution (ABA, 2001). The patient is closely monitored for signs of hypovolemia such as changes in level of consciousness, rapid or thready pulses, decreased blood pressure, or narrowing pulse pressure. Burn injury rarely results in hypovolemic shock in the very early prehospital phase. If evidence of shock is present, then associated internal or external injury must be suspected.

Heat loss occurs rapidly in a major burn injury because the protective covering of skin is lost, thereby allowing heat to escape. Cover the burned patient with a clean, dry sheet and blankets to prevent hypothermia and further contamination of the wounds.

Secondary Survey

The secondary survey in the prehospital setting should be brief and should not delay transport to a hospital. A rapid head-to-toe assessment to rule out any additional trauma is completed as part of the secondary survey (Figure 19-9). Patients with an injury mechanism suggestive of the potential for spinal injury (e.g., jumping from a burning building, electrical injury) have a cervical collar applied and are placed on a backboard before transport. Often, the patient is the most alert during this initial period after the injury. Therefore, an accurate history of the events that led to the burn injury is obtained, including the date and time of injury, the source of burns, and any events leading to the injury. Additionally, acquiring a brief medical history is beneficial, including allergies, current medical problems and medications taken, past surgical procedures and/or trauma, time of last meal, and history of tetanus immunization (ABA, 2001).

In preparation for transport, a short-acting narcotic such as morphine sulfate may be administered

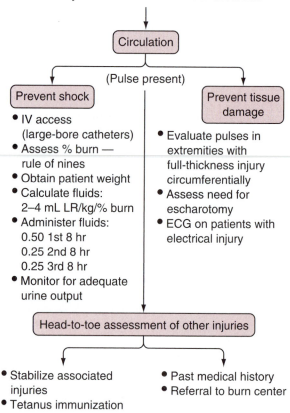

FIGURE 19-9 Major burn injury: secondary survey. *ABG,* Arterial blood gas; *ECG,* electrocardiogram; *IV,* intravenous; *LR,* lactated Ringer's solution.

by the IV route for pain relief. No intramuscular medications are given during the resuscitative phase because perfusion of edematous tissues is poor and produces sporadic narcotic absorption. The patient should not receive anything by mouth before and during transport, to prevent vomiting and aspiration.

RESUSCITATIVE PHASE: EMERGENCY DEPARTMENT AND CRITICAL CARE BURN CENTER

The burn patient is transferred from the injury scene to either a community hospital ED or a burn center. Management goals at either facility continue to be restoration and maintenance of the ABCs and the prevention of burn shock. Caring for a patient with major burn injury is one of the greatest challenges to a critical care nurse.

Transfer to a Burn Center

The care of a patient who has sustained a major burn injury is complex and requires the expertise of a specially trained multidisciplinary health care team. Burn team members include nurses, physicians (plastic and general surgeons), occupational therapists, physical therapists, dietitians, respiratory therapists, infection control specialists, pharmacists, child life specialists, social workers, psychologists, chaplains, injury prevention educators, and physician specialists (e.g., rehabilitation physicians, pediatricians, and neurosurgeons, as indicated). A burn center provides the necessary resources to improve burn patient care and outcome, including a dedicated staff delivering specialized clinical care, prehospital and community education, injury prevention, and research. Small hospitals may not have the personnel or medical supplies needed to provide the specialized care these patients require. Therefore, the American Burn Association has developed guidelines (see Clinical Alert: Guidelines for Burn Center Referral) for determining which burn-injured patients should be referred to a specialized burn center after initial stabilization (ABA, 2001).

When transfer to a burn center is considered, the referring physician must make direct contact with the burn center physician. The burn center physician determines the mode of transportation (by ground ambulance or air) and the treatment necessary to stabilize the patient for transport (ABA, 2001). Transport is optimally done early in the postburn period during the resuscitative phase, based on guidelines provided by the receiving burn center. Accurate and timely communication between the staff at both facilities is essential and can be facilitated by the use of a patient transfer information sheet (Figure 19-10).

Primary Survey

On arrival to either the ED or the burn center, the primary survey is reassessed. Once the patient has arrived in the critical care burn unit, primary and secondary assessments are again performed.

Airway. Ineffective airway clearance related to tracheal edema may occur early, or it may not be apparent until after fluid resuscitation is initiated. Patients with suspected inhalation injuries who are not already intubated must be monitored frequently for hoarseness, stridor, or wheezing. Because massive edema formation is an anticipated response to fluid resuscitation in an extensively burned patient, patients with severe facial burns are prophylactically intubated. The presence of any other symptoms suggestive of inhalation injury (see Clinical Alert: Clinical Indicators of Inhalation Injury) necessitates early intubation to maintain adequate oxygenation and perfusion. Fiberoptic bronchoscopy may be performed to confirm the presence of inhalation injury. If the patient is already intubated, accurate tube position is assessed. It is essential for the nurse to ensure that the endotracheal tube is securely tied (not taped) in place to prevent accidental extubation (Figure 19-11). This measure is especially important with young children, who often require the use of uncuffed endotracheal tubes that can easily dislodge. A dislodged endotracheal tube may be impossible to replace in the presence of massive edema and airway obstruction, thereby necessitating an emergency cricothyroidotomy or tracheostomy. The head of the patient's bed is elevated to reduce facial and airway edema.

Breathing. Assessment for impaired gas exchange related to CO poisoning or inhalation injury is important. Breath sounds, characteristics of respirations, work of breathing, sputum color and consistency, and symmetry of chest wall excursion are evaluated. Arterial blood gases and COHgb are measured when inhalation injury is suspected. Humidified 100% oxygen is administered via face mask or endotracheal tube until COHgb levels are determined. Once COHgb levels have normalized (lower than 5% to 10%), the 100% oxygen is weaned as tolerated by the patient, as demonstrated by maintaining a partial pressure of arterial oxygen greater than 90 mm Hg, pulse oximetry greater than 95%, and unlabored respirations. If the patient has a circumferential full-thickness burn of the thorax, the nurse assesses for adequate ventilatory effort because edema and restrictive eschar may inhibit chest wall expansion. Young children are particularly prone to this complication because their thoracic walls are more pliable. Therefore, an immediate chest wall *escharotomy* may be indicated to facilitate breathing (Figure 19-12). An escharotomy is an incision performed at the bedside through a full-thickness wound to reduce constriction caused by the tight nonelastic band of eschar. This relieves pressure and restores ventilation and/or blood flow. Local anesthesia is not required because the full-thickness burn eschar is painless. This procedure should be done only in consultation with the burn center.

MetroHealth Medical Center
Burn Center Transfer Form

Time: _____ Referring Hospital: _____ Physician: _____

Patient name: _____ Age: _____ Sex: _____

Address: _____ Phone: _____

Next of Kin: _____ Phone: _____ Notified: _____

Time of Burn: _____ Cause of Burn: _____ Treatment: _____

Significant Past Medical History: _____

Allergies: _____

Medications: _____

Height: _____ Weight: _____ Last Tetanus: _____

ASSESSMENT	LABS
	ABG
HEENT/NEURO _____	pH _____
PULMONARY _____	PO_2 _____
CARDIAC/CIRC _____	CO_2 _____
GI/GU _____	O_2 Sat _____
	Bicarb _____
MUSCULOSKELETAL _____	CO Level _____
MEDICATIONS GIVEN _____	O_2 Therapy _____

	X-RAYS
TIME _____	
TEMPERATURE _____	
PULSE _____	
RESPIRATION _____	
BLOOD PRESSURE _____	

INTRAVENOUS THERAPY _____

FLUID
SITE GAUGE _____

FLUID
SITE GAUGE _____

FOLEY _____ OUTPUT _____

NG _____

ET _____ SIZE _____

OTHER INFORMATION _____

FLUID RESUSCITATION - PARKLAND FORMULA
4mL/kg/% Burn

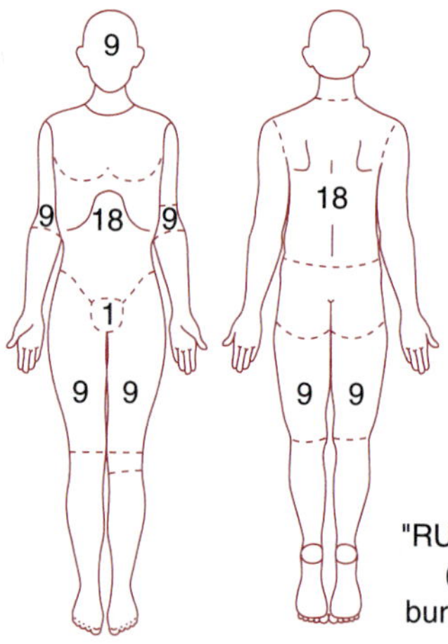

9
9 18 9
1
9 9

18

9 9

"RULES OF NINES"
(Indicate area
burned on diagram)

ESTIMATE % _____

M.D. or NURSE_____

FIGURE 19-10 MetroHealth Medical Center Burn Center Transfer Form. The use of a transfer form to summarize information concerning a burn patient's status promotes good communication between the referring and receiving facilities and ensures continuity of care. *CIRC,* Circulatory; *CO,* carbon monoxide; *ET,* endotracheal tube; *GI/GU,* gastrointestinal/genitourinary; *HEENT,* head, eye, ear, nose, throat; *NG,* nasogastric tube. (Courtesy of MetroHealth Medical Center, Cleveland, OH)

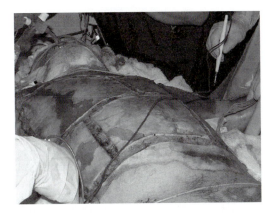

FIGURE 19-12 Escharotomy. In circumferential full-thickness burns of the thorax, edema and restrictive eschar may inhibit chest wall expansion. A chest wall escharotomy performed at the bedside may be indicated to facilitate breathing. An escharotomy is an incision through a full-thickness wound to reduce constriction caused by the nonelastic band of eschar. This relieves pressure and restores ventilation and/or blood flow (Courtesy of University of Michigan Trauma Burn Center, Ann Arbor, MI.)

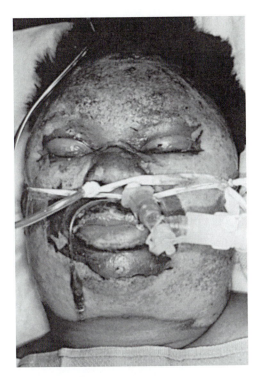

FIGURE 19-11 Facial edema. The massive edema that develops during fluid resuscitation in a major burn victim can lead to potential complications unless it is closely monitored by the critical care nurse. All facial tubes, such as endotracheal and nasogastric tubes, are secured with cloth ties to prevent dislodgment. Care must be taken to prevent ties from placing pressure on burned ears.

Ongoing assessment of breath sounds, arterial blood gases, and ventilatory status is crucial. All patients with inhalation injuries receive assistance with coughing, deep breathing, suctioning, and repositioning at least every 2 hours. Pulse oximetry and end-tidal carbon dioxide monitoring occur continuously as appropriate.

Circulation

Fluid resuscitation. Fluid resuscitation is a critical intervention for burn shock management. To estimate fluid resuscitation requirements, the depth and extent of injury must be assessed. Fluid resuscitation requirements are estimated according to body weight in kilograms, the %TBSA burned, and the patient's age. Historically, one of the most widely used burn resuscitation fluid formulas is the Parkland formula. It provides an approximation of fluid replacement requirements by calculating the amount of lactated Ringer's (LR) to infuse during the first 24 hours postburn at 4 mL LR/kg/%TBSA. Half of the calculated amount is given over the first 8 hours after injury, and the remaining half is given over the next 16 hours. A revised version of the Parkland formula, called the Consensus formula, is the formula taught and advocated by the Advanced Burn Life Support course (ABA, 2001). The Consensus fluid formula outlined in Box 19-1 specifies the fluid requirements for adults and children during the initial 24 hours after the burn. Half of the calculated amount is given over the first 8 hours after the injury, and the second half is given over the next 16 hours. IV fluid resuscitation is instituted in patients with burns greater than 15% to 20% TBSA because these burns are associated with a diffuse capillary leak, large intravascular fluid loss, and ileus. Patients with smaller %TBSA burns may be resuscitated with oral hydration. Two large-bore (14- to 16-gauge) peripheral IV lines are inserted. If an unburned location is not available, the IV lines are placed through burned skin. Cordis or central venous catheters are commonly inserted in patients with major burns to facilitate and accommodate large IV fluid infusion requirements. LR solution is the preferred initial IV fluid for burn resuscitation (ABA, 2001). It is a crystalloid that has an osmolality and electrolyte composition most similar to normal body physiological fluids, and it does not contain dextrose, which can cause a misleading high urine output from glycosuria and osmotic diuresis.

BOX 19-1

Burn Fluid Resuscitation Formula

FIRST 24 HR, ADMINISTER:

ABLS Consensus Formula (Based on the Parkland Formula)

In adults: LR 2 to 4 mL/kg/%TBSA

In children: LR 3 to 4 mL/kg/%TBSA

Half given over the first 8 hr after injury and the remaining half given over the next 16 hr

In infants <12 months and young children: Give fluid with 5% dextrose at a maintenance rate in addition to the resuscitation fluid noted above to prevent hypoglycemia. Maintenance rate is calculated by the following:

For the first 10 kg of body weight: 100 mL/kg over 24 hr

For the second 10 kg of body weight: 50 mL/kg over 24 hr

For each kg of body weight above 20 kg: 20 mL/kg over 24 hr

Titrate fluids to maintain urine output of 30 to 50 mL/hr in adults and 1 mL/kg/hr in children weighing <30 kg

Example: For an adult weighing 75 kg with a 55% TBSA burn and inhalation injury:

4 mL LR × 75 kg × 55%TBSA = 16,500 mL of LR infused over 24 hr

First 8 hr after burn injury: 8200 mL LR infused over 8 hr or 1031.25 mL/hr

Next 16 hr after burn injury: 8200 mL LR infused over 16 hr or 515.6 mL/hr

SECOND 24 HR, ADMINISTER:

Parkland Formula

Dextrose in water, plus potassium to maintain normal electrolyte balance

Colloid-containing fluid at 20% to 60% of calculated plasma volume, which equals an infusion rate of approximately 0.35 to 0.5 mL/kg/%TBSA

LR, Lactated Ringer's solution; *TBSA*, total body surface area.

Additionally, LR contains lactate, which helps to buffer the metabolic acidosis associated with hypoperfusion and burn shock. Because LR is a crystalloid, it does not provide any intravascular protein replacement to increase intravascular oncotic pressure. Hence, in the presence of increased capillary membrane permeability, the intravascular retention of LR is only about 25% of the infused volume, thereby necessitating large fluid volume infusions to maintain circulating blood volume.

Fluid requirements calculated by the Consensus formula serve only as a guide for estimating initial fluid needs. Each patient reacts differently to burn injury and so requires varying amounts of IV fluid to support perfusion and reduce the effects of burn shock. The patient's requirements for fluid resuscitation are affected by several factors including age, depth of burn, concurrent inhalation injury, preexisting disease or comorbidities, delay in burn injury treatment, and associated injuries. Inhalation injuries increase the extent of %TBSA injury, and these patients therefore typically require more resuscitation fluids. Larger fluid resuscitation volumes are also required in patients with electrical injuries, to prevent acute tubular necrosis by clearing the renal

tubules from precipitating myoglobin caused by skeletal muscle damage or *rhabdomyolysis*. Children also require relatively more resuscitation fluid because they have a greater ratio of body surface area to mass than that of adults, thereby having higher evaporative losses. Because evaporative fluid losses continue until burn wounds are closed, these losses are calculated as a part of the total daily maintenance fluid replacement formula.

Colloids, such as albumin, contain proteins and are sometimes used in burn shock resuscitation to increase intravascular oncotic pressure. The increase in intravascular oncotic pressure pulls fluid from the interstitium back into the circulating intravascular volume, thereby reducing edema and combating burn shock. However, during increased permeability, colloids can leak into the interstitium and can contribute to further intravascular fluid loss. Therefore, if colloids are used during burn resuscitation, it is generally advocated that they are not administered within 8 to 12 hours of burn injury when capillary permeability is at its highest level (ABA Evidence-Based Group, 2001).

During the second 24 hours postinjury when capillary permeability has decreased, a fluid formula such as the Parkland (see Box 19-1), which incorporates colloids, dextrose, and electrolyte replacement, is utilized. Colloids and hypertonic dextrose solutions increase oncotic pressure, which helps pull third-spaced fluid from the interstitium back into the circulatory system and restores intravascular volume. Potassium is added to IV fluids to replace potassium losses in the urine.

End-point monitoring. Assessment of fluid volume status related to changes in capillary permeability is essential. The goal of burn resuscitation is to maintain tissue perfusion and organ function while avoiding the complications of inadequate or excessive fluid therapy (ABA, 2001). Resuscitation fluid infusion rates are titrated to specific measured outcomes of patient response, known as physiological end points (Ahrns, 2004). During burn shock resuscitation, IV crystalloids and/or colloids are administered according to Consensus formula guidelines, with normalization of urine output and blood pressure used as the hemodynamic end points to titrate fluids. A urinary catheter is inserted to evaluate resuscitation adequacy. IV infusion rates are adjusted to ensure a urinary output of 30 to 50 mL per hour in adults and 1 mL/kg of body weight per hour in children weighing less than 30 kg. During the resuscitation phase, steady increases or decreases in IV resuscitation rates are performed, rather than administration of fluid boluses (Ahrns, 2004).

Peripheral circulation. Special attention is given to *circumferential* (completely surrounding a body part) full-thickness burns of the extremities. Pressure from bands of eschar or from edema that develops as resuscitation proceeds may impair blood flow to underlying and distal tissue. Therefore, extremities are elevated to reduce edema. Active or passive range-of-motion (ROM) exercises are performed every hour for 5 minutes to increase venous return and to minimize edema. Peripheral pulses are assessed every hour, especially in circumferential burns of the extremities, to confirm adequate circulation. An ultrasonic flow meter (Doppler) is used to auscultate radial, palmar, digital, or pedal pulses. Delayed capillary refill, tense skin, progressively decreasing or absent pulse, and other neurovascular changes (e.g., intense pain, paresthesia, paralysis) indicate impaired blood flow and developing *compartment syndrome.* Compartment syndrome occurs when tissue pressure in the fascial compartments of extremities increases, compressing and occluding blood vessels and nerves. If signs and symptoms of compartment syndrome are present on serial examination, preparation is made for an escharotomy to relieve pressure and to restore circulation.

If decreased perfusion is not quickly detected, ischemia and necrosis with loss of limb may occur. A *fasciotomy* (incision through fascia) may be indicated for deep electrical burns or severe muscle damage to restore blood flow. Escharotomy and fasciotomy sites are treated with a topical antimicrobial agent and are closely monitored for bleeding. Cautery, silver nitrate sticks, or sutures may be indicated to stop continued bleeding.

Secondary Survey

On admission to the ED or burn center, a chest x-ray study is obtained, and other x-ray studies are ordered as indicated by the patient's condition. Spinal immobilization precautions are continued until clinical assessment and radiological studies demonstrate no evidence of vertebral injury. The patient's medical history and the history of the injury event are conveyed to the medical team. The critical care nurse must assess indices or end points of essential organ function to evaluate adequacy of burn shock resuscitation and to prevent complications. Initially, monitoring is performed frequently to detect changes that can rapidly occur during fluid resuscitation. Critical indices monitored at least hourly include blood pressure, heart rate, cardiac rhythm, respiration quality and rate, temperature, peripheral pulse presence and quality, and urinary output. In addition, urine specific gravity, urine glucose and ketones, occult blood tests, and gastric pH levels are typically evaluated every 2 hours. The patient is weighed on admission and daily thereafter until the preburn weight is obtained after diuresis. Pain is closely monitored, and efforts are made to control it adequately. All parameters are documented for analysis of trends. Assessment and intervention in the resuscitative phase focus on early detection and prevention of problems in the systems discussed in the following sections.

Cardiovascular system. Historically, mean arterial pressure greater than 70 mm Hg and the absence of tachycardia (heart rate less than 120 beats per minute) have been standard assessments of adequate burn shock resuscitation (Ahrns, 2004). However, the cardiovascular response of the patient to burn injury warrants special consideration by the critical care nurse. The burn patient often has an elevated baseline heart rate of 100 to 120 beats per minute from postinjury metabolic changes. Compensatory mechanisms do not allow hypotension to develop until significant intravascular volume losses have occurred, thereby rendering decreasing blood pressure a late sign of inadequate perfusion. Both arterial and noninvasive cuff pressure readings may be altered by peripheral tissue edema or by catecholamine and mediator-induced arteriospasm. Changes in heart rate and blood pressure may also be masked or may appear increased from pain, anxiety, or fear rather than from inadequate resuscitation. Therefore, monitoring for a narrowing pulse pressure is helpful, because it provides an earlier indication of shock than assessing systolic blood pressure alone (Mikhail, 1999).

The routine use of pulmonary artery catheters is not supported by the literature (ABA Evidence-Based Group, 2001). However, patients with significant cardiopulmonary disease, the elderly, or those who have unexplained large resuscitation fluid volume requirements may benefit from insertion of a pulmonary artery catheter to assess cardiac function (ABA Evidence-Based Group, 2001; Ahrns, 2004; Mikhail, 1999). If a pulmonary artery catheter is used, low right atrial pressure and pulmonary artery occlusion pressure are reflective of hypovolemia and require intervention. Assessing trends in cardiac output variables and oxygen transport variables can provide useful information to guide burn shock resuscitation.

Local thermal injury, venous stasis, hypercoagulability, and immobility place the burn patient at risk of developing thromboembolic complications such as deep venous thrombosis (DVT) and pulmonary embolism. However, clinical findings indicative of DVT may not be present, or they may be obscured by extremity burn wound pain, edema, or erythema. Data suggest that the incidence of thromboembolic complications in burn patients is dramatically higher than previously thought (Wahl et al., 2002). Therefore, the investigators recommend that immobile burn patients receive routine DVT prophylaxis with sequential compression devices, low-molecular-weight heparin, or another prophylactic modality. The critical care nurse must recognize that the traditional signs of DVT may not present in the burn patient. Therefore, the nurse must closely monitor for sudden respiratory deterioration, which may indicate pulmonary embolism.

Neurological status. Surprisingly, severely injured burn patients are initially awake, alert, and oriented. Monitoring of sensorium is crucial. If a burned patient initially presents with decreased level of consciousness, other injuries or causes should be suspected (e.g., head injury, CO poisoning, drug overdose). The patient's sensorium is evaluated hourly because increased agitation or confusion or a continued decreased level of consciousness may be an indication of hypovolemia and/or hypoxemia. The head of the bed is elevated 30 degrees to prevent cerebral edema during fluid resuscitation.

Renal status. Urine output closely reflects renal perfusion, which is sensitive to decreasing cardiac output and developing shock. Therefore, urinary output is the quickest and most reliable indicator of adequate burn fluid resuscitation. Titration of calculated fluid requirements according to hourly urine output is an essential function of the nurse during resuscitation. Urine output, color, and concentration are also closely monitored. Oliguria may occur if fluid resuscitation is inadequate.

Gastrointestinal system. The GI system is monitored for problems occurring with its initial response to the burn injury (i.e., ileus, Curling's ulcer). It is essential to assess for the presence and quality of bowel sounds, abdominal distention, gastric pH, characteristics of gastric secretions, and the presence of GI bleeding. Because patients with burns greater than 20% TBSA generally develop an ileus, a nasogastric tube is inserted and connected to low suction to prevent vomiting and aspiration. If oral intake is not feasible, enteral feedings by small bowel feeding tube are started early. Antacids and/or H_2 histamine receptor antagonists are administered to protect GI mucosa from erosion and ulceration with associated GI hemorrhaging.

Circumferential torso eschar or bowel edema (from fluid resuscitation and/or the inflammatory response) can cause intraabdominal hypertension. The incidence of this serious complication may be underestimated in burn patients and has been the focus of much recent research (Ahrns, 2004). Intraabdominal hypertension causes compression of intraabdominal contents and leads to renal, gut, and hepatic ischemia (Ivy et al., 2000). If not treated by trunk escharotomies and/or diuresis, intraabdominal hypertension can progress to abdominal compartment syndrome or death. Abdominal compartment syndrome is characterized by the presence of intraabdominal hypertension, decreasing urine output, and difficulty with ventilation (Ivy et al., 2000; Sheridan, 2002). Abdominal compartment syndrome mandates immediate decompression by laparotomy; otherwise, multiple organ dysfunction and death may quickly ensue (see Chapter 18).

Integumentary system. Assessing a burn victim for the first time is frightening and overwhelming to most health care providers. However, other life- or limb-threatening conditions (e.g., airway compromise, burn shock, extremity compartment syndrome) take priority over treating the burn wound during the initial resuscitation phase. Depth and extent of burn injury are assessed to assist with fluid resuscitation predictions. Specific interventions regarding burn wound management and infection control are discussed later in this chapter.

Burn wounds are prone to tetanus, and therefore the patient receives tetanus immunization on ED or burn center admission, if indicated. In general, for major burns, tetanus toxoid immunization is administered if more than 5 years have elapsed since the last received dose, or tetanus hyperimmune globulin and tetanus toxoid are given if the patient's immunization history is unknown (ABA, 2001; Wraa, 2003).

During the resuscitation period, loss of the protective skin layer and administration of large amounts of fluid place the burn patient at risk of developing hypothermia. The patient's temperature is closely monitored. Loss of body heat is minimized by limiting skin exposure and covering the patient with clean, dry sheets and blankets. Fluid/blood warmers are used for IV fluid infusion. The environmental temperature is strictly regulated by increasing the room temperature, closing room doors to prevent air drafts, and using external heat lamps or radiant heat shields.

Blood and electrolytes. Serum electrolyte levels are determined on admission and as dictated by the patient's status. Serum sodium levels typically approach the concentration of the resuscitation fluid being administered. Serum potassium levels may be increased as a result of release from injured tissue. The blood urea nitrogen level may also be increased when excessive protein catabolism occurs, and hyperglycemia may occur as a result of catecholamine release. Arterial blood gas values and serum lactate levels are evaluated frequently because metabolic acidosis can indicate inadequate tissue perfusion (see Laboratory Alerts: Alterations Seen During Acute Care Management of the Burned Patient).

ACUTE CARE PHASE: CRITICAL CARE BURN CENTER

With successful resuscitation, burn shock and its dramatic fluid and protein fluctuations stabilize approximately 48 to 72 hours after injury, and the acute phase of burn care begins. Assessments and interventions during the acute phase of burn recovery are implemented to promote wound healing, to prevent complications, and to improve function of the various body systems.

Respiratory System

Assessment continues for signs of respiratory compromise and pneumonia. Tachypnea, abnormal breath sounds, fever, increased white blood cell count, purulent secretions, and infiltrations on chest x-ray films indicate developing pneumonia. Aggressive pulmonary hygiene including suctioning, positioning and postural draining, coughing, deep breathing, and early ambulation are essential.

Cardiovascular System

As capillary permeability stabilizes, IV fluid requirements decrease. Patients must receive maintenance IV fluid infusions that match overall fluid output. Therefore, monitoring daily weights and intake and output is essential. Increased fluid resuscitation requirements after debridement and grafting operations are often required, because the inflammatory response is triggered by the surgical intervention. Frequent monitoring of vital signs continues.

Neurological Status

Assessment continues to monitor for changes in neurological status, which may indicate hypoxemia, hypoperfusion, or sepsis.

LABORATORY ALERTS: ALTERATIONS SEEN DURING ACUTE CARE MANAGEMENT OF THE BURNED PATIENT

Serum sodium	Levels approach the concentration of fluids being administered
Serum potassium	↑ Related to tissue damage; assess for cardiac dysrhythmias
Blood urea nitrogen	May be ↑ secondary to catabolism or falsely ↑ in hypovolemia; monitor nutrition and volume status
Serum lactate	Level will be ↑ in metabolic acidosis; should ↓ if fluid resuscitation adequate
Carboxyhemoglobin	Present in carbon monoxide poisoning; level is drawn if smoke inhalation suspected; maintain airway and oxygenation

↑, Increased; ↓, decreased.

Renal Status

Urine output assessment continues. Postburn diuresis starts approximately 48 to 72 hours after injury, with urine output ranges of 100 to 600 mL per hour commonly observed. Intake and output assessment remains important. After postburn diuresis, urinary output should correlate with intake of IV and oral fluids. In the absence of diabetes, glycosuria may indicate an early sign of sepsis.

Gastrointestinal System

Assessment of GI function continues. The patient is monitored for developing stress ulcer. Tolerance of enteral feedings is assessed. Nutritional considerations are a treatment priority and are discussed later in this chapter.

Integumentary System

The burn wound becomes the major focus of the acute phase of burn recovery. Assessment continues to include monitoring for burn wound healing, burn wound depth conversion, and signs of infection (see the later discussion of wound management).

Blood and Electrolytes

Although fluid and protein shifts from burn shock stabilize in the acute care phase, blood and electrolyte abnormalities related to other processes may still be observed. Hemodilution with associated decreased hematocrit may result from reentry of fluid into the intravascular compartment and from loss of red blood cells that were destroyed at the burn injury site. Hyponatremia from diuresis may occur, but it usually resolves within 1 week of onset. Inadequate replacement of evaporative water loss may produce hypernatremia. Hypokalemia may develop as potassium reenters the cells. Electrolyte shifts also affect the ability to maintain a proper acid-base balance and may cause metabolic acidosis. Hypoproteinemia and negative nitrogen balance may occur from an increase in metabolic rate and insufficient nutrition. Leukopenia may develop from administration of the topical antimicrobial agent silver sulfadiazine. Infection and/or excessive carbohydrate loading can contribute to hyperglycemia. Additionally, an increase in white blood cells, prolonged coagulation times, and decreased platelet count may result from infection and/or sepsis.

Special Considerations and Areas of Concern

Burns of the face, ears, eyes, hands, feet, major joints, genitalia, and perineum pose distinct concerns for the critical care nurse, because injuries to these areas contribute to overall burn injury severity and require unique management. Certain types of burns (electrical, chemical, and abuse) also mandate special consideration and intervention.

BURNS OF THE FACE

The presence of head or neck burns signals a potential inhalation injury. Associated facial edema may lead to a compromised airway. Close monitoring of the patient's respiratory status is essential. The head of the bed is elevated to facilitate respiratory exchange and edema reabsorption. Special care must be taken during cleansing of facial burns to prevent excessive bleeding and damage to new tissue growth. All hair (except for eyebrows) is shaved from the wound each day. Once the wound is cleaned and debrided, a topical antimicrobial agent is applied per unit protocol. Because of the rich blood supply in the face, partial-thickness burns usually heal quickly as long as infection is prevented. Good oral hygiene is essential.

BURNS OF THE EARS

The ears are especially prone to inflammation and infection of the cartilage (*chondritis*), which can lead to complete loss of ear cartilage. Ear burns are treated with a topical antimicrobial agent. Mafenide acetate (Sulfamylon) is the agent of choice because of its ability to penetrate the cartilage. Mechanical pressure on the ears from dressings or other external sources (tube ties, pillows) must be avoided because the pressure impairs blood flow and contributes to development of chondritis. Cloth ties are used for securing tubes to the face and are monitored frequently to ensure that pressure is not being placed on top of the ears. Pillows are not used for the head. Instead, a foam donut with a hole for the ear to rest in while the patient is in a lateral position is substituted.

BURNS OF THE EYES

Immediate examination of the eyes is necessary on arrival to the hospital because eyelid edema forms rapidly. Eyelid edema can cause the cornea to become exposed as the eyelid retracts. Contact lenses are removed if present. A thorough examination by an ophthalmologist is mandatory for serious injuries. The eyes are stained with fluorescein to rule out corneal injury, and the eyes are irrigated with copious amounts of physiological saline if injury is confirmed. Nursing care involves the frequent application of ophthalmic ointment or artificial tears to protect the cornea and conjunctiva from drying. Careful observation of eyelashes is also necessary because they may invert and scratch the cornea.

BURNS OF THE HANDS, FEET, OR MAJOR JOINTS

Extensive burns of the hands and feet may cause permanent disability, necessitating a long convalescence. An important aspect of critical care nursing care is preservation of function. Burned hands are elevated above the level of the heart on slings or wedges to reduce edema formation. Fingers and toes are wrapped individually during dressing changes with gauze, 4 × 4 bandages, or biological products to keep digits separated to prevent *webbing* (the skin growing together between burned body parts). Occupational therapy and physical therapy staff members are involved in the patient's plan of care from the day of admission to address and evaluate function and mobility parameters. Although ROM exercises may be painful, they must be initiated as soon as possible after the injury and performed frequently throughout each day. Active ROM exercises prevent muscle atrophy, reduce or prevent the shortening of ligaments, and reduce edema. Passive ROM exercises are indicated if patients are unable to move their extremities actively. Burn wounds over joints are prone to scar tissue *contractures* that limit joint ROM. The position of comfort is the position of contracture and deformity development. Therefore, splinting and anti-deformity positioning (e.g., extension of knees and elbows, extension and supination of wrists, abduction of hips and shoulders) are required for the maintenance of function and the prevention of deformities of the affected part. When the patient is ambulating or sitting, an elastic bandage is applied over burn wounds of the feet and legs to prevent venous stasis and pooling of blood. Venous pooling delays wound healing and increases the risk of DVT development. The elastic bandage is removed when the feet are elevated. In establishing a nursing plan of care, the nurse must remember that patients with bilateral burned hands are very dependent on nursing personnel for their physical needs.

BURNS OF THE GENITALIA AND PERINEUM

Patients with perineal burns often require hospitalization for observation of urinary tract obstruction. An indwelling urethral catheter is indicated until the surrounding wounds are healed or grafted. Meticulous wound care is essential because of the high risk of fecal or urine contamination and resulting infection. Perineal hair must be shaved over wound areas. Scrotal edema is common, and the scrotum is elevated on towels or foam.

ELECTRICAL INJURY

Cardiopulmonary arrest is a common complication of high-voltage electrical injury. Other severe complications related to electrical injury are summarized in Box 19-2. Hypoxia may occur secondary to tetanic contractions and resulting paralysis of the respiratory muscles. Oxygen and endotracheal intubation with mechanical ventilation are implemented as indicated. Patients are evaluated for spinal fractures from tetanic contractions or from falls during the injury event. Cervical collars and backboards are used to maintain spinal immobilization until radiological tests and clinical examinations have confirmed the absence of injury. All patients with electrical injury are monitored closely for cardiac dysrhythmias. If present, continuous cardiac monitoring or serial electrocardiographic evaluations continue for at least 24 hours after injury. Pink or dark red or port-colored pigment in the urine indicates the presence of hemochromogens (*myoglobin*) released as a result of severe deep tissue damage in a process called rhabdomyolysis. Accumulation of myoglobin in the renal tubules causes acute renal failure. Therefore, urinary output for these patients is maintained at 75 to 100 mL per hour until the urine becomes clear (ABA, 2001). Resuscitation fluid volumes larger than predicted by the Consensus formula are often required to achieve this high urine output. Sodium bicarbonate and mannitol may be administered at the burn center physician's discretion to increase urine pH and output. Affected extremities are closely monitored for development of compartment syndrome. Often, fasciotomies are required to release compartment pressure.

BOX 19-2

Manifestations and Complications of Electrical Injury

- Cardiac dysrhythmias or cardiopulmonary arrest and death
- Hypoxia secondary to tetanic contractions and paralysis of the respiratory muscles
- Deep tissue necrosis (may not be evident on initial presentation)
- Compartment syndrome of extremities requiring fasciotomy
- Long bone or vertebral fractures from tetanic muscle contractions
- Myoglobinuria and/or acute renal failure due to release of myoglobin from damaged muscle tissue
- Delayed cataract formation
- Neurological deficits, such as: spinal cord paralysis, traumatic brain injury/ischemia, peripheral neuropathy, seizures, deafness, motor and sensory deficits

CHEMICAL INJURY

Treatment of chemical injuries focuses on stopping the burning process while maintaining the safety of the nurse. Protective gear such as plastic gowns, gloves, masks, and goggles are worn by the burn team during decontamination. The patient's clothing is immediately removed. Dry chemicals are brushed off, and the area exposed to chemicals is then continuously flushed with water for at least 30 minutes. The nurse questions the patient and significant others to determine the specific chemical agent involved. Some chemicals, such as alkalis, may require even longer lavage, which can be quite uncomfortable for the patient. Nursing interventions include pain control and minimizing of heat loss caused by continual irrigation. Additionally, patients must be closely monitored for signs of systemic chemical absorption and effects.

ABUSE

Burns are a prevalent form of abuse and can result from either an active intent to injure or from neglect. Vulnerable populations such as children, the elderly, disabled persons, and mentally impaired persons are at increased risk of abuse. The critical care nurse plays a lead role in recognizing and identifying potential abuse or neglect cases, because he or she is in a unique position of being the burn team member that spends the most time interfacing with the patient and significant others. Nurses must elicit the history of the story and circumstances surrounding the injury event, carefully and accurately document wound appearance and pattern of injury (including use of photographs), and observe interactions between the patient and caregivers or family. The reported injury history should correlate with physical findings. Discrepancies between reported accounts of the injury event and physical assessment findings indicate a potential abuse situation. The presence of other injuries (i.e., associated bruising, fractures, abrasions, or other trauma) and the distribution and characteristics of the burn wound also provide revealing and key information on the true cause of the burn injury. For example, a scald burn with a clear demarcation and/or symmetrical wound pattern on extremities without splash mark burns indicates an intentional immersion injury instead of an accidental scald (Figure 19-13). All potential or suspected abuse cases must be reported to the appropriate authorities as governed by state laws. The patient is hospitalized until social workers and protective services have investigated the patient's home environment to determine whether the patient will be safe on discharge. Refer to the recommended readings (Peck &

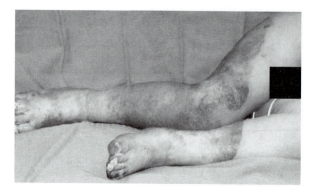

FIGURE 19-13 Child abuse by hot water immersion. The thigh burn wound edges have a clear demarcation line (are in a straight line) and there are no splash marks. The parents delayed seeking medical treatment for the child's burns until 3 days after injury (note the dry, crusty appearance of the wounds). The child also had a forearm fracture and multiple areas of bruising on the body. (Courtesy of University of Michigan Trauma Burn Center, Ann Arbor, MI.)

Priolo-Kapel, 2002) for additional information regarding assessment of abuse injuries.

Pain Control

Jonsson, Holmsten, Dahlstrom, and Jonsson (1998) stated that pain is a tormenting consequence of burn injury, both immediately after the injury and during the healing of the burn wound. Pain experienced during the acute phase of recovery consists of a constant or *resting pain*, as well as a shorter peak of excruciating pain (*procedural or breakthrough pain*) often associated with therapeutic procedures (Carrougher et al., 2003). Many aspects of burn treatment produce pain including dressing changes, debridement, surgical intervention, application of topical antimicrobials, and physical and occupational therapy. This situation illustrates the major paradox of burn pain management: the nurse inflicts pain and then must relieve it.

Adequately treating a burn patient's pain is a challenge to health care professionals. Altered pharmacokinetics secondary to changes in volume distribution and hypermetabolism is associated with burn injury. Additionally, burn patients commonly have histories of regular alcohol consumption or substance use that can further compound pain management and narcotic resistance (Byers, Bridges, Kijek, & LaBorde, 2001; Ilechukwu, 2002). Therefore, quantities of analgesics required by burn patients often exceed those of other disease states (Saffle, 2003). However, inaccurate assessment of a patient's pain or fears of addiction can lead to undermedication. The literature supports that much work needs to be done in improving assessment and intervention of severe burn pain (AHCPR, 1992; Carrougher et al., 2003). A study by Carrougher and colleagues (2003) found that burn patients have realistic expectations of their care and do not expect to be completely free of acute pain; however, a patient's satisfaction with their care was related to the level of pain experienced. Therefore, to control a patient's pain successfully and to achieve increased patient satisfaction, accurate serial pain assessments must occur, and the patient must be involved in creating an individualized analgesic treatment plan (Byers, Bridges, Kijek, & LaBorde, 2001; Carrougher et al., 2003). Pain levels should be assessed frequently as "the fifth vital sign," with additional assessment before, during, and after all procedures or treatments. The nurse serves as the patient's advocate by ensuring that appropriate delivery methods of pain medications and dosages are administered to reduce pain intensity.

Opiates are the most common analgesics used in the treatment of burn pain. Subcutaneous or intramuscular injections are ineffective in the resuscitative phase because of impaired circulation in soft tissue. Absorption is sporadic, leading to risk of undermedication or narcotic overdose. IV morphine is the drug and route of choice. A continuous IV infusion of morphine may be useful in maintaining a consistent level of analgesia, but it is typically used only in critically ill patients requiring mechanical ventilation. Patients have expressed increased satisfaction in being able to have some "control" over their pain (Sim, Hwang, Chan, & Seah, 1996). Therefore, use of a patient-controlled analgesic may be beneficial in providing adequate pain relief. Analgesic medications can be given safely by oral route once the patient is hemodynamically stable and the ileus has resolved. Although pain is reduced as wounds are covered with temporary dressings or skin grafts, frequent surgical procedures and wound care procedures produce episodic periods of pain and anxiety until permanent wound closure or healing is completed. Itching that occurs during the healing process also contributes to the patient's overall discomfort. Several medications and soothing emollients can assist in controlling pruritus.

The entire burn care and treatment experience produces anxiety, which can further exacerbate pain (Byers, Bridges, Kijek, & LaBorde, 2001). Consequently, the ideal pain management regimen must incorporate treatment of both pain and anxiety. Fear and a loss of control over their lives and schedules increase patients' anxiety. Therefore, the critical care nurse must provide frequent and repeated explanations of care plans, interventions, and procedures

at an age-appropriate level. Patients are encouraged to participate as much as possible in their wound care, medication administration, feeding, and exercise therapy. Anxiolytics and benzodiazepines are commonly administered in the acute care phase. Psychological techniques, such as simple relaxation and guided-imagery techniques, can also serve as useful adjuncts for reducing anxiety and enhancing pain relief. In summary, accurate pain and anxiety assessment, close monitoring, and individualized dosing of medications are essential for successful pain control (Saffle, 2003).

Infection Control

Burn patients have a high risk of infection related to altered skin integrity and altered immune response. When the skin's natural mechanical barrier protection is lost, the patient's susceptibility to infection increases. Additionally, other host defense mechanisms are impaired, and immunosuppression develops. Although great strides have been made in the management of infection, it remains a predominant determinant in the outcome of the burn-injured patient (ABA, 2002; ABA Evidence-Based Group, 2001). The incidence of infection among burn patients is higher than in any other patient group, and the incidence is particularly high in injuries greater than 30% TBSA (Weber, 1998). Invasive monitoring and treatment procedures such as urinary catheters, IV catheters, and endotracheal tubes also provide a source of infection. Therefore, the control of infection is an important nursing intervention in the care of burn patients.

The goals of infection control in burn care are as follows:

- Prevention of transmission of exogenous organisms to patients or personnel
- Control of the transfer of endogenous organisms (normal flora) to sites at increased risk of infection
- Protection and support of existing defenses in patients with seriously impaired resistance (Weber, 1998).

Infection control in the burn patient is dependent on the following strategies:

- Aseptic management of the wound and the environment of the patient
- Knowledgeable use of topical antibacterial agents
- Aggressive wound management with close monitoring for changes in wound appearance
- Judicious use of systemic antibiotics
- Maintenance of adequate nutrition
- Close monitoring of laboratory and clinical signs of impending sepsis

Although infection control policies differ among burn units, all policies stress standard precautions, including the use of barrier techniques, strict hand washing, and appropriate garb when caring for a burn-injured patient.

Wound Management

Patient outcomes from burn injury are optimized by focusing on the goals of wound infection prevention and treatment and expedited burn wound closure. Interventions performed to obtain these goals are wound cleansing, debridement, topical antimicrobial and/or biological-biosynthetic dressing therapy, and definitive surgical wound closure. Burn wound care protocols and procedures vary among burn centers across the country. However, the underlying goals of wound care are the same: removal of nonviable tissue to promote reepithelialization and prompt coverage via skin grafts when necessary.

WOUND CARE

To promote prevention of infection and healing of the burn wound, the nurse must focus on performing meticulous wound care. Wound care is typically done once or twice a day, depending on the healing status of the wound, the topical agents or dressing used, and the number of days postoperatively from grafting. Before initiating wound care, the nurse carefully explains the procedure to the patient and significant others and encourages participation as able. Analgesics are administered (and sedatives if indicated) before starting the procedure. All wounds are cleansed with a mild soap or surgical detergent disinfectant and are then rinsed with warm tap water. The patient is not immersed in water, because immersion has a significant potential for cross-contamination of wounds. Instead, water is allowed to flow over the wounds and immediately drained away. This regimen is best accomplished in a shower or hydrotherapy stretcher, but bed baths may also be used for hemodynamically unstable patients. All previously applied topical agents, necrotic tissue, exudate, and fibrous debris are removed from the wound to expose healthy tissue, to control bacterial proliferation, and to promote healing. Loose eschar and wound debris are *debrided* (removed) with washcloths or gauze sponges, scissors, and forceps. Mechanical trauma and damage from aggressive cleansing of newly formed epithelial skin buds or healing granulation tissue must be avoided. Hair in and immediately surrounding the wound bed is shaved (except eyebrows) to eliminate a medium for bacterial growth and to facilitate wound assessment. All wounds are inspected closely, with wound location, size, color, texture, and drainage carefully documented so any changes in appearance or developing signs of infection are noted.

The patient's core body temperature is closely monitored. Hydrotherapy and room temperature must be maintained to prevent chilling and excessive body heat loss.

TOPICAL AGENTS AND DRESSINGS

Recent years have witnessed a proliferation of new topical wound care agents and biosynthetic dressings. Newer products have broader antimicrobial actions, interact with the wound growth factors and collagen fibers to accelerate healing and to stop the zone of stasis from expanding, help to fill in defects, and may even reduce scarring. All these actions can positively affect outcomes in patients with burn injury by reducing infection, shortening healing time, preventing wound conversion to full-thickness depth, and improving long-term cosmetic appearance and scarring. After each hydrotherapy session, the unhealed or unexcised burn wound is covered with an antimicrobial topical agent and/or dressing. Table 19-3 describes the most commonly used agents and related nursing considerations. The selection of an agent and dressing is determined by burn depth, anatomical location, frequency of wound visualization desired, and presence and type of microorganisms identified. The ideal antimicrobial agent demonstrates broad-spectrum activity against microorganisms and penetrates eschar. At the same time, the agent should not interfere with wound healing (Jordan & Harrington, 1997). The burn center physician orders the antimicrobial agent, the frequency of application, and the method of application.

Many advances have been made in the development of wound dressings and skin substitutes to provide coverage for major burns. Temporary wound coverings are classified as either biological or biosynthetic (a combination of biological and synthetic properties). Table 19-4 provides descriptions of the most common types and uses for biological and biosynthetic coverings. Biological or biosynthetic dressings are commonly used as temporary wound coverings for freshly excised (surgically debrided) burn wounds until autograft skin is available (Integra, AlloDerm, xenograft, or allograft are commonly used for this indication). Biological or biosynthetic products may also be used as a dressing for partial-thickness burns, meshed autograft skin, or donor sites to promote healing (TransCyte, BioBrane, allograft, or xenograft are typically used for this type of application). Temporary wound coverings have the added benefits of controlling heat loss, decreasing infection risk, stimulating healing, and increasing patient comfort.

Enzymatic agents such as collagenase, papain/urea, or sutilains are also sometimes used for debridement of smaller necrotic tissue areas on deep partial- and

TABLE 19-3

Topical Antimicrobial Agents for Burn Wound Management

Agent	Indications	Nursing Considerations
Mafenide acetate (Sulfamylon)	Active against most gram-positive, gram-negative, and pseudomonas pathogens; drug of choice for ear burns; penetrates thick eschar and ear cartilage	Apply once or twice daily. Strong carbonic anhydrase inhibitor that can cause metabolic acidosis: monitor respiratory rate, electrolyte values, and arterial blood gases. Hydroscopic (draws water out of tissue) and can be painful/burning for 15 to 60 min after application. It tends to slow eschar separation.
Silver-coated dressings (Acticoat, Aquacel Ag, Silverlon)	Silver-coated, flexible, nonadhesive wound dressings; as long as dressing is moist, provides continuous release of silver ions for 3 to 14 days (depending on product used); effective broad-spectrum coverage for numerous pathogens commonly associated with burn wound infections (gram-negative bacteria, gram-positive bacteria, antibiotic-resistant bacteria, yeast, and mold); an alternative for patients allergic to sulfa drugs	Apply new dressing every 1 to 7 days, by (1) applying to moist open wound, with wound exudate maintaining silver activation until drainage stops on wound healing; (2) applying to wound, rewetting with sterile water q4-6h to keep dressing moist (not wet). Use sterile water to moisten dressings; saline renders silver ions ineffective. A decrease in the number of required dressing changes increases patient comfort and cost-effectiveness. Aquacel Ag does not require wetting and converts to a gel with wound exudate absorption.
Silver nitrate	Effective against a wide spectrum of common wound pathogens; acts on surface microorganisms only; poor eschar penetration; used in patients with toxic epidermal necrolysis syndrome or sulfa allergy	Apply 0.5% solution wet dressing two or three times daily; rewet the dressing q2h to ensure that it remains moist. Hypotonic solution causes leeching of electrolytes; monitor for hyponatremia, hypochloremia, hypocalcemia, and hypokalemia; administer supplements as ordered. Must be kept in a light-resistant container. Stains easily: protect walls, floors, and equipment with plastic.
Silver sulfadiazine (SSD, Silvadene)	Active against a wide spectrum of gram-negative, gram-positive, and *Candida albicans* pathogens; acts only on cell wall and membrane; does not penetrate thick eschar	Apply once or twice daily. May wrap wounds or leave as an open dressing. Can cause leukopenia; monitor the white blood cell count.
Clotrimazole cream or nystatin (Mycostatin)	Fungal colonization of wounds	Apply once or twice daily. Use in conjunction with an antibacterial topical agent. May cause skin irritation.

full-thickness burns. Topical enzymatic agents are proteolytic enzyme ointments that act as potent digestants of nonviable protein matter or necrotic tissue, but they are harmless to viable tissue. Enzymatic agents do not have antimicrobial properties; therefore, wounds must be closely monitored for infection.

Burn wounds can be treated in one of two ways: open or closed methods. The decision of which method to use depends on the location, size, and depth of the burn, as well as on specific burn unit protocols. Each method has advantages and disadvantages. With the open method, the burn wounds are left open to

TABLE 19-4	
Biological and Biosynthetic Dressings	
Type of Dressing	**Definition**
Biological dressing:	Temporary wound cover from human or animal species tissue
Allograft (homograft) skin	Graft of skin transplanted from another human, living or dead
Xenograft (heterograft) skin	Graft of skin, usually pigskin, transplanted between animals of different species
Biosynthetic dressing:	A wound covering composed of both biological and synthetic materials
AlloDerm	Transplantable tissue consisting of human cryopreserved allogenic dermis from which the epidermal, fibroblasts, and endothelial cells targeted for immune response have been removed
Integra	Skin replacement dressing system composed of two layers: (1) a "dermal" layer made of animal collagen and glycosaminoglycan that interfaces with the wound and functions as a dermal matrix for cellular growth and collagen synthesis, and (2) a temporary outer synthetic "epidermal" layer made of Silastic that acts as barrier to water loss and bacteria; dermal layer biodegrades within months as new wound collagen matrix is synthesized; silastic epidermal layer removed in 14-21 days and replaced with a thin autograft
TransCyte	Temporary skin substitute composed of an outer synthetic layer and an inner collagen base layer of human neonatal fibroblasts; interacts with the wound to amplify tissue regeneration: fibroblasts secrete growth factors, matrix proteins, human fibronectin, and collagen
Apligraf	Bilayer allogenic (from another human) skin substitute cultured from neonatal foreskin, consisting of (1) an outer multilayered "epidermal" barrier of cultured epidermal keratinocytes and (2) a "dermal" collagen matrix gel layer embedded with fibroblasts
Composite Cultured Skin (CCS or OrCel)	Similar to Apligraf. Allogenic skin substitute made from neonatal foreskin cultured onto a bovine collagen matrix sponge into two layers: (1) an outer "epidermal" layer of cultured allogenic epidermal keratinocytes placed on top of a sponge; (2) a "dermal" layer of fibroblasts cultured onto bottom and within the collagen sponge

air after the antimicrobial agent is applied. The open method provides increased wound visualization and more opportunities for observation, eliminates dressing supplies, and improves joint mobility normally limited by the presence of restrictive dressings. However, the open method allows direct contact between the wound and the environment. The applied topical antimicrobial agent may rub off on clothing, bedding, or equipment. Furthermore, the open method increases wound exposure time and the risk of hypothermia. The open method is commonly used on superficial burns to the face treated with the topical agent bacitracin. With the closed method, the wound is covered with gauze dressings that have been saturated with a topical antimicrobial agent, or a gauze dressing is placed over an agent that was applied directly to the wound. The closed method reduces heat loss and pain or sensitivity from wound exposure, and it assists in protecting wounds from external mechanical trauma.

The dressings applied may also assist with debridement. However, the closed method requires a dressing change to assess the wound, and the presence of dressings may impair ROM. The closed method is commonly used on full-thickness burns treated with silver sulfadiazine and new grafts.

A unique dressing system has been developed for treatment of grafts, partial-thickness burns, and deep surgical wounds (as seen in the nonburn injury necrotizing fasciitis). The vacuum-assisted closure (VAC) device consists of a sponge and suction tubing placed on the wound bed and covered with an occlusive dressing (Figure 19-14*A*). The device then creates a negative-pressure dressing to decompress edematous interstitial spaces and increase local perfusion, to help draw wound edges closed uniformly, to remove wound fluid, and to provide a closed, moist wound healing environment (Figure 19-14*B*). VAC also allows the collection and quantification of wound drainage.

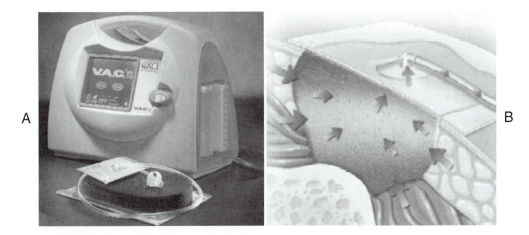

FIGURE 19-14 A, Vacuum-assisted closure (VAC) device. **B,** The device creates a negative-pressure dressing to decompress edematous interstitial spaces and to increase local perfusion, help draw wound edges closed uniformly, remove wound fluid, and provide a closed, moist wound healing environment. (Courtesy of Kinetic Concepts, Inc., San Antonio, TX.)

VAC therapy is showing promising results. It has been associated with lower wound bacterial counts, reduction in graft loss, and earlier reepithelialization (Scherer, Shiver, Chang, Meredith, & Owings, 2002).

SURGICAL EXCISION AND GRAFTING

Full-thickness burns are nonvascular and therefore will not heal without skin grafting for closure. Deep partial-thickness burns are also commonly grafted to decrease the risk of infection by achieving earlier wound closure and to improve cosmetic appearance (Sheridan, 2002). *Excision* is surgical debridement by scalpel or electrocautery to remove *necrotic* (dead) tissue until a layer of healthy, well-vascularized tissue is exposed. *Skin grafting* is placing skin on the excised burn wound (Figure 19-15*A*). Several types of skin can be used for skin grafting, including *allograft,* which is also called *homograft* (skin from another human, e.g., cadaver skin), *xenograft* (skin from another animal, e.g., pigskin), or *autograft* (skin from oneself that is transferred to a new location on the same individual's body, i.e., the patient's own skin). Autografts are the only permanent type of skin grafting (Table 19-5). Homografts and xenografts are temporary biological dressings (see Table 19-4). With autografts, a partial-thickness wound called a *donor site* is created where the skin was *harvested* or removed from the patient.

Excision and grafting are performed in the operating room and are typically initiated within the first week after burn injury. Early excision within the first 1 to 3 days is advocated because it has been associated with decreased mortality and morbidity (Barret & Herndon, 2003a and b; Sheridan, 2002). Advantages reported include modulation of the hypermetabolic response, reduced infection and wound colonization rates, increased graft take, and decreased length of hospitalization (Barret & Herndon, 2003a). Depending on the size of burn and the presence of infection, sequential or repeated surgical debridements and grafting may be required. In major burns, it is often not possible to graft all full-thickness wound areas initially either because of the patient's instability from the size and severity of burned areas or because of a lack of donor sites to provide adequate coverage. Priority areas for autograft skin application include the face, the hands, the feet, and over joints. In addition, other temporary and permanent synthetic products have been developed to substitute for a person's own skin (see Table 19-4). These products allow early burn wound coverage, while delaying grafting until previously used donor sites have healed and can be reharvested.

Autograft skin can be applied as meshed grafts or as sheet grafts. Sheet (nonmeshed) grafts are often used on the face and hands for better cosmetic results. Meshed grafts are commonly used elsewhere on the body (Figure 19-15*B*). A meshed graft is created by using a tool that places multiple tiny slits or holes in the piece of skin that was harvested from the donor site. The wider the mesh of the graft is, the larger the area that can be covered with the autograft skin. However, wider mesh grafts also typically contribute to more scarring and a less cosmetically pleasing appearance (Figure 19-15*C*). Table 19-5 summarizes the types of skin autografts used, along with nursing care requirements. Splitting of graft sites

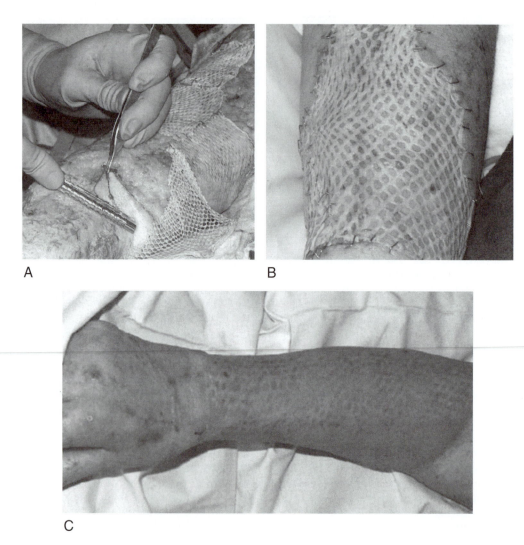

A

B

C

FIGURE 19-15 Excision and autografting. **A,** Surgical debridement (excision) with meshed autograft placement in the operating room. **B,** Meshed autograft 2 days postoperatively. **C,** Comparison of sheet autograft (on hand) versus meshed autograft (on forearm) 3 weeks postoperatively. Use of meshed autograft allows larger body surface area coverage, but it also typically leads to more scarring and a less cosmetically pleasing appearance. (Courtesy of University of Michigan Trauma Burn Center, Ann Arbor, MI.)

may be indicated to prevent movement and shearing of the grafts until healing is complete. Extremities are elevated to prevent pooling of blood and edema, which can lead to increased pressure and graft loss.

Many types of dressings can be used on donor sites (Table 19-6), but the product chosen must promote healing of the donor site within 8 to 14 days. Donor sites can be reused or reharvested once healed.

When patient donor sites are limited because of the severity of the burn injury, cultured epithelium autograft (CEA) can also be used to provide coverage

for a major burn injury. With CEA, a biopsy is obtained from the patient's skin and is sent to a laboratory where keratinocytes are cultured and grown. The process usually takes 2 to 3 weeks and results in small pieces of skin. These fragile pieces of skin are then surgically applied to a clean, excised burn wound bed. The disadvantage of CEA is its fragility, partly the result of the lack of the durable dermis. Researchers have been investigating the development of a different type of cultured skin substitute that incorporates CEA with a dermal layer (Boyce & Warden, 2002).

TABLE 19-5		
Autograft Skin: Nursing Implications		
Type of Autograft	**Definition**	**Nursing Implications**
Split-thickness sheet skin graft	Sheet of skin composed of the epidermis and a variable portion of the dermis that is harvested at a predetermined thickness. Sheet kept intact (not meshed) to improve cosmetic appearance; often used on face and hands.	Grafted area must be immobilized; pockets of serous/serosanguinous fluid must be evacuated by needle aspiration or rolling of the fluid with a cotton tip applicator toward the skin edges; if fluid is not evacuated, graft adherence is compromised.
Split-thickness meshed skin graft	Split-thickness sheet graft that is cut by a mesh dermatome, to expand the graft from 1.5 to 9 times its original size before being placed on a recipient bed of granulation tissue; used to cover large surface areas	Grafted area is immobilized, often in splints; skin graft is covered with fine mesh gauze, then coarse mesh gauze, and then wrapped with absorbent gauze roll before being placed in a splint; dressings must be kept moist—with an antimicrobial solution or biological dressing—but not saturated, to prevent desiccation and to promote epithelialization of the interstices of the meshed skin; first dressing change is in 3-5 days.
Full-thickness skin graft	A skin graft that contains the full thickness of the skin down to the subcutaneous tissue, typically used for eyelids or later reconstructive procedures	Requires the same care as a sheet skin graft.
Cultured epidermal autograft (CEA)	Layered sheets of human epidermal cells grown in the laboratory by use of tissue culture techniques to expand keratinocytes derived from a small skin biopsy specimen; allows for the potential of covering extensive wound areas more quickly without having to wait for healing of limited donor site skin surfaces. Epidermal layer replacement only. Epicel is trade name of CEA made by an outside company instead of on-site at the burn center	In the first 7-10 days after surgery, daily dressing changes involve only the outer layer of fluffy gauze; underlying coarse mesh gauze and petroleum jelly gauze, which are sutured over the graft, are not to be disturbed. Outer dressing must remain dry; many topical antimicrobial agents are toxic to the CEA skin and should not come in contact with the graft dressings. Once the petroleum jelly gauze is loose (7-10 days), it can be removed, and wet saline dressings are used until approximately 21 days after grafting, when the skin graft is usually well adherent. Gentle passive range-of-motion exercises can begin once the petroleum jelly gauze is removed.

Burn units vary in their protocols to treat grafted areas and donor sites. However, basic wound care principles are applied, and prevention of infection is always the primary goal. Although the critical care nurse may not actually develop the wound care plan, involvement by the entire burn team to promote compliance with the plan is essential for positive patient outcomes. A method of documenting wound treatment that facilitates day-to-day team communication of care requirements should be used.

Inherent in all wound care management is the necessity to improve and maintain function.

TABLE 19-6

Types of Donor Site Dressings

Dressing	Description
Fine mesh gauze	Cotton gauze placed directly on a donor site; a crust or "scab" is formed as the gauze dries and epithelialization of the wound occurs under the dressing; gauze peels away easily as the wound heals
Scarlet Red	Cotton gauze is impregnated with a blend of lanolin, olive oil, petrolatum, and the red dye "scarlet red"; healing occurs as with fine mesh gauze dressing
Xeroform	Fine mesh gauze containing 3% bismuth tribromophenate in a petrolatum blend; promotes healing as with other mesh gauze dressings
Op-Site	A thin elastic film that is occlusive, waterproof, and permeable to moisture, vapor, and air; fluid under dressing may need to be evacuated
DuoDerm	A hydrocolloid dressing that interacts with moisture on skin, and creates a bond that makes it adhere
N-terface	A translucent, nonabsorbent, and nonreactive surface material used between the burn wound and the outer dressing
Vigilon	A colloidal suspension on a polyethylene mesh support that provides a moist environment and is permeable to gases and water vapor
Kaltostat	Hydrophilic, nonwoven fiber that converts to a firm gel when it is activated by wound exudates; creates a warm, moist environment that is nonadherent to the wound
BioBrane	Bilaminate wound dressing composed of nylon mesh embedded with a collagen derivative with an outer silicone rubber membrane; permeable to wound drainage and topical antimicrobial agents; peels away as wound heals
Silver-coated dressings	Acticoat, Aquacel Ag, and Silverlon. Silver-coated, flexible dressings that provide continuous release of silver ions for 3-14 days while dressing is moist

Occupational and physical therapists are essential members of the burn team and are consulted on the day of admission. Often, the position of comfort for the patient is one that leads to dysfunction or deformity. Specialized splints and exercises are required for the prevention of future complications.

Nutritional Considerations and Metabolism

Adequate nutrition plays a critical role in the survival of extensively burned patients. A major burn injury produces a stress-induced hypermetabolic-catabolic response that is greater than that of any other disease process or injury. Skeletal muscle is the major protein store in the body. Postburn hypermetabolism can lead to deleterious consequences including significant skeletal muscle breakdown with protein degradation, body weight loss, marked delays in wound healing, skin graft loss, impaired immunological responsiveness, sepsis, or even death if adequate nutrition is not provided and an anabolic or positive nitrogen balance is not achieved (Barret & Herndon, 2003b; Wraa, 2003; Wray, Mammen, &

Hasselgren, 2002). Furthermore, muscle weakness and atrophy contribute to prolonged mechanical ventilation and delayed ambulation (Wray, Mammen, & Hasselgren, 2002). Thus, nutritional therapy must be instituted immediately after the burn injury to meet energy demands, to maintain host defense mechanisms, to replenish body protein stores, and to curtail progressive loss of lean body mass. The nurse collaborates with the patient, the registered dietitian, and the physician to coordinate a nutritional plan. If the patient is able to tolerate an oral diet, a high-calorie, high-protein diet with supplements is instituted with daily calorie counts performed to monitor dietary intake closely. If oral intake is not tolerated or caloric intake is insufficient, enteral tube feedings are begun. Early enteral feedings, within the first 24 hours after burn injury, have been shown to decrease the production of catabolic hormones, to improve nitrogen balance, to maintain gut integrity, to lower incidence of diarrhea, and to decrease hospital stay (Rose & Herndon, 1997; Sheridan, 2002). Research efforts have focused on methods of pharmacological intervention

Text continued on page 717

Nursing Care Plan: Resuscitative and Acute Care Phases of Major Burn Injury

NURSING DIAGNOSIS: *Ineffective airway clearance and impaired gas exchange related to tracheal edema or interstitial edema secondary to inhalation injury and/or circumferential torso eschar manifested by hypoxemia and hypercapnia*

Patient Outcomes	Interventions	Rationales
Partial pressure of arterial oxygen, >90 mm Hg; partial pressure of arterial carbon dioxide, <45 mm Hg; oxygen saturation, >95%; carboxyhemoglobin, <10%	Assess: respiratory rate, character, and depth q1h; breath sounds q4h; level of consciousness q1h. If the patient is not intubated, assess for stridor, hoarseness, and wheezing q1h.	Airway obstruction or dysfunction leads to inadequate oxygenation of vital tissues and organs.
Respirations 16 to 20 breaths/min and unlabored; breath sounds present and clear in all lobes; chest wall excursion symmetrical and adequate	Evaluate the need for chest escharotomy during fluid resuscitation.	Circumferential torso eschar can restrict lung expansion and decrease ventilation; releasing eschar by escharotomy improves ventilation and oxygenation.
Mentation clear; patient will mobilize secretions, which are clear to white in color	Administer humidified oxygen as ordered.	Expedites elimination of carbon monoxide and prevents or treats hypoxemia. Humidification assists with ease of breathing and patient comfort.
	Monitor oxygen saturation q1h, arterial blood gases and carboxyhemoglobin as needed, and the chest x-ray study as ordered.	Assists in modifying the treatment plan and interventions according to patient response and status.
	Assist the patient in coughing and deep breathing q1h while awake. Suction q1-2h or as needed. Monitor sputum characteristics and amount. Turn the patient q2h to mobilize secretions. The patient is out of bed as tolerated.	Promotes lung expansion, assists with ventilation, clearing of secretions, and in maintaining a clear airway.
	Elevate the head of the patient's bed.	Decreases edema of the face, neck, mouth and facilitates lung expansion.
	Schedule activities to avoid fatigue.	Fatigue can contribute to dyspnea and decreased ventilatory effort.

NURSING DIAGNOSIS: *Deficient fluid volume secondary to fluid shifts into the interstitium and evaporative loss of fluids from the injured skin*

Patient Outcomes	Interventions	Rationales
Weight gain based on volume of fluids administered in first 48 hr, followed by moderate diuresis over next 8-10 days	Titrate calculated fluid requirements in the first 48 hr to maintain acceptable urinary output and hemodynamic stability. Monitor vital signs q1h until stable. Monitor mental status q1h for at least 48 hr.	Fluid resuscitation assists restoration of intravascular volume. Clinical indices or end points serve as guide for adjusting fluid replacement.
Hourly urine output, 30 to 50 mL/hr; 75 to 100 mL/hr		

Continued

Nursing Care Plan: Resuscitative and Acute Care Phases of Major Burn Injury—cont'd

Patient Outcomes	Interventions	Rationales
in those with electrical injury	Obtain and record weights daily. Record hourly intake and output measurements and evaluate trends.	Assists with evaluation of fluid loss and replacement.
Specific gravity normal except during diuresis; urine negative for glucose and ketones		
Heart rate 80-120 beats/min; blood pressure adequate in relation to pulse and urine output		
Sensorium clear		
Serum laboratory values within normal limits	Monitor electrolyte, hematocrit, serum glucose, blood urea nitrogen, creatinine levels at least twice daily for the first 48 hr and then as required by patient status.	Evaluates the need for electrolyte and fluid replacement associated with large fluid and protein shifts.

NURSING DIAGNOSIS: *Decreased cardiac output related to decreasing blood volume from fluid shifts and/or release of myocardial depressant mediators*

Patient Outcomes	Interventions	Rationales
Optimal tissue perfusion		
Cardiac output, 4-8 L/min; heart rate, 60-120 beats/min; mean arterial pressure, 70-105 mm Hg; systemic vascular resistance, 900-1200 dynes/sec/cm^{-5}; central venous pressure and pulmonary artery occlusion pressure at upper ends of normal range; partial pressure of arterial oxygen, >90 mm Hg; partial pressure of arterial carbon dioxide, <45 mm Hg; oxygen saturation >95%	Monitor cardiac output, central venous pressure, pulmonary artery occlusion pressure, and systemic vascular resistance if a pulmonary artery catheter is present. Monitor oxygen saturation q1h and arterial blood gases as needed. Monitor vital signs and cardiac rhythm q1h until stable.	Evaluates tissue perfusion and circulation adequacy to determine the need for further fluid replacement or pharmacological intervention.
Hourly urine output, 30 to 50 mL/hr; 75 to 100 mL/hr in those with those with electrical injury	Monitor urine output hourly. Titrate fluid resuscitation as indicated; administer colloids as ordered.	Urine output closely reflects renal perfusion and overall adequacy of tissue perfusion.
Absence of dysrhythmias		
Mentation clear	Monitor mental status q1h for at least 48 hours.	Mental status is a sensitive indicator of oxygenation status.
Normal capillary refill; nonburned skin warm and pink		

Nursing Care Plan: Resuscitative and Acute Care Phases of Major Burn Injury—cont'd

NURSING DIAGNOSIS: *Ineffective tissue perfusion related to compression and impaired vascular circulation in extremities with circumferential burns*

Patient Outcomes	Interventions	Rationales
No tissue injury in extremities secondary to inadequate perfusion from edema or eschar Peripheral pulses present and strong	Assess peripheral pulses q1h for 72 hr. Notify the physician of changes in pulses, capillary refill, or pain sensation. Be prepared to assist with escharotomy or fasciotomy. Elevate the upper extremities (with intravenous poles or on pillows); elevate the lower extremities with pillows or blankets.	Assesses the status of peripheral perfusion and the need for escharotomy. Escharotomy or fasciotomy releases a band of constricting eschar, allows for edema expansion, and permits peripheral perfusion. Decreases edema formation.

NURSING DIAGNOSIS: *Acute pain related to burn trauma*

Patient Outcomes	Interventions	Rationales
Identifies factors that contribute to pain; verbalizes improved comfort level Physiological parameters returned to normal Respirations adequate and hemodynamic stability achieved after administration of narcotic analgesia	Use valid assessment tools to assess pain and anxiety; assess for nonverbal cues. Monitor for physiological responses to pain, such as increased blood pressure and heart rate and restlessness. Administer analgesic and/or anxiolytic medication as ordered; administer intravenously during critical care phases. Medicate the patient before bathing, dressing changes, and major procedures, as needed. Minimize open exposure of wounds. Reduce anxiety: explain all activities before initiating them; talk to the patient while performing activities; use nonpharmacological pain-reducing methods as appropriate; encourage participation in care activities. Monitor and document the patient's response to analgesics or other interventions.	Pain responses are variable and unique to each patient. Facilitates pain relief. Intramuscular medications are not consistently absorbed during resuscitation and critical care acute phases because of edema and decreased tissue perfusion. Medications given before treatments assist the patient to perform at higher level of function. Exposed nerve endings increase pain. Educating the patient about care plans assists with decreasing anxiety and fear of the unknown, increases the patient's control over the situation, and decreases anxiety. Pain level is best determined by the patient. This evaluates the effectiveness of pain-relieving interventions.

Continued

Nursing Care Plan: Resuscitative and Acute Care Phases of Major Burn Injury—cont'd

NURSING DIAGNOSIS: *Risk for infection related to loss of skin, impaired immune response, and invasive therapies*

Patient Outcomes	Interventions	Rationales
No inflamed burn wound margins No evidence of burn wound or donor site infection or invasive catheter site infection Autograft or allograft skin adherent to granulation tissue Sputum, blood, and urine cultures negative Body temperature 98.6°-101° F White blood cell counts within normal limits Glycosuria, vomiting, ileus, and/or change in mentation absent	Assess the burn wound and invasive catheter sites; assess and document the characteristics of urine and sputum. Assess and record the temperature and vital signs q1-4h as appropriate. Monitor the white blood cell count. Provide protective isolation appropriate to the method of wound care. Provide meticulous wound care with antimicrobial topical agents as ordered. Shave hair (except eyebrows) at least 1 inch around burn wounds. Adhere to guidelines issued by Centers for Disease Control and Prevention for invasive catheter care. Instruct visitors in burn unit guidelines. Obtain wound, sputum, urine, and blood cultures as ordered.	Facilitates early detection of developing infections to initiate prompt treatment. Facilitates prevention of infection by reducing exposure to pathogens. Hair is a medium for microorganism growth. Proper hand washing and use of protective barriers decrease contamination. Determines the source of infection and the specific invading microorganism to guide topical and/or systemic antimicrobial therapy appropriately.

NURSING DIAGNOSIS: *Impaired skin integrity related to burn wound and/or the consequences of immobility*

Patient Outcomes	Interventions	Rationales
No evidence of pressure ulcers or other injury present in unburned skin No evidence of progressive burn wound or donor site injury Burn wound, donor site healing, and skin graft adherence occurring within appropriate time frames	Elevate the patient's extremities and the head of the bed. Assess the skin over pressure areas, burn wounds, donor sites, pressure points under splints, and dependent areas. Pad pressure areas: heels, elbows, sacrum, scapulae, and burned ears. Assess the need for special beds or mattresses. Remove blood pressure cuff from areas of burned skin. Assess the circulation of digits in splinted extremities. Monitor securing devices for the endotracheal tube to ensure that devices do not put pressure on ears. Promote drying of donor sites as appropriate: keep heat lamps at a safe distance to prevent injury. Immobilize skin graft sites for 3 to 7 days after grafting per unit protocols. Roll sheet grafts as ordered to promote adherence.	Reduces edema; edematous skin is at higher risk of injury. Regular monitoring of high-risk areas facilitates early detection of further skin loss from pressure or mechanical trauma. Facilitates graft adherence and take. Movement can cause shearing or dislodging of the graft. Fluid collections underneath the graft impede graft adherence.

Nursing Care Plan: Resuscitative and Acute Care Phases of Major Burn Injury—cont'd

Patient Outcomes	Interventions	Rationales
	Assess wound healing status.	Evaluates the effectiveness of treatments and interventions and facilitates early detection of developing infectious processes that would further impair skin integrity.

NURSING DIAGNOSIS: *Ineffective tissue perfusion of bowel related to hypovolemia manifested by ileus; risk for injury: gastrointestinal bleeding related to stress response*

Patient Outcomes	Interventions	Rationales
Decreased gastric motility and ileus resolved; enteral feedings absorbed and tolerated	Place a nasogastric tube in patients with >20% TBSA burns. Administer H_2 blockers and/or antacids as ordered to keep gastric pH >5.	Gastric decompression is required to prevent nausea, emesis, and aspiration from ileus. Gastrointestinal prophylaxis prevents the development of stomach and duodenal ulcers.
No evidence of gastrointestinal hemorrhaging	Assess the nasogastric aspirate for color, quantity, pH, and guaiac; monitor stool guaiac. Assess the abdomen and bowel sounds. Initiate enteral feeding per orders, and evaluate tolerance.	Facilitates early detection of stomach and duodenal ulcers that can lead to frank hemorrhaging. Evaluates resolution of decreased gastric motility and ileus.

NURSING DIAGNOSIS: *Imbalanced nutrition: less than body requirements related to increased metabolic demands secondary to physiological stress and wound healing*

Patient Outcomes	Interventions	Rationales
Daily requirement of nutrients consumed, based on formulas for appropriate calorie calculation Positive nitrogen balance Progressive wound healing 90% of preburn weight maintained	Record all oral intake. Count calories as needed. Activate the enteral/parenteral feeding protocol; Provide high-calorie/protein supplements as needed. Monitor weights daily or biweekly. Assess the abdomen and bowel sounds q8h. Monitor characteristics and quantity of output from the nasogastric tube and from stools. Provide adaptive devices to facilitate self-feeding. Have family members assist at meal time. If the patient has an oral diet, schedule interventions and activities to avoid interrupting feeding times.	Caloric and protein intake must be adequate to maintain a positive nitrogen balance and to promote healing. Evaluates weight loss from inadequate caloric intake and fluid volume changes, and it assesses tolerance and response to feeding interventions. Encourages the patient to increase intake. Pain, fatigue, or sedation interferes with a desire to eat.

Continued

Nursing Care Plan: Resuscitative and Acute Care Phases of Major Burn Injury—cont'd

NURSING DIAGNOSIS: *Impaired physical mobility and self-care deficit related to therapeutic splinting, immobilization requirements after skin graft, and/or contractures*

Patient Outcomes	Interventions	Rationales
No evidence of permanent decreased joint function from preburn status unless directly related to trauma Vocation resumed without functional limitations, or adjustment to new vocation based on functional limitations	Perform active and passive range-of-motion exercises to all extremities q2h while the patient is awake. Increase the patient's activity as tolerated. Maintain proper joint alignment with splints; maintain antideformity positioning. Elevate the patient's extremities. Provide pain relief measures before physical and/or occupational therapy. Promote the use of adaptive devices.	Assists with preventing loss of movement, function; prevent contracture development. Edema interferes with range of motion and mobility. Medications given before treatments and therapy facilitate mobility and assist the patient to perform at a higher level of function. Decreases dependency on caregivers.

NURSING DIAGNOSIS: *Risk for hypothermia related to loss of skin and/or external cooling*

Patient Outcomes	Interventions	Rationales
Rectal/core temperature 98.6°-101° F	Monitor and document rectal/core temperature q1-2h; assess for shivering. Minimize skin exposure; maintain environmental temperatures. For a temperature of less than 98.6° F, institute rewarming measures.	Evaluates the status of body heat loss. Increased exposure and cool environment increase the rate of body heat evaporative and conductive losses. Hypothermia is associated with serious complications and must be prevented or immediately treated.

NURSING DIAGNOSIS: *Risk for ineffective individual coping and disabled family coping related to acute stress of critical injury and potential life-threatening crisis.*
Interrupted family processes related to critical injury and potential lifestyle or family role changes

Patient Outcomes	Interventions	Rationales
Patient and family verbalizing goals of treatment regimen Patient and family demonstrating knowledge of support systems Patient and family able to express concerns and fears	Support adaptive and functional coping mechanisms. Orient the patient and family to unit and support services and reinforce information frequently. Involve the patient and family in the plan of care. Use interventions to reduce patient fatigue and pain.	Involvement and knowledge decrease fear and anxiety and enhance feelings of control and self-worth. Adequate pain control and rest facilitate patient coping.

Nursing Care Plan: Resuscitative and Acute Care Phases of Major Burn Injury—cont'd

Patient Outcomes	Interventions	Rationales
Patient and family's coping functional and realistic for phase of hospitalization; family processes at precrisis level	Promote the use of group support sessions. Consult the social worker for assistance in discharge planning and psychosocial assessment issues. Consult psychiatric services for inadequate coping skills or for treatment of substance abuse.	Assists the patient and family in understanding experiences and reactions after burn injury and methods of dealing with trauma. Uses the entire burn team to provide expert consultation and intervention.

NURSING DIAGNOSIS: *Deficient knowledge related to burn injury, treatments, and wound healing*

Patient Outcomes	Interventions	Rationales
Verbalizing understanding of plan of care Demonstrating ability to care for burn wounds Discharge planning initiated on admission	Explain procedures, interventions, and tests in clear, simple, age-appropriate language. Reinforce the proper use and importance of splints and antideformity positioning compliance. Provide unit guidelines, written information, and/or instructions to which the patient and family can refer. Begin multidisciplinary discharge planning on the day of patient admission.	The patient will more likely participate and adhere to the treatment plan if the purpose is understood. Reinforces verbal information provided to the patient and family. Facilitates patient and family participation in the plan of care and smoothes the discharge process.

TBSA, total body surface area.

to regulate the hypermetabolic-catabolic response to burn injury (Saffle, 2003). Please refer to Chapter 5 for additional information.

Psychosocial Considerations

Burn injury is one of the most psychologically devastating injuries to patients and their families. Not only is there a very real threat to survival, but psychological and physical pain, fear of disfigurement, and uncertainty of long-term effects of the injury on the future can precipitate a crisis for the patient and family. Before appropriate functioning returns, the patient may exhibit stages of psychological adaptation (Box 19-3). A patient may not manifest every stage, but support and therapy are necessary for any patient and family experiencing major burn injury.

To facilitate a person's emotional adjustment to burn trauma, it is first necessary to consider the complex interaction of preinjury personality, extent of injury, social support systems, and home environment. For example, many burn injuries are the result of suicide attempts, abuse, assaults, or arson. The patient may be dealing with loss of loved ones in the fire, nightmare or injury event flashbacks, loss of home and/or belongings, job or financial concerns, or fear of assailants or the patient may even be facing criminal charges. Additionally, preinjury psychiatric disorders such as depression, mood disorders, psychoses, and alcohol and drug abuse frequently exist in the burn patient population (Ilechukwu, 2002). Therefore, the critical care nurse must assess the patient's and family's support systems, coping mechanisms, and potential for development of

BOX 19-3

Stages of Postburn Psychological Adaptation

SURVIVAL ANXIETY

This is often manifested by lack of concentration, easy startle response, tearfulness, social withdrawal, and inappropriate behavior. Instructions need to be repeated, and the patient has to be allowed time to verbalize concerns and fears. Increased reports of pain are frequently associated with high levels of anxiety.

SEARCH FOR MEANING

During this phase, the patient repeatedly recounts the events leading to the injury and tries to determine a logical explanation that is emotionally acceptable. It is important to avoid judging the patient's reasoning and to listen actively and to participate in the discussions with the patient.

INVESTMENT IN RECUPERATION

This is a period of increased cooperation with the treatment regimen. The patient is motivated to be independent and takes pride in small accomplishments. The nurse should educate the patient concerning discharge goals and should involve the patient and family in planning for a program of increased self-care. The patient requires much praise and verbal encouragement in this phase.

INVESTMENT IN REHABILITATION

As self-confidence increases, the patient is focused on achieving as much preburn function as possible. Depression may occur as new losses in function are realized. Staff support is limited in this phase, which usually occurs after the patient is discharged from the hospital and is undergoing outpatient rehabilitation. Praise, support, and continued information are beneficial.

REINTEGRATION OF IDENTITY

The patient accepts losses and recognizes that changes have occurred. Adaptation is completed, and staff involvement is terminated.

Modified from Watkins, P., Cook, E., May, S., & Ehleben, C. (1988). Psychological stages in adaptation following burn injury: A method for facilitating psychological recovery of burn victims. *Journal of Burn Care Rehabilitation, 9*(4), 376-384.

posttraumatic stress disorder. Inadequate coping may be demonstrated by changes in behavior, manipulation, regression, sleep deprivation, or depression. Interventions based on individual assessments are the most beneficial and may require assistance from support personnel such as chaplains, clinical nurse specialists, child life specialists, psychiatrists, and social workers. As the patient moves out of the critical care unit, support mechanisms and continuity of care must persevere because psychosocial recovery can take months, years, or a lifetime.

Geriatric Considerations

As a group, older patients are more prone to and more adversely affected by burns (Redlick et al., 2002). Diminished manual dexterity, reaction time, vision, hearing, and judgment render the elderly vulnerable to burn injuries. Many older people live alone and are often physically or mentally unable to respond appropriately to an emergency. Additionally, elderly skin is much less resilient to mechanical trauma. The physiological and psychosocial trauma of a burn injury in the elderly patient provides a tremendous challenge for the burn team.

Many variables influence outcome of the elderly burn victim, including preinjury health, burn severity, and postinjury complications (see Geriatric Assessment). Complications of thermal injury significantly affect outcomes in elderly patients, especially when there is more than one major complication (Covington, Wainwright, & Parks, 1996). Preexisting cardiovascular, renal, or pulmonary disorders contribute to difficulties in providing adequate fluid resuscitation and to a higher mortality. Older patients with heart failure may require administration of positive inotropic medications to increase cardiac contractility and circulate resuscitation fluid volumes. Elderly patients with inhalation injury frequently require mechanical ventilation support and are more prone to episodes of pneumonia and sepsis. Prolonged immobilization and ongoing physiological stress also contribute to a significant morbidity related to inhalation injury. Wound care presents a challenge in managing the elderly burn patient. Skin changes associated with aging, such as flattened dermal-epidermal junction and loss of dermal and subcutaneous mass, manifest as skin thinning and predispose this group to deeper burn wounds and to poor or delayed healing. This situation affects not only the healing of the original burn wounds, but also the skin graft recipient beds and donor sites. A decline in immune system functioning increases susceptibility to infectious complications in this group as well. Moreover, older patients have a diminished physiological reserve and capacity

Geriatric Assessment

- Preexisting cardiovascular, renal, and pulmonary diseases lead to challenges in fluid resuscitation.
- Fluid administration may be guided by hemodynamic monitoring.
- Determine as early as possible in care if the patient has an advanced directive.
- Physiological changes in the skin from aging predispose the elderly to deeper burn wounds and poor or delayed wound healing. Burn wounds, grafts, and donor sites must be monitored carefully.
- Decline in immune system functioning contributes to increased susceptibility to infection.
- Elderly patients have reduced physiological reserves and capacity to respond to the metabolic stress of burn injury.
- Mechanical ventilation contributes to a higher risk of pneumonia, sepsis, and complications of immobility. Ventilator weaning may be prolonged because of muscular weakness.
- Reduced renal and hepatic functioning predisposes elderly patients to delayed clearance of medications (antibiotics, analgesics) and increased potential for toxicity or overdose.
- Elderly patients have greater morbidity and mortality compared with younger patients with similar percentages of total body surface area burn (Redlick et al., 2002).

to respond to the metabolic stress and bacterial challenge after a burn injury.

Advances in technology and treatment have improved survival after burn injury (Barret & Herndon, 2003a; Brigham & Quinn, 2003; Redlick et al., 2002; Wraa, 2003). However, data suggest that advanced age continues to be a major determinant of mortality after thermal injury (Brandt, Ahrns, & Wahl, 2003). Therefore, the decision to proceed with resuscitation in elderly patients with large burns and concomitant inhalation injury should be carefully considered, with advanced directives, next of kin, and/or durable power of attorney consulted (Sheridan, 2001). Poor outcomes after injury highlight that prevention of burn injuries in the elderly is of utmost importance. Recognition and regulation, or avoidance, of high-risk activities by the elderly and their caregivers should occur. Cooking, hot bathing water, smoking materials, and home heating devices are often reported as sources of burn injuries in this group (Redlick et al., 2002).

Nonburn Injury

The experience of the burn team in providing excellent wound and critical care leads to burn unit admissions of patients with a variety of other severe exfoliative and necrotizing skin disorders such as toxic epidermal necrolysis, staphylococcal scalded skin syndrome, and necrotizing fasciitis. These conditions create a clinical wound picture like that of a burn wound and require similar patient management and wound care. Management of these patients in a burn center has been associated with a marked increase in survival (ABA, 2001; Saffle, 2003).

SEVERE EXFOLIATIVE DISORDERS

Toxic epidermal necrolysis (TEN), Stevens-Johnson syndrome, and erythema multiforme are similar conditions in which the body sloughs its epidermal layer in response to some causative agent. The skin separation occurs at the epidermal-dermal junction, with varying degrees of dermal involvement. Clinically, it is difficult to diagnose these similar disorders; assessment of the extent of cutaneous involvement and skin biopsy for histopathology are required for differential diagnosis. However, nursing diagnoses and interventions are the same for all severe exfoliative disorders. TEN is the most extensive form of severe exfoliative disorder and is therefore discussed. The most common cause of TEN is drug reaction, particularly from sulfa drugs, phenobarbital, and phenytoin. However, some cases have no apparent cause. A multiinstitutional burn center study found that TEN was associated with a mortality rate of 32% (Palmieri, Greenhalgh, & Saffle, 2002). Patients present with fever and flulike symptoms, and erythema and blisters develop within 24 to 96 hours. As large bullae develop, the skin and mucous membranes slough, resulting in a significant and painful partial-thickness injury. TEN is also associated with mucosal wound involvement of conjunctival, oral, GI tract, and/or urogenital areas (ABA, 2001; Sheridan, 2002; Palmieri et al., 2002). Immune suppression occurs and contributes to life-threatening complications such as sepsis and pneumonia. Optimal wound treatment consists of early coverage of cutaneous wounds with biological dressings. Severe exfoliative disorders typically require intensive critical care management to provide fluid resuscitation and nutritional support. Prevention of infection is crucial to stop progression of wounds to full-thickness depth.

NECROTIZING SOFT TISSUE INFECTIONS

Staphylococcal Scalded Skin

Staphylococcal scalded skin (SSS) syndrome occurs primarily in children and often presents with a clinical picture similar to that of toxic epidermal necrolysis. SSS syndrome is caused by a reaction to a staphylococcal toxin with *intraepidermal* splitting (unlike *epidermal-dermal* separation in TEN) resulting in skin sloughing. The differential diagnosis is made by microscopic examination of the denuded skin to determine the level of skin separation (ABA, 2001). SSS syndrome is limited to epidermal involvement and does not affect the mucous membranes. A low mortality (5%) exists with this condition in children, although mortality may be as high as 60% in adults (Patel & Finlay, 2003). SSS syndrome is best treated with antibiotic therapy and wound care management.

Necrotizing Fasciitis

Necrotizing fasciitis occurs more frequently in adults and is associated with a 23% mortality rate (Faucher, Morris, Edelman, & Saffle, 2001). Necrotizing fasciitis is caused by toxin-producing organisms, often introduced from minor skin disruptions such insect bites or cuts, that lead to widespread fascial and muscle necrosis. Diabetes, obesity, and age are risk factors for the development of necrotizing fasciitis (Faucher, Morris, Edelman, & Saffle, 2001). Necrotizing fasciitis typically has a subtle initial presentation of a localized painful edematous area with increasing erythema. The pain is severe and out of proportion to cutaneous findings. Early diagnosis, aggressive surgical excision and wound care, and antibiotics are essential for a positive outcome.

Discharge Planning

Discharge planning for critically ill burned patients or those who have sustained a nonburn injury must begin on the day of admission. Assessments are made regarding patient survival, the potential or actual short-term or long-term functional disabilities secondary to the burn or nonburn injury, the financial resources available, the family roles and expectations, and the psychological support systems. Patient and family education is essential to prepare for transfer from the critical care unit and eventual discharge from the hospital. Patients and families who are returning home must understand how to manage their physical requirements, as well as care for their psychological and social needs. Nurses play an important role in multidisciplinary discharge planning by providing patient and family education and by evaluating the need for additional resources to meet patient long-term rehabilitative and home care requirements.

Burn Prevention

Burn injuries are tragic because most could have been avoided. It is estimated that as many as 90% of burns and fire-related injuries are preventable (Wraa, 2003). Critical care nurses play an active and vital role in teaching prevention concepts and in promoting fire safety legislation that assists in preventing fires and burn injury. The incidence of burn injuries has been successfully decreased with government-mandated regulations on industrial environments, products, and home safety (e.g., hot water heater temperature, fire-retardant children's sleepwear, and mandatory smoke detectors) (Saffle, 2003; Sheridan, 2002). Box 19-4 lists strategies for preventing burn injuries.

BOX 19-4

Strategies for Preventing Burn Injuries

COOK WITH CARE

Turn pot handles toward the back of the stove.

Keep appliances with long cords toward the back of the counter.

Always use cooking mitts, and never carry more than you can safely handle.

Never wear loose sleeves or other loose clothing while cooking.

Always set a kitchen timer to remind you to turn off burners and the oven.

If a pan of food catches fire, carefully slide a lid over the pan and turn off the burner.

Never throw water on a grease or electrical fire; turn off the heat source and, if necessary, use a smothering substance such as flour.

Stir microwave foods to distribute heat, and test all heated foods before giving to a child.

Create a safety zone for children by using gates, playpens, and highchairs to keep them at a safe distance from all hot items.

BOX 19-4

Strategies for Preventing Burn Injuries—cont'd

HOT LIQUIDS CAUSE SCALDS

Never hold an infant or child while pouring or drinking hot liquids.

Many injuries occur when hot liquids are pulled from the microwave, especially by a child.

Bath water is a potentially dangerous hot liquid; turn your water heater down to 120° F; use a bath thermometer to check water temperature before touching bath water.

HOME PRECAUTIONS

Teach children the stop, drop, and roll procedure.

Small children often use their teeth to pull apart plugs; keep electrical cords out of reach, and teach safety.

Keep all matches and lighters out of the reach of children.

Teach children to stay away from high-voltage utilities.

Teach older children how to use appliances safely and about the dangers of electricity near water.

Do not overload outlets.

Use only UAL-approved portable space heaters, and keep space heaters 3 feet away from everything, including yourself; do not use them with extension cords.

Be safe when smoking: use large, deep ashtrays, and dispose of ashes in the toilet; do not smoke while lying down or in bed (quitting smoking is the best safety precaution of all).

There is only one acceptable use of gasoline: fueling an engine.

Put sunscreen on you and your children.

Be prepared for a fire emergency: practice escape routes with your children and your babysitter; small children could become frightened and hide when faced with an unfamiliar emergency situation.

Keep all flame sources away from home oxygen.

Acknowledge that alcohol, drugs, and some medications impair your balance, judgment, and reaction time; use caution around fire sources.

Closely supervise burning candles, and keep them out of reach of children and pets who may knock them over; never have candles burning while you are sleeping.

Never store flammable liquids (gasoline, propane, cleaners, paint solvents) near fire sources such as a furnace or a pilot light.

FIRE EXTINGUISHERS AND SMOKE DETECTORS

Fire extinguishers must be easily accessible (near exits).

Learn how to use your fire extinguisher.

Smoke detectors are burn prevention tools; they can prevent injury and save lives.

Install several smoke detectors and check batteries monthly.

OCCUPATION-RELATED PRECAUTIONS

Always wear all safety equipment and personal protection gear.

Fatigue contributes to carelessness and accidents; take breaks to prevent accidents.

Know the location of emergency exits, fire extinguishers, safety showers and eye washers, and main electrical and/or gas shutoff valves.

Be familiar with potential chemical hazards in your workplace; review Material Safety Data Sheets.

 ## Case Study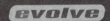

Mrs. J. is a 70-year-old woman who sustained a thermal burn injury in a house fire. An electric heater ignited her bedspread while she was asleep. She was trapped in the room for approximately 15 minutes before being rescued by firefighters.

QUESTIONS

1. Once Mrs. J. is removed from the fire, what priorities are essential in her initial management?
2. She has singed nose hair and is coughing up sooty sputum. The emergency department is 15 minutes away. Based on this assessment, what should the paramedics do?
3. What diagnostic tests and assessments do you anticipate once Mrs. J. reaches the emergency department?
4. Mrs. J weighs 65 kg. She has burned an estimated 30% of her body. What is her estimated fluid requirement during the first 24 hours?
5. How much fluid will be given in the first 8 hours after the injury?
6. Given Mrs. J's age, what are important assessments during aggressive fluid resuscitation?
7. Mrs. J has circumferential, white, leathery burn wounds on both arms. What type of burn wound does she have? What assessments should be performed? What type of surgical treatment and wound care should be expected during the resuscitative phase, and later in the acute care phase?
8. What type and route of pain medication should be administered to Mrs. J?

SUMMARY

The physiological response to a major burn injury is one of a biphasic pattern of multiorgan system hypofunction followed by hyperfunction. A major goal of resuscitative care is the prevention of burn shock. The critical care nurse's observations of patient responses are crucial for the prevention of complications related to increased capillary permeability and massive resuscitation fluid therapy. In the acute phase, therapeutic goals include prevention of further tissue loss, maintenance of function, prevention of infection, and wound closure. As the patient progresses through various stages of wound care management, the nurse must not only provide skilled care but also monitor the patient and family's responses to the treatment regimen. Psychosocial support is integral to the entire process. Although providing care to the burned patient is a team effort, it is the critical care nurse who is with the patient 24 hours a day. The skill and support of the nurse make the critical difference in the patient's outcome.

CRITICAL THINKING QUESTIONS

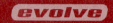

1. Explain why patients with burns need extensive fluid resuscitation even though they are extremely edematous.
2. What interventions would you use to meet the high caloric needs of burn patients who can take foods by mouth?
3. What interventions can be used in the critical care unit to promote early rehabilitation of a burned patient?
4. Many burned patients must be treated at institutions far away from home. What interventions can be used to meet the psychosocial needs of these patients and their families?

REFERENCES

Agency for Health Care Policy and Research (AHCPR). (1992). *Clinical practice guideline. Acute pain management: Operative or medical procedures and trauma* (No. 92-0032). Rockville, MD: U.S. Department of Health and Human Services.

Ahrns, K.S. (2004). Trends in burn resuscitation: Shifting the focus from fluids to adequate endpoint monitoring, edema control, and adjuvant therapies. *Critical Care Nursing Clinics of North America, 16*(1), 75-98.

Ahrns, K. S., & Harkins, D. R. (1999). Initial resuscitation after burn injury: Therapies, strategies, and controversies. *AACN Clinical Issues, 10*(1), 46-60.

American Burn Association (ABA). (2001). *Advanced burn life support course: Instructor's manual.* Chicago: American Burn Association.

American Burn Association (ABA), Evidence-Based Guidelines Group. (2001). Practice guidelines for burn care. *Journal of Burn Care and Rehabilitation, 22*[2 Suppl], S1-S67.

American Burn Association (ABA). (2002). *National burn repository: 2002 report.* Chicago: American Burn Association.

Barret, J. P., & Herndon, D. N. (2003a). Effects of burn wound excision on bacterial colonization and invasion. *Plastic and Reconstructive Surgery, 111*(2), 744-752.

Barret, J. P., & Herndon, D. N. (2003b). Modulation of inflammatory and catabolic responses in severely burned children by early burn wound excision in the first 24 hours. *Archives of Surgery, 138*(2), 127-132.

Boyce, S. T., & Warden, G. D. (2002). Principles and practices for treatment of cutaneous wounds with cultured skin substitutes. *American Journal of Surgery, 183*(4), 445-456.

Brandt, M. M., Ahrns, K. S., & Wahl, W. L. (2003). Elderly burn patients: Poorer outcome at what cost? *Journal of Burn Care and Rehabilitation, 24*(2), S47.

Brigham, P. A., & Quinn, A. H. (2003). Recent estimates of burn incidence and mortality based on national data sources. *Journal of Burn Care and Rehabilitation, 24*(2), S150.

Byers, J. F., Bridges, S., Kijek, J., & LaBorde, P. (2001). Burn patients' pain and anxiety experiences. *Journal of Burn Care and Rehabilitation, 22*(2), 144-149.

Carrougher, G. J., Ptacek, J. T., Sharar, S. R., et al. (2003). Comparison of patient satisfaction and self-reports of pain in adult burn-injured patients. *Journal of Burn Care and Rehabilitation, 24*(1), 1-8.

Cope, D., & Moore, F. D. (1947). The redistribution of body water in the fluid therapy of the burn patient. *Annals of Surgery, 126*, 1010-1018.

Covington, D. S., Wainwright, D. J., & Parks, D. H. (1996). Prognostic indicators in the elderly patient with burns. *Journal of Burn Care and Rehabilitation, 17*(2), 222-230.

Demling, R. H., Mazess, R. B., Witt, R. M., & Wolberg, W. H. (1978). The study of burn wound edema using dichromatic absorptiometry. *Journal of Trauma, 18*(2), 124-128.

Faucher, L. D., Morris, S. E., Edelman, L. S., & Saffle, J. R. (2001). Burn center management of necrotizing soft-tissue surgical infections in unburned patients. *American Journal of Surgery, 182*(6), 563-569.

Hart, D. W., Wolf, S. E., Mlcak, R., et al. (2000). Persistence of muscle catabolism after severe burn. *Surgery, 128*(2), 312-319.

Ilechukwu, S. T. (2002). Psychiatry of the medically ill in the burn unit. *Psychiatric Clinics of North America, 25*(1), 129-147.

Ivy, M. E., Atweh, N. A., Palmer, J., Possenti, P. P., Pineau, M., & D'Aiuto, M. (2000). Intra-abdominal hypertension and abdominal compartment syndrome in burn patients. *Journal of Trauma, 49*(3), 387-391.

Jonsson, C. E., Holmsten, A., Dahlstrom, L., & Jonsson, K. (1998). Background pain in burn patients: Routine measurement and recording of pain intensity in a burn unit. *Burns, 24*(5), 448-454.

Jordan, B. S., & Harrington, D. T. (1997). Management of the burn wound. *Nursing Clinics of North America, 32*(2), 251-273.

Koumbourlis, A. C. (2002). Electrical injuries. *Critical Care Medicine, 30*[11 Suppl], S424-S430.

Maass, D. L., White, J., & Horton, J. W. (2002). IL-1beta and IL-6 act synergistically with TNF-alpha to alter cardiac contractile function after burn trauma. *Shock, 18*(4), 360-366.

Mikhail, J. (1999). Resuscitation end points in trauma. *AACN Clinical Issues, 10*(1), 10-21.

Palmieri, T. L., Greenhalgh, D. G., Saffle, J. R., (2002). A multicenter review of toxic epidermal necrolysis treated in U.S. burn centers at the end of the twentieth century. *Journal of Burn Care and Rehabilitation, 23*(2), 87-96.

Patel, G. K., & Finlay, A. Y. (2003). Staphylococcal scalded skin syndrome: Diagnosis and management. *American Journal of Clinical Dermatology, 4*(3), 165-175.

Pruitt, B. A., Jr., Goodwin, C. W., & Cioffi, W. G. (1995). Thermal injuries. In J. H. David & G. G. Sheldon (eds.). *Surgery: A problem solving approach.* St. Louis: Mosby.

Redlick, F., Cooke, A., Gomez, M., Banfield, J., Cartotto, R. C., & Fish, J. S. (2002). A survey of risk factors for burns in the elderly and prevention strategies. *Journal of Burn Care and Rehabilitation, 23*(5), 351-356.

Rose, J. K., & Herndon, D. N. (1997). Advances in the treatment of burn patients. *Burns, 23*[Suppl 1], S19-S26.

Saffle, J.R. (2003). What's new in general surgery: Burns and metabolism. *Journal of the American College of Surgeons, 196*(2), 267-289.

Scherer, L. A., Shiver, S., Chang, M., Meredith, J. W., & Owings, J. T. (2002). The vacuum assisted closure device: A method of securing skin grafts and improving graft survival. *Archives of Surgery, 137*(8), 930-934.

Sheridan, R. L. (2002). Burns. *Critical Care Medicine, 30*[11 Suppl], S500-S514.

Sheridan, R. L. (2001). Comprehensive treatment of burns. *Current Problems in Surgery, 38*(9), 657-756.

Sim, K. M., Hwang, C., Chan, Y. W., & Seah, C. S. (1996). Use of patient-controlled analgesia with alfentanil for burn dressing procedures: A preliminary report of five patients. *Burns, 22*(3), 238-241.

Wahl, W. L., Brandt, M. M., Ahrns, K. S., et al. (2002). Venous thrombosis incidence in burn patients: Preliminary results of a prospective study. *Journal of Burn Care and Rehabilitation, 23*(2), 97-102.

Weber, J. M. (1998). Epidemiology of infections and strategies for control. In G. J. Carrougher (ed.). *Burn care and therapy.* St. Louis: Mosby.

Wraa, C. (2003). Burns. In L. Newberry (ed.). *Sheehy's emergency nursing principles and practice.* 5th ed. St. Louis: Mosby.

Wray, C. J., Mammen, J. M. V., & Hasselgren, P. (2002). Catabolic response to stress and potential benefits of nutrition support. *Nutrition, 18*(11/12), 971-977.

RECOMMENDED READINGS

Jones, I., Currie, L., & Martin, R. (2002). A guide to biological skin substitutes. *British Journal of Plastic Surgery, 55*(3), 185-193.

Osborn, K. (2003). Nursing burn injuries. *Nursing Management, 34*(5), 49-56.

Peck, M. D., & Priolo-Kapel, D. (2002). Child abuse by burning: A review of the literature and an algorithm for medical investigations. *Journal of Trauma, 53*(5), 1013-1022.

evolve *Did you remember to check out the bonus material, including free self-assessment exercises, on the Evolve Web site at http://evolve.elsevier.com/Sole/ and on the CD-ROM?*